OXFORD HILLS INTERNAL
MEDICINE GROUP
193 MAIN STREET SUITE 1
NORWAY, ME 04268

Feigenbaum's Echocardiography

Sixth Edition

Feigenbaum's Echocardiography

Sixth Edition

Harvey Feigenbaum, MD

Distinguished Professor of Medicine
Indiana University School of Medicine
Krannert Institute of Cardiology
Indianapolis, Indiana

William F. Armstrong, MD

Professor of Medicine
Director, Echocardiography Laboratory
University of Michigan
Ann Arbor, Michigan

Thomas Ryan, MD

Professor of Medicine
Director, Duke Heart Center
Duke University Health System
Durham, North Carolina

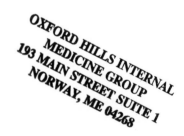

OXFORD HILLS INTERNAL
MEDICINE GROUP
193 MAIN STREET SUITE 1
NORWAY, ME 04268

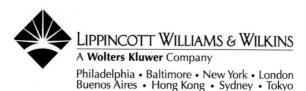

LIPPINCOTT WILLIAMS & WILKINS
A **Wolters Kluwer** Company
Philadelphia • Baltimore • New York • London
Buenos Aires • Hong Kong • Sydney • Tokyo

Acquisitions Editor: Ruth Weinberg
Developmental Editor: Joyce Murphy
Production Editor: Alicia Jackson
Manufacturing Manager: Benjamin Rivera
Marketing Manager: Kathy Neely
Cover Designer: Larry Didona
Compositor: Graphic World, Inc.
Printer: Quebecor World Taunton

© 2005 by LIPPINCOTT WILLIAMS & WILKINS
530 Walnut Street
Philadelphia, PA 19106 USA
LWW.com

Printed in the USA
Fifth Edition, 1994 © Williams & Wilkins
Fourth Edition, 1986 © Lea & Febiger
Third Edition, 1981 © Lea & Febiger
Second Edition, 1976 © Lea & Febiger
First Edition, 1972 © Lea & Febiger

Library of Congress Control Number

2004108538

Care has been taken to confirm the accuracy of the information presented and to describe
generally accepted practices. However, the authors, editors, and publisher are not responsible for
errors or omissions or for any consequences from application of the information in this book
and make no warranty, expressed or implied, with respect to the currency, completeness, or
accuracy of the contents of the publication. Application of this information in a particular
situation remains the professional responsibility of the practitioner.

The authors, editors, and publisher have exerted every effort to ensure that drug selection
and dosage set forth in this text are in accordance with current recommendations and practice at
the time of publication. However, in view of ongoing research, changes in government
regulations, and the constant flow of information relating to drug therapy and drug reactions, the
reader is urged to check the package insert for each drug for any change in indications and
dosage and for added warnings and precautions. This is particularly important when the
recommended agent is a new or infrequently employed drug.

Some drugs and medical devices presented in this publication have Food and Drug
Administration (FDA) clearance for limited use in restricted research settings. It is the
responsibility of the health care provider to ascertain the FDA status of each drug or device
planned for use in their clinical practice.

10 9 8 7 6 5 4 3 2

To our children and grandchildren, who make it all worthwhile - Steve, Tom, Lyle, Andrew, Russell, Megan, Katie, Patrick, Tess, Olivia, Jake, and Lucy

CONTENTS

PREFACE

This latest edition of *Echocardiography* represents a major transition not only in the field of echocardiography but in the history of this publication. As with previous editions there have been numerous important advances which warrant an updated review of the field. A more fundamental change is that echocardiography has now become the backbone of cardiac imaging. It is an integral part of clinical cardiology. With the introduction of digital acquisition and display of echocardiograms, the images and reports have become ubiquitous, with clinicians having access to the recordings throughout the clinical environment. It is now possible to access reports and images of echocardiograms from almost anywhere including the emergency room, office, outpatient facility and even from home or a hotel.

There are very few situations in clinical cardiology where an echocardiogram is not of significant value. Therefore virtually all physicians who care for cardiology patients have to be familiar with echocardiography. Furthermore, the description and understanding of cardiologic problems almost always involves the echocardiographic findings. As a result of this fundamental change in the role of echocardiography, the sixth edition is much more clinical in nature. A brief review of the clinical problem in which echocardiography is useful is provided in every chapter. How echocardiography integrates with clinical practice is emphasized far more than it has been in previous editions.

In past editions a large percentage of the illustrations were borrowed from the literature. This edition represents a major departure from this practice. First of all it is far more difficult to reproduce illustrations from prior publications. But more importantly, virtually all of the illustrations in this edition were acquired digitally. This practice enhances the quality of the illustrations. More significantly, it provides a real-time moving display of the two-dimensional and color Doppler images. Thus, a DVD-ROM with extensive moving images is provided with this text. Since echocardiography is an imaging technique, an exhaustive number of illustrations is essential for a proper understanding of this diagnostic modality.

Probably the most important deviation from prior editions is that the sixth edition is no longer principally a single-author textbook. The first three editions of the book were entirely written by me. However, the fourth edition had a chapter written by William Armstrong and the fifth edition had a chapter by Tom Ryan. This sixth edition is being written by all three of us. The bulk of the writing, with rare exception, has been by Bill and Tom. This change in authorship was done for various reasons. First of all it is almost impossible now for a single author to cover the entire field of echocardiography satisfactorily. The developments in the field have been too numerous, and the role that echocardiography plays in clinical cardiology requires almost a mini cardiology textbook. Furthermore this text represents an example of a "changing of the guard." In my judgment Bill and Tom represent the next generation of senior authorities in this field.

Despite the fact that this book technically is a multi-author textbook, we have made a great effort for it to read as if it were written by a single person. This feature has always been important to me because I feel that it is a much better educational experience for the reader if all of the chapters are integrated and written in a similar style. Since both Bill and Tom have contributed to previous editions, it is natural for them to be the principal authors of this newest edition. All three of us have read every chapter and made editorial comments. We have made every effort for the chapters to be similar so that one cannot tell who actually wrote the chapter. Bill and Tom began their careers in echocardiography at Indiana University, so our understanding of the technique has the same basic foundation. The other major necessity for this text to come from multiple institutions is the fact that since almost all of the illustrations are original, it would be very difficult for any one institution to have appropriate illustrations for everything in the field of echocardiography. Thus the illustrations come from all three institutions and cover the field extremely well.

In past editions I made an effort for the references to be exhaustive so that the textbook could be used as a reference library. In this day of the Internet and ready access to multiple references, this need is no longer present. As a result the references are not nearly as extensive, but we attempt to give the reader some guidance as to where more references can be found in the literature.

Harvey Feigenbaum, MD

ACKNOWLEDGMENTS

A project such as this would be impossible without the assistance and support of many people. Although it is impractical to thank them all individually, the authors wish to express their gratitude to the sonographers, fellows, and colleagues who contributed ideas, suggestions, and illustrations. We especially want to acknowledge Allison Thodoroff and David Adams for their superb help with the text and illustrations. Among other things, Allison and David created most of the illustrations and digital loops for the text. Their contribution to the final product is immeasurable. Several colleagues read portions of the text and made substantive suggestions, particularly Sidney Edelman, PhD, who provided extremely helpful suggestions in the chapter on physics and instrumentation. Finally, the secretarial support of Cheryl Childress, Karen Spirl, Joyce Price, Hope Odzak, and Pam King is warmly recognized.

Feigenbaum's Echocardiography

Sixth Edition

Chapter 1

History of Echocardiography

Harvey Feigenbaum, M.D.

Many histories of diagnostic ultrasound, and cardiac ultrasound in particular, have been written.[1–6] They all seem to address this field from a different perspective. One can begin the history in the twentieth century, Roman times, or any of the centuries in between. It is stated that a Roman architect, Vitruvius, first coined the word *echo*.[7] A Franciscan friar, Marin Mersenne (1588–1648), is frequently called the "father of acoustics" because he first measured the velocity of sound.[7] Another early physicist, Robert Boyle (1627–1691), recognized that a medium was necessary for the propagation of sound.[7] Abbe Lazzaro Spallanzani (1727–1799) is frequently referred to as the "father of ultrasound."[8] He demonstrated that bats were blind and in fact navigated by means of echo reflection using inaudible sound. In 1842, Christian Johann Doppler (1803–1853) noted that the pitch of a sound wave varied if the source of the sound was moving.[9] He worked out the mathematical relationship between the pitch and the relative motion of the source and the observer. The ability to create ultrasonic waves came in 1880 with the discovery of piezoelectricity by Curie and Curie.[10,11] They noted that if certain crystalline materials are compressed, an electric charge is produced between the opposite surfaces. They then noted that the reverse was also true. If an electrical potential is applied to a crystal, it is compressed and decompressed depending on the polarity of the electric charge, and thus very high frequency sound can be produced. In 1912, a British engineer, L. F. Richardson, suggested that an echo technique could be used to detect underwater objects. Later during World War I, Paul Langevin was given the duty of detecting enemy submarines using sound, which culminated in the development of sonar.[3] Sokolov[12] described a method for using reflected sound to detect metal flaws in 1929. In 1942, Floyd Firestone,[13] an American engineer, began to apply this technique and received a patent. It is this flaw detection technique that ultimately was used in medicine.

An Austrian, Karl Dussik,[14] was probably the first to apply ultrasound for medical diagnosis in 1941. He initially attempted to outline the ventricles of the brain. His approach used transmission ultrasound rather than reflected ultrasound. After World War II, many of the technologies developed during that war, including sonar, were applied for peaceful and medical uses. In 1950, W. D. Keidel,[15] a German investigator, used ultrasound to examine the heart. His technique was to transmit ultrasonic waves through the heart and record the effect of ultrasound on the other side of the chest. The purpose of his work was to try to determine cardiac volumes. The first effort to use pulse-reflected ultrasound, as described by Firestone, to examine the heart was initiated by Dr. Helmut Hertz of Sweden. He was familiar with Firestone's observations and in 1953 obtained a commercial ultrasonoscope, which was being used for nondestructive testing. He then collaborated with Dr. Inge Edler who was a practicing cardiologist in Lund, Sweden. The two of them began to use this commercial ultrasonoscope to examine the heart. This collaboration is commonly accepted as the beginning of clinical echocardiography as we know it today.[16]

The original instrument (Fig. 1.1) was quite insensitive. The only cardiac structures that they could record initially were from the back wall of the heart. In retrospect, these echoes probably came from the posterior left ventricular wall. With some modification of their instrument, they were able to record an echo from the anterior leaflet of the mitral valve. However, they did not recognize the source of this echo for several years and originally attributed the signal to the anterior left atrial wall. Only after some autopsy investigations did they recognize the echo's true origin. Edler[17] went on to perform a number of ultrasonic studies of the heart. Many of the cardiac echoes currently used were first described by him. However, the principal clinical application of echocardiography developed by Edler was the detection of mitral stenosis.[18] He noted that there was a difference between the pattern of motion of the anterior mitral leaflet in patients who did or did not have mitral stenosis. Thus, the early

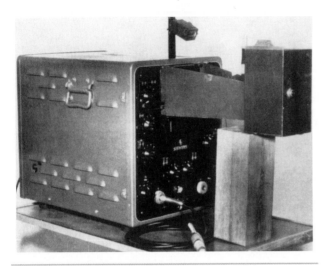

FIGURE 1.1. Ultrasonoscope initially used by Edler and Hertz for recording their early echocardiograms. (From Edler I, Ultrasoundcardiography. Acta Med Scand Suppl 370 1961;170:39, with permission.)

studies published in the mid-1950s and early 1960s primarily dealt with the detection of this disorder.

The work being done in Sweden was duplicated by a group in Germany headed by Dr. Sven Effert.[19,20] Their publications began to appear in the late 1950s and were primarily duplications of Edler's work describing mitral stenosis. One notable observation made by Effert and his group[20] was the detection of left atrial masses. Schmitt and Braun[21] in Germany also began working with ultrasound cardiography and published their work in 1958, again repeating what Edler and Effert had been doing. Edler and his co-workers[22] developed a scientific film that was shown at the Third European Congress of Cardiology in Rome in 1960[22]. Edler et al.[23] also wrote a large review of cardiac ultrasound as a supplement to *Acta Medica Scandinavica*, which was published in 1961, and remained the most comprehensive review of this field for more than 10 years. In the movie and the review, Edler and his co-investigators described the ultrasonic techniques for the detection of mitral stenosis, left atrial tumors, aortic stenosis, and anterior pericardial effusion.

Despite their initial efforts at using ultrasound to examine the heart, neither Edler nor Hertz really anticipated that this technique would flourish. Helmut Hertz was primarily interested in being able to record the ultrasonic signals. In the process, he developed ink jet technology and only spent a few years in the field of cardiac ultrasound. He devoted most of the rest of his career to ink jet technology, for which he held many important patents. He also advised Siemens Corporation, who provided their first ultrasonic instrument, that they should not enter the field of cardiac ultrasound because he personally did not feel that there was a great future in this area (Effert, personal communication, 1996). Edler too did not develop any further

techniques in cardiac ultrasound. He retired in 1976 and until then was primarily concerned with the application of echocardiography for mitral stenosis and, to a lesser extent, mitral regurgitation. He never became involved with any of the newer techniques for pericardial effusion or ventricular function.

China was another country where cardiac ultrasound was used in the early years. In the early 1960s, investigators both in Shanghai and Wuhan were using ultrasonic devices to examine the heart. They began initially with an A-mode ultrasound device and then developed an M-mode recorder.[24,25] The investigators duplicated the findings of Edler and Effert with regard to mitral stenosis.[26] Unique contributions of the Chinese investigators included fetal echocardiography[27] and contrast echocardiography using hydrogen peroxide and then carbon dioxide.[28]

In the United States, echocardiography was introduced by John J. Wild, HD Crawford, and John Reid[29] who examined the excised heart. They were able to identify a myocardial infarction and published their findings in 1957 in the *American Heart Journal*. Neither Wild nor Reid was a physician. Reid was an engineer who subsequently went to the University of Pennsylvania for his doctorate degree. While there, he wanted to continue his interest in examining the heart ultrasonically. He joined forces with Claude Joyner, who was a practicing cardiologist in Philadelphia. Reid proceeded to build an ultrasonoscope, and Joyner and he began duplicating the work on mitral stenosis that was described by Edler and Effert. This work was published in *Circulation* in 1963 and represents[30] the first American clinical effort using pulsed reflected ultrasound to examine the heart.[30]

I became interested in echocardiography in the latter part of 1963. While operating a hemodynamic laboratory and becoming frustrated with the limitations of cardiac catheterization and angiography, I saw an ad from a now defunct company that was claiming that it had an instrument that could measure cardiac volumes with ultrasound. This claim ultimately proved to have no basis. However, when I first saw the ultrasound instrument displayed at the American Heart Association meeting in Los Angeles in 1963, I placed the transducer on my chest and saw a moving echo, which had to be coming from the posterior wall of my heart. This signal undoubtedly was the same echo that Hertz and Edler had noted approximately 10 years earlier. I had the people from the company explain the principles by which such a signal might be generated. I asked them whether fluid in back of the heart would give a different type of a signal, and they said that fluid would be echo free. When I returned to Indiana, I found that the neurologists had an ultrasonoscope that they used for detecting the midline of the brain. Fortunately for me, the instrument was rarely being used and I was able to borrow it. I proceeded to examine more individuals, and again I was able to record an echo from the back wall of the left ventricle. I looked for a patient with pericardial effusion. As predicted, there were now two echoes separated by an echo-free space. The more posterior echo no longer moved, whereas the more anterior echo moved with cardiac motion. We went to the animal laboratory to confirm these findings and thus began my personal career in cardiac ultrasound. This initial paper on pericardial effusion was published in the *Journal of the American Medical Association* in 1965.[31]

Although this phase of the history of echocardiography is commonly considered the origins of the early practice of echocardiography, it should be mentioned that Japanese investigators were working simultaneously using ultrasound to examine the heart. In the mid-1950s, several Japanese investigators such as Satomura, Yoshida, and Nimura at Osaka University were using Doppler technology to examine the heart. They began publishing their work in the mid-1950s.[32,33] These efforts laid the basis for much of what we do today with Doppler ultrasound.

The field of cardiac ultrasound has evolved with the efforts of numerous individuals over the past 50 years. This development is an outstanding example of collaboration between physicists, engineers, and clinicians. Each of the cardiac ultrasonic techniques has its own individual history. Even the name echocardiography has a story of its own. Edler and Hertz first called this technique *ultrasound cardiography* with the abbreviation being UCG. Ultrasound cardiography was a somewhat cumbersome name. The most common use of medical diagnostic ultrasound in the late 1950s and early 1960s was an A-mode technique to detect the midline of the brain. This midline echo would shift if there were an intracranial mass. The technique was known as echoencephalography, and the instrument was an echoencephalograph. It was such an instrument that I borrowed from the neurologists. If the ultrasonic examination of the brain is echoencephalography, then an examination of the heart should be echocardiography. Unfortunately, the abbreviation for an echocardiogram would be ECG, which was already preempted by electrocardiography. We could not use the abbreviation "echo" because it did not differentiate from an echoencephalogram. The reason the term echocardiography finally caught on was because echoencephalography disappeared. No other diagnostic ultrasound technique used the term echo except for the examination of the heart. So the abbreviation echo" now stands only for echocardiography and is not confused with any other ultrasonic examination.

DEVELOPMENT OF VARIOUS ECHOCARDIOGRAPHIC TECHNOLOGIES

The story of echocardiography involves the evolution and development of its many modalities such as A-mode, M-mode, contrast, two-dimensional, Doppler, transesophageal, and intravascular applications. The Doppler story is truly lengthy and international. The Japanese began working with Doppler ultrasound in the mid-1950s.[32,33] American workers, such as Robert Rushmer in Seattle, were early investigators using Doppler techniques.[34] Dr. Rushmer was a recognized expert in cardiac physiology. John Reid later moved to Seattle and joined Rushmer and his group in developing Doppler technology. One of the engineers, Donald Baker, was in that group and developed one of the first pulsed Doppler instruments.[35] Eugene Strandness was a vascular surgeon in Seattle using Doppler for peripheral arterial disease.[36] European investigators were also very active in using Doppler technology. Several early French workers, namely Peronneau[37] and later Kalmanson,[38] wrote extensively on the use of Doppler ultrasound to examine the cardiovascular system. A major development in Doppler ultrasound came when Holen[39] and then Hatle[40] demonstrated that one could derive hemodynamic information from Doppler ultrasound. They noted that one could use a modified version of the Bernoulli equation to detect gradients across stenotic valves. The report that the pressure gradient of aortic stenosis could be determined with Doppler ultrasound was probably the development that established Doppler echocardiography as a clinically important technique.

The field of contrast echocardiography began with an unexpected observation by Gramiak et al.[41] at the University of Rochester. They apparently were doing an ultrasonic examination on a patient undergoing an indicator dilution test using indocyanine green dye. Much to their surprise, they noticed a cloud of echoes introduced into the cardiovascular system with the injection of dye. Apparently, Joyner had noticed a similar observation with the injection of saline but did not report the finding. I heard Gramiak present his group's work at a meeting and promptly used that technique to help establish the echocardiographic identity of the left ventricular cavity.[42] Workers at the Mayo Clinic headed by Jamil Tajik and Jim Seward went on to use this contrast technique in a very eloquent way to identify right-to-left shunts.[43] Contrast agents have evolved to the current commercial products, which are manufactured. The tiny echo-producing bubbles are small enough to pass through capillaries so that a peripheral injection can be seen on the left side of the heart.[44]

Two-dimensional echocardiography has a lengthy and fascinating history. As with almost every aspect of cardiac ultrasound, there is an international flavor to this story. Two-dimensional ultrasonic scanning dates back to early workers such as Douglass Howry when he began using compound scanning for various parts of the body. One of his early compound scanners used a transducer that was mounted on a ring from a B29 gun turret.[45] The Japanese introduced a variety of ultrasonic devices to create two-dimensional recordings of the heart.[46] They used elaborate water baths and scanning techniques (Fig. 1.2). Gramiak and co-workers[47] at the University of Rochester used reconstructive two-dimensional M-mode techniques

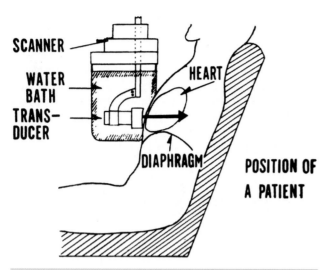

FIGURE 1.2. Relatively early system using a mechanical sector scanner and a water bath to obtain cross-sectional echograms of the heart. (From Ebina T, Oka S, Tanaka N, et al. The ultrasono-tomography of the heart and the great vessels in living human subjects by means of the ultrasonic reflection technique. Jpn Heart J 1967;8:331, with permission.)

to create ultrasonic "cinematography" (Fig. 1.3). Donald King[49] in New York developed a stop-action type of technique for creating a reconstructed two-dimensional image of the heart (Fig. 1.4).

A major breakthrough occurred when an engineer, Nicholas Bom, in Rotterdam, developed a linear scanner (Fig. 1.5).[49] By using multiple crystals, he could create a

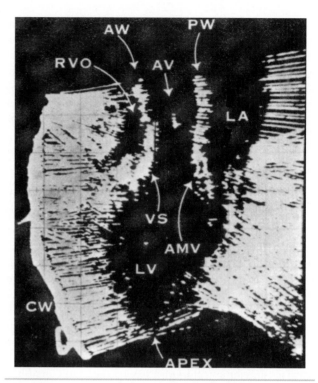

FIGURE 1.4. Compound, electrocardiograph-gated cross-sectional examination of the heart. RVO, right ventricular outflow tract; AW, anterior wall of the aorta; AV, aortic valve; PW, posterior wall of the aorta; LA, left atrium; VS, interventricular septum; AMV, anterior mitral valve leaflet; LV, left ventricle; CW, chest wall. (From King DL, Steeg CN, Ellis K. Visualization of ventricular septal defect by cardiac ultrasonography. Circulation 1973;48:1215, with permission.)

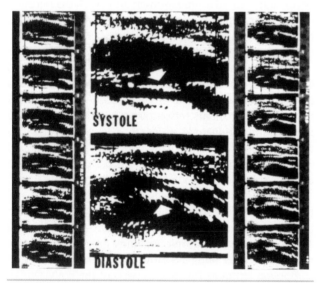

FIGURE 1.3. Frames from a movie film using a spatially oriented reconstruction of the M-mode echogram to produce a pseudo real-time, cross-sectional examination of the mitral valve motion. The two enlarged frames show the position of the mitral valve (arrow) in systole and diastole. (From Gramiak R, Waag R, Simon W. Cine ultrasound cardiography. Radiology 1973;107:175, with permission.)

rectangular image of the heart in real time. Although this technique ultimately never proved to be useful in examining the heart, partially because of the rib shadows, this technique did show the virtue of real-time imaging. It ultimately proved to be a leading form of two-dimensional imaging in other parts of the body but not the heart. Real-time two-dimensional echocardiography became practical by using a sector scan rather than a linear scan. Initially, the scan devices were mechanical. Griffith and Henry[50] at the National Institutes of Health developed a mechanical device that rocked the transducer back and forth. The device was handheld; however, the ability to manipulate the transducer was very limited. Reggie Eggleton, who originally worked at the University of Illinois with Robert, Frank, and Elizabeth Frye, moved to Indiana and developed a mechanical two-dimensional scanner (Fig. 1.6). Interestingly enough, his first prototype was actually a modified Sunbeam electric toothbrush. This early mechanical scanner was the first commercially successful real-time two-dimensional device.[51] Eventually, mechanical sector scanners were replaced by phased-array technology, which was initially developed by Fritz Thurstone and Olaf vonRamm at Duke University.[52]

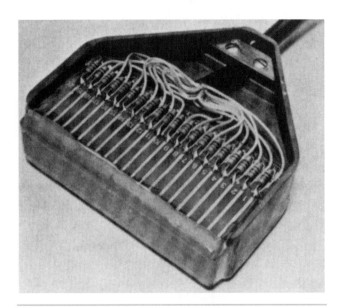

FIGURE 1.5. Photograph of a multielement transducer that provides an electronic linear scan of the heart. This probe consists of 20 individual piezoelectric elements. (From Bom N, Lancee CT, Van Zwienten G, et al. Ultrascan echocardiography. I. Technical description. Circulation 1973;48:1066, with permission.)

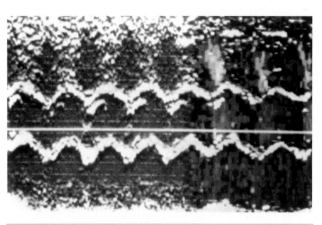

FIGURE 1.7. Combined M-mode and Doppler recording whereby the Doppler signal is superimposed on the M-mode tracing. The direction and velocity of the Doppler signal are displayed in varying colors. This particular recording shows the right ventricular outflow tract (RVOT) and aorta. (From Brandestini MA, Eyer MK, and Stevenson JG. M/Q: M/Q-mode echocardiography. The synthesis of conventional echo with digital multigate Doppler. In: Lancee CT, ed. Echocardiography. The Hague, Netherlands: Martinus-Nijhoff, 1979, with permission.)

Color flow Doppler or two-dimensional Doppler ultrasound dates back to the late 1970s. A group headed by Brandestini working at the University of Washington in Seattle showed how one could use an M-mode recording of a multigated Doppler signal (Fig. 1.7).[53] They encoded the Doppler signal with color to indicate the direction of

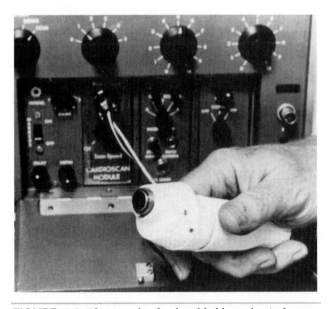

FIGURE 1.6. Photograph of a hand-held mechanical sector scanner. (From Eggleton RC, Feigenbaum H, Johnston KW, et al. Visualization of cardiac dynamics with real-time B-mode ultrasonic scanner. In: White D, ed. Ultrasound in Medicine. New York: Plenum Publishing, 1975:1385, with permission.)

flow. This principle was later more fully developed by Japanese workers including Kasai et al.[54] The key to the development of their two-dimensional color display was the autocorrelation detection of the Doppler velocities. They were now able to provide an excellent real-time two-dimensional display of color flow. Omoto, a Japanese cardiovascular surgeon, and co-workers[55] helped to popularize the clinical value of two-dimensional color Doppler imaging.

The origin of transesophageal echocardiography also dates back to the 1970s. Lee Frazin, a cardiologist in Chicago, placed an M-mode transducer at the tip of a transesophageal probe and demonstrated how one could obtain an M-mode recording of the heart via the esophagus.[56] This technique never became clinically popular. However, both Japanese and European investigators began working with this technology.[57,58] They all attempted to obtain two-dimensional images with a transesophageal probe. Initially, the devices were mechanical and later became electronic. Hisanaga and co-workers[57] were among the Japanese engineers, and Jacques Souquet was a European engineer who made a major contribution to transesophageal electronic probes in 1982.[59] Most of the early clinicians who demonstrated the utility of transesophageal echocardiography were European.

The versatility of ultrasound is exemplified by the fact that one can devise ultrasonic imaging techniques using very large or very small transducers. An exquisite ultrasonic imaging device used to examine the entire body was developed by an Australian engineer, George Kossoff. He developed an instrument called an Octoson. It consisted of eight very large transducers that rotated around the body. The instrument produced images that were of excellent resolution and clarity. The other extreme is the ability to put a tiny transducer on the tip of a catheter that can be inserted in the cardiovascular system. Reggie Eggleton devised a catheter-based imaging system in the 1960s as did Ciezynski in Europe and Omoto in Japan. In the early 1970s, Nicholas Bom and colleagues[60] described a real-time intracardiac scanner using a circular array of 32 elements at the tip of a catheter. This technology developed further to the point that catheter-tipped transducers could be placed on an intracoronary device. Such instruments have been used clinically and for investigational purposes for many years now. Possibly the clinician who used intracoronary ultrasound to its greatest extent is Steven Nissen, who currently is at the Cleveland Clinic. He has used this technique to revolutionize our understanding of coronary atherosclerosis.[61]

There has been interest in three-dimensional echocardiography for many years. Numerous efforts at using compound two-dimensional scans to produce three-dimensional imaging have been demonstrated.[62,63] Some of these compound three-dimensional devices have been used clinically. There has been active investigation using real-time three-dimensional ultrasound. Among the leaders in this effort is Olaf vonRamm and his group.[64]

Handheld echocardiographs date back to 1978.[65] This early device did not have sufficient image quality to be useful. However, now several such instruments are available and increasing in popularity.

RECORDING ECHOCARDIOGRAMS

Along with developing instruments to create images and physiologic information of the heart, there has been a simultaneous history of developing techniques for recording this information. From the very beginning, Helmut Hertz was primarily interested in recording rather than creating ultrasonic images. In so doing, he developed ink jet technology, which proved to be extremely important. When I first began using ultrasound in the early 1960s, a Polaroid camera was the principal recording technique for A-mode and M-mode echocardiograms (Figs. 1.8 and 1.9). This approach was extremely limited and had many problems. Some investigators, such as Gramiak, used 35 mm film to record their M-mode echocardiograms. Much of my early efforts were to get commercial companies to provide strip chart recorders for our M-mode echocardiograms. The variety of strip chart recorders that became available has its own history. With the advent of two-dimensional echocardiography, we had to work out a scheme for recording these real-time two-dimensional

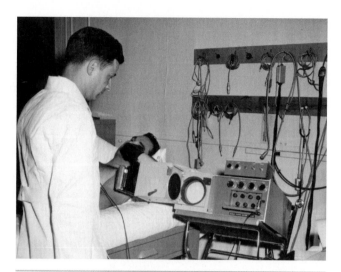

FIGURE 1.8. Early M-mode echocardiograph using a Polaroid camera to record an echocardiogram.

images. At our own institution, we first used super 8 movie film as our recording medium. We would direct a movie camera at the oscilloscope and generate movies. The use of movie film was short-lived and we soon went to videotape. Initially, we used reel-to-reel tape recorders. Then a variety of recorders with cassettes became available. A popular tape recorder in the early years was produced by Sanyo. Unfortunately, analyzing a study frame by frame was very tedious. One had to turn a small button-like control and could not view images backward. Finally, Panasonic developed a tape recorder that permitted easy forward and backward viewing as well as frame-by-frame analysis.

Because of the dominance of two-dimensional echocardiography in the clinical use of echocardiography, videotape became the standard means of recording echocardiogram for decades. Unfortunately, videotape also has major limitations. Looking at serial studies with videotape is problematic. The accessibility of videotape is inconvenient. One cannot make measurements from videotaped images. Copies of videotaped images are always degraded. Digital recording of echocardiograms began in the early 1980s. Interest in using digital techniques has been accelerating ever since. There are numerous advantages to using a digital recording. Side-by-side comparisons are facilitated. One can make measurements easily, and the images are more accessible. Initially, the digital images were generated by grabbing the video signal either from the instrument or by digitizing the videotape. In recent years, a direct digital output from ultrasonic instruments has become available. Digital recording standards using DICOM have facilitated the use of digital imaging and have become a major factor in the general utility of this approach.

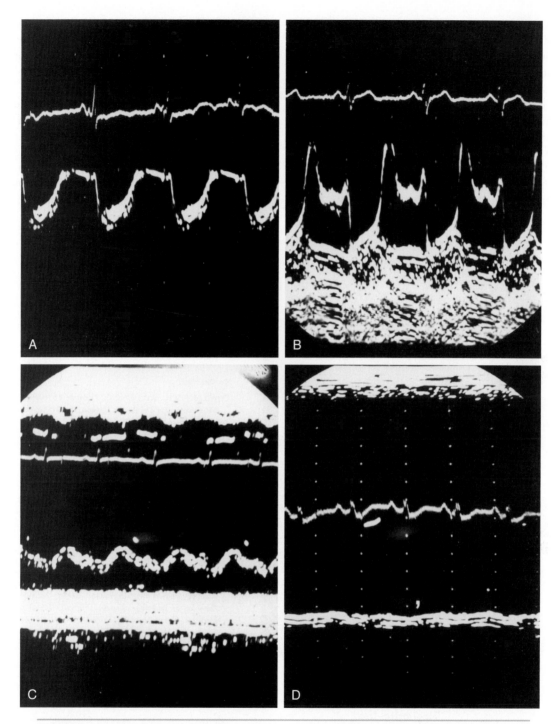

FIGURE 1.9. Early Polaroid recordings of M-mode echocardiogram. **A:** Mitral stenosis, **B:** normal mitral valve, **C:** pericardial effusion, **D:** dilated nonmoving left ventricle.

CARDIAC SONOGRAPHERS

Early in my experience with cardiac ultrasound, it became apparent that the technique would become fairly popular. Performing the echocardiograms myself became a fairly time-consuming activity. Being a clinical cardiologist with responsibilities for patient care, including car-

diac catheterization, I clearly felt that I could not continue to be the principal person to obtain echocardiograms. We also did not have sufficient physicians interested in the technique to provide a complement of physicians to do the echocardiograms throughout the day. As a result, I believed that it would be possible to train a nonphysician to do an echocardiogram. There was considerable skepticism among the few physicians active in the field of ultrasound at the time as to whether this approach was feasible. The first nonphysician hired to perform echocardiograms was Charles Haine.

Our second cardiac sonographer was Sonia Chang. Her skills in obtaining an M-mode echocardiogram were so outstanding that with my encouragement she eventually published a book on the M-mode echocardiographic examination. It was a major publication from which many of the early users of M-mode echocardiography learned their technical skills. Most of the visitors who came to Indiana in the early days learned how to do echocardiograms from Sonia. Sonia left Indiana just after the introduction of two-dimensional echocardiography. She went to Emory University in Atlanta to work with Dr. Willis Hurst, who was the Chairman of Cardiology at the time.

Virtually every echocardiographic laboratory in the United States has a sonographer who excels in the ability to obtain an echocardiogram. Cardiac sonographers have been a major factor in making echocardiography a cost-effective examination. Using a nonphysician to create echocardiograms is not a worldwide concept. In most countries, echocardiograms are still obtained by physi-

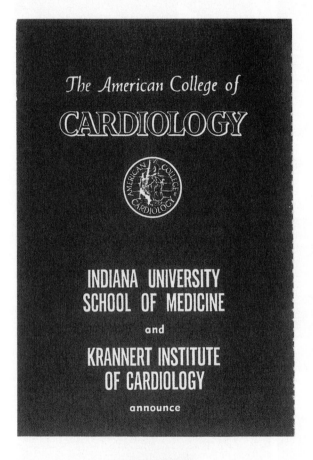

FACULTY

Program Director:

HARVEY FEIGENBAUM, M.D., Associate Professor of Medicine, Indiana University School of Medicine; Research Associate, Krannert Institute of Cardiology, Indianapolis, Ind.

Co-Director:

CHARLES FISCH, M.D., F.A.C.C., Professor of Medicine and Director, Cardiovascular Division, Indiana University School of Medicine; Director, Krannert Institute of Cardiology, Indianapolis, Ind.

INGE EDLER, M.D., Department of Cardiology, University Hospital, Lund, Sweden

CHARLES L. HAINE, Senior Ultrasound Technician, Heart Reseach Center, Indiana University School of Medicine, Indianapolis, Ind.

CLAUDE R. JOYNER, JR., M.D., F.A.C.C., Associate Professor of Medicine, University of Pennsylvania School of Medicine, Philadelphia, Pa.

BERNARD J. OSTRUM, M.D., Associate, Division of Radiology, Albert Einstein Medical Center; Assistant Professor of Radiology, Temple University School of Medicine, Philadelphia, Pa.

RICHARD L. POPP, M.D., Cardiology Fellow, Indiana University School of Medicine, Indianapolis, Ind.

JOHN M. REID, Ph.D., Research Assistant Professor, Department of Physiology and Biophysics, University of Washington School of Medicine, Seattle, Wash.

BERNARD SIGEL, M.D., Associate Professor of Surgery, Woman's Medical College of Pennsylvania, Philadelphia, Pa.

DONALD E. STRANDNESS, JR., M.D., Chief, Peripheral Vascular Service, Veterans Administration Hospital; Associate Professor of Surgery, University of Washington School of Medicine, Seattle, Wash.

WILLIAM L. WINTERS, JR., M.D., F.A.C.C., Associate Professor of Medicine, Division of Cardiology, Temple University School of Medicine, Philadelphia, Pa.

FIGURE 1.10. The program for the first course devoted to diagnostic ultrasound and cardiovascular disease held in Indianapolis in January 1968.

cians. One exception is England, where there is a somewhat different situation. Their cardiac sonographers are probably more highly trained individuals than our sonographers. They come closer to being a physician's assistant and have a greater formal education in cardiac physiology and anatomy. They also perform interpretations with a higher degree of frequency than do sonographers in the United States.

ECHOCARDIOGRAPHIC EDUCATION AND ORGANIZATIONS

The first meeting dedicated solely to cardiac ultrasound was in Indianapolis in January 1968 (Fig. 1.10). Among the faculty were Drs. Edler, Joyner, Reid, and Strandness (Fig. 1.11). There were approximately 50 people who attended that course, one of whom was Raymond Gramiak. At that meeting, Dr. Edler showed the movie that he had created for the 1960 European Congress of Cardiology Meeting in Rome. Another member of the faculty was Richard Popp, who was a cardiology fellow at Indiana at the time. Bernard Ostrum, who was a radiologist at Albert Einstein Medical Center, presented data on abdominal aortas. Chuck Haine was an integral part of the program and demonstrated some of our ultrasonic techniques at Indiana.

The American Society of Echocardiography was also created in Indianapolis in 1975. The decision to create the society was made at a postgraduate meeting in Indianapolis. The *Journal of the American Society of Echocardiography* began in 1988 and the first annual American Society of Echocardiography scientific meeting was held in Washington, DC in 1990. There are now several worldwide echocardiography organizations, publications, and meetings.

Echocardiography has come a long way since its beginnings in the mid-1950s. Although there are many new, highly sophisticated imaging technologies being developed, there is every reason to believe that the clinical utility and popularity of echocardiography will continue to grow. This diagnostic tool is amazingly versatile. It is still very cost-effective compared with competing technologies and has many new possibilities as to how this examination can be improved and provide more and better information. Thus, the future of echocardiography should be as productive and exciting as have been the previous five decades.

REFERENCES

1. Feigenbaum H. Echocardiography. 1st Ed. Philadelphia: Lea & Febiger, 1972.
2. Holmes JH. Diagnostic ultrasound during the early years of A.I.U.M. J Clin Ultrasound 1980;8:299–308.
3. Wild PW. Early history of echocardiography. J Cardiovasc Ultrasonogr 1996;5:2.
4. Goldberg P, Kimmelman BA. Medical Diagnostic Ultrasound: A Retrospective on its 40th Anniversary. Rochester, NY: Eastman Kodak Co., 1988.
5. Feigenbaum H. Evolution of echocardiography. Circulation 1996; 93:1321.
6. Roelandt JRTC. Seeing the invisible: a short history of cardiac ultrasound. Eur J Echocardiogr 2000;1,8–11.
7. Miller DC. Anecdotal History of the Science of Sound. New York: Macmillan, 1935.
8. Talbott JH. A Biographical History of Medicine. New York: Grune & Stratton, 1935:290.
9. Feldman A, Ford P. Scientists and Inventors. New York: Facts on File, 1979.
10. Curie P, Curie J. Developpement, par pression de l'electricite polaire dans les cristaux hemiedres a faces inclines. Comptes Rendus 1880;91:291–295.
11. Curie P, Curie J. Lois du degagement de l'electricite par pression, dans la tourmaline. Comptes Rendus 1881;92:186.
12. Sokolov SY. Means for indicating flaws in materials. U.S. Patent 2. 1937;164:1125.
13. Firestone FA: Flaw detecting device and measuring instrument. U.S. Patent 1.1942;280:226.
14. Dussik KT. Uber die Moglichkeit Hochfrequente Mechanische schwingungen als Diagnostisches Hilfsmittel zu Verwerten. Z Neurol 1941;174:153.
15. Keidel WD. Uber eine Methode zur Registrierung der Volumanderungen des Herzens am Menschen. Z Kreislaufforsch 1950;39:257.
16. Edler I, Hertz CH. Use of ultrasonic reflectoscope for the continuous recording of movements of heart walls. Kungl Fysiogr Sallsk Lung Forth 1954;24:40.
17. Edler I. The diagnostic use of ultrasound in heart disease. Acta Med Scand Suppl 1955;308:32.
18. Edler I. Ultrasound cardiogram in mitral valve disease. Acta Chir Scand 1956;111:230.
19. Effert S, Erkens H, Grosse-Brockoff H. The ultrasound echo method in cardiological diagnosis. Ger Med Mo 1957;2:325.
20. Effert S, Domanig E. The diagnosis of intra-atrial tumor and thrombi by the ultrasonic echo method. Med Meth 1959;4:1.
21. Schmidt W, Braun H. Ultrasonic cardiograph in mitral defect and in non-pathological heart. Z Kreislaufforsch 1958;47:291.
22. Edler I, Gustafson A, Karlefors T, et al. The movements of aortic and mitral valves recorded with ultrasonic echo techniques (motion picture). Presented at the III European Congress of Cardiology, Rome, Italy, 1960.

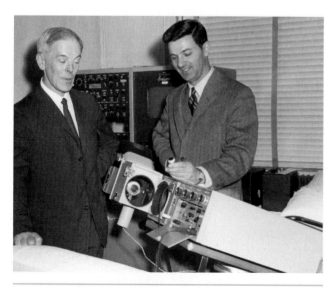

FIGURE 1.11. Photograph of Drs. Edler and Feigenbaum demonstrating an M-mode echocardiograph at the 1968 meeting of cardiac ultrasound in Indianapolis.

23. Edler I, Gustafson A, Karlefors T, et al. Ultrasoundcardiography. Acta Med Scand Suppl 370 1961;170:5–123.
24. Hsu CC. Ultrasonic diagnostics. Shang Sci Tech Press 1961:167.
25. Hsu CC. Preliminary studies on ultrasonics in cardiological diagnosis, I. Experimental observations on cardiac echo valves. II. The use of A-scope ultrasound apparatus in the diagnosis of heart disease. Acta Acad Med Prim Shanghai 1964:2:251.
26. Gao Y, Wang XF, Gao RY, et al. The characteristics of normal echocardiography and its changes in patients with mitral stenosis (in Chinese). Chin J Int Med 1965;13:710.
27. Wang XF, Xiso JP, et al. Fetal echocardiography—method for pregnancy diagnosis. Chin J Obstet Gynecol 1964;10:267–269.
28. Wang XF, et al. Contrast echocardiography with hydrogen peroxide. I. Experimental study. Chin Med J 1979;92:595.
29. Wild JJ, Crawford HD, Reid JM. Visualization of the excised human heart by means of reflected ultrasound or echography. Am Heart J 1957;54:903.
30. Joyner CR Jr, Reid JM, Bond JP. Reflected ultrasound in the assessment of mitral valve disease. Circulation 1963;27:503–511.
31. Feigenbaum H, Waldhausen JA, Hyde LP. Ultrasound diagnosis of pericardial effusion. JAMA 1965;191:711–714.
32. Satomura S, Matsubara, Yoshioka M. A new method of mechanical vibration and its applications. Mem Inst Sci Ind Re 1955;13:125.
33. Yoshida T, Mori M, Nimura Y, et al. Study of examining the heart with ultrasonics, IV: clinical applications. Jpn Circ J 1956;20:228.
34. Rushmer RF, Baker DW, Stegall HF. Transcutaneous Doppler flow detection as a non-destructive technique. J Appl Physiol 1966;21:554–566.
35. Baker DW, Rubenstein SA, Lorch GS. Pulsed Doppler echocardiography: principles and applications. Am J Med 1977;63:69–80.
36. Strandness DE, Schultz RD, Summner DS, et al. Ultrasonic flow detection: a useful technique in the evaluation of peripheral vascular disease. Am J Surg 1967;113:311–320.
37. Peronneau EPA, Deloche A, Bui-Meng-Hung, et al. Debitmetre ultrasonore: developpmements et applications experimentale. Eur Surg Res 1969;1:147.
38. Kalmanson D, Veyrat C, Derai C, et al. Non-invasive technique for diagnosing atrial septal defect and assessing shunt volume using directional Doppler ultrasound: correlations with phasic flow velocity patterns of the shunt. Br Heart J 1972;34:981–991.
39. Holen J, Simonsen S. Determination of pressure gradient in mitral stenosis with Doppler echocardiography. Br Heart J 1979;41:529–535.
40. Hatle L, Angelsen B, Tromsdal A. Noninvasive assessment of aortic stenosis by Doppler ultrasound. Br Heart J 1979;43:284–292.
41. Gramiak R, Shah PM, Kramer DH. Ultrasound cardiography: contrast studies in anatomy and function. Radiology 1969;92:939–938.
42. Feigenbaum H, Stone JM, Lee DA, et al. Identification of ultrasound echoes from the left ventricle using intracardiac injections of indocyanine green. Circulation 1979;41:615–621.
43. Seward JB, Tajik AJ, Spangler JG, et al. Echocardiographic contrast studies: initial experience. Mayo Clin Proc 1975;50:163–192.
44. Feinstein SB, Cheirif J, Ten Cate FJ, et al. Safety and efficacy of new transpulmonary ultrasound contrast agent: initial multicenter clinical results. J Am Coll Cardiol 1990;16:316–324.
45. Howry DH, Holmes JH, Cushman RR, et al. Ultrasonic visualization of living organs and tissues, with observations on some disease processes. Geriatrics 1955;10:123.
46. Ebina T, Oka S, Tanaka M, et al. The ultrasono-tomography of the heart and great vessels in living human subjects by means of the ultrasonic reflection technique. Jpn Heart J 1967;8:331–353.
47. Gramiak R, Waag R, Simon W. Cine ultrasound cardiography. Radiology 1973;107:175–180.
48. King DL. Cardiac ultrasonography. Radiology 1972;103:837.B
49. Bom N, Lancee CT, Honkoop J, et al. Ultrasonic viewer for cross-sectional analyses of moving cardiac structures. Biomed Eng 1971;6:500.
50. Griffith JM, Henry WL. A sector scanner for real-time two-dimensional echocardiography. Circulation 1974;49:1147–1152.
51. Eggleton RC, Feigenbaum H, Johnston KW, et al. Visualization of cardiac dynamics with real-time B-mode ultrasonic scanner. In: White D, ed. Ultrasound in Medicine. New York: Plenum Publishing, 1975.
52. Thurstone FL, vonRamm OT. A new ultrasound imaging technique employing two dimensional electronic beam steering. In: Green PS, ed. Acoustical Holography. New York: Plenum Publishing, 1974:149–159.
53. Brandestini MA, Eyer MK, Stevenson JG. M/Q-mode echocardiography: the synthesis of conventional echo with digital multigate Doppler. In: Lancee CT, ed. Echocardiography. The Hague, Netherlands: Martinus-Nijhoff, 1979.
54. Kasai C, Namekawa K, Koyano A, et al. Real-time two-dimensional blood flow imaging using an autocorrelation technique. IEEE Trans Sonics Ultrason 1985;32:460–463.
55. Omoto R, Yokote Y, Takamoto S, et al. The development of real-time two-dimensional Doppler echocardiography and its clinical significance in acquired valvular regurgitation. Jpn Heart J 1984;25:325–340.
56. Frazin L, Talano JV, Stephanides L, et al. Esophageal echocardiography. Circulation 1976;54:102–108.
57. Hisanaga K, Hisanaga A, Nagata K, et al. Transesophageal cross-sectional echocardiography. Am Heart J 1980;100:605–609.
58. Schluter M, Henrath P. Transesophageal echocardiography: potential advantages and initial clinical results. Pract Cardiol 1983;9:149.
59. Souquet J, Hanrath P, Zitelli L, et al. Transesophageal phased array for imaging the heart. IEEE Trans Biomed Eng 1982;29:707.
60. Bom N, Lancee CT, Egmond van FC. An ultrasonic intracardiac scanner. Ultrasonics 1972;10:72–76.
61. Nissen SE, Gurley JC, Grines CL, et al. Intravascular ultrasound assessment of lumen size and wall morphology in normal subjects and patients with coronary artery disease. Circulation 1991;84:1087.
62. Wollschlager H. Transesophageal echo computer tomography: a new method for dynamic three-dimensional imaging of the heart. In: Computers in Cardiology 1989. IEEE Computer Society, 1990:39.
63. Roelandt J, ten Cate FJ, Bruining N, et al. Transesophageal rotoplane echo-CT. A novel approach to dynamic three-dimensional echocardiography. Thoraxcentre J 1993;6:4–8.
64. vonRamm OT, Smith SW, Pavy HG Jr. High-speed ultrasound volumetric imaging system. Part II. Parallel processing and image display. IEEE Trans Ultrason Ferroelectr Freq Control 1991;38:109–115.
65. Roelandt J, Wladiniroff JW, Baars AM. Ultrasonic real-time imaging with a hand-held scanner. Ultrasound Med Biol 1978;4:93.

Chapter 2

Physics and Instrumentation

Sound is a mechanical vibration transmitted through an elastic medium. When it propagates through the air at the appropriate frequency, sound may produce the sensation of hearing. *Ultrasound* includes that portion of the sound spectrum having a frequency greater than 20,000 cycles per second (20 KHz), which is considerably above the audible range. The use of ultrasound to study the structure and function of the heart and great vessels defines the field of echocardiography. The production of ultrasound for diagnostic purposes involves physical principles and instrumentation that are both complex and sophisticated. As technology has evolved, a thorough understanding of these principles mandates an extensive background in physics and engineering. Fortunately, the use of echocardiography for clinical purposes does not require a complete mastery of the physics and instrumentation involved in the creation of the ultrasound image. However, a basic understanding of these facts is necessary to take full advantage of the technique and to appreciate the strengths and limitations of the technology.

This book is intended principally as a clinical guide to the broad field of echocardiography, to be used by clinicians, students, and sonographers concerned more about the practical application of the technology than the underlying physics. For this reason, an extensive description of the physics and engineering of ultrasound is beyond the scope of this book. Instead, this chapter focuses on those aspects of physics and instrumentation that are relevant to the understanding of ultrasound and its practical application to patient care. In addition, many of the newer technical advances in ultrasound instrumentation are presented briefly, primarily to provide the reader a sense of the changing and ever-improving nature of echocardiography.

PHYSICAL PRINCIPLES

Ultrasound (in contrast to lower, i.e., audible, frequency sound) has several characteristics that contribute to its diagnostic utility. First, ultrasound can be directed as a beam and focused. Second, as ultrasound passes through a medium, it obeys the laws of reflection and refraction. Finally, targets of relatively small size reflect ultrasound and can therefore be detected and characterized. A major disadvantage of ultrasound is that it is poorly transmitted through a gaseous medium and attenuation occurs rapidly, especially at higher frequencies. As a wave of ultrasound propagates through a medium, the particles of the medium vibrate parallel to the line of propagation, producing *longitudinal waves*. Thus, a sound wave is characterized by areas of more densely packed particles within the medium (an area of compression) alternating with regions of less densely packed particles (an area of rarefaction). The amount of reflection, refraction, and attenuation depends on the acoustic properties of the various media through which an ultrasound beam passes. Tissues composed of solid material interfaced with gas will reflect most of the ultrasound energy, resulting in poor penetration. Very dense media also reflect a high percentage of the ultrasound energy. Soft tissues and blood allow relatively more ultrasound energy to be propagated, thereby increasing penetration and improving diagnostic utility. Bone also reflects most ultrasound energy, not because it is dense but because it contains so many interfaces.

The ultrasound wave is often graphically depicted as a sine wave in which the peaks and troughs represent the areas of compression and rarefaction, respectively (Fig. 2.1). Microscopic pressure changes occur within the medium, corresponding to these areas, and result in tiny oscillations of particles, although no actual particle motion occurs. Depicting ultrasound in the form of a sine wave has some limitations but allows the demonstration of several fundamental principles. The sum of one compression and one rarefaction represents one *cycle*, and the distance between two similar points along the wave corresponds to *wavelength* (see Table 2.1 for definitions of commonly used terms). Over the range of diagnostic ultrasound, wavelength varies from approximately 0.15 to 1.5 mm in soft tissue. The *frequency* of the sound wave is

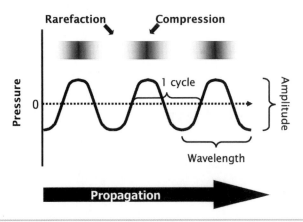

FIGURE 2.1. This schematic illustrates how sound can be depicted as a sine wave whose peaks and troughs correspond to areas of compression and rarefaction, respectively. As sound energy propagates through tissue, the wave has a fixed wavelength that is determined by the frequency and amplitude that is a measure of the magnitude of pressure changes. See text for further details.

the number of wavelengths per unit of time. Thus, wavelength and frequency are inversely related and their product represents the velocity of the sound wave:

$$v = f \times \lambda \qquad \text{[Eq. 2.1]}$$

where v is velocity, f is frequency (in cycles per second or hertz) and λ is wavelength. Velocity through a given medium depends on the density and elastic properties or stiffness of that medium. Velocity is directly related to stiffness and inversely related to density. Ultrasound travels faster through a stiff medium, such as bone. Velocity also varies with temperature, but because body temperature is maintained within a relatively narrow range, this phenomenon is of little significance in medical imaging. Table 2.2 provides a comparison of average velocity values in various types of tissues. Within soft tissue, velocity of sound is fairly constant at approximately 1,540 m/sec (or 1.54 m/msec, or 1.54 mm/µsec). Thus, to find the wave-

▌ **TABLE 2.1 Definitions of Basic Terms**

Term	Definition
Absorption	The transfer of ultrasound energy to the tissue during propagation
Acoustic impedance	The product of the density of the medium and the velocity of sound; differences in AI between 2 media determine the ratio of transmitted versus reflected sound at the interface
Amplitude	The magnitude of the pressure changes along the wave; also, the strength of the wave (in decibels)
Attenuation	The net loss of ultrasound energy as a wave propagates through a medium
Cycle	The combination or sum of 1 compression and 1 rarefaction of a propagating wave
Dead time	The time in between pulses that the echograph is not emitting ultrasound
Decibel	A logarithmic measure of the intensity of sound, expressed as a ratio to a reference value (dB)
Duty factor	The fraction of time that the transducer is emitting ultrasound, a unitless number between 0 and 1
Far field	The diverging conical portion of the beam beyond the near field
Frequency	The number of cycles per second, measured in Hertz (Hz)
Half-layer value	The distance an ultrasound beam penetrates into a medium before its intensity has attenuated to one-half the original value
Intensity	The concentration or distribution of power within an area, often the cross-sectional area of the ultrasound beam, analogous to loudness
Longitudinal wave	A cyclic disturbance in which the energy propagation is parallel to the direction of particle motion
Near field	The proximal cylindrical-shaped portion of the ultrasound beam before divergence begins to occur
Period	The time required to complete 1 cycle, usually expressed in microseconds (µsec)
Piezoelectricity	The phenomenon of changing shape in response to an applied electric current, resulting in vibration and the production of sound waves; the ability to produce an electric impulse in response to a mechanical deformation; thus, the interconversion of electrical and sound energy
Power	The rate of transfer over time of the acoustic energy from the propagating wave to the medium, measured in Watts
Pulse	A burst or packet of emitted ultrasound of finite duration, containing a fixed number of cycles traveling together
Pulse length	The physical length or distance that a pulse occupies in space, usually expressed in millimeters (mm)
Pulse repetition frequency	The rate at which pulses are emitted from the transducer, ie, the number of pulses emitted within a period of time, usually 1 second
Resolution	The smallest distance between 2 points that allows the points to be distinguished as separate
Sensitivity	The ability of the system to image small targets at a given depth
Ultrasound	A mechanical vibration in a physical medium, characterized by a frequency > 20,000 Hz
Velocity	The speed at which sound moves through a given medium
Wavelength	The length of a single cycle of the ultrasound wave; a measure of distance, not time

▶ **TABLE 2.2 Velocity of Sound in Air and Various Types of Tissues**

Medium	Velocity (m/sec)
Air	330
Fat	1450
Water	1480
Soft tissue	1540
Kidney	1560
Blood	1570
Muscle	1580
Bone	4080

length of a 3.0-MHz transducer, the solution would be given by:

$$v = f \times \lambda \qquad \text{[Eq. 2.1]}$$
$$\lambda = v \div f$$
$$\lambda = 1{,}540 \text{ m/sec} \div 3{,}000{,}000 \text{ cycles/sec} \approx 0.51 \text{ mm}$$

A simpler version of this equation is given by λ (in millimeters) = 1.54/f, where f is the transducer frequency (in megahertz). This converts 1,540 m/sec to 1.54 mm/μsec, expresses frequency in megahertz, and yields wavelength in millimeters. Thus,

$$\lambda = v \div f$$
$$\lambda = 1.54 \div 3.0 \approx 0.51 \text{ mm}$$

If an ultrasound wave encounters an area of higher stiffness, for example, velocity will increase. Because frequency does not change, wavelength will also increase. As is discussed later, wavelength is a determinant of resolution: the shorter the wavelength is, the smaller the target that is able to reflect the ultrasound wave and thus the greater the resolution.

Another fundamental property of sound is *amplitude*, which is a measure of the strength of the sound wave (Fig. 2.1). It is defined as the difference between the peak pressure within the medium and the average value, depicted as the height of the sine wave above and below the baseline. Amplitude is measured in *decibels*, a logarithmic unit that relates acoustic pressure to some reference value. The primary advantage of using a logarithmic scale to display amplitude is that a very wide range of values can be accommodated and weak signals can be displayed along side much stronger signals. Of practical use, an increase of 6 dB is equal to a doubling of signal amplitude, and 60 dB represents a 1,000-fold change in amplitude or loudness. A parameter closely related to amplitude is *power*, which is defined as the rate of energy transfer to the medium, measured in watts. For clinical purposes, power is usually represented over a given area (often the beam area) and referred to as *intensity* (watts per centimeter squared or W/cm²). This is analogous to loudness. Inten-

sity diminishes rapidly with propagation distance and has important implications with respect to the biologic effects of ultrasound, which are discussed later.

INTERACTION BETWEEN ULTRASOUND AND TISSUE

These basic characteristics of ultrasound have practical implications for the interaction between ultrasound and tissue. For example, the higher the frequency of the ultrasound wave (and the shorter the wavelength), the smaller the structures that can be accurately resolved. Because precise identification of small structures is a goal of imaging, the use of high frequencies would seem desirable. However, higher frequency ultrasound has less penetration compared with lower frequency ultrasound. The loss of ultrasound as it propagates through a medium is referred to as *attenuation*. This is a measure of the rate at which the intensity of the ultrasound beam diminishes as it penetrates the tissue. Attenuation has three components: absorption, scattering, and reflection. Attenuation always increases with depth and is also affected by the frequency of the transmitted beam and the type of tissue through which the ultrasound passes. The higher the frequency is, the more rapidly it will attenuate. Attenuation may be expressed as the "half-value layer" or the "half-power distance," which is a measure of the distance that ultrasound travels before its amplitude is attenuated to one half its original value. Representative half-power distances are listed in Table 2.3. As a rule of thumb, the attenuation of ultrasound in tissue is between 0.5 and 1.0 dB/cm/MHz. This approximation describes the expected loss of energy (in decibels) that would occur over the round-trip distance that a beam would travel after being emitted by a given transducer. For example, if a 3-MHz transducer is used to image an object at a depth of 12 cm (24-cm round trip), the returning signal could be attenuated as much as 72 dB (or nearly 4,000-fold). As expected, attenuation is greater in soft tissue compared with blood and is even greater in muscle, lung, and bone.

The velocity and direction of the ultrasound beam as it passes through a medium are a function of the acoustic impedance of that medium. Acoustic impedance (Z, measured in rayls) is simply the product of velocity (in meters per second) and physical density (in kilograms per cubic meter). As impedance increases, a greater acoustic mismatch is created and relatively more ultrasound energy will be reflected rather than transmitted. Within a homogeneous structure, the density of the medium primarily determines these parameters. In such a structure, sound would travel in a straight line at a constant velocity, depending on the density and stiffness. Within the body, the tissues through which an ultrasound beam passes have different acoustic impedances. When the

▶ **TABLE 2.3** **Representative Half-Power Distances Relevant to Echocardiography**

Material	Half-power distance (in cm)	
Water	380	Less attenuation
Blood	15	
Soft tissue (except muscle)	1–5	
Muscle	0.6–1	
Bone	0.2–0.7	
Air	0.08	
Lung	0.05	More attenuation

beam crosses a boundary between two media, a portion of the energy is reflected, a portion is refracted, and a portion continues in a relatively straight line (Fig. 2.2A). These interactions between the ultrasound beam with acoustic interfaces form the basis for ultrasound imaging. The phenomena of *reflection* and *refraction* obey the laws of optics and depend on the angle of incidence between the transmitted beam and the acoustic interface as well as the *acoustic mismatch*, i.e., the magnitude of the difference in acoustic impedance. Small differences in velocity also determine refraction. These properties explain the importance of using an acoustic coupling gel during transthoracic imaging. Without the gel, the air-tissue in-

terface at the skin surface results in more than 99% of the ultrasonic energy being reflected at this level. This is primarily due to the very high acoustic impedance of air. The use of gel between the transducer and the skin surface greatly increases the percentage of energy that is transmitted into and out of the body, thereby allowing imaging to occur.

As the ultrasound beam is transmitted through tissue, it encounters a complex array of large and small interfaces and targets, each of which affect the transmission of the ultrasound energy. These interactions can be broadly categorized as *specular echoes* and *scattered echoes* (Fig. 2.2B). Specular echoes are produced by reflectors that are large relative to ultrasound wavelength, such as the endocardial surface of the left ventricle. Such targets reflect a relatively greater proportion of the ultrasound energy in an angle-dependent fashion. The spatial orientation and the shape of the reflector determine the angles of specular echoes. Examples of specular reflectors include endocardial and epicardial surfaces, valves, and pericardium.

Targets that are small relative to the wavelength of the transmitted ultrasound produce *scattering*, and such objects are sometimes referred to as *Rayleigh scatterers*. The resultant echoes are diffracted or bent and scattered in all directions. Because the percentage of energy returning to the transducer from scattered echoes is considerably less than that resulting from specular interactions, the ampli-

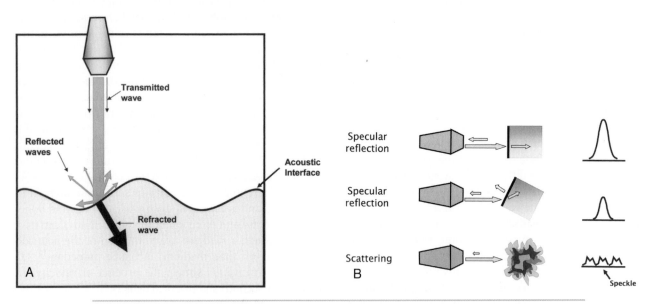

FIGURE 2.2. **A:** A transmitted wave interacts with an acoustic interface in a predictable way. Some of the ultrasound energy is reflected at the interface and some is transmitted through the interface. The transmitted portion of the energy is refracted, or bent, depending on the angle of incidence and differences in impedance between the tissues. **B:** The interaction between an ultrasound wave and its target depends on several factors. A specular reflection occurs when ultrasound encounters a target that is large relative to the transmitted wavelength. The amount of ultrasound energy that is reflected to the transducer by a specular target depends on the angle and the impedance of the tissue. Targets that are small relative to the transmitted wavelength produce a scattering of ultrasound energy, resulting in a small portion of energy being returned to the transducer. This type of interaction results in "speckle" that produces the texture within tissues.

tude of the signals produced by scattered echoes is very low (Fig. 2.2B). Despite this fact, scattering has important clinical significance (and forms the basis for Doppler imaging). Scattered echoes contribute to the visualization of surfaces that are parallel to the ultrasonic beam and also provide the substrate for visualizing the texture of gray-scale images. The term *speckle* is used to describe the tissue-ultrasound interactions that result from a large number of small reflectors within a resolution cell. Without the ability to record scattered echoes, the left ventricular wall, for example, would appear as two bright linear structures, the endocardial and the epicardial surfaces, with nothing in between.

From the above discussion, it is evident that the interaction between an ultrasound beam and a reflector depends on the relative size of the targets and the wavelength of the beam. If a solid object is submerged in water, for example, whether reflection of ultrasound occurs depends on the size of the object with respect to the wavelength of the transmitted ultrasound. Specifically, the thickness or profile of the object relative to the ultrasound beam must be at least one-fourth the wavelength of the ultrasound. Thus, as the size of the target decreases, the wavelength of the ultrasound must decrease proportionately to produce a reflection and permit the object to be recorded. This explains why higher frequency ultrasound

allows smaller objects to be visualized. In clinical practice, echocardiography typically employs ultrasound with a range of 2,000,000 to 8,000,000 cycles per second (2–8 MHz). At a frequency of 2 MHz, it is generally possible to record distinct echoes from interfaces separated by approximately 1 mm. However, because high-frequency ultrasound is reflected by many small interfaces within tissue, resulting in scattering, much of the ultrasonic energy becomes attenuated and less energy is available to penetrate deeper into the body. Thus, penetration is reduced as frequency increases. Similarly, as the medium becomes less homogeneous, the degree of reflection and refraction increases, resulting in less penetration of the ultrasound energy.

THE TRANSDUCER

The use of ultrasound for imaging became practical with the development of piezoelectric transducers. The principles of piezoelectricity are illustrated in Figure 2.3. Piezoelectric substances or crystals rapidly change shape or vibrate when an alternating electric current is applied. It is the rapidly alternating expansion and contraction of the crystal material that produces the sound waves. Equally important is the fact that a piezoelectric crystal will pro-

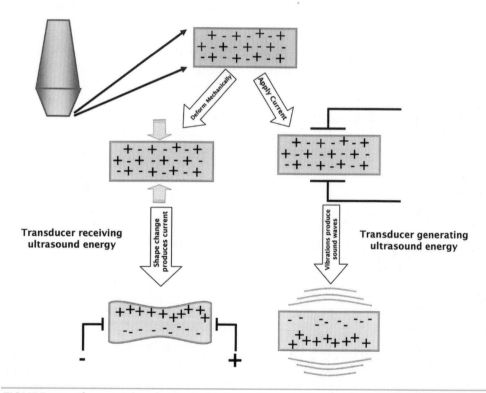

FIGURE 2.3. The principles of piezoelectricity are illustrated in this schematic. A piezoelectric crystal will vibrate when an electric current is applied, resulting in the generation and transmission of ultrasound energy. Conversely, when reflected energy encounters a piezoelectric crystal, the crystal will change shape in response to this interaction and produce an electrical impulse. See text for further details.

duce an electric impulse when it is deformed by reflected sound energy. Such piezoelectric crystals form the critical component of ultrasound transducers. Although a variety of piezoelectric materials exist, most commercial transducers employ ceramics, such as ferroelectrics, barium titanate, and lead zirconate titanate. The creation of an ultrasound pulse thus requires that an alternating electric current be applied to a piezoelectric element. This results in the emission of sound energy from the transducer, followed by a period of quiescence during which the transducer "listens" for some of the transmitted ultrasound energy to be reflected back (known as "dead time"). The amount of acoustic energy that returns to the transducer is a measure of the strength and depth of the reflector. The time required for the ultrasound pulse to make the round-trip from transducer to target and back again allows calculation of the distance between the transducer and reflector.

An ultrasound transducer consists of many small, carefully arranged piezoelectric elements that are interconnected electronically (Fig. 2.4). The frequency of the transducer is determined by the thickness of these elements. Each element is coupled to electrodes, which transmit current to the crystals, and then record the voltage generated by the returning signals. An important component of transducer design is the dampening (or backing) material, which shortens the ringing response of the piezoelectric material after the brief excitation pulse. An excessive ringing response (or "ringdown") lengthens the ultrasonic pulse and decreases range resolution. Thus, the dampening material both shortens the ringdown and provides absorption of backward and laterally transmitted acoustic energy. At the surface of the transducer, matching layers are applied to provide acoustic impedance matching between the piezoelectric elements and the body. This increases the efficiency of transmitted energy by minimizing the reflection of the ultrasonic wave as it exits the transducer surface.

Transducer design is critically important to optimal image creation. An important feature of ultrasound is the ability to direct or focus the beam as it leaves the transducer. This results in a parallel and cylindrically shaped beam. Eventually, however, the beam diverges and becomes cone shaped (Fig. 2.5). The proximal or cylindrical portion of the beam is referred to as the *near field* or Fresnel zone. When it begins to diverge, it is called the *far field* or Fraunhofer zone. For a variety of reasons, imaging is optimal within the near field. Thus, maximizing the length of the near field is an important goal of echocardiography.

The length of the near field (*l*) is described by the formula:

$$l = r^2/\lambda \qquad \text{[Eq. 2.2]}$$

where *r* is the radius of the transducer and λ is the wavelength of the emitted ultrasound. Either decreasing the wavelength (increasing the frequency) or increasing the size of the transducer will lengthen the near field. These relationships are illustrated in Figure 2.6. From the above formula, one might conclude that optimal ultrasound imaging would always employ a large-diameter, high-frequency transducer to maximize the length of the near field. Several factors prevent this approach from being practical. First, the transducer size is predominantly limited by the size of the intercostal spaces. A transducer that is too large will not be able to image between the ribs. Second, although higher frequency does lengthen the near field, it also results in greater attenuation and lower penetration of the ultrasound energy, thereby limiting its usefulness. These tradeoffs must be balanced to maximize imaging performance. Even when the near field length is maximized, most targets will still lie in the far field. To improve imaging in this area, the rate of beam divergence must be minimized. To decrease the amount of divergence in the far field, a large-diameter, high-frequency transducer is optimal. As discussed previously, focusing of

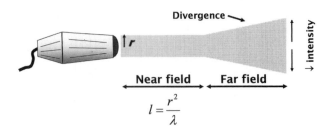

FIGURE 2.5. When ultrasound is emitted from a transducer, the shape of the beam obeys particular physical principles. If the transducer face is round, the transmitted beam will remain cylindrical for a distance, defined as the near field. After a particular distance of propagation, the beam will begin to diverge and become cone shaped. This region of the beam is referred to as the far field. Within this portion of the beam, a decrease in intensity occurs. The length of the near field is determined by the radius of the transducer face and the wavelength or frequency of the transmitted energy. See text for details.

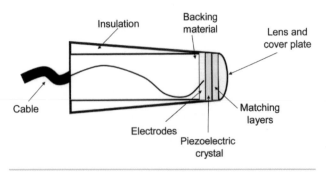

FIGURE 2.4. A schematic diagram of a transducer is provided. See text for details.

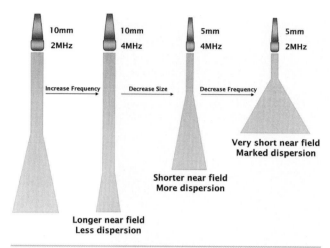

FIGURE 2.6. The length of the near field depends on transducer frequency and transducer size, as illustrated in these four examples. On the left, a transducer with a 10 mm diameter emits ultrasound at 2.0 MHz. This determines both the length of the near field and the rate of divergence in the far field. If the same size transducer emits energy at 4 MHz, the length of the near field increases and the rate of dispersion is less. A transducer half that size (5 mm) transmitting at 4.0 MHz will have a shorter near field. Finally, a 5 mm transducer that transmits at 2 MHz will have the shortest near field and the greatest rate of dispersion in the far field.

the transmitted beam tends to improve imaging in the near field but will increase the rate or angle of divergence in the far field (Fig. 2.7). Focusing is accomplished through the use of an acoustic lens placed on the surface of the transducer or by constructing the piezoelectric crystal in a concave shape. Thus, transducer frequency, size, and focusing all interact to affect image quality in

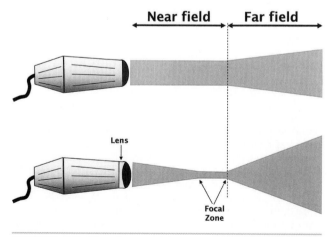

FIGURE 2.7. The ultrasound beam emitted by a transducer can be either unfocused **(top)** or can be focused by use of an acoustic lens **(bottom)**. Focusing results in a narrower beam but does not change the length of the near field. An undesirable effect of focusing is that the rate of dispersion in the far field is greater.

the near and far fields. Tradeoffs exist that must be taken into account to create optimal images. Figure 2.8 is an example of the effects of varying transducer frequencies on image quality and appearance. On the left, a short-axis view is recorded using a 3.0-MHz transducer. On the right, a similar image is captured using a 5.0-MHz probe. Note how the higher frequency results in improved resolution and detail, especially within the myocardium.

MANIPULATING THE ULTRASOUND BEAM

For most clinical applications, the ultrasound beam is both focused and steered electronically. Although beam manipulation can be done mechanically, with modern equipment, it is primarily achieved through the use of phased-array transducers, which consist of a series of small piezoelectric elements interconnected electronically (Fig. 2.9). In such transducers, the wave front of the beam consists of the sum of the individual wavelets produced by each element. By manipulating the timing of excitation of individual elements, both focusing and steering are possible. If all elements are excited simultaneously, each one will produce a circular wavelet that combines to generate a longitudinal wave front that is parallel to the face of the transducer and propagates in a direction perpendicular to that face. By adjusting the timing of excitation, as shown in Figure 2.10A, the beam can be steered. Further adjustments in the timing allow the beam to be steered through a sector arc, resulting in a two-dimensional image. Using a similar approach, electronic transmit focusing of the beam is also possible (Fig. 2.10B). For example, by exciting the outside elements first and then progressively activating the more central elements, the individual wavelets form a curved front that allow focusing at a particular distance within the near field. This can either be fixed or adjustable, and the process is referred to as *dynamic transmit focusing*.

It should be recognized that the ultrasound beam is a three-dimensional structure that, in the case of a phased-array transducer, is roughly rectangular in cross section (Fig. 2.11). The dimensions of the beam are referred to as axial (along the axis of wave propagation) and lateral (parallel to the face of the transducer, sometimes called azimuthal). The lateral dimension is further divided into a vertical and horizontal component. Acoustic focusing through a lens will change the shape in the vertical and horizontal dimensions equally. Electronic focusing will narrow the beam in one of these two dimensions, resulting in a "thinner" sector slice. Transducers that employ anular phased-array technology have the capacity to focus in both dimensions, resulting in a compact, high-intensity beam profile.

Another type of transducer uses a *linear array* of elements. Such transducers have a rectangular face with

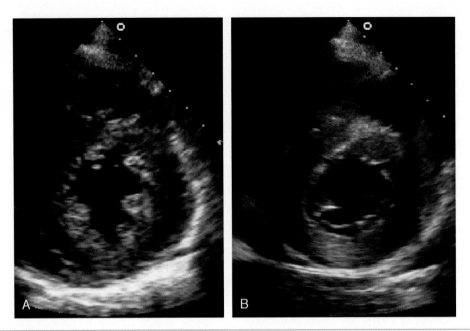

FIGURE 2.8. The effects of different transducer frequencies on image quality and appearance are demonstrated. **A:** A 3.0-MHz transducer is used to record a short-axis view. **B:** The same image is recorded using a 5.0-MHz transducer.

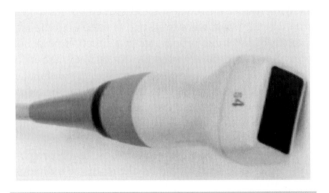

FIGURE 2.9. A phased-array ultrasound transducer is shown.

crystals aligned parallel to one another along the length of the transducer face. Unlike phased-array transducers, the elements are excited simultaneously so the individual scan lines are directed perpendicular to the face and remain parallel to each other. This results in a rectangle-shaped beam that is unfocused. Linear-array technology is often used for abdominal, vascular, or obstetric applications. Alternatively, the face of a linear transducer can be curved to create a sector scan. This innovative design is now being used in some handheld ultrasound devices.

Focusing has the effect of concentrating the acoustic energy into a smaller area, resulting in increased intensity at the point of focus. Intensity also varies across the lateral dimensions of the beam, being greatest at the center and decreasing in intensity toward the edges. When the shape of the ultrasonic beam is diagrammed, it is con-

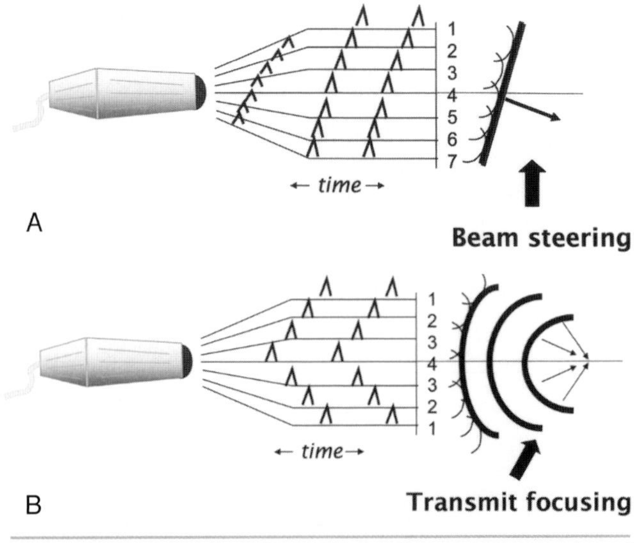

Beam steering

Transmit focusing

FIGURE 2.10. **A:** Phased-array technology permits steering of the ultrasound beam. By adjusting the timing of excitation of the individual piezoelectric crystals, the wave front of ultrasound energy can be directed, as shown. Beam steering is a fundamental feature of how two-dimensional images are created. **B:** By adjusting the timing of excitation of the individual crystals within a phased-array transducer, the beam can be focused. In this example, the outer elements are fired first, followed sequentially by the more central elements. Because the speed of sound is fixed, this manipulation in the timing of excitation results in a wave front that is curved and focused. This is called transmit focusing.

Single Crystal

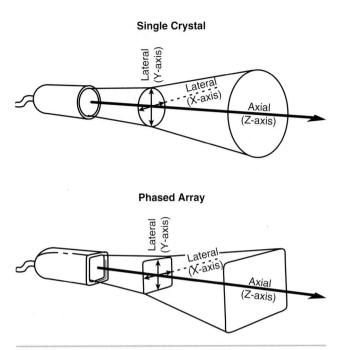

Phased Array

FIGURE 2.11. The ultrasound beam can be represented as a three-dimensional structure. A single-crystal transducer **(top)** will emit a cylindrically shaped beam. If the transducer face is rectangular shaped **(bottom)**, the beam will also have a rectangular shape. The various beam axes are labeled in the two drawings.

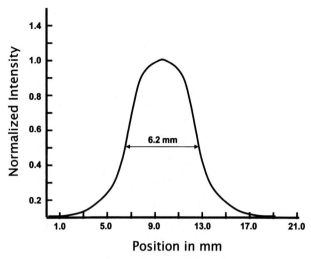

FIGURE 2.12. A transaxial beam plot is demonstrated. The beam width or lateral resolution is a function of the intensity of the ultrasonic beam. The beam width is commonly measured at the half-intensity level, and, in this case, the beam width would be reported as 6.2 mm.

ventional to draw the edge of the beam to the half-value limit of the beam plot. An example of a transaxial beam plot is illustrated in Figure 2.12. This diagram illustrates the important relationship between intensity and beam width. At its peak intensity, the beam may be as narrow as 1 mm. At its weakest intensity, however, beam width may be as great as 12 mm. For purposes of comparison, it is customary to measure the beam width at its half amplitude or intensity. In the example shown, the beam width would be reported as 6.2 mm. Finally, it should be remembered that gain setting will affect these values in a predictable manner. At high gain settings, the weaker portion of the ultrasound beam is recorded and beam width is greater. Conversely, at low gain settings, the beam width would be narrower.

As is apparent from the previous discussion, focusing of the ultrasonic beam is generally desirable. By increasing beam intensity within the near field, the strength of returning signals is enhanced. An undesirable effect of focusing is its effect on beam divergence in the far field. Because focusing results in a beam with a smaller radius, the angle of divergence in the far field is increased. However, because beam divergence begins from a small cross-sectional area of a focused beam, the net effect is variable. The result of these relationships is a tradeoff between resolution at the point of focus and depth of field. Divergence

also contributes to the formation of important imaging artifacts such as side lobes (discussed later).

RESOLUTION

Resolution is the ability to distinguish between two objects in close proximity. Because echocardiography depends on its ability to image small structures and provide detailed anatomic information, resolution is one of its most important variables. Furthermore, because echocardiography is a dynamic imaging technique, resolution has at least two components: spatial and temporal. Spatial resolution is defined as the smallest distance that two targets can be separated for the system to distinguish between them. It, too, has two components: *Axial resolution* refers to the ability to differentiate two structures lying along the axis of the ultrasound beam (i.e., one behind the other) and *lateral resolution* refers to the ability to distinguish two reflectors that lie side by side relative to the beam (Fig. 2.13).

The primary determinants of axial resolution are the frequency of the transmitted wave and, more importantly, its effect on pulse length. Higher frequency is associated with shorter wavelength, and the size of the wave relative to the size of the object determines resolution. In addition to frequency, pulse length or duration also affects axial resolution. The shorter the train of cycles is, the greater the likelihood that two closely positioned targets can be resolved. Because a higher frequency and/or broad bandwidth transducer delivers a shorter pulse, it is also associated with higher resolution.

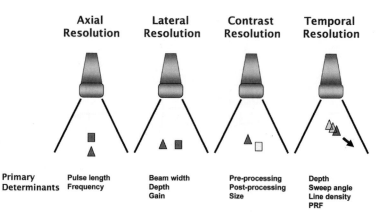

| Primary Determinants | Pulse length Frequency | Beam width Depth Gain | Pre-processing Post-processing Size | Depth Sweep angle Line density PRF |

FIGURE 2.13. The different types of resolution are demonstrated in this schematic. See text for details.

Lateral resolution varies throughout the field of imaging and is affected by several factors. The width or thickness of the interrogating beam, at a given depth, is the most important determinant. Ideally, the ultrasonic beam should be very narrow to provide a thin "slice" of the heart. Recall that the beam has finite width, even in the near field, and tends to diverge as it propagates. The importance of beam width stems from the fact that the system will display all targets within the path of the beam along a single line represented by the central axis of the beam. In other words, the echograph displays structures within the image as if the beam were infinitely narrow. Thus, lateral resolution diminishes as beam width (and depth) increases. The distribution of intensity across the beam profile will also affect lateral resolution. As illustrated in Figure 2.14, both strong and weak reflectors can be resolved within the central portion of the beam, where intensity is greatest. At the edge of the beam, however, only relatively strong reflectors may produce a signal. Furthermore, the true size and position of such objects may be distorted by the width of the beam, resulting in significant beam width artifacts. This is illustrated in Figure 2.15. This observation also explains the importance of overall system gain and its effect on lateral resolution. *Gain* is the amplitude, or the degree of amplification, of the received signal. When gain is low, weaker echoes from the edge of the beam may not be recorded and the beam appears relatively narrow. If system gain is increased, weaker and more peripheral targets are recorded and beam width appears greater. Thus, to enhance lateral resolution, a minimal amount of system gain should be employed. Figure 2.16 illustrates how changes in gain setting can drastically alter lateral resolution and anatomic information.

A third component of resolution is called *contrast resolution*. Contrast resolution refers to the ability to distinguish and to display different shades of gray within the image. This is important both for the accurate identification of borders and for the ability to display texture or detail within the tissues. To convert the returning radio frequency (RF) information into a gray-scale image, pre- and post-processing of the data are performed. These steps in image formation rely heavily on contrast resolution. From a practical standpoint, contrast resolution is necessary to differentiate tissue signals from background noise. Contrast resolution is also dependent on target size. A higher degree of contrast is needed to detect small structures compared with larger targets.

Temporal resolution, or frame rate, refers to the ability of the system to accurately track moving targets over

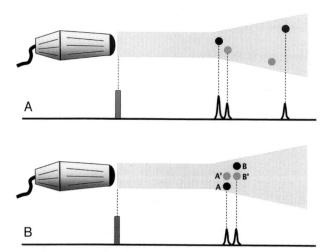

FIGURE 2.14. This schematic illustrates the interrelationship between beam intensity and acoustic impedance. The center of the beam has higher intensity compared with the edges. **A:** Whether an echo is produced, and with what amplitude it is recorded, depends on the relationship between intensity and acoustic impedance. Objects with higher impedance (black dots) produce stronger echoes and can therefore be detected even at the edges of the beam. Weaker echo-producing targets (gray dots) only produce echoes when they are located in the center of the beam. **B:** The effect of beam width on target location is shown. Objects A and B are nearly side by side with B slightly farther from the transducer. Because of the width of the beam, both objects are recorded simultaneously. The resulting echoes suggest that the two objects are directly behind each other (A' and B') rather than side by side.

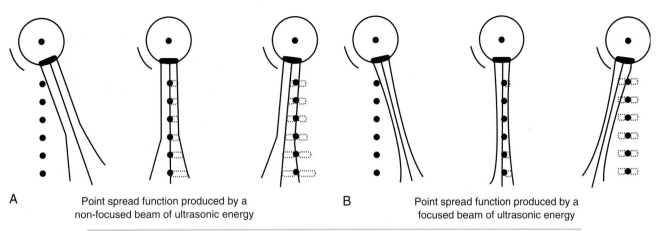

A   Point spread function produced by a
non-focused beam of ultrasonic energy

B   Point spread function produced by a
focused beam of ultrasonic energy

FIGURE 2.15. These diagrams demonstrate how beam width distorts the image in a two-dimensional sector scan **(A)** and how a focused beam can reduce this distortion **(B)**. The true image should be a series of dots; beam width, however, distorts the image into a series of dashes.

time. It is dependent on the amount of time required to complete a scan, which in turn is related to the speed of ultrasound and the depth of the image as well as the number of lines of information within the image. Generally, the greater the number of frames per unit of time, the smoother and more aesthetically pleasing the real-time image. Factors that reduce frame rate, such as increasing depth of field, will diminish temporal resolution. This is particularly important for structures with relatively high velocity, such as valves. Temporal resolution is the main reason that M-mode echocardiography is still a useful

clinical tool. With sampling rates of 1,000 to 2,000 images per second, temporal resolution of this modality is much higher than that of two-dimensional imaging.

CREATING THE IMAGE

The instrument used to create an ultrasound image is called an *echograph*. It contains the electronics and circuitry needed to transmit, receive, amplify, filter, process, and display the ultrasound information. The essential

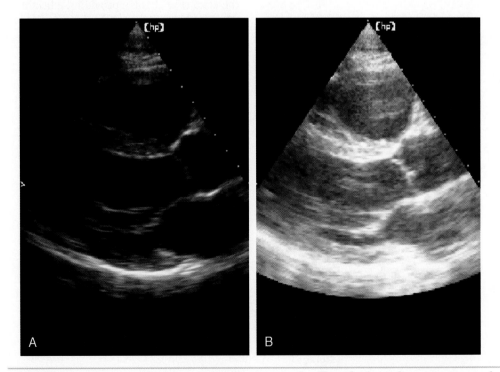

FIGURE 2.16. Parasternal long-axis images demonstrate the effect of gain on the appearance on the echocardiographic image. **A:** Gain is adjusted appropriately to allow recording of all relevant information. **B:** Too much gain is used, distorting the image, reducing resolution, and increasing noise.

components of the system are illustrated in Figure 2.17. As a first step, the returning energy is converted from sound waves to voltage signals. These are very low amplitude, high-frequency signals that must be amplified and, because they arrive slightly out of phase, realigned in time. In modern instrumentation, this realignment is accomplished using a digital beam former to allow proper summation and phasing of all the channels. Because the signals are still very high frequency at this point, the scan lines are referred to as RF data. The complexity of the information at this stage is in part due to the wide range of amplitudes and the inclusion of background noise. Logarithmic compression and filtering are performed to render the RF data more suitable for processing.

The polar scan line data at this point consist of sinusoidal waves, and each ultrasound target is represented as a group of these high-frequency spikes. Each group of high-frequency RF data is consolidated into a single envelope through a curve-fitting process called envelope detection. The resulting signal is then referred to as the polar video signal. This is sometimes called R-theta, indicating that each point in a polar map can be defined by its distance (R) and angle (theta) from a reference point. The next very important step involves digital scan conversion and refers to the complex task of converting polar video data into a cartesian or rectangular format. The image formed at this stage can be either stored in digital format or converted to analog data for videotape storage and display.

Figure 2.18 displays these different forms of imaging data as energy is received and processed by the echo-

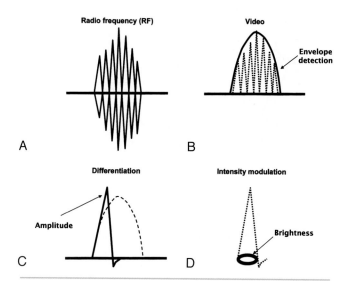

FIGURE 2.18. Some of the key steps in image creation are illustrated graphically. See text for details.

graph. The energy created by excitation of the piezoelectric elements is an RF signal (Fig. 2.18A). As discussed in the previous section, for the signal to be in a form that can be displayed visually, it must be converted to a video signal. This is accomplished by outlining (envelope detection) the outer edge of the upper portion, or positive deflection, of the RF signal (Fig. 2.18B). Differentiation of the video signal effectively accentuates the leading edge of the echo (Fig. 2.18C), providing a brighter signal and improving the ability to differentiate closely spaced targets. This is sometimes referred to as A-mode, for amplitude,

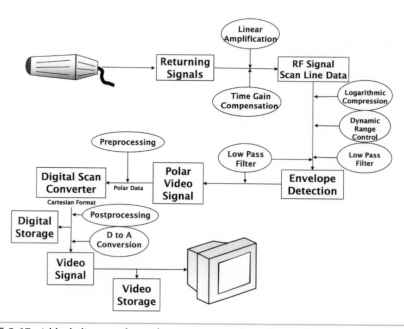

FIGURE 2.17. A block diagram shows the components of an echograph. The various steps needed to create an image, beginning at the transducer and continuing to the display, are included. See text for details.

imaging. Finally, intensity modulation converts the height or amplitude of the signal to a corresponding brightness level for video display (Fig. 2.18D). This is often called B-mode, for brightness, imaging and forms the basis of both M-mode and two-dimensional imaging display. How these various signal formats are used to create a visual display is covered in greater detail in a later section.

TRANSMITTING ULTRASOUND ENERGY

For most clinical applications, ultrasound is emitted from the transducer as a brief pulse of energy. A fundamental control feature is power output, which is simply the amount of ultrasound energy within each emitted pulse. In general, the higher the power output, the higher the amplitude of the returning signal. The pulse, which is a collection of cycles traveling together, is emitted at fixed intervals (Fig. 2.19). The time between pulsing is referred to as the *dead time* and is largely a function of depth. During the dead time, the transducer is "listening" for returning signals. The duration of the ultrasound pulse is sometimes referred to as *pulse length*, and the *pulse repetition period* represents the total of one pulse length plus one dead time. To image at a greater depth, the dead time is lengthened, allowing the ultrasound system to listen for reflections arising from greater depths before returning to the transducer. *Duty factor*, or the percentage of time that the transducer is pulsing, is simply the pulse duration divided by the pulse repetition period. This is a very small number, in the range of 0.1%, indicating that the system is "on" for a brief time and "off," or listening, for the majority of time. Each pulse of ultrasound energy results in the reception of a single line of ultrasound data.

Pulsing in ultrasound is necessary to obtain range resolution, that is, to localize reflectors accurately along the axis of the beam. In theory, an emitted pulse must travel to the target and be reflected back to the transducer before a second pulse can be emitted to prevent interference and range ambiguity. Pulses are typically quite short, usually less than 5 microseconds. Unlike continuous-wave ultrasound, pulsed ultrasound results in a relatively broad frequency spectrum. The shorter the pulse duration is, the broader the frequency spectrum is (Fig. 2.20). This means that the distribution of frequencies occurs over a predictable range that are centered on a central frequency. This is referred to as *bandwidth*, and such a transducer is said to deliver a *band of frequencies*. Bandwidth has important effects on the texture of the image and the resolution. Transducers that deliver a wider bandwidth will provide higher axial resolution, primarily because the pulse length is shorter.

To obtain an image, ultrasound must be transmitted, reflected, and received. A brief current of electricity intermittently excites the piezoelectric elements. This results in a pulse or burst of ultrasound that travels into the body while the transducer waits for the returning signal. Commercial echographs have repetition rates between 200 and 5,000 per second. To perform M-mode examinations, pulse repetition rates of between 1,000 and 2,000 per second are used. For two-dimensional imaging, repetition rates of 3,000 to 5,000 per second are necessary to create the 90-degree sector scan. This does not mean, however, that temporal resolution is higher for two-dimensional imaging. In fact, the opposite is true. Although the pulse repetition rate is lower for M-mode, because all the pulses are devoted to a single raster line, the temporal resolution is actually much higher for M-mode compared with two-dimensional echocardiography. Diagnostic echographs are extremely sensitive receivers and can detect a signal

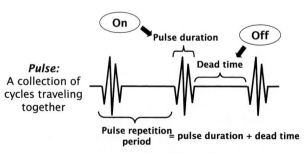

FIGURE 2.19. Ultrasound energy is usually emitted from the transducer in a series of pulses, each one representing a collection of cycles. Each pulse has a duration and is separated from the next pulse by the dead time. The diagram is not drawn to scale. In reality, dead time is much greater than pulse duration. See text for details.

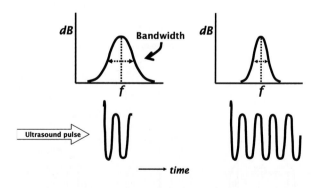

FIGURE 2.20. The diagram demonstrates the relationship between pulse duration, or length, and bandwidth. With increasing pulse length, the bandwidth becomes narrower, thereby reducing resolution. Therefore, to improve resolution, a short pulse length should be employed.

that is greatly attenuated, which is necessary because less than 1% of the emitted ultrasound energy is typically reflected back to the transducer.

Figure 2.21 demonstrates how one can use ultrasound to obtain an image of an object. In this illustration, a transducer placed on the side of a beaker of water sends out short pulses of ultrasound. These pulses travel through the homogeneous water and are reflected at the interface between the water and the opposite beaker wall (part A). The pulse retraces its original path and strikes the transducer, which, functioning as a receiver, converts the mechanical vibration of the impact into an electric signal that is registered on the oscilloscope of the echograph. Because the velocity of the sound wave traveling through the water is known, the time it takes for the echo to leave the transducer and return to excite the crystal, sometimes called *time of flight*, can be measured and used to calculate the distance between the transducer and the opposite wall of the beaker. Although the echograph is actually measuring a "time" variable, the value can automatically be converted to "distance." The various options for displaying this information, including A-, B-, and M-modes, are shown in the drawings.

If an object, such as a rod, is placed in the center of the beaker, the same ultrasound beam would now first strike the rod, which is closer to the transducer than the far side of the beaker (2.21B). In this case, some of the acoustic energy is reflected back from the rod, while a portion of the beam continues on to the far beaker wall before returning to the transducer. Both returning echoes would be recorded on the oscilloscope, indicating the position of the two targets relative to the transducer. Finally, if the rod is moved slowly within the beaker in a direction parallel to the sound beam, the distance between it and the transducer is constantly changing (2.21C). Each pulse of ultrasonic energy will strike the rod at a different position relative to the transducer, and its motion can be graphed over time. How well the motion is visualized depends in part on the repetition rate of the ultrasound pulse, also known as the sampling rate or pulse repetition frequency (PRF) of the echograph. The higher the repetition rate is, the more precisely the motion of the rod is tracked. Some of the important implications of PRF are discussed in greater detail in the next section.

DISPLAY OPTIONS

In the previous section, the concept of signal processing of the returning ultrasound energy is discussed. The raw RF energy is sequentially converted to various forms, including an amplitude signal and a brightness form (Fig. 2.18). Returning to Figure 2.21, if the motion of the rod is visualized on the oscilloscope, it would appear as a bright signal moving back and forth on the scope. This motion could be recorded by filming the oscilloscopic image. The motion could also be displayed using the technique of intensity modulation. This technique converts the amplitude of the echo (displayed as a spike) to intensity (displayed as a bright dot). In the amplitude mode (also known as A-mode), the height of the spike corresponds to the amplitude of the returning echo. In the brightness mode (known as B-mode), the intensity of the signal corresponds to the brightness of the dot.

Because the heart is a moving object, one can record that motion by introducing time as the second dimension. For example, if the tracing is swept from bottom to top, as is shown in Figure 2.21 (bottom panels), a wavy line is inscribed to demonstrate the motion of the rod. This is how an M-mode recording is created. In this case, M stands for motion and allows a single dimension of anatomy to be graphed against time. The intensity of any given echo within that display is represented as the density or thickness of the line, as is shown in the figure.

By definition, the M-mode presentation depicts anatomy along a single dimension corresponding to the ultrasound beam creating what has been called the "ice-pick" view of the heart. The relationship among these display formats, as they relate to cardiac imaging, is illustrated in Figure 2.22.

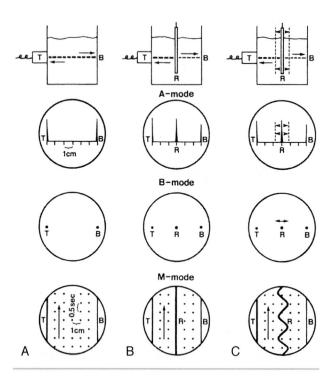

FIGURE 2.21. The basic principles of pulsed ultrasound are demonstrated in this schematic. See text for details. T, transducers; B, beaker; R, rod. (From Feigenbaum H, Zaky A. Use of diagnostic ultrasound in clinical cardiology. J Indiana State Med Assoc 1966;59:140, with permission.)

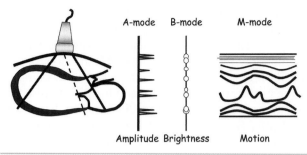

FIGURE 2.22. Echocardiography provides several display options. **Left:** A transducer is applied to the chest wall, and an ultrasound beam is directed through the heart at the level of the mitral valve. The returning ultrasound information can be displayed in amplitude mode (A-mode) in which the amplitude of the spikes corresponds to the strength of the returning signal. Amplitude can be converted to brightness (B-mode), in which the strength of the echoes at various depths is depicted as relative brightness. Motion can be introduced by plotting the B-mode display against time. This is the basis of M-mode echocardiography.

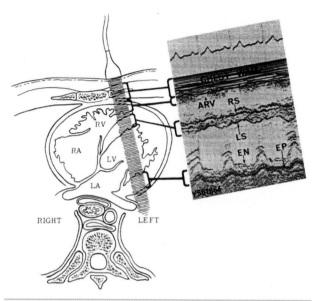

FIGURE 2.23. M-mode echocardiography is often described as an "ice-pick" view of the heart. The diagram shows the relationship of the transducer to the structures of the chest wall and heart. The corresponding M-mode echocardiogram provides relative anatomic information along a single line of information. ARV, anterior right ventricular wall; RS, right septum; LS, left septum; EN, posterior left ventricular endocardium; EP, posterior left ventricular epicardium; RA, right atrium: RV, right ventricle; LV, left ventricle; LA, left atrium.

Figure 2.23 shows how the echocardiographic system can record an M-mode tracing of the heart. In this example, the beam is directed toward the left ventricle. The ultrasonic beam also intersects a small portion of the right ventricular cavity. In the illustration, the M-mode recording was created using a strip chart recorder. The beam first passes through the chest wall structures, which are stable and unmoving. They appear as a series of straight lines. The echoes reflected by the anterior right ventricular wall are poorly visualized and recorded as a fuzzy band of reflections that are thicker during systole and thinner in diastole. The relatively echo-free space between the right ventricular wall and right side of the interventricular septum is a portion of the right ventricular cavity. The band of echoes running through the middle of the tracing represents the interventricular septum (right and left sides). Note that the left side of the interventricular septum moves downward in systole and upward in diastole. Next, echoes are seen originating from the posterior left ventricular wall with the endocardial echo having higher amplitude during systole than the epicardial echo. The less echogenic space between the endocardial and epicardial reflectors is the myocardium. The echo-free space between the septum and the posterior left ventricular wall is the cavity of the left ventricle. Within this space, echoes from the mitral valve apparatus are intermittently recorded.

In the early years, M-mode scanning formed the backbone of clinical echocardiography. By positioning the transducer over different acoustic "windows" of the chest wall, single dimensional images of cardiac structures could be recorded and inferences about structure, dimensions, and function could be made. Conversely, the B-mode display when held stationary to represent a one-

dimensional format offered little in the way of useful diagnostic information. It was soon recognized, however, that a B-mode scan swept through a sector arc could provide a cross-sectional image that depicted structure and function in real time. This technique was originally called *cross-sectional echocardiography* and is now widely referred to as *two-dimensional echocardiography*.

Figure 2.24 compares the M-mode imaging examination with a two-dimensional sector scan. The object being recorded is a sphere moving as a pendulum within a beaker of fluid. Using the M-mode technique, the oscilloscope display shows a series of wavy lines that primarily depict the leading and trailing edges of the sphere as it moves relative to the transducer within the beaker. Because the one-dimensional beam actually has a finite width or thickness, multiple secondary, less intense echoes are also recorded. Thus, the M-mode image provides an assessment of the dimensions of the object and its motion relative to the ultrasound beam. No information about motion in the orthogonal direction is provided and a complete recording of the object's shape is lacking.

If the same recording is created using two-dimensional imaging, more structural information is provided. Still, however, complete knowledge of the object is impossible because only two of the three spatial dimensions are included. In addition, two-dimensional imaging provides a more precise understanding of the true motion pattern

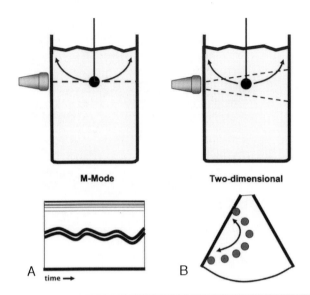

FIGURE 2.24. The relationship between M-mode and two-dimensional echocardiography is demonstrated. **A:** A black circular object swings through a beaker of water on a string. The motion of the ball can be recorded using M-mode echocardiography, as shown. Only motion in a single dimension, relative to the transducer, is recorded. **B:** The same motion is visualized using two-dimensional imaging. In this case, motion in two dimensions is recorded.

compared with the M-mode recording. In the example, the simplistic M-mode recording suggests that the object is moving back and forth, whereas the two-dimensional recording confirms that the object is moving in an arc. Motion outside the plane of the scan is still not recorded, even with two-dimensional imaging. A key assumption in the discussion is that the rate of scanning through the sector arc (the PRF of the system) is sufficiently high relative to the movement of the object to record the motion accurately. Even more recently, real-time three-dimensional imaging has been developed. This technology is discussed in detail in Chapter 3. By rapidly scanning through a pyramid-shaped field, more complete analysis of both shape and motion is accomplished.

TRADEOFFS IN IMAGE CREATION

Imaging a moving object, such as the heart, in real time creates a series of challenges. Not only must each "snapshot" be acquired rapidly enough to avoid blurring and distortion, but each successive snapshot must be captured at a sufficient rate to record the nuances and subtlety of motion smoothly and accurately. Then, each individual picture can be assembled into a motion picture that is the essence of real-time imaging. Because ultrasound travels at a fixed and relatively slow velocity through tissue, the ultimate rate at which imaging information can be ac-

quired and assembled is limited. Thus, tradeoffs and constraints exist that must be recognized.

The variables to consider include the desired depth of examination, the line density, the PRF, the sweep angle, and the frame rate. Constructing a complex, real-time image begins with emission of an ultrasound pulse that penetrates the body and returns information from varying depths. Because the velocity of sound in the body is essentially fixed, the time required to send and receive information is a function of depth of view. Again, the rate at which individual pulses are transmitted is referred to as the PRF. Each pulse allows a single line of ultrasonic data to be recorded. To go from a single line of ultrasonic data to a two-dimensional image, the beam must be swept through an angle that typically varies from 30 to 90 degrees. The larger the angle is, the more lines are needed to fill the sector with data. Because line density is an important determinant of image quality, it is desirable to acquire as many ultrasonic lines as possible. The term *line density* refers to the number of lines per degree of sweep. A line density of approximately two lines per degree is necessary to construct a high-quality image.

Another important factor in image quality is frame rate. Depending on the speed of motion of the structure of interest, a higher or lower frame rate will be necessary to construct an accurate and aesthetically pleasing "movie" of target motion. For example, the aortic valve can move from the closed to the open position in less than 40 milliseconds. At an imaging rate 30 frames per second, it is likely that the valve will appear closed in one frame and open in the next, with no appearance of motion because intermediate positions were not captured. If one wished to record the aortic valve in an intermediate position, a very high frame rate must be employed. However, to increase the frame rate, additional compromises must be accepted. Specifically, increasing the frame rate generally results in a decrease in line density and degradation in image quality.

It should be appreciated that modern echocardiographic instruments use scan converters and forms of digital manipulation to convert the image into an aesthetically pleasing display format. Individual raster lines are thereby eliminated so that the appearance of individual lines radiating like spokes from the apex of the scan are no longer present. Instead, images are displayed on a television screen using the concept of *fields* and *frames*. A field is the total ultrasonic data recorded during one complete sweep of the beam. A frame is the total sum of all imaging data recorded and generally implies that new information is superimposed on previously recorded data. With television technology, two fields are interlaced (to improve line density) to produce one frame. Using this approach, the frame rate would be half of the corresponding sweep rate.

SIGNAL PROCESSING

When the transducer is acting as a receiver, the piezoelectric elements convert the returning ultrasonic energy to an electric impulse in the form of RF data. As previously discussed, the RF data are processed and converted to a video signal in which signal strength corresponds to brightness. Because of attenuation, signals returning from the most distant reflectors (i.e., structures at greater depth) will be the weakest or least bright echoes. By selectively amplifying echoes from greater depths, using a method referred to as time gain compensation, images of uniform brightness are created. This device allows returning signals from different depths to be selectively suppressed or amplified to provide relatively uniform signal strength (Fig. 2.25). Some control of depth compensation is provided on virtually all commercially available echocardiographic instruments. Although this is one of the most useful and important image control features, it is also a source of distortion and misuse. If one remembers that the purpose of this device is to compensate for the loss of ultrasonic energy (i.e., attenuation) as the beam propagates through the body, then one better understands how the controls should be used. The primary purpose is to enhance the far echoes and suppress near echoes, without creating distortion or artifact.

A late and very important stage in image creation involves the use of gray scale to display anatomic data. The challenge here results from discordance between the wide range of signal strength of the returning echoes and the limitations of the human eye to perceive differences in gray scale. The range of voltages generated during data acquisition extends over several log units, whereas the human eye is able to distinguish only approximately 30 shades of gray. The ultrasound instrument, using an operation called preprocessing, must reduce the range of the voltage signals to a more manageable number. *Dynamic range* is the extent of useful ultrasonic signals that can be processed (Fig. 2.26). It is expressed in decibels and is defined as the ratio of the largest to smallest signals measured at the point of input to the display. At the low end, noise and undesired weak echoes exist that can be eliminated using a reject control. At the high end, signal saturation occurs and these echoes are also suppressed. In between, it is desirable to preserve as large a dynamic range as possible to ensure that all clinically important returning signals are included in the image. For example, scattered echoes are by definition much weaker than specular echoes, yet both are important in image construction. A mechanism to accommodate both is necessary, and this is accomplished through the use of a proper dynamic range. Through the technique of nonlinear compression, a wide dynamic range can be handled for processing by the scan converter.

The second challenge is how to convert the wide range of input signals into a manageable range of gray scales.

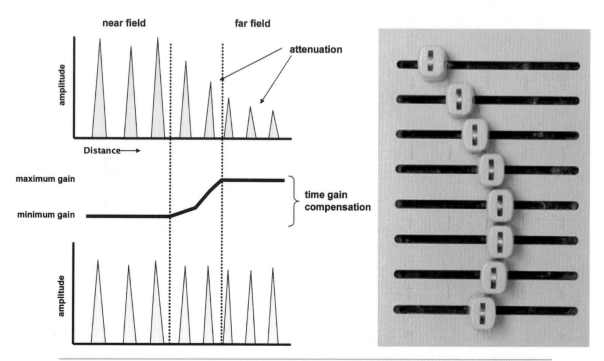

FIGURE 2.25. The amplitude of returning signals is plotted against distance, or depth, from the transducer. Time gain compensation can be used to enhance the amplitude of the weaker signals returning from targets at greater depth and permits similar targets at different depths to be displayed accurately. On the right, the time gain compensation controls from an ultrasound machine are shown.

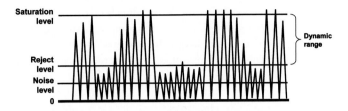

FIGURE 2.26. The schematic illustrates the concept of dynamic range. See text for details.

With the exception of color flow imaging, echocardiography is essentially a black and white medium. An image is constructed of very small pixels that are assigned a gray level ranging from absolute white to absolute black. This is accomplished using a digital approach in which the range of brightness is divided into either 128 or 256 levels of gray (Fig. 2.27). The process of remapping the digital output of the scan converter to the range of gray scale values used in the video display is called *post-processing*. This step permits manipulation of the imaging data to enhance the visual quality of the display.

TISSUE HARMONIC IMAGING

In the course of propagation of the ultrasound wave, the transmitted, or fundamental, frequency of the signal may be altered due to nonlinear interactions with the tissue. The net effect of such interactions is the generation of frequencies not present in the original signal. These new frequencies are integer multiples of the original frequency and are referred to as *harmonics*. The returning signal contains both fundamental and harmonic frequencies. By suppressing or eliminating the fundamental component, an image is created primarily from the harmonic energy. Unlike the harmonic technique that is so important to contrast echocardiography, in which the interaction of the ultrasound energy and the microbubbles produces vibrations that occur at multiple (harmonic) frequencies, tissue harmonics are generated during propagation by gradual conversion of energy from one frequency to another. The development of tissue harmonics can be compared with an ocean wave that changes shape and speed as it approaches the beach. Thus, the strength of the harmonic frequency actually increases as the wave pene-

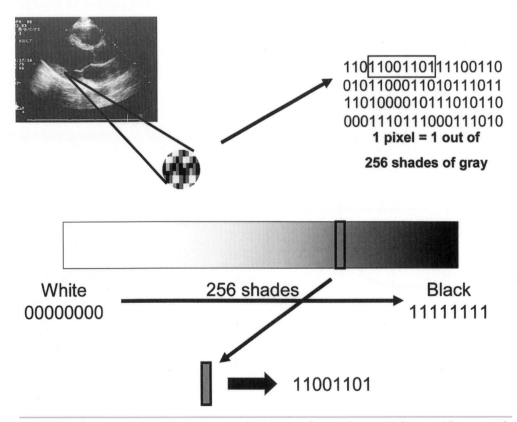

FIGURE 2.27. Gray scale is a key concept in the creation of a two-dimensional image. The gray scale refers to the number of shades that can possibly be displayed between the two extremes of white and black. In the example, 256 shades are depicted. Each pixel is assigned one of these shades. In a digital system in which imaging data are stored as a binary code, eight bits are required to encode one of the 256 shades of gray.

trates the body. This is profoundly different from the fate of the fundamental frequency wave that attenuates constantly during propagation (Fig. 2.28A). This difference in behavior has important and practical implications for imaging. Close to the chest wall, where many of the troublesome imaging artifacts are generated, there is very little harmonic signal. For this reason, imaging that exploits the harmonic frequency avoids many of the near field artifacts that affect fundamental imaging. At depths of 4 to 8 cm, the relative strength of the harmonic signal is near its maximum, whereas the fundamental frequency has diminished considerably. Thus, the harmonic signal is strongest at distances that are most relevant to transthoracic imaging.

A second feature of tissue harmonic imaging, again the result of nonlinear interactions, relies on the fact that strong fundamental signals produce intense harmonics and weak fundamental signals produce almost no harmonic energy. This phenomenon further reduces the artifact generation during harmonic imaging because most such artifacts result from weak fundamental signals. By producing images from the harmonic frequency reflections, the weak signals that cause many artifacts are disproportionately suppressed. The net result is that harmonic imaging reduces near field clutter and many of the other sources of imaging artifact that plague fundamental frequency imaging. The signal-to-noise ratio is improved and image quality is enhanced, especially in patients with poor fundamental frequency images. A consistent finding in most studies has been improved endocardial border definition. However, an important side effect of tissue harmonic imaging is that strong specular echoes, such as those arising from valves, appear "thicker" than they would on fundamental imaging. This is particularly true

in the far field and can lead to false-positive interpretations. To avoid such pitfalls but to take advantage of the benefits of harmonic imaging, most clinical studies should include both fundamental and harmonic imaging in the course of the examination.

A recent application of harmonic imaging involves *pulse inversion technology*. Unlike tissue harmonic imaging, in which the fundamental signal is filtered, pulse inversion harmonic imaging takes a different approach to eliminating the fundamental frequency. In the pulse inversion mode, the transducer sequentially emits two pulses with similar amplitude but with inverted phase (Fig. 2.28B). When backscattered from a linear reflector such as tissue, and then summed, these pulses cancel each other, resulting in almost complete elimination of the fundamental frequency signal, called *destructive interference*. The remaining harmonic energy can then be selectively amplified, producing a relatively pure harmonic frequency spectrum. The result is an image with many of the potential advantages previously attributed to tissue harmonic imaging. How much additional benefit can be ascribed to pulse inversion technology remains to be determined.

ARTIFACTS

The complexity of image creation using either mechanical or phased-array transducer technology is evident. Therefore, it should not be surprising that a variety of artifacts can occur that have a significant impact on image quality and diagnostic potential. One of the most important of these artifacts involves the generation of side lobes. Side lobes occur because not all the energy produced by the transducer remains within the single, central beam. In-

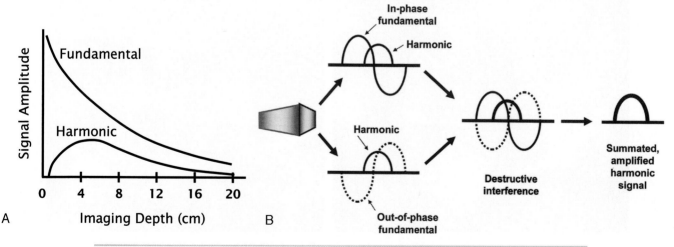

FIGURE 2.28. A: Unlike fundamental frequencies, harmonic frequencies increase in strength as the wave penetrates the body. At the chest wall, where many artifacts are generated, very little harmonic signal is present. At useful imaging depths (4–8 cm), the relative strength of the harmonic signal is at its maximal. See text for details. **B:** The concept of pulse inversion technology is demonstrated. See text for details.

stead, a portion of the energy will concentrate off to the side of the central beam and propagate radially, a phenomenon known as edge effect. A side lobe may form where the propagation distance of waves generated from opposite sides of a crystal differs by exactly one wavelength. Side lobes are three-dimensional artifacts, and their intensity diminishes with increasing angle. The artifact created by side lobes occurs because all returning signals are interpreted as if they originated from the main beam. Hence, a weak-intensity echo originating from a laterally positioned target (but recorded via the off-axis side lobe) will be displayed as if it were located along the central axis of the main beam. It should be emphasized that side lobes are considerably weaker than the main beam so the returning echoes produced by a side lobe are also weaker. Side lobe reflections usually become evident when they do not conflict with real echoes. A prerequisite for a dominant side lobe artifact is that the source of the artifact must be a fairly strong reflecting target. The atrioventricular groove and the fibrous skeleton of the heart are examples of good sources of side lobe echoes (Fig. 2.29). When strong, these artifactual echoes can lead to significant problems in interpretation. Lesser degrees of side lobe artifact merely increase the general noise level of the system.

A second important source of artifacts in echocardiography is reverberations. To understand how these occur, it is helpful to return to the example of a transducer held against a beaker of water (Fig. 2.21). In this case, the strongest reflector of the beam is the opposite beaker wall. As the reflected ultrasound returns to the transducer, it is likely that a portion of the returning signal undergoes a second reflection at the near beaker wall interface. This portion of the acoustic energy again reflects off the far wall and is finally returned to the transducer. With each step, the signal becomes weaker but may still be within the range of detection by the transducer. Most of the signal correctly identifies the far beaker wall as the primary reflector. That portion of the signal that makes two round-trips to the far wall also registers a signal. In this case, the pulse required twice as long as the original pulse to be detected and therefore incorrectly places the target at twice the distance from the transducer. This secondary echo represents a reverberation and occurs because of secondary reflection at the near beaker wall or at the surface of the transducer. In the clinical situation, such artifacts not only result from the beam reflecting from the transducer but also may originate from other strong echo-producing structures within the heart or chest (Fig. 2.30). Typically, a reverberation artifact that originates from a fixed reflector will not move with the motion of the heart. It appears as one or more echo targets directly behind the reflector, often at distances that represent multiples of the true distance. In some cases, the source of reverberations is not apparent. These are particularly troublesome and frequently result in misinterpretation of the image.

Another potential artifact is shadowing. Its appearance, in some ways, is the opposite of a reverberation. That is, instead of a series of echoes behind the source of the artifact, shadowing results in the *absence* of echoes directly behind the target (Fig. 2.31). Shadowing occurs when one attempts to visualize structures beyond a region of unusually high attenuation, such as a strong reflector.

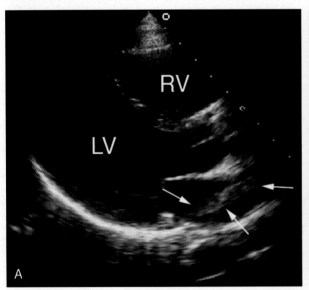 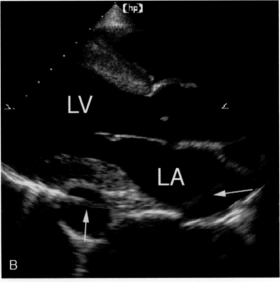

FIGURE 2.29. Two examples of side lobes are shown. **A:** The strong echoes produced by the posterior mitral anulus and atrioventricular groove produce a side lobe artifact that appears as a mass within the left atrium. **B:** Bright echoes within the pericardium produce a linear artifact that appears within the descending aorta and left atrium (arrows). LA, left atrium; LV, left ventricle; RV, right ventricle.

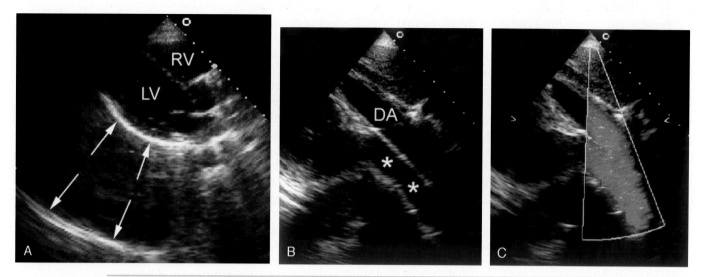

FIGURE 2.30. Reverberation artifacts are demonstrated. **A:** The source of the artifact is the posterior pericardium, which is a very strong reflector. This creates the illusion of a second structure behind the heart. In this case, the second line of echoes (far arrows) is twice the distance from the transducer as the actual pericardial echoes. **B:** A second lumen appears just distal to the descending aorta (DA) in this subcostal view. The illusion of a second vessel was apparent with two-dimensional imaging (*, **B**) and color Doppler imaging **(C)**. LV, left ventricle; RV, right ventricle.

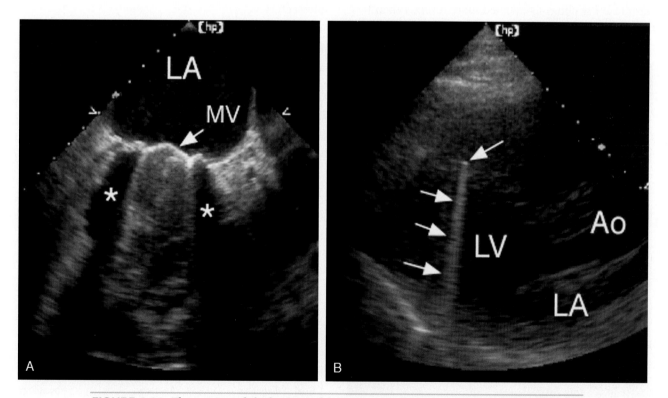

FIGURE 2.31. The concept of shadowing is demonstrated and compared with reverberations. **A:** A St. Jude mitral prosthesis (MV) is present. The echo-free space beyond the sewing ring (*) represents shadowing behind the strong echo-reflecting sewing ring. The cascade of echoes directly beyond the prosthetic valve itself that extend into the left ventricle (LV) represent reverberations. **B:** A shotgun pellet within the heart (arrow) casts a series of reverberations into the left ventricle. Ao, aorta; LA, left atrium.

Because only a very small portion of the ultrasound beam can propagate beyond such a reflector, an acoustic shadow is created from which no reflections are produced. Perhaps the most relevant example of shadowing occurs in the setting of prosthetic valves. Such mechanical devices create strong reflectors behind which imaging is quite limited. Native structures that become heavily calcified are additional sources of shadowing. In this case, the presence of shadowing can be useful to identify the existence of strong reflectors, such as calcium. Contrast containing blood also produces shadowing, which significantly limits its utility.

One additional source of artifact is termed *near field clutter*. This problem, also referred to as "ringdown artifact," arises from high-amplitude oscillations of the piezoelectric elements. This only involves the near field and has been greatly reduced in modern-day systems. The artifact is troublesome when trying to identify structures that are particularly close to the transducer, such as the right ventricular free wall or left ventricular apex. This artifact is illustrated in Figure 2.32.

DOPPLER ECHOCARDIOGRAPHY

Despite being clinically adopted more recently than two-dimensional imaging, Doppler imaging is an integral and indispensable part of the echocardiographic examination. Knowledge of basic Doppler imaging principles is essential to fully understand the value and limitations of these techniques. Although Doppler imaging can be regarded as being complementary to two-dimensional imaging, the principles and instrumentation underlying this technique are substantially different. Used primarily to examine the flow of blood, Doppler imaging is concerned with the direction, velocity, and then pattern of blood flow through the heart and great vessels. The differences between B-mode or imaging echocardiography and Doppler imaging are fundamental (Table 2.4). The primary targets of the anatomic echocardiographic examination are the myocardium and valves of the heart. For Doppler imaging, the primary target is the red blood cells. Whereas echocardiography provides information on structure, Doppler imaging provides information on function. Thus, echocardiography can be regarded as an imaging technique that focuses on anatomy, whereas Doppler imaging focuses on physiology and hemodynamics. Finally, whereas echocardiography functions optimally when the beam and the target are at right angles, the Doppler equations rely on a more parallel alignment between the beam and the flow of blood. Thus, echocardiography and Doppler imaging provide diagnostic data that are largely complementary.

Principles of Doppler Ultrasound

The Doppler principle is based on the work of the Austrian physicist Christian Doppler, first published in 1842. He studied the phenomenon that the apparent pitch of sound was affected by motion either toward or away from the listener. If the source of sound were stationary, then the pitch or frequency of that sound was constant. If, however, the source of sound moved toward the listener, the frequency increased and the pitch appeared to rise. Conversely, if the sound source was moving away from the listener, the frequency of the sound decreased relative to the listener and the pitch appeared lower.

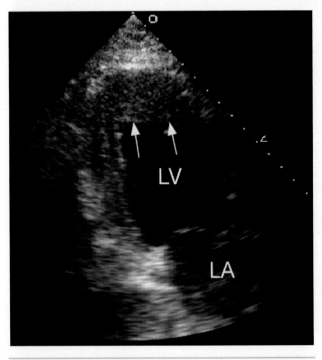

FIGURE 2.32. This apical two-chamber view demonstrates an artifact called near field clutter (arrows). This is the result of high-amplitude oscillations emitted by the transducer and is a common source of misinterpretation. LA, left atrium; LV, left ventricle.

▶ **TABLE 2.4 A Comparison of Two-Dimensional Echocardiography and Doppler**

	Two-dimensional echocardiography	*Doppler*
Ultrasound target	Tissue	Blood
Goal of diagnosis	Anatomy	Physiology
Type of information	Structural	Functional
Optimal alignment between beam and target	Perpendicular	Parallel
Preferred transducer frequency	High	Low

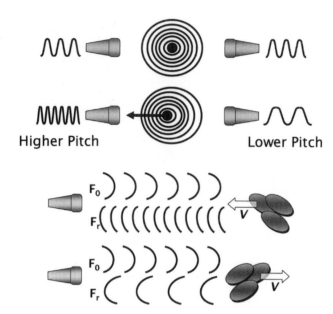

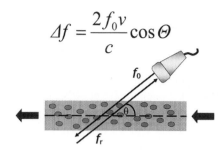

$$\Delta f = \frac{2f_0 v}{c} \cos \Theta$$

FIGURE 2.34. Calculation of the Doppler shift requires knowledge of the transmitted frequency (f_0), the reflected frequency (f_r), the angle of incidence (θ), and the speed of sound. See text for details.

FIGURE 2.33. The basic principles of the Doppler phenomenon are illustrated. **Top:** A stationary source of sound produces a given pitch or frequency. If the sound is moving toward a recorder, the pitch appears increased and if the sound is moving away from a recorder, the pitch appears decreased. **Bottom:** This same concept is applied to blood flow. If the red blood cells are moving toward the transducer at a given velocity (v), the reflected frequency (F_r) will be higher than the emitted frequency (F_0). If the red blood cells are moving away from the transducer, the opposite will occur.

The application of this phenomenon to blood flow measurement is illustrated in Figure 2.33. In this example, ultrasound is emitted from a transducer and reflected from a moving target such as a red blood cell. If that target is stationary, the frequency and wavelength of the emitted and reflected ultrasound are identical. If the target is moving toward the transducer, the reflected frequency is "shifted" upward proportional to the velocity of the target relative to the transducer. Conversely, movement of the target away from the transducer results in the reflected ultrasound having a lower frequency than the emitted ultrasound, a downward shift in frequency. The increase or decrease in frequency due to relative motion between the transducer and the target is referred to as the *Doppler shift.*

In addition to the qualitative observation of the frequency shift, Christian Doppler also described the mathematical relationship between the magnitude of the frequency shift and the velocity of the target relative to the source. As can be seen in Figure 2.34, the Doppler shift (Δf) depends on the transmitted frequency of the ultrasound, the speed of sound, the intercept angle between the interrogating beam and the flow, and, finally, the velocity of the target.

$$\Delta F = \frac{2f_0 v}{c} * \cos \Theta \qquad \text{[Eq. 2.3]}$$

Because the velocity of sound and the transmitted frequency are known, the Doppler shift depends on the velocity of blood and the angle of incidence, θ.

$$\Delta f \propto v * \cos \Theta \qquad \text{[Eq. 2.4]}$$

Thus, the velocity of blood flow (the unknown variable) is directly related to the Doppler shift (what is actually measured by the instrument) corrected for the angle θ. This angle correction actually depends on the cosine of θ, which has a predictable and critically important effect on the calculation of velocity. Because the cosine of 0 degrees = 1, this correction (i.e., multiplying by 1) has no net effect on the calculation of the Doppler shift. Thus, the derived blood flow velocity is the true velocity. As the angle between the beam and the blood flow direction increases from 0 toward 90 degrees, the cosine θ decreases from 1 toward 0. The relationship between θ and cosine θ is shown in Figure 2.35A. For any angle other than 0, multiplying by the cosine θ results in a *decrease* in calculated velocity. Consequently, misalignment of the interrogating beam will lead to underestimation but never overestimation of true velocity. For practical purposes, this only becomes significant beyond approximately 20 degrees. As can be seen in the graph, if θ equals 10 degrees, cosine θ equals approximately 0.98 and the degree of underestimation is trivial. As θ increases to 30 degrees, cosine θ becomes 0.83 and the true velocity is underestimated by 17%. As the angle increases further, the rate of underestimation increases rapidly. The effect of angle θ on the accuracy of the Doppler gradient calculation is illustrated in Figure 2.35B. For example, if a jet with a peak velocity of 5 m/sec is properly aligned, an accurate pressure gradient of 100 mm Hg will be measured. If the same jet is recorded at an incident angle (θ) of 30 degrees, the calculated gradient will be approximately 75 mm Hg, a significant underestimation.

Another important component of the Doppler equation is the transducer or carrier frequency, which is a primary determinant of the maximal blood flow velocity that can

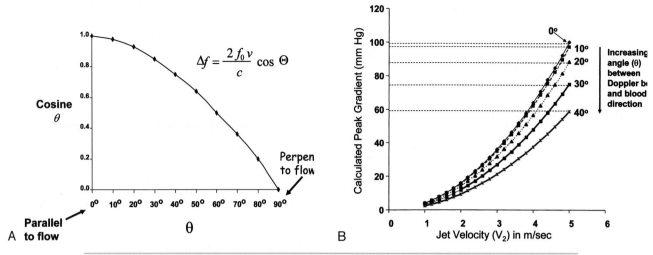

FIGURE 2.35. **A:** The effect of intercept angle on the Doppler equation is shown. See text for details. **B:** The intercept angle has an important effect on the accuracy of velocity measurement. This effect is magnified at higher velocity and becomes increasingly important as the intercept angle increases from 0 to 40 degrees, as shown by the different curves. See text for details.

be resolved. The relationship between the Doppler shift and blood flow velocity at four different transmitted frequencies is illustrated in Figure 2.36. A high flow velocity such as 5 m/sec is more readily recorded using a low carrier frequency such as 1 MHz compared with a high transducer frequency such as 5 or 10 MHz because of the corresponding Doppler shift. In this respect, Doppler imaging is the opposite of echocardiographic imaging. With echocardiography, a higher transducer frequency is desirable because it is associated with higher resolution. With Doppler imaging, a lower frequency is advantageous because it allows high flow velocity to be recorded.

The primary job of the Doppler instrument is to measure the Doppler shift, and from this measurement, velocity can be calculated. The Doppler shift is defined as the difference in frequency between the transmitted and received or backscattered signal. In cardiac imaging, values

are generally in the 5 to 20 kHz range, well within the audible range of human hearing. The process of determining the Doppler shift is a complex one, referred to as *spectral analysis*. This involves a comparison of the actual waveforms of the transmitted and received frequencies using a method called fast Fourier transform analysis. The net result of this analysis is a spectral display of the entire range of velocities.

Doppler Formats

For cardiovascular applications, there are five basic types of Doppler techniques: continuous wave Doppler, pulsed wave Doppler, color flow imaging, tissue Doppler, and duplex scanning. Pulsed wave Doppler imaging is similar to echocardiography. Short, intermittent bursts of ultrasound are transmitted into the body. Although targets at multiple points along the beam may reflect the transmitted ultrasound, the pulsed Doppler instrument only "listens" at a fixed and very brief time interval after transmission of the pulse (Fig. 2.37). This permits returning signals from one specific distance from the transducer to be selectively received and analyzed, a process called *range resolution*. By adjusting the timing between transmission and reception, different ranges or depths can be evaluated. This effectively creates a sample volume at a specified point along the transmitted beam that can be positioned within the field of view to permit blood flow velocity information to be sampled. Using a superimposed two-dimensional image for purposes of localization, pulsed wave Doppler imaging interrogates the distribution of blood flow values within a relatively limited region.

An important limitation of pulsed Doppler imaging is the maximal velocity that can be accurately resolved. This

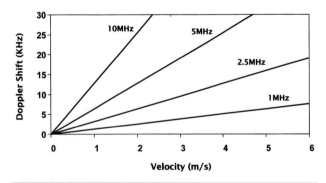

FIGURE 2.36. The relationship between the Doppler shift and blood flow velocity for four different transducers is shown. The graph demonstrates that lower frequency transducers are capable of resolving higher velocity flow. See text for details.

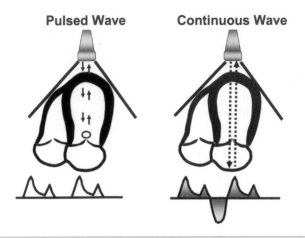

FIGURE 2.37. The differences between pulsed and continuous wave Doppler imaging are illustrated. See text for details.

occurs because of the phenomenon referred to as *aliasing*. The number of pulses transmitted from a Doppler transducer each second is called the PRF. Sampling rate is an important determinant of how accurately the system re-

solves frequency information. To accurately represent a given frequency, it must be sampled at least twice, that is

$$PRF = 2 \times f_{DOP}. \qquad [Eq.\ 2.5]$$

This formula establishes the limit (Nyquist limit) below which the sampling rate is insufficient to characterize the Doppler frequency. This key concept is demonstrated in Figure 2.38. In Figure 2.38A, a sine wave of fixed wavelength is tracked at three different sampling rates. In the top panel, the sampling rate is sufficiently high relative to the wavelength (17 times in four wavelengths or 4.25 per cycle) that the frequency can be reasonably estimated. This is indicated by how well the dashed line (sampling rate) tracks the solid line (the ultrasound wave). In the middle panel, a lower sampling rate (11 times every four wavelengths) results in a less precise tracking of the true frequency. In the bottom panel, by sampling only seven times over the four cycles, it is impossible to accurately characterize the frequency of the wave. The relevance of this phenomenon to pulsed wave Doppler imaging is shown in Figure 2.38B. In each

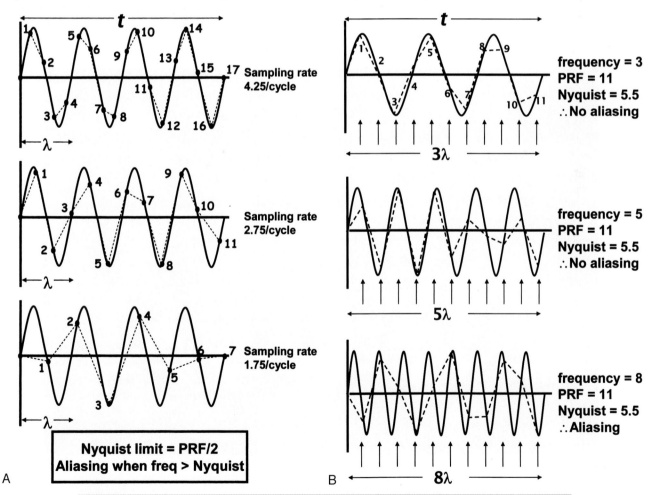

FIGURE 2.38. The concept of aliasing is demonstrated graphically in this schematic. See text for details.

panel, a constant sampling rate, or PRF (11 times over time *t*, indicated by the vertical arrows), is maintained. This results in a Nyquist limit of 5.5. In the top panel, this sampling rate is adequate to characterize the relatively low frequency wave (a frequency of three cycles per time *t*). As the frequency increases, the sampling rate will eventually become too slow to follow the frequency. For example, in the middle panel, the frequency has increased to five cycles per time *t*. This frequency is still below the Nyquist limit, so aliasing does not occur and the true frequency is accurately resolved. In the bottom panel, at a frequency of eight per time *t*, the Nyquist limit of 5.5 has now been exceeded and aliasing occurs. Practically speaking, aliasing is the inability of a pulsed wave Doppler system to detect the higher frequency Doppler shifts. The upper limit of frequency that can be detected by a given pulsed system is the Nyquist limit, which is defined as one-half the PRF.

Figure 2.39 shows a sample volume at the level of the mitral valve in a patient with mitral regurgitation. High velocity flow occurs in systole and is directed away from the transducer. Because this velocity exceeds the Nyquist limit, the Doppler signal aliases and appears to wrap around the baseline. Aliasing creates confusion as to the

direction of flow and prevents an accurate measure of maximal velocity. Figure 2.40 illustrates the relationship between sample volume depth, or range, and the maximal velocity that can be resolved. Note that the relationship again depends on the transducer frequency. As the depth increases, the maximal velocity that can be accurately detected decreases. However, for any given depth, a lower frequency transducer permits higher velocities to be resolved compared with a higher frequency transducer.

Continuous wave Doppler imaging differs in a fundamental way from pulsed wave Doppler imaging and echocardiography. Rather than sending out intermittent pulses of information, continuous wave Doppler imaging simultaneously transmits and receives ultrasound signals continuously. This can be accomplished in one of two ways. One type of transducer employs two distinct elements: one to transmit and the other to receive (Fig. 2.41). Alternatively, with phased-array technology, one crystal within the array is dedicated to transmitting while another is simultaneously receiving. Because the transmitted signal is not pulsed, range resolution is impossible and the reflected signals all along the ultrasound beam are sampled simultaneously. Thus, it is impossible to know where along the sample beam that any recorded ve-

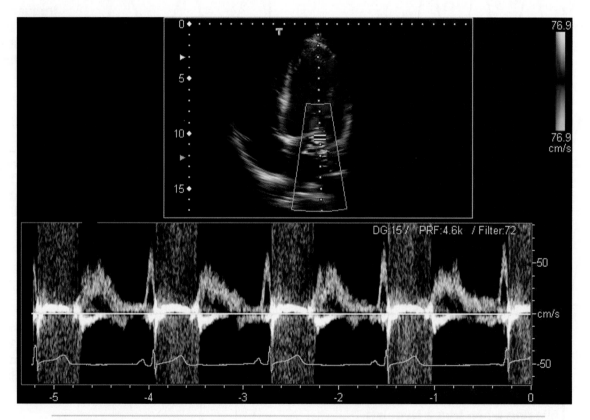

FIGURE 2.39. An example of aliasing is provided. Using pulsed wave Doppler imaging, the sample volume is placed in the left atrium, just beyond the mitral valve. In systole, mitral regurgitation produces a high velocity jet that cannot be resolved with the pulsed wave Doppler technique. Aliasing of the jet is the result.

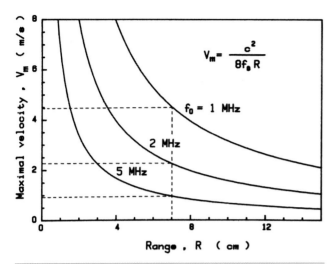

FIGURE 2.40. This graph demonstrates the relationship between range, or depth, and the maximal velocity that can be resolved, using two different transducer frequencies. The relationship is given by the equation. In both cases, as depth increases, the maximal velocity that can be recorded decreases. However, for any given depth, the lower frequency transducer is capable of resolving higher velocities compared with the higher frequency transducer. V_{max}, maximal velocity; c, velocity of ultrasound; f_0, transducer frequency; R, range. (From Hatle L, Angelsen B. Doppler Ultrasound in Cardiology: Physical Principles and Clinical Applications. 2nd Ed. Philadelphia: Lea & Febiger, 1985, with permission.)

locity signal arises. Using a variety of amplification and signal-processing techniques, however, both the direction and the velocity spectrum of blood flow are recorded. A major advantage of continuous wave Doppler imaging is that aliasing does not occur and very high velocities can be accurately resolved. The combination of pulsed and continuous wave Doppler imaging forms a powerful tool for clinical applications.

High PRF Doppler imaging is a technique that combines features of both pulsed and continuous wave Doppler imaging. Using pulsed wave Doppler imaging, velocity within a single sample volume is determined by receiving signals only at the point in time that corresponds to that depth. However, the listening window will also capture returning signals from twice that depth that were emitted by the previous ultrasound pulse. Using this approach, velocity information from the primary sample volume as well as integer multiples of that depth can all be analyzed during a single listening event. If the sample volume is placed at one-half of the actual depth of interest, velocity information from both sites can be recorded over two consecutive pulses. Because the use of the shallower sample volume depth is associated with a higher PRF, higher velocities can also be analyzed without aliasing. Although some degree of range ambiguity is inherent, this has limited practical effects. By positioning multiple sample gates along the beam, a significant increase in

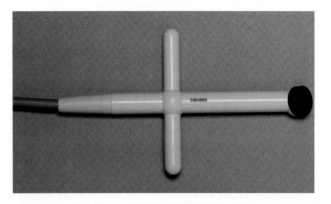

FIGURE 2.41. A nonimaging, or Pedoff, continuous wave Doppler transducer is shown. The transducer contains two elements: one for transmitting and one for receiving.

PRF is achieved, allowing relatively high velocities to be resolved with a modest loss of range resolution.

Because Doppler imaging provides information on direction and velocity of flow, it is useful to display this information graphically by plotting instantaneous flow velocity against time. By convention, velocity is displayed on the vertical axis with flow toward the transducer above the baseline and flow away from the transducer below the baseline (Fig. 2.42). In the illustration, aortic flow accelerates toward the transducer in systole, with very little flow occurring during diastole. A relatively thin envelope of the Doppler signal indicates that the flow is essentially *laminar*. Under physiologic conditions, most examples of blood flow in the cardiovascular system are laminar,

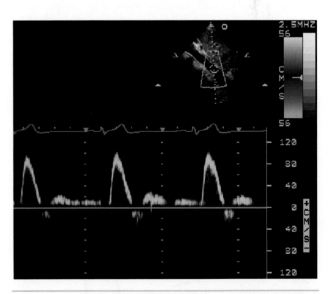

FIGURE 2.42. Laminar, pulsatile flow in the abdominal aorta is recorded with pulsed wave Doppler imaging. The signal demonstrates a narrow envelope during systole. The maximal velocity of the flow is approximately 100 cm/sec. Note, however, that the ultrasound beam is not parallel to the flow direction.

meaning that individual blood cells are traveling at approximately the same speed in approximately the same direction parallel to the walls of the chamber or vessel. Of course, some range of velocities naturally occurs. For example, velocity tends to be higher in the center of a vessel and lower near the vessel wall, as predicted by basic hydraulic principles (Fig. 2.43). As shown in the schematic, a flat, laminar profile is characteristic of large straight vessels. Flow tends to become more parabolic (i.e., less flat) as vessel size decreases. Flow through a curved vessel is characterized by higher velocities along the outside wall and lower velocities nearer the inside. Flow through a bifurcation produces eddy currents along the inner side of the branches, but relatively laminar flow along the outer walls. Blood flow through a U-shaped vessel, such as the aortic arch, is complex, depending on the profile of flow entering the arch, the angle of curvature, and the centrifugal forces acting on the blood. Even within the heart itself, flow remains generally laminar and occurs over a relatively narrow range of velocities. In pathologic situations, such as valve abnormalities or congenital defects, flow tends to become turbulent, often with abnormally high velocity.

Doppler instrumentation depends on an ability to record and display the range of velocities and directions within a region of interest. By digitizing a snapshot of Doppler shift information and then applying a complex mathematical technique called fast Fourier transform, the instantaneous flow velocity spectrum can be displayed. At each instant, the range of velocities determines the width of the Doppler signal and the frequency distribution of each individual velocity is represented by the gray scale. In the cardiovascular system, most flow is pulsatile.

Purely laminar flow has a narrow envelope of velocities, indicating that most of the blood cells travel over a narrow range of velocity. With increasing turbulence, both the direction and the range of velocities increase, and this leads to a widening of the spectral pattern as shown in Figure 2.44. Thus, a narrow spectral envelope indicates the presence of laminar flow, whereas spectral broadening is consistent with turbulence. It should be emphasized that this distinction is only possible when using pulsed wave Doppler imaging. Because continuous wave Doppler imaging samples at multiple sites along the beam, a narrow spectral envelope almost never occurs.

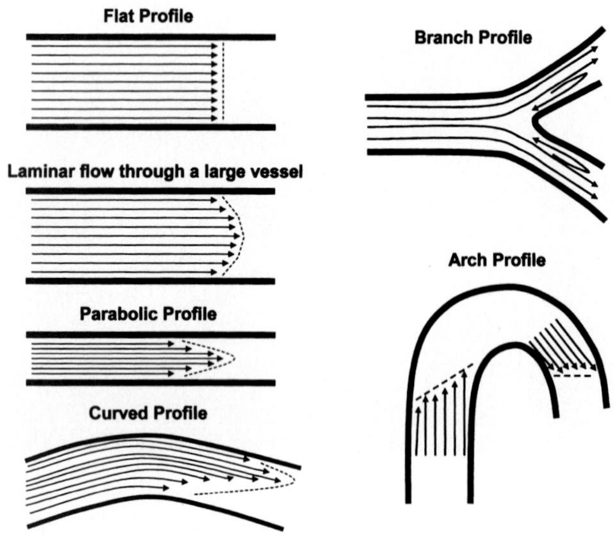

Color Flow Imaging

Color flow imaging is a form of pulsed wave Doppler imaging that uses multiple sample volumes along multiple raster lines to record the Doppler shift, based on principles described earlier for pulsed wave and high PRF Doppler imaging. By overlaying this information on a two-dimensional or M-mode template, the color flow image is created. Constructing the color flow image is complex. Each pixel represents a region of interest in which the flow characteristics must be measured. Rather than analyzing the entire velocity spectrum within one of these small regions (which would require several seconds for each image if a complete Fourier transform were performed), some compromises are necessary and only mean frequencies and frequency spreads (variance) are calculated.

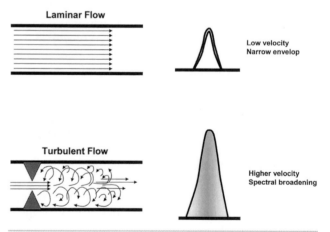

FIGURE 2.44. Top: A laminar flow profile occurs when most of the red blood cells are traveling in approximately the same direction at approximately the same velocity. In a pulsatile system, this results in a Doppler signal that has a narrow envelope, as shown on the right. This would be typical of systolic flow through the aortic valve. **Bottom:** The changes seen in the setting of turbulent flow as might occur with aortic stenosis are shown. In this case, blood accelerates through a narrow orifice and becomes disturbed distal to the site of obstruction. This has two primary effects on the Doppler signal: velocity increases (as flow accelerates) and spectral broadening occurs.

FIGURE 2.43. Various types of flow patterns are shown. See text for details.

As a first step, for each pixel, the strength of the returning echo is determined. If it is above a predetermined threshold, it is painted a shade of gray and displayed as a two-dimensional echocardiographic data point. If it is below the threshold, it is analyzed as Doppler information. By repetitive sampling, an average value for mean velocity and variance is determined with greater accuracy. The flow velocity, direction, and a measure of variance are then integrated and displayed as a color value (Fig. 2.45). By performing such operations extremely rapidly over the entire range of the Doppler overlay, a color pattern is created that provides information on flow characteristics. By using a color reject threshold, only flow above a given velocity level is displayed as color. This limits the potential for "information overload" and allows the observer to integrate the Doppler and gray scale image information in a meaningful way. A color algorithm can be constructed to display these multiparametric data. For example, the direction of flow can be displayed using red (toward) and blue (away). The brightness of these primary colors encodes the magnitude of the mean velocity. High variance, or turbulence, is coded green, which, when mixed with red or blue, yields yellow or cyan, respectively, often with a mosaic appearance.

Technical Limitations of Color Doppler Imaging

By "visualizing" the velocity of flow in a two-dimensional format, color Doppler imaging has been used extensively to assess abnormal flow patterns such as valvular regurgitation. Although this is done routinely, the technical limitations of this technique are considerable. As described previously, the instrumentation needed to construct a color flow map is complex and involves several compromises and manipulations. Because no two manufacturers approach the problem in exactly the same way, one of the fundamental problems of color Doppler imaging is the difficulty in comparing images from different ultrasound systems.

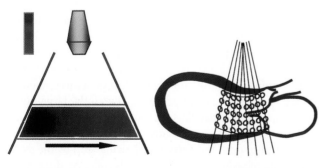

Color Encoding of Flow Direction   Multiple Pulsed Doppler Sampling Sites

FIGURE 2.45. The basic principles of color flow imaging are illustrated. See text for details.

It is tempting to equate color flow imaging with angiography and assume that color jets are a direct visualization of regurgitant flow. Although color Doppler imaging is a very sensitive technique for detecting regurgitation, the relationship between jet size and regurgitation severity is complex. First, remember that jets are three-dimensional entities that can never be completely captured in a two-dimensional format. The primary determinant of jet size is jet momentum, which depends on both flow rate and velocity. Thus, factors that affect velocity, including blood pressure, will also affect jet size. If color Doppler imaging is performed when blood pressure is either very high or very low, this clinical information should be noted and taken into account when the study is interpreted. Chamber constraint is another factor that determines jet size. This is particularly true of eccentric jets that become entrained along a wall, making them appear smaller than they actually are. For similar reasons, chamber size can also influence the apparent area of a color flow jet.

Among the most important determinants of jet size are instrument settings. By adjusting the color scale, PRF is altered, and jet size can change dramatically. By lowering the scale (or Nyquist limit), the lower velocity blood at the periphery of the jet becomes encoded and displayed, making the jet appear larger. In general, the color scale should be set as high as possible for a given depth. Increasing the wall filter will have the opposite effect; this will reduce the jet size by excluding velocities at the periphery. Power and instrument gain will also alter jet size. Increasing these settings will increase jet area. To optimize the settings, color gain should be increased until color pixels appear within the tissues, then the gain should be reduced slightly. Finally, transducer frequency has a complex effect on color jet area. The jet size will tend to increase with high carrier frequency because of the relationship between velocity and the Doppler shift. On the other hand, greater attenuation at higher frequency will make jets appear smaller. Obviously, instrument settings can profoundly affect the clinical utility of color flow imaging. It is recommended that most settings related to color imaging should be optimized when the machine is first set up and then left unchanged, to the degree possible, to maximize consistency.

The differences between color Doppler imaging and angiography are noteworthy. If contrast is injected into the left ventricle of a patient with mitral regurgitation, any contrast that appears in the left atrium must come through the mitral valve in the form of regurgitation. The amount of contrast that is visualized in the atrium, although impossible to quantify, correlates with the regurgitant flow volume. Doppler imaging, however, records velocity rather than flow. Thus, the color jet that is seen in the left atrium includes not only red blood cells that regurgitate through the mitral valve but also blood that was already in the atrium and is essentially being moved by the incoming jet. This has been called the "billiard ball effect" and is illustrated in Figure 2.46. In the upper diagram, the blood in the left ventricle is depicted by the triangles and the left atrial blood by the circles. In the lower panel, some left ventricular blood has entered the left atrium through the incompetent mitral valve (filled triangles). This blood displaces the left atrial blood, transferring some of its energy and forcing the atrial blood to accelerate away from the regurgitant orifice (filled circles). If the velocity of this left atrial blood is sufficiently high, it will be detected by color Doppler imaging, just as the blood that accelerated through the regurgitant orifice is similarly detected. Thus, Doppler imaging records velocity, not flow. It cannot distinguish whether the moving left atrial blood originated in the ventricle (the filled triangles) or atrium (the filled circles), simply that it has sufficient velocity to be detected. Unlike angiography, the Doppler jet consists of both atrial and ventricular blood, all of which is moving faster than a predetermined velocity.

The important difference between velocity and flow is further illustrated in Figure 2.47. This schematic demonstrates yet another limitation of using color Doppler imaging for regurgitant flow quantification. The regurgitant orifice area (ROA) is perhaps the most fundamental meas-

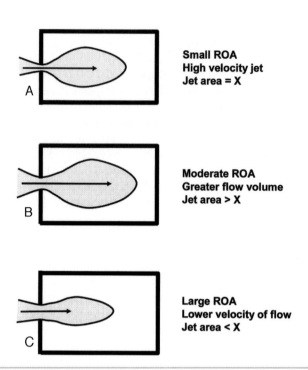

FIGURE 2.47. This diagram demonstrates how turbulent flow through a regurgitant orifice relates to color Doppler signal. See text for details. ROA, regurgitant orifice area.

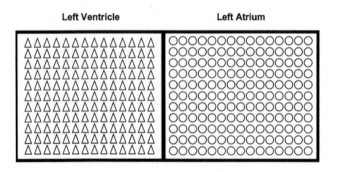

FIGURE 2.46. **Top:** This is a schematic depiction of mitral regurgitation, with the triangles representing blood within the left ventricle, and the circles indicating left atrial blood. **Bottom:** Mitral regurgitation is demonstrated by some of the triangles moving through the orifice into the left atrium. The effect of those cells on the left atrial blood (circles) is shown. Because of the increase in velocity, some of the triangles and some circles are encoded and displayed by the color Doppler signal (filled triangles and circles). See text for details.

ure of regurgitation severity. In this example, three different sizes of ROA are shown, along with their corresponding jet areas. As the ROA increases, flow rate increases and more blood enters the chamber and is detected by the Doppler method (middle panel). However, because velocity is inversely related to orifice area, as the ROA increases, the velocity of the regurgitant jet may decrease (if the pressure gradient is less). Because Doppler imaging records velocity, this larger (but lower velocity) flow may be recorded as a smaller color jet (lower panel).

Despite these limitations, color flow imaging can provide a semiquantitative approach to regurgitation severity. When viewed in real-time, with proper instrument settings, jet area and regurgitant volume are correlated. Analyzing such images, however, can be confusing. Color Doppler imaging aliases at a low velocity, so jets change color frequently, in part because of changes in velocity and in part because of changes in location relative to the transducer (Fig. 2.45). Because of the low frame rate of color Doppler imaging, rapidly moving structures, such as valves, can produce color artifacts. Due to the large number of operations that must be rapidly performed to construct each color image, any one frame can contain artifacts or ghosts. For this reason, using stop-frame techniques to measure jet dimensions should be done very cautiously. Real-time viewing tends to filter out much of the insignificant artifacts seen on stop-frame analysis. By integrating information over many cardiac cycles, useful

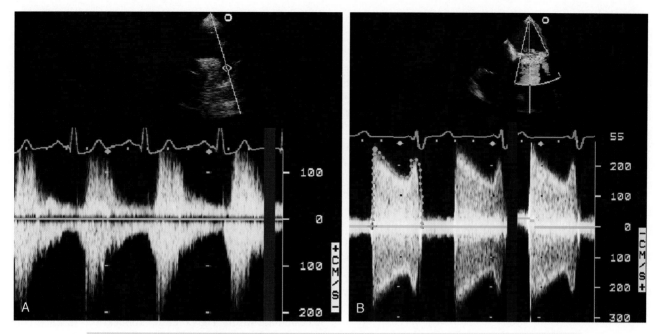

FIGURE 2.48. Two examples of mirror image artifact are demonstrated. **A:** descending aortic flow appears to occur both above and below the baseline. **B:** A stenotic porcine mitral valve is recorded with pulsed wave Doppler imaging. The intensity of the signal results in a classic mirror image artifact.

diagnostic data are available. On the other hand, a single color frame can never convey a complete depiction of the true jet dimensions and often results in the measurement of artifact or noise rather than real flow information.

Doppler Artifacts

As is the case with two-dimensional imaging, the creation of the Doppler image involves the production of a variety of potential artifacts. Some of these are related directly to the Doppler principle. For example, aliasing occurs when pulsed wave Doppler techniques are applied to flow velocities that exceed the Nyquist limit. This topic has already been covered in detail. A commonly encountered artifact is called *mirror imaging*, also called *crosstalk*. As the name suggests, this is the appearance of a symmetric spectral image on the opposite side of the baseline from the true signal. Such mirror images are usually less intense but similar in most other features to the actual signal (Fig. 2.48). These artifacts can be reduced by decreasing the power output and optimizing the alignment of the Doppler beam with the flow direction.

Beam width artifacts are common to all forms of ultrasound imaging. With pulsed Doppler imaging, it must be remembered that the sample volume(s) has finite dimensions that tend to increase with depth. A sample volume placed in the far field is large enough to straddle more than one flow jet. For example, left ventricular inflow and outflow can often be recorded simultaneously from the apical four-chamber view. This is because the

sample volume at that depth is broad enough to simultaneously record both flow patterns. This is sometimes desirable, permitting the timing and velocity of different flow patterns to be compared (Fig. 2.49). However, beam width artifact often has less desirable effects. For example, a large sample volume may hinder one's ability to distinguish aortic stenosis from mitral regurgitation.

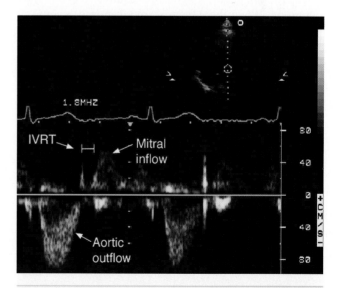

FIGURE 2.49. Beam width artifacts in Doppler imaging can be clinically useful. In this case, the thickness of the Doppler beam allow simultaneous recording of both aortic outflow and mitral inflow. This permits the isovolumic relaxation time to be determined. IVRT, isovolumic relaxation time.

Color Doppler imaging can be affected by several types of artifacts. Shadowing may occur, masking color flow information beyond strong reflectors. Ghosting is a phenomenon in which brief swathes of color are painted over large regions of the image. Ghosts are usually a solid color (either red or blue) and bleed into the tissue area of the image (Fig. 2.50). These are produced by the motion of strong reflectors such as prosthetic valves. They tend to be very transient and do not correspond to expected flow signals. Ghosting is most problematic when color flow images are frozen to analyze or planimeter a jet.

Finally, it should be remembered that color Doppler imaging is very gain dependent. Too much gain can create a mosaic distribution of color signals throughout the image. Too little gain eliminates all but the strongest Doppler signals and may lead to significant underestimation of jet area. With experience, the operator learns to adjust the gain settings to eliminate background noise, without oversuppression of actual flow information.

Tissue Doppler Imaging

A unique and relatively recent application of the Doppler principle is tissue Doppler imaging. By adjusting gain and reject settings, the Doppler technique can be used to record the motion of the myocardium rather than the blood within it. To apply Doppler imaging to tissue, two important differences must be recognized. First, because the velocity of the tissue is much lower than blood flow, the machine must be adjusted to record a much lower range of velocities. Second, because the tissue is a much stronger reflector of the Doppler signal compared with blood, additional adjustments are required to avoid oversaturation. When these factors are taken into account, a semiquantitative approach to myocardial velocity analysis is possible. An example of tissue Doppler imaging is provided in Figure 2.51. Note how this early systolic frame displays the direction and relative velocity of the different myocardial segments. One obvious limitation is that the incident angle between the beam and the direction of target motion varies from region to region. This limits the ability of the technique to provide absolute velocity information, although direction and relative changes in tissue velocity are displayed.

One potentially important derivation of this technique involves *strain rate imaging*. Strain is a measure of the deformation that occurs when force is applied to tissue. Strain rate is simply its temporal derivative. By measuring instantaneous velocity at two closely positioned points within the myocardium and knowing the initial distance between two points, both strain and strain rate can be determined. The Doppler tissue imaging technique has been used successfully to derive the velocity information needed to calculate strain. The potential applications of these concepts are discussed more fully in Chapters 3 and 6.

BIOLOGIC EFFECTS OF ULTRASOUND

Some of the success and popularity of echocardiography can be attributed to the safety and risk-free nature of ultrasound. In addition to being completely noninvasive, the biologic effects of ultrasound, as used in routine clinical situations, pose minimal risks to the patient. Ultrasonic examination of many parts of the body, including such potentially sensitive tissues as a developing fetus and the eye, have been performed on millions of patients without docu-

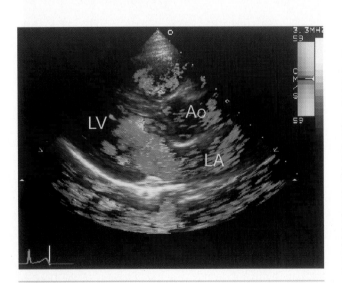

FIGURE 2.50. Ghosting occurs when brief displays of color are painted over regions of tissue, as shown in the illustration. See text for details. Ao, aorta; LA, left atrium; LV, left ventricle.

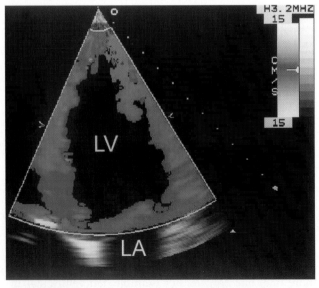

FIGURE 2.51. An example of tissue Doppler imaging is provided. See text for details. LA, left atrium; LV, left ventricle.

mentation of a single serious adverse event. Still, the question of safety when an external energy source is transmitted into the body must be considered. Newer applications and instruments may involve higher levels of energy, so the potential impact of such approaches should also be examined.

The biologic effects of ultrasound depend on the total energy applied to a given region. Thus, both the intensity of the ultrasound beam and the duration of exposure are important factors. Acoustic energy is measured in joules, which is defined as the amount of heat generated by the transmission of ultrasound. Recall that power is the amount of acoustic energy per unit of time and intensity is the acoustic power per unit of area. For example, the power level is 1 W if 1 J of energy is produced in 1 second. A milliwatt is 0.001 W. The biologic effects of ultrasound are generally discussed in terms of power, and the units of power are in the milliwatt range. Intensity is usually expressed as watts per meter squared (W/m^2) or in milliwatts per centimeter squared (mW/cm^2). The actual measure of intensity is complex in biologic systems and typically reported as spatial peak intensity, spatial average intensity, or intensity at a particular point. As discussed previously, intensity varies spatially across the ultrasound beam. Thus, spatial average (SA) intensity is equal to the total power emitted by the transducer divided by the cross-sectional area of the ultrasound beam. If the power output is 2.0 mW and the beam area is 1.0 cm^2, then SA intensity would be 2.0 mW/cm^2. Spatial peak (SP) intensity will usually occur at the center of the beam where power is most concentrated.

Measuring the intensity of the beam in a pulsed mode system is more complicated. When ultrasound is transmitted in pulses, the intensity will vary both spatially and temporally, depending on the pulsing sequence. This latter factor depends on both the pulse duration and the pulse repetition period. To calculate the energy from a pulsed ultrasonic beam, it is necessary to know the duty factor, which is a measure of the fraction of time during which the transducer emits ultrasound (i.e., is "on"). If the duration is 1.5 microseconds and the pulse repetition rate is 1,000/sec, then the pulse repetition would be 1,000 microseconds or 1 millisecond. In this case, the duty factor would be 1.5 divided by 1,000 or 0.0015. This means that the transducer is transmitting only 0.15 % of the time. The average power of a pulsed echocardiograph would be the peak power multiplied by the duty factor. If the peak power were 10 W and the duty factor were 0.0015, then the average power would be 0.015 W or 15 mW.

When discussing intensity in pulsed-mode systems, a common measurement is the spatial averaged, temporal averaged intensity, which is obtained by measuring the power of the transducer over the pulse repetition period and then dividing it by the surface area of the transducer. This measure, frequently quoted by manufacturers, is the lowest of the various intensities measured

with a pulsed system. The spatial averaged, temporal peak intensity is a measure of average power divided by the transducer surface area that occurs when the transducer is emitting. The SP intensity is usually two to three times greater than the SA intensity. Of course, the highest measure of intensity would be the spatial peak, temporal peak intensity, which uses peak intensity that occurs when the transducer is "on." Commercial ultrasound instruments operating in pulsed mode for two-dimensional imaging have spatial peak, temporal averaged intensities ranging from 0.001 to more than 200 mW/cm^2. Pulsed Doppler imaging, however, may have a spatial peak, temporal average as high as 1,900 mW/cm^2, considerably greater than 100 mW/cm^2 level that has been most extensively studied and has never been shown to produce a biologic effect.

The biologic effects of ultrasound energy are related primarily to the production of heat (a goal of ultrasonic therapy). With pulsed ultrasound, it is extremely unlikely that the duty factor is high enough for significant heat to be generated within the body. Heat is generated whenever ultrasound energy is absorbed, and the amount of heat produced depends on the intensity of the ultrasound, the time of exposure, and the specific absorption characteristics of the tissue. It should also be noted that the flow of blood and specifically the perfusion of tissue have a dampening effect on heat generation and physically allow heat to be carried away from the point of energy transfer.

The relatively short periods of pulsing, coupled with the fact that the transducer is constantly moving so that no single area is imaged for a long period, contribute to the low likelihood of delivering significant heat to the tissue. With transesophageal imaging, however, this is not always the case. For example, during intraoperative imaging, the probe may remain nearly stationary for extended periods. The heat generated by the transducer itself must also be considered. Although there are no reports of significant injury resulting from even prolonged intraoperative transesophageal echocardiography, attention to these issues is recommended. Limited imaging time, occasional repositioning of the probe, and constant monitoring of the probe temperature will all help to ensure an impeccable safety record.

Another physical effect of ultrasound is cavitation. This term refers to the formation and behavior of gas bubbles produced when ultrasound penetrates into tissue. It is very difficult to measure or even detect the phenomenon of cavitation *in vivo*. Because of the relatively high viscosity of blood and soft tissue, significant cavitation is unlikely. An important aspect of cavitation concerns its effect during the injection or infusion of contrast microbubbles. It is now well established that ultrasound energy causes such microbubbles to resonate, resulting in cyclical changes in bubble diameter and stability.

A variety of other physical forces may also be produced by ultrasound energy. These include oscillatory, sheer, radiation, pressure, and microstreaming. Although each of these effects can be demonstrated *in vitro*, there is no evidence that any of these physical phenomena has a significant biologic effect on patients. Despite considerable study, virtually no clinically important biologic effects attributable to ultrasound at diagnostic power levels have been demonstrated. However, a few reports have suggested that some changes might occur at the chromosomal level that would be relevant to the developing fetus. These observations have caused considerable concern within the field of fetal echocardiography. The overwhelming evidence, however, supports the relative safety of ultrasound even in this critically sensitive arena.

Research will continue in this important area. All evidence to date suggests that diagnostic ultrasound, particularly that used in echocardiography, is an extremely safe tool with no demonstrated adverse effects even with the use of newer technology and more powerful instrumentation. Although this is reassuring and justifiably inspires continued confidence in ultrasound imaging, the desire for more and better diagnostic information should never occur at the expense of patient safety. Therefore, keeping the scan time to a minimum, especially when performing Doppler imaging, should always be a consideration. It is likely that ongoing reassessment of the safety of echocardiography will continue for the foreseeable future.

SUGGESTED READINGS

Adler L, Hiedemann EA. Determination of the nonlinearity parameter b/a for water and m-xylene. J Acoust Soc Am 1962;34:410–412.

Aggarwal KK, Moos S, Philpot EF, et al. Color velocity determination using pixel color intensity in Doppler color flow mapping. Echocardiography 1989;6:473–483.

Asberg A. Ultrasonic cinematography of the living heart. Ultrasonics 1967;5:113–117.

Averkiou MA, Hamilton MF. Measurements of harmonic generation in a focused finite-amplitude sound beam. J Acoust Soc Am 1995;98:3439–3442.

Baker DW, Rubenstein SA, Lorch GS. Pulsed Doppler echocardiography: principles and applications. Am J Med 1977;63:69–80.

Baker ML, Dalrymple GV. Biological effects of diagnostic ultrasound: a review. Radiology 1978;126:479–483.

Barnett SB, Kossoff G. Temporal peak intensity as a critical parameter in ultrasound dosimetry. J Ultrasound Med 1984;3:385–389.

Becher H, Tiemann K. Improved endocardium imaging using modified transthoracic echocardiography with the second harmonic frequency (tissue harmonic imaging). Herz 1998;23:467–473.

Bom K, de Boo J, Rijsterborgh H. On the aliasing problem in pulsed Doppler cardiac studies. J Clin Ultrasound 1984;12:559–567.

Bom N, Lancee CT, van Zwieten G, et al. Multiscan echocardiography. I. Technical description. Circulation 1973;48:1066–1074.

Burns PN. The physical principles of Doppler and spectral analysis. J Clin Ultrasound 1987;15:567–590.

Burns PN. Harmonic imaging with ultrasound contrast agents. Clin Radiol 1996;51(Suppl 1):50–55.

Burns PN, Wilson SR, Simpson DH. Pulse inversion imaging of liver blood flow: improved method for characterizing focal masses with microbubble contrast. Invest Radiol 2000;35:58–71.

Carstensen EL, Duck FA, Meltzer RS, et al. Bioeffects in echocardiography. Echocardiography 1992;9:605–623.

Edler I. Diagnostic use of ultrasound in heart disease. Acta Med Scand 1955;308–332.

Edvardsen T, Gerber BL, Garot J, et al. Quantitative assessment of intrinsic regional myocardial deformation by Doppler strain rate echocardiography in humans: validation against three-dimensional tagged magnetic resonance imaging. Circulation 2002;106:50–56.

Eggleton RC, et al. Visualization of cardiac dynamics with real-time B-mode ultrasonic scanner. In: White D, ed. Ultrasound in Medicine. New York: Plenum Publishing, 1975.

Feigenbaum H. Use of echocardiography in evaluating left ventricular function. Presented at the Second World Congress on Ultrasonics in Medicine. Excerpta Medica, 1973;June.

Feigenbaum H, Zaky A. Use of diagnostic ultrasound in clinical cardiology. J Indiana State Med Assoc 1966;59:140.

Fry WJ. Mechanism of acoustic absorption in tissue. J Acoust Soc Am 1952;24:412.

Goldman DE, Jueter TF. Tabular data of the velocity and absorption of high-frequency sound in mammalian tissues. J Acoust Soc Am 1956;28:35.

Goss SA, Frizzell LA, Dunn F. Ultrasonic absorption and attenuation in mammalian tissues. Ultrasound Med Biol 1979;5:181–186.

Gramiak R, Waag RC, Simon W. Cine ultrasound cardiography. Radiology 1973;107:175–180.

Greenberg NL, Firstenberg MS, Castro PL, et al. Doppler-derived myocardial systolic strain rate is a strong index of left ventricular contractility. Circulation 2002;105:99–105.

Gregg EC, Palagallo GL. Acoustic impedance of tissue. Invest Radiol 1969;4:357–363.

Griffith JM, Henry WL. A sector scanner for real time two-dimensional echocardiography. Circulation 1974;49:1147–1152.

Griffith JM, Henry WL. An ultrasound system for combined cardiac imaging and Doppler blood flow measurement in man. Circulation 1978;57:925–930.

Hatle L, Angelson B. Doppler Ultrasound in Cardiology: Physical Principles and Clinical Applications. 2nd Ed., Philadelphia: Lea & Febiger, 1985.

Hertz CH. Ultrasonic engineering in heart diagnosis. Am J Cardiol 1967;19:6–17.

Hertz CH, Lundstrom K. A fast ultrasonic scanning system for heart investigation. Presented at the 3rd International Conference on Medical Physics, Gotenburg, Sweden, 1972.

Huntsman LL, Gams E, Johnson CC, et al. Transcutaneous determination of aortic blood-flow velocities in man. Am Heart J 1975;89:605–612.

King DL. Cardiac ultrasonography. Cross-sectional ultrasonic imaging of the heart. Circulation 1973;47:843–847.

Kisslo JA, vonRamm OT, Thurstone FL. Cardiac imaging using a phased array ultrasound system. II. Clinical technique and application. Circulation 1976;53:262–267.

Kisslo JA, vonRamm OT, Thurstone FL. Dynamic cardiac imaging using a focused, phased-array ultrasound system. Am J Med 1977;63:61–68.

Kornbluth M, Liang DH, Paloma A, et al. Native tissue harmonic imaging improves endocardial border definition and visualization of cardiac structures. J Am Soc Echocardiogr 1998;11:693–701.

Kossoff G. Diagnostic applications of ultrasound in cardiology. Aust Radiol 1966;10:101–106.

Light LH. Transcutaneous observation of blood velocity in the ascending aorta in man. Biol Cardiol 1969;26:214–221.

Macintosh IJ, Davey DA. Relationship between intensity of ultrasound and induction of chromosome aberrations. Br J Radiol 1972;45:320–327.

Mason WP. Piezoelectric Crystals and Their Application to Ultrasonics. New York: Van Nostrand, 1950.

Matsumoto M, Matsuo H, Ohara T, et al. Use of kymo-two-dimensional echoaortocardiography for the diagnosis of aortic root dissection and mycotic aneurysm of the aortic root. Ultrasound Med Biol 1977;3:153–162.

Melton HE Jr, Thurstone FL. Annular array design and logarithmic processing for ultrasonic imaging. Ultrasound Med Biol 1978;4:1–12.

Miller DL. Ultrasonic detection of resonant cavitation bubbles in a flow tube by their second-harmonic emissions. Ultrasonics 1981;19:217–224.

Miyatake K, Okamoto M, Kinoshita N, et al. Clinical applications of a new type of real-time two-dimensional Doppler flow imaging system. Am J Cardiol 1984;54:857–868.

Morgan CL, Trought WS, Clark WM, et al. Principles and applications of a dynamically focused phased array real time ultrasound system. J Clin Ultrasound 1978;6:385–391.

Murai N, Hoshi K, Nakamura T. Effects of diagnostic ultrasound irradiated during fetal stage on development of orienting behavior and reflex ontogeny in rats. Tohoku J Exp Med 1975;116:17–24.

Omoto R. Color Atlas of Real-Time Two-Dimensional Doppler Echocardiography. Tokyo: Shindan-To-Chiryo, 1984.

Pye SD, Wild SR, McDicken WN. Adaptive time gain compensation for ultrasonic imaging. Ultrasound Med Biol 1992;18:205–212.

Reid J. A review of some basic limitations in ultrasonic diagnosis. In: Grossman CC, Holmes JH, Joyner C, et al., eds. Diagnostic Ultrasound. Proceedings of the First International Conference, University of Pittsburgh, 1966. New York: Plenum Publishing, 1965.

Roelandt J, van Dorp WG, Bom N, et al. Resolution problems in echocardiology: a source of interpretation errors. Am J Cardiol 1976;37:256–262.

Rushmer RF, Baker DW, Stegall HF. Transcutaneous Doppler flow detection as a nondestructive technique. J Appl Physiol 1966;21:554–566.

Skorton DJ, Collins SM, Greenleaf JF, et al. Ultrasound bioeffects and regulatory issues: an introduction for the echocardiographer. J Am Soc Echocardiogr 1988;1:240–251.

Spencer KT, Bednarz J, Mor-Avi V, et al. The role of echocardiographic harmonic imaging and contrast enhancement for improvement of endocardial border delineation. J Am Soc Echocardiogr 2000;13:131–138.

Spencer KT, Bednarz J, Rafter PG, et al. Use of harmonic imaging without echocardiographic contrast to improve two-dimensional image quality. Am J Cardiol 1998;82:794–799.

Stewart HD, Stewart HF, Moore RM Jr, et al. Compilation of reported biological effects data and ultrasound exposure levels. J Clin Ultrasound 1985;13:167–186.

Taylor KJ. Current status of toxicity investigations. J Clin Ultrasound 1974;2:149–156.

Vancon AC, Fox ER, Chow CM, et al. Pulse inversion harmonic imaging improves endocardial border visualization in two-dimensional images: comparison with harmonic imaging. J Am Soc Echocardiogr 2002;15:302–308.

Veluchamy V. Medical ultrasound and its biological effects. J Clin Eng 1978;3:162–166.

Vogel J, Bom N, Ridder J, et al. Transducer design considerations in dynamic focusing. Ultrasound Med Biol 1979;5:187–193.

vonRamm OT, Thurstone FL. Cardiac imaging using a phased array ultrasound system. I. System design. Circulation 1976;53:258–262.

Waggoner AD, Bierig SM. Tissue Doppler imaging: a useful echocardiographic method for the cardiac sonographer to assess systolic and diastolic ventricular function. J Am Soc Echocardiogr 2001;14:1143–1152.

Wells PNT. Physics. In: Leech G, Sutton G, eds. An Introduction to Echocardiography. London: MediCine Ltd., 1978.

Wild JJ, Reid JM. Application of echoranging techniques to the determination of structure of biological tissues. Science 1952;115:226.

Chapter 3

Specialized Echocardiographic Techniques and Methods

Cardiac ultrasound or echocardiography is a diagnostic technique by which ultrasound is used to display anatomic and physiologic characteristics of the cardiovascular system. The basic principles of interaction of ultrasound with tissue and blood and the basic mechanisms by which an image is created are discussed in Chapter 2 . Echocardiography consists of several different imaging "domains" or display methodologies. The commonly used clinical imaging domains are listed in Table 3.1. Each of these ultrasound methodologies has specific strengths and weaknesses, and there are specific clinical arenas in which one technique may play a predominant role. Each imaging modality uses the same basic principle of reflection of sound in the ultrasonic frequency range to register data, conveying information regarding the presence and location of a reflective boundary or the direction and velocity of a moving target such as red blood cells or tissue. Information from any of these methodologies can be gathered using ultrasound transducers of varying capabilities and delivering diagnostic ultrasound to cardiac structures via a variety of routes.

IMAGING DEVICES AND METHODS

M-Mode Echocardiography

The earliest ultrasound image was obtained using a single interrogation beam from a dedicated transducer. Basically, ultrasound energy is sent out from the transducer as an ultrasound packet that is then reflected back to the transducer. Transmission of ultrasound from the transducer is not continuous but rather interrupted, with the nontransmit time being used to receive the signal. When used in this method and directed into the thorax, the ultrasound along the single line of interrogation is reflected from cardiac structures and registered as a series of reflective interfaces. If the location and strength of these interfaces are then plotted over time, typically by recording the continuous returning signal on a strip-chart recorder

▶ **TABLE 3.1 Imaging Domains for Clinical Echocardiography**

Anatomic imaging domain
  Single-line interrogation
    M-mode echocardiography
  Multiple-line interrogation
    Two-dimensional echocardiography
  Multiple-dimensional imaging
    Three-dimensional imaging
      Reconstructed
      Real-time three-dimensional imaging
Doppler domains
  Pulsed Doppler methods
    Single-interrogation volume
    Multiple-interrogation volume
    Saturated-interrogation volume area
      Color flow imaging
      M-mode color interrogation
Continuous wave Doppler
Analysis domains
  Frequency shift
  Power spectrum
  Variance
  Correlation methods
  Tissue velocity imaging
  Strain rate imaging

or scrolling video screen, then an M-mode echocardiogram is recorded (Fig. 3.1). The term M-mode refers to the motion that is derived from the time component. Some older references have referred to this methodology as a time-motion mode (T-M mode). Because M-mode echocardiography interrogates only along a single line, it does not provide a rapid anatomic screening method. Another limitation is that the true orientation of the beam with respect to accurate cardiac anatomy is often not known if a stand-alone transducer is used. Advantages of M-mode interrogation include high temporal resolution (1,000–3,000 Hz compared with 20–60 Hz for traditional

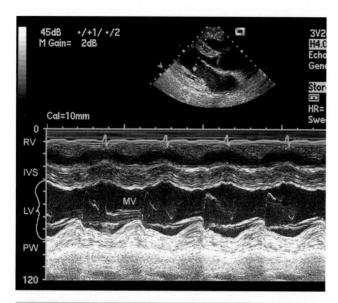

FIGURE 3.1. M-mode echocardiogram recorded through the left ventricle at the level of the mitral valve tips.

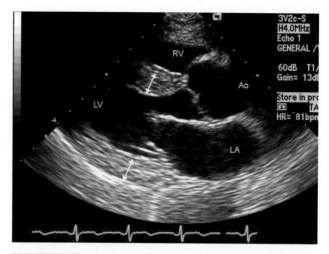

FIGURE 3.2. Transthoracic two-dimensional echocardiogram recorded in a parasternal long-axis view revealing the right ventricle, left ventricle, left atrium, and proximal aorta as well as septal and posterior wall thickness (*double-headed arrows*).

two-dimensional echocardiography). Additionally, the spatial resolution along the single line of interrogation is higher than that of two-dimensional echocardiography. This was of clinical relevance when using earlier generation two-dimensional ultrasound devices. Current devices using harmonic imaging or high-frequency transducers provide spatial resolution clinically equivalent to that available from M-mode echocardiography. They do not, however, provide the temporal resolution of M-mode echocardiography, which is suited to identifying brief rapid motion or fine oscillatory motion, such as that seen with mitral valve diastolic flutter in patients with aortic insufficiency, aortic valve systolic notching in dynamic outflow obstruction, and subtle abnormalities of wall motion as seen in conduction disturbances.

Two-Dimensional Echocardiography

Two-dimensional echocardiography provides an expanded view of cardiac anatomy by imaging not along a single line of interrogation but along a series of lines typically spanning a 90-degree arc (Fig. 3.2). In modern scanners, any of the additional domains of imaging such as M-mode and Doppler can be simultaneously performed and superimposed on the two-dimensional image or otherwise simultaneously displayed.

Color B-mode Scanning

For routine two-dimensional imaging (B-mode), the image typically is displayed in gray scale. Although first-generation scanners were limited to 16 shades of gray and

later scanners to 64 shades, current instruments display 256 shades of gray. This degree of gray-scale range exceeds the eye's ability to discern differences. An alternate mode of display is to convert the gray scale assignments to a range of color or of hue within a color (color B-mode) (Figs. 3.3 and 3.4). Studies have suggested that this may enhance detection of subtle soft-tissue density targets.

DOPPLER INTERROGATION

Whereas two-dimensional structural imaging relies on analysis of the time of transit and intensity of a returning ultrasound signal to identify an anatomic structure, Doppler interrogation relies on analysis of a change in the frequency of the transmitted ultrasound. Initially, this was displayed as the actual frequency shift. The magnitude of frequency shift is in the kilohertz range. This frequency shift can be converted to velocity of the interrogated target by the Doppler equation. Virtually all modern instrumentation provides this computation online, and it is the actual velocities that are displayed rather than frequency shifts. Doppler is used in multiple different formats.

The first Doppler format to be clinically used was a spectral display of the returning frequency shifts, which, as noted previously, is converted to velocity on all modern clinical scanners. This is typically displayed with reference to a *zero crossing line*. Any signal above that line represents motion toward the transducer, and any signal below the line represents motion away from the transducer. The magnitude of the frequency shift is directly related to velocity by the Doppler equation.

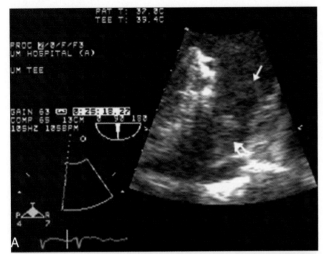

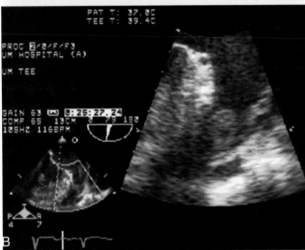

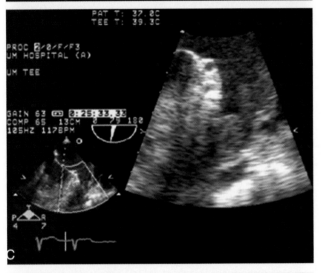

FIGURE 3.3. Transesophageal echocardiogram concentrating on the left atrial appendage in a patient with atrial fibrillation, demonstrating the effect of B-mode color. **Top:** This image was recorded in routine gray scale; **middle and bottom:** B-mode color was used. Note the more obvious nature of the left atrial appendage thrombus and associated spontaneous contrast in the B-mode color images.

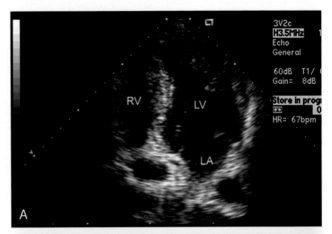

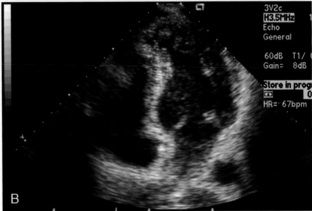

FIGURE 3.4. Apical four-chamber view recorded in a patient with the apical variant of hypertrophic cardiomyopathy in routine gray scale **(top)** and with B-mode color **(bottom)**. Note the more obvious nature of the apical hypertrophy in the B-mode color image.

Any of the Doppler methodologies can be simultaneously performed with anatomic two-dimensional imaging by sharing the computational resources of the ultrasound instrument. The spectral Doppler display can then be displayed simultaneously with the two-dimensional image. Early instrumentation did not have the computational power to perform both of these analyses simultaneously, and often anatomic imaging was suspended during Doppler interrogation. Modern instrumentation overcomes this shortcoming and can simultaneously display real-time, two-dimensional imaging and Doppler interrogation (Fig. 3.5).

Spectral Doppler imaging is acquired through two different methods, continuous and pulsed wave (Fig. 3.6). As the name implies, continuous wave Doppler imaging continuously transmits and receives the ultrasound signal. Because it is continuously transmitting and receiving, the ability to determine the time of transit is lost and only the frequency shift of the returning signal is calculated. This results in a phenomenon known as range ambiguity, in which the precise velocity of motion can be calculated but not the precise location at which that velocity occurred.

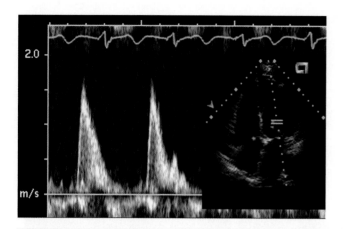

FIGURE 3.5. Pulsed Doppler of the mitral valve inflow derived from an apical four-chamber view. The small inset is the simultaneously obtained apical four-chamber view showing the location of the sample volume at the tips of the mitral valve.

In contrast, pulsed wave Doppler imaging interrogates velocity of motion by way of discrete ultrasound packets sent out at a predefined rate, the pulse repetition frequency. Transmit and receipt timing are employed so that the location from which the frequency shift arises can be calculated from the time of transit. This allows the sample volume to be steered along both its longitudinal and lateral axes. Because sampling is not continuous, there are limitations on the maximal velocity that can be determined, which is related to the pulse repetition frequency. The maximal obtainable velocity is known as the Nyquist limit. Using pulsed wave Doppler imaging, one can obtain a recording of velocity at any specific point within the cardiac anatomy, but the maximal velocity that can be displayed will be limited by the Nyquist limit and defines the total velocity range that can be measured, i.e., is the sum of velocity in both directions.

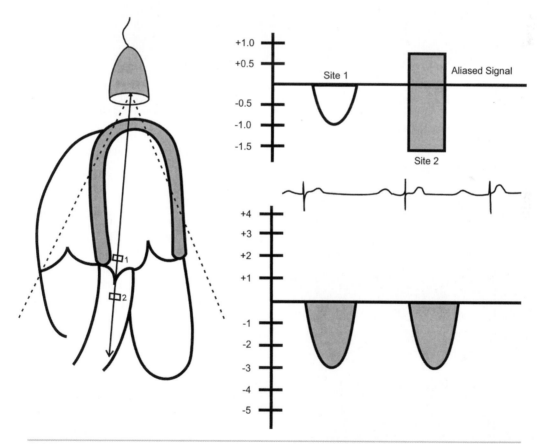

FIGURE 3.6. Schematic representation of pulsed wave **(top right)** and continuous wave **(bottom right)** imaging in a hypothetical case of mild aortic stenosis. Using pulsed wave Doppler imaging, it is possible to record a spectral signal from a precise location along the line of interrogation. If recorded at site 1 in the left ventricular outflow tract where velocities are low, the maximal velocity of approximately 1.0 m/sec is clearly demonstrated. If the sample volume is moved to site 2, which is downstream from the stenotic aortic valve, the Nyquist limit is exceeded and an aliased signal results, from which it is not possible to determine the true maximal velocity. Using continuous wave Doppler imaging **(bottom right)**, the true maximal velocity along the line of interrogation can be determined, but the precise location of obstruction is not known from the spectral recording.

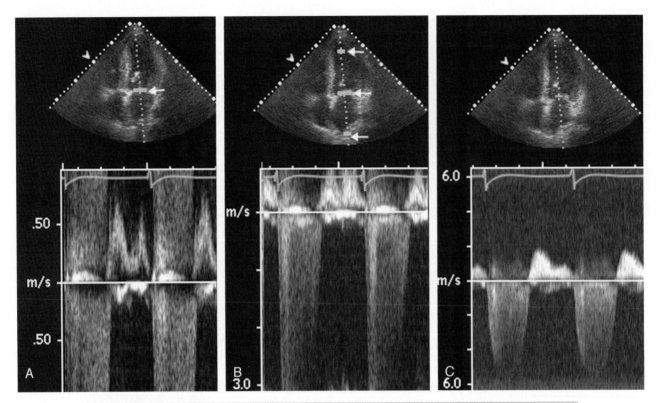

FIGURE 3.7. Example of three different Doppler methods recorded in the same patient with mitral regurgitation. **Left:** Standard pulsed wave Doppler imaging was used with a single sampling gate (*arrow*). Note that the Nyquist limit has been exceeded at approximately 1 m/sec in either direction so that aliasing occurs. **Middle:** Three simultaneous gates have been opened that effectively increase the Nyquist limit such that a maximal velocity of 4 m/sec could be recorded. **Right:** This image was recorded using continuous wave Doppler imaging from which the true maximal velocity of the mitral regurgitation can be easily determined.

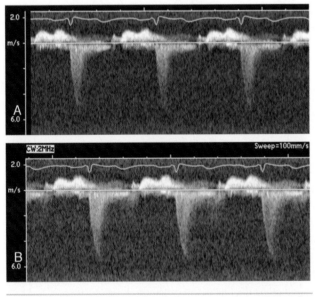

FIGURE 3.8. Color B-mode application to spectral Doppler imaging. **Top:** A faint spectral Doppler signal of mitral regurgitation was recorded in gray scale. **Bottom:** The same signal (with the same gain settings) displayed in B-mode color. Note the enhanced ability to identify the full spectral Doppler envelope in the colorized image.

A variation on pulsed wave Doppler imaging is multigate Doppler imaging in which multiple (typically two to five) Doppler interrogation points are simultaneously opened (Fig. 3.7). Interrogation of multiple points effectively increases the pulse repetition frequency and therefore the Nyquist limit. It preserves much of the ability to locate the site of the maximal velocity and allows a recording of velocities approaching that seen with continuous wave Doppler imaging. Early instrumentation did not allow simultaneous continuous wave Doppler imaging and two-dimensional imaging and did not allow steering of a continuous wave interrogation beam. Multigate Doppler was initially developed as a solution to this limitation. All current-generation equipment allows simultaneous steerable continuous wave Doppler imaging, and hence the clinical utility and need for multigate Doppler have diminished substantially.

As with two-dimensional imaging, the Doppler spectral display, which is typically displayed as a gray-scale image, can be displayed in various color hues (Fig. 3.8). This type of processing may make faint spectral signals more easily discernible.

Color Flow Doppler Imaging

Color flow imaging or color Doppler imaging is a variation of pulsed Doppler imaging and shares all its limitations. The result of this technique is to provide a colorized image representing the velocity and direction of blood flow in a region of interest, superimposed over a real-time, two-dimensional image (Fig. 3.9). The technique has shown tremendous clinical utility for the evaluation of regurgitant valvular lesions and detection of intracardiac shunts. It should be remembered that this is a pulsed Doppler technique and has all the limitations of pulsed Doppler imaging including relatively limited maximal velocities due to a low Nyquist limit. Because of the tremendous number of pulsed Doppler gates that are open simultaneously, color Doppler imaging has a lower frame rate than two-dimensional structural imaging (typically, 15–30 Hz with a region of interest typically used for mitral regurgitation).

Color flow imaging is obtained by simultaneous assessment of multiple Doppler interrogation regions within an area of interest. In modern scanners, the number of interrogation regions can range to as much as several hundred, depending on the size of the area of interrogation. At each of the interrogation sites, a pulsed Doppler interrogation is performed and analyzed. Rather than display each of these pulsed sample interrogation sites as a spectral display (which obviously is impossible when interrogating several hundred sites simultaneously), the frequency shift at each site is converted into a color and then the pixel at that interrogation site encoded with that color. Traditional color flow maps encode negative velocities (i.e., indicating flow away from the transducer) in varying shades of blue and flow toward the transducer in varying shades of red. Either the intensity or the hue of the individual color is then directly related to the magnitude of the Doppler shift, indicating velocity. Because of a relatively low Nyquist limit (typically <1.5 m/sec), even normal physiologic flow velocities frequently exceed the Nyquist limit and aliasing occurs in which flow may be encoded in its opposite color. The original method for determining the color and hue was to use a look-up table. Because the computational power required to calculate specific color hues is substantial, the computationally less intensive solution of a look-up table in which the anticipated velocities are compared with returning velocities and then matched with a predetermined color is employed. In instances in which there is a threshold level of variance from the look-up table because of mixed velocities, the color is inscribed as a variance reading, typically encoded in orange or yellow. Detection of substantial variance or variation in velocity and direction is a manifestation of turbulent flow, typically at a high velocity. These colors are then superimposed over the two-dimensional image and provide a simultaneous assessment of ventricular function and blood flow within the area of interest. There are numerous color flow maps that correspond to the different Doppler domains such as velocity, power, and energy.

Color Doppler M-Mode Imaging

Color Doppler M-mode imaging is a technique in which pulsed Doppler interrogation is done along a single line of interrogation, analogous to M-mode echocardiography. Unlike M-mode echocardiography, in which the location and intensity of a reflective spectral signal are recorded, the Doppler velocity shift is recorded and then subsequently color encoded and superimposed on the traditional M-mode image (Fig. 3.10). This provides high temporal resolution data regarding the timing and direction of flow events. Because this is a pulsed Doppler technique, velocity resolution is limited as it is with routine color Doppler imaging; however, the single-line interrogation provides a high level of spatial and temporal resolution along the interrogation line. Figure 3.10A is an example of color Doppler M-mode imaging recorded from the apex of the left ventricle. From this imaging position, characteristics of mitral valve inflow can be evaluated. Another clinical instance in which color Doppler M-mode imaging plays a role is in the determination of the width of an aortic insufficiency jet (Fig. 3.10B) and duration of mitral regurgitation. The high temporal resolution of this technique has been used to assist in determining the velocity

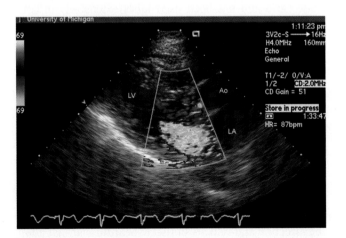

FIGURE 3.9. Transthoracic parasternal long-axis echocardiogram with color flow Doppler imaging recorded in a patient with moderate to severe mitral regurgitation. Note the pyramid-shaped region of interest in which color Doppler imaging is performed, superimposed on the parasternal long-axis view of the left ventricle. Also note the frame rate of 16 Hz, which is substantially slower than the frame rate of 58 Hz recorded for this image without color Doppler imaging.

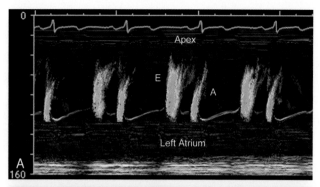

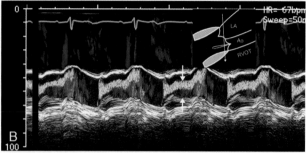

FIGURE 3.10. Color Doppler M-mode echocardiograms recorded from the left ventricular apex demonstrate normal mitral inflow **(top)** and aortic insufficiency from a transesophageal echocardiogram **(bottom)**. The image orientation is as noted in the inserted schematic.

of propagation (V_p) of left ventricular inflow. This issue is discussed further in Chapters 6 and 17.

DOPPLER TISSUE IMAGING

Routine Doppler imaging typically targets blood flow and hence the receiver characteristics, including the frequency filters that determine the range of velocities to be interrogated, are set to maximize the shifts anticipated with moving blood and to exclude the velocity shifts that would be seen with slower moving structures. Because red blood cells are relatively weak reflectors and tissue is a fairly intense reflector, filters are also adjusted to exclude highly reflective objects and to maximize less reflective objects when using conventional Doppler (Fig. 3.11). Doppler tissue imaging uses the same principles; however, the target is tissue rather than red blood cells. For this purpose, filters are set to parameters opposite those needed to accurately detect red blood cell motion. Because tissue has a greater reflectivity and slower motion, instrumentation filters are set to exclude high velocities and low-intensity reflectors. With this technique, either the myocardium or fibrous skeleton of the heart can be targeted and weaker reflections from the higher velocity blood cells relatively excluded.

One of the initial applications of this technique was to use color flow imaging display methodology and to saturate an area of interest with Doppler interrogation. The color Doppler signal from the moving tissue was then superimposed on the two-dimensional gray-scale image. An example of this use is seen in Figure 3.12. Using traditional blue-red encoding for direction of motion, this results in dissimilar color encoding even when walls are moving at a similar velocity. The normally moving ventricular septum will be encoded in blue (motion away from the transducer), and the normal anterior motion of the posterior wall will be encoded in red. This results in opposite color encoding of opposing walls, which each have normal directional motion. The color encoding scheme can be changed to be unidirectional, recording only velocity irrespective of direction, in the same color. This has the disadvantage of encoding a dyskinetic wall with the same color as a normally contracting wall. This technique has substantial potential in that it would allow superimposing information regarding velocity and direction of motion on the anatomic image. It is limited in its applicability by relatively low frame rates and the inability to fully saturate the signal. Other limitations include potential aliasing of the color signal with higher velocity motion and limited registration of velocity information at an angle of incidence (θ) exceeding 30 degrees. Signal-to-noise ratios are typically relatively low, and in poor-quality images, there may be substantial bleeding of the color signal from the tissue into the blood pool.

The initial attempts at color encoding and Doppler tissue imaging used standard Doppler shifts of velocity. The Doppler signal in the power or energy domain can also be encoded. The power domain refers to the registration of the intensity or amplitude of the reflected Doppler shifts rather than just their velocity (Fig. 3.13). In theory, this format may be of benefit because of its higher signal-to-noise ratio and has been used fairly extensively in contrast echocardiography.

Complete saturation of the image with color signal has seen little clinical acceptance because of the limitations of frame rate and saturation with an adequate signal-to-noise ratio. It should be recognized that the original source signal is actually pulsed Doppler information, acquired from a wide area of interest and targeted to tissue motion. A greater degree of acceptance has been seen by displaying the spectral signal of velocity and extracting quantitative information from localized areas using this technique. Analogous to the use of a sample volume in blood flow imaging, a sample volume can be placed within the myocardium or mitral or tricuspid anulus and the direction and velocity of the myocardium at that point in space accurately determined (Fig. 3.14).

A variation on Doppler tissue imaging is to acquire color-encoded images of tissue motion along an M-mode interrogation line. This represents a combination of M-mode echocardiography, color Doppler imaging, and quantitative Doppler tissue imaging. An example of this technique is shown in Figure 3.15. Color tissue Doppler M-mode imaging is a high temporal and spatial resolution

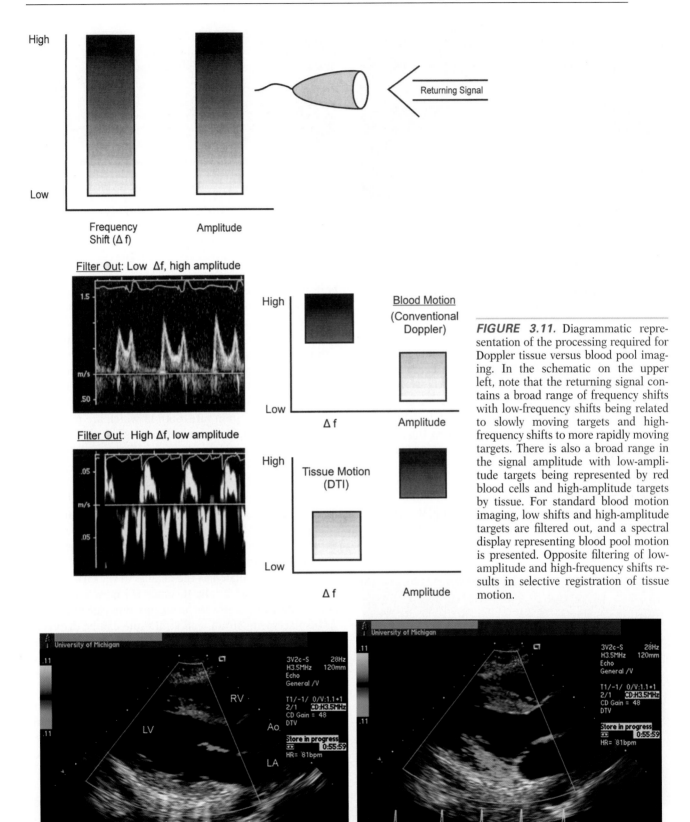

FIGURE 3.11. Diagrammatic representation of the processing required for Doppler tissue versus blood pool imaging. In the schematic on the upper left, note that the returning signal contains a broad range of frequency shifts with low-frequency shifts being related to slowly moving targets and high-frequency shifts to more rapidly moving targets. There is also a broad range in the signal amplitude with low-amplitude targets being represented by red blood cells and high-amplitude targets by tissue. For standard blood motion imaging, low shifts and high-amplitude targets are filtered out, and a spectral display representing blood pool motion is presented. Opposite filtering of low-amplitude and high-frequency shifts results in selective registration of tissue motion.

FIGURE 3.12. Transthoracic parasternal long-axis view of the left ventricle using color Doppler tissue imaging to saturate the myocardial signature. **Left:** Recorded in diastole; **right:** recorded at end-systole. Note that as the septum moves posteriorly, it is encoded in blue, and as the posterior wall moves anteriorly in systole, it is encoded in red.

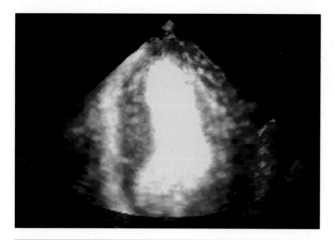

FIGURE 3.13. Power Doppler image recorded at the time of contrast echocardiography using a perfluorocarbon-based agent. Note the excellent signal-to-noise ratio and the marked discrimination between the blood pool and the wall with this imaging method.

technique for investigating myocardial mechanics, and the information thus extracted can secondarily be employed for determining velocity gradients between adjacent points or more recently for strain rate imaging.

Figure 3.16 outlines the "evolution" of data, which can be derived from Doppler tissue imaging. As Doppler imaging inherently detects motion and determines velocity, this is the fundamental parameter available. From this displacement of the tissue, the distance traveled can be determined as the product of velocity and time. More complex derivatives of the velocity determination include the calculation of the velocity gradient between two points and strain or strain rate imaging, which are mea-

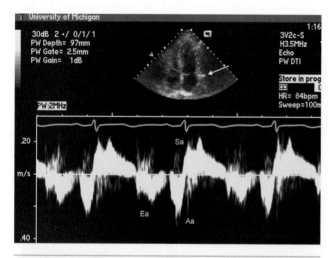

FIGURE 3.14. Doppler tissue imaging using a spectral display and a single area of interest targeted to the lateral mitral valve anulus. The location of the sample volume is noted by the arrow and in this instance is in the lateral anulus. The systolic motion of the anulus (S_a) and the diastolic anular motion (E_a and A_a) are as noted.

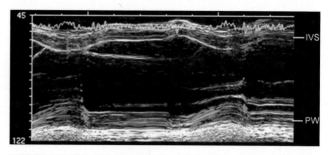

FIGURE 3.15. M-mode color Doppler tissue imaging recorded from a parasternal transducer position. With systole, the septum moves posteriorly and is colored in blue and the posterior wall with normal anterior motion is colored in red. Note the excellent temporal resolution of this technique.

sures of tissue deformation. The simplest calculation that can be derived from two-point analysis is the absolute difference in velocities. This has had clinical applicability in determining the gradient between endocardial and epicardial velocities, which may be a more sensitive indicator of myocardial ischemia than an absolute decrease in velocity across the entire myocardial wall (Fig. 3.17).

More complex derivatives of these measurements include strain and strain rate, both of which are more load independent than parameters such as ejection fraction and wall motion and provide a more direct assessment of myocardial contractility. Because strain rate refers to the first derivative of motion (i.e., velocity change), it is more directly derived from Doppler tissue imaging, which inherently is a velocity calculation. As noted in Figure 3.16, strain is defined as the change in distance between two points divided by the initial length (L_0). Mathematically, it is a unitless number. Strain rate is the first derivative of strain and is calculated as the change in velocity between two points divided by the distance (L) between the two points. Mathematically, the units of strain rate are 1/s.

Displacement, strain, and strain rate can be displayed in several formats. The easiest to understand is a graphic output of either of these parameters over time, as demonstrated in Figures 3.16, 3.18, and 3.19. One or more discrete regions of interest can be identified and simultaneously graphed for comparison of displacement, strain, or strain rate at any given time point. Because these parameters are derived from tissue Doppler imaging, which has high spatial resolution, it is often beneficial to simultaneously display these values for multiple points throughout the ventricular myocardium or for all points along a continuous line drawn through the myocardium. Display of this type of information requires a different format than a simple x/y graph as is appropriate for a single point. The solution to this display dilemma has been to create a "curved" M-mode display in which time is conventionally displayed on the x axis, distance around the ventricle on the y axis, and the value of displacement, strain, or strain

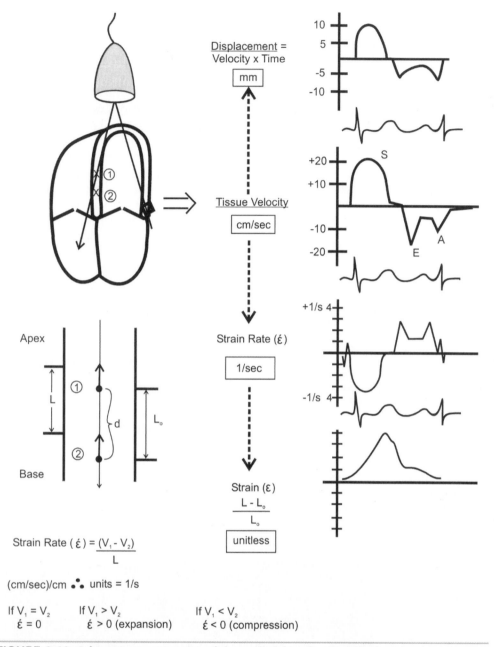

FIGURE 3.16. Schematic representation of the methodology for obtaining Doppler tissue imaging (DTI) of the mitral anulus or of two adjacent points for calculation of myocardial strain or strain rate. Each of the derived parameters is also schematized on the right. (See text for details.)

rate in color (Fig. 3.19). This is analogous to the display of Doppler velocity data in a color M-mode but obviously incorporates the third dimension of location within the heart.

Numerous studies have demonstrated that Doppler imaging–derived myocardial gradients as well as strain and strain rate provide a higher resolution evaluation of myocardial mechanics than evaluation of wall motion, myocardial thickening, or tissue velocities alone. This issue is further discussed in Chapter 6.

TISSUE CHARACTERIZATION

Tissue characterization refers to the ultrasound determination of myocardial texture. It has been employed for investigational purposes for more than 20 years, initially using dedicated, specifically designed ultrasound units that evaluated the complete returning radio frequency signal for cyclical changes in image intensity (backscatter) and "signature." This was necessary because the generation of clinically used ultrasound equipment at that time did not

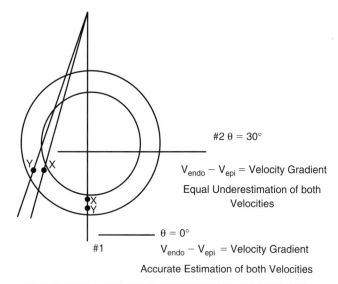

$V_{endo} - V_{epi}$ = Velocity Gradient

Equal Underestimation of both Velocities

$\theta = 0°$

$V_{endo} - V_{epi}$ = Velocity Gradient

Accurate Estimation of both Velocities

FIGURE 3.17. Schematic demonstrates the mechanism for determining an endocardial-epicardial gradient. For the interrogation line with an angle of incidence (θ) of 0 degrees, no correction would be necessary for accurate velocity determination. For the example with an angle of incidence of 30 degrees, systematic underestimation of velocity would be anticipated. However, because both points X and Y, representing endocardial and epicardial regions of interest, are interrogated with the same angle of incidence, calculation of the velocity gradient, as a relative measure, is unaffected.

have the dynamic range to allow a similar analysis to be undertaken from the clinically used image. In the normally contracting myocardium, there is a cyclic variation in the intensity of the signal being reflected from the myocardium such that reflected intensities are lower in systole

and greater in diastole. With ischemia, the normal pattern of systolic thickening is lost and with it the magnitude of cyclic variation in backscatter is diminished. This technique was demonstrated to be a sensitive indicator of both myocardial infarction and ischemia. Subsequent to its initial development, advances in routine ultrasound instrumentation have made available a tremendous increase in dynamic range and availability of the radio frequency signal on some commercially available clinical instruments. Many of these instruments also contain algorithms for determining image intensity from digitally captured loops and can be used to determine the cyclic variation of myocardial image intensity and texture (Fig. 3.20). As with the earlier dedicated investigational instruments, several investigators have demonstrated a lack of cyclic variation in integrated backscatter in the presence of myocardial ischemia and myocardial infarction. Some studies have suggested that the tissue signature obtained in this way may also be an accurate marker of reperfused myocardium, which has not yet recovered function.

ACQUISITION OF CARDIAC ULTRASOUND INFORMATION

The acquisition of the actual cardiac ultrasound examination involves using a transducer to deliver and subsequently receive ultrasound energy from the cardiac structures. Since its inception, a number of different routes for acquisition of information and strategies for delivering, receiving, and analyzing the reflected information have been developed. These are listed in Table 3.2 and are discussed in Chapter 5.

FIGURE 3.18. Myocardial strain image recorded in a normal and abnormal segment of the left ventricle from an apical four-chamber view. The two regions of interest are noted by ovals superimposed on the myocardium. For the normal segment, note the negative strain during systole, and for the abnormal segment, the systolic expansion is noted by a positive wave form.

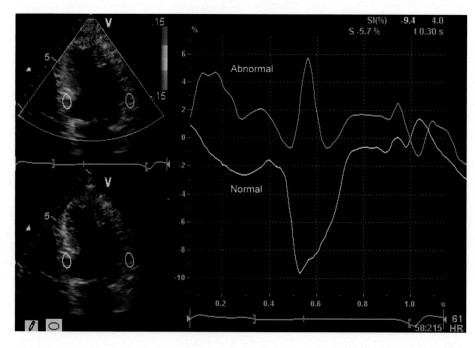

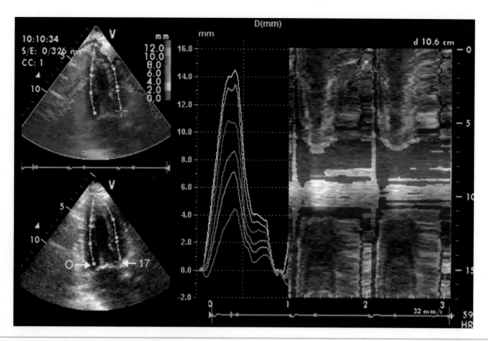

FIGURE 3.19. Demonstration of displacement recorded from Doppler tissue imaging in a normal individual. **Left:** Note the curved line through the ventricular myocardium, which is used to create the curved M-mode signal on the far right. Discrete regions of interest can also be individually plotted over time as noted by the individual displacement lines **(middle). Right:** The curved M-mode representation of myocardial displacement is shown. Note in the two-dimensional echocardiogram on the left, the location of the region of interest that stretches from the basal inferior wall (point 0) to the anterior base (point 17) with the apex being located at approximately point 9. Two consecutive cardiac cycles are represented, and the color at any point denotes the degree of displacement from end diastole (defined by the QRS) versus its location along the region of interest within the ventricular myocardium.

Transthoracic Echocardiography

The majority of echocardiographic examinations are performed via the transthoracic route, for which a transducer is placed on the surface of the chest and the ultrasound beam aimed through intercostal or other nonreflective anatomic spaces to deliver and receive ultrasound. The typical two-dimensional imaging transducer has a "footprint" ranging from 5 × 10 mm to 15 × 20 mm (Fig. 3.21). High-frequency transducers designed for pediatric work may have a smaller footprint. The standard transthoracic transducer is the mainstay of the

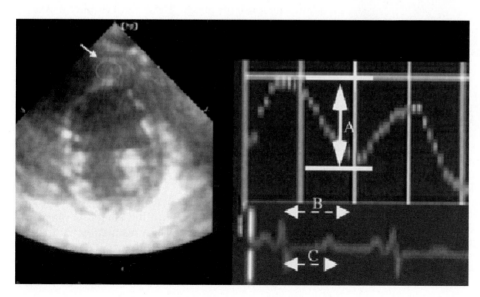

FIGURE 3.20. Analysis of integrated backscatter. **Left:** A parasternal short-axis view with an area of interest in the anterior septum (arrow). **Right:** A graphic demonstration of the cyclic variation of integrated backscatter. (From Iwakura K, et al. Detection of TIMI-3 flow before mechanical reperfusion with ultrasonic tissue characterization in patients with anterior wall acute myocardial infarction. Circulation 2003;107:3159–3164, with permission.)

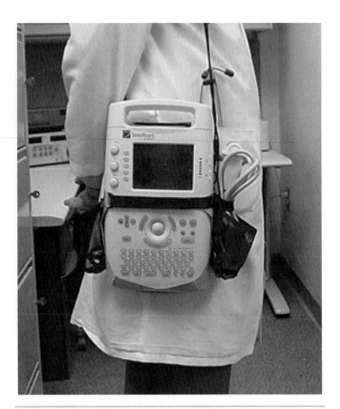

FIGURE 3.22. Hand-carried portable two-dimensional ultrasound device. Note the overall size of the device and its easy portability.

▶ TABLE 3.2 Diagnostic Ultrasound Delivery Routes

Transthoracic window
　　Left parasternal
　　Apical
　　Subcostal
　　Right parasternal
　　Suprasternal
　　Posterior thoracic
Transesophageal
Intravascular
　　Intracardiac
　　Intracoronary
Epicardial

examination and in modern instrumentation provides all the modalities discussed previously.

Hand-Carried Ultrasound

There have been efforts made to create clinically useful ultraportable or hand-carried ultrasound units since the 1970s. More recently, several manufacturers have produced and marketed small, lightweight (<10 lb), battery-powered ultrasound units (Fig. 3.22). These devices provide wide-angle two-dimensional imaging and often spectral Doppler, M-mode echocardiography, and color

Doppler imaging. The robustness of color Doppler imaging has typically lagged behind the other modalities. In their basic configuration, they provide no or only limited capacity for image storage. The two-dimensional image provided by these units (Figs. 3.23 and 3.24) is not equivalent to that obtained with full-service platforms, but in several small trials, it has been shown to be of diagnostic quality in most instances. These devices play a role in rapid scanning, bedside teaching, and targeted evaluation for pericardial effusion and global left ventricular function but generally fall short of providing an accurate, comprehensive examination comparable with that obtained with full-service platforms.

Dedicated Single-Line Interrogation Transducers

The earliest echocardiograms were recorded using single-beam transducers, originally intended for transcranial ultrasound. These transducers consist of a single crystal propagating energy perpendicular to the face of the transducer. Technologically, they are the simplest transducer and provide the highest rates of transmission and receipt and hence the highest temporal resolution. Dedicated M-mode echocardiography, as performed in the early days of clinical cardiac ultrasound, was performed using this type

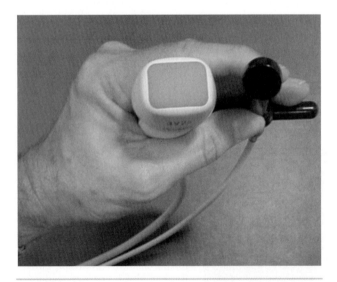

FIGURE 3.21. A standard adult transthoracic two-dimensional echocardiography probe (on the left) capable of two-dimensional imaging, spectral and color flow Doppler imaging, and all other modalities discussed in this text and the stand-alone Pedoff probe designed exclusively for continuous wave Doppler imaging. Note the smaller circular footprint of the dedicated continuous wave probe that allows it to be placed in tighter intercostal interspaces or other anatomic areas such as the suprasternal notch, which are not easily approached with the larger full-function probe.

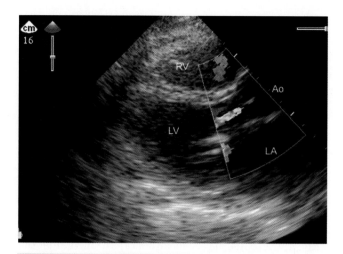

FIGURE 3.23. Two-dimensional echocardiogram with color Doppler imaging recorded in a patient with mild aortic insufficiency using a hand-carried ultrasound scanner.

of transducer. In contemporary practice, it is unusual to use a dedicated transducer for M-mode recording because the M-mode extracted from the two-dimensional transducer is typically of equivalent quality and allows precise localization of the interrogation beam. Dedicated transducers with single-line interrogation are most often used in clinical practice for continuous wave Doppler interrogation. They have the advantage of a very small footprint (typically <8 mm diameter), which can be placed easily within intercostal spaces or in the suprasternal notch (Fig. 3.21). The dedicated nature of these transducers, through which all computational resources of the instrument are dedicated to providing a spectral display, may provide a higher fidelity recording of Doppler shifts than transducers using shared technology in which the primary purpose of the transducer is image acquisition and only secondarily Doppler acquisition. There are few clinical situations in which the higher fidelity of the stand-alone transducer compensates for the loss of anatomic reference points; however, its remarkably small footprint may allow acquisition of Doppler signals from an angle of interrogation not available with the large footprint of a standard two-dimensional transducer.

Transesophageal Echocardiography

The techniques for transesophageal echocardiography involve incorporating an ultrasound transducer on the tip of a gastroscope-like device. The early transesophageal echocardiographic probes were actually modified gastroscopes. Current transesophageal probes have been specifically manufactured for echocardiographic purposes. The method by which ultrasound is propagated from the transducer and returning signals processed is identical to

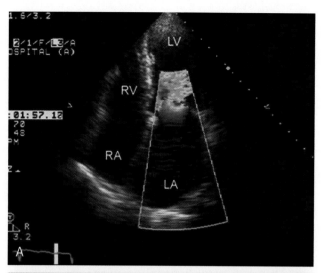

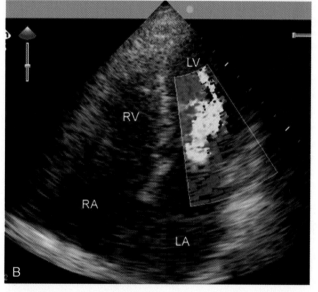

FIGURE 3.24. Apical four-chamber view recorded with a full-function, current-generation ultrasound platform **(top)**, and the same patient recorded with a handheld ultrasound unit **(bottom)**. Image quality is generally superior with the full-function system; however, note the ability to identify the significant pathology with the hand-carried system including the dilated left atrium, thickened mitral valve, and color Doppler imaging evidence of mitral stenosis.

that for transthoracic echocardiography. The transducer face is obviously smaller than a transthoracic probe, and hence there are fewer channels available for transmission. There have been four generations of transesophageal echocardiographic probes. The first was a single dedicated M-mode transducer that saw brief use in the early 1970s. The first functional transesophageal probes were single-plane devices typically using phased-array methodology, although several early devices used a rotating mechanical scanner. These monoplane probes were rapidly replaced by biplane devices that had two separate ultrasound transducers with perpendicular orientation of the two imaging planes. The current-generation probes are all multiplane devices (Fig. 3.25). These devices use an array of ultrasound crystals either in a square or circular configuration and phased-array technology to steer the ultrasound examining plane through a 180-degree arc. This effectively provides 360-degree "panoramic" image of the heart. All the modalities discussed including M-mode, spectral, color flow Doppler imaging, and color M-mode typically can be obtained using a modern multiplane transesophageal scanner. Doppler tissue imaging and second harmonic imaging are also provided on some of the most recent-generation instrumentation. Transesophageal probes operate at multiple frequencies, typically 3.5 to 7.0 MHz. In view of the unobstructed window for interrogation and the intrinsically high frequencies, the potential benefit of tissue harmonic imaging is probably less than that of transthoracic imaging. Pediatric transesophageal probes are smaller in diameter (5–7 mm), often limited to biplane imaging, and provide higher frequency (5–10 MHz) imaging. Their smaller size is more appropriate for children and infants. The greater flexibility of the probe may reduce control over imaging planes. For these reasons, they are not typically used in adult patients. As for transthoracic echocardiography, the transesophageal echocardiogram provides a family of related views of cardiac anatomy (see Chapter 5).

There are distinct advantages and disadvantages as well as risks associated with transesophageal echocardiography. Its advantages are unimpeded ultrasound visualization of virtually all areas of the heart, allowing a highly accurate diagnosis of the majority of anatomic cardiac problems. The combination of unobstructed visualization and high-resolution scanning makes it an ideal technique for identifying fine anatomic detail such as valve chordae, small masses such as valvular papillomas, detection of vegetations in patients with suspected endocarditis, detection of left atrial appendage thrombus, and evaluation of the thoracic portions of the aorta. There are several clinical situations in which transesophageal echocardiography plays a unique and clearly incremental role compared with transthoracic echocardiography (Table 3.3).

There are distinct risks and disadvantages associated with transesophageal echocardiography, including the fact that it is a mildly invasive procedure. In general, it carries all the elements of risk and patient discomfort associated with any upper endoscopic procedure. The potential risks of transesophageal echocardiography are outlined in Table 3.4. There are several absolute and relative contraindications to performing the examination, which are also listed. Transesophageal echocardiography is performed after obtaining informed consent. The operator should ensure that no contraindications to the procedure exist and should always specifically query the pa-

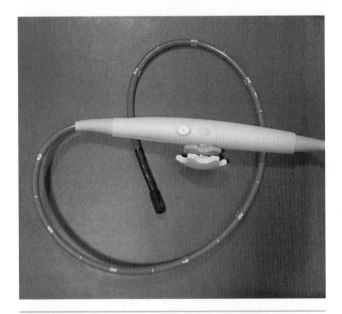

FIGURE 3.25. A commercially available standard multiplane transesophageal probe. The knobs on the handle allow lateral flexion in both directions and anteflexion and retroflexion of the probe. The button on the handle controls the rotation of the imaging plane from 0 to 180 degrees.

▶ **TABLE 3.3   Unique Data from Transesophageal Echocardiography**

Atrial thrombi/masses
  Left atrial appendage clot
  Left atrial appendage spontaneous contrast
  Clot in body of left atrium
  Right atrial thrombus
  Thrombus/mass on pacemaker wire or indwelling catheter
Mitral valve
  Precise mechanism of mitral regurgitation
  Refined suitability for valvotomy in severe mitral stenosis
  Define eccentric jets
  Function of prosthetic valve
Aorta
  Detection/characterization of dissection
  Detection of atheroma
Aortic trauma/transection
Chambers
  Refinement (minor) of patent foramen ovale characteristics
Online monitoring
  Intraoperative left ventricular size/function
  Monitoring interventional procedures
    Atrial septostomy
    Balloon valvotomy
    Pulmonary vein/left atrial interventions
Endocarditis
  Detect aortic abscess
  Identify smaller vegetations

▶ TABLE 3.4 **Risks of Transesophageal Echocardiography**

Topical anesthesia
  Allergic reactions
  Toxic methemoglobinemia
Conscious sedation
  Respiratory compromise/hypoxia
  Hypotension
  Paradoxical hypertension
  Paradoxical agitation
  Idiosyncratic reactions
Probe insertion: immediate
  Oral trauma
  Dental trauma
  Esophageal perforation
  Vagal reaction
Probe insertion: delayed
  Aspiration
  Tachycardia
    Paroxysmal supraventricular tachycardia
    Ventricular tachycardia
Contradictions
  Absolute
    Recent esophageal trauma/surgery
    Recent esophageal bleed
  Relative
    Poorly cooperative patient

tient regarding previous esophageal disease, dysphagia, or other swallowing difficulty. If a patient has a history suggesting any of these conditions, it is often advisable to have the patient evaluated and cleared by a gastroenterologist before proceeding.

In most instances, transesophageal echocardiography is performed using a combination of topical oral and pharyngeal anesthetizing agents such as topical benzocaine and viscous lidocaine and intravenous conscious sedation, typically with a short-acting anxiolytic and a narcotic agent. In rare instances, general anesthesia has been required for uncooperative patients such as children with congenital heart disease or patients with cognitive defects.

Transesophageal echocardiography should be performed only by individuals with specific training in the technique and experience sufficient to be able to independently recognize and diagnose expected abnormalities. The American Society of Echocardiography, the American Heart Association, and the American College of Cardiology have all addressed the issue of appropriate training for performance of transesophageal echocardiography. Unlike transthoracic echocardiography, in which a suboptimal or incomplete examination can be easily repeated by a second more experienced observer, transesophageal echocardiography should be viewed as a one-time procedure during which all clinical information will be obtained and that no "second chance" will be available.

Three-Dimensional Echocardiography

Three-dimensional echocardiography is a technique currently in evolution. The eventual goal is a real-time, three-dimensional display of cardiac anatomy including all the modalities mentioned above including Doppler flow imaging, M-mode echocardiography, and Doppler tissue imaging. Several approaches have been taken to acquire and display three-dimensional information. The basic problems with three-dimensional echocardiography can be divided into those of acquisition of the three-dimensional data set and subsequent display of the three-dimensional images. A limitation has been that the information either acquired or reconstructed into a three-dimensional data set must subsequently be displayed as a two-dimensional video image.

There have been two basic approaches to the acquisition of a three-dimensional data set. The first has been to acquire a series of two-dimensional images that are then stored, typically encoded with registration of the precise angle at which the heart is interrogated as well as electrocardiographic and respiratory gating information. An entire sequence of images is thus obtained, through either a transthoracic or transesophageal route, that is stored and then reconstructed into a three-dimensional data set (Fig. 3.26).

From a transthoracic approach, this has required some mechanism for determining the precise location of the transducer and hence the location of the ultrasound beam within the thorax. In the past, this was accomplished either by attachment of a mechanical arm to the transducer, which then through either a series of position sensors or a spark gap or magnetic location device determines the exact position and orientation of the transducer. The localization device provides triangulation information that is encoded simultaneously with the echocardiographic images into a three-dimensional data set. Because of the cumbersome nature of this localization method and the complex nature of reconstruction, there has been little enthusiasm for this approach in clinical practice and it is currently not used.

Three-dimensional echocardiography from a transesophageal approach capitalizes on the rotational ability of the multiplane transducer. From the transesophageal approach, the transducer position remains fixed, and the multiplane rotational ultrasound beam is automatically rotated at 2- to 5-degree increments, creating a 360-degree panoramic view of the cardiac structures. It is obviously important that the transducer position and orientation within the esophagus remain absolutely stable. Even slight motion of the transducer, due either to patient or operator motion results in marked deterioration in image quality. A three-dimensional data set is then obtained from the series of rotational images. Typically, 3 to 7 minutes are required to obtain a complete three-dimensional

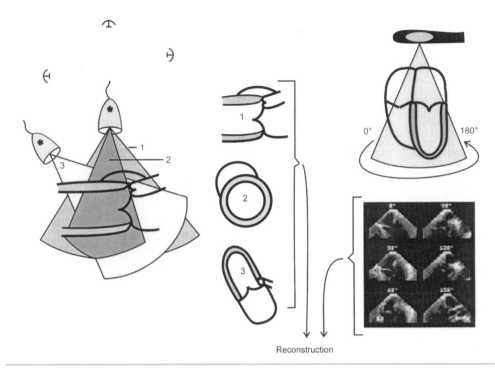

Reconstruction

FIGURE 3.26. Schematic demonstration of two methods for collection of two-dimensional echocardiograms for subsequent reconstruction into a three-dimensional data set. **Left:** Transthoracic imaging is depicted in which a transducer is either mounted with a spark-gap detector and surrounded by three sensors or is controlled by a positioning arm. In this schematic, three separate imaging planes have been collected, timed to the QRS, and subsequently merged into a three-dimensional data set (Fig. 3.31). **Right:** The methodology involved in three-dimensional reconstruction from the transesophageal echocardiographic approach using a multiplane rotational image. The two-dimensional image is rotated at 3- to 5-degree increments, and a series of images is then collected. Six representative images are demonstrated. These images are then merged into a three-dimensional data set for subsequent reconstruction.

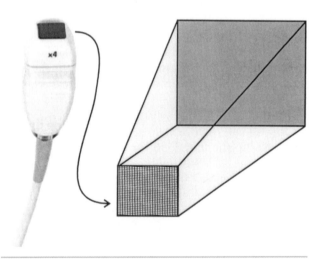

FIGURE 3.27. A three-dimensional volumetric probe. Note the relatively square footprint of the probe compared with a standard two-dimensional probe. The face of the probe consists of a nearly rectangular matrix of crystals that results in a pyramidal scan profile, as depicted in the schematic on the right.

data set with this approach. More recently, a similar approach has been undertaken by mounting the rotational transesophageal imaging probe on a handheld transthoracic device that can be used to acquire a three-dimensional data set in exactly the same manner as that for transesophageal echocardiography.

The second and more promising method of acquisition of three-dimensional echocardiographic data is "volumetric" imaging. In this technique, a transducer is constructed with a rectangular (vs. linear) ultrasound array of transmit/receive crystals (Fig. 3.27). This allows collection of a pyramidal image data set, representing real-time, three-dimensional acquisition of data.

The current (2004) generation of ultrasound platforms that provide real-time, three-dimensional imaging does not have the computational power to acquire an entire volume of data sufficient to encompass all cardiac structures in an adult in one cycle. For acquisition of a complete volume of cardiac data, four sequential cardiac cycles are typically captured and added to create a complete volume of information (full volumetric scanning) (Fig. 3.28). Alternately, a smaller partial volume scan can be created that may encompass 20% to 50% of overall car-

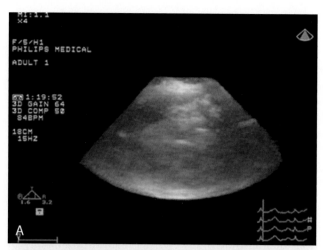

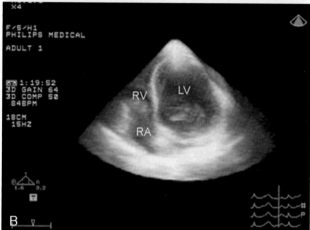

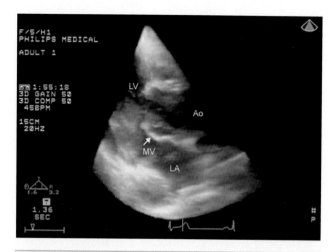

FIGURE 3.29. Real-time, three-dimensional image recorded in a parasternal long-axis view. With this method, the volumetric scan is set to incorporate an approximate 90-degree sector that is approximately 20 degrees in elevation. This provides real-time, three-dimensional visualization of the cardiac structures as noted.

FIGURE 3.28. Real-time volumetric scan from a transthoracic echocardiogram. This methodology involves a volumetric scan that collects four consecutive cardiac cycles and merges all data into a three-dimensional volume set. **Top:** The three-dimensional volume set for the four cardiac cycles (note electrocardiogram). Note that this large three-dimensional volume set does not reveal any interior cardiac anatomy and is not identifiable as a cardiac structure. **Bottom:** The full three-dimensional volume has been cropped (Fig. 3.31) so that the interior of the three-dimensional volume has now been exposed. This three-dimensional volume was collected from an apical transducer position, and when "sliced open," the left ventricle and right atrium and ventricle are "exposed." A three-dimensional volume set can be "opened" in any imaging plane, providing both long- and short-axis views of cardiac structures.

diac anatomy, which can be displayed online in real time (Fig. 3.29). It should be emphasized that this is a limitation of computational power and processor speed and in all likelihood will improve over time. Either approach avoids the intermediate steps of "image reconstruction" necessary with the previously mentioned techniques. Use of the volumetric probe also allows the option for simultaneous acquisition of true real-time biplane echocardiograms in which any two planes can be simultaneously imaged. Figure 3.30 is a real-time, two-dimensional image

acquired from a parasternal transducer position. Notice that both parasternal long- and short-axis images are simultaneously recorded and that each image represents the exact same cardiac cycle.

Once acquired, the three-dimensional data set must then be viewed and analyzed. Several display formats have been used (Fig. 3.31). The first is simply to display the entire three-dimensional data set on a grid with several intersecting interrogation lines. The two-dimensional image along any of the interrogation lines can then be displayed (Figs. 3.31–3.33). Although not providing a true three-dimensional image, this methodology allows precise location of a two-dimensional plane along either typical or atypical orientations to maximize accuracy for measurement of complex structures and so on.

A second method of display is to slice the full-volume data set to "expose" the interior. This provides a three-dimensional perspective of what is otherwise a two-dimensional image (Figs. 3.28B, 3.31, and 3.34). The most recent generation of real-time, three-dimensional scanning can also acquire color Doppler information that can be processed in an identical manner (Fig. 3.35).

Although in theory, only providing a different two-dimensional plane, three-dimensional echocardiography has the advantage of ensuring precise alignment of a two-dimensional interrogation plane in atypical orientations. It also provides a more complete spatial orientation. This may be very useful for identification of small ventricular septal defects, assessment of the size of an atrial septal defect, and creating imaging planes that are not feasible using a single two-dimensional plane such as an *en face* view of the atrial septum for visualization of the fossa ovalis or an atrial septal defect. A major ad-

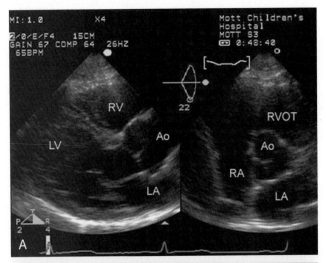

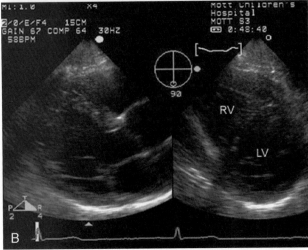

FIGURE 3.30. Real-time biplane imaging using a three-dimensional probe. Both images were recorded from the parasternal transducer position. Note the ability to simultaneously visualize any two planes. **Top:** Parasternal long- and short-axis views at the base of the heart, revealing the proximal aorta, are demonstrated. **Bottom:** The second plane has been adjusted to intersect the left ventricle at the level of the mitral valve. In each image set, both images are simultaneously visualized in real time.

vantage is in the evaluation of complex congenital abnormalities. Three-dimensional echocardiography has also shown promise in assessing the mechanism of mitral regurgitation and in precise identification of flail leaflets. Another area in which reconstructed three-dimensional echocardiography has shown substantial promise is in evaluating prosthetic valves for paravalvular regurgitation. It is frequently difficult to precisely identify the location and determine the size of a paravalvular leak, even with transesophageal echocardiography. Three-dimensional reconstruction of the face of the anulus frequently provides superb visualization of the entire circumference of the anulus and localization of multiple paravalvular leaks. Finally, quantitative accuracy for chamber volume determination is greater for three-dimensional than for two-dimensional echocardiography (Figs. 3.36 and 3.37). This advantage is most obvious when dealing with irregularly shaped chambers such as the right ventricle or abnormal left ventricles. This is discussed further in Chapter 6 on the evaluation of left ventricular size and function.

Additional imaging formats have been proposed for three-dimensional echocardiography including real-time, three-dimensional holographic displays of the three-dimensional data set. The feasibility of this approach has been demonstrated; however, the clinical availability of equipment to produce these images is limited. A final approach has been to create physical three-dimensional models from the ultrasound data set. This relies on the technology used in plastics manufacturing and can provide a solid or hollow model of a three-dimensional data set from cardiac images.

Epicardial Imaging

The fidelity of image registration is greatest when the amount of intervening tissue is minimal. For this reason, application of an ultrasound probe directly to the cardiac structures provides a high-resolution, nonobstructive view of cardiac structures. Because the very near field of most ultrasound transducers is subject to distortion, probes have been designed specifically for epicardial application. Because these probes are placed directly on the beating heart or vasculature, they must be either sterilized or more commonly placed in a sterile insulating sheath before use. Additionally, because there is no intervening tissue, the focusing characteristics of the probe are engineered to maximize rear-field quality. Imaging from these probes provides remarkably high-resolution, high-fidelity images of cardiac structures. They are infrequently used because of the limited applicability of this technique and the fact that the majority of information can be obtained by either transthoracic or intravascular ultrasound. Before the widespread use of intraoperative transesophageal echocardiography, direct epicardial imaging had been used for evaluating atheroma along the course of the ascending aorta and arch at the time of cardiovascular surgery in an effort to identify the most appropriate site for either cannula or vein graft insertion. Although it could be used as a substitute for intraoperative transesophageal echocardiography, the complexity of epicardial imaging, combined with the added potential risk of contaminating a sterile operative field, generally has caused it to be abandoned in favor of transesophageal imaging.

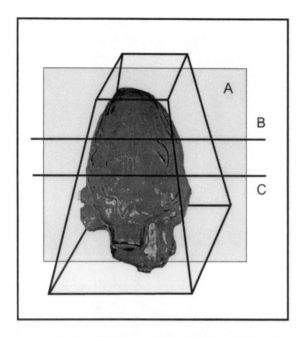

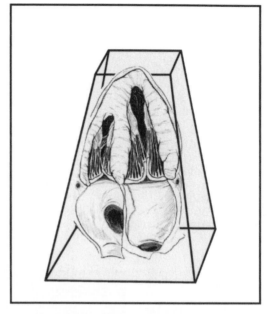

Unprocessed Full Volume   "Cropped" Full Volume Data Set

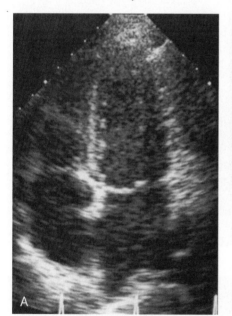
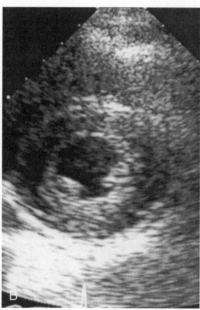
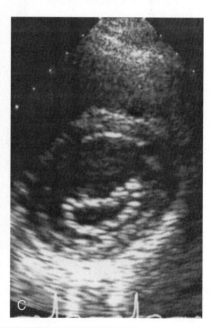

FIGURE 3.31. Schematic demonstrates various methods for processing real-time, three-dimensional, full-volume data sets. **Upper left:** Schematic represents the total volume in a pyramidal scan that contains all four cardiac chambers. Note, as in the top of Figure 3.28, that distinct cardiac structures are not visualized. **Upper right:** A "cropped" full-volume data set in which the full-volume data set has been "sliced" through its midpoint. This effectively exposes the middle of the three-dimensional data set in the cropped plane. In this example, this results in a three-dimensional image of an apical four-chamber view. The lower three images represent extracted two-dimensional images from the full-volume data set. Each has been created by extracting a discrete imaging plane along either the long- (*A*) or short-axis (*B and C*) plane of the three-dimensional data set. In reality, an infinite number of imaging planes could be selected from the three-dimensional data set, resulting in creation of any of the traditional or nontraditional two-dimensional imaging planes.

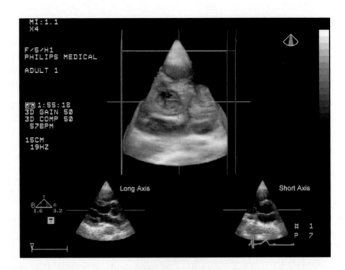

FIGURE 3.32. Full-volume, three-dimensional data set from which a long-axis view and a short-axis view of the left ventricle have been extracted. **Top:** The full-volume, three-dimensional data set that has been cropped is shown. The horizontal and vertical lines denoting the direction of the extracted imaging planes are demonstrated. **Bottom:** Long- and short-axis two-dimensional images extracted from the full volume data set.

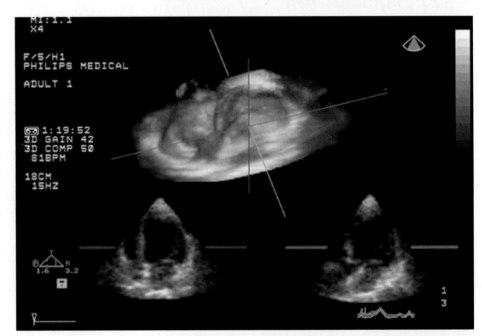

FIGURE 3.33. Real-time, three-dimensional image from the apex of the heart. Two orthogonal imaging planes **(top)** have been selected from which traditional apical four- and two-chamber views have been extracted **(bottom)**.

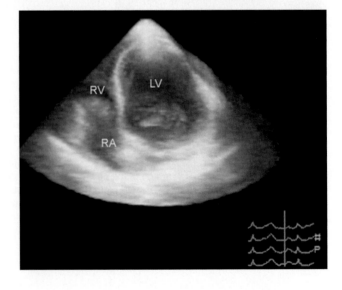

FIGURE 3.34. Cropped full-volume, three-dimensional data set recorded in a patient with ischemic cardiomyopathy. The data set has been cropped through the midpoint of the left ventricle and shows a dilated hypokinetic left ventricle.

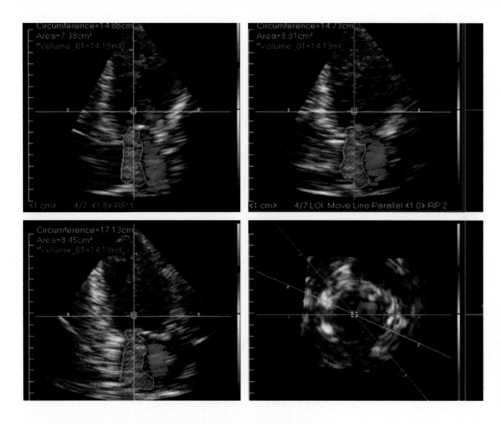

FIGURE 3.35. Four different two-dimensional echocardiograms with color flow Doppler imaging extracted from a three-dimensional data set revealing different perspectives on a mitral regurgitation jet.

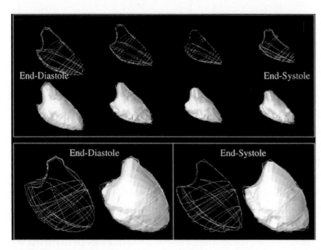

FIGURE 3.36. Wire frame– and volume-rendered reconstructions of a heart with normal function are displayed from end-diastole to end-systole **(top)** and of a dilated cardiomyopathy at end-diastole and end-systole from which diastolic and systolic volumes and ejection fraction were obtained **(bottom)**. (From Hibberd MG, Chuang ML, Beaudin RA, et al. Accuracy of three-dimensional echocardiography with unrestricted selection of imaging planes for measurement of left ventricular volume and ejection fraction. Am Heart J 2000;140:469–475, with permission.)

Intracardiac Echocardiography

Catheter-based transducers for intracardiac (vs. intracoronary) echocardiography have recently been developed (Fig. 3.38). This technology involves a single-plane,

high-frequency transducer (typically 10 MHz) on the tip of a steerable intravascular catheter, typically 9 to 13 French in size. The catheter can be steered in both directions laterally and can be retroflexed and anteflexed. There is a 64-element, single-plane ultrasound transducer mounted at the tip that provides high-resolution, two-dimensional imaging as well as color flow imaging and Doppler spectral imaging.

This technique is obviously applicable only in the cardiac catheterization laboratory and requires large-bore intravascular access. To date, it has been used predominantly in the venous circuit and provides remarkably high-resolution views of the right atrium including the fossa ovalis area. The depth of penetration is such that visualization of the left atrium and the base of the heart is likewise available as is visualization of left ventricular function. This technique has seen greatest use for monitoring complex interventional procedures such as percutaneous atrial septal defect closure, atrial septostomy, and pulmonary vein isolation for treatment of atrial fibrillation. Figures 3.39 and 3.40 were acquired using a commercially available intracardiac ultrasound probe.

Intravascular Ultrasound (IVUS)

Intracoronary ultrasound was developed before the intracardiac probes noted previously. Typically, these are ultraminiaturized ultrasound transducers mounted on

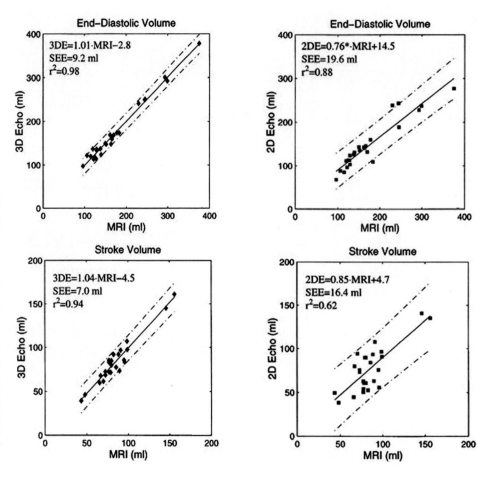

FIGURE 3.37. Graphic demonstration of the relationship of end-diastolic volume and stroke volume as determined by either two- or three-dimensional echocardiography and cardiac magnetic resonance imaging (MRI). For both end-diastolic volume and stroke volume, the correlation with the standard of MRI is substantially greater with three-dimensional echocardiography than it is with MRI. (From Hibberd MG, Chuang ML, Beaudin RA, et al. Accuracy of three-dimensional echocardiography with unrestricted selection of imaging planes for measurement of left ventricular volume and ejection fraction. Am Heart J 2000;140: 469–475.),

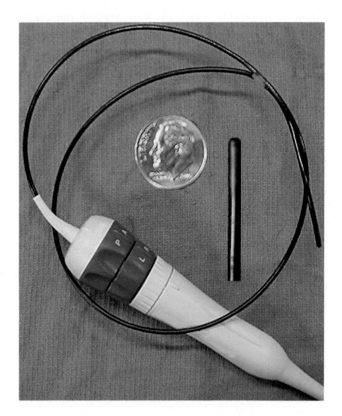

modified intracoronary catheters. Both phased-array and mechanical rotational devices have been developed. These devices operate at frequencies of 10 to 30 MHz and provide circumferential 360-degree imaging. Because of the high frequencies, the depth of penetration is relatively low and the field of depth is limited to usually less than 1 cm. Most devices provide only anatomic imaging and do not provide Doppler information. Intracoronary ultrasound is by definition performed in the cardiac catheterization laboratory and in the majority of instances is performed by an invasive cardiologist rather than a dedicated echocardiographer. The technique provides high-resolution images of the proximal coronary arteries and can identify calcification and plaque and further characterize plaque (Figs. 3.41–3.43). The technique was instrumental in determining the optimal methods for intracoronary stent deployment. It is usually most often used to define the

FIGURE 3.38. Dedicated single-plane, two-dimensional probe developed for intracardiac ultrasound. The two blue rings on the white handle allow flexion of approximately 60 degrees in two different planes. The middle image is an expanded view of the tip of the catheter. The probe is approximately 10 French in size.

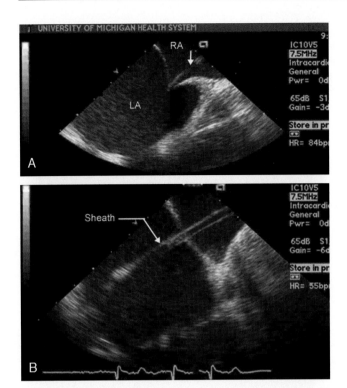

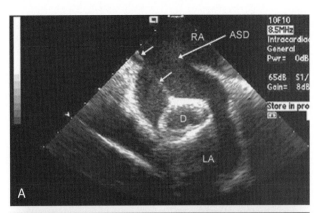

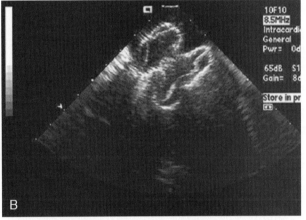

FIGURE 3.39. Images from an intracardiac two-dimensional imaging device recorded at the time of atrial septal puncture for performance of an electrophysiologic procedure. **Top:** The transseptal needle (*arrow*) as it is puncturing the atrial septum near the foramen ovale. Note that at the time of puncture, it is "tenting" the atrial septal tissue. **Bottom:** Recorded after passing a sheath from the right to the left atrium for subsequent passage of electrophysiologic catheters.

FIGURE 3.40. Intracardiac ultrasound recorded from the right atrium in a patient undergoing percutaneous closure of an atrial septal defect (Amplatzer device). Note the ability to clearly visualize the path of the closure device through the defect. **Bottom:** Recorded after deployment of the left atrial side of the occlusion device.

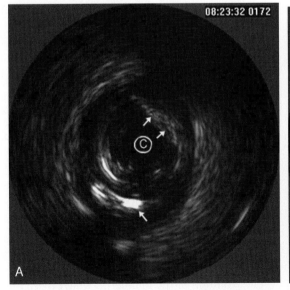

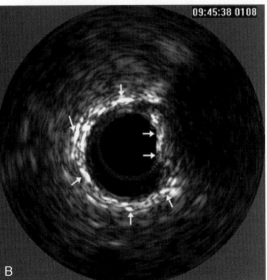

FIGURE 3.41. Intracoronary ultrasound recorded in two patients. The catheter (*C*) is the dark circle in the center of the image. **Left:** Recorded in a patient with moderate intraluminal atheroma (*arrows*) and also calcific atheroma creating a bright echo and shadow (*lower arrow*). **Right:** Recorded in a patient who had undergone coronary stenting. The individual wire mesh of the stent is clearly seen as a sequence of bright echoes at the periphery of the artery. From roughly 1 o'clock to 5 o'clock, there is nonobstructive intimal hyperplasia/recurrent atheroma within the lumen of the artery.

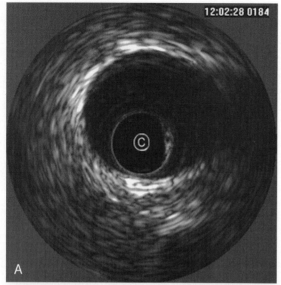

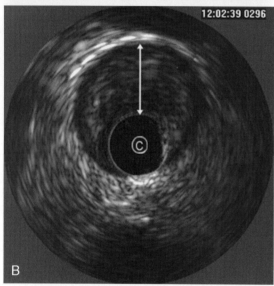

FIGURE 3.42. Intracoronary ultrasound image recorded in a patient with a tight stenosis of the left anterior descending coronary artery. **Top:** Image was recorded distal to the occlusion and reveals a widely patent lumen. **Bottom:** Image was recorded at the area of maximal obstruction. Note the crescent-shaped atheroma, the maximal dimension of which is noted by the *double-headed arrow*. Note also that the diameter of the residual lumen is essentially equal to that of the imaging catheter.

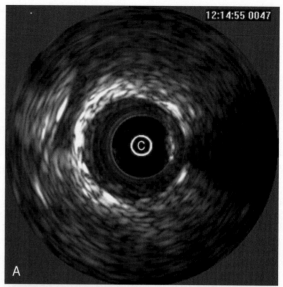

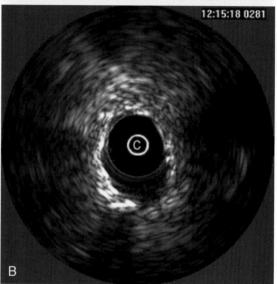

FIGURE 3.43. Intracoronary ultrasound image demonstrates incomplete stent deployment. **Top:** Image was recorded at an area of complete stent deployment. Note the bright matrix of echoes representing the actual stent at the periphery of the lumen. **Bottom:** Image was recorded at an area of incomplete stent deployment. Note the oval versus circular shape of the stent representing incomplete deployment.

true anatomic severity of "intermediate" coronary lesions noted on angiography or for highly precise evaluation of coronary arterial wall anatomy.

Separate Doppler flow wires are available that provide intracoronary Doppler information. Data from intracoronary Doppler flow wires can be used to assess the integrity of hyperemic reverse by determining flow characteristics under basal conditions and after vasodilatation. It provides another method for defining the physiologic significance of a coronary stenosis.

THE DIGITAL ECHO LABORATORY

Cardiac ultrasound examinations generate a tremendous amount of information consisting of moving gray-scale images, color images, and static images. There has been a rapid evolution of the manner in which these images are acquired, stored, and analyzed. During the early days of echocardiography, only M-mode tracings were available, and these were typically recorded on a strip-chart recorder and stored as light-sensitive paper output. With the advent of two-dimensional echocardiography, the need arose to store moving video images. For approximately two decades, these images were stored using standard video technology and reviewed from videotape. Although this provides "full-disclosure" registration and review of all available information, it is an inefficient method for reviewing studies, results in the need for substantial storage and archiving space, and has the disadvantage of the degradation of video information over time. In the early 1980s, high-speed digitizing devices became available that allowed analog data to be converted to a digital format and stored as such. The limitation of these early attempts was the relatively slow speed of computer processors and the limitations in both speed and cost of computer memory. Over time, there has been a dramatic reduction in cost and improvement in speed and reliability, so that storage of large amounts of digital information is now within the reach of virtually all echocardiography laboratories. Finally, all modern ultrasound scanners are intrinsically "digital" platforms. The information collected from the transducer face is done so in a digital format, processed as digital information, and displayed by a computer processor as digital information. It is converted to analog format only for purposes of recording on videotape. As such, the original, nondegraded digital images are available for both review and storage if the appropriate offline systems are made available.

Digital archiving systems are now available from a number of ultrasound and third-party vendors, all of which are capable of providing transfer from current-generation ultrasound platforms to a file server (and subsequently to bulk storage devices) and retrievable to standard computer workstations. A major breakthrough in digital medical imaging came with the advent of the DICOM standard (digital imaging and communication in medicine). The DICOM standard was negotiated among major medical manufacturers, regulatory bodies, and professional organizations in an effort to ensure that medical imaging information would be available in a standardized nonproprietary format so that it could be easily transferred from institution to institution and platform to platform for storage and analysis. Virtually all current-generation ultrasound platforms provide output of echocardiographic images in a DICOM-compatible format that can be archived to and retrieved from offline analysis systems. The DICOM committee has also standardized image formats and recommended standards for image compression. Because a complete ultrasound examination may include 30 to 100 image clips and static images, it represents a substantial file size. In an effort to reduce file size, image clips are typically compressed. Compression can be either lossless (no information lost) or lossy, with the potential for image degradation. The DICOM committee has recommended motion JPEG, which provides as much as 20:1 compression as the accepted compression method of video images.

The modern digital echocardiography laboratory has several components as noted in Figure 3.44. In a typical installation, ultrasound platforms are connected to a file server by either a local area network (LAN) or Internet connection. Depending on the size of the laboratory, the "file server" may be an enhanced desktop computer or a standard file server with a high-speed hard drive capacity of several hundred gigabytes. In either instance, the ultrasound platform can be configured to either automatically or on command transmit the DICOM format ultrasound images to the file server for storage. Reading stations typically are desktop personal computers that can retrieve images for analysis and report generation. Because all information is digital and communicated over a computer network, echocardiograms recorded in remote sites can be transmitted almost instantaneously to the file server for review at the interpreting laboratory. Additionally, physicians can retrieve images at any appropriately equipped desktop computer, including physician offices, hospital ward stations, and catheterization laboratories.

The method for long-term storage of digital information is currently in evolution and can result in substantially more expense than the initial outlay for a basic digital echocardiography laboratory. Most hospital and regulatory agency stipulations require that medical information be stored with several layers of redundancy, and, as such, a "purely digital" laboratory must be prepared to provide storage at a minimum of two separate sites along with tape backup to ensure guaranteed access to medical information, even in the event of catastrophic failure at one site. In view of this, many laboratories that rely heavily on digital imaging still record standard analog videotape as a means of long-term archiving for regulatory purposes.

In migrating to a digital echo laboratory, it is important to recognize that even with the enhanced speed and availability of large-scale memory, it is still not feasible to record 20 to 40 minutes of continuous video information in digital format for high-volume laboratories. In view of this, the digital laboratory must develop a protocol for acquisition of select images that may be specific to the clinical presentation or disease being investigated. Typically, a digital echocardiographic examination will comprise 30 to 100 individual clips consisting of real-time, two-dimensional imaging, color Doppler flow imaging, and static images of M-mode echocardiography, spectral Doppler display, and so on. The precise images to be acquired are a matter of individual laboratory preference and policy, but, as a general rule, it should be possible to acquire representative clips of each of the standard views typically required during videotaping of an echocardiogram within the stipulated 30- to 100-image volume.

Once digitally acquired and archived, the images can be retrieved from any appropriately equipped computer including standard office desktops, laptops, and hospital workstations (Figs. 3.45–3.47). A typical full-function

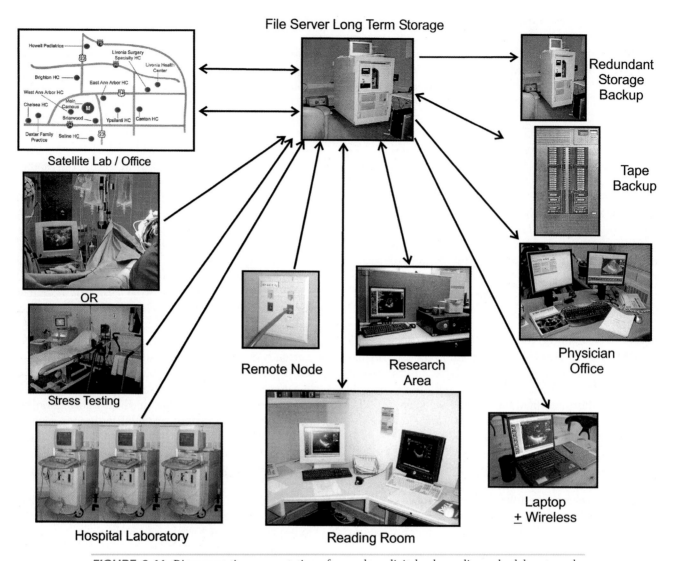

File Server Long Term Storage

Satellite Lab / Office

OR

Stress Testing

Hospital Laboratory

Remote Node

Research Area

Reading Room

Redundant Storage Backup

Tape Backup

Physician Office

Laptop ± Wireless

FIGURE 3.44. Diagrammatic representation of a modern digital echocardiography laboratory denoting the multiple components for image analysis and storage as well as the diversity of sites from which images can be transferred or viewed.

FIGURE 3.45. Typical review station screen of a digital laboratory workstation. On the left is a series of "thumbnail" clips that can be selected for viewing in the larger window. The toolbar at the top activates a variety of other functions including measurement and report-generation packages as well as configuration details. The series of small icons at the top allows instantaneous contouring of the screen for image size, side-by-side comparison, and altering playback speed as well as image quality.

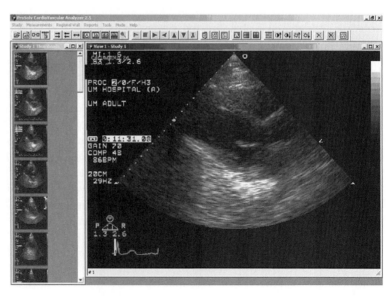

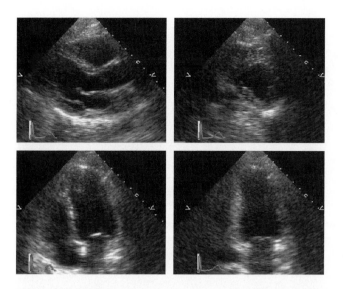

FIGURE 3.46. Typical quad screen image format available from a digital echo review station. In this image, four different views from a resting two-dimensional echocardiogram are viewed in a quad screen format allowing immediate comparison of wall motion in all 16 segments.

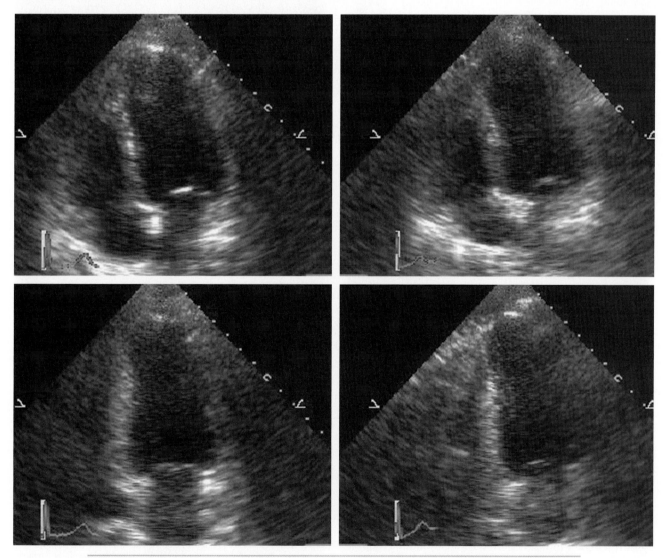

FIGURE 3.47. Quad screen view of apical four- and two-chamber views recorded at rest **(left)** and with stress **(right)**. The resting images are identical to the images presented in Figure 3.46 and have been "scrambled" to allow side-by-side comparison of rest and stress images.

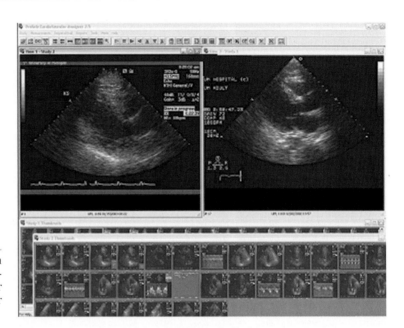

FIGURE 3.48. Alternate viewing format in which serial studies are visualized side by side. Most modern digital review stations allow retrieval of two or more studies and subsequent display side by side for comparison of two points in time.

workstation has the ability to retrieve and review studies, make multiple measurements, and generate reports. Additionally, in a fully digital hospital environment, it is anticipated that all other medical images including catheterization data, results of nuclear medicine studies, and electrocardiograms, will also be available in a DICOM format. Most vendors of digital archiving and review stations provide access for non-echocardiographic images. The review stations can be configured as either review-only systems or full-function analysis and report-generation systems. Typically, a laboratory that is heavily invested in the digital echocardiographic laboratory may have a number of view-only stations for use by requesting physicians, emergency department physicians, the operating room, among others, with a more limited number of more sophisticated workstations for measurement and report generation.

A major advantage of the digital environment is the ability to pull up and compare in a side-by-side format multiple studies (Figs. 3.47 and 3.48). This allows a side-by-side display of equivalent images recorded at two different points in time for evaluation of serial changes and has particular relevance with respect to evaluating resolution of wall motion abnormalities after acute myocardial infarction, serial changes in valvular insufficiency, or serial changes in left ventricular function. This ability to rapidly evaluate echocardiograms recorded at different points in time in a side-by-side fashion has been a major advantage of the digital echocardiography laboratory. Finally, the digital image is played as a continuous loop of anywhere from one to three cardiac cycles. Because this is a controllable digital loop, the reviewer has the ability to evaluate wall motion, valvular function, and other parameters on a frame-by-frame basis and provide a highly detailed temporal resolution of cardiac events, which is typically not feasible when reviewing video images.

Although the cost of instituting a digital archiving and review system can be significant, the majority of laboratories that have migrated from videotape to a digital environment have found that the improved efficiency of analyses and the cost-saving achieved by not archiving videotape substantially mitigates the increased cost of a digital laboratory.

The techniques and methods of echocardiography should not be viewed in isolation. All the techniques are interrelated, and, in theory, all the different imaging modalities such as two-dimensional imaging, M-mode imaging, color flow imaging, and spectral Doppler imaging are available from any given single transducer. Limitations in computational power and transducer design of necessity may limit the information at this time from any one device.

SUGGESTED READINGS

Ahmad M, Xie T, McCulloch M, et al. Real-time three-dimensional dobutamine stress echocardiography in assessment of ischemia: comparison with two-dimensional dobutamine stress echocardiography. J Am Coll Cardiol 2001;37:1303–1309.

Balestrini L, Fleishman C, Lanzoni L, et al. Real-time 3-dimensional echocardiography evaluation of congenital heart disease. J Am Soc Echocardiogr 2000;13:171–176.

Bruce CJ, Packer DL, Seward JB. Transvascular imaging: feasibility study using a vector phased array ultrasound catheter. Echocardiography 1999;16:425–430.

Bruce CJ, O'Leary P, Hagler DJ, et al. Miniaturized transesophageal echocardiography in newborn infants. J Am Soc Echocardiogr 2002;15:791–797.

Chuang ML, Parker RA, Riley MF, et al. Three-dimensional echocardiography improves accuracy and compensates for sonographer inexperience in assessment of left ventricular ejection fraction. J Am Soc Echocardiogr 1999;12:290–299.

Collins M, Hsieh A, Ohazama CJ, et al. Assessment of regional wall motion abnormalities with real-time 3-dimensional echocardiography. J Am Soc Echocardiogr 1999;12:7–14.

Donovan CL, Armstrong WF, Bach DS. Quantitative Doppler tissue imaging of the left ventricular myocardium: validation in normal subjects. Am Heart J 1995;130:100–104.

Edvardsen T, Gerber BL, Garot J, et al. Quantitative assessment of intrinsic regional myocardial deformation by Doppler strain rate echocardiography in humans: validation against three-dimensional tagged magnetic resonance imaging. Circulation 2002;106:50–56.

Goodkin GM, Spevack DM, Tunick PA, et al. How useful is hand-carried bedside echocardiography in critically ill patients? J Am Coll Cardiol 2001;37:2019–2022.

Hibberd MG, Chuang ML, Beaudin RA, et al. Accuracy of three-dimensional echocardiography with unrestricted selection of imaging planes for measurement of left ventricular volume and ejection fraction. Am Heart J 2000;140:469–475.

Iwakura K, Ito H, Kawano S, et al. Detection of TIMI-3 flow before mechanical reperfusion with ultrasonic tissue characterization in patients with anterior wall acute myocardial infarction. Circulation 2003;107:3159–3164.

Jiang L, Vazquez de Prada JA, Handschumacher MD, et al. Three-dimensional echocardiography. In vivo validation for right ventricular volume and function. Circulation 1994;89:2342–2350.

Lee D, Fuisz AR, Fan PH, et al. Real-time 3-dimensional echocardiographic evaluation of left ventricular volume: correlation with magnetic resonance imaging—a validation study. J Am Soc Echocardiogr 2001;14:1001–1009.

Lin LC, Kao HL, Wu CC, et al. Alterations of myocardial ultrasonic tissue characterization by coronary angioplasty in patients with chronic stable coronary artery disease. Ultrasound Med Biol 2001;27:1191–1198.

Main ML, Grayburn PA. Clinical applications of transpulmonary contrast echocardiography. Am Heart J 1999;137:144–153.

Marcovitz PA, Bach DS, Segar DS, et al. Impact of B-mode color encoding on rapid detection of ultrasound targets: an *in vitro* study. J Am Soc Echocardiogr 1993;6:382–386.

Marcus RH, Bednarz J, Coulden R, et al. Ultrasonic backscatter system for automated on-line endocardial boundary detection: evaluation by ultrafast computed tomography. J Am Coll Cardiol 1993;22:839–847.

Milunski MR, Mohr GA, Perez JE, et al. Ultrasonic tissue characterization with integrated backscatter. Acute myocardial ischemia, reperfusion, and stunned myocardium in patients. Circulation 1989;80:491–503.

Oemrawsingh PV, Mintz GS, Schalij MJ, et al. Intravascular ultrasound guidance improves angiographic and clinical outcome of stent implantation for long coronary artery stenoses: final results of a randomized comparison with angiographic guidance (TULIP Study). Circulation 2003;107:62–67.

Packer DL, Stevens CL, Curley MG, et al. Intracardiac phased-array imaging: methods and initial clinical experience with high resolution, under blood visualization: initial experience with intracardiac phased-array ultrasound. J Am Coll Cardiol 2002;39:509–516.

Pandian NG, Nanda NC, Schwartz SL, et al. Three-dimensional and four-dimensional transesophageal echocardiographic imaging of the heart and aorta in humans using a computed tomographic imaging probe. Echocardiography 1992;9:677–687.

Quinones MA, Douglas PS, Foster E, et al. ACC/AHA clinical competence statement on echocardiography: a report of the American College of Cardiology/American Heart Association/American College of Physicians-American Society of Internal Medicine Task Force on Clinical Competence. J Am Coll Cardiol 2003;41:687–708.

Ren JF, Schwartzman D, Callans DJ, et al. Intracardiac echocardiography (9 MHz) in humans: methods, imaging views and clinical utility. Ultrasound Med Biol 1999;25:1077–1086.

Ren JF, Marchlinski FE, Callans DJ, et al. Clinical use of AcuNav diagnostic ultrasound catheter imaging during left heart radiofrequency ablation and transcatheter closure procedures. J Am Soc Echocardiogr 2002;15:1301–1308.

Sagar KB, Pelc LR, Saeian K, et al. Ultrasonic tissue characterization of normal and ischemic myocardium. Echocardiography 1990;7:11–19.

Salustri A, Spitaels S, McGhie J, et al. Transthoracic three-dimensional echocardiography in adult patients with congenital heart disease. J Am Coll Cardiol 1995;26:759–767.

Senior R, Soman P, Khattar RS, et al. Improved endocardial visualization with second harmonic imaging compared with fundamental two-dimensional echocardiographic imaging. Am Heart J 1999;138: 163–168.

Seward JB, Khandheria BK, Freeman WK, et al. Multiplane transesophageal echocardiography: image orientation, examination technique, anatomic correlations, and clinical applications. Mayo Clin Proc 1993;68:523–551.

Spencer KT, Bednarz J, Rafter PG, et al. Use of harmonic imaging without echocardiographic contrast to improve two-dimensional image quality. Am J Cardiol 1998;82:794–799.

Spencer KT, Anderson AS, Bhargava A, et al. Physician-performed point-of-care echocardiography using a laptop platform compared with physical examination in the cardiovascular patient. J Am Coll Cardiol 2001;37:2013–2018.

Sun JP, Stewart WJ, Yang XS, et al. Automated echocardiographic quantification of left ventricular volumes and ejection fraction: validation in the intensive care setting. J Am Soc Echocardiogr 1995;8: 29–36.

Takuma S, Zwas DR, Fard A, et al. Real-time, 3-dimensional echocardiography acquires all standard 2-dimensional images from 2 volume sets: a clinical demonstration in 45 patients. J Am Soc Echocardiogr 1999;12:1–6.

Urheim S, Edvardsen T, Torp H, et al. Myocardial strain by Doppler echocardiography. Validation of a new method to quantify regional myocardial function. Circulation 2000;102:1158–1164.

Contrast Echocardiography

Ultrasound contrast agents were first used in conjunction with clinical echocardiography in the mid-1970s. Early agents consisted of either agitated saline or agitated saline stabilized with indocyanine green dye. Injections were done both intravenously and more centrally at the time of cardiac catheterization. The resultant cloud of microbubbles was used to define cardiac borders and detect shunts. Early contrast echocardiography studies were essential for determining the nature of reflective tissue targets and identifying the endocardial border and other structures with echocardiography (Fig. 4.1). It became rapidly apparent that these early contrast agents, after intravenous injection, were isolated to the right heart and that their appearance in the left heart was evidence of a right-to-left shunt.

SOURCE OF ULTRASOUND CONTRAST

The source of ultrasound contrast is now established to be microbubbles, either purposefully injected into the circulation or as a side effect of an intravenous injection. Initial theories that the microbubble targets were created by cavitation at the time of injection have been dispelled. Although it is possible to create microbubbles due to a cavitation effect, the pressure with which fluid must be injected to create a cavitation effect is well beyond that encountered in routine clinical practice. Contrast occurring spontaneously at the time of an intravenous injection is more likely due to air contamination in the injection apparatus than to creation by the injection process.

Gas-containing microbubbles are intense ultrasound reflectors and typically reflect ultrasound at a level several orders of magnitude greater than non–gas-containing structures. Current ultrasound agents contain a variety of gases including air, or, more recently, perfluorocarbons. It should be emphasized that the increased reflectivity from a microbubble target is due to the differential reflection of the contained gas compared with surrounding blood and tissue.

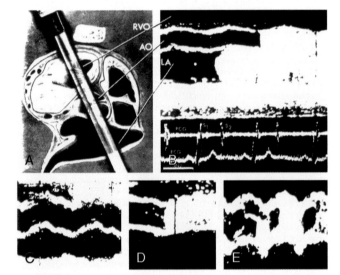

FIGURE 4.1. Early M-mode contrast echocardiograms recorded in the cardiac catheterization laboratory. **A:** The orientation of the M-mode ultrasound beam. **B:** Image was recorded after injection of contrast into the left atrium and shows subsequent appearance of contrast in the aorta. **C:** Contrast injected into the right ventricular outflow tract is shown. **D:** Contrast appears in the aorta after a left ventricular injection. **E:** Image was recorded after a supravalvular injection into the aorta. Contrast is seen exclusively in diastole with a contrast-free area due to competitive flow during aortic valve opening. (From Gramiak R, Shah PM, Kramer DH. Ultrasound cardiography: contrast studies in anatomy and function. Radiology 1969;92:939–948, with permission.)

CONTRAST AGENTS

The simplest ultrasound contrast agent consists of saline microbubbles. Effective right heart contrast can be obtained by forcefully agitating a solution of saline between two 10-mL syringes, each of which contains 5 mL of saline and 0.1 to 0.5 mL of room air (Fig. 4.2). Forceful agitation through a three-way stopcock creates a population of microbubbles that are highly variable in size and have a tendency to rapidly coalesce. After generation by

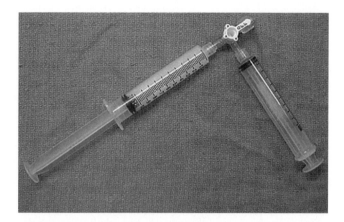

FIGURE 4.2. Two-syringe and three-way stopcock apparatus for preparation of agitated saline contrast for intravenous injection. The total volume in the syringe on the left is approximately 10 mL, which consisted initially of 9.5 mL of saline and 0.5 mL of room air. The contrast was prepared by forcefully injecting the solution from one syringe to the other through the three-way stopcock. Turbulence within the stopcock results in the creation of a large number of microbubbles that are suitable for intravenous injection. For opacification of right heart structures, a typical intravenous "dose" of contrast prepared in this manner ranges from 1.0 to 5.0 mL.

agitation, they should be injected immediately to limit the time available for coalescence. These microbubbles, however, are intense echo reflectors and can be detected in the right atrium and right ventricle (Fig. 4.3). Their size is prohibitive of passage through the pulmonary capillary bed, and their appearance in the left heart implies a pathologic right-to-left shunt. By analyzing the timing and location of appearance, the nature of this shunt can often be determined as being a patent foramen ovale, atrial septal defect, or pulmonary arteriovenous malformation (AVM). Creation of ultrasound contrast by this technique is widely used in clinical practice and has had an excellent safety profile.

Early attempts to create a more stable population of microbubbles involved reduction of surface tension. Surface tension is the physical characteristic that increases the inward pressure of a bubble and is responsible for the tendency of a microbubble to collapse on itself. This tendency to spontaneously decrease in size due to bubble wall surface tension results in a progressive increase in the pressure within the microbubble, which in turn increases the driving force for the contained gas to diffuse out of the bubble. These factors lead to an acceleration in the rate at which the microbubble shrinks and eventually disappears. By reducing and stabilizing surface tension, bubbles undergo less spontaneous collapse and a population of stabilized, longer lasting microbubbles can be created. Several agents including surfactant and indocyanine green dye have been used to reduce surface tension and create a population of smaller, more stable microbubbles.

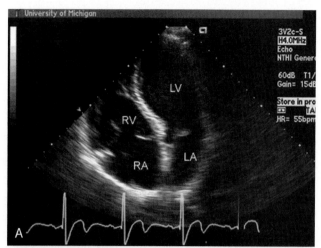

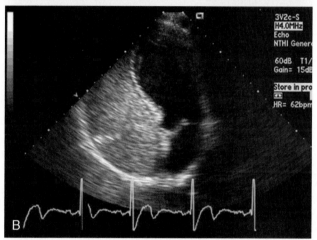

FIGURE 4.3. Apical four-chamber view recorded in a patient before **(top)** and after **(bottom)** injection of saline into a left upper extremity vein. Note the absence of contrast in any of the four chambers. After injection of intravenous contrast, there is uniform opacification of the right atrium and right ventricle with no appearance of contrast in the left heart.

Many of the early fundamental observations in contrast echo were made using indocyanine green dye–stabilized microbubbles (Fig. 4.1). For practical purposes, there is little need to stabilize saline microbubbles. Because their size is relatively large, they do not pass the pulmonary capillary bed, and the safety record of this easily prepared agent has been remarkable. Beginning in the early 1980s, a number of attempts were made to engineer and manufacture microbubbles that would be uniform in size, have stability with respect to coalescence and size, and provide a homogeneous and reproducible degree of contrast.

Recognition that high-intensity sonication resulted in populations of microbubbles was a major breakthrough in contrast echocardiography. The stability of the resultant contrast agent was dependent on the solution being sonicated and the contained gas. Through trial and error, it was recognized that sonication of 5% human albumin resulted in creation of a relatively homogeneous population of small microbubbles consisting of a denatured albumin shell containing air. These microbubbles were small enough to allow transpulmonary passage, resulted in an intense contrast effect, and could be commercially prepared as a sterile solution providing reproducible contrast effect. The major limitations of the early air-containing contrast agents were their relatively large size and inability to pass the pulmonary capillary bed in all patients. Refinements in the sonication process included replacement of the contained gas with a high-density perfluorocarbon instead of air and in some agents replacement of the albumin shell by a lipid membrane. A number of other approaches to the manufacture of microbubbles have also been undertaken including saccharide particles that form gas microbubbles on their surface and engineered microbubble shells of various size and composition. In general, the commercially available microbubbles have an initial size of 1.1 to 8.0 μm and are prepared at a concentration of 5×10^8 to 1.2×10^{10} microbubbles/mL, depending on the agent. As such, the number of microbubbles injected per "dose" is substantially greater than that seen with agitated saline. Because of their stability (in a low ultrasound intensity field), they have substantial persistence and a single injection will provide a usable contrast effect for 3 to 10 minutes.

An engineered microbubble has two basic components, the outer shell and contained gas, the effects of which are reflective characteristics, duration of contrast effect, and biological activity (Fig. 4.4). Bubble shells can be designed to be either rigid or flexible and to have varying resistance to collapse at high pressure. Recognition of these phenomena allows creation of microbubble populations that can be highly resistant to ultrasound destruction and therefore provide persistent contrast effect or can be easily destroyed in the ultrasound beam, resulting in simulated acoustic emission and enhanced detectability by this mechanism. The shell can be designed to allow varying degrees of permeability and outward diffusion of the contrast gas. Finally, the composition of the shell can be altered to include nonreflective therapeutic compounds. Application of the latter hypothetically includes the ability to deliver chemotherapeutic or biologically active agents, including gene transfection vectors, to targeted tissue.

The gas contained within the shell also affects the intensity and duration of the effect. Because the gas-blood interface is such a potent reflector, the intensity of contrast effect is substantially greater for any of the current generation of commercially available agents than that seen with agitated saline, largely because of the greater concentration of microbubbles. As is discussed subsequently, many ultrasound techniques either purposefully or incidentally disrupt the microbubble shell, allowing the gas to escape into the blood pool. Gases such as oxygen, nitrogen, and room air will rapidly diffuse down a concentration gradient, resulting in rapid loss of contrast effect. High-density perfluorocarbons diffuse more slowly and therefore provide a longer lasting contrast effect even after bubble shell disruption.

CLINICAL USE

The use of contrast echocardiography can be divided into four broad categories. Detection of right-to-left shunts by detection of contrast targets in the left heart remains a primary use of contrast echocardiography. Left-to-right shunts also can be detected if a negative contrast effect is noted in the right heart. As noted elsewhere in this text, contrast echocardiography remains the standard for the diagnosis of a patent foramen ovale. This diagnosis is established using agitated saline, which does not pass through the pulmonary capillary bed as the contrast agent is cleared by the pulmonary capillaries.

Because of their small size and stability, commercially available perfluorocarbon-based contrast agents pass through the pulmonary capillary bed relatively unimpeded and subsequently opacify the left ventricular

FIGURE 4.4. Schematic representation of a microbubble depicts its contents and various shell characteristics. See text for details.

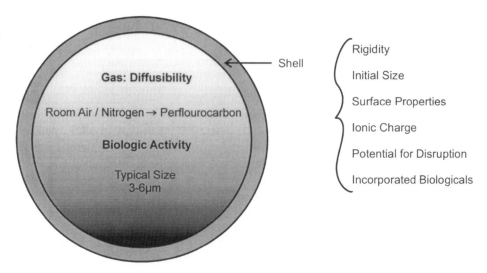

cavity. This results in enhanced visualization of the left ventricular border and provides increased accuracy for border detection, chamber volume determination, evaluation of regional wall motion, and detection of mural thrombi. Because these newer agents cross the pulmonary capillary bed, their appearance in the left heart is not indicative of a pathologic shunt. Additionally, the new generation of contrast agents is capable of opacification of the left ventricular myocardium. When used for this purpose, the contrast agent parallels myocardial blood volume and can be used as a marker of normal and abnormal perfusion.

Finally, contrast agents can be used to enhance Doppler signals. This has had clinical utility for enhancing the tricuspid regurgitation signal for assessing right heart hemodynamics (saline contrast) and, less often, for enhancing a weak aortic stenosis jet or pulmonary vein flow signals. The use of contrast agents during color Doppler interrogation results in marked signal deterioration and is counterproductive.

ULTRASOUND INTERACTION WITH CONTRAST AGENTS

Microbubbles interact with the ultrasound beam in a variety of ways including direct reflection at the fundamental frequency and resonance with creation of harmonic frequencies. The frequency at which a bubble has maximal reflectance is related to the diameter of the bubble. For any given ultrasound frequency, the amplitude of reflection from a microbubble decreases as the bubble diameter decreases. All bubbles have a diameter at which reflectance is maximal (the resonant diameter). Below the resonant diameter of the bubble, the amplitude of reflection again diminishes with the cube of the diameter. It is a fortuitous occurrence that bubbles having a diameter that allows transpulmonary passage have excellent reflectance when interacting with ultrasound clinically relevant transmission frequencies.

Interaction of microbubbles with the ultrasound beam has three phases (Fig. 4.5). In its simplest form, ultra-

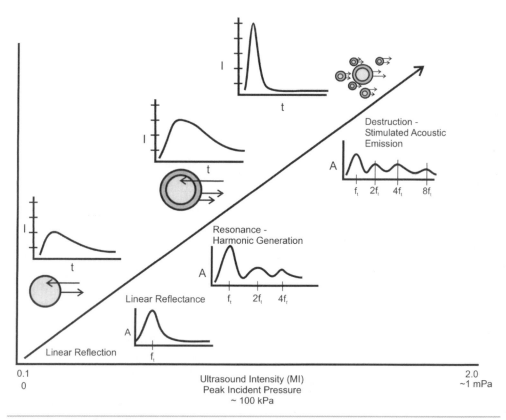

FIGURE 4.5. Schematic representation of various microbubble responses to increasing ultrasound intensity. Above the diagonal line, depicting increasing intensity, is a graphic representation of image intensity at each level of ultrasound intensity and below the line a stylized depiction of the frequency response noted with each technique. At low intensity, a linear response can be obtained that results in detection of a returning frequency identical to the transmit frequency (f_t). At higher incident pressures, bubble resonance occurs, resulting in the generation of a nonlinear or harmonic response such that signal is returned at the fundamental transmitted frequency as well as a series of its harmonics (e.g., f_t). At higher ultrasound intensities, bubble integrity is disrupted resulting in a subpopulation of smaller bubbles with a broad range of resonant frequencies. Because bubble destruction occurs at the higher insonating pressure, the duration of contrast effect is substantially less.

sound interacts with a microbubble by pure reflection of the ultrasound beam at its fundamental (i.e., transmitted) frequency. Maximal reflection from the microbubble is dependent on the relationship of the frequency and diameter as noted previously. At higher ultrasound imaging intensities, microbubbles are not pure reflectors but begin to resonate. A resonating bubble will reflect ultrasound not only at the fundamental insonating frequency (f_t) but also at harmonics of that frequency. In this instance, a microbubble insonated with a 2-MHz interrogating beam will reflect back the 2-MHz fundamental frequency but also resonate, creating reflected frequencies at 4, 8, and 16 MHz. Each of these subsequent harmonic frequencies doubles in frequency and diminishes in amplitude. In routine clinical practice, only the first harmonic (i.e., twice the fundamental frequency) is typically used for anatomic imaging. Contrast-specific imaging often relies on either multiple harmonic frequencies or subharmonics of the first harmonic (i.e., four and eight times the fundamental frequency). This provides a more contrast-specific signal.

At increasing ultrasound energy levels, the bubbles are physically destroyed by the insonating ultrasound beam. The process of destruction results in the creation of subpopulations of bubbles of variable diameters. The highly variable diameter subpopulations result in a broad range of reflection of harmonic frequencies. By this destructive bubble technique, a large amount of acoustic energy is generated both as reflected ultrasound and as multiple Doppler shifts that can be detected. This final phenomenon in which microbubbles are destroyed, thereby creating detectable ultrasound targets, is referred to as stimulated acoustic emission. This phenomenon can be maximized by the use of a microbubble with a fragile shell and containing nitrogen, which diffuses rapidly, resulting in a rapid loss of the contrast effect after shell disruption.

DETECTION METHODS

Interaction of a microbubble with the ultrasound beam is complex and can be divided into three types of interaction: fundamental reflection, harmonic creation and detection, and stimulated acoustic emission. The receiving characteristics of the ultrasound instrument can then be altered to capitalize on any of these three phenomena. Table 4.1 outlines the different ultrasound domains (e.g., B-mode vs. Doppler) and several commonly used acquisition or capturing modalities. Virtually any of the different ultrasound domains can be linked to any of the acquisition methods to register the contrast-enhanced image. The exact combination of ultrasound domain and acquisition protocol will depend on the nature of the examination (e.g., left ventricular border vs. myocardial perfusion)

▶ **TABLE 4.1 Imaging Modalities for Contrast Detection**

Ultrasound Domain	Acquisition Mode
B-mode	**Continuous**
Fundamental	
Harmonic	**Triggered**
High mechanical index (MI)	Fixed interval
Low mechanical index (MI)	Variable, incremental interval
	Triggered sequential
Doppler	**Destruction/Detection image**
Harmonic vs. fundamental	**sequence**
Frequency shift	
Power spectrum	
Correlation techniques	

as well as the characteristics of the available contrast agent and imaging platform.

The simplest method for contrast detection is routine B-mode ultrasound. As noted previously, microbubbles are intense reflectors of ultrasound and the amount of reflected energy is substantially greater than that of the surrounding tissue or blood. Because of this, routine B-mode scanning is highly sensitive for the detection of isolated microbubble targets. This routine imaging technology is sufficient for detection of intracardiac shunts such as atrial septal defect using agitated saline. When used with newer perfluorocarbon-based agents, detection is markedly facilitated by the use of second harmonic imaging (Fig. 4.6).

Intermittent Imaging

It was recognized in the mid-1990s that the routine interrogating ultrasound beam destroyed ultrasound targets (Figs. 4.7–4.9). This was a fortuitous observation made when investigators recognized the absence of contrast effect in the left ventricular cavity or myocardium during continuous imaging, which was then markedly enhanced after brief interruption of scanning. This led to the technique of intermittent imaging in which ultrasound interrogation is triggered to the electrocardiogram. In between triggered imaging, no ultrasound energy is delivered, allowing time for restitution of the contrast effect and its subsequent detection when imaging is resumed. Obviously with intermittent imaging, the ability to analyze wall motion is lost, and this imaging technique is typically used for evaluation of myocardial perfusion. Similar studies also demonstrated a direct relationship between microbubble destruction, measured as loss of contrast effect, and the intensity of delivered ultrasound (Fig. 4.9).

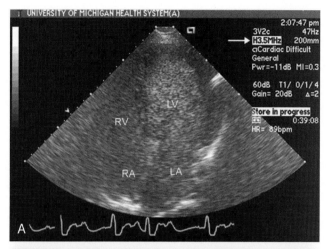

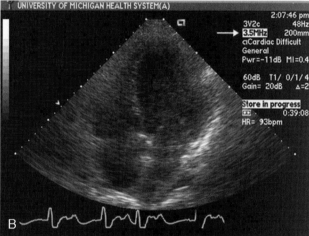

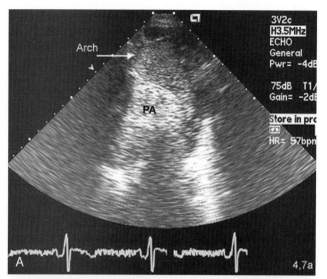

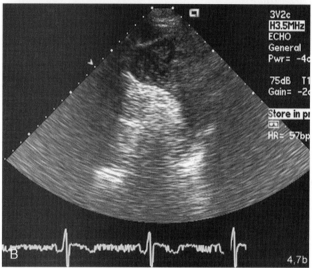

FIGURE 4.6. Four-chamber view recorded in a patient during harmonic **(top)** and fundamental **(bottom)** imaging. Note that with harmonic imaging, there is smooth opacification of the cavity and detection of contrast in all four cardiac chambers. **Bottom:** Recorded in the same patient using fundamental rather than harmonic imaging (*arrows* denote imaging mode). Note the lack of contrast detection with fundamental imaging.

Low Mechanical Index Imaging

Having recognized that the interrogating ultrasound beam is responsible for accelerated microbubble destruction and that continuous imaging results in the loss of contrast effect, algorithms for continuous imaging at a low mechanical index have been developed. The mechanical index is a measure of the power of an ultrasound beam and is defined as peak negative acoustic pressure/f_t, where f_t is the transmitted frequency. Routine B-mode scanning for anatomy and function typically is undertaken at a mechanical index of 0.9 to 1.4, which results in optimal tissue signature but variable degrees of contrast destruction, especially in the near field. Typically, at a mechanical index of 1.3 and above, all perfluorocarbon-based ultrasound contrast agents are rapidly destroyed in

FIGURE 4.7. Suprasternal view of a normal aorta after intravenous injection of ultrasound contrast. The electrocardiogram is provided for timing. **Top:** A systolic frame in which contrast is clearly identified in the arch of the aorta. **Bottom:** The diastolic portion of the same cardiac cycle, in which far less contrast is detected, is shown. In the real-time image, note the phasic appearance and disappearance of the contrast in the aorta. Note that, during systole, a "fresh bolus" of contrast is ejected into the arch from an area out of the plane of imaging. During diastole, when there is less flow in the aorta, there is more time for ultrasound interaction with the contrast agent and it is progressively destroyed.

the ultrasound beam. Although this results in an instantaneous burst signal due to stimulated emission, the ongoing destruction of the agent results in the inability to detect any contrast effect. At a lower mechanical index (<0.4), continuous imaging of the blood pool containing contrast can be undertaken with substantially less bubble destruction (Fig. 4.10). This allows homogeneous detection of contrast effect in the blood pool and to a lesser degree in the ventricular myocardium.

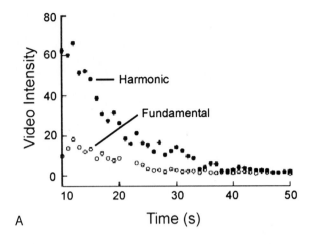

A

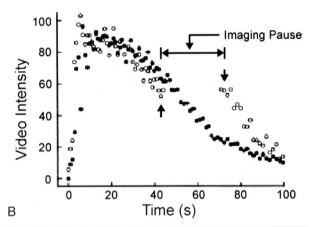

B

FIGURE 4.8. Graphic demonstration of the effect of the imaging method and duration on the detection of contrast. **Top:** The time intensity curve in an *in vitro* model of a steady-state concentration of contrast agent. Note that, with harmonic imaging, the intensity is substantially greater because of a higher intensity ultrasound transmission as well as more sensitive detection. **Bottom:** The impact of interrupted imaging is shown. The *dark circles* represent the time intensity curve of a steady-state concentration of contrast during continuous imaging. The *white dots* represent the contrast intensity with an imaging pause. Note that, during the pause in imaging, there is no further loss of contrast effect. When imaging is reinstituted, contrast intensity is at precisely the point that it was when imaging was paused, providing indirect evidence of bubble destruction by ultrasound. (From Wei K, et al. Interactions between microbubbles and ultrasound: *in vitro* and *in vivo* observations. J Am Coll Cardiol 1997;29:1081–1088, with permission.)

Other Mechanical Factors Affecting Contrast Detection

In addition to mechanical index, there are other machine settings that have an impact on detection of ultrasound contrast. In general, anything that increases delivery of the ultrasound energy to the contrast agent results in a greater degree of destruction and consequently a decrease

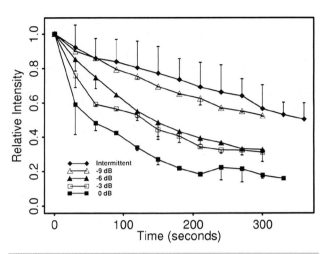

FIGURE 4.9. Impact of intermittent imaging and continuous imaging at four different ultrasound intensities in an *in vitro* model. Note the progressive decline in ultrasound contrast intensity with increasing ultrasound power from −9 to 0 dB. (From Villarraga HR, Foley DA, Aeschbacher BC, et al. Destruction of contrast microbubbles during ultrasound imaging at conventional power output. J Am Soc Echocardiogr 1997;10: 783–791, with permission.)

in the degree of contrast effect. As such, high frame rates will result in greater ultrasound contrast destruction than low frame rates. There can be selective destruction of contrast at the point at which a transmit focal zone has been set. Because of increased ultrasound energy at shallow imaging depths, the near field is more susceptible to contrast agent destruction than is the far field.

Doppler Imaging

Because bubbles interact with the ultrasound beam, they create a range of frequency shifts in the reflected beam that can be detected as a Doppler shift. These Doppler shifts are dependent not only on motion of the bubbles but also on their resonance in a stationary field. Within the Doppler domain, several different parameters can be used to detect and quantify the contrast effect. Both the Doppler shift itself and the power of the Doppler spectrum, which is directly related to the number of targets being interrogated, can be registered and quantified. One of the more promising methods for detection of contrast effects is the use of phase correlation techniques, in which an automatic correlation of the insonating and reflected frequencies is undertaken. Because microbubbles are nonlinear reflectors and result in variable Doppler shifts, the characteristics of reflected ultrasound from two sequential pulses will contain different reflected frequency spectra and frequency shifts. This nonlinear response is not seen after interaction with tissue where the characteristics of two sequential ultrasound pulses will be iden-

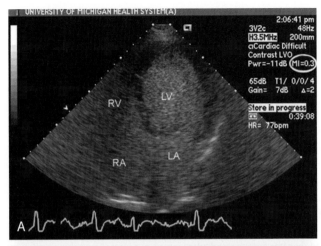

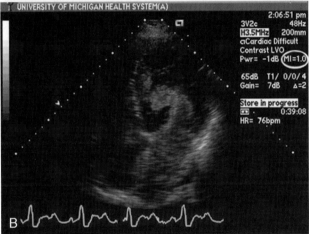

FIGURE 4.10. Apical four-chamber view recorded in a patient demonstrating the impact of mechanical index on contrast appearance. **Top:** Image was recorded with a mechanical index of 0.3 and reveals smooth opacification of all four cardiac chambers. **Bottom:** Image was recorded 10 seconds later with a mechanical index of 1.0. Note the complete lack of contrast in the near field and the swirling nature of the partial filling in the far field.

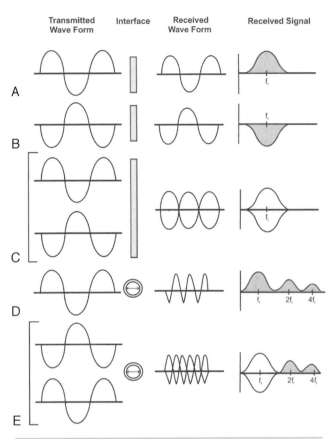

FIGURE 4.11. A simplified version of phase analysis is presented in which only sequential pulses 180 degrees out of phase are diagrammed. In reality, both phase and amplitude may be altered in the sequential pulses. **A:** A transmitted wave interacts with a linear reflector (*solid bar*). The received wave is identical in configuration to the transmitted wave but will have less amplitude because of attenuation. The received signal is centered on the transmit frequency (f_t). **B:** The identical frequency transmitted 180 degrees out of phase with that in **A. C:** The interaction of two sequential pulses each of which is 180 degrees out of phase with the other (A + B transmitted nearly simultaneously) is depicted. When received and summed, the waveform is as demonstrated and the received signal consists of identical positive and negative amplitudes that result in zero signal, as denoted by the absence of shading. **D:** The interaction of a transmitted wave with a microbubble is depicted. Because microbubbles contract and expand at different rates, they alter the contour of the transmitted wave. The received waveform has components of the fundamental frequency and harmonic frequencies at two and four times the transmit frequency. It is also altered in contour as noted. **E:** The interaction of two closely spaced pulses, 180 degrees out of phase (identical to the transmitted pulses in **C**), which then interact with a microbubble is represented. Because the two pulses interact in opposite manners with the microbubble, they result in a more complex received waveform. The fundamental frequencies are returned 180 degrees out of phase, and the harmonic signals are preserved. This results in a relatively contrast-specific signal.

tical. This methodology can be referred to as phase image analysis. For phase image analysis two ultrasound signals are sent out with close temporal proximity (Fig. 4.11). The second pulse is 180 degrees out of phase with the first pulse and may have a different amplitude. When the two reflected signals are then received, they are summed, and the summed ultrasound signal is then displayed. If each of these signals is reflected from a linear, nonharmonic reflector, such as tissue or blood, they are then received back at the transducer precisely 180 degrees out of phase (exactly as transmitted), and when summed, they cancel each other to create zero signal. Conversely, if the signals interact with microbubbles, each signal is shifted in phase. Additionally, because microbubbles compress and expand at different rates in the ultrasound field, the contour of the reflected signal is altered compared with the transmitted signal. When summed, cancellation no longer occurs, and a signal is preserved. In theory, this provides a highly specific methodology for the detection of ultrasound contrast. This type of analysis is typically performed using the harmonic frequencies and provides a highly contrast-specific signal.

CONTRAST ARTIFACTS

Appropriate and successful use of ultrasound contrast requires careful attention to technical detail and machine capabilities and imaging algorithms that often differ from those used for routine clinical scanning. Even with meticulous attention to detail, there are a number of pitfalls and artifacts that can diminish the clinical yield of contrast echocardiography. Contrast artifacts can be divided into two broad categories: those due to the agent and its interaction with the ultrasound beam and physiologic artifacts, both of which may interfere with interpretation (Table 4.2).

As contrast agents are very potent reflectors of ultrasound, they will result in nearly complete attenuation of ultrasound penetration if present in high concentration. This phenomenon is particularly prominent when using the newer, more highly reflective perfluorocarbon-based agents. Attenuation occurs when there is an abnormally high concentration of ultrasound targets in the near field, beyond which the ultrasound beam cannot penetrate (Figs. 4.12 and 4.13). This results in detection only of the initial layer of contrast-enhanced blood, with all areas of the heart behind this area being effectively shadowed. Attenuation is common during bolus injections of perfluorocarbon-based agents. It can be avoided by delaying scanning until later in the infusion protocol, after the peak contrast effect has declined, or preferably by the use of a smaller bolus or lower concentration of the ultrasound agent.

As noted previously, the intensity of the insonating ultrasound beam is directly related to the amount of microbubble destruction. Although the microbubbles generated by agitated saline are relatively resistant to the

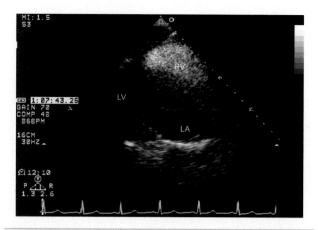

FIGURE 4.12. Parasternal long-axis view recorded immediately after injection of ultrasound contrast. Note the significant attenuation of ultrasound signal behind the dense bolus of contrast in the right ventricular outflow tract which precludes visualization of any posterior structures.

destruction of the ultrasound beam, the newer generation of perfluorocarbon-based agents can be exquisitely sensitive to ultrasound disruption. At a mechanical index used for typical anatomic imaging (0.9–1.4), microbubbles will be rapidly destroyed in the blood pool, resulting in a dramatic reduction in the ultrasound contrast. By reducing the transmit intensity to a mechanical index (0.3–0.6), this phenomenon is reduced and the ultrasound contrast effect is preserved (Fig. 4.10). Inadvertent imaging at an inappropriately high mechanical index results in the destruction of contrast, predominantly in the near field, and the appearance of a contrast defect in that region.

Another well-recognized artifact is that created by shadowing from a papillary muscle when imaging in the four-chamber view. The shadow created at the proximal boundary of the contrast with the papillary muscle extends toward the left atrium in a straight line. This shadow can be confused with the lateral endocardial border (Fig. 4.14).

Shadowing from a papillary muscle is not the only source of an artifactual, contrast-free region within the left ventricular cavity. If a patient has areas of dense fibrosis or calcification between the transducer and the blood pool, a shadow will occur behind the echoreflective focal area mimicking a contrast-free area. Figure 4.15 was recorded in a patient with a chronic apical aneurysm with areas of intramural calcification. Note the two separate areas of apparent lack of contrast effect that radiate down from the apex into the cavity of the blood pool. These are the result of shadowing from calcific deposits in an apical aneurysm.

Because the contrast agent interacts with ultrasound, irrespective of the analysis made, it has a profound impact on the appearance and validity of color Doppler flow

▶ TABLE 4.2 Contrast Artifacts

Agent/ultrasound related
Attenuation
Shadowing
Apical destruction
Physiologic
Competitive flow
SVC − IVC
Marginated flow
Eustachian valve

IVC, inferior vena cava; SVC, superior vena cava.

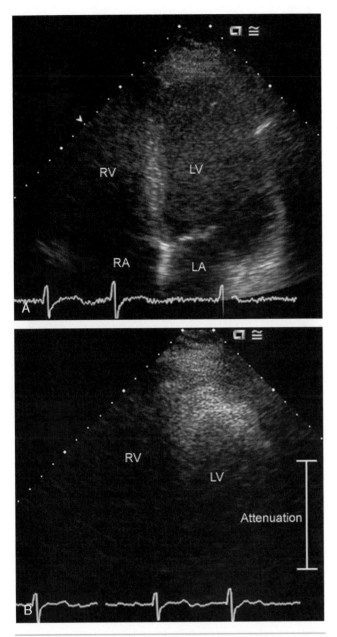

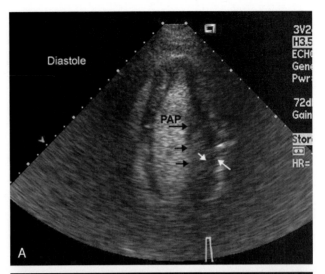

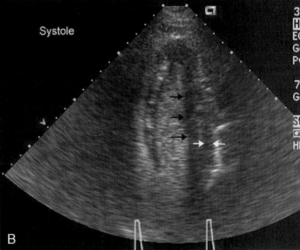

FIGURE 4.13. Apical four-chamber view recorded before **(top)** and after **(bottom)** intravenous injection of a perfluoro-carbon-based contrast agent demonstrating an excessive bolus effect at the apex of the left ventricle, resulting in attenuation and shadowing behind the apical third of the left ventricle.

FIGURE 4.14. Apical four-chamber view demonstrates a papillary muscle shadow. **Top:** Image was recorded in diastole. Note the location of the papillary muscle (*black arrows*) and the faint shadow behind it. Also note the true location and thickness of the lateral wall (*white arrows*). **Bottom:** Image was recorded in systole and demonstrates a more exaggerated papillary muscle shadow. Mistaking the papillary muscle shadow for the lateral wall will result in dramatic underestimation of the size of the left ventricle.

signals (Figs. 4.16 and 4.17). For this reason, if use of a contrast is anticipated, the operator should collect all required color Doppler images before using intravenous contrast. Imaging of even limited amounts of contrast markedly distorts the color Doppler signal and results in erroneous registration of data.

Physiologic artifacts include competitive flow and marginated flow. Because the contrast agent is contained within the bloodstream of the vessel into which it has been injected, its appearance will parallel that of the na-

tive vessel blood flow. If there is competing flow from another vessel that is not contrast enhanced, there will be a negative contrast effect created within the chamber. This is commonly seen after intravenous injection of saline contrast for evaluating an atrial septal defect (Fig. 4.18). In this instance, superior vena caval flow (assuming an arm injection) enters the right atrium as a homogeneous bolus that interacts with the non–contrast-enhanced flow from the inferior vena cava. This creates a swirling matrix of contrast and non–contrast-enhanced blood, which is

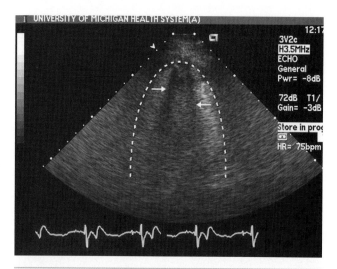

FIGURE 4.15. Apical four-chamber view recorded after intravenous injection of a perfluorocarbon-based contrast agent in a patient with an apical aneurysm and focal calcification in the apex. Note the two distinct shadows arising from the apex in the otherwise smooth homogeneous filling of the left ventricular cavity. The *dotted lines* represent the true cavity boundary.

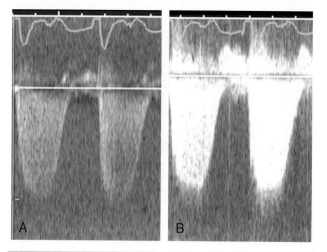

FIGURE 4.16. Continuous wave spectral recording of tricuspid regurgitation demonstrating the effect of contrast on signal intensity. Note the dramatic increase in spectral signal strength in the right-hand signals recorded after intravenous injection of a perfluorocarbon-based contrast agent compared with the baseline signal on the left.

often maximal along the interatrial septum. This effect may be accentuated in a high-flow state where there is greater than usual inferior *vena caval* flow such as chronic hepatic disease or pregnancy. On occasion, this effect has been confused with a pathologic shunt at the atrial level. Another similar phenomenon occurs when a prominent eustachian valve is present in the right atrium. This results in margination of superior vena caval flow in the atrium and may either mimic or mask the presence of an atrial shunt (Fig. 4.19).

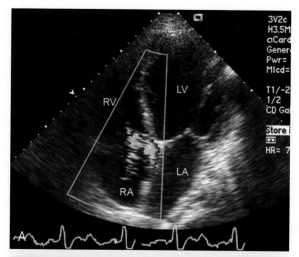

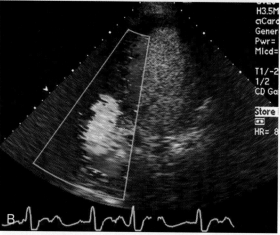

FIGURE 4.17. Apical four-chamber view recorded in a patient with mild tricuspid regurgitation before **(top)** and after **(bottom)** injection of a perfluorocarbon-based contrast agent. **Top:** Note the relatively disorganized tricuspid regurgitation jet consistent with mild regurgitation. **Bottom:** Note the dramatic increase in the size and intensity of the color flow signal jet when intracavitary contrast is present.

DETECTION AND UTILIZATION OF INTRACAVITARY CONTRAST

Detection of contrast in the cardiac chambers was the first clinical use of ultrasound contrast (Fig. 4.1). It remains a valuable adjunct to the clinical examination for detection of shunts and more recently for enhanced visualization of left ventricular wall motion. The new generation of perfluorocarbon-based microbubbles easily passes through the pulmonary circulation in quantities sufficient to fully opacify the left ventricular cavity. As noted previously, scrupulous attention to machine settings and technique is necessary to optimize contrast visualization for left ventricular opacification. Numerous studies have demonstrated the enhanced visualization of the left ventricular endocardial border after intravenous contrast in-

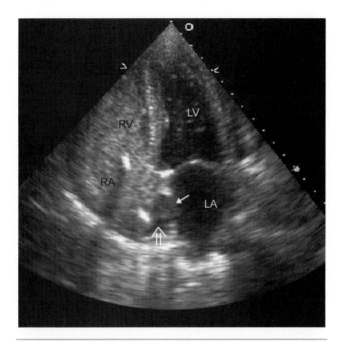

FIGURE 4.18. Apical four-chamber view recorded in a patient after injection of agitated saline into an upper extremity vein. Note the area of absent contrast effect (*large arrow*) along the most superior portion of the atrial septum, which is due to competitive flow from non–contrast-enhanced inferior vena caval blood flow. Such an area of absent contrast could be confused with a true negative contrast effect due to an atrial septal defect. This position of the atrial septum is noted by the *smaller arrow*.

jection and the ability to "salvage" echocardiograms that otherwise may have been suboptimal for diagnostic purposes.

Figures 4.20 through 4.22 represent examples of contrast echocardiograms in which a perfluorocarbon-based agent has been used to enhance endocardial definition. Opacification of the left ventricular cavity with the newer generation of contrast agents not only improves definition of the endocardial border but also has been demonstrated to improve reproducibility for both wall motion analysis and volumetric measurements (Fig. 4.23).

There are several limitations of this approach for edge definition including attenuation, shadowing, and apical destruction, which were noted previously and illustrated in previous figures. Selection of patients for left ventricular opacification should be based on the need for incremental information. When the full extent of the endocardial border is completely visualized, there is little incremental yield from the use of left ventricular contrast agents. Similarly, if the echocardiogram is technically limited to the point of nonvisualization of any of the cardiac structures, it is unlikely that an intravenous contrast agent will provide a fully diagnostic image. The maximal yield of contrast for left ventricular opacification appears to be in individuals in whom 20% to 60% of the endocardial border is suboptimally visualized at baseline.

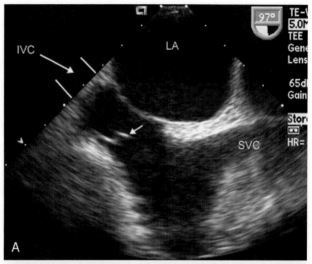

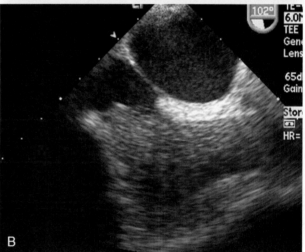

FIGURE 4.19. Transesophageal echocardiogram demonstrating a prominent eustachian valve and margination of contrast-enhanced blood flow. **Top:** Image was recorded before injection of contrast into an upper extremity vein. Note the prominent eustachian valve adjacent to the inferior vena cava (*arrow*). **Bottom:** Image was recorded after injection of contrast agent into an upper extremity vein. Note the appearance of contrast in the superior vena cava and the main portion of the right atrium but the absence of contrast in the area delineated by the eustachian valve. This absence of contrast could be confused with a negative contrast effect due to an atrial septal defect.

In addition to identifying the border of the left ventricular cavity for assessment of left ventricular chamber size and function, left ventricular contrast can be used for a number of other less common purposes including detection or exclusion of intracavitary thrombus, identification of unusual entities such as ventricular noncompaction, diagnosis of atypical forms of hypertrophic cardiomyopathy, and detecting abnormal communication to the ventricular chamber.

In marginal quality studies, one occasionally encounters an apparently hypokinetic or akinetic apex with

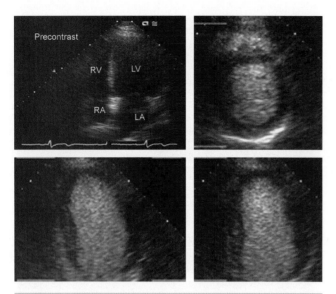

FIGURE 4.20. Example of left ventricular opacification after intravenous injection of a perfluorocarbon-based contrast agent. **Top left:** A baseline apical four-chamber view. Note the poor visualization of the apex and lateral wall. The other three panels were recorded after intravenous injection of a perfluorocarbon-based contrast agent. Note the excellent delineation of the left ventricular cavity, and (apical four-chamber view) the complete cavity opacification and the ability to fully identify the apex and lateral walls **(bottom left)**.

vague, ill-defined echoes that may suggest the presence of an apical thrombus. Use of high-frequency, short-focus transducers or color B-mode imaging can occasionally resolve the issue. An additional mechanism for confirming the presence or absence of left ventricular thrombus is to use contrast for left ventricular opacification. Once completely and homogeneously opacified, the true boundary of the left ventricle can be identified and a thrombus, if present, will appear as a filling defect (Fig. 4.24). Similarly, if there is complete filling of the ventricular apex, the source of the vague echo density is likely to be artifact (Fig. 4.25).

An additional entity that results in vague, confusing echoes in the left ventricle is ventricular noncompaction. This is a form of congenital cardiomyopathy in which the embryologic myocardium, which is naturally filled with sinusoidal spaces, does not "compact" into normally structured myocardium. This results in a network of sinusoids within the ventricular myocardium and is associated with a dilated cardiomyopathy. With routine two-dimensional scanning, one encounters vague, irregular thickening of the apical and lateral walls, although the distribution of noncompaction can be highly variable. The differential diagnosis of the echo appearance is that of complex thrombi versus ventricular noncompaction. Injection of intravenous contrast and opacification of the left ventricular cavity will allow identification of the multiple sinusoidal cavities within the apparently "spongy"

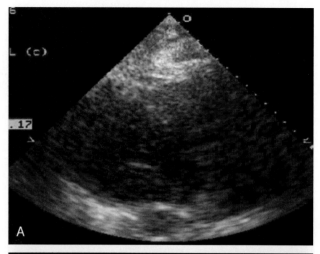

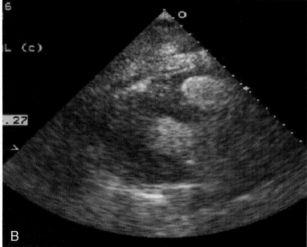

FIGURE 4.21. Parasternal long-axis echocardiogram recorded in a morbidly obese patient in an intensive care unit undergoing mechanical ventilation. **Top:** Image was recorded before injection of a perfluorocarbon-based contrast agent. Even in the real-time image, it is difficult to identify any cardiac structures. **Bottom:** Image was recorded after intravenous injection of a perfluorocarbon-based agent, also in a parasternal long-axis view. Note the excellent opacification of the right ventricular outflow tract and left ventricular cavity. In the real-time image, note the normal left ventricular size and systolic function.

myocardium, confirming the diagnosis of myocardial noncompaction (Fig. 4.26).

The apical variant of hypertrophic cardiomyopathy is occasionally missed on routine two-dimensional scanning. Because the hypertrophied muscle is of relatively low density and by definition in the near field when the heart is examined from an apical transducer position, the true thickness of the myocardium may not be appreciated. The ultrasound beam, especially if using low-frequency transducers, may "burn through" the apical myocardium leading to the impression that the epicardial boundary is the endocardial border. As for suspicious thrombus, use of

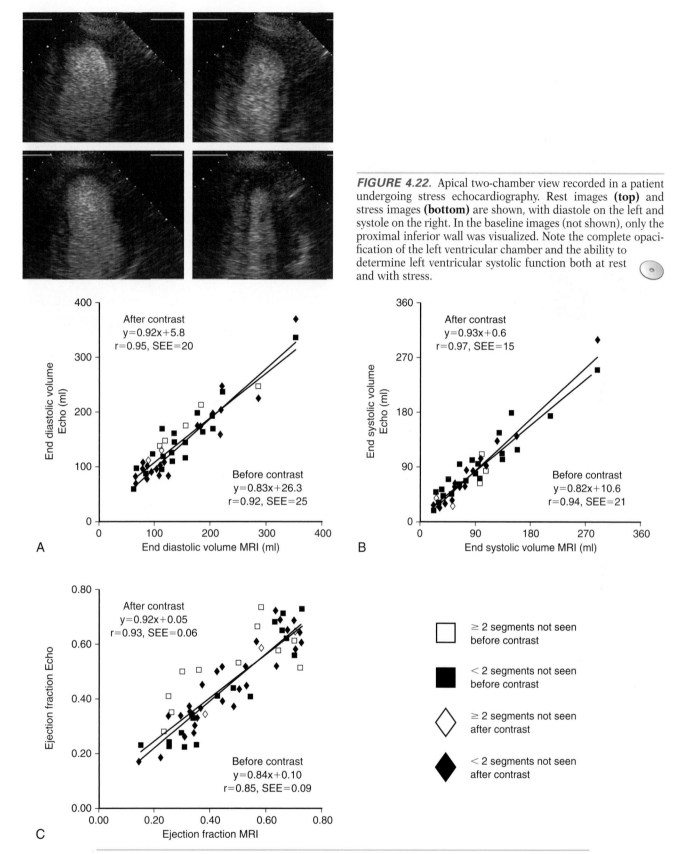

FIGURE 4.22. Apical two-chamber view recorded in a patient undergoing stress echocardiography. Rest images **(top)** and stress images **(bottom)** are shown, with diastole on the left and systole on the right. In the baseline images (not shown), only the proximal inferior wall was visualized. Note the complete opacification of the left ventricular chamber and the ability to determine left ventricular systolic function both at rest and with stress.

FIGURE 4.23. Graphic demonstration of the impact of left ventricular opacification by contrast echocardiography on diastolic and systolic volumes and left ventricular ejection fraction as compared with magnetic resonance imaging (MRI). As noted in the lower right of the figure, individual patients are distinguished based on the number of segments not clearly identified either before or after contrast. Note that for each measured parameter, there is an increase in the correlation with MRI after left ventricular opacification by contrast. (From Hundley WG, et al. Administration of an intravenous perfluorocarbon contrast agent improves echocardiographic determination of left ventricular volumes and ejection fraction: comparison with cine magnetic resonance imaging. J Am Coll Cardiol 1998;32:1426–1432, with permission.)

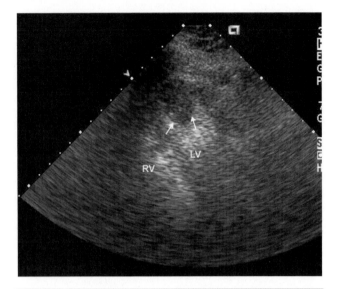

FIGURE 4.24. Apical view recorded in a patient with a vague echo density on noncontrast imaging. After intravenous injection of a perfluorocarbon-based agent, a distinct spherical filling defect is noted in the apex, consistent with a pedunculated apical thrombus (*arrows*).

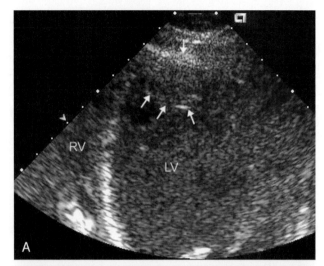

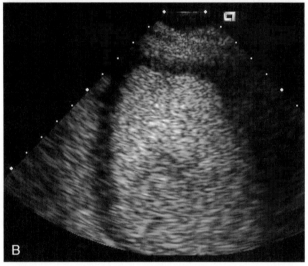

FIGURE 4.25. **Top:** Apical four-chamber view recorded in a patient with a dilated cardiomyopathy and a vague echo density in the left ventricular apex (*arrows*) noted on a non–contrast-enhanced image. Note the position of the anatomic apex (*downward-pointing arrow*). **Bottom:** Image was recorded after injection of a perfluorocarbon-based contrast agent and demonstrates complete opacification of the left ventricular cavity. Note that, with contrast, the entire left ventricular cavity is filled, confirming that the vague echo density in the apex was not a true mural thrombus.

high-frequency, short-focus length transducers, or B-mode color scanning may resolve this issue, as will scrupulous attention to technical detail. Left ventricular opacification with contrast is a very effective mechanism for identifying the true endocardial boundary in this situation and may allow confident establishment of this diagnosis in otherwise confusing instances (Fig. 4.27).

A final use of contrast for left ventricular opacification is in determining the nature of abnormal communications to the left ventricular cavity. Ventricular pseudoaneurysms can occasionally be difficult to visualize with respect to the orientation of the communication to the left ventricular cavity, and on occasion one identifies an extracardiac space, for which it is unclear whether there is a communication between the space and the left ventricular cavity. Occasionally, the issue can be resolved with color Doppler flow imaging. Use of contrast for left ventricular opacification can also be helpful in this situation (Fig. 4.28).

Spectral Doppler Enhancement

The interaction of ultrasound with contrast agents results in a substantially higher magnitude of Doppler signal than interaction with red blood cells or tissue structures. It is assumed that the frequency shift itself remains stable as a microbubble is insonated and that it is only the intensity (power or energy) of the reflected signal that is increased. Therefore, the frequency shift and calculated velocities will accurately reflect the physiologic state; however, the intensity of the signal will increase dramati-

cally. Low concentrations of contrast agents can be used to intensify Doppler signal strength in instances in which there is a suboptimal spectral signal. Excessive contrast effect will result in substantial noise in the signal and may be counterproductive. The first use of this was on the right side of the heart for enhancing the tricuspid regurgitation jet (Fig. 4.29). The new transpulmonary agents can provide a similar degree of enhancement for pulmonary vein flow (Fig. 4.30) or for increasing the spectral image intensity of a relatively weak aortic stenosis jet.

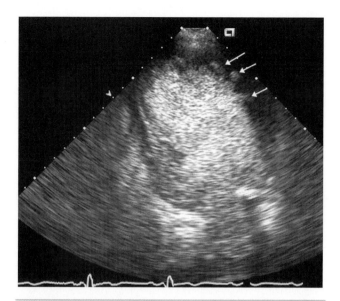

FIGURE 4.26. Contrast echocardiogram for left ventricular opacification (perfluorocarbon-based agent) recorded in a patient with a dilated cardiomyopathy and irregular thickening of the apical and lateral walls. After injection of contrast, note the contrast-filled areas within the thickened left ventricular wall, which represent sinusoids characteristic of ventricular noncompaction.

Because the ultrasound contrast agent interacts with all forms of Doppler imaging, caution should be exercised when color flow imaging is employed. The addition of even very low concentrations of ultrasound contrast to the blood pool results in a substantially greater color flow area than would be recorded without contrast present (Fig. 4.17). Because the color flow jet area is commonly used to estimate volumetric flow and regurgitation severity, the apparent increase in jet area caused by interaction with contrast will result in systematic overestimation of regurgitation severity.

Shunt Detection

Detection of right-to-left shunts was one of the earliest uses of contrast echocardiography and a use for which agitated saline remains the agent of choice because of its low cost, long safety record, and lack of need for contrast opacification of the left heart structures. When evaluating a patient for right-to-left shunt, an agent that appears in the left ventricle because of transpulmonary passage would not be appropriate. Right-to-left shunts that can be documented by intravenous injection of agitated saline include atrial septal defects of all types, patent foramen ovale, and pulmonary arteriovenous malformations. Larger ventricular septal defects may allow some right-to-left shunting during diastole when pressure in the two ventricles is relatively equal.

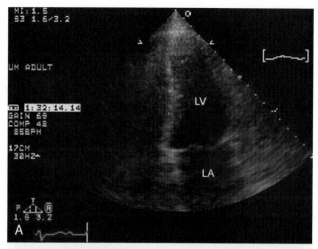

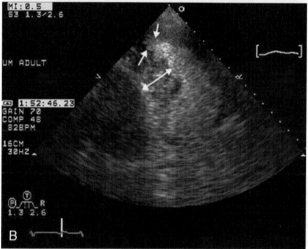

FIGURE 4.27. Apical two-chamber view recorded in a patient with ventricular arrhythmias. **Top:** Image was recorded before injection of intravenous contrast. **Bottom:** Image recorded after left ventricular opacification. **Top:** Note the poorly defined ventricular apex. **Bottom:** After opacification of the left ventricular cavity, note the fairly characteristic "spade-like" geometry of the left ventricular cavity and the ability to identify the marked hypertrophy of the inferior septum in this patient with an apical variant of hypertrophic cardiomyopathy.

Intravenous contrast injection of saline remains one of the primary diagnostic tools for detecting an atrial septal defect and, in smaller defects, may provide crucial information as to the presence of a potential shunt that is not directly visualized or has not resulted in a right ventricular volume overload (Fig. 4.31). The detection of a right-to-left shunt on contrast echo is indirect evidence of an atrial septal defect or a larger patent foramen ovale. When clinically indicated, additional studies such as transesophageal echocardiography may be appropriate. Typically, the right-to-left shunt of a large atrial septal defect may be nearly continuous, whereas for smaller atrial septal defects, the appearance of contrast in the left atrium

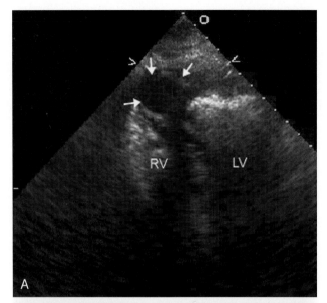

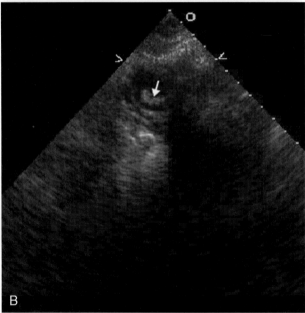

FIGURE 4.28. Off-axis apical view recorded in a patient with a small apical pseudoaneurysm. **Top:** Note the nearly spherical echo-free space at the left ventricular apex. Contrast has already opacified the body of the left and right ventricles. **Bottom:** Frame recorded one cardiac cycle later. Note the appearance of a small amount of contrast (*arrow*) within the cavity, confirming its communication with the left ventricular cavity.

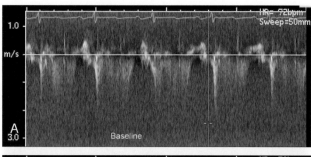

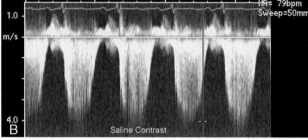

FIGURE 4.29. Contrast enhancement of a faint tricuspid regurgitation jet by agitated saline injected into an upper extremity vein. In the spectral images at the top, note the faint tricuspid regurgitation signal from which it is not possible to ascertain the complete spectral profile or maximal velocity. The spectral profiles at the bottom were recorded after enhancement of the jet with agitated saline. Note the substantially more robust signal and the ability to identify the maximal velocity with confidence.

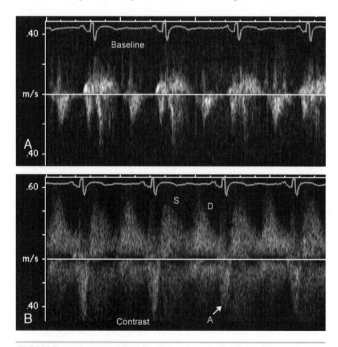

FIGURE 4.30. Example of enhancement of pulmonary vein spectral Doppler imaging with intravenous contrast. The spectral signals **(top)** were recorded from an apical view. Note the very poorly defined pulmonary vein inflow signal. **Bottom:** Image recorded in the same patient after injection of a perfluorocarbon-based intravenous agent demonstrates marked enhancement of the spectral signal of pulmonary vein flow. Note that both the systolic (*S*) and diastolic (*D*) antegrade flows as well as the retrograde A-wave flow (*A*) are clearly seen after contrast enhancement.

may be phasic, coordinated with the respiratory cycle. During inspiration, right heart filling increases, thus increasing the flow of contrast into the right atrium and the likelihood and magnitude of right-to-left shunting also increases. On occasion, an atrial septal defect will be associated almost exclusively with a left-to-right shunt. In these instances, evaluating the appearance of contrast in the right atrium along the atrial septum may allow detec-

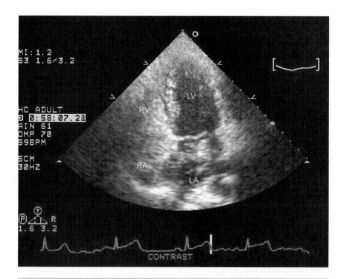

FIGURE 4.31. Apical four-chamber view recorded in a patient with an atrial septal defect after intravenous injection of contrast agent. Note the opacification of the right atrium and the right ventricle and the significant amount of contrast appearing in the left atrium, consistent with a right-to-left shunt at the atrium level, subsequently confirmed to be a secundum atrial defect.

tion of a negative contrast effect (Fig. 4.32). The negative contrast effect occurs when non–contrast-enhanced blood from the left atrium flows across the atrial septal defect into the right atrium, displacing contrast-enhanced blood.

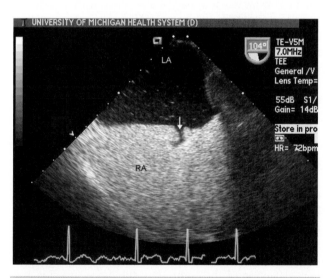

FIGURE 4.32. Transesophageal echocardiogram recorded in a longitudinal view concentrating on the atrial septum. Agitated saline has been injected into an upper extremity vein and has completely filled the right atrium. Note a small number of individual contrast targets in the left atrium consistent with a limited right-to-left shunt. Also note the small negative contrast effect (*arrow*) arising from the atrial septum and projecting into the contrast-enhanced right atrium. This effect occurs due to flow of non–contrast-enhanced blood from the left atrium through a small (4 mm) secundum atrial septal defect into the contrast-filled right atrium.

Caution is advised when making this analysis because there will naturally be non–contrast-enhanced blood flowing from the inferior vena cava that should not be confused with a negative jet arising in the left atrium (Fig. 4.18). Because inferior vena caval flow is directed more toward the atrial septum than is superior vena caval flow, injection of contrast into a lower extremity vein may increase the likelihood of detecting a right-to-left shunt.

A patent foramen ovale can be reliably detected with contrast echocardiography, again using agitated saline (Fig. 4.33). A patent foramen ovale represents an unsealed overlap of the foraminal valve with the more basal portion of the atrial septum. Variations of patent foramen include small fenestrations, which may be multiple. Atrial septal aneurysms are often associated with one or more small perforations (Fig. 4.34). Because left atrial pressure typically exceeds right atrial pressure, only a small and hemodynamically inconsequential left-to-right shunt is typically present in patients with patent foramen ovale. The magnitude of this shunt is below that which can be documented with oximetry or dye dilution techniques. Additionally, the shunt is often phasic with the respiratory cycle. Maneuvers such as Valsalva and cough, which transiently increase right heart pressure, may allow the occult right-to-left shunt component of a patent foramen ovale to become manifest with contrast echocardiography. Patients are best evaluated for a patent foramen ovale in the apical four-chamber or subcostal view with one or more contrast injections performed during quiet respiration, cough, and Valsalva. Using this fairly vigorous approach, 30% to 40% of individuals with otherwise structurally normal hearts may be demonstrated to have

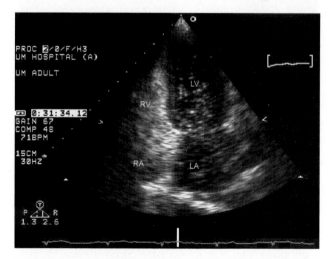

FIGURE 4.33. Apical four-chamber view recorded in a 30-year-old patient with a recent neurologic event. Agitated saline has been injected into an upper extremity vein and has opacified the right atrium and right ventricle. A small amount of contrast is seen in the left atrium and left ventricle consistent with a patent foramen ovale with right-to-left shunting.

trivial degrees of right-to-left shunting through a patent foramen ovale. Data are accumulating that show that it is only those patients with a larger patent foramen ovale, with more substantial degrees of right-to-left shunting, who are at risk of cardioembolic disease.

A prominent eustachian valve may result in a negative contrast effect within the right atrium, leading to the false impression that a defect with left-to-right shunting is present (Fig. 4.19). Because the eustachian valve marginates flow in the right atrium, it may result in only inferior vena caval blood flow (i.e., not contrast enhanced if the injection is into an upper extremity view) coming in contact with the atrial septum in the area of an atrial septal defect or patent foramen ovale. This may result in a false-negative evaluation for right-to-left shunting. When essential, injection of a contrast agent into a lower extremity vein will circumvent this problem.

A final right-to-left shunt that can be detected by contrast echocardiography is the pulmonary arteriovenous malformation (AVM). This can be seen in the presence of end-stage liver disease but also occur as part of several medical syndromes. The classic contrast echocardiographic appearance of an AVM is that of a delayed right-to-left shunt in which contrast appears in the left atrium after a delay of five to 15 cardiac cycles (Fig. 4.35). This typically represents the time required for a transit of the contrast agent through the pulmonary arterial bed and the AVM, and into the pulmonary veins. On occasion, a large AVM may result in more rapid appearance of contrast in the left heart. Other characteristics of a pulmonary AVM include the tendency of the contrast to build up persistently and slowly over time in the left heart and the lack of phasic appearance of contrast in the left atrium, which is more characteristic of an atrial level shunt. In the presence of larger or multiple AVMs, the magnitude of the right-to-left shunt can be substantial and may be associated with hypoxia. In these larger shunts, it is common to see contrast intensity continue to build in the left atrium and left ventricle at a time when it is diminishing in the right heart. This pattern of contrast appearance is virtually pathognomonic of an AVM. Finally, direct inspection of pulmonary veins can often identify contrast targets in the pulmonary veins and thereby establish the diagnosis as well (Fig. 4.36).

DETECTION OF MISCELLANEOUS CONDITIONS

Occasionally contrast echocardiography, typically using intravenous agitated saline, is useful for delineating abnormal extracardiac communications. Injection of agitated saline into a lower extremity vein in an individual with azygous continuation of the inferior vena cava allows detection of the contrast in the more superior portion of the right atrium, confirming the presence of this congenital anomaly. A more common scenario is to identify a patient with a dilated coronary sinus, typically best visualized in a parasternal long-axis view (Fig. 4.37). The differential diagnosis of a dilated coronary sinus includes chronic elevation of right heart pressure due to chronic volume or pressure overload and persistence of a left superior vena cava with drainage directly into the coronary

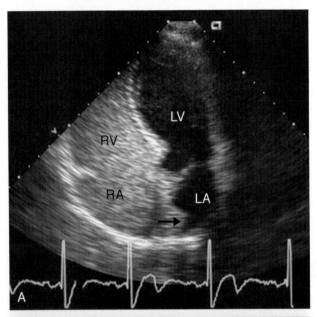

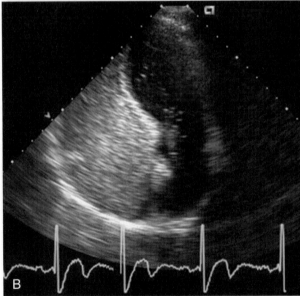

FIGURE 4.34. Apical four-chamber view recorded in a patient with an atrial septal aneurysm after intravenous injection of agitated saline. **Top:** Note the complete opacification of the right atrium and right ventricle and the bulging of the atrial septal aneurysm (*arrow*) into the left atrium. **Bottom:** Image was recorded later in the same cardiac cycle and demonstrates a small amount of contrast in the left atrium consistent with an associated patent foramen ovale.

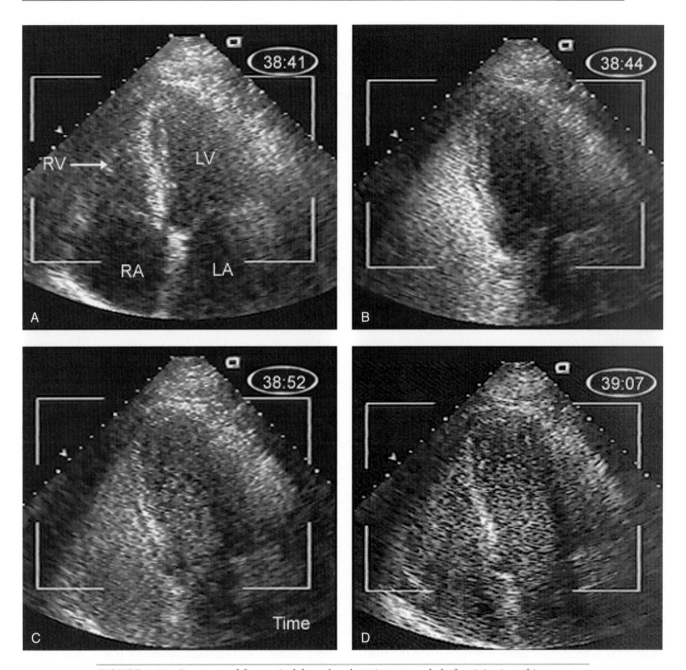

FIGURE 4.35. Sequence of four apical four-chamber views recorded after injection of intravenous contrast agent into an upper extremity vein in a patient with end-stage liver disease and a pulmonary arteriovenous malformation (AVM). **Top left:** Image was recorded before injection of contrast. **Top right:** Image was recorded after opacification of the right heart by contrast. **Bottom left:** Image was recorded 8 seconds after the appearance of contrast and shows continuous contrast appearance in the left heart. **Bottom right:** Image was recorded 23 seconds after the initial appearance of contrast in the right heart and shows contrast intensity in the left heart equivalent to that in the right heart. Both the delayed appearance of contrast and the buildup of contrast in the left heart as it is clearing from the right heart are characteristic of a pulmonary AVM.

sinus. The later anomaly can be documented by injecting agitated saline into a left upper extremity vein after which it will opacify the dilated coronary sinus before draining into the right atrium (Fig. 4.37).

MYOCARDIAL PERFUSION CONTRAST

Detection and quantitation of myocardial perfusion have been a goal of echocardiography since the ability to

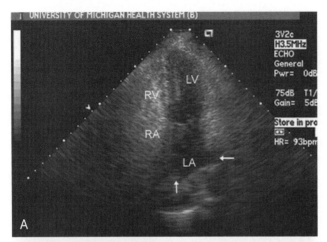

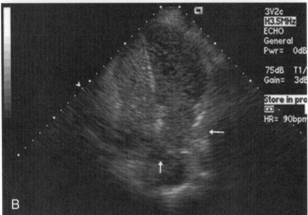

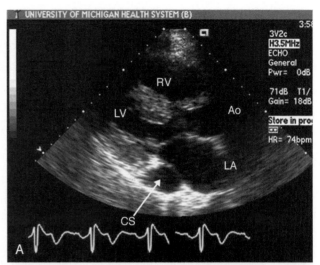

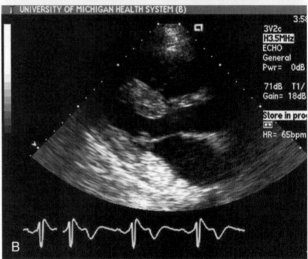

FIGURE 4.36. Apical four-chamber view recorded in a patient with a pulmonary arteriovenous malformation. **Top:** Saline contrast has been injected and has fully opacified the right atrium and right ventricle. Note a small amount of contrast in a right pulmonary vein (*upward-pointing arrow*) and the absence of contrast in the left pulmonary vein (*horizontal arrow*). **Bottom:** Image was recorded several seconds later and shows significant buildup of contrast in the left atrium and left ventricle as well as definite contrast in both visualized pulmonary veins.

FIGURE 4.37. **Top:** Parasternal long-axis view recorded in a healthy young patient. In the parasternal long-axis view, note the dilated circular structure bordered by the mitral anulus and left atrium. This structure has a relatively thin wall and represents dilated coronary sinus. **Bottom:** Image was recorded after injection of agitated saline into a left upper extremity vein and reveals prompt opacification of this structure before the appearance in the right ventricle, confirming that it represents a persistent left superior vena cava connecting directly to the coronary sinus. In the real-time image, note the early appearance of contrast in the right ventricle as well.

opacify the myocardium was first recognized in the 1980s. Early animal laboratory work confirmed that contrast distribution paralleled myocardial blood flow and furthermore confirmed that the absence of a contrast effect in the presence of a coronary stenosis accurately reflected the ultimate size of a myocardial infarction in an animal model of coronary occlusion (Fig. 4.38). Subsequent work demonstrated that the newer contrast agents could be used to identify coronary collateral circulation and that a preserved contrast effect in the myocardium was evidence of microvascular integrity and blood flow to the area (Fig. 4.39). The presence of microvascular blood flow was shown to correlate with recovery of function after myocardial infarction (Fig. 4.40).

The contrast effect can be seen in the cavity and as a fainter effect within the myocardium. It also can be di-

rectly visualized in either epicardial or intramural coronary arteries (Fig. 4.41). When there is evidence of contrast perfusing the intramural coronary arteries, this is excellent evidence of their patency. This finding has been correlated with the presence of a patent epicardial artery after coronary intervention. Contrast within these intramural arteries can also be used to enhance Doppler flow signals.

These observations were an "all-or-none phenomenon" based on the injection of an ultrasound contrast agent into a coronary artery or the aortic root. Similar observa-

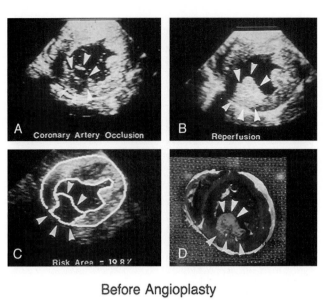

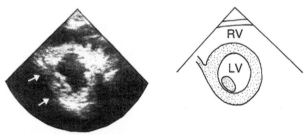

Before Angioplasty

After Angioplasty

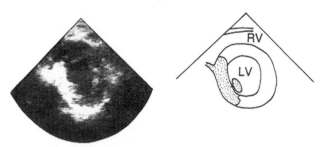

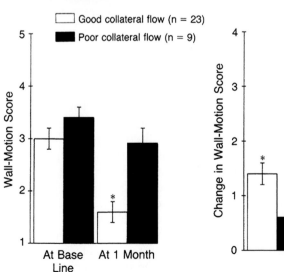

FIGURE 4.38. Contrast echocardiogram demonstrates myocardial contrast effect in an animal model of acute myocardial infarction. **Top left:** A short-axis image immediately after occlusion of a coronary artery. Note the opacification of the majority of the myocardium and the absence of contrast effect in the posterior wall (*arrowheads*). **Top right:** Image was recorded immediately after release of the coronary occlusion (brief occlusion) and demonstrates hyperemic flow in the previously occluded zone. Note the dramatic increase in contrast intensity in the previously occluded zone compared with the contrast intensity in the remaining myocardium. **Bottom left:** Image was recorded in the chronic phase of coronary occlusion and again demonstrates a distinct contrast-free zone in the posterior wall. **Bottom right:** The corresponding anatomic specimen shows excellent correlation between the anatomic location and extent of myocardial infarction and that predicted by absence of flow with contrast echocardiography.

FIGURE 4.39. Contrast echocardiograms recorded after intracoronary injection of a contrast agent in a patient with acute inferior wall myocardial infarction and good collateral flow to the infarct territory. **Top:** Image was recorded after injection of contrast into the left coronary artery in a patient with a totally occluded right coronary artery. Note the robust opacification of the left anterior descending and circumflex coronary artery territories and the definite contrast effect in the distribution of the right coronary artery. This pattern is consistent with occlusion of the right coronary artery with good collateral flow protecting that region. **Bottom:** Image was recorded after reperfusion of the right coronary territory by angioplasty. Injection of the right coronary artery demonstrates a robust contrast effect in the inferior wall. (From Sabia PJ, et al. An association between collateral blood flow and myocardial viability in patients with recent myocardial infarction. N Engl J Med 1992;327:1825–1831, with permission.)

FIGURE 4.40. Graphic representation of the impact of collateral flow in the setting of acute myocardial infarction. The graph on the left depicts the wall motion score at baseline and at 1 month in patients with either good or poor collateral flow. Note the equivalent wall motion scores at baseline and the dramatic improvement in systolic wall motion seen at 1 month in those patients with good collateral flow. The bar graph on the right depicts the change wall motion score from baseline to 1 month based on good or poor collateral flow. (From Sabia PJ, et al. An association between collateral blood flow and myocardial viability in patients with recent myocardial infarction. N Engl J Med 1992;327:1825–1831, with permission.)

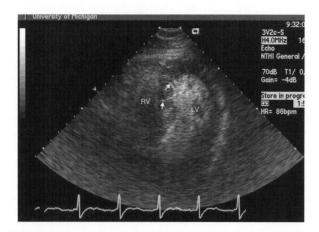

FIGURE 4.41. Apical two-dimensional echocardiogram recorded after injection of a perfluorocarbon-based contrast agent. Note the opacification of intramural vessels within the ventricular septum (*small arrows*).

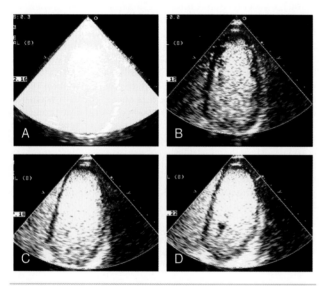

FIGURE 4.42. Apical four-chamber view recorded after intravenous injection of a perfluorocarbon-based contrast agent for the purpose of myocardial perfusion echocardiography. **Top left:** Image was recorded at the time of a high mechanical index "burst." **Top right:** Image was recorded immediately after the burst and demonstrates the diminished contrast effect both in the cavity and especially in the ventricular myocardium. **Bottom left:** Frame was recorded four cardiac cycles later and demonstrates restitution of contrast effect in the left ventricular cavity and a faint contrast effect developing within the ventricular myocardium. **Bottom right:** Frame was recorded 10 cardiac cycles after the burst and demonstrates further opacification of the left ventricular myocardium.

tions were subsequently made after intravenous injection of the newer generation of microbubbles. When assessing only the presence or absence of contrast within the myocardium, the time of appearance is of less importance than if one is attempting to identify lesser degrees of flow reduction. Detailed analysis of myocardial flow characteristics requires different imaging methodology than does

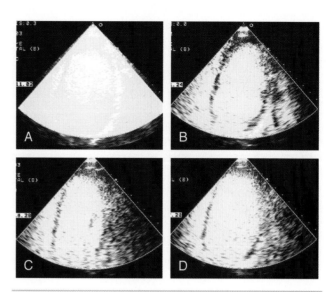

FIGURE 4.43. Apical four-chamber view recorded in the same patient depicted in Figure 4.42 at the time of hyperemia due to dipyridamole infusion. The format and timing are identical to those for Figure 4.42. In the presence of a hyperemic state, note the increase in the contrast effect in the ventricular myocardium and the more rapid development of significant contrast effect in the ventricular myocardium.

the simple detection of contrast within the myocardium. To create a time of appearance curve requires a bolus effect in the coronary circulation, which can be obtained in several ways. After intravenous injection of a contrast agent, the microbubbles will appear first on the right side of the heart, then in the left heart, and last in the aorta, the coronary arteries, and myocardial capillaries. Thus, a single intravenous injection results in the ability to record a single time appearance curve in the myocardium. For detailed evaluation, multiple time appearance curve analyses are necessary, often targeted to different regions of interest or performed under basal conditions and after vasodilator stress. Obviously, in view of the persistence of the newer contrast agents, one would need to wait 10 minutes or more before repeating an intravenous injection to obtain a second bolus. An alternate strategy for obtaining multiple bolus effects is to rely on purposeful destruction of the contrast agent. This can be accomplished by delivering a burst of high-intensity (high mechanical index) ultrasound to the image field (Figs. 4.42 and 4.43). This has the effect of destroying contrast that is present in relatively low concentration in the myocardium and reducing the contrast intensity in the myocardium to near zero. Imaging is then continued either in a continuous or intermittent format while myocardial replenishment occurs, from which a time intensity curve can be generated. If ultrasound contrast is present in the bloodstream at a steady-state concentration, this technique allows the creation of multiple "pseudo-boluses" for the evaluation of different regions of interest from different views or of repeated analysis under basal and stress conditions.

Analysis of myocardial perfusion with ultrasound contrast requires specific acquisition algorithms. As mentioned previously, interaction of the high-intensity ultrasound with a contrast agent results in bubble destruction and lack of contrast effect; therefore, if one wishes to detect contrast within the myocardium, standard imaging algorithms will be counterproductive. The two commonly used methods for detecting contrast, without resulting in counterproductive destruction, are continuous low mechanical index imaging and intermittent triggered imaging. Either of these methods may be used with any of the ultrasound domains including B-mode imaging, harmonic or ultraharmonic imaging, power Doppler imaging, and phase correlation techniques. Continuous low mechanical index imaging is the easiest to understand because it provides continuous imaging of all targeted cardiac structures with real-time visualization of wall motion, ventricular function, and myocardial thickening simultaneously with the ability to observe contrast flow into the myocardium (Figs. 4.42 and 4.43). Note in the real-time images for Figures 4.42 and 4.43 the instantaneous burst that represents purposeful destruction of ultrasound contrast, followed by the progressive appearance of contrast within the myocardium. This imaging format allows simultaneous evaluation of left ventricular systolic function and regional wall motion. If this method for myocardial contrast analysis is used, generation of a curve can be undertaken either by continuous frame-by-frame analysis within regions of interest or by analyzing only a fixed time point with reference to the electrocardiogram in sequential images after the burst. The advantage of analyzing intensity only at one time point at each cardiac cycle is that it typically results in less motion artifact and hence a smoother appearance curve.

A second method for detecting contrast in the myocardium without its destruction is to use intermittent triggered imaging. As mentioned previously, continuous high mechanical index imaging results in continuous destruction of microbubbles. By imaging only intermittently, time is allowed for replenishment of the ultrasound contrast agent within the myocardium, and, hence, it can be detected with each subsequent ultrasound pulse. Intermittent imaging capitalizes on this phenomenon by imaging, triggered to the QRS, at progressively longer intervals. If one images with each cardiac cycle, there is fairly continuous destruction of ultrasound in the myocardium and little time for contrast replenishment in the myocardium. As such, only a faint amount of contrast is detected. If the imaging interval is doubled, there will be twice as much time for replenishment, and, hence, each subsequent pulse detects twice the contrast effect. Similarly, if the triggering interval is increased further to 1:4, 1:8, 1:16, and so on, then progressively longer periods of time will be provided for replenishment. With progressively longer triggering intervals, a greater myocardial

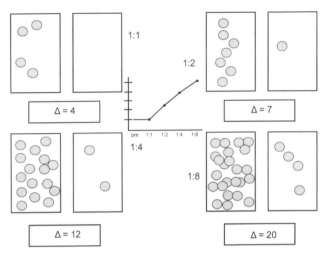

FIGURE 4.44. Graphic demonstration of the intermittent imaging technique for creating a time intensity curve. Four pairs of images are presented. For each, the schematic on the left represents the amount of contrast before imaging and on the right the amount of contrast after contrast imaging. In each instance, there is a decrease in the amount of contrast due to interaction with the ultrasound beam. **Top left:** Imaging is occurring with each cardiac cycle, which allows little time for replenishment of contrast within the target zone. As such, a relatively small amount of contrast is detected with each imaging pulse, and all contrast is destroyed by the subsequent imaging pulse. **Top right:** This example (ratio of 1:2) depicts the effect of imaging every other cardiac cycle. This allows for a greater degree of replenishment of contrast within the target zone, not all of which is destroyed by the ultrasound beam. **Bottom:** Imaging at ratios of 1:4 and 1:8, which allow for progressively greater amounts of contrast replenishment and hence a greater contrast image intensity is shown. These results are presented graphically in the center.

contrast intensity will be noted (Fig. 4.44). Although not allowing a simultaneous assessment of function and flow, triggered imaging may provide a more visibly obvious contrast effect. With either technique, one or more regions of interest can be drawn in the myocardium and the intensity of contrast tracked either continuously or at each level of sequential imaging. Either method results in an appearance curve demonstrating a baseline low level of myocardial contrast effect, a slope of appearance, and a plateau phase from which various parameters can be extracted that directly relate to myocardial blood volume and flow (Fig. 4.45).

It has now been well established that the intensity of contrast in the myocardium is directly related to myocardial blood volume and not coronary blood flow. The flow rate is related to the slope of appearance. As with any indicator technique, a contrast time appearance curve can be generated and multiple parameters of such a curve can be correlated with myocardial perfusion. Recording accurate myocardial contrast perfusion curves requires specialized ultrasound instrumentation for registration and

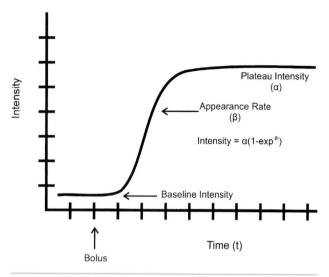

FIGURE 4.45. Stylized time appearance curve of contrast within the ventricular myocardium depicting the different parameters of a contrast appearance curve. (See text for details.)

analysis of contrast effect, as noted in previous sections of this chapter. Once curves are generated, either by continuous low mechanical index imaging or intermittent imaging, analysis can be undertaken for determination of myocardial blood volume and flow. Figures 4.45 and 4.46 schematize stylized contrast echo appearance curves and the different characteristics of the curve that can be related to coronary blood flow. The two most important features of the curve are α, which is the intensity at which the contrast effect plateaus, and β, which is the time constant of contrast appearance. α is directly related to myocardial blood volume, whereas β is related to flow rate. The product of α and β (α × β) is directly proportional to myocardial blood flow. Under basal conditions, all areas of ventricular myocardium have roughly equivalent contrast intensity. Because of far-field attenuation and shadowing, the apparent contrast effect may be less in the more basal portions of the heart depending on the imaging plane. Subtraction techniques may assist in demonstrating the contrast effect in these areas. In the absence of a significant coronary stenosis, infusion of a vasodilator increases the flow rate (β), whereas the absolute myocardial blood volume as reflected by α does not change significantly. In the presence of a total coronary occlusion, there will be a diminished or absent contrast effect. Generally speaking, a coronary stenosis of less than 90% is not flow restrictive at rest and results in normal contrast appearance kinetics under basal conditions. The addition of a vasodilator such as dipyridamole or adenosine results in an increase in flow velocity only in those areas not perfused by a stenosed artery, and the appearance of the contrast curves will therefore differ in the normal and diseased beds. By comparing characteristics of the flow curve including α, β, and their product, which is directly related to myocardial blood flow volume, a hyperemic ra-

tio can be calculated by comparison of basal and vasodilator contrast injections. Figure 4.46 outlines stylized contrast appearance curves in normal arteries and with various degrees of coronary obstruction.

Although not yet (2004) approved by the U.S. Food and Drug Administration for this purpose, several clinical studies have demonstrated the technical feasibility of using myocardial perfusion contrast echo to identify areas

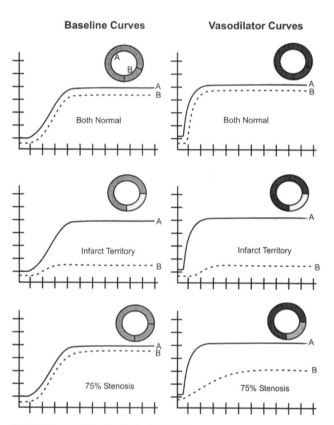

FIGURE 4.46. Stylized time appearance curves depict normal coronary flow and different disease states. The curves on the left are all depictions of baseline appearance curves and those on the right are the anticipated appearance curves at the time of vasodilator stress. Two separate coronary territories representing a normal reference area (*A*) and an area of coronary obstruction (*B*) are depicted as *solid lines* and *dotted lines*, respectively. **Top:** In the two graphs, both territories A and B are normal and have virtually identical contrast appearance curves. Note that during vasodilation, both curves have a plateau (α) equivalent to that seen at baseline, but the rate of increase of contrast effect (β) is substantially steeper. **Middle:** The appearance curves in the presence of a total coronary occlusion and myocardial infarction in area B are depicted. Note that curve A is identical to that at baseline but that curve B has a substantially blunted contrast effect. After vasodilatation, there is no change in curve B and curve A behaves as a normal flow territory. **Bottom:** The impact of a significant coronary stenosis in area B is shown. After vasodilatation, territory A has an increased rate of appearance, whereas both the rate of appearance and plateau contrast intensity for area B are significantly diminished compared with baseline.

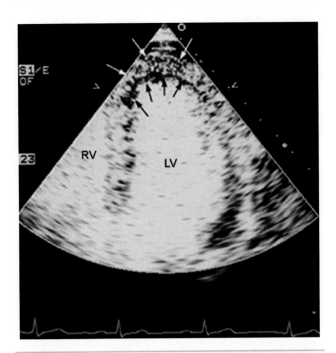

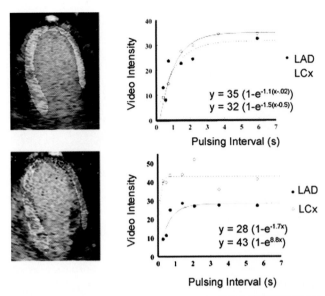

FIGURE 4.47. Myocardial contrast echocardiogram performed using a continuous infusion in continuous low mechanical index imaging. This frame was recorded approximately 20 cardiac cycles after the burst phase (Fig. 4.40) and reveals the absence of contrast effect in the left ventricular apex and a robust myocardial contrast effect in the remaining walls. This patient was subsequently demonstrated to have a total occlusion of the distal left anterior descending coronary artery.

FIGURE 4.49. Myocardial contrast echocardiogram recorded in a patient with a significant left anterior descending coronary obstruction. **Top:** Image was recorded under basal conditions. **Bottom:** Image recorded after vasodilatation. Note the equivalent opacification and time appearance curves of the two coronary territories under basal conditions. **Bottom:** Images were recorded with a vasodilator and reveal diminished contrast effect in the lateral wall on the myocardial contrast image. Note the increase in β with only a slight increase in α in the circumflex territory and the decreased α and β values in the obstructed left anterior descending territory. Note that these curves are similar to those schematized for the coronary stenosis example depicted in Figure 4.46 (bottom). (From Wei K, et al. Noninvasive quantification of coronary blood flow reserve in humans using myocardial contrast echocardiography. Circulation 2001;103: 2560–2565, with permission.)

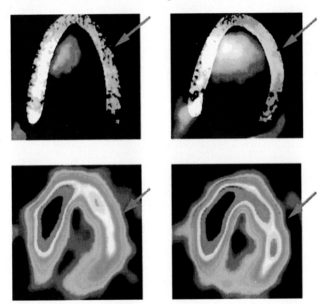

FIGURE 4.48. Example of a partially reversible defect in the lateral wall (*arrows*) in an apical four-chamber view on myocardial contrast echocardiography **(top)** and single-photon emission computed tomography **(bottom)**. The post-dipyridamole images are on the left and the baseline images are on the right. The lateral defect in the postdipyridamole images (left) is partially resolved in the baseline images (right). (From Kaul S, et al. Detection of coronary artery disease with myocardial contrast echocardiography: comparison with 99mTc-sestamibi single-photon emission computed tomography. Circulation 1997;96: 785–792, with permission.)

of nonperfused myocardium when compared with thallium scintigraphy or known coronary artery anatomy (Figs. 4.47 and 4.48) or to provide data regarding relative flow in coronary territories (Fig. 4.49). It should be emphasized that, although myocardial contrast perfusion echocardiography has shown tremendous promise and has demonstrable accuracy in rigorously controlled animal experiments, its ability to detect coronary stenoses in a wide range of patients is still undergoing validation.

A final use of myocardial contrast echocardiography is in monitoring transcatheter alcohol septal ablation performed for treatment of obstructive hypertrophic cardiomyopathy. This is a newly developed interventional technique in which a catheter is placed, typically in the first septal perforator of the left anterior descending coronary artery. Alcohol is then injected to create a controlled myocardial infarction for reduction of the proximal septal mass. This has the effect of reducing the magnitude of a dynamic left ventricular outflow tract obstruction and has shown tremendous promise for nonoperative treatment of patients with obstructive hypertrophic cardiomyopathy. The goal of this therapy is

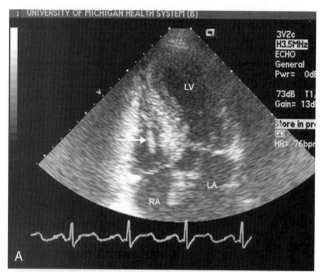

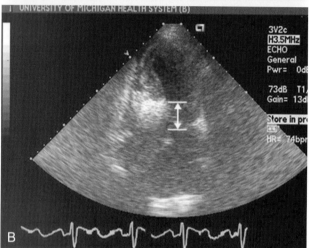

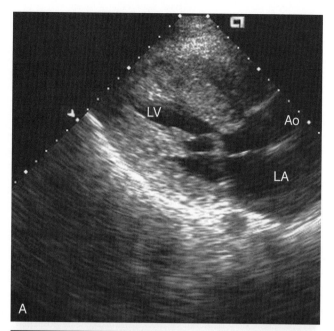

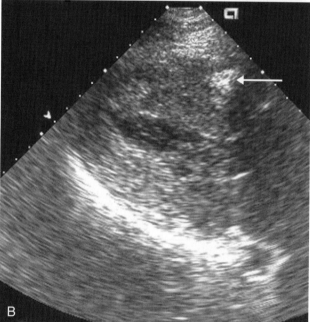

FIGURE 4.50. Apical four-chamber view recorded in a patient with a hypertrophic cardiomyopathy undergoing alcohol septal reduction therapy. **Top:** Image recorded under basal conditions. There is a pacemaker catheter in the right ventricle (*arrow*) and systolic anterior motion of the mitral valve. Note the marked hypertrophy of the ventricular septum. **Bottom:** Image was recorded after injection of a diluted perfluorocarbon-based contrast agent into a septal perforator artery in the cardiac catheterization laboratory. Note the distinct contrast in the proximal ventricular septum maximum at the area of mitral valve contact with the septum in systole. This patient subsequently underwent successful reduction therapy for treatment of hypertrophic cardiomyopathy.

FIGURE 4.51. Parasternal long-axis view recorded in a patient with hypertrophic cardiomyopathy being considered for alcohol septal reduction therapy. **Top:** Image was recorded at baseline. Note the hypertrophy of the ventricular septum and the systolic anterior motion of the mitral valve. **Bottom:** Image was recorded after injection of a diluted perfluorocarbon-based contrast agent into a septal perforator artery. Note the absence of contrast effect in the ventricular septum but the appearance of contrast in the right and left ventricular cavity and the marked contrast effect in right ventricular muscle trabeculae (*arrow*) **(bottom).** This patient was not considered a candidate for alcohol septal reduction therapy and the procedure was not performed.

controlled septal mass reduction. Contrast echocardiography, with the agent injected directly into the septal perforator, plays a major role in determining the feasibility of the procedure and in following its progress (Figs. 4.50–4.51). Before injection of ethanol, dilute ultrasound contrast agent is injected into the selected artery. This serves two purposes. The first is to ensure that there is no significant reflux of the contrast into the body of the left anterior coronary descending artery or into the bloodstream itself. Additionally, in some individuals, there may be a significant amount of contrast that appears in the right ventricular cavity. In any of these noted instances, one would anticipate that injection of ethanol into the selected artery would result in the ethanol being delivered, not to the localized area of myocardium, but more diffusely to the myocardium or the right ventricle. In these instances, the procedure may not be feasible with injection into the selected artery. The second role that contrast plays is to confirm the presence and size of the perfused bed. The goal of this procedure is that the proximal septum and ideally the area resulting in dynamic obstruction is selectively "reduced." Because the contrast serves as a marker of the eventual route of the destructive ethanol injection, myocardial contrast echo serves as an excellent guide for monitoring this procedure.

SUGGESTED READINGS

Agrawal DI, Malhotra S, Nanda NC, et al. Harmonic power Doppler contrast echocardiography: preliminary experimental results. Echocardiography 1997;14:631–636.

Armstrong WF, Mueller TM, Kinney EL, et al. Assessment of myocardial perfusion abnormalities with contrast-enhanced two-dimensional echocardiography. Circulation 1982;66:166–173.

Bommer WJ, Shah PM, Allen H, et al. The safety of contrast echocardiography: report of the Committee on Contrast Echocardiography for the American Society of Echocardiography. J Am Coll Cardiol 1984;3:6–13.

Camarano G, Jones M, Freidlin RZ, et al. Quantitative assessment of left ventricular perfusion defects using real-time three-dimensional myocardial contrast echocardiography. J Am Soc Echocardiogr 2002;15:206–213.

Castello R, Bella JN, Rovner A, et al. Efficacy and time-efficiency of a "sonographer-driven" contrast echocardiography protocol in a high-volume echocardiography laboratory. Am Heart J 2003;145:535–541.

Christiansen JP, Leong-Poi H, Klibanov AL, et al. Noninvasive imaging of myocardial reperfusion injury using leukocyte-targeted contrast echocardiography. Circulation 2002;105:1764–1767.

Cohen JL, Cheirif J, Segar DS, et al. Improved left ventricular endocardial border delineation and opacification with OPTISON (FS069), a new echocardiographic contrast agent. Results of a phase III multicenter trial. J Am Coll Cardiol 1998;32:746–752.

Gramiak R, Shah PM, Kramer DH. Ultrasound cardiography: contrast studies in anatomy and function. Radiology 1969;92:939–948.

Heinle SK, Noblin J, Goree-Best P, et al. Assessment of myocardial perfusion by harmonic power Doppler imaging at rest and during adenosine stress: comparison with (99m)Tc-sestamibi SPECT imaging. Circulation 2000;102:55–60.

Hundley WG, Kizilbash AM, Afridi I, et al. Administration of an intravenous perfluorocarbon contrast agent improves echocardiographic determination of left ventricular volumes and ejection fraction: comparison with cine magnetic resonance imaging. J Am Coll Cardiol 1998;32:1426–1432.

Kaul S, Senior R, Dittrich H, et al. Detection of coronary artery disease with myocardial contrast echocardiography: comparison with 99mTc-sestamibi single-photon emission computed tomography. Circulation 1997;96:785–792.

Kaul S, Ito H. Microvasculature in acute myocardial ischemia: part I: evolving concepts in pathophysiology, diagnosis, and treatment. Circulation 2004;109:146–149.

Lim YJ, Nanto S, Masuyama T, et al. Visualization of subendocardial myocardial ischemia with myocardial contrast echocardiography in humans. Circulation 1989;79:233–244.

Lindner JR, Song J, Xu F, et al. Noninvasive ultrasound imaging of inflammation using microbubbles targeted to activated leukocytes. Circulation 2000;102:2745–2750.

Main ML, Magalski A, Chee NK, et al. Full-motion pulse inversion power Doppler contrast echocardiography differentiates stunning from necrosis and predicts recovery of left ventricular function after acute myocardial infarction. J Am Coll Cardiol 2001;38:1390–1394.

Main ML, Magalski A, Morris BA, et al. Combined assessment of microvascular integrity and contractile reserve improves differentiation of stunning and necrosis after acute anterior wall myocardial infarction. J Am Coll Cardiol 2002;40:1079–1084.

Masugata H, Peters B, Lafitte S, et al. Quantitative assessment of myocardial perfusion during graded coronary stenosis by real-time myocardial contrast echo refilling curves. J Am Coll Cardiol 2001;37: 262–269.

Nagueh SF, Vaduganathan P, Ali N, et al. Identification of hibernating myocardium: comparative accuracy of myocardial contrast echocardiography, rest-redistribution thallium-201 tomography and dobutamine echocardiography. J Am Coll Cardiol 1997;29:985–993.

Nakatani S, Imanishi T, Terasawa A, et al. Clinical application of transpulmonary contrast-enhanced Doppler technique in the assessment of severity of aortic stenosis. J Am Coll Cardiol 1992;20: 973–978.

Nanda NC, Kitzman DW, Dittrich HC, et al. Imagent improves endocardial border delineation, inter-reader agreement, and the accuracy of segmental wall motion assessment. Echocardiography 2003;20: 151–161.

Porter TR, Xie F, Li S, et al. Increased ultrasound contrast and decreased microbubble destruction rates with triggered ultrasound imaging. J Am Soc Echocardiogr 1996;9:599–605.

Porter TR, Xie F, Silver M, et al. Real-time perfusion imaging with low mechanical index pulse inversion Doppler imaging. J Am Coll Cardiol 2001;37:748–753.

Price RJ, Skyba DM, Kaul S, et al. Delivery of colloidal particles and red blood cells to tissue through microvessel ruptures created by targeted microbubble destruction with ultrasound. Circulation 1998;98:1264–1267.

Ragosta M, Camarano G, Kaul S, et al. Microvascular integrity indicates myocellular viability in patients with recent myocardial infarction. New insights using myocardial contrast echocardiography. Circulation 1994;89:2562–2569.

Reilly JP, Tunick PA, Timmermans RJ, et al. Contrast echocardiography clarifies uninterpretable wall motion in intensive care unit patients. J Am Coll Cardiol 2000;35:485–490.

Rose GC, Armstrong WF, Mahomed Y, et al. Atrial level right to left intracardiac shunt associated with postoperative hypoxemia: demonstration with contrast two-dimensional echocardiography. J Am Coll Cardiol 1985;6:920–922.

Sabia PJ, Powers ER, Jayaweera AR, et al. Functional significance of collateral blood flow in patients with recent acute myocardial infarction. A study using myocardial contrast echocardiography. Circulation 1992;85:2080–2089.

Sabia PJ, Powers ER, Ragosta M, et al. An association between collateral blood flow and myocardial viability in patients with recent myocardial infarction. N Engl J Med 1992;327:1825–1831.

Shimoni S, Frangogiannis NG, Aggeli CJ, et al. Identification of hibernating myocardium with quantitative intravenous myocardial contrast echocardiography: comparison with dobutamine echocardiography and thallium-201 scintigraphy. Circulation 2003;107:538–544.

Sklenar J, Camarano G, Goodman NC, et al. Contractile versus microvascular reserve for the determination of the extent of myocardial salvage after reperfusion. The effect of residual coronary stenosis. Circulation 1996;94:1430–1440.

Skolnick DG, Sawada SG, Feigenbaum H, et al. Enhanced endocardial visualization with noncontrast harmonic imaging during stress echocardiography. J Am Soc Echocardiogr 1999;12:559–563.

Spencer KT, Bednarz J, Mor-Avi V, et al. The role of echocardiographic harmonic imaging and contrast enhancement for improvement of endocardial border delineation. J Am Soc Echocardiogr 2000;13:131–138.

Swinburn JM, Lahiri A, Senior R. Intravenous myocardial contrast echocardiography predicts recovery of dysynergic myocardium early after acute myocardial infarction. J Am Coll Cardiol 2001;38: 19–25.

Thanigaraj S, Schechtman KB, Perez JE. Improved echocardiographic delineation of left ventricular thrombus with the use of intravenous second-generation contrast image enhancement. J Am Soc Echocardiogr 1999;12:1022–1026.

Thomson HL, Basmadjian AJ, Rainbird AJ, et al. Contrast echocardiography improves the accuracy and reproducibility of left ventricular remodeling measurements: a prospective, randomly assigned, blinded study. J Am Coll Cardiol 2001;38:867–875.

Tiemann K, Becher H, Bimmel D, et al. Stimulated acoustic emission nonbackscatter contrast effect of microbubbles seen with harmonic power Doppler imaging. Echocardiography 1997;14:65–70.

Tuchnitz A, von Bibra H, Sutherland GR, et al. Doppler energy: a new acquisition technique for the transthoracic detection of myocardial perfusion defects with the use of a venous contrast agent. J Am Soc Echocardiogr 1997;10:881–890.

Villanueva FS, Glasheen WP, Sklenar J, et al. Characterization of spatial patterns of flow within the reperfused myocardium by myocardial contrast echocardiography. Implications in determining extent of myocardial salvage. Circulation 1993;88:2596–2606.

Villanueva FS, Klibanov A, Wagner WR. Microbubble-endothelial cell interactions as a basis for assessing endothelial function. Echocardiography 2002;19:427–438.

Wei K, Skyba DM, Firschke C, et al. Interactions between microbubbles and ultrasound: *in vitro* and *in vivo* observations. J Am Coll Cardiol 1997;29:1081–1088.

Wei K, Ragosta M, Thorpe J, et al. Noninvasive quantification of coronary blood flow reserve in humans using myocardial contrast echocardiography. Circulation 2001;103:2560–2565.

Wu CC, Feldman MD, Mills JD, et al. Myocardial contrast echocardiography can be used to quantify intramyocardial blood volume: new insights into structural mechanisms of coronary autoregulation. Circulation 1997;96:1004–1011.

Yong Y, Wu D, Fernandes V, et al. Diagnostic accuracy and cost-effectiveness of contrast echocardiography on evaluation of cardiac function in technically very difficult patients in the intensive care unit. Am J Cardiol 2002;89:711–718.

Yu EH, Skyba DM, Sloggett CE, et al. Determination of left ventricular ejection fraction using intravenous contrast and a semiautomated border detection algorithm. J Am Soc Echocardiogr 2003;16: 22–28.

Chapter 5

The Echocardiographic Examination

The ability to record high-quality echocardiographic images and obtain accurate Doppler flow recordings are essential determinants of the overall value of the echocardiographic examination. As such, echocardiography is highly operator dependent. It is difficult to overemphasize the critical role of the person who performs the imaging. Echocardiography can also be regarded as a partnership between the individual who obtains the data and the one who interprets the study. To obtain a comprehensive and accurate echocardiogram, the operator must understand the anatomy and physiology of the cardiovascular system, have a thorough knowledge of the ultrasound equipment to optimize the quality of the recording, know the specific diagnostic questions that are being asked, and be able to apply the technology to the individual patient so that optimal imaging can be achieved.

Echocardiography is a highly versatile technique that can be applied in variety of clinical settings. Patients are usually referred for an echocardiogram to investigate symptoms or abnormalities found on a physical examination, to evaluate a known or suspected clinical condition, or to screen a subject for the possibility of disease. The value of the diagnostic information depends on the quality of the study and the likelihood that the results will provide new information that will have an impact on the patient's management or well-being. Guidelines have been published jointly by the American Heart Association, the American College of Cardiology, and the American Society of Echocardiography that critically evaluate the strength of evidence for the use of echocardiography in various clinical situations. Throughout this book, the recommendations provided by these guidelines are highlighted. These guidelines are based on the weight of evidence that supports the utility of the test and the consensus of a panel of experts. The recommendations concerning the use of echocardiography use the following classification system:

Class I: Conditions for which there is evidence and/or general agreement that a given procedure is useful and effective.

Class II: Conditions for which there is conflicting evidence and/or a divergence of opinion about the usefulness/efficacy of a procedure.

Class IIa: Weight of evidence/opinion is in favor of usefulness/efficacy.

Class IIb: Usefulness/efficacy is less well established by evidence/opinion.

Class III: Conditions for which there is evidence and/or general agreement that the procedure is not useful/effective and in some cases may be harmful.

An example of this classification system provides a guide for the general use of echocardiography for the evaluation of patients with a heart murmur (Table 5.1).

Most echocardiographic examinations are comprehensive. That is, a thorough and fairly standardized approach is undertaken with the goal of recording a complete array

▶ **TABLE 5.1 Indications for Echocardiography in the Evaluation of Heart Murmurs**

	Class
1. A murmur in a patient with cardiorespiratory symptoms	I
2. A murmur in an asymptomatic patient if the clinical features indicate at least a moderate probability that the murmur is reflective of structural heart disease	I
3. A murmur in an asymptomatic patient in whom there is a low probability of heart disease but in whom the diagnosis of heart disease cannot be reasonably excluded by the standard cardiovascular clinical evaluation	IIa
4. In an adult, an asymptomatic heart murmur that has been identified by an experienced observer as functional or innocent	III

Adapted from Cheitlin MD, Alpert JS, Armstrong WF, et al. ACC/AHA Guidelines for the Clinical Application of Echocardiography : a report of the American College of Cardiology/American Heart Association Task Force on Practice Guidelines (Committee on Clinical Application of Echocardiography) developed in collaboration with the American Society of Echocardiography. Circulation 1997;95:1686-1744, with permission.

of images and Doppler data that address the full spectrum of possible diagnoses (Table 5.2). Occasionally, a more targeted or focused examination is undertaken that is only concerned with a specific diagnostic issue, often comparing the current situation with a recent examination. In other situations, an entirely different approach is required, such as when evaluating an infant with suspected complex congenital heart disease. Clearly, echocardiography requires an individualized approach and each patient represents a unique set of problems and challenges. The technical details involved in obtaining a high-quality echocardiogram are unique, and the examination must be customized for each patient. It is not feasible to simply place the transducer at routine locations on the chest and expect standardized, high-quality images to be available in each patient. The examiner must rely on experience, persistence, and creativity to record the most comprehensive and highest quality data. Additional factors, including transducer selection, instrument settings, patient comfort and positioning, and even the patient's breathing pattern will also affect the quality of the recording.

TABLE 5.2 Transthoracic Echocardiographic Views

Two-Dimensional Imaging	Doppler Imaging
Parasternal	**Parasternal**
Long-axis	MR, AR, VSD
Medially angulated long axis	RV inflow, TR
Short-axis (multiple levels)	AR, TR, PS, PR, VSD
Basal	MR
MV level	
Papillary muscle level	
Apical	
Apical	**Apical**
Four-chamber	Mitral, tricuspid inflow; MR, TR
Two-chamber	Mitral inflow, MR
Long-axis	MR, AR, AS, LVOT
Five-chamber	LV outflow, AR, AS, IVRT
Subcostal	**Subcostal**
Four-chamber	RV inflow, TR, ASD
Short-axis	
Basal	TR, PS, PR
Mid-ventricular	IVC, hepatic veins
Suprasternal	**Suprasternal**
Aortic arch in long-axis	Ascending/descending aortic flow,
Aortic arch in short-axis	AR, PDA, SVC
Right parasternal	**Right parasternal**
Ascending aorta	AS

AR, aortic regurgitation; AS, aortic stenosis; ASD, atrial septal defect; IVC, inferior vena cava; IVRT, isovolumic relaxation time; LV, left ventricle; LVOT, left ventricular outflow tract; MR, mitral regurgitation; MV, mitral valve; PDA, patent ductus arteriosus; PR, pulmonic regurgitation; PS, pulmonic stenosis; RV, right ventricle; SVC, superior vena cava; TR, tricuspid regurgitation; VSD, ventricular septal defect.

SELECTING THE TRANSDUCERS

Most ultrasound systems are equipped with a selection of transducers with a range of capabilities and limitations. With the exception of dedicated continuous wave Doppler (called nonimaging or Pedoff) transducers, most probes are capable of performing M-mode, two-dimensional, and Doppler imaging (Fig. 5.1). It is rare that one transducer is ideal for every aspect of a given examination. For instance, a high-frequency imaging transducer may provide optimal resolution for near-field imaging (such as the right ventricular free wall or the cardiac apex) but will offer inadequate penetration to allow imaging of the far field. In a large patient, the apical window may place the left atrium as far as 20 cm from the transducer. For adequate visualization, a relatively low frequency transducer will be necessary. The best Doppler studies are generally obtained with lower frequency transducers. It may be necessary to switch from one transducer to another to take advantage of the capabilities of each. Some modern transducers provide a range of frequencies or allow selection of different frequencies as an added convenience. The frequency of the transducer used for cardiac imaging often depends on body habitus and patient size. For large patients or thick-chested individuals, a 2.0- or 2.5-MHz transducer may be necessary to provide adequate penetration. Children and smaller adults can generally be adequately imaged using a 3.5- or even 5.0-MHz transducer. For infants and children, a 7.0- or 7.5-MHz transducer is often ideal.

In addition to transducer frequency, transducer size or "footprint" is also a consideration. The footprint refers to the dimensions of the surface area coming in contact with the patient's skin. Because of the relatively narrow spaces between the ribs, the footprint can be a limiting factor in transducer selection (Fig. 5.2). In this illustration, the distal septum and posterior left ventricular wall are obscured

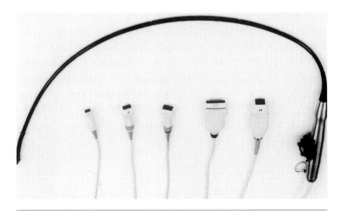

FIGURE 5.1. A variety of transducers are available for use in clinical echocardiography. A transesophageal transducer and five transthoracic probes are illustrated.

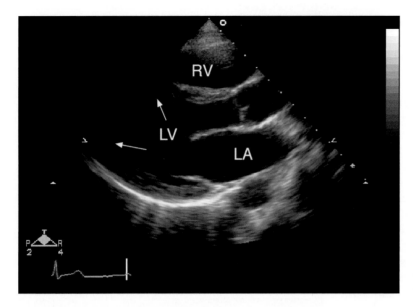

FIGURE 5.2. An example of rib shadowing is demonstrated (*arrows*). The presence of the rib relative to the transducer footprint obscures the distal septum and posterior wall of the left ventricle (*LV*). LA, left atrium; RV, right ventricle.

by the rib shadow along the left side of the image. If the transducer surface is too big to fit between ribs or to maintain continuous contact with the skin, suboptimal imaging will be obtained.

PATIENT POSITION

The transthoracic examination can be performed with the echocardiographer (or sonographer) sitting on the patient's left or right side. This is largely a matter of personal preference, comfort, and custom. When seated to the right side of the patient, scanning is performed with the right hand. If the left side is used, usually the operator scans with his or her left hand and manipulates the machine settings with the right hand. Developing experience

scanning from both sides is recommended. Not only does this minimize the risk of repetitive-use injury, but it prepares the sonographer for room situations where only one side of the bed may be available for approaching the patient.

One of the goals of the echocardiographic examination is to obtain the highest quality images without creating unnecessary discomfort or anxiety for the patient. Because transthoracic echocardiography can take as long as an hour, the comfort and well-being of both the examiner and the patient are important. The transthoracic echocardiographic examination usually requires more than one patient position. For most adult patients, imaging is performed with the patient either supine and/or tilted in the left lateral decubitus position (Fig. 5.3). By tilting the patient to the left, the heart is brought forward to the chest

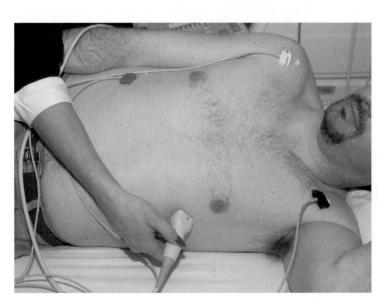

FIGURE 5.3. Proper positioning for the echocardiographic examination is demonstrated. The transducer is placed over the apical window, and the patient is tilted in the left lateral decubitus position.

wall and more to the left of the sternum thereby improving the ultrasound windows. The degree to which the patient should be rotated to the left must be individualized, and occasionally excellent images can be obtained with the patient supine.

Additional patient positions are often necessary. Tilting the patient into the right lateral decubitus position may be necessary in some forms of congenital disease or to record aortic valve flow (Fig. 5.4). To facilitate subcostal imaging, a supine position with the legs flexed at the knees generally provides the greatest relaxation of the abdominal muscles so that the transducer can be properly positioned (Fig. 5.5). To use the suprasternal notch as an ultrasound window, it is often necessary to place a pillow behind the patient's shoulders so that the neck can be comfortably hyperextended, thereby creating an opening for transducer placement (Fig. 5.6). Finally, even the sitting position may sometimes be required, especially for some forms of congenital heart disease.

Patient cooperation is an important consideration in the echocardiographic examination. Explaining the purpose of the examination, ensuring the patient's comfort, and stressing the safety and noninvasive aspects of ultrasound will alleviate anxiety and enhance cooperation. In children and infants in whom anxiety and lack of cooperation can be anticipated, special approaches are necessary. Enlisting the assistance of a parent is frequently adequate, although sedation may occasionally be necessary to complete the examination.

PLACEMENT OF THE TRANSDUCER

Figure 5.7 illustrates the various locations for placement of a transthoracic transducer for examination of the

heart and great vessels. The goal of the transthoracic echocardiographic examination is to acquire a complete two-dimensional interrogation from all the available ultrasonic windows. In doing so, the heart can be visualized in multiple orthogonal planes, allowing tomographic data to be integrated in a coherent manner. The transducer locations endorsed by the American Society of Echocardiography for transthoracic imaging in the adult include the left and right parasternal locations, the cardiac apex, the subcostal window, and the suprasternal notch location. The examination is frequently begun with the patient lying supine, rotated into the left lateral decubitus position, and the transducer located at the left parasternal position. Depending on body habitus, the presence or absence of lung disease, and the position of the heart within the thorax, the optimal intercostal space

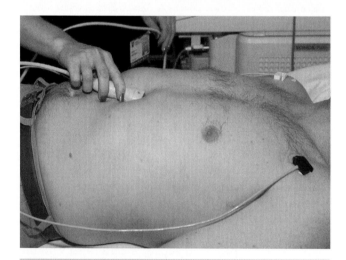

FIGURE 5.5. The transducer is applied to the subcostal window, with the patient supine.

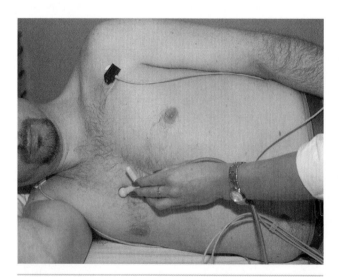

FIGURE 5.4. The right lateral decubitus position is shown, and a Pedoff transducer is applied to record ascending aortic flow.

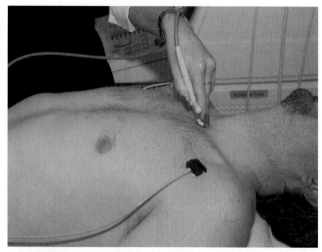

FIGURE 5.6. To record aortic flow from the suprasternal notch, it is often necessary to elevate the shoulders using a pillow to tilt the head backward.

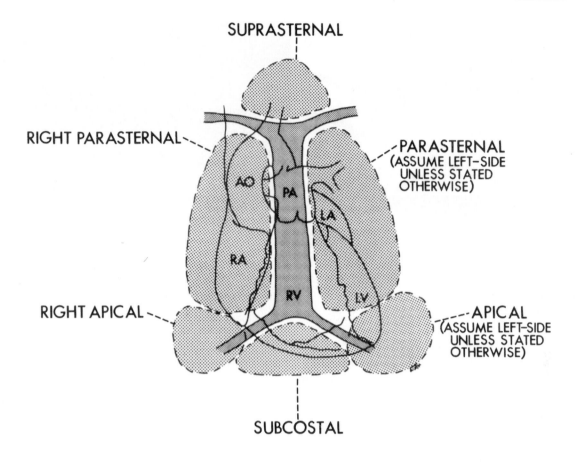

NOMENCLATURE FOR TRANSDUCER LOCATION

FIGURE 5.7. This diagram demonstrates the various transducer locations used in echocardiography. Ao, aorta; PA, pulmonary artery; LA, left atrium; RA, right atrium; RV, right ventricle; LV, left ventricle. (From Henry WL, DeMaria A, Gramaik R, et al. Report of the American Society of Echocardiography Committee on Nomenclature and Standards in Two-Dimensional Echocardiography. Circulation 1980;62:212–217, with permission.)

for recording the "parasternal views" will vary. Imaging from the cardiac apex frequently requires tilting the patient into a steep left lateral decubitus position. By palpation, the point of maximal impulse is located and used as the starting point for apical imaging. The subcostal approach is particularly important in patients with advanced lung disease or thick chest walls and provides the unique opportunity to view the inferior vena cava, hepatic veins, and many of the important congenital anomalies. The suprasternal notch is most useful to visualize the great vessels and left atrium.

Less commonly used windows include the right parasternal location. This position is useful to examine the aorta or interatrial septum and in patients with congenital malposition of the heart, such as dextrocardia. It plays a major role in the assessment of aortic stenosis. This approach usually requires positioning the patient in the right lateral decubitus position. The right apical, right supraclavicular fossa, and even the back are potential

acoustic windows that must occasionally be used. For example, the right supraclavicular examination often provides the best opportunity to visualize the superior vena cava.

It should be emphasized that the standard patient positions and transducer locations serve only as a general guide, applicable to the majority of patients. In patients with chest deformities, such as pectus excavatum, or those with chronic obstructive lung disease, these standard approaches may be inadequate. Likewise, some anomalies within the thorax, including dextrocardia, pleural effusion, and pneumothorax may also render the standard approaches ineffective. In such cases, it is the experience and creativity of the examiner that will often determine the value of the information derived from the transthoracic study. Using the transducer as an exploratory camera will occasionally reveal unexpected acoustic windows that will yield important diagnostic information.

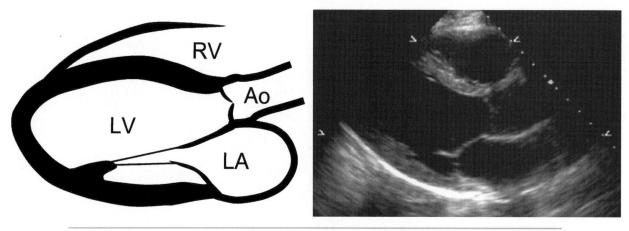

FIGURE 5.8. The parasternal long-axis view is shown. Ao, aorta; LA, left atrium; LV, left ventricle; RV, right ventricle.

AN APPROACH TO THE TRANSTHORACIC EXAMINATION

A comprehensive transthoracic echocardiographic examination will include two-dimensional imaging, Doppler imaging, and M-mode imaging. It is customary to start with the two-dimensional examination, which provides orientation and a frame of reference for the other components (Table 5.2). In most laboratories, the parasternal window serves as a starting point for the study. Beginning at the third left intercostal space, the transducer is applied and rotated to record the parasternal long-axis view. To optimize the image, it may be necessary to move up or down one or two intercostal spaces and to rotate the patient into a left lateral decubitus position. When properly recorded, this view depicts the mid portion and base of the left ventricle, both leaflets of the mitral valve, the aortic valve and

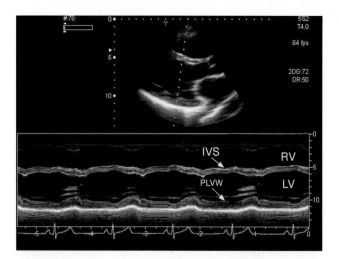

FIGURE 5.9. From the two-dimensional image, an M-mode display at the mid ventricular level is derived. IVS, interventricular septum; LV, left ventricle; PLVW, posterior left ventricular wall; RV, right ventricle.

aortic root, the left atrium, and the right ventricle (Fig. 5.8). The left ventricular apex is rarely visualized from this window. The transducer position should be adjusted so that the scanning plane is parallel to the major axis of the left ventricle and passes through the center of the left ventricular chamber. This is the point where the minor-axis diameter is maximal and the mitral valve leaflet excursion is greatest. This is best accomplished by gradual medial to lateral angulation until left ventricular size is at its maximum. From this view, an M-mode cursor can be placed to record minor-axis dimensions (Fig. 5.9). This orientation will record the full excursion of the mitral valve, aortic valve opening and closing, right ventricular free wall motion, and the left ventricular septal and posterior wall motion. The coronary sinus will be visualized in the posterior atrioventricular groove, just below the base of the posterior mitral leaflet. An example of this is shown in Figure 5.10, which demonstrates the normal relationship between the coronary sinus, the atrioventricular groove, and the descending aorta. Behind the left atrium, a portion of the descending aorta will often be recorded. This view is also ideal to confirm the presence or absence of a pericardial effusion. A narrow, echo-free space *behind* the posterior left ventricular wall, but *anterior* to the descending aorta is strongly suggestive of pericardial fluid.

PARASTERNAL LONG-AXIS VIEWS

An imaging plane aligned parallel to the long axis of the left ventricle will not, in most cases, be exactly parallel to the left ventricular outflow tract and aortic root. This is illustrated in Figure 5.11, which demonstrates that slight counterclockwise rotation of the transducer is needed to follow the long axis of the left ventricle into the long axis of the aorta. In this illustration, the true dimensions of the proximal aorta are underestimated in the left panel, which shows a properly aligned parasternal long-axis

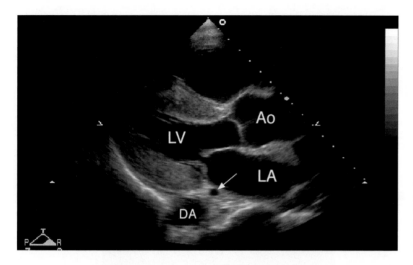

FIGURE 5.10. This parasternal long-axis view illustrates the relationship between the coronary sinus (*arrow*) and the descending aorta (*DA*). Ao, aorta; LA, left atrium; LV, left ventricle.

view. By slightly rotating the transducer (right panel), the aortic root is "opened up" and the true long axis of the aorta is demonstrated. In most patients, some angulation of the scan plane from medial to lateral is required to obtain a complete interrogation of the aortic valve, including the leaflets, anulus, and sinuses.

An important advantage of the parasternal long-axis view is that it orients many of the structures of interest perpendicular to the ultrasound beam, which improves target definition by increasing resolution. By moving the transducer to a lower interspace, the left ventricular apex can be included in the field of view and an apical long-axis plane can be recorded. The advantage of this view is, of course, the ability to include the apex. The major disadvantage is that major structures, particularly the walls of the left ventricle, now lie more parallel to the transducer beam, thereby reducing endocardial definition and making wall motion analysis more difficult. This issue is covered in detail later in this chapter.

Starting from the parasternal long-axis view, medial angulation of the scan plane affords an opportunity to examine the right atrium and right ventricle (Fig. 5.12). As the plane is swept under the sternum, the posterior segment of the interventricular septum is recorded, as is the posteromedial papillary muscle, and eventually the right ventricular inflow tract. Because the right ventricular inflow tract is not parallel to its left ventricular component, slight clockwise rotation of the transducer is generally required. In this plane, the important landmark is the tricuspid valve and the plane is considered optimized when the full excursion of the anterior and septal tricuspid leaflets is recorded and the right ventricular dimension is greatest. This recording permits the inferior portion of the right atrium, including the eustachian valve and occasionally the inferior vena cava, to be visualized. By further rotation of the transducer, a plane that records the right ventricular outflow tract, pulmonary valve, and main pulmonary artery is obtained (Fig. 5.13A). In this example, the entire length of the main pulmonary artery is seen and trivial pulmonary regurgitation is demonstrated. To record the bifurcation of the main pulmonary artery, either this view or the basal short-axis view (Fig. 5.13B) is ideal.

Doppler evaluation of the parasternal long-axis view is useful to record blood flow through the mitral and aortic valves (Fig. 5.14). Because the flow of blood is not parallel to the ultrasound beam, quantitation of flow velocities is generally not possible. However, color flow Doppler from this view is routinely used to detect aortic or mitral regurgitation. In this example, a systolic frame demonstrates acceleration of blood in the left ventricular outflow tract, toward the aortic valve. No evidence of mitral regurgitation is recorded. Slight medial angulation provides an excellent opportunity to detect flow through a ventricular septal defect. Further medial angulation permits Doppler recording of tricuspid valve inflow and both qualitative and quantitative assessment of tricuspid regurgitation.

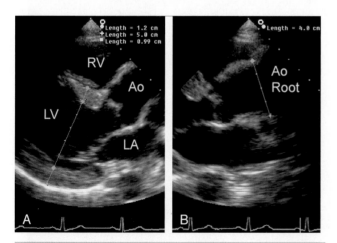

FIGURE 5.11. **A:** The parasternal long-axis view is adjusted so that the scan plane is parallel to the long-axis of the left ventricle (*LV*). In this plane, the proximal aorta (*Ao*) appears normal. **B:** The plane is rotated slightly counterclockwise to better align with the long axis of the ascending aorta. By doing so, the true dimension of the aortic root is apparent. LA, left atrium; RV, right ventricle.

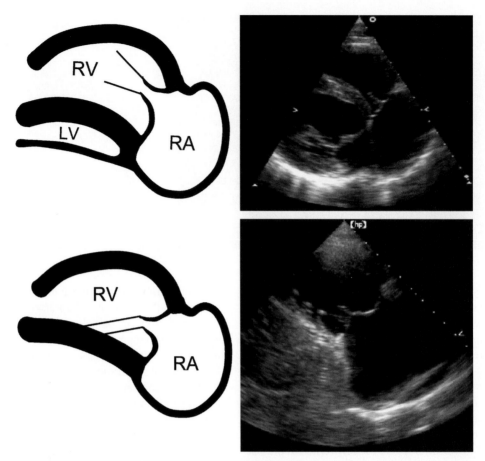

FIGURE 5.12. Two examples of the right ventricular (*RV*) inflow view are shown. **Top:** A portion of the left ventricle (*LV*) is preserved within the scan plane. **Bottom:** Further angulation excludes the left ventricle and only the right atrium (*RA*) and right ventricle remain.

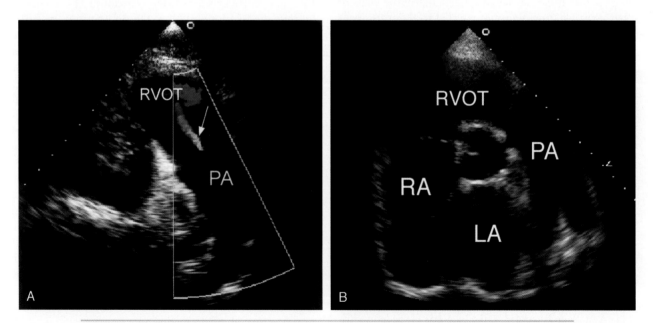

FIGURE 5.13. A: The right ventricular outflow view records the right ventricular outflow tract (*RVOT*) and the main pulmonary artery (*PA*). Trivial pulmonary valve regurgitation (*arrow*) is illustrated. **B:** The bifurcation of the main pulmonary artery is seen from the basal short-axis view. LA, left atrium; RA, right atrium.

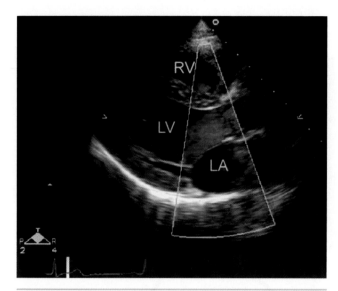

FIGURE 5.14. The parasternal long-axis view with color flow imaging is shown. LA, left atrium; LV, left ventricle; RV, right ventricle.

PARASTERNAL SHORT-AXIS VIEWS

From the parasternal long-axis transducer position, clockwise rotation of the transducer approximately 90 degrees moves the imaging plane to the short-axis view. By rotating the transducer clockwise, the patient's lateral wall is placed to the observer's right and the medial wall is to the observer's left. Although theoretically an infinite number of short-axis planes exist between the base and apex of the heart, in practice, three or four representative views are recorded from this general transducer position. Because these different planes span several centimeters, some repositioning of the transducer is necessary, requiring moving from the second through the fourth intercostal spaces and tilting the transducer at various angles. The relationship of the various short-axis planes to the long-axis view is demonstrated in Figure 5.15.

A useful reference point to begin the short-axis examination is the tip of the anterior mitral valve leaflet. By rotating the transducer slightly and adjusting the tilt of the plane, the left ventricle can be made to appear circular and both leaflets of the mitral valve will demonstrate maximal excursion (Fig. 5.16A). As in all short-axis views, the left ventricle is displayed as if viewed from the apex of the chamber. When properly recorded, the short-axis view in this plane corresponds roughly to the mid left ventricular level and allows optimal recording of mitral leaflet excursion, mid left ventricular wall motion, and visualization of a portion of the right ventricle. The normal interventricular septal curvature can be appreciated and any abnormalities of septal position, shape, or motion can be assessed. Minor base-to-apex angulation is useful to record the orifice of the mitral valve, the coaptation of the

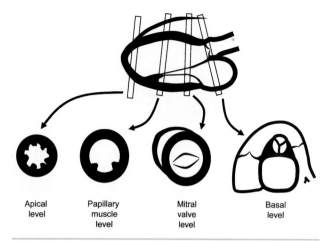

FIGURE 5.15. This schematic demonstrates the various short-axis planes that can be derived from the parasternal long-axis view. Note that the planes are not exactly parallel but provide views of anatomy from apex to base.

leaflets, and the mitral chordae and their insertion into the anterolateral and posteromedial papillary muscles.

Moving to a more basal plane, the short-axis view approaches the level of the aortic anulus and allows simultaneous visualization of several important structures (Fig. 5.16B). In addition to the anulus, the aortic valve, coronary ostia, left atrium, interatrial septum, right atrium, tricuspid valve, right ventricular outflow tract, pulmonary valve, and proximal pulmonary artery can also be recorded. Occasionally, the left atrial appendage also can be visualized from this plane. When properly aligned, the three cusps of the aortic valve can be seen to open and close in systole and diastole, respectively. Immediately superior to the anulus, the ostia of the left and right coronary arteries can be seen. If the anulus is regarded as a clock face, the left main artery originates at approximately 4 o'clock and the right coronary artery at 11 o'clock (Fig. 5.17). The nearly orthogonal relationship between the aorta and the pulmonary artery and the relative positions of the aortic and pulmonary valves can be appreciated. With slight superior angulation, the pulmonary artery can be followed to its bifurcation and both the right and left branches identified (Fig. 5.13B).

By moving the transducer to a lower interspace and angling the scan plane more apically, the image will sweep through the papillary muscle level and then the left ventricular apex (Fig. 5.18). This series of views is ideal for assessing the contractile pattern of the left ventricle at the midventricular and apical levels. When recording these views, adjustments are aimed at maintaining the near-circular appearance of the left ventricular cavity as the overall cavity size decreases toward the apex.

The Doppler evaluation of the various parasternal short-axis views serves several purposes. At the base of the heart, the scan plane can be adjusted so that blood flow is

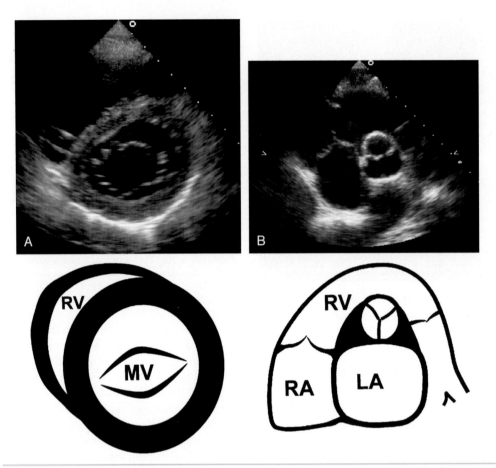

FIGURE 5.16. Two short-axis views are provided. **A:** The short-axis view at the level of the mitral valve (*MV*) is demonstrated. **B:** A basal short-axis projection is shown at the level of the aortic valve. LA, left atrium; RA, right atrium; RV, right ventricle.

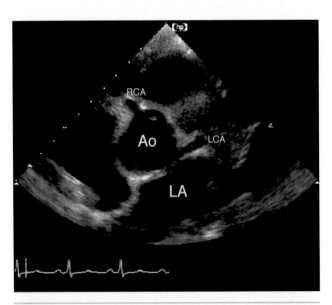

FIGURE 5.17. From the basal short-axis view just above the aortic valve, the origins of the left (*LCA*) and right (*RCA*) coronary arteries can be recorded. Ao, aorta; LA, left atrium.

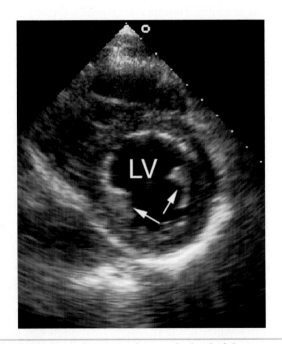

FIGURE 5.18. A short-axis plane at the level of the papillary muscles (*arrows*) is shown. LV, left ventricle.

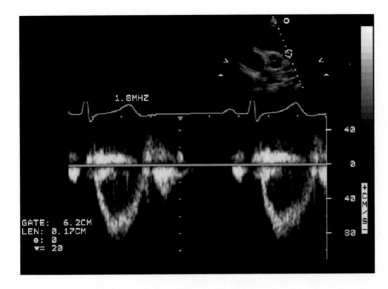

FIGURE 5.19. The basal short-axis view is ideal to record flow through the pulmonary valve using pulsed Doppler imaging.

oriented nearly parallel to the ultrasound beam through both the tricuspid and pulmonary valves. Both tricuspid inflow and tricuspid regurgitation can be recorded from this position. Slight angulation permits a similar assessment of the pulmonary valve from the same basal view (Fig. 5.19). Conversely, aortic flow is nearly perpendicular to the scan plane, therefore quantitative Doppler assessment of aortic flow is not possible. However, color flow imaging just below the aortic valve (at the level of the left ventricular outflow tract) may allow visualization of the aortic regurgitant jet as it emerges from the regurgitant orifice (Fig. 5.20). An assessment of regurgitant jet area at this level is useful. By moving to the mitral valve level, a similar approach using color flow imaging to assess the

mitral regurgitant jet is also possible (Fig. 5.21). This may be of particular value to localize the source of mitral valve regurgitant jets. By scanning carefully through the plane of the mitral leaflets, the location and extent of the regurgitant orifice can often be identified.

APICAL VIEWS

With the patient rotated to the left and the transducer placed at the cardiac apex, a family of long-axis images is available. A useful starting point for this part of the examination is the apical four-chamber view, illustrated in Figure 5.22. Once the apical window is located, the trans-

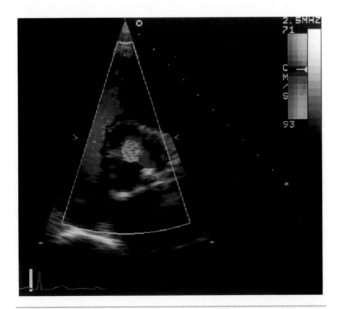

FIGURE 5.20. Color flow imaging from the short-axis view in diastole, just below the aortic valve, records an aortic regurgitation jet in cross section as it emerges from the valve.

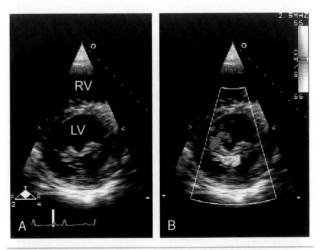

FIGURE 5.21. At the level of the tips of the mitral leaflets, the short-axis view permits the mitral regurgitation jet to be recorded. **A:** Two-dimensional imaging shows thickened mitral leaflets. **B:** Color flow imaging shows the extent of the regurgitant jet at the same level. LV, left ventricle; RV, right ventricle.

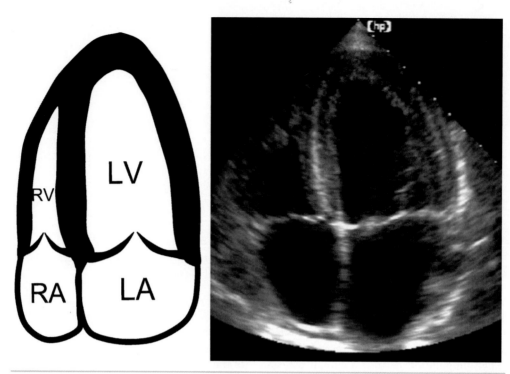

FIGURE 5.22. The apical four-chamber view is shown. LA, left atrium; LV, left ventricle; RA, right atrium; RV, right ventricle.

ducer is pointed in the general direction of the right scapula and then rotated until all four chambers of the heart are optimally visualized. This occurs when the full excursion of both mitral and tricuspid valves is recorded and the "true" apex of the left ventricle lies in the near

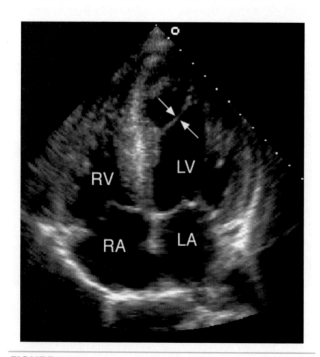

FIGURE 5.23. An example of a false tendon (*arrows*) in the left ventricular (*LV*) apex is demonstrated. LA, left atrium; RA, right atrium; RV, right ventricle.

field. The normal true apex can be identified by its relatively thin walls and lack of motion. Incorrect transducer position will lead to foreshortening of the left ventricle and failure to visualize the true apex. A common variant seen in normal hearts is the false tendon in the left ventricular apex (Fig. 5.23). Such structures are benign anomalies but must be differentiated from pathologic findings, including a thrombus or tumor. When properly adjusted, this image includes the four chambers, both atrioventricular valves, and the interventricular and interatrial septa. Examining the crux of the heart, it should be noted that the insertion of the septal leaflet of the tricuspid valve is several millimeters more apical than the insertion of the mitral leaflet. In a properly oriented four-chamber view, the anterior mitral leaflet is recorded medially and the smaller posterior leaflet is seen as it arises from the lateral margin of the atrioventricular ring. On the right side, the septal leaflet of the tricuspid valve inserts medially and the larger anterior leaflet arises laterally. Confirming this relationship is useful for orientation of the image and is critical in diagnosing several congenital conditions, such as Ebstein anomaly and endocardial cushion defects. The moderator band is often seen in the right ventricular apex (Fig. 5.24), and the descending aorta can frequently be visualized behind the left atrium. Although the left atrium lies in the far field, the junction of the pulmonary veins into the posterior wall of the chamber often can be seen.

By tilting the transducer into a shallower angle relative to the chest wall, resulting in a more anterior scan plane,

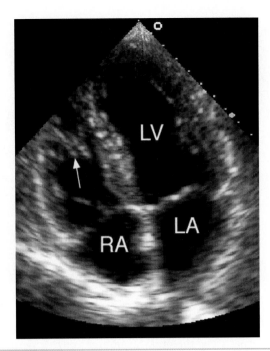

FIGURE 5.24. An apical four-chamber view demonstrates a moderator band (*arrow*) in the right ventricular apex. LA, left atrium; RV, right ventricle; RA, right atrium.

the left ventricular outflow tract, aortic valve, and aortic root can be recorded (Fig. 5.25). This is frequently referred to as the "five-chamber view," recognizing the obvious inaccuracy of the term. Despite the unfortunate ter-

minology, the view has several practical uses. It places both the left ventricular inflow and left ventricular outflow roughly parallel to the ultrasound beam, permitting quantitative Doppler assessment of both patterns simultaneously (Fig. 5.26). In addition, both aortic and mitral regurgitation can be detected from this view, and it is often the best perspective to distinguish between subvalvular and valvular aortic stenosis.

Using the apical four-chamber view as a reference, the other apical views are readily derived. By rotating the transducer counterclockwise approximately 60 degrees, an apical two-chamber view is recorded (Fig. 5.27). The intent here is to completely exclude the right atrium and ventricle from the recording so that only the left ventricle, left atrium, and mitral valve are visualized. The two-chamber view is also similar in orientation to the right anterior oblique (RAO) angiographic view. For this reason, it is sometimes referred to as the RAO equivalent. Although not truly orthogonal to the four-chamber view, the apical two-chamber image records different walls of the left ventricle and the combination of these two views often provides an accurate representation of left ventricular size, shape, and function. The two views are often used in combination for biplane quantitative approaches to left ventricular function. This view also permits the left atrial appendage to be recorded in some patients (Fig. 5.28). Although transesophageal echocardiography will always be superior for this purpose, this is one of the few opportunities on transthoracic imaging to visualize this structure.

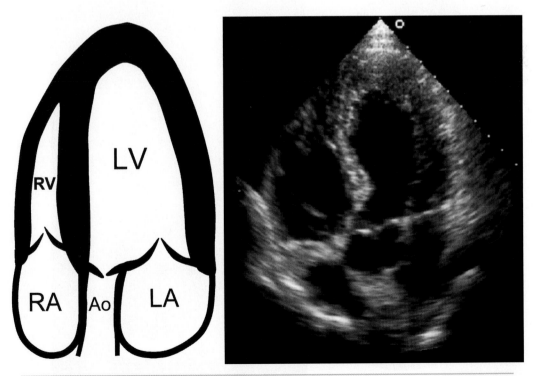

FIGURE 5.25. Starting from the four-chamber view, the transducer can be tilted to a shallower angle to produce a plane that includes the left ventricular outflow tract and proximal aorta (*Ao*). LA, left atrium; LV, left ventricle; RA, right atrium; RV, right ventricle.

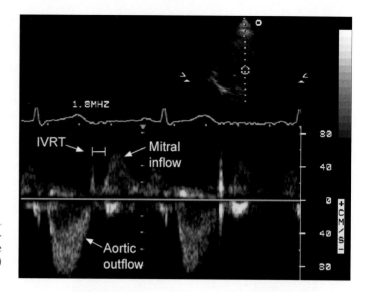

FIGURE 5.26. From the apical five-chamber view, simultaneous recording of aortic outflow and mitral inflow can be performed. This permits isovolumic relaxation time (IVRT) to be measured.

If the transducer position is returned to the four-chamber orientation and then rotated clockwise approximately 60 degrees, an apical long-axis view is recorded, characterized by the presence of both the mitral and aortic valves in the same plane (Fig. 5.29). This is a similar plane to the parasternal long-axis view except recorded from the apex. An important difference between the two long-axis views is the relationship between the endocardial surface and the ultrasound beam. From the parasternal view, the endocardium is roughly perpendicular to the beam, thereby facilitating endocardial definition. From the apical window, the left ventricular walls and the ultrasound beam are more parallel, which in some cases results in endocardial dropout and poorer visualization of wall motion. An advantage of this view is its utility in detecting and quantifying aortic valvular

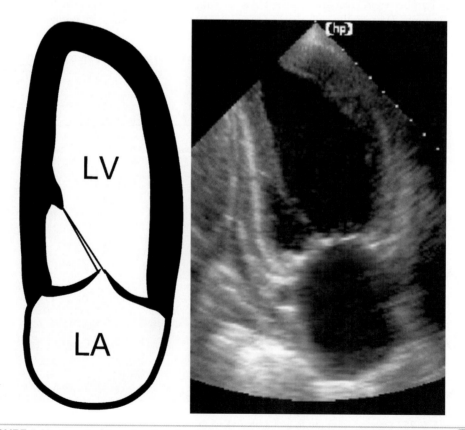

FIGURE 5.27. An apical two-chamber view is demonstrated. LA, left atrium; LV, left ventricle.

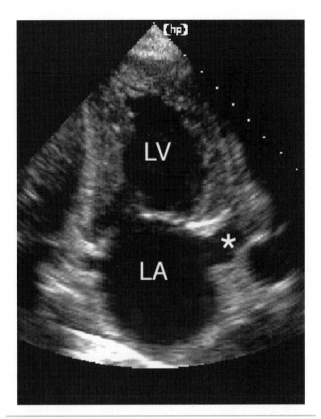

FIGURE 5.28. The two-chamber view sometimes allows the left atrial appendage (*) to be visualized. LA, left atrium; LV, left ventricle.

and subvalvular obstruction, including hypertrophic cardiomyopathy.

It is sometime helpful to relate these three apical views as relative positions on a clock face (Fig. 5.30). Starting with the four-chamber view, the left ventricular walls are imaged at the 10 o'clock and 4 o'clock positions. The two-chamber view records left ventricular walls at the 2 o'clock and 8 o'clock positions, whereas the apical long-axis bisects the left ventricle at approximately 12 o'clock and 6 o'clock. These are only approximate guidelines but serve to orient the three views and underscore the fact that each records different segments of the left ventricle.

Doppler evaluation from the apical views has several important applications. The orientation of blood flow relative to the scan plane permits recording of mitral, aortic, and pulmonary venous blood flow profiles from the apex. From the four-chamber view, the Doppler sample volume is first placed at the tips of the mitral leaflets to record mitral inflow (Fig. 5.31). An analogous approach can be taken to sample tricuspid inflow. Aortic outflow is then recorded from the five-chamber view, with the sample volume positioned at the level of the aortic anulus (Fig. 5.32). Pulsed Doppler interrogation of pulmonary venous flow is usually obtained from the apical four-chamber view, despite the considerable distance between the transducer and target (Fig. 5.33). Using a low-velocity scale and keeping the wall filters at a low level, the sample volume is placed within the mouth of the pulmonary vein. In the ex-

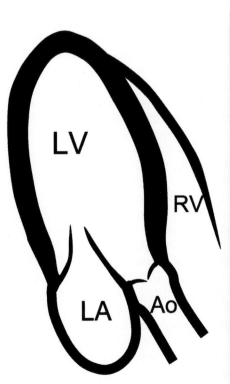

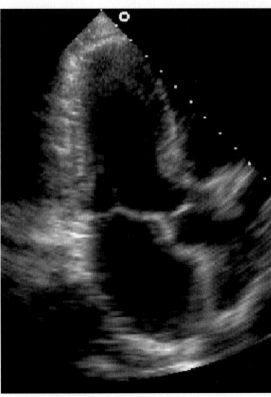

FIGURE 5.29. The apical long-axis view is similar to the parasternal long-axis view but is recorded from a lower interspace. Ao, aorta; LA, left atrium; LV, left ventricle; RV, right ventricle.

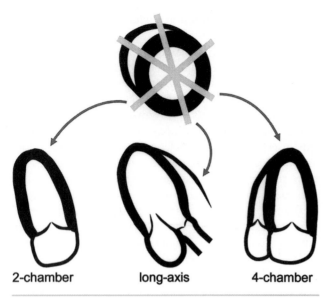

2-chamber   long-axis   4-chamber

FIGURE 5.30. The relationship among the various apical long-axis views and the parasternal short-axis is demonstrated. See text for details.

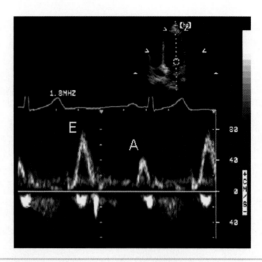

FIGURE 5.31. The apical four-chamber view is ideal to record mitral inflow using pulsed Doppler imaging. In this normal example, the E- and A-waves are demonstrated.

ample shown, the systolic and diastolic filling waves and the slight retrograde flow during atrial systole are all clearly recorded. Finally, from the apical views, color Doppler imaging should be routinely performed to assess for regurgitation of the mitral, aortic, or tricuspid valve.

Tissue Doppler imaging of the mitral anulus is being performed with increasing regularity to aid in the assessment of diastolic function and filling pressures. To record anular velocities, use a small sample volume and adjust gain and filter settings to a low level. From the four-chamber view, position the sample volume over the mitral anulus medially in the area of the septum (Fig. 5.34). Anular velocities in the region of the lateral wall should also be recorded. The velocity scale should be turned to its lowest level. Motion of the anulus throughout the cardiac cycle can be recorded in most patients. Finally, color M-mode recording of mitral inflow and left ventricular filling is being used increasingly as a novel approach to diastolic function (Fig. 5.35). Using routine color flow imaging for orientation, the M-mode cursor is placed in the center of the inflow jet. The M-mode display reveals the acceleration of blood in early diastole through the mitral valve toward the apex. The slope of the red-blue interface represents the propagation velocity of left ventricular inflow and correlates with the rate of chamber relaxation.

THE SUBCOSTAL EXAMINATION

In most patients, placement of the transducer in the subcostal location provides an opportunity to record a four-chamber and a series of short-axis planes. The subcostal

four-chamber view is similar to the corresponding apical view with two exceptions. First, the ultrasound beam is oriented perpendicular to the long axis of the left ventricle and thus often provides better endocardial definition of the ventricular walls. Second, because of the position of the transducer relative to the cardiac apex, foreshortening or inability to visualize the left ventricular apex is more likely from the subcostal position (Fig. 5.36). Because of the orientation of the interventricular and interatrial septa relative to the scan plane, this view is particularly useful to examine these structures and to search for septal defects. In adult patients, this is frequently the only echocardiographic view that visualizes the superior portion of the atrial septum, permitting sinus venosus defects to be detected. The proximity of the right ventricular free wall to the transducer also makes this view ideal for assessing right ventricular free wall thickness and motion and may be helpful in evaluating abnormal wall motion in patients with suspected pericardial tamponade (Fig. 5.37).

From the four-chamber view, the transducer can be rotated approximately 90 degrees counterclockwise to record a series of short-axis images. Figure 5.38A demonstrates a short-axis plane at the papillary muscle level. The plane can usually be adjusted to provide an excellent view of the right ventricular outflow tract, pulmonary valve, and proximal pulmonary artery (Fig. 5.38B). This is a useful alternative to the parasternal short-axis view for the assessment of these structures. The orientation of blood flow parallel to the ultrasound beam facilitates quantitative Doppler analysis. From this view, inferior angulation of the transducer can provide multiple short-axis views of the left and right ventricles moving from base to apex. The subcostal view is also useful for direct recording of the inferior vena cava and hepatic veins by modifi-

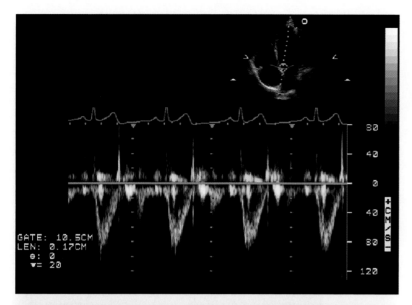

FIGURE 5.32. The apical five-chamber view allows recording of aortic outflow using the pulsed Doppler technique.

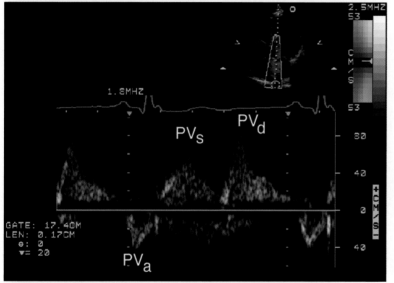

FIGURE 5.33. From the apical four-chamber view, pulsed Doppler imaging can often be used to record pulmonary venous flow by positioning the sample volume at the junction of the pulmonary vein and left atrium. In this example, pulmonary venous flow has three phases: a systolic phase (PV_s), a diastolic phase (PV_d), and a small wave of flow reversal during atrial systole (PV_a).

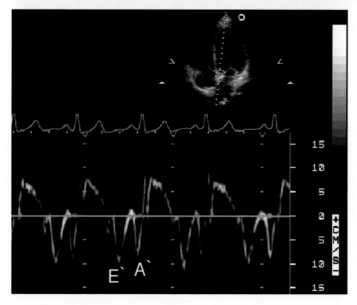

FIGURE 5.34. Tissue Doppler imaging of the medial mitral anulus demonstrates velocity away from the transducer in systole and two waves toward the transducer (*E'* and *A'*) in diastole.

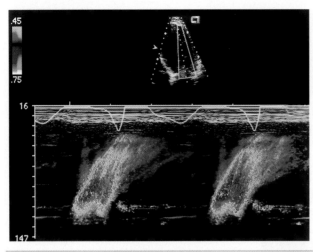

FIGURE 5.35. Color M-mode recording of mitral inflow during diastole, recorded from the apical window.

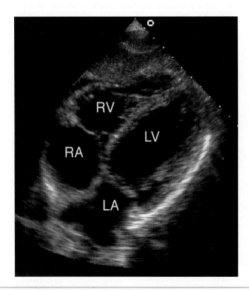

FIGURE 5.36. A subcostal four-chamber view is demonstrated. LA, left atrium; LV, left ventricle; RA, right atrium; RV, right ventricle.

cation of the short-axis plane (Fig. 5.39). The dimensions of the inferior vena cava and its response to "sniffing" should be analyzed. Hepatic vein flow is recorded using pulsed Doppler imaging. To record flow in the hepatic veins, it is first necessary to visualize the inferior vena cava, a few centimeters below the diaphragm. Then, using color Doppler imaging, the liver can be interrogated until a vein is identified oriented parallel to the ultrasound beam. Pulsed Doppler imaging can then be used to record flow velocities within the hepatic vein. For maximal value, hepatic vein flow must be assessed in conjunction with the respiratory cycle.

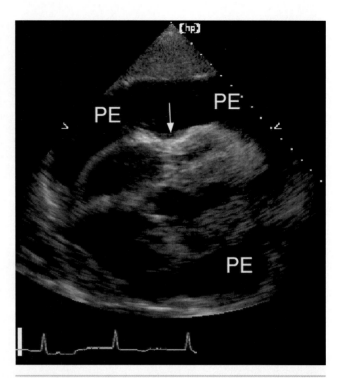

FIGURE 5.37. A subcostal four-chamber view from a patient with a large pericardial effusion (*PE*) is provided. From this window, diastolic right ventricular free wall collapse (*arrow*) can be demonstrated.

SUPRASTERNAL VIEWS

The primary use of the suprasternal views is to examine the great vessels. Extending and rotating the patient's head can position the transducer so that the aortic arch is readily recorded. Orientation of the scan plane is based on the position of the arch relative to the ultrasound beam. Although a variety of terms have been used to define the various transducer positions, describing the imaging plane as either parallel or perpendicular to the arch is most intuitive.

When the plane is oriented parallel to the aortic arch, it is often possible to visualize both ascending and descending segments of the aorta as well as the origin of the innominate, left common carotid, left subclavian, and right pulmonary arteries (Fig. 5.40). Because of the proximity of the arch to the transducer, a 90-degree sector may not be wide enough to simultaneously record both ascending and descending segments of the aorta. Angulation of the transducer is necessary for a complete recording in such patients. From this position, the transducer can be rotated 90 degrees to provide the perpendicular plane, which demonstrates the arch in short-axis orientation. From this view, the right pulmonary artery and left atrium can usually be recorded. By adjusting the scan plane leftward and slightly anteriorly, the superior vena cava can also be visualized. Figure 5.41 illustrates the

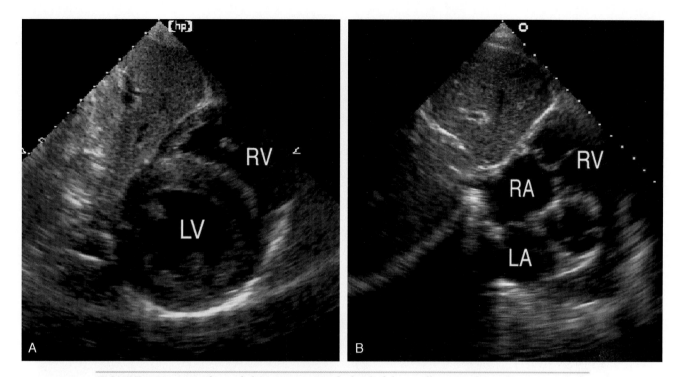

FIGURE 5.38. **A:** A subcostal short-axis view at the level of the papillary muscles is shown. **B:** A short-axis view at the base is shown. This view provides a clear recording of the interatrial septum and the right ventricular outflow tract, pulmonary valve, and main pulmonary artery. LA, left atrium; LV, left ventricle; RA, right atrium; RV, right ventricle.

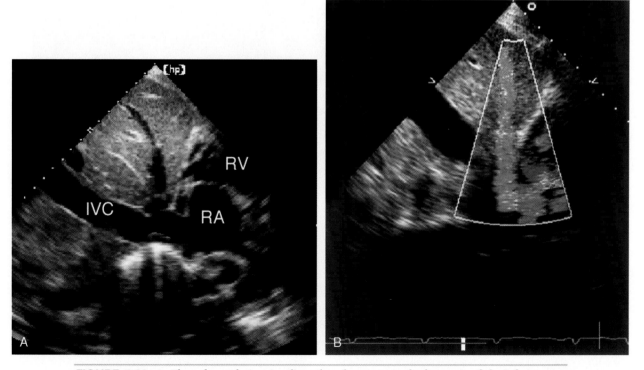

FIGURE 5.39. **A:** The subcostal view is adjusted to demonstrate the long-axis of the inferior vena cava (*IVC*) joining the right atrium (*RA*). **B:** Color flow imaging of hepatic vein flow is demonstrated. RV, right ventricle.

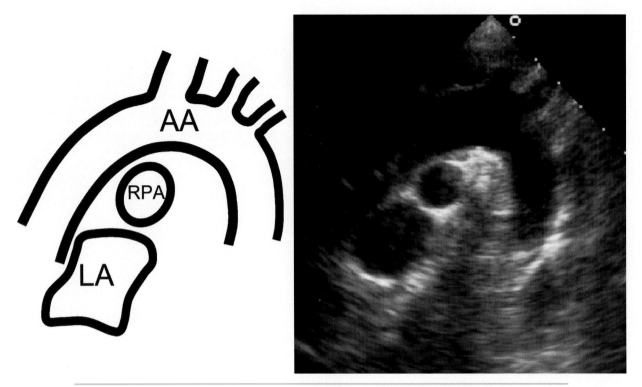

FIGURE 5.40. From the suprasternal notch, the imaging plane is aligned parallel to the aortic arch (*AA*). The relationship among the arch, right pulmonary artery (*RPA*), and left atrium (*LA*) is demonstrated.

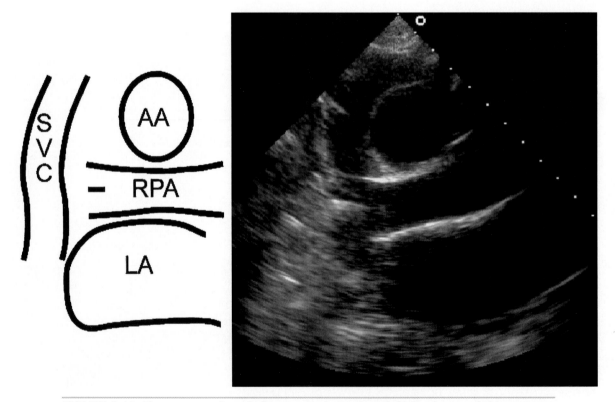

FIGURE 5.41. The suprasternal notch also permits the aortic arch (*AA*) to be recorded in cross section. This plane allows visualization of the superior vena cava (*SVC*) and demonstrates the right pulmonary artery (*RPA*) coursing below the arch and above the left atrium (*LA*).

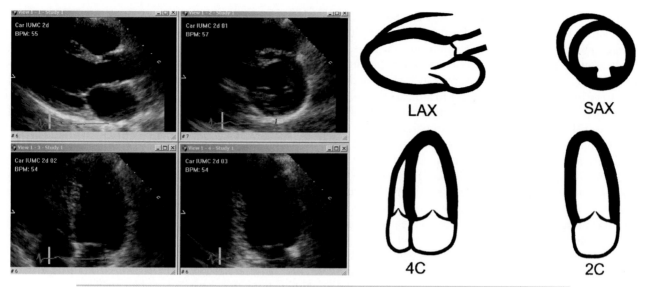

FIGURE 5.42. In a quad screen format, the four views most often included are the parasternal long- and short-axis and the apical four- and two-chamber views. LAX, long axis; SAX, short axis; 4C, four chamber; 2C, two chamber.

suprasternal short-axis view, demonstrating the aortic arch in cross section, and, below it, the right pulmonary artery and left atrium can be seen.

It should be clear from the previous sections that numerous echocardiographic views can and should be routinely recorded. Using digital techniques, it is common to display multiple views in a single quad screen format. Although any views can be included in the four quadrants, it has become customary to display the parasternal long- and short-axis and the apical four- and two-chamber views (Fig. 5.42). This format has several advantages, including providing a thorough display of the left ventricular walls. This makes it particularly useful for wall motion analysis and in stress echocardiography. These topics are covered in later chapters.

ORIENTATION OF TWO-DIMENSIONAL IMAGES

Orientation of the echocardiographic image has been addressed by the American Society of Echocardiography. In the parasternal long-axis view, for example, the aorta is positioned to the right side of the sector scan. In the short-axis view, the right ventricle is displayed to the left side, as if the observer were viewing the heart from the apex. From the apex, the four-chamber view is most often displayed with the right heart to the left of the screen and the left heart to the right. In some laboratories, this is reversed, as illustrated in Figure 5.43. There are no particular advantages or disadvantages of either approach, therefore consistency and standardization among different laboratories should be the priority. Another variation is to invert the apical images so that the atria are displayed at the top of

the screen and the ventricular apex at the bottom. This may be regarded as more anatomically "correct" and is favored by most pediatric echocardiographers. As a result, several of the illustrations in the chapter on congenital heart diseases (Chapter 18) follow this convention.

To account for the multiple possibilities with respect to orientation, the American Society of Echocardiography has recommended a standardized approach to two-

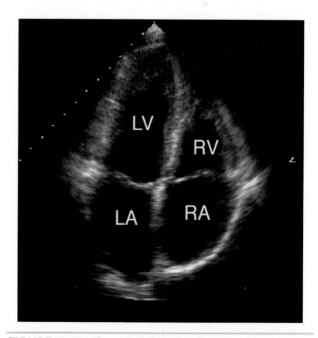

FIGURE 5.43. The apical four-chamber view is sometimes recorded with this orientation that places the right heart on the right side of the display. LA, left atrium; LV, left ventricle; RA, right atrium; RV, right ventricle.

dimensional echocardiographic imaging. The Society further suggests that all two-dimensional imaging transducers have an index mark that clearly indicates the edge of the ultrasonic plane, i.e., the direction in which the ultrasound beam is swept. It is conventional for this index mark to be located on the transducer to indicate that edge of the image that will appear on the right side of the display screen (Fig. 5.44). For example, in parasternal long-axis examination, the index mark should be oriented in the direction of the aorta and the aorta should appear to the observer's right of the image display. Furthermore, it is recommended that the index mark should point in the direction of either the patient's head or his or her left side. The effect of this convention is to position the parasternal long-axis view so that the aorta is to the right, the short-axis view so that the right ventricle is to the left side, and the apical four-chamber view so that the left heart is to the right. Finally, the subcostal four-chamber view shows the two ventricles to the right of the screen. These conventions are followed throughout this text.

TWO-DIMENSIONAL ECHOCARDIOGRAPHIC MEASUREMENTS

Two-dimensional echocardiography lends itself to quantitation, and routine measurements should be a part of most comprehensive echocardiographic examinations. A list of standard measurements available with transthoracic echocardiography is provided in Table 5.3. Recently, the American Society of Echocardiography has made recommendations regarding the measurements and descriptive items that constitute a standard report of an adult transthoracic echocardiogram (Gardin, et al, 2002). This document offers a comprehensive listing of the various features that should be routinely analyzed. The goal of such a listing is to encourage standardization of echocardiographic reports and to ensure that examinations are thorough and comprehensive. Guidelines for performing and interpreting such measurements are provided in the chapters corresponding to the chamber or valve being analyzed.

LEFT VENTRICULAR WALL SEGMENTS

Although the left ventricle could be divided into any number of segments, the American Society of Echocardiography has adopted a set of standards and recommended terminology. The scheme begins by dividing the left ventricle into thirds along the major axis from base to apex (Fig. 5.45). The most basal third of the left ventricle extends from the atrioventricular groove to the tip of the papillary

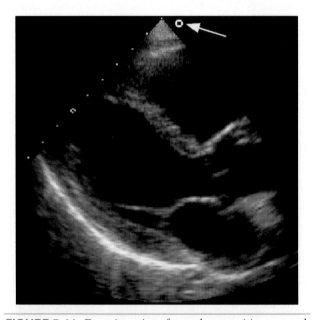

FIGURE 5.44. For orientation of transducer position, most ultrasound manufacturers provide an index mark along one side of the transducer. It is conventional that this index mark be located on the transducer to indicate that edge of the image that will appear to the right side of the display screen (*arrow*).

▶ **TABLE 5.3 Two Dimensional Echocardiographic Measurements**

Direct Measurement	Derived Data
Linear measurements	
LVd (minor axis dimension at end-diastole)	Fractional shortening (%)
LVs (minor axis dimension at end-systole)	
Left atrial dimension (at end-systole)	
IVSh (Interventricular septal wall thickness at end-diastole)	LV mass
PWh (posterior LV wall thickness at end-diastole)	
LVOTd (left ventricular outflow tract dimension, systole)	Stroke volume, aortic valve area
Area measurements	
SAXd (LV short-axis area at end-diastole)	Fractional area change (%)
SAXs (LV short-axis area at end-systole)	
Left atrial area (at end-systole)	Left atrial volume
LVVd (left ventricular volume, apical view, end-diastole)	
LVVs (left ventricular volume, apical view, end-systole)	LV ejection fraction (%)
MVa (mitral valve area, early diastole)	Mitral stenosis severity

LV, left ventricle.

muscles. The middle third is identified as that portion of the left ventricle containing the papillary muscles, and the apical third begins at the base of the papillary muscle and extends to the apex. The Society also identifies the left ventricular outflow tract as the area extending from the free edge of the anterior mitral leaflet to the aortic valve anulus.

The next step is to divide each region into segments around the circumference of the minor axis. The basal and mid thirds are customarily divided into six segments each, and the apical region is divided into four segments, as illustrated in Figure 5.46. The result is the creation of 16 segments that comprise the left ventricle. The rationale for this approach was intended to reconcile the short-axis planes at each level with the three corresponding longitudinal views: the parasternal long-axis, the apical four-chamber, and the apical two-chamber views. In addition, this segmentation approach was intended to acknowledge the importance of coronary artery anatomy to wall motion analysis. As is discussed in Chapter 15, this scheme provided a logical and rational correlation between coronary distribution and left ventricular segmentation.

As is seen in Figure 5.46, one practical advantage of this approach is that each segment can be visualized in both a long-axis and a corresponding short-axis projection. Using three short-axis planes (one corresponding to each of the thirds of the left ventricle) and the three longitudinal projections, a total of six basal, six mid, and four apical segments are recorded. Thus, whether one assesses the left ventricular segments from a series of three short-axis planes or three longitudinal projections, the total number of segments and their interrelationships are preserved. This occurs because the parasternal long-axis view does not visualize the apex, thereby accounting for the fact that there are only four segments in the apical short-

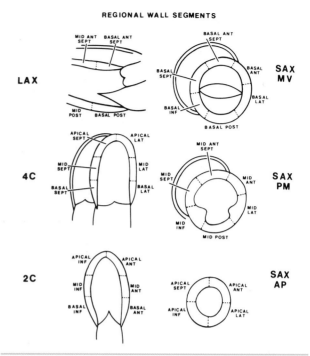

REGIONAL WALL SEGMENTS

FIGURE 5.46. The 16-segment model for left ventricular segmentation is demonstrated. See text for details. LAX, parasternal long-axis; 4C, apical four chamber; 2C, apical two chamber; SAX MV, parasternal short-axis view at the level of the mitral valve; SAX PM, parasternal short-axis view at the papillary muscle level; SAX AP, apical short-axis view.

axis projection. Even so, the apex is relatively overrepresented in this scheme. This is commonly referred to as the 16-segment model and has become the standard approach for assessing regional left ventricular function and wall motion analysis.

More recently, in an attempt to standardize terminology among the various imaging modalities and to improve consistency with respect to left ventricular segmentation, a task force representing various organizations has recommended a 17-segment model of the left ventricle. This document (Cerqueira et al., 2002) addresses nomenclature and segmentation in an effort to reconcile differences among echocardiography, nuclear imaging, and the newer cardiac modalities such as computed tomography, magnetic resonance imaging, and positron emission tomography. The major recommendation of this document was to identify the apex as a separate (the 17th) segment (Fig. 5.47). The impact of this document on the general practice of echocardiography remains to be determined.

M-MODE EXAMINATION

With the development of two-dimensional and Doppler echocardiography, the M-mode examination has been subjugated to a supporting role. Although it is rarely, if

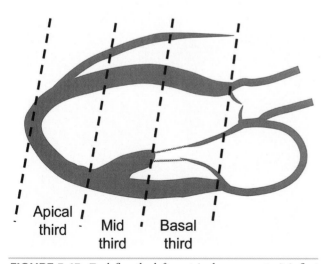

FIGURE 5.45. To define the left ventricular segments, it is first necessary to divide the left ventricle into apical, mid, and basal thirds, as shown in the schematic.

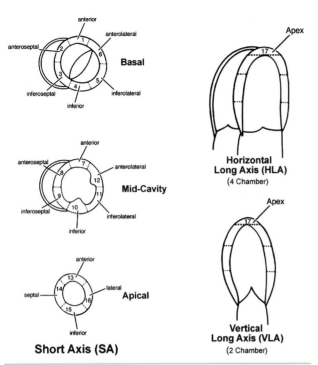

FIGURE 5.47. An alternative approach to segmenting the left ventricle suggests identifying the apex as a separate (17th) segment. See text for details. (From Cerqueira MD, Weissman NJ, Dilsizian V, et al. Circulation 2002;105:539–542, with permission.

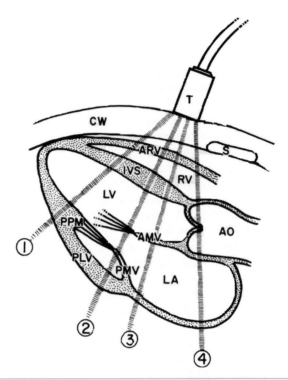

FIGURE 5.48. With a transducer (*T*), placed on the chest wall (*CW*) in the parasternal window, a variety of possible M-mode views can be recorded. See text for details. ARV, anterior right ventricular wall; Ao, aorta; AMV, anterior mitral valve leaflet; PMV, posterior mitral valve leaflet; IVS, interventricular septum; LA, left atrium; LV, left ventricle; PLV, posterior left ventricular wall; PPM, posterior papillary muscle; RV, right ventricle; S, sternum. (From Feigenbaum H. Clinical applications of echocardiography. Prog Cardiovasc Dis 1972;14:531–558, with permission.)

ever, performed as a freestanding study, the ancillary information provided by M-mode echocardiography still has a role to play in many clinical situations. To obtain an M-mode image, a single raster line from the two-dimensional image is selected and displayed. Distance, or depth, is displayed along the vertical axis and time along the horizontal axis. One of the strengths of M-mode echocardiography is the very high temporal resolution that it provides. This yields a very rapid sampling rate and affords the ability to record subtle and/or high-frequency motion.

Figure 5.48 demonstrates four M-mode positions that can be obtained from the parasternal window. In each case, the ultrasound first penetrates the chest wall, then the right ventricular cavity, and finally into the left heart structures. Depending on the level selected, different left heart structures are recorded, from apex to base in the figure. Because of the high rate of sampling, some rapidly moving structures may be optimally imaged with this technique. For example, abnormalities of interventricular septal motion, such as those due to left bundle branch block, right ventricular volume overload, or other abnormal right ventricular filling patterns, can be readily demonstrated. Subtle abnormalities of mitral valve motion can only be seen using the M-mode technique. These include the fine fluttering associated with aortic regurgitation and the B bump caused by elevated left ventricular diastolic pressure. Figure 5.49 demonstrates a B bump

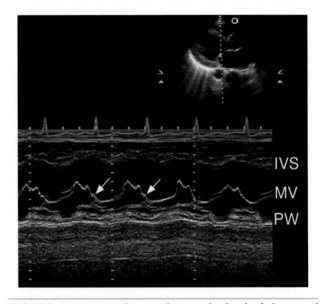

FIGURE 5.49. M-mode recording at the level of the mitral valve is shown. A B bump is indicated by the *arrows*. IVS, interventricular septum; MV, mitral valve; PW, posterior wall.

from a patient with dilated cardiomyopathy. The subtlety and brief duration of the B bump make it impossible to appreciate with two-dimensional imaging. Abnormalities of posterior wall and/or interventricular septal motion, as would occur in patients with constrictive pericarditis, can also be detected.

It is clear that M-mode echocardiography has a limited role to play in the modern comprehensive echocardiographic examination. However, several specific clinical situations are optimally assessed using this modality. For example, the early diastolic right ventricular free wall collapse that occurs in patients with tamponade is best recorded using an M-mode view that simultaneously demonstrates right ventricular free wall motion and motion of one of the cardiac valves. Including valve motion in the scan allows precise timing and identification of early diastole. If the right ventricular wall motion is collapsing during this time, evidence of a hemodynamically significant effusion has been demonstrated.

Another important application of M-mode echocardiography involves the study of hypertrophic cardiomyopathy. Several of the subtle hemodynamic abnormalities of this condition, such as partial mid-systolic closure of the aortic valve due to subvalvular obstruction and systolic anterior motion of the mitral valve, are demonstrated best using M-mode echocardiography. Partial mid-systolic closure of the aortic valve may be the best way to differentiate subvalvular from valvular aortic stenosis (Fig. 5.50). M-mode also provides unique information on the pulmonary valve. An example of a pulmonary valve M-mode echocardiogram is shown in Figure 5.51. The small letters indicate the various motions of a normal pulmonary

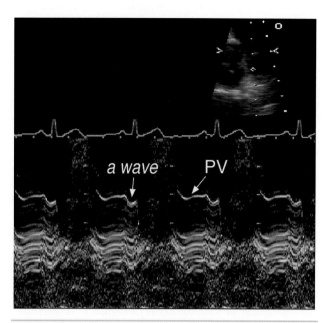

FIGURE 5.51. An M-mode recording of pulmonary valve (*PV*) motion is shown. The A-wave, corresponding to right atrial systole, is indicated.

leaflet. For example, the downward motion labeled *a* corresponds to atrial contraction and corresponds to the A-wave of mitral valve Doppler inflow. One of the earliest echocardiographic signs associated with valvular pulmonary stenosis was an exaggerated A-wave. Another finding, mid-systolic notching of pulmonary valve echo, is indicative of pulmonary hypertension. This was a valuable finding before the availability of Doppler imaging and was often the only echocardiographic indication of elevated pulmonary artery pressure. More recently, the accurate quantitative information provided by the Doppler approach has relegated this M-mode application to historic interest only.

Although less important now than in the past, one of the earliest advantages of M-mode echocardiography was its use for quantifying chamber sizes and function. Much of this has now been supplanted by two-dimensional echocardiography, which provides better spatial orientation for proper alignment of the measurements. In some laboratories, M-mode measurements are still performed, particularly the measurements of chamber dimension, left ventricular wall thickness, and left ventricular fractional shortening. Several other specific applications of M-mode echo continue to play a role in the practice of echocardiography. These are discussed in the respective chapters dealing with valvular and congenital heart diseases.

TRANSESOPHAGEAL ECHOCARDIOGRAPHY

Although transesophageal echocardiography has become an integral part of echocardiography, it is most often per-

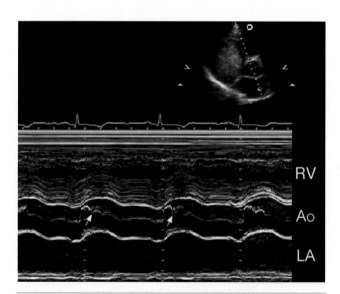

FIGURE 5.50. An M-mode recording of the aortic valve is provided, demonstrating mid systolic partial closure of the valve due to subaortic obstruction. Ao, aorta; LA, left atrium; RV, right ventricle.

formed as a separate examination. Since becoming popular in the late 1980s, transesophageal echocardiography has changed the diagnostic approach to several cardiovascular diseases. It is complementary to transthoracic echocardiography in some situations (such as in the evaluation of infective endocarditis) and has clearly supplanted the transthoracic approach in others (such as the detection of left atrial thrombi). Today, approximately 5% to 10% of all echocardiographic studies are transesophageal.

The clinical success of transesophageal echocardiography is the result of several factors. First, the close proximity of the esophagus to the posterior wall of the heart makes this approach ideal for examining several important structures. The closeness and absence of intervening tissues, such as bone or lung, allow the use of high-frequency transducers and ensure high-quality imaging in the majority of patients. Second, the ability to position the transducer in the esophagus or stomach for extended periods provides an opportunity to monitor the heart over time, such as during cardiac surgery. Third, although more invasive than other forms of echocardiography, the technique has proven to be extremely safe and well tolerated so that it can be performed in critically ill patients and very small infants.

Transesophageal echocardiography has proven to be a safe and generally well-tolerated procedure. Because of the invasive nature of the procedure and the unusual views that can potentially be recorded, special training is required of the operator as well as the nurse monitor. Transesophageal echocardiography is essentially a form of upper endoscopy. Complications are rare but include aspiration, arrhythmia, perforation of the esophagus, laryngospasm, and hematemesis. Complications may also arise from the effects of the medications that are administered as part of the examination, such as hypotension, hypertension, or hypoxia (see later). Death can occur but is very rare.

Preparation of the patient is critical to a successful procedure. A list of contraindications to transesophageal echocardiography is provided in Table 5.4. First, the patient should be thoroughly informed about the indications and procedure. Informed consent should be obtained. The patient should fast for at least 4 to 6 hours before undergoing transesophageal echocardiography. Any history of dysphagia or other forms of esophageal abnormalities should be sought. All patients should have intravenous access and both supplemental oxygen and suction should be available in all cases. Before intubation, the use of a topical anesthetic to numb the posterior pharynx is recommended. Either lidocaine or cetacaine is typically used for this purpose. Although safe and well tolerated, rare cases of toxic methemoglobinemia have been reported and should be considered whenever significant oxygen desaturation complicates the procedure. Treat-

▶ **TABLE 5.4 Contraindications to Transesophageal Echocardiography**

Esophageal pathology
   Severe dysphagia
   Esophageal stricture
   Esophageal diverticula
   Bleeding esophageal varices
   Esophageal cancer
Cervical spine disorders
   Severe atlantoaxial joint disorders
   Orthopedic conditions that prevent neck flexion

ment of this condition is intravenous administration of methylene blue, usually given in a dose of 1 mg/kg as a 1% solution over 5 minutes. Various intravenous agents are also frequently used for light sedation, for pain prevention, and as an anxiolytic. The combination of midazolam and fentanyl is popular in many laboratories. Bacteremia induced by upper endoscopy during transesophageal echocardiography is very rare. Although such decisions should always be made on an individual basis, the routine use of antibiotic prophylaxis has generally been abandoned.

To perform the procedure, the patient is placed in the left lateral decubitus position (Fig. 5.52). The head of the bed is elevated approximately 30 degrees to improve comfort and help avoid aspiration. If the patient has dentures, these should be removed, and in most patients, a bite block is placed between the teeth to prevent damage to the probe. After the probe has been lubricated with surgical jelly, it is introduced into the oropharynx and gradually advanced while the patient is urged to "swallow" to facilitate intubation. Once the probe has passed into the esophagus, a complete examination can usually be per-

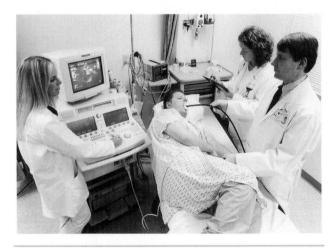

FIGURE 5.52. Patient, sonographer, nurse, and physician positioning for performing transesophageal echocardiography is demonstrated. See text for details.

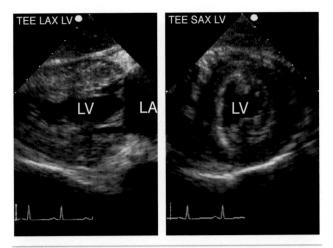

FIGURE 5.53. A biplane transesophageal echocardiogram is shown. The long-axis view of the left ventricle (*LV*) with the transducer located in the patient's stomach is shown **(left)**. The orthogonal view demonstrating a short-axis plane is shown **(right)**. LA, left atrium.

formed in 10 to 30 minutes. During this time, monitoring by a nurse is considered the standard of care. Special attention should be paid to the patient's blood pressure, heart rate and rhythm, and oxygen saturation. Suctioning of the oropharynx is often required, and additional intravenous medications may be needed to maintain the proper level of conscious sedation and comfort.

Early transesophageal echocardiographic transducers were capable of imaging from only one tomographic plane in the transverse orientation and were called monoplane devices. The second-generation instruments had biplane capability and were able to record images in both the transverse and longitudinal orientations (Fig. 5.53). Using these transducers, the various transesophageal views were obtained by moving the transducer to various levels of the esophagus and stomach and by flexing the tip of the transducer via hand controls on the device. Most current-generation transesophageal echocardiographic transducers have multiplane capability. The image is rotated, either electronically or mechanically, around a 180-degree arc to yield an infinite number of possible imaging planes. This development not only increased the number of planes that could be recorded but reduced the need for extreme flexion of the transducer tip to record all necessary information.

TRANSESOPHAGEAL ECHOCARDIOGRAPHIC VIEWS

Transesophageal echocardiography does not lend itself to standardization of views as readily as transthoracic echocardiography. As with any technique, a clear awareness of potential pitfalls and normal variants is essential.

Because the examination is often oriented toward answering a specific question or making a particular diagnosis, care must be taken to perform a thorough assessment and avoid missing important ancillary findings. The targeted nature of the test, together with the constraints imposed by the esophagus and its relation to the heart, limit our ability to define and describe standard views using this modality. Despite these limitations, some degree of standardization is both appropriate and beneficial to ensure a complete and comprehensive examination. This is accomplished by advancing the probe to the level of the superior portion of the left atrium and then recording a series of transverse and longitudinal views at sufficient levels to provide a comprehensive assessment of the entire heart.

A useful starting point is the four-chamber view, which is recorded with the transducer positioned immediately superior and posterior to the left atrium and flexed in a way to provide a long-axis plane through all four chambers (Fig. 5.54). Because of the relationship between the heart and esophagus, a true long-axis plane is often difficult to achieve. However, with proper transducer positioning, an image that approximates the apical four-chamber view (recorded upside down) can usually be obtained (Fig. 5.55). This perspective provides similar information to the corresponding transthoracic view, seen from the opposite direction. Because of the different perspectives of the two modalities, it is important to point out that each has its advantages and limitations. For example, the transthoracic four-chamber view places the

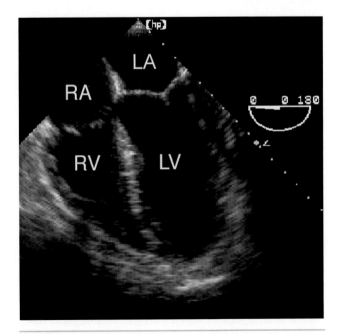

FIGURE 5.54. With the transducer positioned in the esophagus, a four-chamber view is illustrated. LA, left atrium; LV, left ventricle; RA, right atrium; RV, right ventricle.

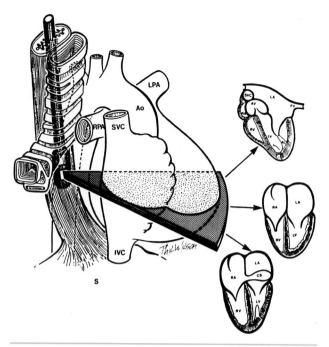

FIGURE 5.55. Three of the echocardiographic views that can be obtained with the horizontal probe in the mid esophageal location. LPA, left pulmonary artery; Ao, aorta; RPA, right pulmonary artery; SVC, superior vena cava; IVC, inferior vena cava; S, stomach; LA, left atrium; PV, pulmonary vein; AV, aortic valve; LV, left ventricle; RV, right ventricle; RA, right atrium; CS, coronary sinus.

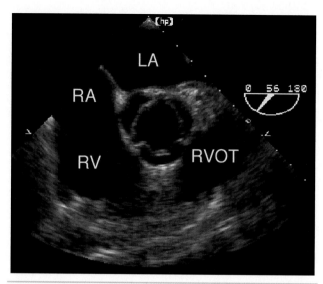

FIGURE 5.56. From the esophagus, the probe can be flexed to yield a basal short-axis projection. LA, left atrium: RA, right atrium: RV, right ventricle; RVOT, right ventricular outflow tract.

left ventricular apex in the near field and is ideally suited to detect apical thrombi. In contrast, the transesophageal four-chamber view places the left atrium in the near field and is ideally suited for assessing left atrial and mitral valve pathology.

By anteflexing the probe tip, the long-axis orientation can be gradually converted into a more short-axis view for evaluation of the left ventricular outflow tract and aortic valve (Fig. 5.56). This view is similar to a parasternal basal short-axis view obtained from the chest wall. By gently flexing and relaxing the probe, the aortic root, aortic valve, and left ventricular outflow tract can be thoroughly assessed (Fig. 5.57). By rotating the array angle from 0 degrees (transverse) to approximately 90 degrees, a two-chamber view can be obtained (Fig. 5.58). Further angle rotation, to approximately 135 degrees, will approximate a left ventricular long-axis view (Fig. 5.59). This plane is closely aligned to the long axis of the heart and provides an excellent assessment of the aortic valve and aortic root. Rotation of the probe clockwise will sweep the imaging plane toward the right heart, eventually recording the bicaval view in which the right atrium, right atrial appendage, and inferior and superior vena cava are visualized (Fig. 5.60). This view also provides a thorough assessment of the atrial septum and is especially helpful to

interrogate the superior portion of the atrial septum for sinus venosus defects.

The left atrial appendage, a frequent target of transesophageal echocardiography, can be visualized in several of the views just described. The basal short-axis view at approximately 45 degrees is often ideal for this purpose. A more vertical plane (approximately 90–120 degrees) with leftward rotation of the probe will also record the appendage (Fig. 5.61). By withdrawing the probe slightly and adjusting to a more horizontal plane (approximately 0 degrees), the bifurcation of the main pulmonary artery can be visualized adjacent to the ascending aorta (Fig. 5.62). The thoracic aorta, another structure uniquely suited to transesophageal echocardiographic inspection, lies in close proximity to the esophagus and on the opposite side from the heart (Fig. 5.63). With the array angle at 0 degrees, the transducer itself is rotated 180 degrees to view the aorta in short axis. Beginning distally, gradual withdrawal of the transducer will follow the descending aorta in a retrograde manner up toward the arch (Fig. 5.64). Some degree of rotation is often required to maintain visualization, but the entire course of the vessel can generally be recorded. At any point, adjusting the array angle to a vertical plane will provide a corresponding longitudinal view. At the level of the aortic arch, the origin of the branch vessels can be recorded (Fig. 5.65). Then, by rotating the transducer and gradually advancing the probe further into the esophagus, a portion of the ascending aorta can be recorded. Because of the interposition of the trachea, some portion of the ascending aorta will not be seen in most patients. These series of views provide an excellent opportunity to detect aortic aneurysm, dissection, and atherosclerosis.

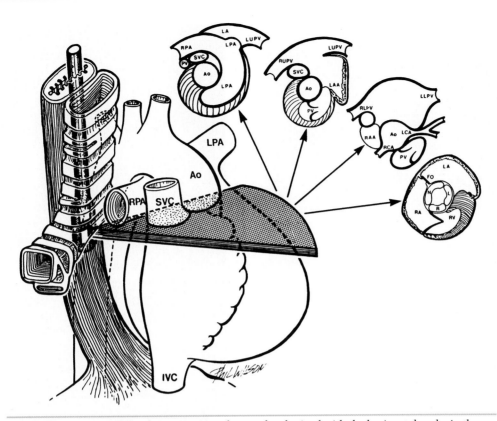

FIGURE 5.57. Four of the short-axis views that can be obtained with the horizontal probe in the upper esophagus. LPA, left pulmonary artery; Ao, aorta; SVC, superior vena cava; RPA, right pulmonary artery; IVC, inferior vena cava; S, stomach; LA, left atrium; LUPV, left upper pulmonary vein; RUPV, right upper pulmonary vein; LAA, left atrial appendage; PV, pulmonary valve; RAA, right atrial appendage; LCA, left coronary artery; RCA, right coronary artery; FO, foramen ovale; RV, right ventricle; N, noncoronary cusp; R, right coronary cusp.

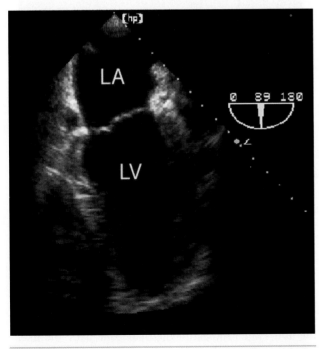

FIGURE 5.58. By adjusting the array angle to approximately 90 degrees, a two-chamber view is recorded. LA, left atrium; LV, left ventricle.

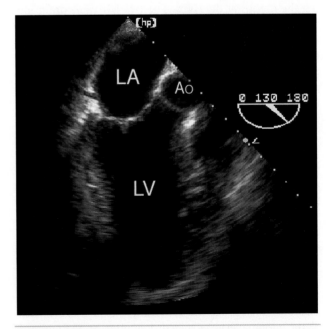

FIGURE 5.59. By increasing the array angle to approximately 130 degrees, the left ventricular outflow tract, aortic valve, and proximal aorta (*Ao*) can be included in the plane, yielding a long-axis view. LA, left atrium; LV, left ventricle.

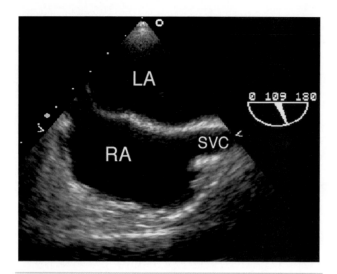

FIGURE 5.60. With the probe relatively high within the esophagus, a vertical plane allows both atria and the interatrial septum to be recorded. This plane is called the bicaval view and also records the entrance of the superior vena cava (*SVC*) into the right atrium (*RA*). LA, left atrium.

The junction of the four pulmonary veins and the posterior wall of the left atrium often can be visualized with transesophageal echocardiography. To record the left pulmonary veins, the transducer angle is adjusted to approximately 100 degrees and the transducer is rotated to the far leftward plane (counterclockwise rotation of the probe). Color flow imaging can be used to assist in locating the mouth of the veins. The two left veins drain into the left atrium in close proximity to each other, and the left upper pulmonary vein is often recorded adjacent to the left atrial appendage (Fig. 5.66). To record the right pulmonary veins, adjust the transducer angle to 50 to 60 degrees and rotate the probe to the patient's far right. Again, the two veins appear to originate together, sometimes as a bifurcation.

The transducer can also be advanced into the patient's stomach to provide a family of views from this unique perspective. Beginning from the transverse plane (0 degrees), extreme anteflexion and gradual withdrawal of the probe will bring the transducer in contact with the superior portion of the stomach, with the ultrasound beam directed upward toward the heart. A series of short-axis views of the ventricles can then be recorded by sequential anteflexion and retroflexion to visualize the various levels of short axis planes (Fig. 5.67). Often, some angle adjustment is required to optimize the true short-axis view. Then, by increasing the array angle to a more vertical plane, a long-axis view is recorded, often providing excellent visualization of the left ventricular outflow tract and aortic valve.

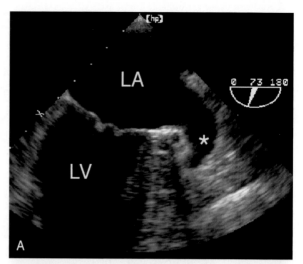

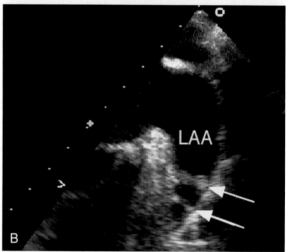

FIGURE 5.61. A: A vertical plane from the mid esophagus demonstrates the left atrial appendage (*LAA*, *). **B:** Pectinate muscles (*arrows*) within the LAA are illustrated. These may be confused with thrombi. LA, left atrium; LV, left ventricle.

ECHOCARDIOGRAPHY AS A SCREENING TEST

The availability, utility, and noninvasive nature of echocardiography have fostered its popularity as a diagnostic test. In this chapter, an approach to the echocardiographic examination that yields accurate and potentially important information in a variety of clinical situations is described. When properly applied, the diagnostic and prognostic utility of echocardiography are unmatched. As with any procedure, however, the potential for overuse exists, and the decision to perform an echocardiogram must always be balanced by the expected value of the results. These should be judged in terms of the anticipated impact of the diagnostic data, the likelihood that the results will alter management, or the prognostic value of the results to reassure or persuade a pa-

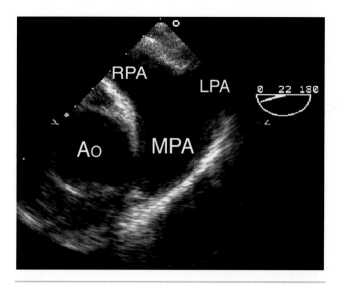

FIGURE 5.62. From a high esophageal position, the horizontal plane will permit the relationship between the main pulmonary artery (*MPA*) and aorta (*Ao*) to be recorded. This view also allows the bifurcation of the MPA into the right (*RPA*) and left (*LPA*) pulmonary arteries to be demonstrated. The ascending aorta is shown in cross section.

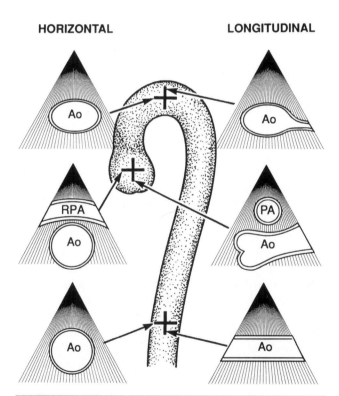

FIGURE 5.63. The various horizontal and longitudinal views of the aorta that can be obtained with transesophageal echocardiography. Ao, aorta; RPA, right pulmonary artery; PA, pulmonary artery.

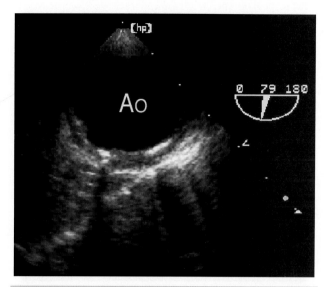

FIGURE 5.64. A cross-sectional view of the descending aorta (*Ao*) is shown.

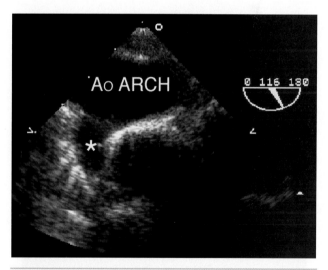

FIGURE 5.65. The distal aortic arch can often be recorded from a vertical plane. In this example, the origin of the left subclavian artery can be seen (*).

tient in a given situation. Thus, the more specific and targeted the question being asked, the more likely it is that the test will provide useful new information. If applied too widely, the yield of the test will be offset by the cost and potential for misleading information.

When used as a screening tool, the benefits of echocardiography depend on the specific situation, some of which are listed in Table 5.5. It should be clear from the preceding discussion that echocardiography is not an appropriate test to screen the general population for heart disease. Although some important positive results might be found, the low yield and the potential for false-positive findings

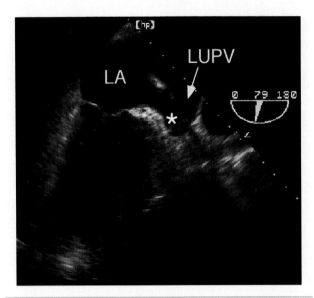

FIGURE 5.66. This view demonstrates the relationship between the left atrial appendage (*) and the left upper pulmonary vein (*LUPV*) from the two-chamber view.

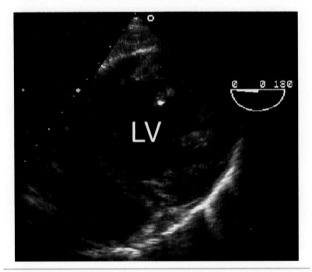

FIGURE 5.67. Transgastric imaging demonstrates a short-axis view at the mid left ventricular (*LV*) level.

▶ **TABLE 5.5 Indications for Echocardiography to Screen for the Presence of Cardiovascular Disease**

	Class
1. Patients with a family history of genetically transmitted cardiovascular disease	I
2. Potential donors for cardiac transplantation	I
3. Patients with phenotypic features of Marfan syndrome or related connective tissue diseases	I
4. Baseline and reevaluations of patients undergoing chemotherapy with cardiotoxic agents	I
5. First-degree relatives of patients with unexplained dilated cardiomyopathy in whom no etiology has been identified	I
6. Patients with systemic disease that may affect the heart	IIb
7. The general population	III
8. Competitive athletes without clinical evidence of heart disease	III
9. Routine screening echocardiogram for participation in competitive sports in patients with normal cardiovascular history, electrocardiogram, and examination	III

Adapted from Cheitlin MD, Alpert JS, Armstrong WF, et al. ACC/AHA Guidelines for the Clinical Application of Echocardiography : a report of the American College of Cardiology/American Heart Association Task Force on Practice Guidelines (Committee on Clinical Application of Echocardiography) developed in collaboration with the American Society of Echocardiography. Circulation 1997;95:1686-1744, with permission.

TRAINING IN ECHOCARDIOGRAPHY

As the field of echocardiography has continued to grow, the need for guidelines for training and proficiency has become apparent. Several documents have attempted to address these issues. Recently, a revision of the recommendations for training in cardiovascular medicine (Core Cardiology Training II or COCATS 2) has been published (Beller et al., 2002). The document addresses fellowship training as well as supplemental training for physicians in practice. It defines three levels of expertise based on the duration, volume, and breadth of experience (Table 5.6). In addition to the recommendations for general transthoracic echocardiography, the guidelines also address special procedures, such as transesophageal, contrast, stress, intraoperative, and intravascular echocardiography. A joint task force of several organizations has recently issued updated guidelines for clinical competence in echocardiography (Quinones, et al, 2003). This comprehensive document focuses on training requirements for the various echocardiographic modalities and techniques. It includes recommendations regarding competency standards for several of the emerging methodologies, such as handheld and intracardiac ultrasound.

argue against this approach. In other situations, however, screening with echocardiography is clearly justified based on clinical evidence. As is always the case, the specific decision to perform the test is predicated on several factors. First, the ordering physician must understand the expected value of the results and be able to apply the new information to the patient. The patient must be informed, both of the expected utility of the test results and the potential for inaccurate or incomplete results. Finally, the study must be performed and interpreted in an expert manner by professionals aware of the question being posed.

▶ **TABLE 5.6 Summary of Training Requirements in Echocardiography**

Level	Duration of Training (mo)	Cumulative Duration of Training (mo)	Minimal Total No. of TTE Examinations Performed	Minimal Total No. of TTE Examinations Interpreted	TEE and Special Procedures
1	3	3	75	150	Yes[a]
2	3	6	150	300	Yes[b]
3	6	12	300	750	Yes

[a]Initial exposure to transesophageal echocardiography and other special procedures
[b]Completion of level 2 and additional special training needed to achieve full competence in transesophageal echocardiography and special procedures.
TEE, transesophageal echocardiography; TTE, transthoracic echocardiography.
Adapted from Beller GA, Bonow RO, Fuster V. ACC revised recommendations for training in adult cardiovascular medicine. Core Cardiology Training II (COCATS 2) (Revision of the 1995 COCATS training statement). J Am Coll Cardiol 2002;39:1242-1246, with permission.

SUGGESTED READINGS

Beller GA, Bonow RO, Fuster V. ACC revised recommendations for training in adult cardiovascular medicine. Core Cardiology Training II (COCATS 2). (Revision of the 1995 COCATS training statement). J Am Coll Cardiol 2002;39:1242–1246.

Cerqueira MD, Weissman NJ, Dilsizian V, et al. Standardized myocardial segmentation and nomenclature for tomographic imaging of the heart: a statement for healthcare professionals from the Cardiac Imaging Committee of the Council on Clinical Cardiology of the American Heart Association. Circulation 2002;105:539–542.

Chan KL, Cohen GI, Sochowski RA, et al. Complications of transesophageal echocardiography in ambulatory adult patients: analysis of 1500 consecutive examinations. J Am Soc Echocardiogr 1991;4:577–582.

Cheitlin MD, Alpert JS, Armstrong WF, et al. ACC/AHA Guidelines for the Clinical Application of Echocardiography: a report of the American College of Cardiology/American Heart Association Task Force on Practice Guidelines (Committee on Clinical Application of Echocardiography) developed in collaboration with the American Society of Echocardiography. Circulation 1997;95:1686–1744.

Daniel WG, Erbel R, Kasper W, et al. Safety of transesophageal echocardiography. A multicenter survey of 10,419 examinations. Circulation 1991;83:817–821.

DeMaria AN, Crawford MH, Feigenbaum H, et al. 17th Bethesda conference: adult cardiology training. Task Force IV: training in echocardiography. J Am Coll Cardiol 1986;7:1207–1208.

Djoa KK, Lancee CT, De Jong N, et al. Transesophageal transducer technology: an overview. Am J Card Imaging 1995;9:79–86.

Feigenbaum H. Clinical applications of echocardiography. Prog Cardiovasc Dis 1972;14:531–558.

Feigenbaum H, Waldhausen JA, Hyde LP. Ultrasound diagnosis of pericardial effusion. JAMA 1965;191:711–714.

Feigenbaum H, Zaky A, Waldhausen JA. Use of ultrasound in the diagnosis of pericardial effusion. Ann Intern Med 1966;65:443–452.

Gardin JM, Adams DB, Douglas PS, et al. Recommendations for a standardized report for adult transthoracic echocardiography: a report from the American Society of Echocardiography's Nomenclature and Standards Committee and Task Force for a Standardized Echocardiography Report. J Am Soc Echocardiogr 2002;15:275–290.

Henry WL, DeMaria A, Gramiak R, et al. Report of the American Society of Echocardiography Committee on Nomenclature and Standards in Two-Dimensional Echocardiography. Circulation 1908;62:212–217.

Nagueh SF, Middleton KJ, Kopelen HA, et al. Doppler tissue imaging: a noninvasive technique for evaluation of left ventricular relaxation and estimation of filling pressures. J Am Coll Cardiol 1997;30:1527–1533.

Nanda NC, Pinheiro L, Sanyal RS, et al. Transesophageal biplane echocardiographic imaging: technique, planes, and clinical usefulness. Echocardiography 1990;7:771–788.

Pearlman AS, Gardin JM, Martin RP, et al. Guidelines for physician training in transesophageal echocardiography: recommendations of the American Society of Echocardiography Committee for Physician Training in Echocardiography. J Am Soc Echocardiogr 1992;5:187–194.

Perry GJ, Helmcke F, Nanda NC, et al. Evaluation of aortic insufficiency by Doppler color flow mapping. J Am Coll Cardiol 1987;9:952–959.

Pollick C, Taylor D. Assessment of left atrial appendage function by transesophageal echocardiography. Implications for the development of thrombus. Circulation 1991;84:223–231.

Quinones MA, Douglas PS, Foster E, et al. ACC/AHA clinical competence statement on echocardiography: a report of the ACC/AHA/ACP-ASIM Task Force on Clinical Competence. J Am Coll Cardiol 2003;41:687–708.

Popp RL, Fowles R, Coltart DJ, et al. Cardiac anatomy viewed systematically with two dimensional echocardiography. Chest 1979;75:579–585.

Richardson SG, Pandian NG. Echo-anatomic correlations and image display approaches in transesophageal echocardiography. Echocardiography 1991;8:671–674.

Sahn DJ, DeMaria A., Kisslo J, et al. Recommendations regarding quantitation in M-mode echocardiography: results of a survey of echocardiographic measurements. Circulation 1978;58:1072–1083.

Schiller NB, Maurer G, Ritter SB, et al. Transesophageal echocardiography. J Am Soc Echocardiogr 1989;2:354–357.

Schiller NB, Shah PM, Crawford M, et al. Recommendations for quantitation of the left ventricle by two-dimensional echocardiography. American Society of Echocardiography Committee on Standards, Subcommittee on Quantitation of Two-Dimensional Echocardiograms. J Am Soc Echocardiogr 1989;2:358–367.

Schneider AT, Hsu TL, Schwartz SL, et al. Single, biplane, multiplane, and three-dimensional transesophageal echocardiography. Echocardiographic-anatomic correlations. Cardiol Clin 1993;11:361–387.

Settle HP, Adolph RJ, Fowler NO, et al. Echocardiographic study of cardiac tamponade. Circulation 1977;56:951–959.

Seward JB, Khandheria BK, Oh JK, et al. Transesophageal echocardiography: technique, anatomic correlations, implementation, and clinical applications. Mayo Clin Proc 1988;63:649–680.

Stoddard MF, Liddell NE, Longaker RA, et al. Transesophageal echocardiography: normal variants and mimickers. Am Heart J 1992;124:1587–1598.

Tajik AJ, Seward JB, Hagler DJ, et al. Two-dimensional real-time ultrasonic imaging of the heart and great vessels. Technique, image orientation, structure identification, and validation. Mayo Clin Proc 1978;53:271–303.

Thomas JD, Garcia MJ, Greenberg NL. Application of color Doppler M-mode echocardiography in the assessment of ventricular diastolic function: potential for quantitative analysis. Heart Vessels Suppl 1997;12:135–137.

Weyman AE. Pulmonary valve echo motion in clinical practice. Am J Med 1977;62:843–855.

Evaluation of Systolic and Diastolic Function of the Left Ventricle

GENERAL PRINCIPLES

Since its inception as a clinical tool, echocardiography has been used to assess left ventricular systolic function. With the advent of Doppler methodology for determining intracardiac blood flow and tissue motion, it has evolved into a valuable technique for assessing diastolic function as well. Virtually all forms of acquired organic heart disease are associated with abnormalities of systolic and/or diastolic function to varying degrees. Assessment of systolic and diastolic function provides valuable prognostic information as well. In nearly all instances, an assessment of left ventricular systolic function should be part of the routine examination. The need to routinely assess diastolic function is less well established. However, for patients with systolic dysfunction or for patients with hypertension, congestive heart failure, or cardiomyopathy, an assessment of diastolic function should be undertaken as well.

Initial attempts to assess left ventricular function included only linear measurements, such as the left ventricular internal dimension in diastole and systole, from which parameters such as fractional shortening and velocity of circumferential shortening could be derived. With the advent of two-dimensional echocardiography, area measurements and their derived volume calculations were also employed. Doppler echocardiography, by providing information on intracardiac blood flow, provides valuable information on systolic flow parameters and more recently diastolic function. There are several recently developed Doppler methodology based algorithms, such as strain rate imaging, that are substantially more sophisticated with respect to determining ventricular function.

Although conceptually simple, M-mode derived linear measurements have the disadvantage of only determining ventricular function along a single interrogation line. In the presence of normal geometry and symmetric function, linear measurements provide an adequate assessment of ventricular function. They are limited, however, in acquired heart disease, in which there may be substantial regional variation in function, and are subject to error with respect to determining true minor-axis dimensions. Two-dimensional imaging allows correction for off-axis interrogation and also for determination of the spatial heterogeneity of function. For this reason, measurements derived from two-dimensional echocardiography, whether linear or area based, have supplanted M-mode measurements in most laboratories.

LINEAR MEASUREMENTS

As mentioned, the first attempts to quantitate left ventricular function involved linear measurements of the minor-axis dimension from a dedicated M-mode echocardiogram. In most centers, measurement directly from two-dimensional echocardiography or two-dimensionally directed M-mode echocardiography has supplanted isolated M-mode recordings. The resolution of M-mode echocardiography for precise identification of timing is superior to that of two-dimensional echocardiography. Although the argument can be advanced that the spatial resolution of a dedicated M-mode beam is superior to that of two-dimensional echocardiography, in general, the ability to visualize the entire left ventricle and to ensure a true minor-axis dimension mitigates these potential advantages.

The precise point at which linear measurements are made has varied over time as the resolution of ultrasound instrumentation has improved. Initial ultrasound equipment had relatively poor resolution and gray-scale registration. As such, the precise boundary between the blood pool and tissue was often difficult to determine. The first approach to linear measurements involved a "leading-edge" technique. With this technique, the boundary was defined as the leading edge of the reflective echo. Using this technique, the septal thickness was defined as the leading edge of the septum on its right ventricular side to

▶ TABLE 6.1 **Linear Measurements of Left Ventricular Size and Function**

Parameter	*Formula*	*Abbreviation*	*Units*
LV internal dimension in diastole		LVIDd	mm
LV internal dimension in systole		LVIDs	mm
Fractional shortening	(LVIDd − LVIDs)/LVIDd	FS	% or 0.XX
Meridional wall stress in systole	PR/h	σ_m	mm Hg or dyne-cm^2
Cubed LV volume in diastole	(LVIDd)^3		cm^3 or ml
Cubed LV + myocardial volume	(IVS + LVIDd + PW)^3		cm^3 or ml
Velocity of circumferential shortening[a]	(LVIDd − LVIDs)/(LVIDd × ET)	VCf	circumference/sec

[a]Measured from the apical four-chamber view.
ET, ejection time; IVS, intraventricular septal thickness; LV, left ventricle; PR, pressure × radius; PW, posterior wall thickness.

the leading edge of bright endocardial echoes on the left ventricular side of the ventricular septum. Depending on the gray scale, image intensity, and resolution, the leading edge of the endocardial echo could be as much as 1 or 2 mm in thickness. Refinements in image processing have allowed greater levels of gray-scale registration with a substantially refined visualization of both the right and left sides of the ventricular septum and the blood pool—the tissue boundary. It is now common practice to measure the actual visualized thickness of the ventricular septum and other chamber dimensions as defined by the actual tissue-blood interface rather than the distance between the leading edge echoes.

Table 6.1 outlines many of the linear measurements that can be made for assessment of left ventricular function. This includes measurement of the dimension of the

left ventricular outflow tract, septal and posterior wall thickness, and the internal dimension of the left ventricle in its minor axis in diastole and systole. The location of these measurements is schematized in Figure 6.1 and further demonstrated in Figure 6.2.

There are several limitations of linear measurements of the left ventricle for determining ventricular performance. One of the most obvious is that many forms of acquired heart disease, especially coronary artery disease, will result in regional variation in ventricular function. By definition, an M-mode assessment provides information regarding size and contractility along a single line. This may either underestimate the severity of dysfunction if only a normal region is interrogated or overestimate the abnormality if the M-mode beam transits through the wall motion abnormality exclusively. A sec-

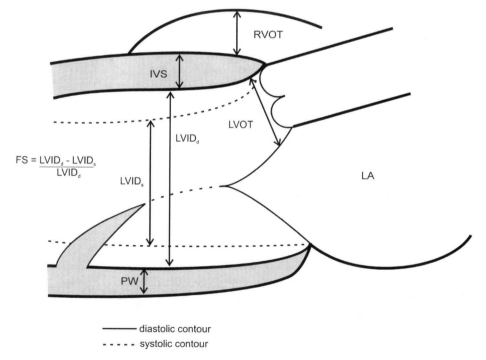

FIGURE 6.1. Schematic representation of a parasternal long-axis view of the left ventricle depicting linear measurements. By convention, linear measurement of the left ventricle is made at the level of the mitral valve chordae. From the linear internal dimension of the left ventricle in diastole and systole, fractional shortening can be calculated as noted. When measuring ventricular septal thickness, caution is advised to avoid measuring the most proximal portion of septum, which is frequently an area of isolated hypertrophy and angulation that does not truly represent ventricular wall thickness.

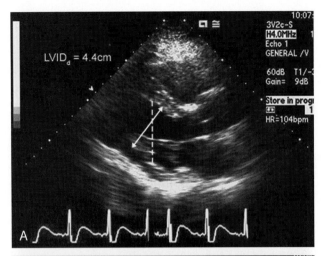

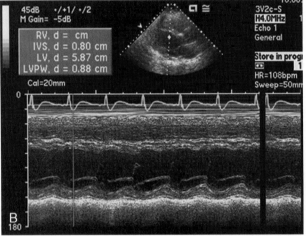

FIGURE 6.2. **Top:** A parasternal long-axis view recorded in diastole demonstrates the effect of cardiac angulation on M-mode measurements. Because the M-mode beam must conform to one of the two-dimensional interrogation lines, it frequently will intersect the left ventricle in a tangential manner (*dotted line*). This results in overestimation of the true minor-axis dimension, which in this example can be seen to be 4.4 cm (*solid arrow*). **Bottom:** The M-mode image from this view is presented and because of the tangential measurement has overestimated the internal dimension as 5.87 cm.

ond limitation of the M-mode assessment is that it often does not reflect the true minor-axis dimension. This phenomenon is illustrated in Figure 6.2 and is very common in elderly patients in whom there is angulation of the ventricular septum. In this instance, an M-mode beam traverses the ventricle in a tangential manner and often overestimates the true internal dimension. Even by using two-dimensionally guided M-mode measurements, it may not be possible to align the beam truly perpendicular to the long axis of the ventricle so that it reflects the true minor-axis dimension. When comparisons are made between M-mode and two-dimensional minor-axis dimensions, the M-mode dimension typically overestimates the true minor-axis of the left ventricle by 6 to 12

mm. For any given patient, one can generally assume that the degree of off-axis interrogation will remain stable over time. When used serially to follow progression of disease, this overestimation will remain constant for any given patient, and differences in serial measurements retain their clinical validity although the actual dimension may be incorrect.

Minor-axis linear measurement can play a different role when obtained directly from the two-dimensional image rather than from a two-dimensionally guided M-mode measurement. When measuring the minor axis of the left ventricle at the valve level, the measurement intersects the interventricular septum very close to its attachment to the aorta. Thus, the measurement is a minor axis of the base of the left ventricle. With a symmetrically contracting left ventricle, the diastolic measurement is a reasonable assessment of the size of the left ventricle and the resultant fractional shortening is an index of systolic function. In a patient with regional wall motion abnormalities, fractional shortening is a specific marker of left ventricular basal contractility and does not necessarily reflect global left ventricular function.

There are several additional parameters of ventricular performance that can be derived from linear measurements. In many instances, this requires digitization of an M-mode for calculation of derived parameters. These include rates of systolic wall thickening of the posterior wall and calculation of velocity of circumferential shortening. For the latter calculation, the minor axis is assumed to represent a circle of known diameter from which the circumference can be calculated and the rate of change of circumference determined. This measurement is typically standardized by normalizing to heart rate.

An additional linear measurement that has been employed in the past is the *descent of the base*. During ventricular contraction, the base of the heart moves toward the apex and the magnitude of this motion is directly proportional to systolic function. Typically, M-mode interrogation is undertaken of the lateral mitral valve anulus, and the amount of excursion toward the transducer is then determined (Fig. 6.3). There is a relative linear correlation between the degree of anular excursion during systole and global systolic function. This technique is rarely used today, having given way to direct measures of ventricular volume and ejection fraction. Of note, this is the same principle used in Doppler tissue imaging (DTI) of the anulus for determination of diastolic and systolic function.

Indirect M-Mode Markers of Left Ventricular Function

Several indirect signs of left ventricular systolic dysfunction can be noted on M-mode echocardiography. These include an increased E-point septal separation and gradual

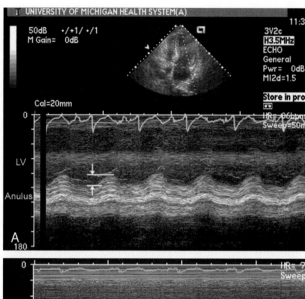

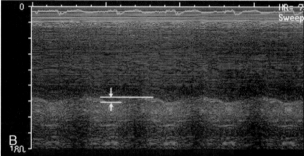

FIGURE 6.3. Apical view recorded in two patients demonstrates the measurement of the descent of the base with M-mode echocardiography. The M-mode interrogation beam has been directed from the apex of the heart through the lateral anulus. **Top:** Note the approximate 1 cm of anular motion toward the apex in systole. **Bottom:** Recording in a patient with severe systolic dysfunction reveals substantially decreased anular motion in systole.

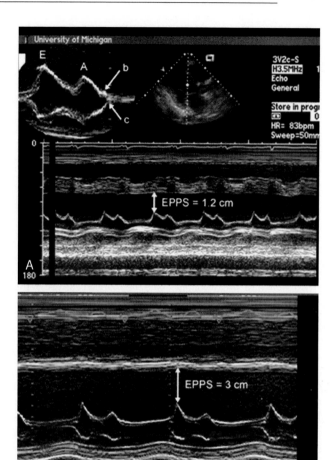

FIGURE 6.4. M-mode echocardiograms recorded in two patients with significant systolic dysfunction. **Top:** An E-point septal separation (EPSS) of 1.2 cm (normal, <6 mm). **Bottom:** Recording in a patient with more significant left ventricular systolic dysfunction in which the EPSS is 3.0 cm. Also note the interrupted closure of the mitral valve with a B bump **(top)**, indicating an increase in the left ventricular end-diastolic pressure.

closure of the aortic valve during systole. The magnitude of opening of the mitral valve, as reflected by E-wave height, correlates with transmitral flow and, in the absence of significant mitral regurgitation, with left ventricular stroke volume. The internal dimension of the left ventricle correlates with diastolic volume. As such, the ratio of mitral excursion to left ventricular size reflects the ejection fraction. Normally, the mitral valve E point (maximal early opening) is within 6 mm of the left side of the ventricular septum. In the presence of a decreased ejection fraction, this distance is increased (Fig. 6.4).

Inspection of the aortic valve opening pattern can also provide indirect evidence regarding systolic function of the left ventricle. If left ventricular forward stroke volume is decreased, there may be a gradual reduction in forward flow in late systole, which results in gradual closing of the aortic valve in late systole. This results in a rounded appearance of the aortic valve in late systole (Fig. 6.5). Many of these observations and calculations have been fully supplanted by more direct measures of ventricular size and performance available from modern ultrasound plat-

forms. The high temporal resolution of M-mode echocardiography may still be useful in select situations.

TWO-DIMENSIONAL MEASUREMENTS

Two-dimensional echocardiography provides inherently superior spatial resolution for determining left ventricular size and function. Its role in obtaining linear measurements has already been discussed. A number of different two-dimensional echocardiographic views have been used to provide information regarding ventricular systolic function, some of which rely exclusively on area measurements and others of which rely on calculation of volume from the two-dimensional image. Table 6.2 outlines commonly used two-dimensional measurements

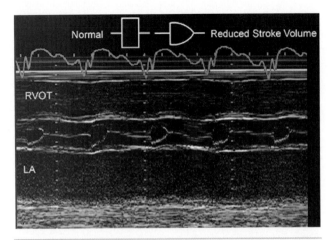

FIGURE 6.5. M-mode echocardiogram recorded through the aortic valve in a patient with reduced cardiac function and decreased forward stroke volume. Note the rounded closure of the aortic valve, indicating decreasing forward flow at the end of systole. Normal and abnormal aortic valve opening patterns are noted in the schematic superimposed on the figure.

and their derived calculations. One of the simpler two-dimensional measures of left ventricular function is the determination of a fractional area change. This is calculated in the short-axis view of the left ventricle by comparing the diastolic area with the systolic area. The area change then represents the difference of these two values divided by the diastolic volume. For a symmetrically contracting ventricle, fractional area change directly reflects global ventricular function. Its obvious limitation is that it assesses ventricular function only at the level being interrogated. If regional dysfunction is present, which is not in the interrogation plane, it may result in a misleading estimate of global ventricular function.

More commonly, two-dimensional images are used to determine ventricular volume, from which stroke volume and ejection fraction are then calculated. Figure 6.6 schematizes several of the geometric assumptions and formulas that have been used in the past for calculating ventricular volume. The advantage of the geometric assumption techniques was that they required only limited visualization for calculation of ventricular volume. Area and length methods provide a volume based on a long-axis dimension from an apical view in combination with a short-axis area, which is either directly determined from two-dimensional echocardiography or calculated based on an M-mode dimension. These formulas only work in a symmetrically contracting ventricle, but they may be particularly useful when the parasternal short-axis view is technically better than the apical views. There are several variations on area-length formulas (e.g., truncated ellipse, "bullet" formula, cylinder and cone) for determining left ventricular volume, each of which includes different assumptions regarding the anticipated geometric shape and/or incorporates regression equations to refine the calculation accuracy.

A simplified method for calculation of ejection fraction involves determining the minor-axis dimension in diastole and systole at the base, mid, and distal left ventricle. These values are combined with a qualitative assessment of apical function (-5% to $+15\%$) to derive the ejection fraction (Fig. 6.7). This methodology has correlated well with standard methods for determination of the ejection fraction.

All the geometric formulas are based on the assumption that the ventricle will adhere to a predictable shape, and if regional abnormalities are present, the accuracy of these methods decreases. The advent of high-resolution, 90-degree, two-dimensional echocardiography as well as the computational capacity of quantitation packages has reduced reliance on geometric formulas for determining volumes, in favor of a more direct assessment. The most common method for determining ventricular volumes is the Simpson rule or the "rule of disks." This technique requires recording an apical, four- or two-chamber view from which the endocardial border is outlined in end-

▶ **TABLE 6.2 Area-/Volume-Based Measurements for Ventricular Size and Function**

Parameter	Abbreviations	Formula	Units
Short axis diastolic area (at mid LV)	ASx_d		cm²
Short axis systole area (at mid LV)	ASx_s		cm²
Fractional area change	FAC	$(ASx_d - ASx_s)/ASx_d$	% or 0.XX
Four-chamber LV area in diastole	ALV_{4c-d}		cm²
Four-chamber LV area in systole	ALV_{4c-s}		cm²
LV volume in diastole[a]	LVV_d		ml
LV volume in systole[a]	LVV_s		ml
Stroke volume	SV	$LVV_d = LVV_s$	ml
Ejection fraction	EF	SV/LVV_d	% or 0.XX

[a]Determined by the Simpson rule, area length method, etc.
LV, left ventricle.

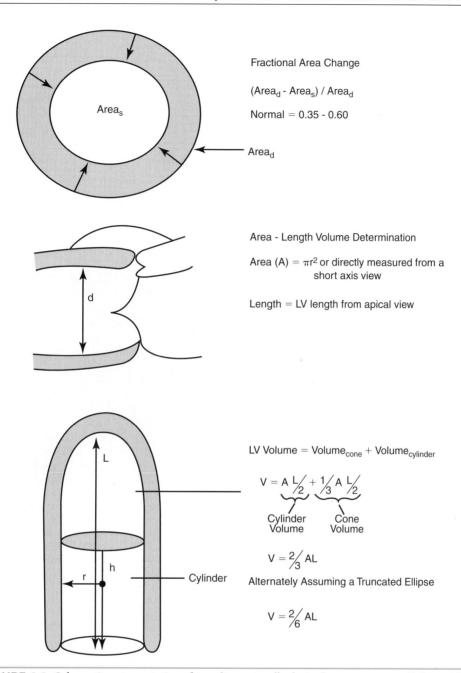

FIGURE 6.6. Schematic representation of two-dimensionally derived measurements of left ventricular systolic function. **Top:** The methodology for determining fractional area change, which is defined by the formula in the figure. **Middle** and **bottom:** Using the geometric assumption that the left ventricular cavity represents a cylinder and cone configuration, the volume of each separate component can be calculated as noted. The overall left ventricular volume equals the sum of the two volumes. See text for further details.

diastole and end-systole. The ventricle is then mathematically divided along its long axis into a series of disks of equal height. Individual disk volume is calculated as height × disk area where height is assumed to be the total length of the left ventricular long axis ÷ the number of segments or disks. The surface area of each disk is determined from the diameter of the ventricle at that point. The ventricular volume is then represented by the sum of

the volume of each of the disks, which are equally spaced along the long axis of the ventricle. This methodology is illustrated in Figure 6.8. If a ventricle is symmetrically contracting, typically either the four- or two-chamber view will then reflect the true ventricular volume. In clinical practice, the apical two-chamber view is often imaged tangentially, and the volume derived from this view may underestimate the true left ventricular volume. In any

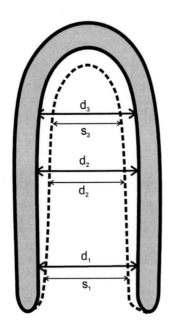

$$EF = K_{apex} + [(d_3^2 - s_3^2) + (d_2^2 - s_2^2) + (d_1^2 + s_1^2)]$$

$$K_{apex} = -5\%, 0, +5\%, +10\% \text{ or } +15\%$$

FIGURE 6.7. Schematic representation of a simplified method for determining the left ventricular ejection fraction from three separate minor-axis dimensions at the base, mid, and distal portion of the left ventricle in an apical view. The contribution of the apex is expressed as a constant (K_{apex}) ranging from −5% to +15%.

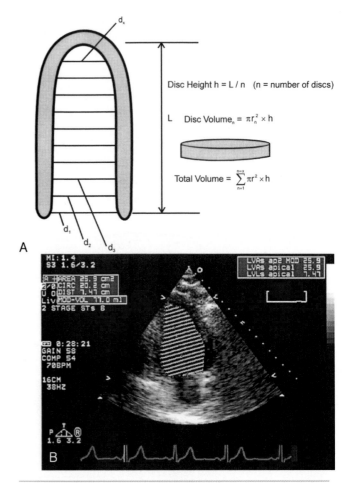

FIGURE 6.8. Method for determining the left ventricular volume from the rule of disks or Simpson rule. **Top:** The left ventricular cavity has been arbitrarily divided into 10 segments ($d_1, d_2, d_3. . .d_n$), each of equal height. The height of each cylinder is defined as overall length divided by the number of disks ($h = L/n$). Individual disk volume is calculated as noted, and the total volume of the ventricle is the sum of the individual disk volumes. **Bottom:** An actual calculation of the left ventricular volume from an apical two-chamber view.

view, foreshortening of the ventricular apex will result in inaccurate assessment of the left ventricular ejection fraction and most often in overestimation of the ejection fraction. If there is asymmetry of the ventricular geometry or a systolic wall motion abnormality, a single-plane view will have reduced accuracy for the reasons previously alluded to. In this instance, a biplane determination of volume will increase accuracy.

Once the diastolic and systolic volumes have been determined, the stroke volume can be calculated as the difference between these two volumes. Forward cardiac output then equals the product of heart rate times stroke volume. Assuming the absence of mitral or aortic insufficiency, this then represents the cardiac output. Because the difference between the diastolic and systolic left ventricular volume represents the total volume pumped by the ventricle (stroke volume), it represents the sum of forward-going stroke volume plus the volume of mitral and

aortic regurgitation, if present. Ejection fraction can be calculated from these volumes as: stroke volume ÷ end diastolic volume.

There are several limitations to using Simpson rule measurements of left ventricular volumes. First, apical views must be used, and myocardial dropout is always a potential problem. The use of tissue harmonic imaging and contrast echocardiography can decrease but not always eliminate this problem. For accurate volume determination, the transducer must be at the true apex and the ultrasonic cross-sectional beam must be through the center of the left ventricle. These conditions are frequently not met, resulting in artifactually small left ventricular volumes. There are several clues that help to determine whether the transducer is at the true apex. In the normal ventricle, the apex does not move from apex to base dur-

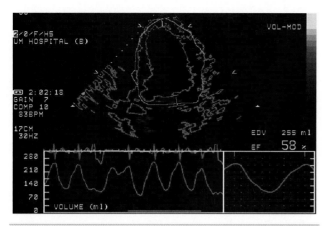

FIGURE 6.9. Automated endocardial border definition used for automatic quantitation (*AQ*) of the instantaneous left ventricular volume. **Top:** The AQ algorithm has been activated and the endocardial border is automatically tracked throughout the cardiac cycle. From this endocardial boundary, the instantaneous left ventricular volume, assuming geometric symmetry of the ventricle, is automatically calculated and plotted versus the QRS ECG. In this instance of a dilated ventricle with normal left ventricular function, the end-diastolic volume (*EDV*) is calculated as 255 mL and the ejection fraction (*EF*) is 58%. In this example, only volume and ejection fraction data have been extracted. A more detailed analysis allows the evaluation of diastolic filling rates as well.

ing filling or emptying of the chamber. Additionally, the true apex is the thinnest area of the left ventricle. If the visualized apex has the same thickness as the surrounding walls and appreciable motion in systole, it is likely to be a tangential cut through the left ventricle rather than a true on-axis view.

In an effort to automate and simplify volume determination, instrumentation is commercially available that will automatically identify and track the endocardial border of the left ventricle. The endocardial borders, which are automatically tracked, are then likewise subject to calculation of volume using the methodology described above, thereby providing an instantaneous ventricular volume display. The stroke volume and ejection fraction can be calculated from the maximal and minimal volumes (Fig. 6.9).

A further refinement of this methodology is the ability to export the instantaneous ventricular volume and then combine it with instantaneous determination of systolic pressure. This allows the creation of a pressure volume loop, which has been shown to provide load-independent information regarding ventricular contractility (Fig. 6.10).

A final refinement in the determination of ventricular volume involves the application of three-dimensional echocardiography. Three-dimensional imaging or reconstruction obviously reduces the limitation on single or biplane imaging, which has the potential to either disproportionately represent or underestimate a wall motion abnormality. By creating a three-dimensional image set, all regions of the ventricular myocardium will be incorporated in the volume determination. The different methodologies for three-dimensional echocardiography are discussed in Chapter 3. Numerous studies have demonstrated the superiority of three-dimensional imaging for determining ventricular volume, especially in abnormally shaped ventricles. Although the accuracy and reproducibility of three-dimensional volumes, when compared with anatomic models or other imaging techniques,

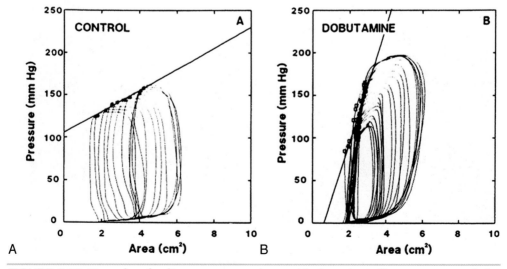

FIGURE 6.10. Examples of online pressure-area loops with the end-systolic pressure-area relation shown immediately before **(A)** and during **(B)** dobutamine infusion at 3 μg/kg body weight/min. (From Gorcsan J 3rd, Romand JA, Mandarino WA, et al. Assessment of left ventricular performance by on-line pressure-area relations using echocardiographic automated border detection. J Am Coll Cardiol 1994;23:242–252, with permission.)

are superior to those of two-dimensional imaging, often the magnitude of improvement falls below levels for which clinical decisions are made. The major technical limitation of three-dimensional volume determination has been the cumbersome nature of reconstruction techniques, which have relied on acquisition of multiple two-dimensional image sets. From a more practical perspective, it is often difficult to obtain complete endocardial definition in all images that is sufficient to result in an accurate reconstruction of cardiac chambers. Even minor

changes in transducer position, due either to patient or transducer motion, result in significant image degradation. Equipment is now available that allows real-time acquisition of a three-dimensional data set. This dramatically reduces the complexity of and time required for calculation of three-dimensional volumes. Figures 6.11 and 6.12 are examples of three-dimensional reconstruction of the left ventricle. Figure 6.13 demonstrates the relative accuracy of two- versus three-dimensional imaging for precise volume determination.

Determination of Left Ventricular Mass

Echocardiography was one of the first imaging modalities used clinically for determination of left ventricular mass. It has received widespread acceptance in epidemiologic studies of hypertension and valvular heart disease in which the presence of hypertrophy has been associated with worsened outcomes and its regression has been a goal of therapy. Left ventricular mass can be determined using a number of echocardiographic formulas and algorithms and has been shown to carry substantial prognostic importance in virtually all forms of heart disease.

The earliest methodology for determining left ventricular mass was based on M-mode measurement of septal and posterior wall thickness and the left ventricular internal dimension. M-mode calculations assume a predefined ventricular geometry, and their accuracy will diminish in

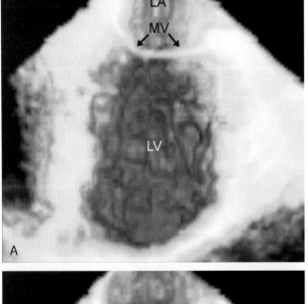

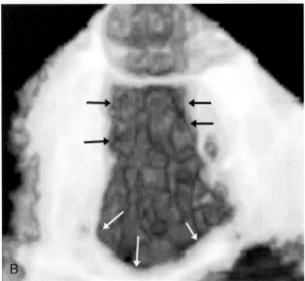

FIGURE 6.11. Three-dimensional reconstruction obtained from a transesophageal echocardiogram recorded in a patient with a large anterior apical aneurysm. **Top:** A still frame at end-diastole. Note the lack of tapering at the apex and the dilated left ventricular chamber. **Bottom:** Recorded at end-systole. Note the preserved function at the base of the heart and the dyskinesis of the aneurysmal apical segments at end-systole.

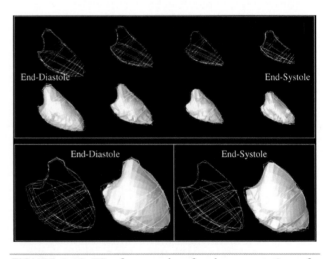

FIGURE 6.12. Wire frame and surfaced representations of a healthy left ventricle **(top)** and a dilated cardiomyopathy **(bottom)**. Four evenly spaced time points, from *ED* to *ES*, are shown for the healthy left ventricle. The dilated cardiomyopathy **(bottom)** is shown only at *ED* and *ES*. Actual volume computations were performed with contours (Fig. 6.13). (From Hibberd MG, Chuang ML, Beaudin RA, et al. Accuracy of three-dimensional echocardiography with unrestricted selection of imaging planes for measurement volumes and ejection fraction. Am Heart J 2000;140:469–475, with permission.)

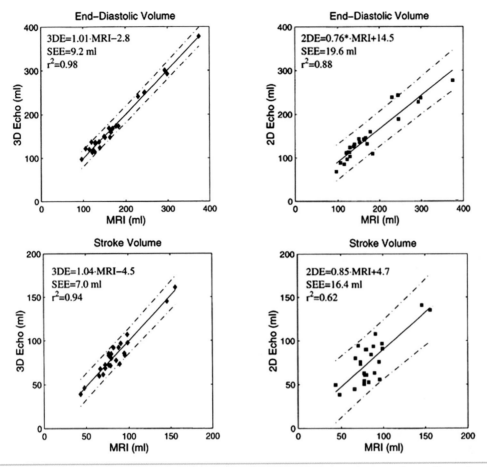

FIGURE 6.13. Graphic demonstration of the relationship between three- and two-dimensional echocardiographic volumes versus the standard of magnetic resonance imaging (MRI). Note that for both diastolic volume and stroke volume (calculated as the difference between end-diastolic and end-systolic volumes) there is a significantly greater correlation between MRI and the echocardiographic technique when three-dimensional imaging is employed compared with standard two-dimensional imaging. (From Hibberd MG, Chuang ML, Beaudin RA, et al. Accuracy of three-dimensional echocardiography with unrestricted selection of imaging planes for measurement volumes and ejection fraction. Am Heart J 2000;140:469–475, with permission.)

instances in which the left ventricular shape is abnormal. One of the methods for determining left ventricular mass is the so-called cubed (Teichholz) formula, which assumes that the left ventricle is a sphere. The diameter of this sphere is the interior dimension of the left ventricle and the sphere wall thickness is that of ventricular myocardium. The formula calculates the outer dimensions of the sphere and then the inner dimension, the difference being the presumed left ventricular myocardial volume. The cubed formula is expressed as left ventricular mass = (interventricular septum + left ventricular interior dimension + posterior wall)^3 − left ventricular interior dimension^3 (Fig. 6.14). This then gives the volume of the stylized sphere of the myocardium, which, when multiplied by the specific gravity of muscle (1.05 g/cm^3), provides an estimate of left ventricular mass. Several investigators subsequently modified this approach using regression analysis. This cubed volume approach has the

obvious limitation of determining ventricle size and wall thickness only along a single line. Although the regression equations allow calculation of a mass that correlates well with autopsy specimens, there can be substantial variation in individual subjects. The cubed methodology has been widely used, especially in serial evaluations, because for any given patient, the magnitude and direction of the error would be expected to remain constant and therefore the technique could be used for evaluating serial changes.

A more accurate determination of left ventricular mass can be obtained with two-dimensional echocardiography. When using two-dimensional echocardiography, geometric assumptions of the ventricular shape are typically still employed but the assumption is that of a bullet-shaped ventricle rather than a sphere. Additionally, mean left ventricular wall thickness is determined rather than wall thickness at only one point on the septum and posterior wall. Mean wall thickness can be calculated by determin-

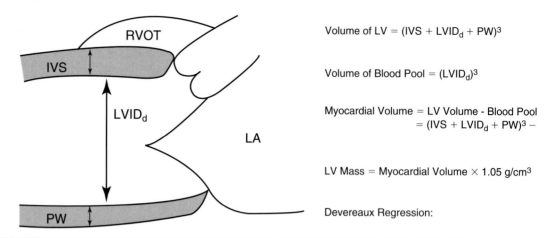

Volume of LV = $(IVS + LVID_d + PW)^3$

Volume of Blood Pool = $(LVID_d)^3$

Myocardial Volume = LV Volume - Blood Pool
= $(IVS + LVID_d + PW)^3 -$

LV Mass = Myocardial Volume $\times$ 1.05 g/cm^3

Devereaux Regression:

FIGURE 6.14. Schematic representation of the cubed formula for determining left ventricular mass. All measurements can be taken from either a two-dimensional or an M-mode echocardiogram of the minor axis of the left ventricle. The formula for calculation of left ventricular mass is as noted. Based on comparison with anatomic specimens, several regression equations have been developed that are variations on the basic cubed formula.

ing the epicardial and endocardial areas of the short axis of the left ventricle at the mid cavity level. The difference between these two areas then represents myocardial area. The left ventricular area can then be calculated either by an area length method or by assuming a truncated ellipse geometry. Figure 6.15 depicts this approach and provides the formulas used for calculation of left ventricular mass with this technique.

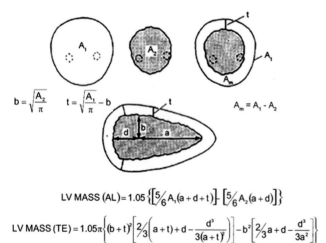

LV MASS BY AREA LENGTH (AL) AND TRUNCATED ELLIPSOID (TE)

$b = \sqrt{\dfrac{A_2}{\pi}}$ $t = \sqrt{\dfrac{A_1}{\pi}} - b$ $A_m = A_1 - A_2$

$$LV\ MASS\ (AL) = 1.05\left\{\left[\tfrac{5}{6}A_1(a+d+t)\right]-\left[\tfrac{5}{6}A_2(a+d)\right]\right\}$$

$$LV\ MASS\ (TE) = 1.05\pi\left\{(b+t)\left[\tfrac{2}{3}(a+t)+d-\dfrac{d^3}{3(a+t)^2}\right]-b^2\left[\tfrac{2}{3}a+d-\dfrac{d^3}{3a^2}\right]\right\}$$

FIGURE 6.15. Method for determining left ventricular mass using two-dimensional measurements. (From Schiller NB, Shah PM, Crawford M, et al. Recommendations for quantitation of the left ventricle by two-dimensional echocardiography. American Society of Echocardiography Committee on Standards, Subcommittee on Quantitation of Two-Dimensional Echocardiograms. J Am Soc Echocardiogr 1989;2:358–367, with permission.)

Physiologic Versus Pathologic Hypertrophy

Left ventricular hypertrophy is typically characterized as being concentric, eccentric, or physiologic (Fig. 6.16). It should be recognized that the calculation of left ventricular mass is a determination of the actual mass of the ventricular muscle and may not relate to overall cardiac enlargement. Increases in left ventricular mass can occur with chamber enlargement and relatively normal wall thickness (eccentric hypertrophy), as is seen in regurgitant valvular lesions, or secondary to a predominant increase in wall thickness with normal chamber sizes, as is seen in the pressure overload of systemic hypertension. When evaluating patients for left ventricular hypertrophy, it is important to characterize the hypertrophy as being due to either chamber enlargement or increased wall thickness. One additional index of hypertrophy is relative wall thickness defined as (posterior wall thickness + interventricular septal thickness)/left ventricular interior dimension. Relative wall thickness more than 0.45 has been used as a threshold of pathologic left ventricular hypertrophy. An additional form of hypertrophy is the physiologic hypertrophy seen in highly trained athletes. In general, this is a physiologic adaptation in which there is a slight increase in both wall thickness and chamber dimension. Wall thickness more than 13 mm is unusual in physiologic hypertrophy. Because the hypertrophy is a physiologic adaptation to physical training, wall stress tends to be normal. The physiologic hypertrophy seen in athletes regresses relatively quickly after cessation of vigorous training. A final measure of left ventricular mass is the ratio of posterior wall thickness to internal dimension or relative wall thickness. This ratio has been useful in characterizing the physiologic hypertrophy of the athletic heart and distinguishing it from pathologic hypertrophy.

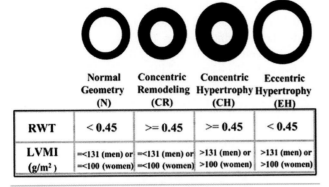

	Normal Geometry (N)	Concentric Remodeling (CR)	Concentric Hypertrophy (CH)	Eccentric Hypertrophy (EH)
RWT	< 0.45	>= 0.45	>= 0.45	< 0.45
LVMI (g/m²)	=<131 (men) or =<100 (women)	=<131 (men) or =<100 (women)	>131 (men) or >100 (women)	>131 (men) or >100 (women)

FIGURE 6.16. Schematic representation of normal geometry and different conditions resulting in left ventricular hypertrophy. (From Yuda S, Khoury V, Marwick TH. Influence of wall stress and left ventricular geometry on the accuracy of dobutamine stress echocardiography. J Am Coll Cardiol 2002; 40:1311–1319, with permission.)

It is exceptionally rare to see wall thickness more than 15 mm in the absence of significant hypertension, hypertrophic cardiomyopathy, or an infiltrative process.

REGIONAL LEFT VENTRICULAR FUNCTION

The most common form of acquired heart disease encountered in modern medicine is coronary artery disease along with its sequelae of myocardial ischemia, infarction, and chronic remodeling. By definition, the early phases of coronary artery disease result in segmental or regional abnormalities rather than global abnormalities. Evaluation of segmental or regional function requires a different set of analysis algorithms and tools different from those used for global function (Table 6.3).

As noted previously, normal ventricular contraction consists of simultaneous myocardial thickening and endocardial excursion toward the center of the ventricle. There is some regional heterogeneity of this motion with the proximal inferoposterior and lateral walls contracting somewhat later than the septum and inferior wall. There is also heterogeneity of the degree of endocardial excursion and myocardial thickening, with greater absolute and percentage changes from diastole to systole at the base when compared with the apex. These changes may be exaggerated with myocardial ischemia (Fig. 6.17).

Abnormal regional wall motion most commonly is the result of coronary artery disease, which interrupts perfusion to fairly well defined territories and hence results in abnormal motion in those segments. There is a gradation of wall motion abnormality that consists progressively of hypokinesis, akinesis, and subsequently dyskinesis in which a wall moves away from the center of the ventricle. Because wall thickening and endocardial motion are intrinsically tied, virtually all regional wall motion abnormalities are expected initially to be associated with abnormalities of thickening as well as endocardial motion.

▌ **TABLE 6.3 Methods for Evaluation of Regional Wall Motion Abnormalities**

Visual/subjective
  Descriptive: normal, hypokinetic, akinetic, dyskinetic
    normal myocardial thickness versus scar
  Location: anterior, lateral, inferior, posterior, apex, basal, mid, apical segments
Semiquantitative
  WMS or WMSI
    Normal = 1
    Hypokinetic = 2   } Scored for each segment
    Akinetic = 3
    Dyskinetic = 4

$$WMSI = \sum_{n=1}^{n=N} WMS \div N$$

Quantitative
  Anatomy based
    Radian change
    Regional area change
    Center-line chordal shortening (applied to short axis or apical views)
  Doppler tissue imaging
    Local velocity
    Velocity gradient (endocardial − epicardial)
    Myocardial displacement
    Myocardial strain
    Strain rate imaging

WMS, wall motion score; WMSI, wall motion score index.

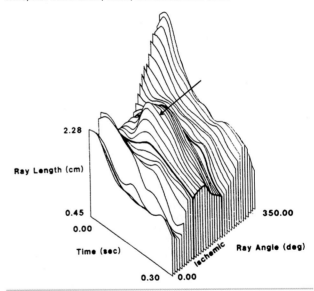

FIGURE 6.17. Three-dimensional display of the time and extent of contraction versus location along 360 degrees of a short-axis view of the left ventricle with an area of ischemic myocardium. Note the regional heterogeneity in radian length and shortening over time. Note also the regional and temporal heterogeneity of radian length shortening over time and the distinct upward motion, with the maximum at approximately 0.1 second (*arrow*) representing dyskinesis of the ischemic segment with subsequent shortening in that segment. (From Weyman AE, Franklin TD Jr, Hogan RD, et al. Importance of temporal heterogeneity in assessing the contraction abnormalities associated with acute myocardial ischemia. Circulation 1984;70:102–112, with permission.).

Figure 6.18 schematizes the currently recommended wall segment model for description of regional wall motion. Most previous schemes have used a 16-segment model, which includes a portion of the true apex in each of the four distal segments. A shortcoming of the 16-segment model is that if an abnormality is isolated to the apex, it is represented in each of four separate segments (segments 13–16), thus resulting in a disproportionate contribution to the wall motion score, especially if the abnormality was limited to the "true" apex.

More recently, a 17th segment has been proposed that represents the true apex. Addition of the 17th segment allows more precise communication with investigators and clinicians dealing with other imaging modalities, which

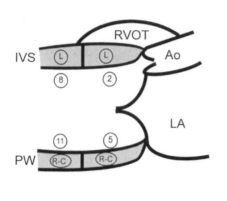

Parasternal Long Axis

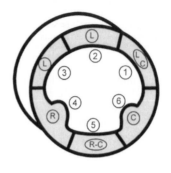

Parasternal Short Axis

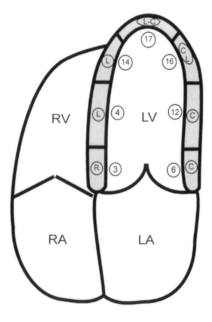

Apical Four Chamber View

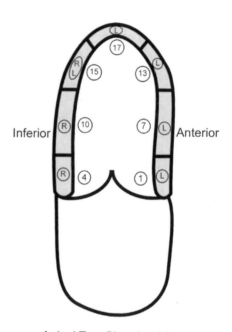

Apical Two Chamber View

L = Left anterior descending coronary artery
R = Right coronary artery
C = Circumflex coronary artery

FIGURE 6.18. Schematic representation of the 16 and 17 segment models of the left ventricle. Parasternal and apical views are depicted. For the standard 16-segment model, each of the distal segments (13–16) incorporates its adjacent portion of the apical segment. The *circled numbers* correspond to the current segment numbers recommended by the American Society of Echocardiography. For each segment, the coronary distribution most likely responsible for wall motion abnormality in that area is noted. When more than one coronary territory is listed, overlap between coronary distributions is anticipated in that segment. The true apex is most often perfused by the left anterior descending coronary artery; however, in the presence of a dominant right or circumflex coronary artery, it may also be perfused by that artery.

have traditionally recognized a true apical segment. Depending on the size of an apical wall motion abnormality, it may either enhance the accuracy of the wall motion score, if the abnormality is confined to the true apex, or result in overestimation if it involves portions of the four distal segments. When portions of the distal segments are involved, they will also be given an abnormal wall motion score, which again may result in disproportionate weighting of an apical wall motion abnormality.

When describing regional wall motion abnormalities, it is important not only to characterize their location but also their extent and severity. When dealing with coronary artery disease, the location of a wall motion abnormality is predictive of the location of the coronary "culprit" lesion. Figure 6.18 also depicts the relationship of the predefined 16 segments of the left ventricle to the traditional distributions of the left anterior descending, circumflex, and right coronary arteries. It should be emphasized that there can be substantial overlap in the more distal distributions of these arteries as well as in the posterior circulation in general. Additionally, after coronary artery bypass surgery, the location of wall motion abnormalities may be atypical, depending on the location of the myocardium perfused by the residual native arteries and by bypass grafts.

The most common type of wall motion analysis to undertake is a segment-by-segment description of wall motion as either being normal, hypokinetic, akinetic, or dyskinetic. A numeric score (1, 2, 3, 4) is then ascribed to each segment, and a score index is calculated by summing the scores and dividing by the number of visualized segments. The techniques for calculating a wall motion score are discussed in Chapter 15. There are several commonly encountered variations on the more typical abnormalities of wall motion that deserve comment.

In clinical practice, one often encounters atypical wall motion abnormalities, one of which is tardokinesis or a segment with delayed systolic contraction. This phenomenon may be difficult to appreciate in real time and is best noted by viewing the segment with M-mode, a frame-by-frame cine loop and trimming the cine loop to display only the first half of systole or with tissue Doppler imaging or strain rate imaging. Another confusing segmental wall motion finding is early relaxation. A given segment appears to relax or move outward before the rest of the chamber. Thus far, this finding has not correlated with any pathology and is generally considered to be a normal variant. It is noted most often with stress echocardiography at high heart rates. The same analysis methods noted for tardokinesis may help identify this wall motion pattern.

There are a number of more quantitative techniques for analyzing left ventricular regional and global function. Many of these have been used for investigational purposes but are rarely if ever used in routine clinical practice. Most quantitative algorithms for assessment of regional wall motion have included measurement of radian

or area shrinkage. Typically, this has been undertaken in the short axis of the left ventricle by describing a series of radians from the center of mass of the ventricle (Figs. 6.19–6.23). The number of radians can range from eight to 100, with each radian defined as the length from the center of mass to the endocardial border in diastole and subsequently in systole. Obviously, normal ventricular motion is represented by a reduction in the length of each of the constructed radians from diastole to systole. Because of rotational motion, there may not be exact correspondence of each radian position in diastole and systole

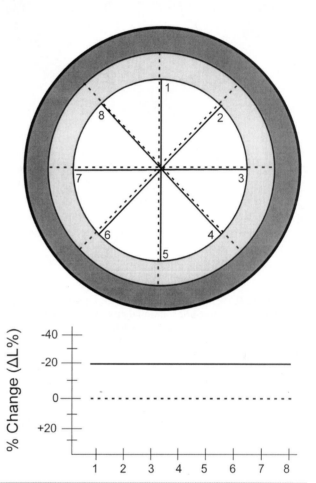

FIGURE 6.19. Schematic diagram of normal endocardial wall motion without translational motion. **Top:** The *outer dark circle* represents the diastolic thickness of the left ventricle and the *inner lighter shaded circle* the extent of systolic contraction. Eight radians from the center of mass have been drawn for both the diastolic (*dotted line*) and systolic (*solid line*) endocardial boundaries. **Bottom:** The percentage of change in length from diastole to systole is schematized. The *dotted line* represents zero change in length and the *solid line* represents the actual percentage of change in length for the normally contracting ventricle, which in this example is a 20% reduction in length. This diagram is subsequently repeated for demonstration of wall motion abnormalities and algorithms for correction of translation motion. In each subsequent similar figure, the *darker outer ring* represents the normal diastolic contour and the *solid line* represents the systolic endocardial contour.

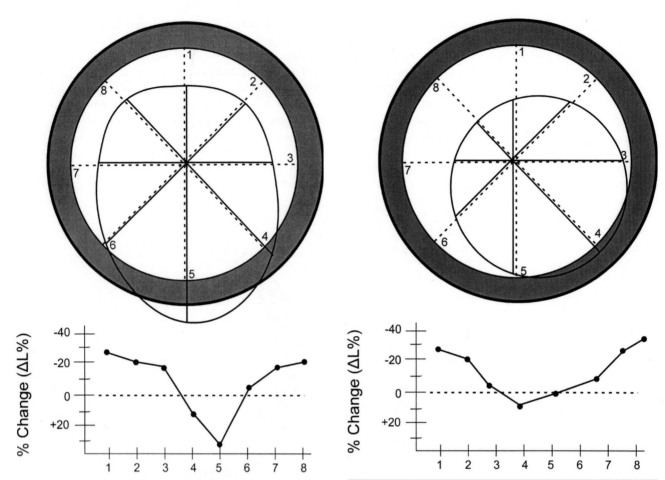

FIGURE 6.20. Schematic demonstration of posterior dyskinesis with no translational or rotational motion using the diastolic center of mass for both systole and diastole. **Top:** The *dark outer ring* represents the contour of the ventricle in diastole and the *inner circle* the endocardial contour in systole. Note the maximal area of dyskinesis at segment five with less dyskinesis at segment four and akinesis at segment six. **Bottom:** The change in radian length from diastole to systole is graphed. Note the hyperkinesis of the noninvolved segments with increased radian shortening compared with normal contraction in Figure 6.19.

FIGURE 6.21. Effect of translational motion in a heart with normal contraction, using the diastolic center of mass for the determination of both diastolic and systolic radian length. Note in the schematic that there has been lateral and posterior motion of the center of the left ventricle with systole. There has been normal symmetric contraction of all eight radians; however, because of translational motion, the apparent length of systolic radians 6, 7, 8, and 9 is shortened, whereas the apparent length from the diastolic center of mass of radians 3, 4, and 5 is artifactually lengthened. If radian lengths are compared using the diastolic center of mass for both comparisons, there will be artifactual dyskinesis, with the maximum at radian 4, as noted in the lower graph. Either readjusting and superimposing (Fig. 6.19) the center of mass or using separate centers of mass will negate this problem in a normally contracting ventricle.

but rather the systolic length of a radian may be compared with the diastolic length of another. A more troublesome issue results from cardiac translation. Because there is motion of the center of the heart from diastole to systole, this results in motion and displacement of the systolic contour compared with the location of the diastolic contour. This has the effect of artificially shortening the radians that lie in the direction of translational motion and lengthening the radians in the opposite direction if the diastolic center of mass is used as a reference (Figs. 6.21 and 6.22). This can be corrected by realigning the center of mass of the contour before radian comparisons are made. When dealing with a normal, symmetrically contracting ventricle, this will correct for the errors attributable to cardiac translation. However, if a wall mo-

tion abnormality is present, the center of mass in diastole and systole will not be equivalent with respect to the distance from either the normal or abnormal walls. If one then corrects by superimposing the center of mass, there will be predictable underestimation of the extent of wall motion abnormality (Fig. 6.23).

In addition to measuring radian length in diastole and systole, the area in each of the segments described by adjacent radian pairs can be quantified and compared in diastole and systole as well. In general, this scheme results in information virtually identical to that from radian

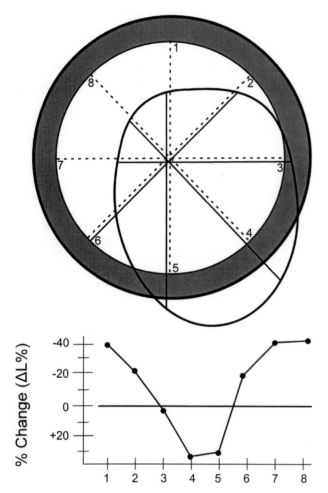

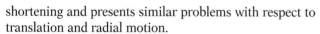

FIGURE 6.22. Schematic representation of posterolateral translation in the presence of a posterolateral wall motion abnormality. In the schematic, the diastolic center of mass has been used for comparison of radian length for both systolic and diastolic contours. Note, in comparison with Figure 6.20, which represents the same degree of posterior dyskinesis, that by using the diastolic center of mass for both contours, in the presence of translational motion there is an overestimation of wall motion extent and severity.

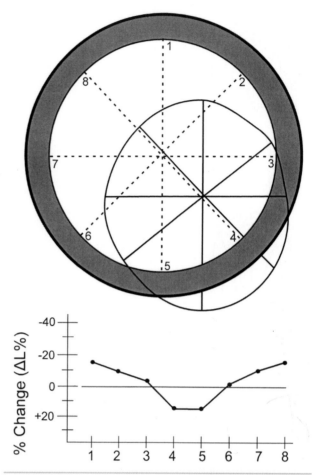

FIGURE 6.23. Schematic representation of posterior dyskinesis with posterolateral translation, using separate diastolic and systolic centers of mass for determining radian length. Note that because there is posterior dyskinesis, the systolic center of mass moves toward the dyskinetic wall, resulting in an apparent reduction in the degree of dyskinesis when separate systolic and diastolic radian lengths are then compared. This results in an artifactual underestimation of the severity of the wall motion abnormality and a simultaneous underestimation of function in the noninvolved zones.

shortening and presents similar problems with respect to translation and radial motion.

Chordal and area shrinkage methods can also be used from the apical four- and two-chamber views (Fig. 6.24). Typically, radians are drawn from the center of mass of the ventricle to the endocardial border and then the diastolic and systolic contours compared in a manner similar to that for short-axis views. As with the short-axis views, problems of rotational and translational motion result in unpredictable errors. Although valuable for detailed quantitative investigational assessment, neither radian nor area shrinkage methods have had widespread acceptance in routine clinical practice.

A final quantitative technique that can be used is center-line chordal shortening. In this technique, both the

epicardial and endocardial border of the ventricle are outlined in diastole and systole. The midpoint between the epicardium and endocardium is then generated. In a short-axis view, this series of midpoints represents a circle parallel to the endocardial and epicardial borders. In the four-chamber view, the chordal midpoint parallels the shape of the left ventricle. After identification of the epicardial and endocardial border and calculation of the midpoint line, a series of chordae (typically 100) is then drawn perpendicular to the center line. Each chorda represents the length from the epicardium to the endocardium (i.e., wall thickness). This measurement is undertaken in diastole and in systole, and the length of each of the 100 chordae is then compared. This method describes myocardial thickness along 100 chordae through-

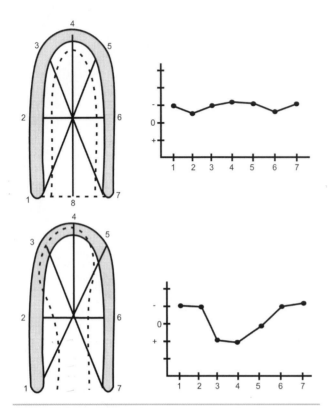

FIGURE 6.24. Schematic representation of radian or area change analysis as applied to an apical view. Normal motion **(top)** and an area of distal septal and apical dyskinesis *(dotted line)* **(bottom)** are depicted. Note that because radians drawn from the center of mass intersect walls at angles ranging from 0 to 30 degrees, the apparent magnitude of endocardial excursion varies with location in the normally contracting ventricle.

out the length of the myocardium being visualized. A normal response is for there to be chordal lengthening, implying myocardial thickening. If a segment is akinetic, the diastolic and systolic chordae will be equal in length and there will be no change in chordal length. If a segment actively thins from diastole to systole, there will be chordal shortening. The change in chordal length can then be plotted versus the location in the left ventricle. Figure 6.25 is a chordal shortening analysis in a patient with an anterior apical myocardial infarction. The graphic demonstration of chordal shortening in the normal contracting heart also demonstrates the regional heterogeneity of contraction in a disease-free state. For any of these quantitative schemes, myocardial tethering will result in a predictable overestimation of actual infarct size. This phenomenon is schematized in Figure 6.26.

Nonischemic Wall Motion Abnormalities

Several conditions result in wall motion abnormalities, unrelated to ischemia or coronary artery disease (Table 6.4). The most commonly encountered are left bundle branch block and the abnormal motion seen after cardiac surgery. Left bundle branch block alters the sequence of activation and hence the sequence of contraction of the left ventricle. Normal electrical activation follows the path of the right and left bundles and the His-Purkinje system. Conduction down the left bundle precedes that down the right bundle by 10 to 20 milliseconds, and hence the initial activation of the heart is in the proximal mid-

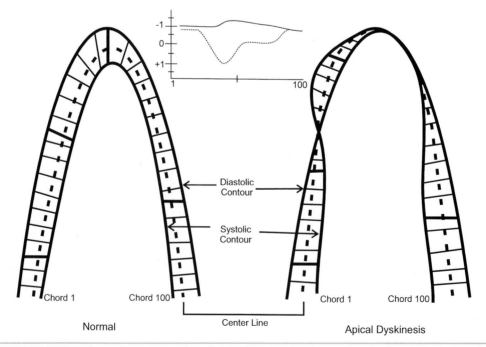

FIGURE 6.25. Schematic representation of centerline chordal shortening. For this method, diastolic and systolic contours of the endocardium are traced. A line midway between the two contours is then created. Equally spaced along this line, perpendicular chordae are drawn connecting the diastolic and systolic contours. The change in chordal length is then plotted as a marker of regional function.

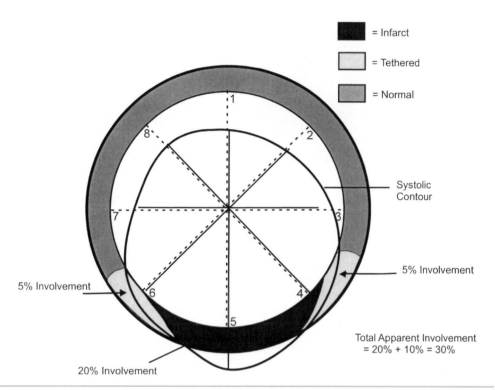

FIGURE 6.26. Schematic representation of horizontal tethering. This diagram represents posterior dyskinesis without translational motion. Note that the true extent of the infarct is as noted in the *darkly shaded area*, encompassing radian five and parts of radians six and four. Note that there is a border zone (*lightly shaded area*) adjacent to the infarct area that is anatomically normal but has abnormal motion due to the tethering effect of posterior dyskinesis. In the schematic, the true anatomic defect represents 20% of the circumference of the left ventricle with the tethered border zone giving an apparent total extent of 30%.

septum on the left ventricular side. In general, after this initial activation, there is relatively smooth progression of activation of contraction. In the presence of a complete left bundle branch block, the initial septal activation sequence is reversed and the right side of the ventricular septum is initially activated. This causes right ventricular and right septal activation before activation of the body of the left ventricle and results in a characteristic wall motion abnormality. This abnormality is often most easily appreciated with M-mode echocardiography (Fig. 6.27).

When imaged from the parasternal window, the abnormality consists of initial downward motion of the ventricular septum followed by anterior or paradoxical septal motion and then subsequent full thickening of the ventricular septum and posterior motion toward the center of the heart. The magnitude of this abnormal motion can be subtle and is often only noted on detailed inspection of an M-mode sweep through the ventricular septum. In other instances, there will be a dramatic "paradoxical" motion of the ventricular septum. This range in activation abnormality is due to the tremendous variation in the degree to which left bundle branch block has resulted in delayed activation, the presence or absence of more distal His-Purkinje system disease, and the impact of concurrent

disease that may either mask or exaggerate the bundle branch block pattern. Another characteristic of the left bundle branch block pattern is that the magnitude of the abnormality is often dramatically increased during phar-

▶ **TABLE 6.4 Nonischemic Regional Wall Motion Abnormality**

Conduction system based
  Left bundle branch block
  Ventricular pacing
  Premature ventricular contractions
  Ventricular preexcitation (Wolf-Parkinson-White syndrome)
Abnormal ventricular interaction
  Right ventricular volume overload
  Right ventricular pressure overload
  Pericardial constriction
Miscellaneous
  After cardiac surgery
  Congenital absence of the pericardium
  Posterior compression
    Ascites
    Hiatal hernia
    Pregnancy

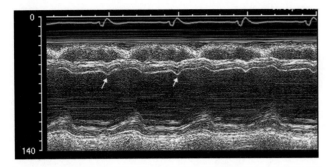

FIGURE 6.27. M-mode echocardiogram recorded in a patient with a left bundle branch block shows an early systolic downward motion of the ventricular septum (*arrows*).

macologic stress with dobutamine. It is less likely to be augmented during the physiologic stress of exercise.

A common scenario is for there to be a left bundle branch block in a patient for whom coronary artery disease is a diagnostic consideration. Separation of the wall motion abnormality due to the bundle branch block from that which can be seen in coronary disease involving the left anterior descending coronary artery can often be problematic, especially for the novice or beginning echocardiographer. Table 6.5 outlines a number of features that can help separate left bundle branch block and other nonischemic abnormalities from an ischemic wall motion abnormality. It should be emphasized that none of these features is absolute, and even in the most experienced hands, the ability to separate left bundle branch block from an ischemic wall motion abnormality is far from absolute. It should also be recognized that bundle branch block may coexist with resting ischemia, myocardial infarction, or inducible ischemia at the time of cardiovascular stress. Perhaps the most valuable observation when attempting to separate bundle branch block from ischemia is myocardial thickening. With bundle branch block, myocardial thickening is typically preserved as is initial early ventricular contraction. By using M-mode echocardiography or confining wall motion analysis to the first half or third of systole, one can often appreciate that systolic thickening is preserved and that there is a component of appropriate downward motion of the septum with systole that is then followed by abnormal mo-

tion. Additional valuable clues regarding ischemia include the fact that ischemia involving the proximal left anterior descending coronary artery, which would be required to result in a proximal septal abnormality, will usually result in abnormalities in the more distal portions of the septum, apex, and anterior wall. In most instances, left bundle branch block does not result in abnormalities in the apex or distal anterior wall as visualized in an apical two-chamber view. This can be a valuable clue to the etiology of the wall motion abnormality. Right bundle branch block does not alter the initial sequence of activation of the left ventricle and hence, unless associated with intrinsic disease of the right heart, will not be associated with appreciable abnormalities of left ventricular wall motion.

Paced Rhythms

The majority of ventricular paced rhythms are done with right ventricular endocardial leads. This results in a left bundle branch block pattern on the electrocardiogram, and a wall motion abnormality similar to that seen in native left bundle branch block. Many of the same rules regarding preservation of thickening and of late systolic endocardial motion discussed previously also pertain to evaluating wall motion in the presence of a paced rhythm. Because most endocardial pacing leads are placed apically, the location of maximal abnormality previously referred to is far less helpful. On occasion, a ventricular pacing lead can be in the more inferior portions of the distal septum and result in a distal inferior wall motion abnormality. Separation of this abnormality from that due to true ischemia can be somewhat more problematic than when dealing with classic lead placement.

It has become standard therapy to use biventricular pacing or, less commonly, left ventricular pacing as a form of resynchronization therapy in patients with systolic dysfunction due to cardiomyopathy and underlying conduction system disease (typically marked left bundle branch). Resynchronization via simultaneous biventricular pacing results in more efficient mechanics of ejection and improved cardiovascular performance. The appearance of regional wall motion abnormalities in these patients will be highly variable and dependent on underlying conduc-

▶ **TABLE 6.5 Ischemic Versus Nonischemic Wall Motion Abnormalities**

Abnormality	*Location*	*Onset*	*Duration*	*Thickening*
Left bundle branch block	Anterior septum	Early systole	Multiphasic	Blunted
Paced rhythm	Distal septum	Early systole	Multiphasic	Blunted
Postoperative motion	Whole heart	Early systole	Whole cycle	Preserved
Ventricular preexcitation (WPW)	Variable	Pre-systolic	Very brief (<50 ms)	Preserved
Constriction	Septum/posterior wall	Diastole	Last 3/4	Preserved
Ischemia/infarction	Distal > proximal	Early systole	All systole	Absent

tion and the relative contributions of the two pacing sites. Caution is advised when attempting to diagnose an ischemic wall motion abnormality in this setting.

Ventricular Preexcitation

Ventricular preexcitation, as typified by the Wolf-Parkinson-White syndrome, also results in segmental wall motion abnormalities. These are often far more subtle than those seen with left bundle branch block or pacing, and whereas the former result in wall motion abnormalities that mimic the distribution of a coronary artery, the abnormalities seen with preexcitation are often in atypical locations that would be highly unlikely to be the effect of coronary artery disease. Ventricular preexcitation results in both electrical and mechanical activation of the ventricular myocardium due to the anomalous bypass connection. Preexcitation of the right ventricular myocardium is rarely if ever detected with echocardiography, and it is more often the septal and posterolateral bypass pathways that are directly noted. Electrical preexcitation results in minor degrees of mechanical motion early in systole often before completion of the QRS. It should be emphasized that normal contraction often begins only after completion of the entire QRS. In most patients with preexcitation, the remaining conduction system is entirely normal, and normal activation through the left bundle branch block and remainder of the left ventricle precedes in an orderly fashion and soon overtakes the wave of the preexcited myocardium. As such, the abnormality associated with ventricular preexcitation is usually fairly localized and of very small magnitude and duration. It is often only appreciated with M-mode echocardiography, which has the ability to detect relatively small degrees of motion that occur over only a 10- or 20-millisecond period (Fig. 6.28).

Postoperative Cardiac Motion

After any form of cardiac surgery in which the pericardium is opened, there is a characteristic abnormality of cardiac motion. This was initially appreciated only as abnormal septal motion on M-mode echocardiography. It is now well established that this motion abnormality is a global phenomenon, involving exaggerated anterior motion of the entire heart within the thorax. The etiology of this wall motion abnormality remains in dispute. The initial descriptions were of patients who had undergone valve replacement surgery, and it was thought to be related only to that procedure. It soon became apparent that coronary artery bypass surgery also resulted in abnormal septal motion. Serial echocardiography during each sequential phase of cardiac surgery has demonstrated that the abnormality becomes apparent for any procedure in which the pericardium is opened. It is as-

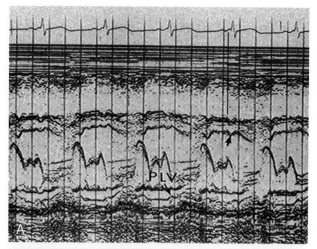
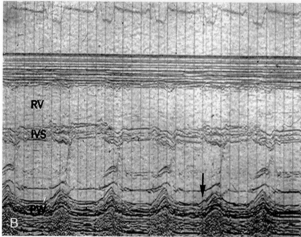

FIGURE 6.28. M-mode echocardiograms recorded in two patients with ventricular preexcitation due to the Wolff-Parkinson-White syndrome. **Top:** A patient with a septal pathway is noted. Note the brief early downward systolic motion of the ventricular septum (*arrow*) slightly before the upstroke of the QRS. **Bottom:** Note the very slight anterior motion of the posterior wall recorded in a patient with a posterolateral pathway due to Wolff-Parkinson-White syndrome.

sumed that the abnormality is due to loss of pericardial constraint. It is typically most obvious after valvular heart disease surgery and may regress over 3 to 5 years. One early observation, which now has little clinical relevance, was that the absence of "paradoxical septal motion" after valve replacement surgery may be an indicator of prosthetic valve dysfunction. There were a number of case examples in which paradoxical septal motion failed to occur in the presence of prosthetic valve dysfunction, presumably due to the concurrent volume overload of the left ventricle that mitigated against the development of abnormal motion. Reliance of this observation is obviously outmoded.

The abnormal postoperative motion on M-mode echocardiography was noted as frank paradoxical motion

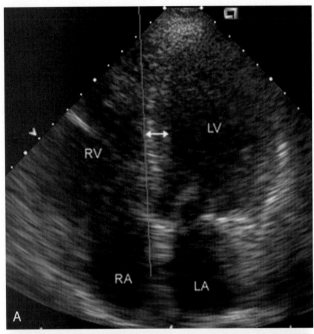

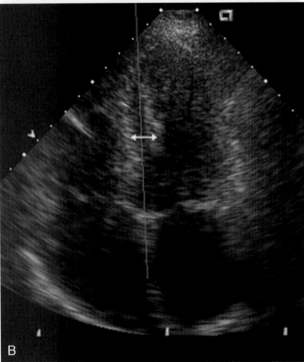

FIGURE 6.29. Apical four-chamber view recorded in a patient after cardiac surgery demonstrates postoperative motion of the entire heart. **Top:** Image was recorded in end-diastole. The *vertical line* marks the position of the right side of the ventricular septum. **Bottom:** Image was recorded in end-systole. Note that, compared with the vertical reference line, there has been overall anterior (leftward) motion of the heart. Note the thickness of the ventricular septum (*double-headed arrow*).

of the ventricular septum with preserved myocardial thickening, but without the initial downward deflection seen with a left bundle branch block. With two-dimensional echocardiography, it is easily appreciated that the center of the left ventricle moves anteriorly during contraction to an exaggerated degree after cardiac surgery. This has the effect of exaggerating apparent motion of the anteroposterior and posterolateral walls and of reducing the apparent motion of the anterior septum. Figure 6.29 was recorded in a patient with paradoxical septal motion after cardiac surgery. Note that septal thickening is preserved even though its motion in the thorax is abnormal.

Evaluation of postoperative wall motion as well as left bundle branch block and paced rhythm is often complicated by the presence of multiple abnormalities including coexistence of any of these three entities plus possible concurrent coronary artery disease with ischemia or myocardial infarction. Combinations of these diseases, all of which can result in septal wall motion abnormalities, obviously make interpretation problematic. Even the most experienced observer often has difficulty determining whether there is a primary ischemic insult when two or more of these factors are present. The single best tool for separating ischemic from nonischemic abnormalities in this setting is to rely heavily on the presence or absence of systolic wall thickening. As mentioned previously, this is often done with directed M-mode echocardiography. Similar results can be obtained by evaluation of a digitized two-dimensional loop on a frame-by-frame basis. Because many of these non-ischemic abnormalities are confined to the latter half of systole, evaluating the two-dimensional echocardiography in a digitized form only during the first half of systole often allows the echocardiographer to demonstrate preserved thickening and initial normal endocardial motion. It is also important to have a firm understanding of the anticipated pathophysiology of underlying coronary artery disease. Many of the abnormalities discussed above result in an "anatomically incorrect" distribution of wall motion abnormalities, and a skilled clinician-echocardiographer should be in a position to recognize that a wall motion abnormality is a result of a non-ischemic process based on its location, behavior, and overall characteristics. It should also be recognized that after successful coronary bypass surgery, the distribution of regional wall motion abnormalities might also be atypical.

Pericardial Constriction

Pericardial constriction results in a variety of wall motion abnormalities. The underlying reason for the abnormalities is exaggerated differential filling and contraction of the right and left ventricles. The predominant effect of this is to alter the sequence and magnitude of septal position and motion. Superimposed on the beat-to-beat abnormality of septal motion can be exaggerated respiratory variation in this abnormality. Initial descriptions of abnormal wall motion in constrictive pericarditis were based on M-mode echocardiography in an attempt to describe one or two septal and posterior wall motion abnormalities (Fig. 6.30). It quickly became apparent that there were a large number of septal motion abnormalities that could be seen, all of which could be described as resulting in early downward deflection of the septum followed by varying degrees of paradoxical motion, with or without subsequent appropriate motion of the ventricular septum. With further experience, it became apparent that there was a continuum of septal wall motion abnormalities, many of which mimic right ventricular volume or pressure overload, septal preexcitation, left bundle branch block, and, less commonly for the experienced observer, myocardial ischemia. This topic is discussed further in Chapter 9.

Premature Ventricular Contractions

As should be anticipated from the previous discussion, a premature ventricular contraction (PVC) will result in segmental wall motion abnormality for the beat in which the left ventricle is activated by the PVC. The mechanical result of the PVC is an abnormal onset of electrical and mechanical activation and subsequent abnormal propagation of the electromechanical impulse through the ventricular myocardium. The most extreme example is a PVC arising in the lateral wall that is temporally and anatomically as remote from normal contraction as possible. In this instance, there will be immediate myocardial thickening and contraction of the lateral wall, occasionally resulting in dyskinesis of the relaxed septum, followed by asynchronous contraction of the left ventricle. High temporal resolution, two-dimensional echocardiography can be used to identify the site of earliest mechanical activa-

tion. In practice, a skilled echocardiographer should rarely be confused by wall motion abnormalities arising from premature ventricular contractions. Scrutiny of the accompanying electrocardiogram is obviously informative, and the nature of the wall motion abnormality is frequently inconsistent with the known distribution of coronary artery disease or any other form of organic heart disease commonly encountered. Appreciation of the secondary effects of PVC is important (Fig. 6.31). After a PVC, there is a "compensatory pause" and the subsequent left ventricular contraction is normally hyperdynamic. It is important to appreciate this phenomenon so as not to then compare beats during normal sinus rhythm and assume that the ventricle is hypokinetic. On occasion, an echocardiogram is performed in a patient with persistent bigeminy or trigeminy. This can result in confusion because each PVC will be accompanied by grossly abnormal activation of the ventricle with abnormal wall motion. The wall motion of the subsequent beat will then be hyperdynamic. The third beat, representing a normally conducted contraction, will then provide the only assessment of true normal ventricular contractility. This issue may be especially problematic when viewing single cardiac cycle cine loops, where the relationship of systole function to rhythm may not be obvious.

DOPPLER EVALUATION OF GLOBAL LEFT VENTRICULAR FUNCTION

Clinicians have used Doppler spectral profiles to evaluate global left ventricular function since the early 1970s. The earliest, conceptually simplest, and still probably one of

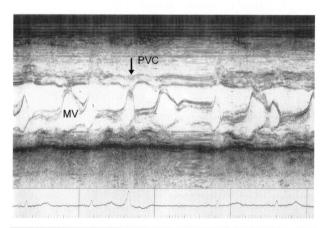

FIGURE 6.31. M-mode echocardiogram recorded in a patient shows the effect of a premature ventricular contraction. Note the early downward motion of the ventricular septum with the premature complex. Note also the truncated mitral valve opening in the preceding diastole and more prolonged opening during the compensatory pause.

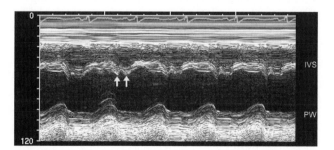

FIGURE 6.30. M-mode echocardiogram recorded in a patient with constrictive pericarditis. Note the relatively flat motion of the posterior wall endocardium and the abnormal multiphasic diastolic motion of the ventricular septum related to an increase in ventricular interdependence.

the more clinically useful methods for following left ventricular function is to evaluate the time velocity integral (TVI) of the left ventricular outflow tract or ascending aorta. The means by which volumetric flow can be determined with this method is discussed in Chapter 8. Basically, the principle is that if the cross-sectional area of the chamber is known, then the product of that cross-sectional area and the mean velocity of flow equals the volumetric flow. In a pulsatile flow system such as the beating heart, in which the flow velocity is confined to mechanical systole, the volume calculated equals the forward ventricular stroke volume in the aorta. This forward stroke volume can then be multiplied by the heart rate to obtain cardiac output. Typically, the areas evaluated for determination of systolic flow and hence global left ventricular performance have been the left ventricular outflow tract, with the Doppler interrogation taking place from the apex of the heart or occasionally the ascending aorta using a right parasternal approach (Figs. 6.32 and 6.33). Using either approach (and in the absence of aortic insufficiency), the calculated stroke volume should accurately reflect actual volume of flow for the analyzed beat.

There are several potential sources of error with this method. First, the methodology assumes a flat velocity profile across the cross-sectional area of the outflow tract or aorta. In reality, the flow profile is parabolic, and thus the average velocity calculated by this technique may not represent the true cross-sectional velocity. In clinical practice, this tends to be a relatively inconsequential effect. A greater source of error is in determining the cross-sectional area of the outflow chamber. This is usually done by obtaining the diameter and then applying the formula area $= \pi r^2$. This assumes circular geometry of the outflow chamber, when in reality it is often elliptical. Several attempts have been made to apply a formula for elliptical geometry or to directly measure the area, each of which has resulted in only minimal improvements in accuracy and has rarely seen widespread clinical acceptance. Because the formula for the cross-sectional area involves the square of the radius, any error in measuring the left ventricular outflow tract may create a substantial error in flow calculation. A 2-mm error in measuring a 2.0-cm diameter outflow tract will result in an approximate 20% error in the flow volume calculation.

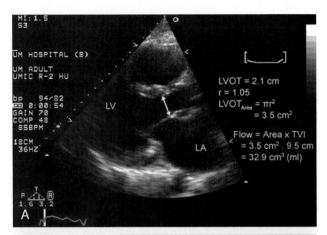

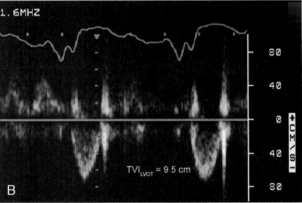

FIGURE 6.33. Example of determining the left ventricular outflow tract stroke volume using the methods depicted in Figure 6.32. **Top:** Parasternal long-axis view from which the left ventricular outflow tract can be measured. **Bottom:** The time velocity integral recorded in the left ventricular outflow tract from an apical transducer position. In this patient with a dilated cardiomyopathy, forward stroke volume is reduced (32.9 mL).

One point that should be emphasized is that, although measurement of the actual outflow tract area may be subject to significant error, there are no commonly encountered disease states in which the area of the outflow tract would be expected to change over a short period. With this in mind, it should be readily apparent that the outflow tract area, which can be considered a constant in most patients, can actually be dropped from the analysis. In this instance, the TVI is the only variable to change over time, and therefore calculation of this value alone can be used to track serial changes. Figure 6.34 was

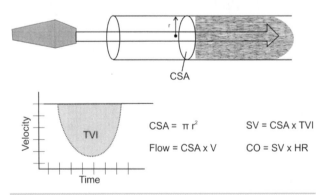

FIGURE 6.32. Schematic representation of the method for determining volumetric flow. This method is applicable for any laminar flow for which the cross-sectional area (*CSA*) of the flow chamber can be determined. The product of cross-sectional area and the time velocity integral (*TVI*) is stroke volume (*SV*). Cardiac output (*CO*) can be calculated as the product of stroke volume and heart rate. See text for further details.

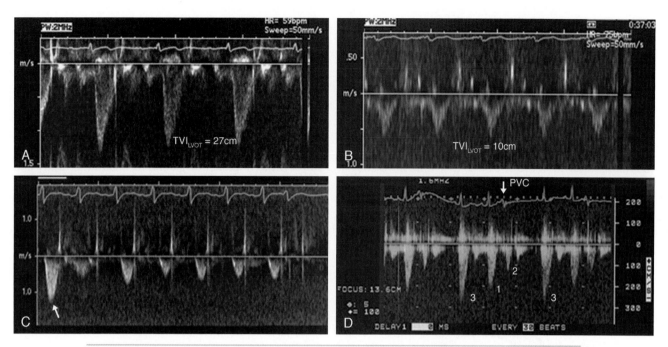

FIGURE 6.34. Time velocity integral (TVI) in the left ventricular outflow tract recorded in four different patients. **Top left:** Note the TVI of 27 cm recorded in a patient with normal cardiac function and a diminished TVI of 10 cm recorded in a patient with a cardiomyopathy and reduced stroke volume **(top right). Bottom left:** The variation in TVI seen in a patient with severe left ventricular systolic dysfunction. The first beat to the left is a post–premature ventricular contraction (PVC) beat showing augmentation. Note the alternating TVIs after this beat, which is the corollary of pulsus alternans. **Bottom right:** Recorded in a patient with mild valvular aortic stenosis. Note the augmented peak velocity and TVI after the compensatory pause after a PVC (complex 3). Note also the marked reduction in both velocity and TVI for the PVC beat. In this instance, only the TVI and peak velocity associated with beat number one represent the true gradient.

recorded from patients with various disease states and shows the range in TVI values that can be encountered. Note in parts C and D that the variation in TVI is due to rhythm disturbances.

In theory, these same principles can be applied to any of the four cardiac valves or outflow or inflow tract dimensions. The right ventricular outflow tract, just below the pulmonic valve, typically is a circular structure and provides information analogous to that for the left ventricular outflow tract. Comparison of the TVI-outflow tract area product at these two sites has been successfully used in congenital heart disease to compare right and left ventricular stroke volume and hence determine shunt ratios in patients with intracardiac shunts. Similar calculations can be performed using either the mitral valve anulus or an average mitral valve area. In practice, determination of the cross-sectional area of the anulus or of the mitral valve orifice is problematic. One exception to this would be patients with mitral stenosis in whom the stenotic area can be directly visualized and planimetered and the flow velocity profile easily calculated. Determination of the true area from an irregularly shaped structure, such as the mitral anulus and the normal mitral orifice, both of which may not adhere to a standard geometric shape in disease states and change in size and shape over the cardiac cycle, introduces substantial error into these calculations. For this reason, they are not commonly used in clinical practice. Only with scrupulous attention to detail in select patients can the left ventricular inflow be used to determine left ventricular stroke volume. Under rigorously controlled circumstances, this measurement has correlated well with standard measures of flow. Because the tricuspid anulus and tricuspid valve assume an irregular and unpredictable shape, there has been little or no success with using this valve for calculation of stroke volume.

Other Techniques for Determination of Left Ventricular Systolic Function

Most clinically used parameters of ventricular function including stroke volume and ejection fraction are afterload dependent, i.e., they are dependent on the pressure developed and impedance against which the left ventricle must contract. Several methods have been proposed for correcting for afterload or creating afterload-independent indices of left ventricular performance.

Closely related to determination of left ventricular volume and ejection fraction is calculation of left ventricular wall stress. These calculations have been used as a measure of myocardial contractility in the investigation of cardiomyopathy and valvular heart disease. By accounting for wall thickness and pressure generation, wall stress is a more afterload-independent measure of contractility than simpler parameters such as fractional shortening or ejection fraction. Left ventricular stress can be calculated either globally or regionally. There are actually three different stress calculations: radial, circumferential, and meridional wall stress, each of which is mutually orthogonal. In its simplest form, meridional stress is defined by the formula: stress = (pressure × radius) ÷ h (where h = wall thickness) (Fig. 6.35). This formula assumes spherical geometry, which obviously is not the case in the left ventricle. As such, while correlating with other measures

of left ventricular stress, it may not truly represent the actual value. Regional stress can be calculated along any of the ventricular segments using a similar equation for which the radius is independently determined for that segment rather than for the left ventricular cavity as a whole. Regional stress varies from apex to base and around the circumference of the left ventricle because of left ventricular–right ventricular interaction and changes in the radius of curvature of the ventricle. Calculation of stress, either regional or global, has had little utility and acceptance in the routine clinical practice of cardiology. Calculation of stress indexed to ventricular volume has been used as an index of ventricular performance in valvular heart disease and cardiomyopathy. In this instance, it is an additional refinement of the determination

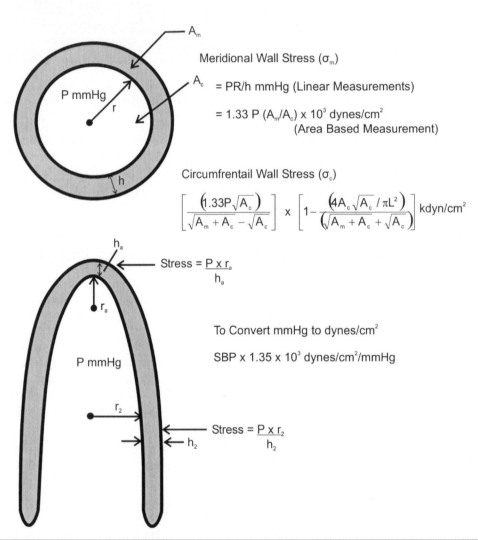

Meridional Wall Stress (σ_m)

= PR/h mmHg (Linear Measurements)

= 1.33 P (A_m/A_c) x 10^3 dynes/cm^2
(Area Based Measurement)

Circumfrentail Wall Stress (σ_c)

$$\left[\frac{\left(1.33P\sqrt{A_c}\right)}{\sqrt{A_m + A_c} - \sqrt{A_c}}\right] \times \left[1 - \frac{\left(4A_c\sqrt{A_c}/\pi L^2\right)}{\left(\sqrt{A_m + A_c} + \sqrt{A_c}\right)}\right] \text{ kdyn/cm}^2$$

Stress = $\dfrac{P \times r_a}{h_a}$

To Convert mmHg to dynes/cm^2

SBP x 1.35 x 10^3 dynes/cm^2/mmHg

Stress = $\dfrac{P \times r_2}{h_2}$

FIGURE 6.35. Schematic representation of the simplified methods for determining left ventricular wall stress. Wall stress can be defined as radial, circumferential, or meridional, all of which are mutually orthogonal. Meridional wall stress is the simplest to calculate. Circumferential wall stress incorporates the length of the left ventricle and is best calculated from the two-dimensional echocardiogram. **Bottom:** The relationship of location to regional stress with respect to variation of wall thickness (h) and local radius of wall curvature (r) is depicted.

of left ventricular reserve and ventricular compensation in either pressure or volume overload states.

Determination of Left Ventricular dP/dt

An additional method for deriving parameters of left ventricular global function is the calculation of left ventricular dP/dt. This represents the rate of increase in pressure within the left ventricle. If confined to the early phases of systole, during isovolumic contraction, this is a relatively load-independent measure of ventricular contractility. dP/dt has long been a standard calculation using a high-fidelity micrometer catheter in the catheterization laboratory.

Using the spectral display of a mitral regurgitation jet, similar information regarding the rate of pressure development within the left ventricle can be derived. If this measurement is undertaken in the early phases of systole while the increasing ventricular pressure is less than the aortic pressure, it is relatively load independent. The method by which this is performed is to record the mitral regurgitation spectral profile at a high sweep speed (typically 100 mm/sec), as shown in Figures 6.36 and 6.37. Examination of the upstroke of the velocity curve can then

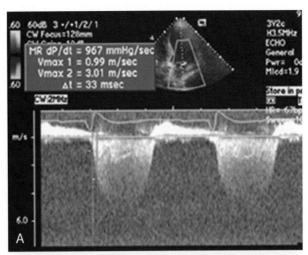

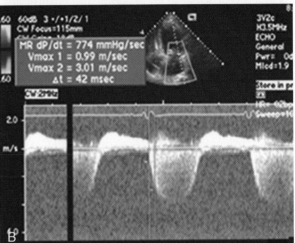

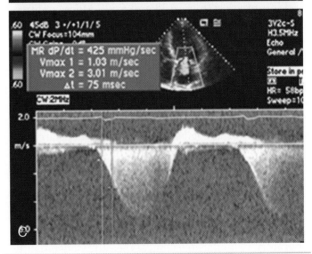

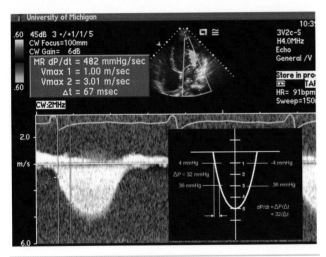

FIGURE 6.36. Schematic representation and example of calculating the left ventricular dP/dt from the continuous wave Doppler mitral regurgitation spectral signal. **Left:** A continuous wave spectral Doppler image recorded in a patient with severe left ventricular systolic dysfunction in which the online measurement of dP/dt is noted to be 482 mm Hg/sec. **Right:** The methodology for this determination, which includes recording continuous wave Doppler imaging of mitral regurgitation at a high sweep speed (150 mm/sec in this example) and defining points for which the mitral regurgitation velocity has reached 1 and 3 m/sec, is depicted. This represents a 32 mm Hg/sec pressure increase in the left ventricle into a low-compliance left atrium, thus making this a relatively load-independent measure of contractility. The time between the two points required to reach 1 and 3 m/sec (Δt) is then divided into the pressure difference (32 mm Hg) for calculation of dP/dt.

FIGURE 6.37. Continuous wave Doppler imaging–derived left ventricular dP/dt in three patients with varying degrees of left ventricular systolic dysfunction. **Top:** Recorded in a patient with relatively mild systolic dysfunction and a dP/dt of 967 mm Hg/sec. **Bottom:** Recorded in a patient with severe systolic dysfunction and a dP/dt of 425 mm Hg/sec.

be used to derive instantaneous pressure measurements. To determine the dP/dt, one calculates the time difference in milliseconds from the point at which the velocity is at 1 m/sec and at 3 m/sec. The time between these two points represents the time that it takes for a 32 mm Hg change to occur in the left ventricular cavity. dP/dt is then calculated as: dP/dt = 32 mm Hg ÷ time (seconds). Determination of dP/dt using this method has been validated against invasive hemodynamic measurements. In addition to determining this parameter in early phases of systole, the negative dP/dt over the analogous pressure change (36 to 4 mm Hg) in diastole can also be calculated and may provide information regarding diastolic function. Either a reduced positive or negative dP/dt carries significant prognostic implications. There are contributors to left ventricular dP/dt in addition to intrinsic myocardial contractility. In the presence of marked mechanical dysynchrony (as typified by left bundle branch block), dP/dt may be reduced, not due to decreased contractility but rather as a consequence of contractile dysynchrony and inefficiency.

Doppler Tissue Velocity

The basic principles of Doppler tissue imaging (DTI) are discussed in Chapter 3. Briefly, this technique relies on altering receiver gains and frequency filters so that the Doppler signal arising from relatively dense, slow-moving targets such as the myocardium and cardiac anulus are interrogated for their velocity. DTI can be displayed as a color display, saturating the typical anatomic structural information (Figs. 6.38 and 6.39). More commonly for the determination of function, a pulsed Doppler sample volume is placed within an area of the myocardium or the anulus and the velocities at that point are then displayed for quantitation (Fig. 6.40). Virtually any area of the myocardium can be evaluated in this manner. DTI has substantial spatial and temporal resolution. The spatial resolution is such that the sample volume can be placed in either the subendocardial or subepicardial regions, and differential velocities in adjacent wall segments can thereby be determined. When evaluating global performance, DTI velocities will show some regional variation based on which area of the mitral anulus is interrogated (septal vs. lateral). Although maximal "accuracy" may be obtained by averaging values, most laboratories standardize clinical measurements to either the septal or lateral anulus to maximize efficiency. The anular velocity in systole has shown a good correlation with the left ventricular ejection fraction over a wide range of ventricular function (Fig. 6.41).

Because there is substantial spatial resolution inherent in the DTI method, velocities can be obtained in adjacent segments. There are several secondary analyses that can then be derived. One of the first to be described was the

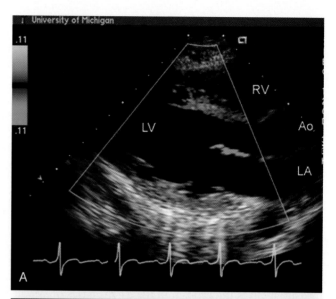

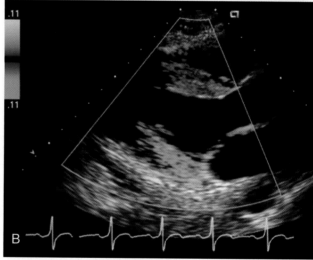

FIGURE 6.38. Parasternal long-axis echocardiogram recorded with superimposed color Doppler tissue imaging. **Top:** The end-diastolic frame; **bottom:** end-systole. Note that by convention, motion toward the transducer is recorded in red and away from it in blue. For this reason, when opposing walls move toward each other, they will be encoded in opposite colors, as noted here.

calculation of the endocardial-epicardial gradient (Fig. 6.42). By placing the DTI sample volume in the subendocardium, the velocities in the inner third of the myocardium can be determined. A similar assessment can then be made of the subepicardial velocities. The difference between these two values is the endocardial-epicardial gradient. Alterations in this gradient with a selective decrease in the subendocardial velocities have shown promise as a very sensitive marker of ischemia. Because the endocardial and epicardial velocities are determined in a single segment with the same angle of interrogation of the Doppler beam, this technique is relatively angle in-

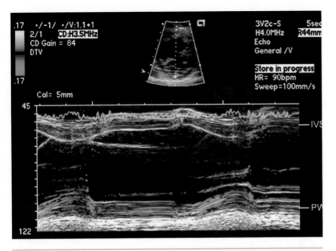

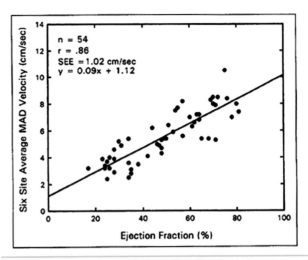

FIGURE 6.39. Color M-mode Doppler tissue imaging of the septum and posterior wall of the left ventricle recorded in an individual with normal contraction. Note that motion toward the transducer is color encoded in red and that oriented away from the transducer is in blue. For this reason, normally contracting walls that move opposing directions are color encoded in opposite colors. Also note the excellent temporal resolution for determining the timing of contraction.

FIGURE 6.41. In this study, Doppler tissue imaging was used to determine the mitral anular velocity at six sites and the average then compared with the left ventricular ejection fraction. Note the excellent correlation between the average velocity of mitral anular motion and the ejection fraction. (Reprinted from Gulati VK, Katz WE, Follansbee WP, et al. Mitral annular descent velocity by tissue Doppler echocardiography as an index of global left ventricular function. Am J Cardiol 1996;77:979–984, with permission.)

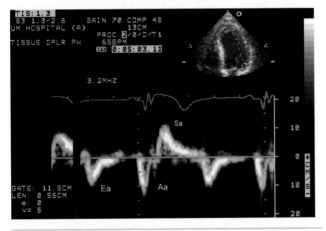

FIGURE 6.40. Doppler tissue imaging of the lateral mitral anulus recorded from an apical four-chamber view. Note the systolic motion of the anulus toward the apex (S_a) and the biphasic diastolic motion (E_a and A_a), which correspond to the mitral valve E- and A-waves.

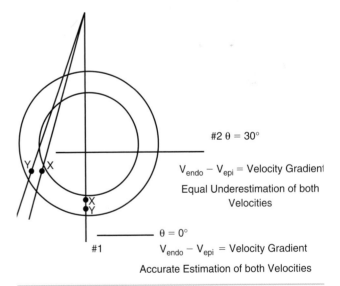

FIGURE 6.42. Schematic demonstrates the mechanism for determining an endocardial-epicardial gradient. For the interrogation line with an angle of incidence (θ) of 0 degrees, no correction would be necessary for accurate velocity determination. For the example with an angle of incidence of 30 degrees, systematic underestimation of velocity would be anticipated. However, because both points X and Y, representing endocardial and epicardial regions of interest, are interrogated with the same angle of incidence, calculation of the velocity gradient, as a relative measure, is unaffected.

dependent because one is comparing the velocities in the two adjacent wall regions interrogated with the identical angle of incidence. Several investigators have demonstrated that this is a more sensitive indicator of ischemia and ventricular dysfunction than are many standard methodologies. Color M-mode DTI (Fig. 6.39) can also be used to assess differential velocities across the left ventricular wall thickness by using an offline analysis system that converts the color assignments to velocity values (Fig. 6.42).

Strain Rate Imaging and Other Derived Doppler Tissue Parameters

DTI determines the direction and velocity of wall motion. There are several additional parameters of systolic function that can be derived from this velocity determination (Fig. 6.43). The simplest to understand is displacement, defined as excursion (in millimeters). This is calculated as the product of systolic velocity and duration of contraction. Figures 6.44 and 6.45 are examples of the myocardial displacement calculation in a normal subject and in the presence of a lateral wall infarction.

Strain rate imaging is a newly developed variation of DTI that provides a high-resolution evaluation of regional myocardial function. Figure 6.43 outlines the methodology for deriving this parameter. For strain rate imaging, DTI is used to simultaneously determine velocities in two adjacent points as well as the relative distance between those two points. Strain rate is defined as the instantaneous rate of change in the two velocities divided by the instantaneous distance between the two points. Positive strain rate represents active contraction and negative values, relaxation or lengthening between the two points. As with the endocardial-epicardial veloc-

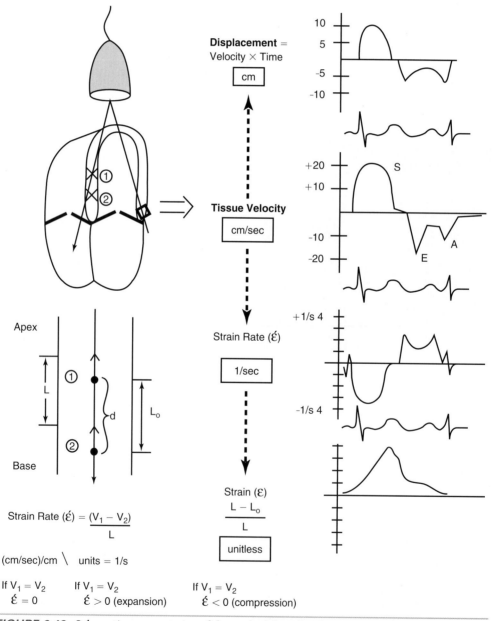

FIGURE 6.43. Schematic representation of the methodology for obtaining Doppler tissue imaging of the mitral anulus or of two adjacent points for calculation of myocardial strain or strain rate. The derived parameters of displacement and strain rate are also graphically displayed. (See text for details.)

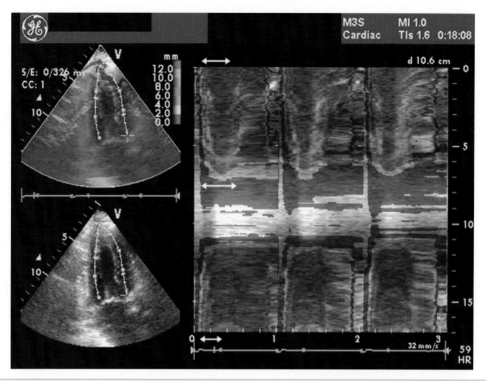

FIGURE 6.44. Color M-mode representation of myocardial displacement derived from Doppler tissue imaging in a normal individual. For this calculation, a center-line region of interest has been drawn extending from the basal inferior wall to the apex and down the anterior wall to the basal anterior anulus (see small two-dimensional images). The format for the color Doppler M-mode imaging includes three consecutive cardiac cycles with time on the X axis and distance along the region of interest on the Y axis. Point 0 is the basal inferior wall and point 17 the basal anterior anulus. Displacement (0.0–12.0 mm) over time is color encoded as noted. In this normal example, note the increasing myocardial displacement during systole *(double head arrow)* and also the lack of motion at the apex.

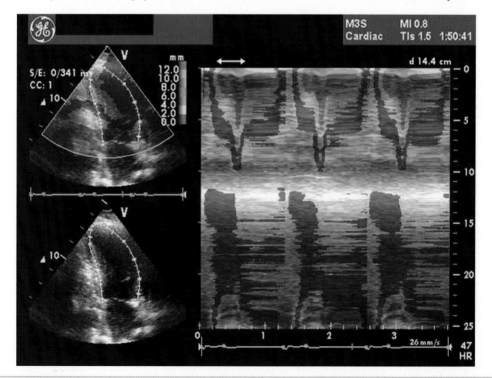

FIGURE 6.45. Myocardial displacement map of the left ventricle recorded in a patient with lateral wall akinesis. Details of the format are given in the legend for Figure 6.44. In this example, note the normal displacement in the septum and a lack of myocardial displacement in the akinetic lateral wall.

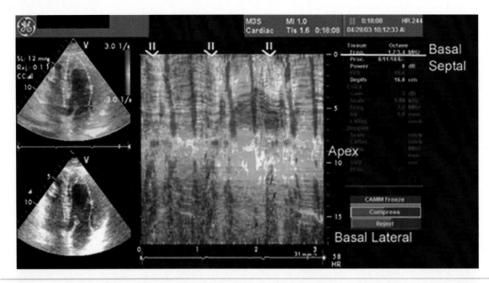

FIGURE 6.46. Curved M-mode representation of myocardial strain rate recorded in a patient with normal ventricular function from an apical four-chamber view. The format for the color demonstration is similar to that for the previous displacement figures. Three consecutive cardiac cycles are displayed along the X axis. Distance from the proximal septum through the apex and down through the lateral wall is displayed on the Y axis as noted. Note the phasic coloration in the septum occuring with mechanical systole *(arrows)*. The signal in the lateral wall is less distinct in large part due to lateral wall dropout.

ity gradient, strain rate has been demonstrated to be a more sensitive and earlier indicator of regional dysfunction than many routine techniques. The images in Figures 6.46 and 6.47 were recorded in a normal subject and in a subject with anterior wall infarction, respectively. Strain rate imaging has tremendous temporal resolution as well and can be used to demonstrate subtle phenomena such as postsystolic contraction. Figure 6.48 is a graphic representation of instantaneous strain rate over time at multiple interrogation points, demonstrating both the temporal and potentially high spatial resolution of this technique.

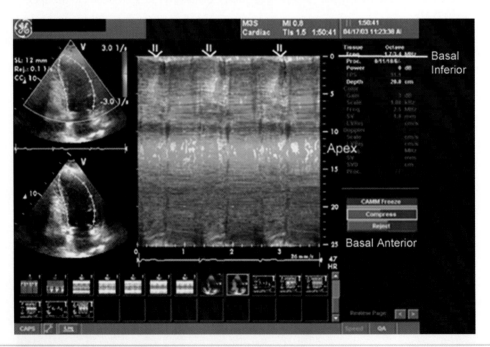

FIGURE 6.47. Strain rate image recorded in a patient with anterior wall hypokinesis. The image format is identical to that presented in Figure 6.46. Again, three consecutive cycles are presented. Note the phasic variation in color of the inferior wall and the lack of phasic coloration, implying neither contraction nor expansion along the anterior wall.

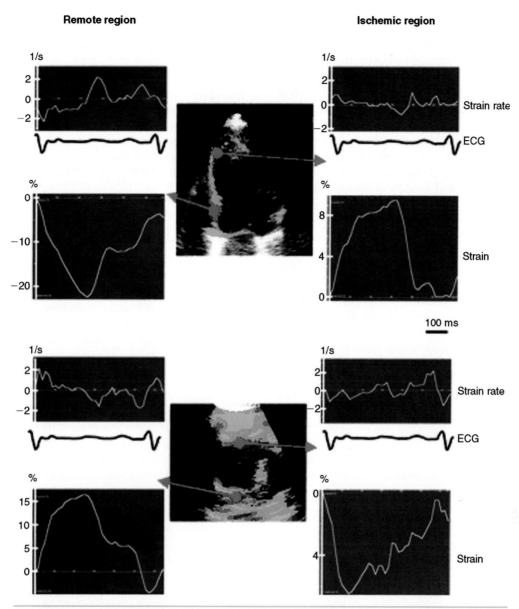

FIGURE 6.48. Demonstration of strain and strain rate recorded in a patient with distal septal ischemia. Both an apical **(top)** and short-axis view **(bottom)** are presented. Note the difference in strain and strain rate contours when comparing the remote and ischemic regions. (From Edvardsen T, Berber BL, Garot J, et al. Quantitative assessment of intrinsic regional myocardial deformation by Doppler strain rate echocardiography in humans: validation against three-dimensional tagged magnetic resonance imaging. Circulation 2002;106:50–56, with permission.)

EVALUATION OF DIASTOLIC FUNCTION

It has become widely recognized that virtually all forms of acquired organic heart disease are associated with a component of left ventricular diastolic dysfunction. This includes obvious entities such as hypertensive cardiovascular disease and hypertrophic cardiomyopathy but also includes coronary artery disease, dilated cardiomyopathy, and many forms of valvular heart disease. Because diastole comprises approximately two-thirds of the cardiac cycle, left ventricular diastolic pressure is transmitted to the left atrium and hence the pulmonary veins for a relatively longer period than is systolic pressure. Transmission of elevated diastolic pressures to the pulmonary venous bed can be a substantial driving force for development of pulmonary hypertension. Because diastole comprises two-thirds of the cardiac cycle, diseases that elevate diastolic pressure are often more likely to be associated with secondary pulmonary hypertension than are diseases with isolated elevation of systolic pressure. A classic example is the propensity to develop secondary pulmonary hypertension in mitral stenosis compared with its lower incidence in mitral regurgitation in which transient left atrial pressures are higher during systole but may remain in the normal range during the longer diastolic period. Diastolic dysfunction is a significant contributor to the development of congestive heart failure. Recent studies have demonstrated that 30% to 40% of patients presenting with congestive heart failure have preserved systolic function of the left ventricle, and the etiology of heart failure is presumed to be diastolic dysfunction. The presence and severity of diastolic function have also been related to prognosis in a wide range of disease states.

A range of findings have been noted in patients with diastolic dysfunction, and the more extreme ranges of this abnormality have been associated with a substantially worsened prognosis (Fig. 6.49). Diastolic function is often categorized as grades 1 through 4, as defined in Figure 6.49. A restrictive pattern confers a substantially worse prognosis than the other grades of dysfunction. Although there are a number of medical and surgical options for patients with systolic overload of the left ventricle such as aortic stenosis, there are fewer options for the treatment of patients with diastolic dysfunction.

Methods for Evaluating Diastolic Function

There are numerous echocardiographic techniques for evaluating left ventricular diastolic function (Table 6.6).

▶ **TABLE 6.6 Methods for Evaluation of Diastolic Dysfunction**

Anatomy based
  Continuous left ventricular volume
    Diastolic filling rate
Flow based
  Mitral valve inflow patterns
    E/A ratio (velocity or area)
    Deceleration time
Isovolumetric relaxation time
Dimensionless myocardial performance index (MPI)
Pulmonary vein flow
Doppler Tissue Imaging
  Mitral anular diastolic velocity (E_A)
  Mitral valve E-wave/E_A ratio

In contemporary practice, Doppler techniques evaluating mitral inflow and pulmonary vein flow and DTI of the mitral anulus have had the most clinical utility. All can be easily evaluated using standard commercially available equipment, and the data can be recorded in most patients presenting for evaluation.

M-Mode Echocardiography

M-mode echocardiography plays little role in the evaluation of diastolic function in contemporary practice. It should be emphasized that evaluation of diastolic dysfunction is most often undertaken when the clinical sit-

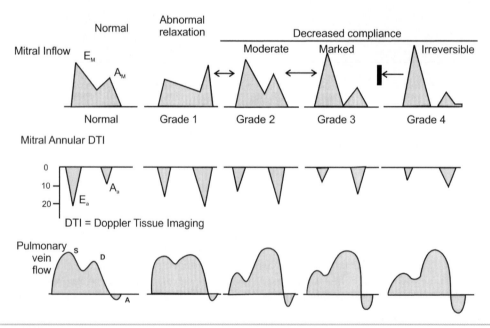

FIGURE 6.49. Schematic representation of mitral inflow **(top)**, mitral anular Doppler tissue imaging **(middle)**, and pulmonary vein flow **(bottom)** in a normal individual and in various grades of diastolic dysfunction.

uation warrants and the appropriate anatomic substrate appears to be present on two-dimensional imaging. M-mode techniques that have previously been used for evaluating diastole include digitization of the posterior wall of the left ventricle from which detailed parameters of contraction and relaxation can be derived. As noted under M-mode evaluation of systolic function, M-mode echocardiography of anular motion recorded from the apex can also provide information regarding the rate of relaxation of the base of the heart. These techniques are infrequently if ever used in contemporary practice and in large part have been replaced by DTI. One M-mode finding that has retained clinical relevance is detection of the so-called B bump of mitral valve closure (Fig. 6.50). Hemodynamic studies have demonstrated that detection of this abnormal closure pattern is seen in patients with elevated left ventricular end-diastolic pressure and that it is the echocardiographic correlate of a rapid increase in left ventricular diastolic pressure during atrial contraction. When present, it is an indication of elevated diastolic pressure; however, it provides no quantitative information.

Two-Dimensional Echocardiography

Two-dimensional echocardiography is an excellent surveillance tool for evaluating all forms of anatomic heart disease because it allows an anatomic description of the underlying organic heart disease and an assessment of systolic function; it plays a confirmatory and exclusionary role in that it can identify, characterize, and quantify diseases that have resulted in diastolic dysfunction.

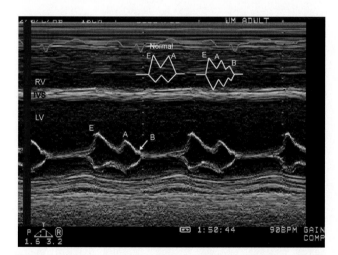

FIGURE 6.50. M-mode echocardiogram recorded in a patient with combined systolic and diastolic left ventricular dysfunction. Note in the M-mode echocardiogram the increased E-point septal separation and the interrupted closure (B bump) of the mitral valve consistent with elevated end-diastolic pressure. Normal and abnormal mitral closure patterns are noted in the schematics superimposed on the figure.

A number of disease entities are associated almost exclusively with diastolic dysfunction, most of which can be diagnosed using two-dimensional echocardiography. The combination of thickened left ventricular walls, left atrial dilation, and absence of mitral valve disease is strong evidence of diastolic dysfunction and elevated left ventricular diastolic pressure. Typically, supplemental Doppler imaging is used to confirm and quantify the degree of diastolic dysfunction. Diseases such as cardiac amyloidosis, which is the prototypical disease causing restrictive cardiomyopathy, nonobstructive hypertrophy cardiomyopathy, and hypertensive cardiovascular disease with preserved left ventricular systolic function are all examples of organic heart disease that can be accurately diagnosed using two-dimensional imaging and for which diastolic dysfunction is well recognized as a major source of symptoms.

Using modern ultrasound platforms, it is possible to calculate instantaneous left ventricular volume. This is typically done to determine stroke volume and ejection fraction. The same technique can be used to determine the serial left ventricular volumes during diastole. These volumes can then be plotted over time (Fig. 6.9) and compared with normal rates of ventricular filling. Although accurate for identifying abnormalities of ventricular filling, as manifest by abnormal patterns of ventricular volume change in early and late diastole, the technique has had little practical application, in large part because of perceived technical difficulty and relatively limited availability of the ultrasound platforms performing these measurements.

Doppler Evaluation of Diastolic Function

It was not until the widespread availability of Doppler echocardiography that evaluation of diastolic function of the left ventricle became a viable clinical tool. There are a number of Doppler approaches for determining diastolic function, including determination of mitral inflow patterns with pulsed Doppler imaging, evaluation of pulmonary vein flow, and the newer technique of DTI, which can be used as a stand-alone technique or combined with mitral inflow patterns. A word of caution is advised when using Doppler parameters as markers of diastolic dysfunction. The accuracy and validity of Doppler markers of diastolic function are greatest in the presence of systolic dysfunction, and individual parameters may lose their validity in the presence of normal systolic function.

Evaluation of Mitral Inflow

For evaluation of diastolic properties of the left ventricle, the mitral inflow pattern is evaluated from an apical transducer position with the sample volume placed at the tips of the mitral valve. Normal mitral inflow consists of biphasic flow from the left atrium into the left ventricle

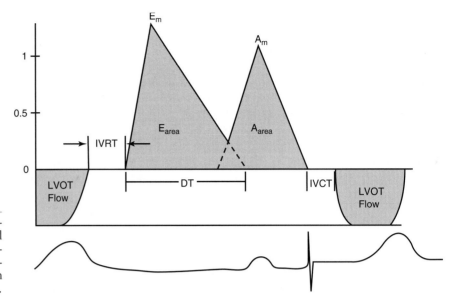

FIGURE 6.51. Schematic representation of different components of mitral valve inflow. See text for details. DT, deceleration time; IVCT, isovolumic contraction time; IVRT, isovolumic relaxation time; LVOT, left ventricular outflow tract.

(Fig. 6.51). In a healthy, disease-free individual, the early flow, coincident with the mitral E-wave, exceeds the later flow, which occurs with atrial systole (the A-wave) both in velocity and volume. The magnitude of these flows, as well as their ratio, varies with age in the normal population. In healthy, young, disease-free individuals the E-wave exceeds the A-wave, and therefore the E/A ratio is more than 1.0. In adolescents and young adults, there may be a disproportionate contribution of active ventricular relaxation to ventricular filling, which results in a markedly accentuated E-wave velocity. In this instance, E/A ratio can exceed a value of 2.0 in a normal, disease-free individual. With advancing age, there is natural stiffening of the ventricle, which results in delayed relaxation. This results in a progressive decrease in E-wave velocity and an increase in A-wave velocity with age so that the an-

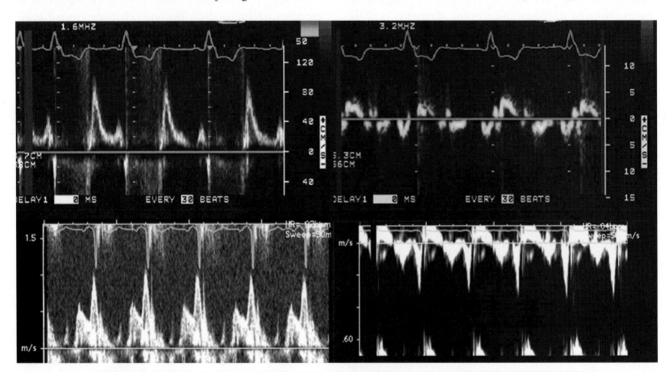

FIGURE 6.52. Mitral inflow **(left)** and mitral anular Doppler tissue velocities **(right)** recorded in two patients with diastolic dysfunction. **Bottom:** Recorded in a patient with grade 1 diastolic dysfunction and a reduced mitral E/A ratio, which is paralleled by the anular E/A ratio. **Top:** Recorded in a patient with grade 3 diastolic dysfunction and evidence of markedly elevated pulmonary capillary pressure. Note the elevated E/A ratio of 2.5 and the pathologically reduced anular E velocity of approximately 3 cm/sec. In the example at the top, the E/E$_a$ ratio exceeds 20, consistent with marked elevation in pulmonary capillary wedge pressure.

ticipated E/A ratio in a disease-free individual older than the age of 60 is often less than 1.0. With pathologic degrees of stiffening of the left ventricular myocardium, a hierarchy of changes can be seen in the mitral inflow patterns. These are schematized in Figure 6.49 and further illustrated in Figure 6.52. This schematic assumes a steady progression of diastolic dysfunction with a component of volume overload at the more extreme ranges. In clinical practice, this steady progression over time is often confounded by concurrent systolic dysfunction or valvular dysfunction.

The appropriate method for measuring mitral valve inflow is to use a two-dimensionally directed pulsed sample volume placed at the tips of the mitral valve. This is the point at which the mitral flow velocities are maximal. If the sample volume is placed closer to the anulus, the measured velocities will be lower (because of a relatively larger cross-sectional area for flow); however, the E/A ratio is accurately reflected. Maximal accuracy and reproducibility of measurement are obtained by evaluating the flow profile at the tips where velocity is maximal. Figure 6.53 shows the change in flow velocities with different sample volume positions.

Figure 6.51 is a detailed schematic of the mitral inflow pattern. There are multiple parameters that can be derived from the inflow pattern including E and A velocities and the time velocity integral of the E-wave and A-wave separately as well as their ratios. An additional commonly used measurement is the deceleration time of the E-wave. With delayed left ventricular relaxation there is a prolongation of deceleration time. In the presence of elevated left ventricular diastolic pressure, as is seen in reduced left ventricular compliance (or a rapid rise in diastolic pressure), the left atrial–left ventricular pressures rapidly equalize, and flow ceases. This results in a shortening of the mitral valve deceleration time.

Measuring the E/A ratio may be problematic at high heart rates in which the E- and A-waves tend to merge. In addition, measurements of deceleration time and the E-to-F slope are problematic when the E-to-F decay curve is not linear. In the majority of these instances, using the mid portion of the E-wave deceleration is most appropriate for determining slope. Many individuals will have a "ski-slope" E-wave in which there is a short rapid decline in E-wave velocity followed by a more gradual slope. In this instance, ignoring the initial steep decline and measuring the mid portion of the E-wave is the appropriate methodology. In most instances, the E-wave velocity does not decline fully to a velocity of 0 m/sec and hence the true time points for deceleration time cannot be determined. Standard practice is to extrapolate the deceleration time from the more proximal portions of the E-wave slope (Fig. 6.51).

There are several "classic" mitral valve inflow patterns that have been attributed in varying degree to

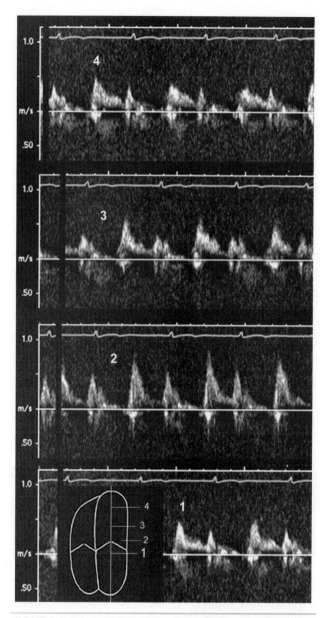

FIGURE 6.53. Demonstration of the effect of sample volume placement on mitral valve inflow patterns. The schematic at the lower left denotes the location of recording of the pulsed sample volume for recording left ventricular inflow velocities. Note the relatively preserved relationship between the E/A ratios but the significant variation in absolute velocities with the maximal velocity and "cleanest" signal noted at position 2, at the tips of the mitral valve leaflets.

diastolic dysfunction. These include delayed relaxation with a reduced E/A ratio and the exaggerated E/A ratio (typically >2.5) with a pathologically short deceleration time that has been ascribed to marked ventricular noncompliance with elevated diastolic pressure, the so-called restrictive physiology pattern. It should be emphasized that these patterns are dependent on intravascular volume status and systolic ventricular function. In many instances, pathologic inflow patterns may be mim-

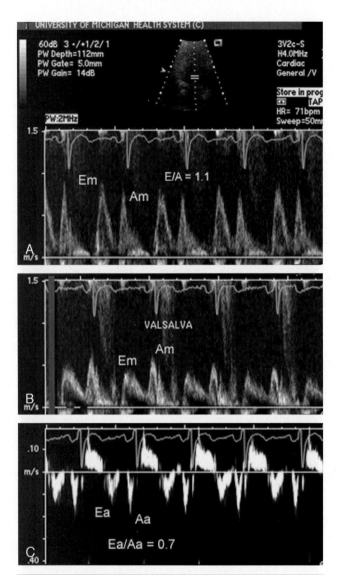

FIGURE 6.54. Pulsed Doppler mitral inflow and anular Doppler tissue imaging recorded in a patient with grade 2 diastolic dysfunction (pseudo-normal pattern). Note the E/A ratio of 1.1 at the top. During the Valsalva maneuver, there is a reversal of the E/A ratio. Note the mitral anular E/A ratio of 0.7, confirming grade 2 diastolic dysfunction.

icked in young, disease-free individuals with normal systolic and diastolic function. The restrictive pattern represents a combination of a stiff, noncompliant ventricle and elevated left ventricular end-diastolic pressure. Maneuvers that alter ventricular volume such as the Valsalva maneuver, lower body negative suction, and leg elevation, can result in dynamic changes in the appearance of the mitral inflow pattern. Scrutiny of Figure 6.49, which schematizes the different mitral inflow patterns and describes them as a hierarchy of change, reveals the intermediate pattern in which diastolic dysfunction is present but mitral inflow patterns are essentially normal. This is the so-called pseudo-normal

pattern and can be seen as a disease process progresses from a point of poor relaxation to pathologic stiffness in a patient with a pathologically stiff ventricle and volume overload as successful diuresis occurs. Monitoring mitral inflow patterns during the Valsalva maneuver, which reduces left ventricular preload, may change the "normal" E/A ratio and unmask evidence of delayed relaxation (Fig. 6.54). There are several other techniques for separating the pseudo-normal from a truly normal pattern, which are discussed subsequently.

Obviously scrutiny of mitral inflow patterns alone will not be adequate in many patients. Evaluation of the E/A ratio requires that the patient be in sinus rhythm, and hence paced rhythms and atrial fibrillation result in an inability to evaluate diastolic function using the mitral inflow pattern alone. The E/A ratio varies with heart rate as well and in a disease-free individual will progressively decrease with higher heart rates. In addition, the E- and A-waves fuse at high heart rates, rendering separation of them for measurement problematic.

Determination of Isovolumic Relaxation Time

The isovolumic relaxation time (IVRT) represents the earliest phase of diastole. It is defined as the time from aortic valve closure to mitral valve opening and normally averages 76 ± 13ms in adults. During this time, systolic contraction has ceased, but left ventricular filling has not yet begun. The IVRT has been used in clinical cardiology for more than three decades and was originally described as a valuable clinical finding using phonocardiography. The determination of IVRT requires knowledge of two separate timing events that may need two different imaging planes. Figures 6.51 and 6.55 illustrate the method for determining IVRT in a clinical echocardiogram. Typically, diseases that result in elevation of left atrial pressure will shorten the IVRT as the crossover point between left atrial and left ventricular diastolic pressure occurs earlier in diastole than in situations in which left atrial pressure is low.

A rapidly determined index of ventricular function has been derived by comparing the total systolic time from mitral valve closure to mitral valve opening with the systolic time involved in actual aortic flow or ejection time. Figures 6.56 and 6.57 illustrate the calculation of this index. The total systolic time is defined as isovolumic contraction time (IVCT) + ejection time + IVRT. The myocardial performance index essentially divides the total isovolumic times (IVCT + IVRT) by the ejection time. This index, referred to as the myocardial performance index (MPI) or Tei index, combines features of both systolic and diastolic function and has been shown to correlate with outcome in ischemic and nonischemic disease states. Normal MPI is less than 0.40 with progressively greater values implying progressively worse ventricular function.

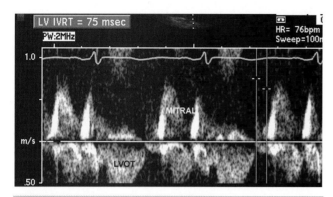

FIGURE 6.55. Example of the calculation of the isovolumic relaxation time from a pulsed wave Doppler image with the sample volume positioned to record mitral inflow and left ventricular outflow simultaneously.

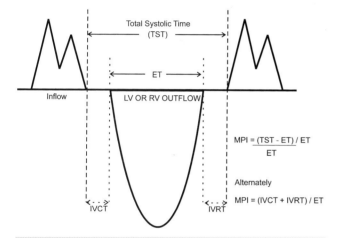

FIGURE 6.56. Schematic representation of the calculation of the myocardial performance index (MPI). The MPI is defined as the ratio of the isovolumic times (IVCT + IVRT) to ejection time. It can be calculated either by measuring each of the three individual times, as noted in the formula at bottom, or by subtracting the ejection time from the total systolic time as a measure of total isovolumic time.

Evaluation of Pulmonary Vein Flow

The same pulsed Doppler techniques used for determining mitral inflow can be used to determine the pattern of pulmonary vein flow into the left atrium. In many clinical echocardiography laboratories, this is not routinely performed because of the presumed difficulty in imaging this flow. In reality, obtaining high-quality pulmonary vein flow tracings is well within the range of virtually all routine clinical laboratories. In exceptionally difficult patients, the use of a transpulmonary contrast agent may allow recording of a more definitive flow profile, although this should be rarely needed for an assessment of diastolic function. Typically, imaging is performed from the apical view. It may be advantageous to saturate the posterior atrial wall with color flow imaging to further identify and

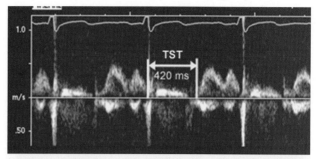

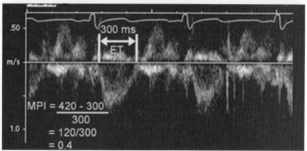

FIGURE 6.57. Pulsed wave Doppler recording of mitral inflow and left ventricular outflow tract flows demonstrates the calculation of the myocardial performance index.

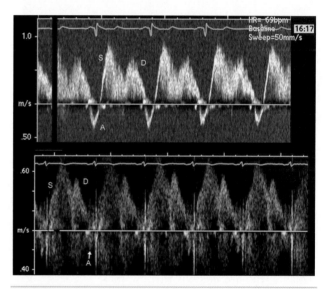

FIGURE 6.58. Pulmonary vein pulsed Doppler imaging recorded from a transesophageal echocardiogram **(top)** and an apical four-chamber view **(bottom)** in patients with normal diastolic function. In each instance, note the systolic predominance of forward flow from the pulmonary veins and relatively narrow pulmonary vein A-wave. Also note the indistinct nature of the pulmonary vein A-wave when recorded by transthoracic echocardiography, making its use as a marker of diastolic function problematic in many individuals.

refine the pulmonary vein origins. Typically from this position, it is the right posterior pulmonary vein that is most easily visualized (Figs. 6.58 and 6.59). The sample volume can then be placed at the orifice of the pulmonary vein and pulsed wave Doppler imaging used to record the flow

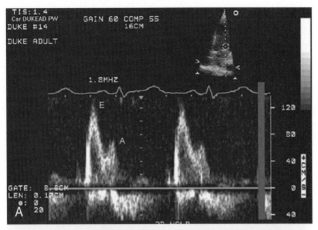

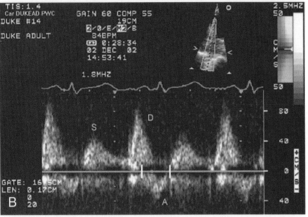

FIGURE 6.59. Pulsed Doppler recording of mitral inflow **(top)** and pulmonary vein flow **(bottom)**. Note in this example the reduced S wave of the pulmonary vein, suggesting diastolic dysfunction. Note also the prominent wide pulmonary vein A-wave.

envelope. Normal pulmonary vein inflow consists of a diastolic and systolic phase as well as atrial reversal. In some instances, there will be two distinct systolic flow phases. In normal, disease-free individuals with normal diastolic properties of the ventricle, the velocity of systolic flow typically equals or exceeds that of diastolic flow. For patients who are in sinus rhythm, there is a short, low-velocity reversal of flow coincident with atrial systole, the so-called pulmonary vein A-wave. With increasing stiffness and decreasing compliance of the left ventricle, emptying of the left atrium becomes incomplete during diastole. Because of this, at the onset of ventricular systole, left atrial volume and pressure are elevated. This results in a reduction of flow volume into the left atrium (from the pulmonary veins) during ventricular systole, which is reflected in a blunting of the systolic flow and a relative increase in the diastolic flow because the overwhelming majority of flow out of the pulmonary veins occurs during ventricular diastole coincident with emptying of the left atrium. The incomplete emptying and increase in atrial pressure also result in an exaggeration of both the veloc-

ity and width of the pulmonary vein A-wave. The pulmonary vein A-wave duration can be compared with the mitral A-wave duration. At least one study has suggested that, if the pulmonary vein A-wave duration exceeds the mitral A-wave duration, the left ventricular end-diastolic pressure exceeds 15 mm Hg in the majority of cases. Accurate recording of the pulmonary vein A-wave can be challenging, making precise measurements of its duration difficult, and for this reason, many laboratories have abandoned this analysis.

Evaluation of pulmonary vein flow should not be considered a stand-alone technique and should be undertaken in conjunction with a detailed evaluation of transmitral flow. Figure 6.49 schematizes different combinations of transmitral flow and pulmonary vein flow in normal and varying disease states. Evaluation of pulmonary vein flow can provide a valuable clue to the presence of pseudo-normalization when a normal mitral inflow E/A ratio has been noted in a situation in which diastolic dysfunction is suspected. In this instance, the pulmonary vein flow will reveal blunted systolic velocities and relatively greater diastolic inflow with accentuation of the A-wave (Fig. 6.59). In many laboratories, analysis of pulmonary vein flow has been largely supplanted by DTI of the mitral anulus for evaluation of diastolic function.

Doppler Tissue Imaging

The methodology for DTI is discussed in Chapter 3 and in the section on determination of systolic function. Using the same interrogation views, DTI can be used to provide information regarding diastolic function. The interrogating sample volume can be placed at any point in the left ventricular wall or the cardiac anulus. Most commonly, DTI of the mitral anulus is employed, and the data used as a marker of global systolic or diastolic function. Disease states that result in delayed myocardial relaxation and delayed filling are associated with abnormal (typically slowed) patterns of anular motion in diastole. Figure 6.49 illustrates these abnormal patterns in patients with abnormal diastolic function. Evaluation of anular motion with DTI has shown promise for providing information regarding global diastolic function and is not affected by atrial fibrillation or rapid heart rates, which obviously confound evaluation of mitral valve inflow patterns. In sinus rhythm, there are two anular motions (E_a and A_a) that parallel the transmitral flow. In normal, disease-free states, E_a is greater than A_a, similar to the relationship of the mitral E- and A-waves (E_m and A_m). With diastolic dysfunction, there is a reduction in E_a such that the anular E/A ratio (E_a/A_a) reverses. The anular velocity is not volume dependent, as opposed to mitral inflow (E), and as such, the anular velocity (E_a) remains depressed in the pressure of a pseudo-normal or restrictive mitral inflow pattern. Comparison of anular and mitral E/A ratios may

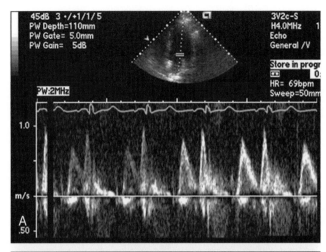

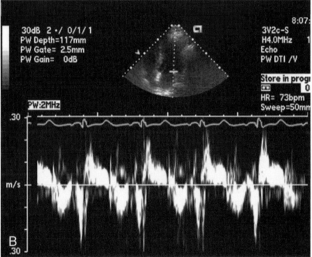

FIGURE 6.60. Pulsed Doppler mitral inflow **(top)** and anular Doppler tissue imaging **(bottom)** recorded in a patient with grade 1 diastolic dysfunction. In the mitral inflow pattern, note the reduced E/A ratio and a parallel decrease in the anular E/A ratio.

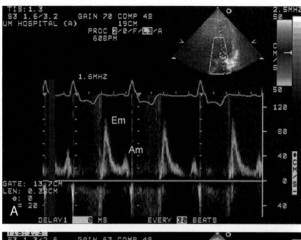

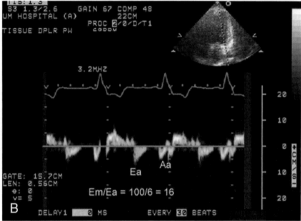

FIGURE 6.61. Pulsed Doppler mitral inflow pattern **(top)** and anular Doppler tissue imaging **(bottom)** recorded in a patient with significant left ventricular systolic dysfunction and elevated left atrial pressures. Note the mitral E/A ratio of approximately 2.5. Also note the ratio of mitral to anular E-wave of 16, suggesting marked elevation in pulmonary capillary wedge pressure.

provide valuable information on the presence and severity of diastolic dysfunction (Figs. 6.49, 6.60, and 6.61).

Several investigators have demonstrated that the combination of mitral E-wave velocity (E) and early diastolic velocities in the anulus (E_a) bear a linear relationship to pulmonary capillary wedge pressure measured with a right heart catheter. This relationship has held in patients with tachycardia, atrial fibrillation, and a broad range of cardiovascular diseases. Figure 6.62 outlines the results of one such study. This observation has been undertaken in relatively small numbers of patients but has encompassed a broad range of clinical diseases and appears to show promise for not only detecting diastolic dysfunction but also predicting intracardiac hemodynamics. Various investigators have used E/E_a ratios of 10, 12, or 15 to stratify pulmonary capillary pressures exceeding thresholds of 18 to 20 mm Hg. Irrespective of the E_m/E_a cutoff used,

there has been a direct correlation between the E/E_a ratio and pulmonary capillary wedge pressure. An elevated E/E_a ratio has also been shown to confer an adverse prognosis in both ischemic and nonischemic left ventricular dysfunction.

Color Doppler M-Mode Imaging

Color Doppler M-mode imaging can be used to provide information on diastolic function. This technique color encodes Doppler velocities along a single M-mode interrogation line. For evaluation of diastolic function, mitral inflow propagation velocity is evaluated from the left ventricular apex. Figure 6.63 is an example of normal color Doppler M-mode propagation velocities (V_p). In situations in which there is delayed filling of the ventricle, this technique can document reduced flow velocities that are manifest as a reduced slope of the color Doppler M-mode sig-

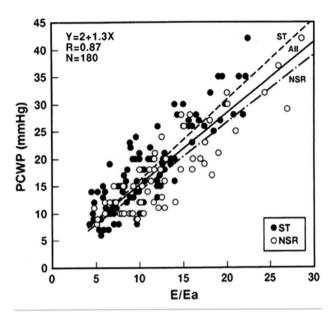

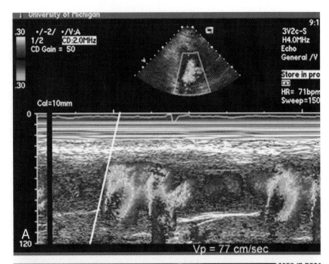

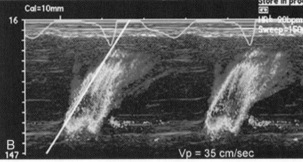

FIGURE 6.62. Graphic representation of pulmonary capillary wedge pressure (PCWP) and mitral E/E_a ratio. Note the direct relationship between PCWP and the ratio E/E_a in which the majority of patients with an E/E_a ratio <10 have a PCWP <15 mm Hg, whereas those with a ratio >20 typically have a PCWP >20 mm Hg. (From Nagueh SF, Kopelen HA, Quinones MA. Assessment of left ventricular filling pressures by Doppler in the presence of atrial fibrillation. Circulation 1998;98:1644–1650, with permission.)

FIGURE 6.63. Color Doppler M-mode image recorded from the apex in a patient with normal diastolic function **(top)** and reduced ventricular compliance **(bottom)**.

nal. Color Doppler M-mode imaging also allows demonstration of not only velocity but also the velocity decay as the left ventricular inflow velocity decreases with propagation toward the apex. Reduction of the depth in the left ventricle to which the mitral flow propagates as organized flow is evidence of diastolic dysfunction. Figure 6.63 at top demonstrates that in a normal situation, there is a rapid slope, implying high velocity of flow (this is similar to a normal or high E-wave slope). Additionally, the organized color flow can be seen to propagate into two-thirds of the depth of the left ventricle. In patients with diastolic dysfunction, the velocity of early filling is reduced (as manifest by a reduced E-wave velocity) and organized propagation of flow does not occur past the mid ventricle. Color Doppler M-mode imaging can demonstrate both of these phenomena simultaneously. Most studies have suggested that detection of a color Doppler M-mode propagation slope less than 45 cm/sec is excellent evidence of diastolic dysfunction with delayed relaxation.

Mitral Flow Dispersion

As noted previously with color Doppler M-mode imaging, propagation of an organized mitral pattern toward the left ventricular apex is reduced in patients with diastolic dysfunction. This same phenomenon can be determined by using a series of pulsed sample volumes. In normal, disease-free individuals, there is preservation of distinct E- and A-waves and a gradual tapering of the E-wave velocity. In the presence of diastolic dysfunction, these velocities do not propagate in an organized fashion to a similar depth, and there is dispersion of the normal mitral inflow pattern when the interrogating sample is moved from the tips of the mitral valve leaflet toward the apex. This technique provides information very similar to that seen obtained with color Doppler M-mode imaging. Both of these techniques retain their validity at varying heart rates and in the presence of atrial fibrillation.

Left Atrial Volume/Size

A final indirect measure of chronic diastolic function is left atrial size, quantified either as area or volume from an apical view (Fig. 6.64). Several recent studies have suggested the prognostic importance of this assessment in both ischemic and nonischemic disease states and suggested that left atrial dilation may supersede the prognostic implication of the other parameters such as mitral inflow patterns.

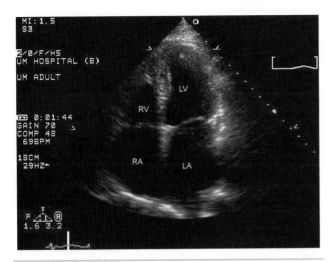

FIGURE 6.64. Apical four-chamber view recorded in an elderly patient with long-standing mild systemic hypertension and congestive heart failure due to predominantly diastolic dysfunction. Note the evidence of significant atrial enlargement, which is a marker of long-standing diastolic dysfunction. LA, Left atrium; LV, left ventricle; RA, right atrium; RV, right ventricle

Overall Evaluation of Diastolic Function

It is imperative that evaluation of diastolic function of the left ventricle not be undertaken in isolation. A comprehensive evaluation of diastolic function includes a thorough anatomic assessment using two-dimensional echocardiography as well as screening for primary and secondary valvular heart disease with color flow imaging and other methodologies. No single Doppler parameter, either spectral Doppler color flow imaging or DTI should be used as a stand-alone indicator of diastolic function. Evaluation of diastolic function requires integration of the anatomic and physiologic information gathered from all the different echocardiographic and Doppler parameters.

SUGGESTED READINGS

Chen C, et al. Continuous wave Doppler echocardiography for noninvasive assessment of left ventricular dP/dt and relaxation time constant from mitral regurgitant spectra in patients. J Am Coll Cardiol 1994;23:970–976.

Chuang ML, et al. Impact of on-line endocardial border detection on determination of left ventricular volume and ejection fraction by transthoracic 3-dimensional echocardiography. J Am Soc Echocardiogr 1999;12:551–558.

Dini FL, et al. Prognostic value of left atrial enlargement in patients with idiopathic dilated cardiomyopathy and ischemic cardiomyopathy. Am J Cardiol 2002;89:518–523.

Edvardsen T, Berber BL, Garot J, et al. Quantitative assessment of intrinsic regional myocardial deformation by Doppler strain rate echocardiography in humans: validation against three-dimensional tagged magnetic resonance imaging. Circulation 2002;106:50–56.

Firstenberg MS, et al. Relationship of echocardiographic indices to pulmonary capillary wedge pressures in healthy volunteers. J Am Coll Cardiol 2000;36:1664–1669.

Garcia MJ, et al. Myocardial wall velocity assessment by pulsed Doppler tissue imaging: characteristic findings in normal subjects. Am Heart J 1996;132:648–656.

Garcia MJ, Thomas JD, Klein AL. New Doppler echocardiographic applications for the study of diastolic function. J Am Coll Cardiol 1998;32:865–875.

Garcia MJ, et al. Color M-mode Doppler flow propagation velocity is a relatively preload-independent index of left ventricular filling. J Am Soc Echocardiogr 1999;12:129–137.

Garcia MJ, et al. Color M-mode Doppler flow propagation velocity is a preload insensitive index of left ventricular relaxation: animal and human validation. J Am Coll Cardiol 2000;35:201–208.

Gillam LD, et al. A comparison of quantitative echocardiographic methods for delineating infarct-induced abnormal wall motion. Circulation 1984;70:113–122.

Gopal AS, et al. Assessment of cardiac function by three-dimensional echocardiography compared with conventional noninvasive methods. Circulation 1995;92:842–853.

Gorcsan J 3rd, Romand JA, Mandarino WA, et al. Assessment of left ventricular performance by on-line pressure-area relations using echocardiographic automated border detection. J Am Coll Cardiol 1994;23:242–252

Hammond IW, et al. Relation of blood pressure and body build to left ventricular mass in normotensive and hypertensive employed adults. J Am Coll Cardiol 1988;12:996–1004.

Hashimoto I, et al. Myocardial strain rate is a superior method for evaluation of left ventricular subendocardial function compared with tissue Doppler imaging. J Am Coll Cardiol 2003;42:1574–1583.

Hibberd MG, Chuang ML, Beaudin RA, et al. Accuracy of three-dimensional echocardiography with unrestricted selection of imaging planes for measurement volumes and ejection fraction. Am Heart J 2000;140:469–475.

Hillis GS, et al. Noninvasive estimation of left ventricular filling pressure by E/e' is a powerful predictor of survival after acute myocardial infarction. J Am Coll Cardiol 2004;43:360–367.

Ilercil A, et al. Reference values for echocardiographic measurements in urban and rural populations of differing ethnicity: the Strong Heart Study. J Am Soc Echocardiogr 2001;14:601–611.

Koren MJ, et al. Relation of left ventricular mass and geometry to morbidity and mortality in uncomplicated essential hypertension. Ann Intern Med 1991;114:345–352.

Kukulski T, et al. Acute changes in systolic and diastolic events during clinical coronary angioplasty: a comparison of regional velocity, strain rate, and strain measurement. J Am Soc Echocardiogr 2002;15:1–12.

Kukulski T, et al. Identification of acutely ischemic myocardium using ultrasonic strain measurements. A clinical study in patients undergoing coronary angioplasty. J Am Coll Cardiol 2003;41:810–819.

Liebson PR, et al. Echocardiographic correlates of left ventricular structure among 844 mildly hypertensive men and women in the Treatment of Mild Hypertension Study (TOMHS). Circulation 1993;87:476–486.

Masuyama T, et al. Pulmonary venous flow velocity pattern as assessed with transthoracic pulsed Doppler echocardiography in subjects without cardiac disease. Am J Cardiol, 1991;67:1396–1404.

McGillem MJ, et al. Modification of the centerline method for assessment of echocardiographic wall thickening and motion: a comparison with areas of risk. J Am Coll Cardiol 1988;11:861–866.

Miyatake K, et al. New method for evaluating left ventricular wall motion by color-coded tissue Doppler imaging: *in vitro* and *in vivo* studies. J Am Coll Cardiol 1995;25:717–724.

Moller JE, et al. Ratio of left ventricular peak E-wave velocity to flow propagation velocity assessed by color M-mode Doppler echocardiography in first myocardial infarction: prognostic and clinical implications. J Am Coll Cardiol 2000;35:363–370.

Municino A, et al. Assessment of left ventricular function by meridional and circumferential end-systolic stress/minor-axis shortening relations in dilated cardiomyopathy. Am J Cardiol 1996;78:544–549.

Nagueh SF, Kopelen HA, Quinones MA. Assessment of left ventricular filling pressures by Doppler in the presence of atrial fibrillation. Circulation 1996;94:2138–2145.

Ommen SR, et al. Clinical utility of Doppler echocardiography and tissue Doppler imaging in the estimation of left ventricular filling pressures: a comparative simultaneous Doppler-catheterization study. Circulation 2000;102:1788–1794.

Palmieri V, et al. Reliability of echocardiographic assessment of left ventricular structure and function: the PRESERVE study. Prospective Randomized Study Evaluating Regression of Ventricular Enlargement. J Am Coll Cardiol 1999;34:1625–1632.

Pearlman JD, et al. Limits of normal left ventricular dimensions in growth and development: analysis of dimensions and variance in the two-dimensional echocardiograms of 268 normal healthy subjects. J Am Coll Cardiol 1988;12:1432–1441.

Quinones MA, et al. A new, simplified and accurate method for determining ejection fraction with two-dimensional echocardiography. Circulation 1981;64:744–753.

Rossvoll O, Hatle LK. Pulmonary venous flow velocities recorded by transthoracic Doppler ultrasound: relation to left ventricular diastolic pressures. J Am Coll Cardiol 1993;21:1687–1696.

Schiller NB, et al. Canine left ventricular mass estimation by two-dimensional echocardiography. Circulation 1983;68:210–216.

Schiller NB, Shah PM, Crawford M, et al. Recommendations for quantitation of the left ventricle by two-dimensional echocardiography. American Society of Echocardiography Committee on Standards, Subcommittee on Quantitation of Two-Dimensional Echocardiograms. J Am Soc Echocardiogr 1989;2:358–367.

Spencer KT, et al. Evaluation of left ventricular diastolic performance using automated border detection. Echocardiography 1999;16:51–62.

Stoylen A, et al. Strain rate imaging by ultrasonography in the diagnosis of coronary artery disease. J Am Soc Echocardiogr 2000;13:1053–1064.

Tei C, Ling LH, Hodge DO, Bailey KR, Oh JK, Rodeheffer RJ, Tajik AJ, Seward JB. New index of combined systolic and diastolic myocardial performance: a simple and reproducible measure of cardiac function—a study in normals and dilated cardiomyopathy, J Cardiol 1995;2(6):357–66.

Vandenberg BF, et al. Estimation of left ventricular ejection fraction by semiautomated edge detection. Echocardiography 1998;15:713–720.

Waggoner AD, Bierig SM. Tissue Doppler imaging: a useful echocardiographic method for the cardiac sonographer to assess systolic and diastolic ventricular function. J Am Soc Echocardiogr 2001;14:1143–1152.

Wang M, et al. Peak early diastolic mitral annulus velocity by tissue Doppler imaging adds independent and incremental prognostic value. J Am Coll Cardiol 2003;41:820–826.

Weyman AE, Franklin TD Jr, Hogan RD, et al. Importance of temporal heterogeneity in assessing the contraction abnormalities associated with acute myocardial ischemia. Circulation 1984;70:102–112

Yamamoto K, et al. Intraventricular dispersion of early diastolic filling: a new marker of left ventricular diastolic dysfunction. Am Heart J 1995;129:291–299.

Yamamoto K, et al. Determination of left ventricular filling pressure by Doppler echocardiography in patients with coronary artery disease: critical role of left ventricular systolic function. J Am Coll Cardiol 1997;30:1819–1826.

Yip G, et al. Clinical applications of strain rate imaging. J Am Soc Echocardiogr 2003;16:1334–1342.

Yuda S, Khoury V, Marwick TH. Influence of wall stress and left ventricular geometry on the accuracy of dobutamine stress echocardiography. J Am Coll Cardiol 2002;40:1311–1319.

Zoghbi WA, et al. Determination of left ventricular volumes with use of a new nongeometric echocardiographic method: clinical validation and potential application. J Am Coll Cardiol 1990;15:610–617.

Left Atrium, Right Atrium, and Right Ventricle

LEFT ATRIUM

In the early history of echocardiography, the left atrium was one of the first cardiac structures to be identified, recorded, and analyzed. A relatively oval-shaped chamber with thin, muscular walls, the left atrium is easily visualized posterior to the aortic root and superior to the left ventricle. With the advent of transesophageal echocardiography, the ability to thoroughly interrogate the left atrium, including its appendage, became possible, and a thorough assessment of its structure and function is now routinely performed.

Left Atrial Dimensions and Volume

The left atrium serves as a reservoir for blood draining the pulmonary veins during ventricular systole and as a conduit for that blood during early diastole. In late diastole, the left atrium becomes a muscular pump to complete the process of left ventricular filling before ventricular contraction and mitral valve closure. Thus, changes in left atrial dimensions and volumes mirror this continuous process of filling and emptying and have been a topic of intense study using two-dimensional echocardiographic techniques. The left atrium can be visualized in a number of echocardiographic views including the parasternal long- and short-axis and the apical four- and two-chamber views (Fig. 7.1). The area, major and minor dimensions, and volumes have been measured from each of these perspectives. Because no single tomographic view conveys complete information about a three-dimensional structure, it is recommended that a combination of two or more imaging planes be used for these purposes.

In each plane, one or more linear dimensions can be measured and the area of the left atrium can be traced. Historically, left atrial size was determined using M-mode echocardiography from the parasternal window (Fig. 7.2). A linear dimension approximating the anteroposterior plane was measured at end-systole, just before mitral valve opening (when the left atrial volume was maximal).

To standardize this approach, the plane should pass through the aortic valve. In most cases this provides a reproducible and accurate reflection of left atrial size. Because the position of the left atrium relative to the scan plane could not be determined with M-mode echocardiography, the assumption that this dimension corresponded to a true anteroposterior measurement represented a significant limitation. For example, if the recording was made from a lower interspace, an oblique dimension was obtained, and the left atrial size was overestimated. This problem can be avoided using two-dimensional echocardiography, ensuring that the measurement plane is properly oriented relative to the chamber. An example of these two approaches to left atrial measurements is provided in Figure 7.3. In A, dimension X (7.0 cm) is correctly aligned relative to the left atrial chamber. If a dimension along a raster line had been used, as would occur with M-mode echocardiography, dimension Y (7.7 cm) would be the result. Figure 7.3B is another example of proper alignment from a patient with a dilated left atrium.

An additional challenge in measuring the left atrial size involves the precise definition of the posterior left atrial wall. In many patients, hazy, amorphous echoes can often be seen lining the posterior wall. These may be due to stagnant blood and can sometimes be eliminated by changing the gain or adjusting the angle of the transducer. Side lobes from a calcified anulus or highly reflective atrioventricular groove can also obscure the location of the posterior left atrial wall.

Although a relationship between this measurement and left atrial volume clearly exists, no single dimension can provide complete information about the true left atrial size. For example, although the left atrium usually dilates as a sphere, asymmetric enlargement can occur. Dilation of the ascending aorta can distort the anteroposterior dimension, whereas dilation of the descending aorta can encroach on the left atrium posteriorly (Fig. 7.4). Additionally, other mediastinal masses can alter left atrial shape and geometry. Figure 7.5 is an example of left atrial compression from a

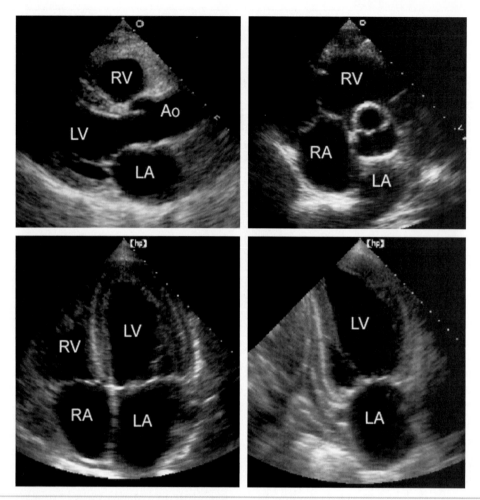

FIGURE 7.1. The left atrium can be visualized from several different echocardiographic views. LA, left atrium; LV, left ventricle; RA, right atrium; RV, right ventricle; Ao, aorta.

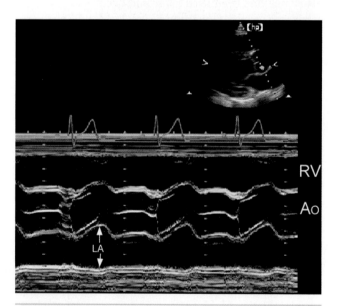

FIGURE 7.2. An M-mode echocardiogram through the base of the heart offers one approach to measuring left atrial (*LA*) size. By convention, the measurement is performed at end-systole when LA volume is greatest. Ao, aorta; RV, right ventricle.

mediastinal lymphoma. The left atrium is completely distorted. The left atrial size cannot be assessed, and the chamber's function is obviously impaired. Thus, an accurate assessment of left atrial size requires visualization of the chamber from multiple views and an appreciation of the limitations of relying on any single plane.

Despite these potential sources of error, left atrial linear dimensions correlate reasonably well with left atrial volume derived from angiography or magnetic resonance imaging. If desired, a more direct measurement of left atrial volume can be obtained. This is typically performed at end-diastole, just before mitral valve opening. A common approach involves the area-length technique from the apical four- and two-chamber views. Using this approach, the area of the left atrium is measured by planimetry of both apical views (Fig. 7.6A). Then, a linear dimension, or length, is measured from the center of the mitral anulus to the superior border of the chamber (and assumed to be the same from both projections). Left atrial volume is then calculated as:

$$\text{Left atrial volume} = (0.85 * A_1 * A_2) \div L \quad \text{[Eq. 7.1]}$$

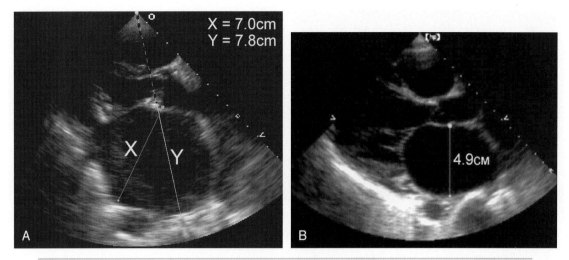

FIGURE 7.3. A limitation of M-mode echocardiography is the lack of spatial orientation. This can result in inaccurate measurement of true left atrial dimension. **A:** Measurement Y (7.7 cm) represents a measurement that would have been recorded using the M-mode approach. The true left atrial dimension is better approximated by measurement X (7.0 cm). Two-dimensional echocardiography provides spatial orientation and avoids the problem of oblique measurements. **B:** Correct orientation of a left atrial minor axis measurement is demonstrated.

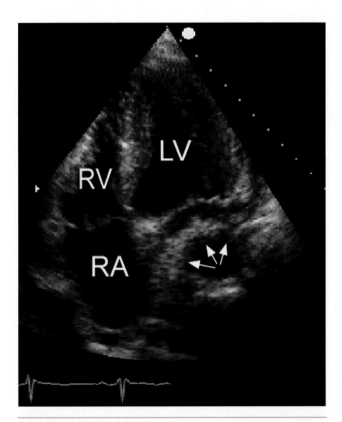

FIGURE 7.4. An apical four-chamber view is shown in a patient with a thoracic aortic aneurysm. The descending aorta (*arrows*) distorts the left atrial shape and creates the appearance of a mass within the chamber. LV, left ventricle; RA, right atrium; RV, right ventricle.

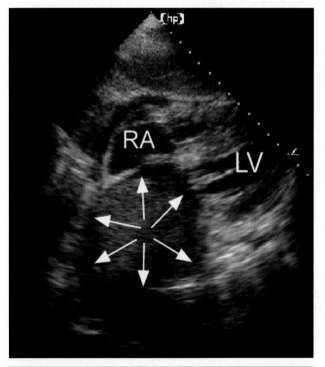

FIGURE 7.5. A subcostal four-chamber view in a patient with a mediastinal lymphoma is shown. External compression of the left atrium by the tumor creates the appearance of a mass (*arrows*). LV, left ventricle; RA, right atrium.

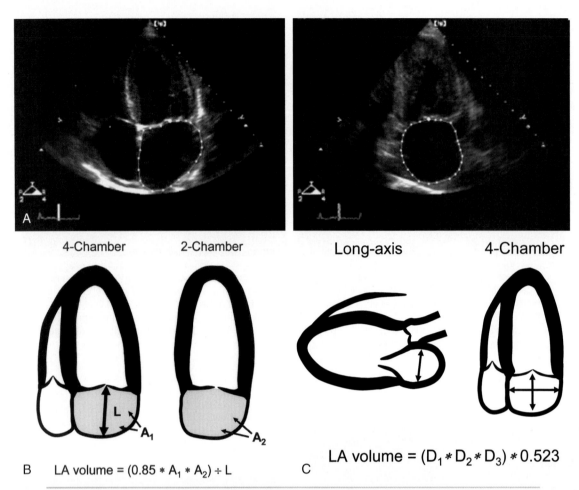

FIGURE 7.6. Left atrial volume can be measured in various ways. **A:** Planimetry of left atrial size from the four- (*left*) and two-chamber (*right*) views. Volume can be determined either using the area-length technique **(B)** or the prolate ellipse method **(C)**. See text for details.

where A_1 is the area in one plane and A_2 is the area in the orthogonal plane, and L is the linear dimension (Fig. 7.6B). Several other formulas have been proposed and most yield similar results. Another practical approach assumes the left atrium can be approximated by a prolate ellipse (Fig. 7.6C). The formula for this structure is

$$\text{Left atrial volume} = (D_1 * D_2 * D_3) * 0.523 \qquad \text{[Eq. 7.2]}$$

The three diameters include the anteroposterior diameter from the parasternal long-axis and two orthogonal diameters from a four-chamber view. Recent studies using these methods confirm the powerful prognostic value of left atrial volume in a variety of situations.

Other indirect measures of left atrial size are also available. For example, the ratio of the aortic root diameter to the left atrial short-axis dimension provides a qualitative estimate that is often used in practice. In normal subjects, the ratio of these two dimensions is approximately 1:1. A significant change in this ratio is a useful visual indicator of an abnormal left atrial size.

Similarly, bowing of the atrial septum into the right atrial cavity indicates left atrial dilation and/or elevated left atrial pressure (Fig. 7.7). This is most easily appreciated using the apical four-chamber view. Finally, isolated dilation of the left atrial appendage has been reported. Although transesophageal echocardiography is most useful for detecting left atrial appendage aneurysms, this abnormality can also be seen from a transthoracic approach.

In summary, some measure of left atrial size should be a part of most echocardiographic examinations. Linear measurements provide limited and potentially misleading data on chamber size but are easy to perform and have traditionally been reported in most clinical studies. Measurements remain useful, provided that the limitations are recognized. If the normally spherical left atrium is distorted, for example, linear dimensions may not accurately reflect chamber size. In the future, more sophisticated approaches that estimate left atrial volume, possibly from three-dimensional imaging, will very likely become a more accepted standard.

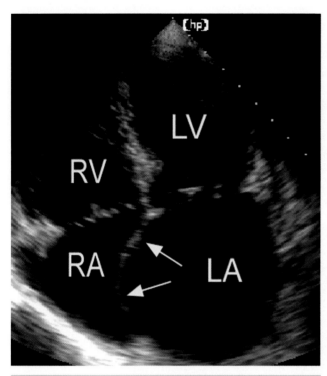

FIGURE 7.7. The interatrial septum reflects the relative pressure difference between the atria. In this example, the septum bows into the right atrial (*RA*) cavity indicating elevated left atrial (*LA*) pressure. LV, left ventricle; RV, right ventricle.

Left Atrial Function

Although not routinely reported, left atrial function has relevance in several disease states and can be assessed using both two-dimensional imaging and Doppler techniques. Contraction of the left atrium, represented by the P-wave on the electrocardiogram, occurs in late diastole and corresponds to the final phase of left ventricular filling before mitral valve closure. This is recorded using Doppler as the A-wave of mitral flow. Both the maximal A-wave velocity and the A-wave time velocity integral correlate with the degree of contractility. Loss of coordinated left atrial contractility, as occurs in atrial fibrillation, is associated with the absence of the mitral A-wave and sometimes the presence of small f waves. Thus, the Doppler A-wave and the P-wave of the surface electrocardiogram represent, respectively, the mechanical and electric manifestations of atrial systole. In most cases, their presence or absence is correlated; both are present in sinus rhythm and both are absent in atrial fibrillation. Figure 7.8 includes three examples of mitral flow from patients with atrial fibrillation before (bottom) and after (top) cardioversion. Note the prominent A-waves in patient C once sinus rhythm is restored. This correlation is not always present, however. For example, immediately after cardioversion, electric activity may return, producing P-waves on the electrocardiogram, before coordinated mechanical function recovers. This results in diminutive or absent Doppler A-waves, as is illustrated by patient B.

With transesophageal echocardiography, left atrial appendage function can also be assessed. Using pulsed Doppler imaging, with the sample volume positioned at the mouth of the appendage, the maximal velocity during atrial contraction can be measured (Fig. 7.9). This velocity corresponds to the force of atrial appendage contraction or emptying. In normal individuals, the left atrial appendage emptying velocity is greater than 50 cm/sec. Significantly lower velocities occur in patients with atrial fibrillation, and this finding has been associated with a predisposition for the development of left atrial thrombus and the risk of thromboembolism (Fig. 7.10).

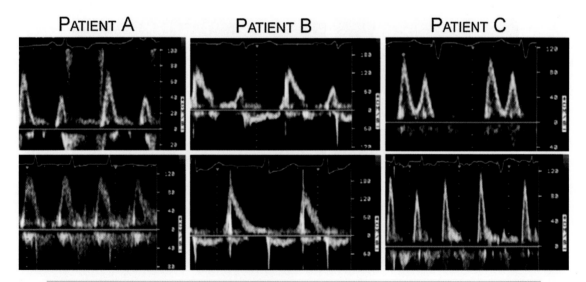

FIGURE 7.8. Three patients with atrial fibrillation are shown before **(bottom)** and after **(top)** cardioversion. Mitral inflow in each case demonstrates the absence of atrial contraction (A-wave) while in atrial fibrillation, but a variable degree of recovery of atrial function after sinus rhythm is restored.

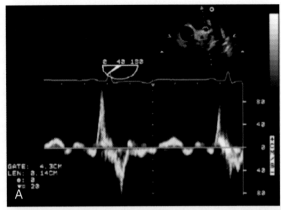

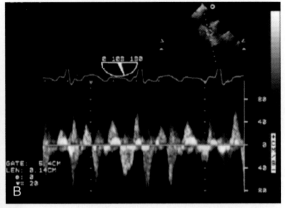

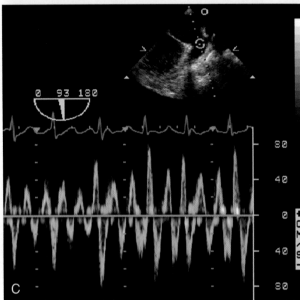

FIGURE 7.9. The left atrial appendage emptying velocity can be recorded using pulsed Doppler imaging. **A:** In a patient in sinus rhythm, the emptying velocity during atrial systole is approximately 60 cm/sec. In atrial fibrillation (**B**), the emptying velocity is variable and much lower, indicating a lack of coordinated contractility. **C:** Another patient during atrial fibrillation. In this case, the velocity is higher.

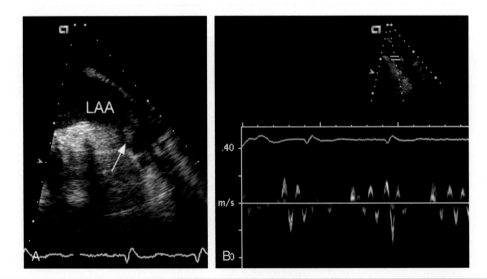

FIGURE 7.10. **A:** A thrombus within the left atrial appendage is shown. The corresponding pulsed Doppler recording demonstrates low left atrial appendage emptying velocity. LAA, left atrial appendage.

Abnormalities of the atrial septum are relatively common and usually congenital in origin. These include a patent foramen ovale (PFO), atrial septal defect (discussed in Chapter 18), and aneurysms of the atrial septum. A PFO is very common, occurring in 25% to 30% of all adults. Unlike atrial septal defect, a PFO represents a failure of the primum and secundum septa to fuse, allowing intermittent blood flow in a bidirectional fashion between the atria. Thus, the septum appears structurally intact, but shunting can be demonstrated by either contrast or color flow imaging. Occasionally, a tunnel-like gap between the two portions of the septa can be intermittently visualized because the transatrial pressure gradient changes with respiration. A PFO is frequently associated with exaggerated mobility of the atrial septum and, in the extreme form, an atrial septal aneurysm. Although a PFO can be seen from transthoracic imaging (Fig. 7.11), transesophageal echocardiography is more sensitive and provides a more complete assessment. To reliably characterize a PFO, the septum must first be thoroughly examined to exclude an atrial septal defect. Then either contrast echocardiography, color Doppler imaging, or both techniques should be performed. Evidence of right-to-left shunting is respiratory cycle dependent and will therefore be intermittent. Once contrast appears in the right atrium, shunting should occur within three or four cardiac cycles. Appearance of contrast in the left atrium after more than four beats is consistent with transpulmonary shunting, usually through an arteriovenous malformation. Figure 7.12 is an example of a small PFO with right-to-left shunting demonstrated using color Doppler imaging. In Figure 7.13, a greater degree of shunting is apparent after contrast venous injection. Although precise quantification of shunting is not possible, contrast echocardiography can provide a rough estimate of the magnitude, based on the number of bubbles that appear in the left atrium within three or four beats of appearance. Figure 7.14 shows a PFO with exaggerated septal mobility and a clearly defined tunnel through which shunting is easily demonstrated.

An atrial septal aneurysm is a redundancy of the mid-portion of the atrial septum that results in excess mobility and billowing of the tissue in this region (Fig. 7.15). Because some motion of the atrial septum is normal, a standardized definition of atrial septal aneurysm requires maximal deviation of the aneurysmal tissue of at least 10 mm from the plane of the septum. The motion of the aneurysm reflects the relative pressure gradient between left and right atria, and thus the outpouching will usually occur in both directions over the course of the cardiac cycle (Fig. 7.16). In the example, redundant tissue in the area of the fossa ovalis billows from left to right, reflecting the changes in relative pressure between the two atria. Figure 7.17 is a similar example, but it also demonstrates a mild degree of shunting through a PFO by color Doppler imaging. In Figure 7.18, an extreme example of atrial septal aneurysm is presented. The redundant aneurysmal tissue nearly protrudes through the tricuspid valve during diastole.

An atrial septal aneurysm can be identified by transthoracic echocardiography from the basal paraster-

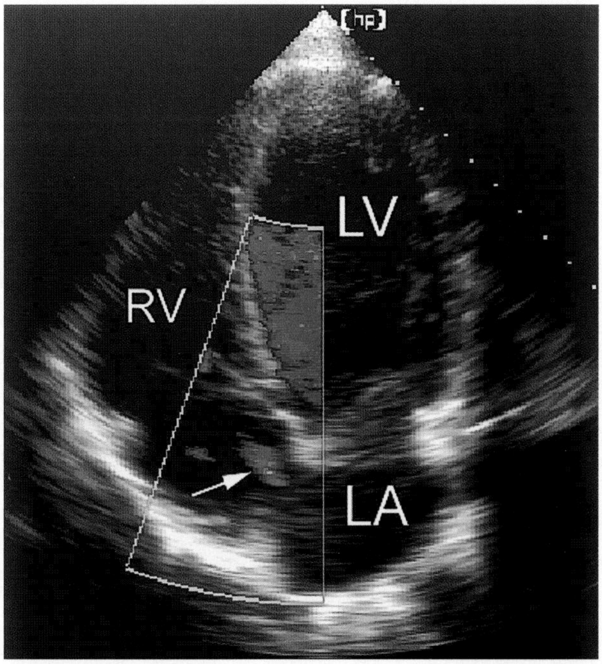

FIGURE 7.11. An apical four-chamber view with color flow mapping reveals a small patent foramen ovale (*arrow*). In this example, left-to-right shunting is demonstrated. LA, left atrium; LV, left ventricle; RV, right ventricle.

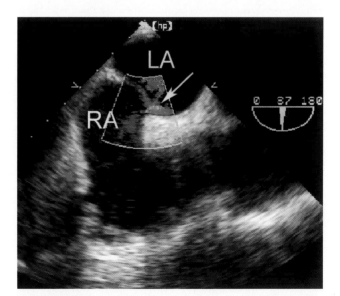

FIGURE 7.12. A transesophageal echocardiogram of the interatrial septum demonstrates a small patent foramen ovale using color Doppler imaging. LA, left atrium; RA, right atrium.

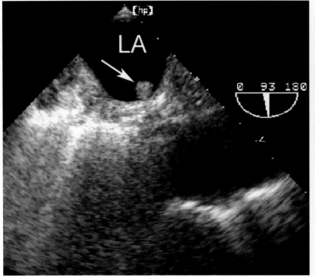

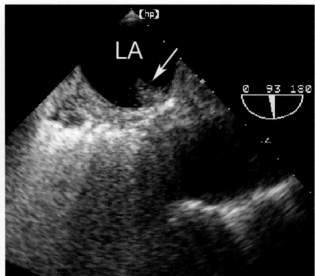

FIGURE 7.13. An example of a patent foramen ovale demonstrated during transesophageal echocardiography by injection of agitated saline into a peripheral vein. Contrast is present in the right atrium. There is intermittent shunting through the patent foramen ovale from right to left. LA, left atrium.

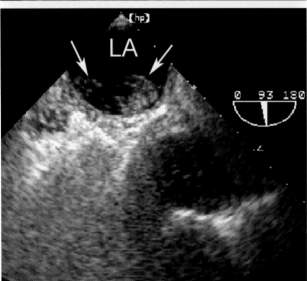

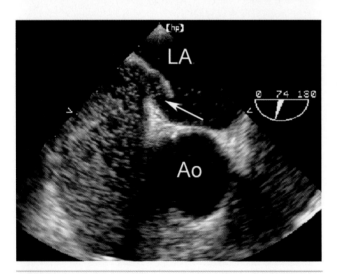

FIGURE 7.14. Contrast injection demonstrates a patent foramen ovale on transesophageal echocardiography. In this case, increased mobility of the atrial septum is present. The tunnel-like gap within the interatrial septum is evident (*arrow*), and bubbles can be seen traversing the patent foramen ovale from right to left. Ao, aorta; LA, left atrium.

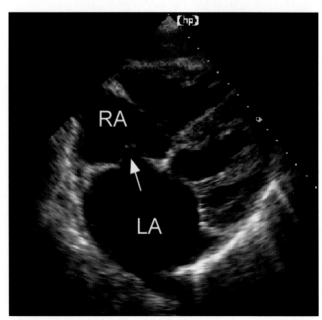

FIGURE 7.15. A subcostal four-chamber view demonstrates an atrial septal aneurysm (*arrow*), bowing into the right atrium (RA). LA, left atrium.

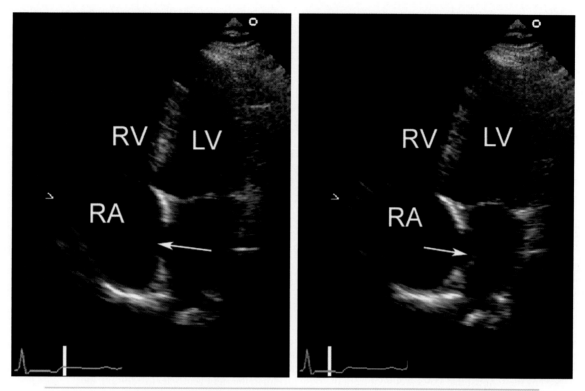

FIGURE 7.16. An atrial septal aneurysm is shown, intermittently bowing into the right (*RA*) and left atria. LV, left ventricle; RV, right ventricle.

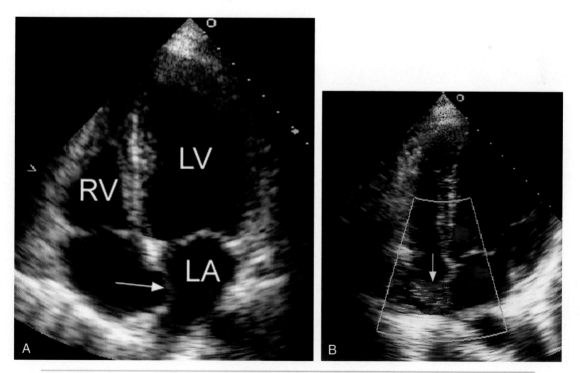

FIGURE 7.17. **A:** An atrial septal aneurysm (*arrow*) is demonstrated from the apical four-chamber view. The mobility of the midportion of the septum is evident. **B:** Color flow imaging confirms a degree of left-to-right shunting through a patent foramen ovale. LA, left atrium; LV, left ventricle; RV, right ventricle.

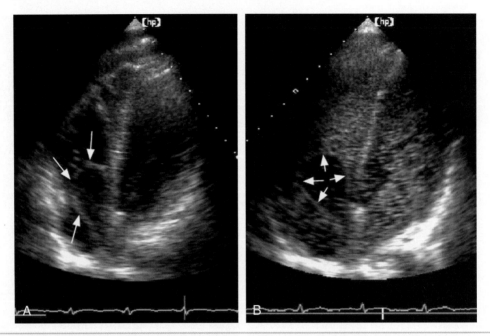

FIGURE 7.18. A: An apical four-chamber view demonstrates an extreme form of an atrial septal aneurysm with a "windsock" appearance of the aneurysmal tissue into the right atrium and partially through the tricuspid valve (*arrows*). **B:** After contrast agent injection, the windsock is outlined by the contrast that flows around it from the right atrium to the right ventricle. In addition, the presence of a patent foramen ovale allows some contrast agent to cross into the left heart.

nal short-axis view or the apical four-chamber view. However, these aneurysms are more readily visualized using transesophageal echocardiography in the four-chamber view. The total excursion of the aneurysmal tissue can be assessed and the presence or absence of an associated shunt can be detected with either color flow imaging or, more accurately, using contrast techniques (Fig. 7.19). Thrombi may form in the pouches created by the septum on either the left or right side and have been associated with thromboembolic events. Atrial septal aneurysms are

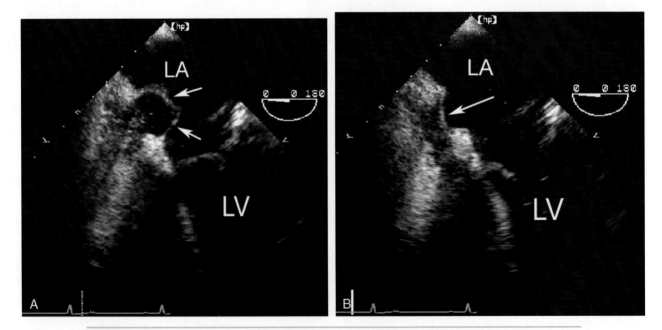

FIGURE 7.19. An example of an atrial septal aneurysm is recorded using transesophageal echocardiography. **A:** The redundant aneurysmal tissue billows into the left atrium (*LA*) (*arrows*). **B:** The *arrow* indicates motion of the tissue back into the right atrium. Theses images were recorded during contrast agent injection, which can be seen filling the right atrium. **B:** A few bubbles are visualized within the LA. This is the result of shunting through a patent foramen ovale. LV, left ventricle.

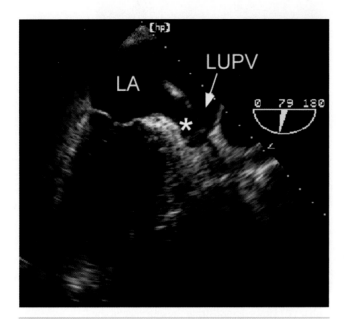

FIGURE 7.20. A transesophageal two-chamber view demonstrates the relationship between the left atrial appendage (*) and the left upper pulmonary vein (*LUPV*). The ridge of tissue separating the two is sometimes mistaken for a mass or a thrombus. LA, left atrium.

The most important pathologic condition affecting the left atrial appendage is the development of a thrombus. This is a common complication of mitral stenosis or atrial fibrillation and is associated with an increased risk of systemic embolic events, especially strokes. Detecting left atrial appendage thrombi is therefore of critical importance and is one of the most common reasons to request an echocardiogram. Transthoracic echocardiography is suboptimal for this purpose and rarely should be relied on to detect or exclude a thrombus in the left atrium. Transesophageal echocardiography, however, is a very accurate technique to interrogate the left atrium for thrombi. From a variety of planes, the appendage can be easily visualized. It lies just below the left upper pulmonary vein and is separated from the vein by a ridge of tissue. This ridge is sometimes quite prominent and may be confused with abnormal masses or thrombi (Fig. 7.20). Color Doppler is often helpful to distinguish the appendage from the pulmonary vein (Fig. 7.21). It should be recalled that the left atrial appendage is frequently multilobed, and therefore multiple views are required for a thorough assessment. To reliably exclude the presence of a thrombus, a thorough inspection of the appendage is required. Because the appendage is multilobed in most patients, multiple views are needed for a complete evaluation. It also contains small pectinate muscles along its surface that must be differentiated from thrombi. This topic is more fully covered in Chapter 21.

Pulmonary Veins

In most normal individuals, four distinct pulmonary veins drain blood from the lungs to the left atrium. These four veins enter the left atrium relatively close together along

associated with either a PFO or an atrial septal defect in as many as 75% of cases. The combination of an atrial septal aneurysm and a PFO has recently been associated with substantial risk of thromboembolism. When an atrial septal aneurysm is detected, it is often appropriate to perform a venous saline contrast injection to search for an associated PFO because its presence may alter management.

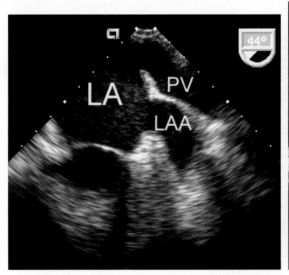
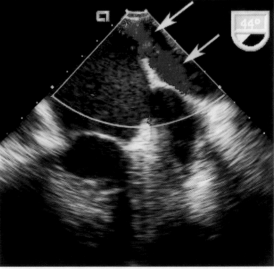

FIGURE 7.21. The relationship between the left atrial appendage (*LAA*) and left upper pulmonary vein (*PV*) is readily demonstrated with transesophageal echocardiography. Differentiating between the two structures can often be accomplished using color flow imaging to document flow within the vein (*arrows*) **(B)**. LA, left atrium.

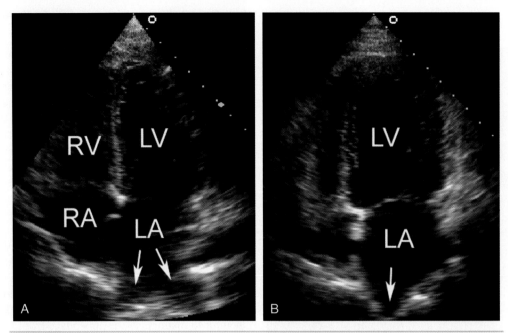

FIGURE 7.22. Apical four-chamber **(A)** and two-chamber **(B)** views demonstrate the entrance of the pulmonary veins (*arrows*) into the superior portion of the left atrium (*LA*). LV, left ventricle; RA, right atrium; RV, right ventricle.

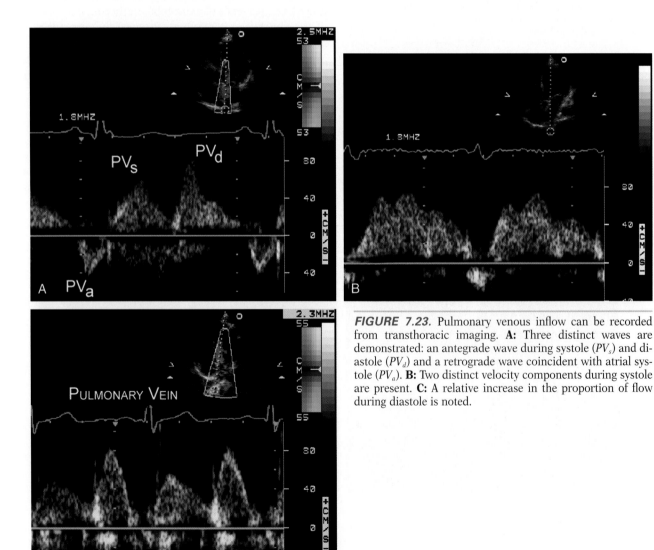

FIGURE 7.23. Pulmonary venous inflow can be recorded from transthoracic imaging. **A:** Three distinct waves are demonstrated: an antegrade wave during systole (PV_s) and diastole (PV_d) and a retrograde wave coincident with atrial systole (PV_a). **B:** Two distinct velocity components during systole are present. **C:** A relative increase in the proportion of flow during diastole is noted.

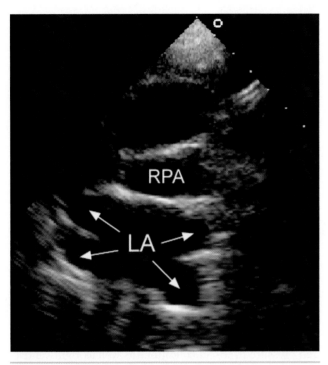

FIGURE 7.24. From the suprasternal notch, a coronal view demonstrates the left atrium (*LA*) just below the right pulmonary artery (*RPA*). Occasionally, the entrance of the pulmonary veins can also be recorded from this view (*arrows*).

from the four-chamber view. An example of this is provided in Figure 7.22. From this same view, a recording of pulmonary venous inflow is possible. This is best accomplished by using color flow imaging to identify one or more veins and then positioning the pulsed Doppler sample volume within the mouth of the vein as it enters the left atrium. Using this approach, pulmonary venous flow patterns can be recorded routinely, and several examples are provided in Figure 7.23. A unique view to record the pulmonary veins is the "crab view," which is recorded from the suprasternal notch with some posterior angulation (Fig. 7.24). Directly below the right pulmonary artery, the posterior wall of the left atrium is visualized and the pulmonary veins occasionally can be recorded.

The entrance of the pulmonary veins into the left atrium is more completely recorded using transesophageal echocardiography. In most patients, all four veins can be visualized. To record the left pulmonary veins, a vertical imaging plane is used and the transducer is rotated to the patient's far left (Fig. 7.25). The atrial appendage may be useful as a landmark to identify the upper vein. Then, by gradually advancing the probe, the lower vein is seen. To record the right veins, set the imaging plane to 45–60 degrees and rotate the shaft of the probe clockwise, to the patient's far right. The right veins are usually seen together, forming a V shape as they drain into the left atrium (Fig. 7.26). Normal pulmonary venous flow has three phases: antegrade flow occurs in systole and early diastole and some retrograde flow occurs after atrial contraction in late diastole (Fig. 7.27A). The ratio of peak flow velocity in systole and diastole and the duration of the retrograde pulmonary venous A-wave are useful pa-

the superior portion of the posterior wall. The veins from the left lung enter laterally, whereas the veins from the right lung enter more medially. It is often possible to visualize the entrance of one or two pulmonary veins into the left atrium using transthoracic echocardiography

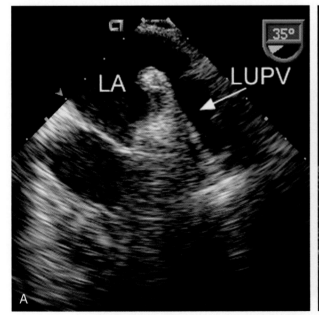

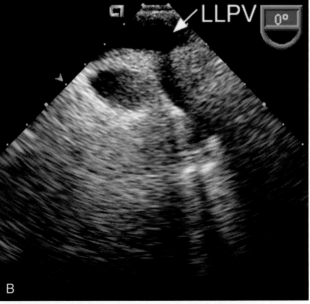

FIGURE 7.25. A transesophageal echocardiogram demonstrates the entrance of the left upper (*LUPV*) (**A**) and left lower (*LLPV*) (**B**) pulmonary veins into the left atrium (*LA*).

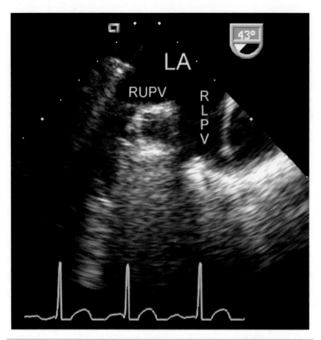

FIGURE 7.26. A transesophageal echocardiogram shows the entrance of the right lower (*RLPV*) and right upper (*RUPV*) pulmonary veins into the left atrium (*LA*).

rameters in the assessment of diastolic dysfunction. This topic is covered in Chapter 6. In addition, retrograde flow into the pulmonary veins in late systole can be observed in patients with severe mitral regurgitation. A variety of pathologic states are also associated with abnormal pulmonary venous flow, including mitral stenosis, constrictive pericarditis, and restrictive cardiomyopathy. Figure 7.27B is an example of abnormal pulmonary venous flow in a patient with ischemic cardiomyopathy and elevated filling pressure. Note that the inflow is almost exclusively during diastole, indicating high left ventricular filling

pressure and restrictive physiology. Figure 7.28 demonstrates increased pulmonary venous flow velocity from a patient with left-to-right shunting through an atrial septal defect. Pulmonary vein stenosis induced by invasive electrophysiologic procedures can also be assessed with transesophageal echocardiography. Finally, transesophageal echocardiography is very useful to demonstrate anomalous pulmonary venous connections, either in isolation or in association with atrial septal defects. This is discussed in detail in Chapter 18.

RIGHT ATRIUM

The right atrium is a thin-walled ovoid structure that receives inflow from the superior and inferior vena cavae and the coronary sinus. It can be visualized in several views and contains several distinct anatomic structures. Right atrial size and function have not been as well studied as the other chambers, although dilation of the right atrium frequently accompanies right ventricular volume and pressure overload conditions as well as right ventricular failure. Measurement of the right atrium is usually performed from the apical four-chamber or subcostal view. Linear dimensions can be determined, and the normal range of right atrial size has been reported. Planimetry of right atrial area can also be performed to more directly assess chamber volume. This method is similar to that described earlier for the left atrium and is illustrated in Figure 7.29. On a clinical basis, visual comparison of left and right atrial size from the apical four-chamber view is routinely performed. A right atrium that appears larger than the left atrium is qualitative evidence of chamber enlargement. Although little information on right atrial volume has been published, three-dimensional echocardiography recently has been used for this pur-

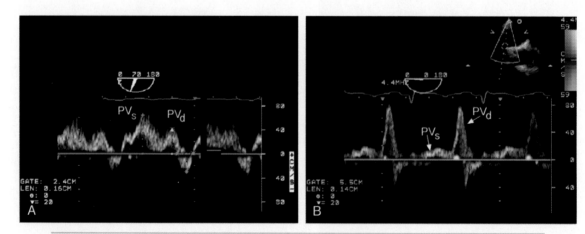

FIGURE 7.27. Pulmonary venous flow is recorded using transesophageal echocardiography. **A:** Normal pulmonary venous flow is demonstrated. **B:** Antegrade systolic flow (*PV$_s$*) is blunted and diastolic flow (*PV$_d$*) is increased in a patient with elevated left atrial pressure due to left heart failure.

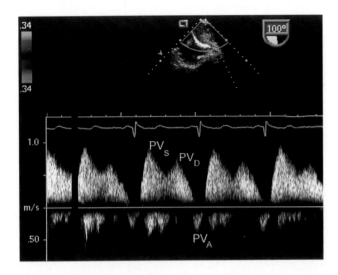

FIGURE 7.28. Flow in the left upper pulmonary vein is recorded from transesophageal echocardiography. In this example, moderately increased flow velocity is the result of a hyperdynamic state.

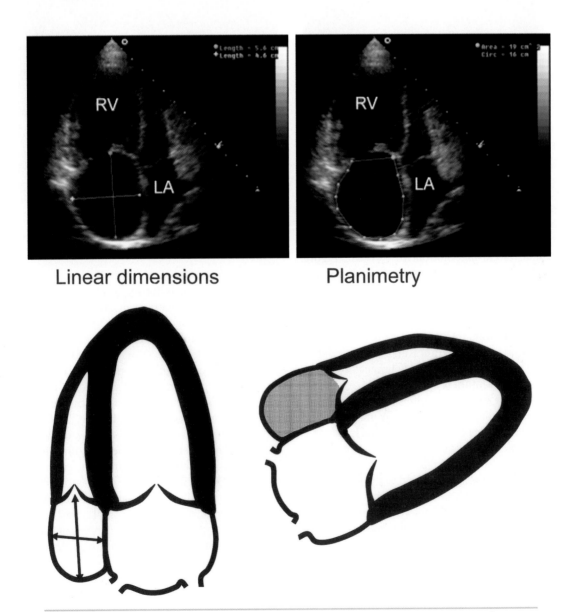

Linear dimensions   Planimetry

FIGURE 7.29. Right atrial size can be assessed using either linear dimensions **(left)** or planimetry **(right)** of the right atrium . LA, left atrium; RV, right ventricle.

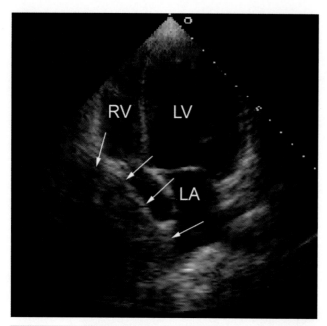

FIGURE 7.30. Compression of the right atrium by a hepatoma (*arrows*) creates the impression of a right atrial mass. LA, left atrium; LV, left ventricle; RV, right ventricle.

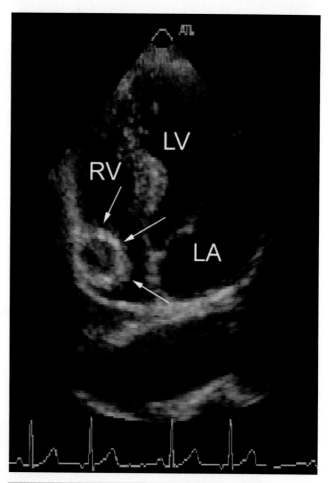

FIGURE 7.31. A cyst attached to the lateral wall of the right atrium is shown (*arrows*). LA, left atrium; LV, left ventricle; RV, right ventricle.

pose. Similar to the left atrium, the right atrium is at risk of compression by extracardiac structures within the liver or mediastinum. Distinguishing extracardiac compression from an intracardiac mass can be difficult. Figure 7.30 is an example of compression of the right atrium by a liver mass. Note how the mass causes distortion of right heart structures and bowing of the atrial septum toward the left. When viewed in real time, the mass was immobile and independent of cardiac motion. In contrast, Figure 7.31 shows a cyst within the right atrium. In this case, the location of the mass within the atrium is apparent. Its motion was linked to motion of the atrioventricular groove, to which it was attached. Figure 7.32 is an example of right atrial myxoma. Although less common than left atrial myxomas, the appearance and characteristics are similar. In the illustration, the attachment of the tumor to the interatrial septum is apparent.

A unique feature of the right atrium is the characteristic anatomic variants, which are occasionally mistaken for pathologic structures. These include the eustachian valve and the Chiari network. The eustachian valve is a remnant of the embryologic valve responsible for directing inferior vena caval blood across the atrial septum to the left atrium. Referred to as the right sinus valve or the valve of the inferior vena cava, this structure normally regresses during embryonic development. Lack of normal regression results in a variety of anomalies that range from a prominent (but physiologically insignificant) eustachian valve to partial or complete septation of the right atrium, a condition inappropriately referred to as *cor triatriatum dexter*. The eustachian valve is a rigid and protuberant structure that

arises along the posterior margin of the inferior vena cava to the border of the fossa ovalis. It is most easily visualized from a medially angulated parasternal long-axis view at the junction of the inferior vena cava and right atrium (Fig. 7.33). The eustachian valve varies considerably in size, from inconspicuous to quite prominent. Although usually immobile, it may occasionally demonstrate independent motion within the right atrium and can be confused with tumors, vegetations, or thrombi (Fig. 7.34). When large, the eustachian valve can divert the flow of blood within the right atrium. An example of nearly complete septation of the right atrium by a very prominent eustachian valve is shown in Figure 7.35. During contrast injection, this can result in both false-negative and false-positive evidence of an atrial septal defect. For example, the streaming effect can result in the appearance of non–contrast-containing blood in the area of the septum, incorrectly suggesting a left-to-right shunt.

A Chiari network is a delicate-appearing, membranous structure arising near the orifice of the inferior vena cava and serving as the valve of the coronary sinus. It is highly

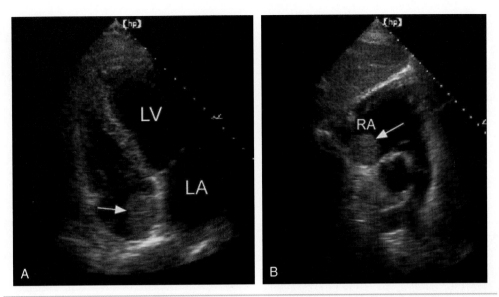

FIGURE 7.32. A right atrial myxoma is demonstrated. **A:** The tumor (*arrow*) is seen attached to the atrial septum in the four-chamber view. **B:** A subcostal short-axis view again demonstrates the tumor attached to the interatrial septum. LA, left atrium; LV, left ventricle; RA, right atrium.

mobile and usually fenestrated, and its site of attachment varies within the chamber (Fig. 7.36). Although sometimes confused with the eustachian valve, a Chiari network is more delicate and more mobile. Like the eustachian valve, it has little clinical significance but may be confused with pathologic structures, such as vegetations or thrombi.

Right Atrial Thrombi

Thrombi can occur either in the body of the right atrium or within the atrial appendage, usually as a consequence of atrial fibrillation. The right atrial appendage is difficult to visualize on transthoracic imaging but can be recorded during transesophageal echocardiography (Fig. 7.37). Be-

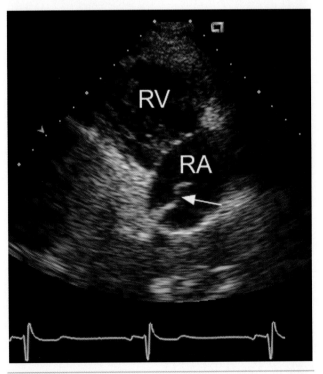

FIGURE 7.33. A medially angulated parasternal view demonstrates the right ventricular (*RV*) inflow tract. In the inferior portion of the right atrium (*RA*), a eustachian valve at the entrance of the inferior vena cava is shown (*arrow*).

FIGURE 7.34. A prominent eustachian valve is demonstrated (*arrow*). RA, right atrium; RV, right ventricle.

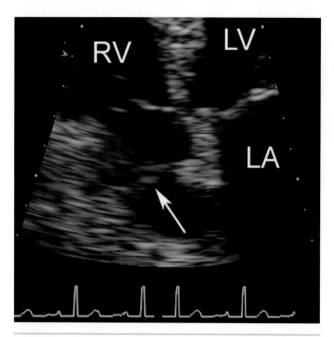

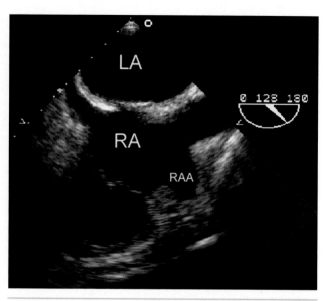

FIGURE 7.37. The bicaval transesophageal echocardiographic view can be used to record the right atrial appendage (*RAA*). From a vertical plane, the probe must be rotated to the right to view this structure. LA, left atrium; RA, right atrium.

FIGURE 7.35. An extreme form of a eustachian valve is demonstrated in this four-chamber view. The prominent ridge of tissue (*arrow*) results in almost complete septation of the right atrium. LA, left atrium; LV, left ventricle; RV, right ventricle.

cause the right atrial appendage is more trabeculated than its left-sided counterpart, distinguishing muscles from thrombi can be challenging. In patients with atrial fibrillation studied before elective cardioversion, an assessment of the right atrial appendage to exclude thrombi should be performed routinely. In most instances, however, when a thrombus develops in the right atrium, it occurs in the main body of the chamber, a consequence of low flow, atrial arrhythmia, or the presence of foreign bodies (such as catheters or pacemaker leads). Thrombi in the right atrium are relatively common (Fig. 7.38). Thromboemboli that arise in lower extremity or pelvic veins may occasionally be seen within the right atrium as a pulmonary embolus in transit. Such masses usually have a multilobulated appearance and are freely mobile. They often have a worm-like shape, a reflection of the lower extremity veins in which they were formed. These thrombi may also be recorded within the inferior vena cava, sometimes extending into the right atrium (Fig. 7.39). A thrombus that formed in the lower extremities and was recorded during transit through the right heart is shown in Figure 7.40. In this example, the thrombus is seen straddling the tricuspid valve. Distinguishing a thrombus from a tumor, especially renal cell carcinoma, may be difficult. Both can extend from the inferior vena cava into the right atrium and have a lobulated, mobile appearance. Other imaging techniques, such as an abdominal computed tomography, may be necessary to differentiate these entities.

Thrombi attached to indwelling catheters may be visualized with transthoracic echocardiography but are much more readily detected with transesophageal techniques.

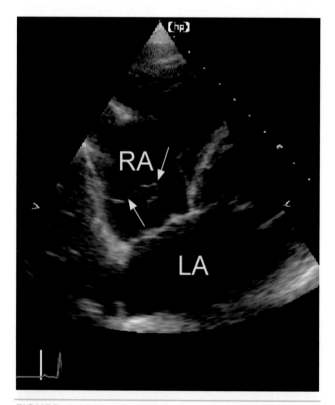

FIGURE 7.36. A subcostal four-chamber view illustrates a Chiari network (*arrows*) within the right atrium (*RA*). In real time, the Chiari network is a highly mobile structure. LA, left atrium; RA, right atrium.

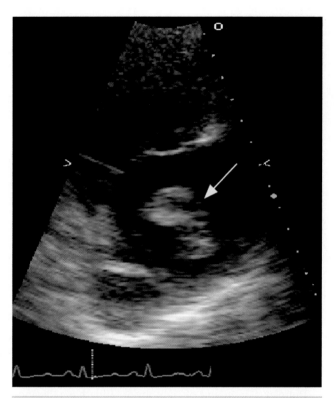

FIGURE 7.38. A magnified view of the right atrium from the parasternal window demonstrates a mobile mass (*arrow*) consistent with a thrombus.

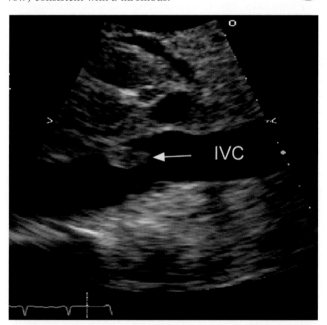

FIGURE 7.39. A subcostal longitudinal recording of the inferior vena cava (*IVC*) demonstrates a mobile mass (*arrow*) consistent with thrombus.

The ability to interrogate the entire right atrium as well as a portion of the superior vena cava is essential to detect such thrombi. Distinguishing a thrombus from vegetation is particularly difficult and may be impossible on echocardiographic grounds alone.

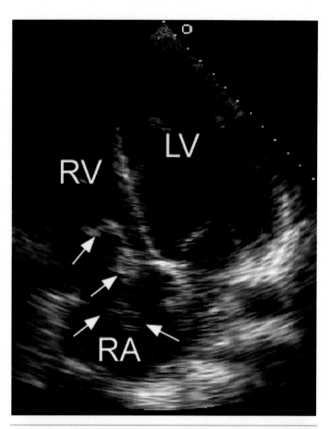

FIGURE 7.40. A multilobed thrombus (*arrows*) is recorded straddling the tricuspid valve from the four-chamber view. The thrombus could be traced to the entrance of the inferior vena cava. LV, left ventricle; RA, right atrium; RV, right ventricle.

Right Atrial Blood Flow

Blood enters the right atrium via the inferior vena cava, superior vena cava, and the coronary sinus. The location and orientation of the inferior vena cava facilitate its visualization from the subcostal views (Fig. 7.41). A highly compliant vessel, the inferior vena cava changes shape and dimensions with changes in central venous pressure and the respiratory cycle. The size and respiratory variation of the inferior vena cava have been used to predict right atrial pressure. Dilation of the inferior vena cava suggests increased central venous pressure and may accompany volume overload states. The diameter of the inferior vena cava normally decreases more than 50% during inspiration. A blunted or absent inspiratory decrease in the inferior vena cava diameter suggests increased right atrial pressure. Both pulsed and color Doppler imaging can be used to record flow within the inferior vena cava. Vena caval flow is occasionally visualized using color Doppler as a streaming effect from the vessel into the inferior portion of the right atrium, extending along the septum. An example of this is shown in Figure 7.42. From the right ventricular inflow view (B), flow is seen emerging from the inferior vena cava, passing around the eustachian valve, and coursing into the right atrium. Such

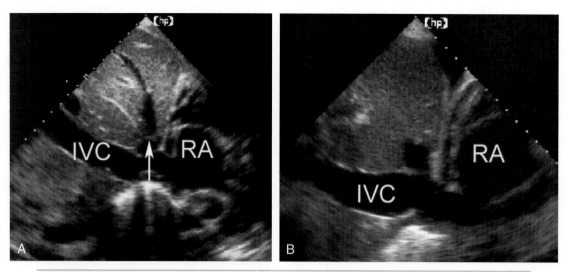

FIGURE 7.41. From the subcostal window, the inferior vena cava (*IVC*) can be recorded as it passes through the diaphragm and enters the right atrium (*RA*). **A:** Hepatic veins can be seen entering the IVC (*arrow*). **B:** The IVC is dilated and does not collapse with inspiration.

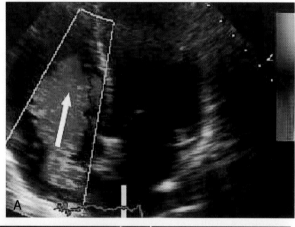

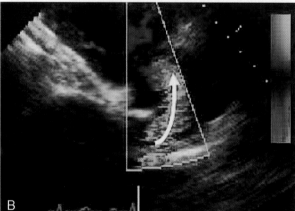

FIGURE 7.42. Inferior vena caval flow can sometimes be recorded with color flow imaging as a streaming effect within the right atrium. The streaming effect is often confused with important pathology such as an atrial septal defect. This is demonstrated from the four-chamber view **(A)** and right ventricular inflow view **(B)**.

a pattern can occasionally be confused with flow through an atrial septal defect.

Doppler assessment of right atrial filling has relevance in several clinical situations. From the subcostal transducer location, alignment of the Doppler beam with inferior vena caval flow is difficult, and it has become customary to substitute hepatic vein flow for this purpose. Because hepatic vein flow and inferior vena caval flow are similar and because it is generally easier to align the Doppler signal with a hepatic vein, this is both useful and practical. An example of normal hepatic vein flow is shown in Figure 7.43. Antegrade flow (toward the right

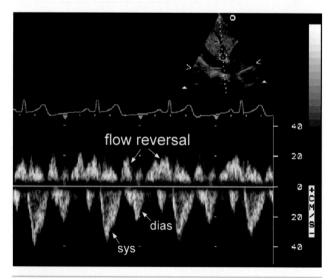

FIGURE 7.43. Hepatic vein flow can be recorded from the subcostal view with pulsed Doppler imaging. See text for details. sys, systole; dias, diastole.

atrium) has two main components: a larger systolic wave and a slightly smaller diastolic wave. Between these two antegrade flow patterns, at end-systole, a small retrograde flow pattern may be recorded. Likewise, during atrial systole, some retrograde flow is also present. Hepatic vein flow is respiratory cycle dependent with increased flow velocity during inspiration and decreased flow velocity (and a greater degree of retrograde flow) during expiration.

Several disease states result in characteristic abnormalities of hepatic vein flow (Fig. 7.44). As a surrogate for inferior vena caval flow, any condition that affects either right atrial pressure or filling will alter hepatic vein flow velocity. For example, increased right atrial pressure has been associated with a decrease in the systolic filling fraction of hepatic vein flow. Thus, as right atrial pressure increases, antegrade systolic hepatic vein flow decreases. Among patients with severe tricuspid regurgitation, flow reversal during ventricular systole is characteristic. As the tricuspid regurgitant jet is transmitted retrograde into the right atrium, the normal antegrade systolic flow is re-

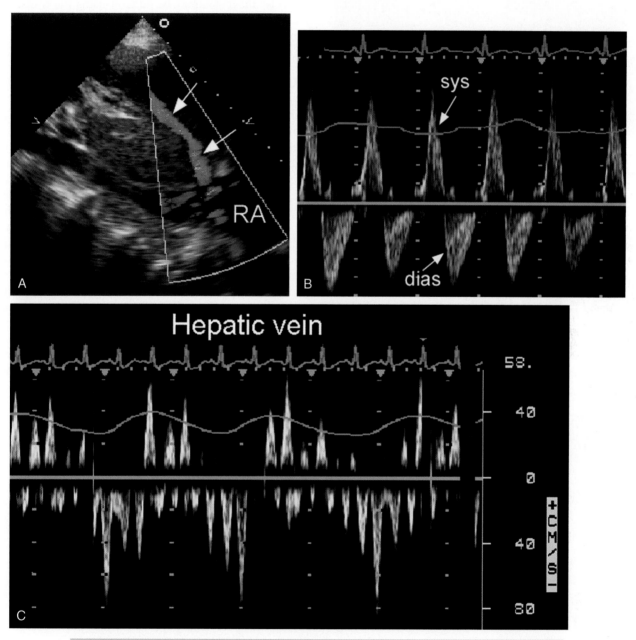

FIGURE 7.44. Examples of Doppler recordings of hepatic vein flow. **A:** Color flow imaging of hepatic vein flow (*arrows*). **B:** A prominent systolic (*sys*) retrograde wave is consistent with significant tricuspid regurgitation. **C:** Variable flow patterns and significant respiratory variation are recorded from a patient with atrial fibrillation. dias, diastole; RA, right atrium.

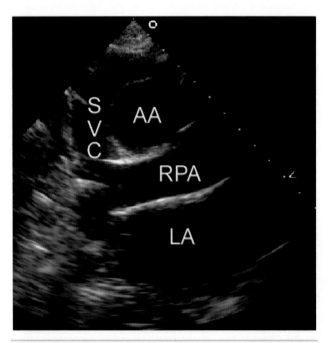

FIGURE 7.45. The superior vena cava can be visualized from the suprasternal notch as a vertical structure just to the right of the aortic arch (*AA*). LA, left atrium; SVC, superior vena cava; RPA, right pulmonary artery.

The superior vena cava can be visualized from the suprasternal notch as a vertical structure just to the right of the aortic arch (Fig. 7.45) but is more readily evaluated using transesophageal echocardiography. Both long- and short-axis views of the vessel are possible (Fig. 7.46). Occlusion or external compression of the superior vena cava is a common clinical problem that can be assessed using echocardiography. The diagnosis can often be established using transthoracic imaging combined with color flow Doppler imaging. Because the underlying pathologic process may result in distorted anatomy, a precise diagnosis may be difficult using the transthoracic approach, and transesophageal echocardiography is often necessary.

RIGHT VENTRICLE

Echocardiographic evaluation of the right ventricle is hampered by its unusual crescent shape, irregular endocardial surface, and complex contraction mechanism. These factors, coupled with the location of the right ventricle almost directly behind the sternum, combine to create formidable problems for the echocardiographer. A dependable characteristic feature of the right ventricle is the moderator band within its apex (Fig. 7.47). This structure helps to identify the morphologic right ventricle and is best appreciated from the apical four-chamber view. The normal right ventricle defies simplified assumptions regarding shape. Along the minor axis, the right ventricle has a characteristic crescent shape. Along the orthogonal long axis, however, the shape is more complex and variable. For this reason, no simple geometric three-dimensional figure accurately represents this chamber. Some simplifications that have been used include a paral-

placed by a prominent retrograde wave. In the setting of atrial fibrillation, retrograde flow during atrial systole and the velocity of systolic antegrade flow are diminished. In contrast, pulmonary hypertension typically results in prominent flow reversal during atrial systole. Analysis of right atrial filling plays an important role in the evaluation of patients with restrictive physiology and constrictive pericarditis. These topics are discussed in Chapters 9 and 17.

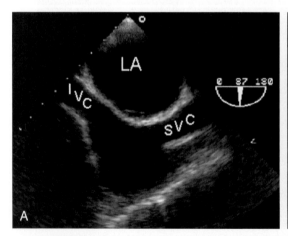
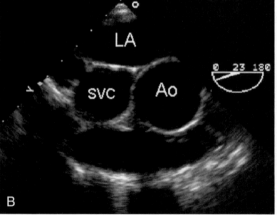

FIGURE 7.46. The superior vena cava (*SVC*) is best recorded with transesophageal echocardiography. **A:** The bicaval view demonstrates both the superior and inferior vena cava (*IVC*). **B:** A transverse plane at the base of the heart demonstrates the relationship between the aorta (*Ao*) and SVC. Posterior to the SVC is the superior portion of the left atrium (*LA*).

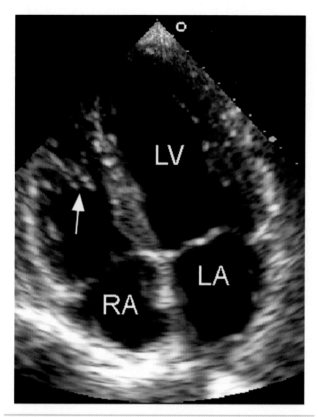

FIGURE 7.47. An apical four-chamber view demonstrates a moderator band (*arrow*) within the right ventricular apex. LA, left atrium; RA, right atrium; LV, left ventricle.

lelepiped (or three-dimensional parallelogram), a prism, and a pyramid with a triangular base.

Contraction of the right ventricle is also complex. The pattern has been compared with the action of a bellows, in which minor axis shortening is combined with signifi-

cant long-axis shortening to draw the tricuspid anulus toward the apex. The low resistance of the pulmonary vascular circuit permits the right ventricle to eject a large volume of blood while performing a minimal degree of myocardial shortening. Relatively small movements of the walls therefore produce large ejection volumes, similar to a bellows.

Right Ventricular Dimensions and Volumes

A qualitative assessment of the right ventricle is a routine part of echocardiography. In the apical four-chamber view, for example, a visual comparison of right and left ventricular area permits a rough estimate of right ventricular volume to be made. Normally, right ventricular size is approximately two-thirds that of the left ventricle. This estimate is based on a comparison of the relative sizes of the two ventricles from multiple views. More quantitative approaches, using two-dimensional echocardiography, are also available. Unlike the left ventricle, however, whose shape lends itself to simple geometric assumptions, the complex shape of the right ventricle greatly complicates volume quantification. This is particularly true of the normally shaped right ventricle. It is fortuitous that in patients with right ventricular enlargement, the chamber's shape becomes more ellipsoid, thereby facilitating the application of these quantitative approaches. Two approaches for the measurement of right ventricular dimensions are shown in Figure 7.48. From the apical four-chamber view, through careful alignment of the imaging plane, a long-axis dimension and a series of short-axis dimensions can be obtained in most patients. Although other views have been used, they are less well suited for this purpose. Figure 7.49 is taken from a patient

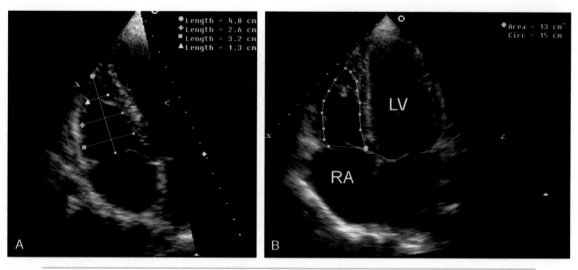

FIGURE 7.48. Two approaches to measuring right ventricular size are illustrated. **A:** A major axis dimension and a series of minor axis dimensions are recorded. **B:** The right ventricle is measured using planimetry from the four-chamber view. RA, right atrium; LV, left ventricle.

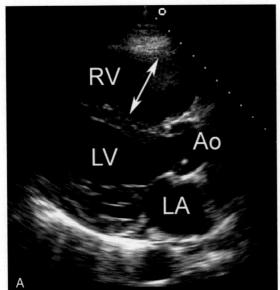

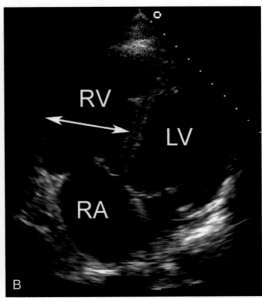

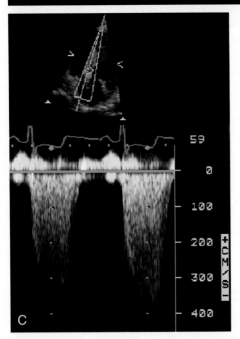

FIGURE 7.49. In this patient, recurrent pulmonary emboli resulted in right ventricular (*RV*) enlargement and pulmonary hypertension. The increase in RV size is apparent in the parasternal long-axis **(A)** and four-chamber **(B)** views. **C:** Doppler recording of tricuspid regurgitation velocity confirms significant pulmonary hypertension. Ao, aorta; LA, left atrium; LV, left ventricle; RA, right atrium.

with recurrent pulmonary emboli. Note the increased right ventricular dimensions, from both the parasternal and apical four-chamber views. The chamber was both enlarged and severely hypokinetic. Doppler imaging demonstrated evidence of severe pulmonary hypertension.

To measure right ventricular volume, simplifying assumptions about shape are necessary. Both area-length and Simpson's rule approaches have been undertaken. The area-length method, for example, employs just two measurements: an estimate of short-axis area (from a mid-ventricular short-axis view) and a linear measure of length (from the apical four-chamber view). An obvious problem with all these methods is the lack of a gold standard for

comparison. Using either angiography or radionuclide techniques, the correlation between echocardiographic volumes and the standard has been variable. More recently, three-dimensional echocardiographic techniques have been applied to this problem. A major advantage of three-dimensional echocardiography is that assumptions about shape are no longer necessary and a complete echocardiographic rendering of the right ventricular cavity can be recorded and analyzed (Fig. 7.50). A limitation of these techniques has been image quality. However, it is clear that one of the important future contributions of three-dimensional imaging will be a more precise approach to quantifying right ventricular volume (Fig. 7.51).

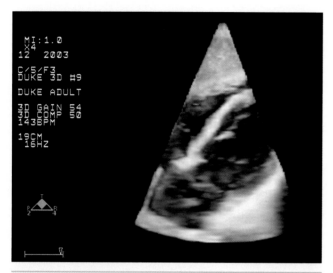

FIGURE 7.50. Three-dimensional echocardiography is now being used to better visualize complex structures such as the right ventricle.

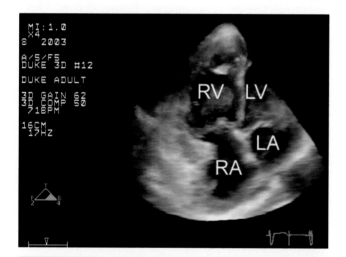

FIGURE 7.51. A dilated, hypokinetic right ventricle (RV) is demonstrated using three-dimensional echocardiography. LA, left atrium; LV, left ventricle; RA, right atrium.

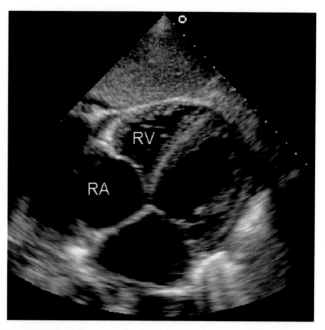

FIGURE 7.52. A subcostal four-chamber view is useful to assess global right ventricular function. In this example, severe right ventricular dysfunction was the result of an acute pulmonary embolus. RA, right atrium; RV, right ventricle.

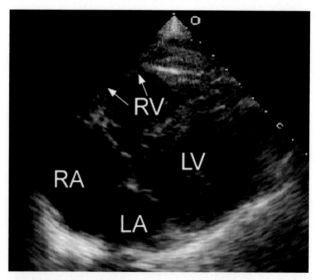

FIGURE 7.53. A segmental wall motion abnormality of the right ventricular free wall (*arrows*) is the result of a right ventricular infarction, complicating an acute inferior myocardial infarction. LA, left atrium; LV, left ventricle; RA, right atrium; LV, left ventricle

Right ventricular systolic function can be evaluated several ways. A subjective assessment of right ventricular contractility can be made from multiple views. Abnormal right ventricular wall motion occurs in several disease states, including inferior myocardial infarction, pulmonary hypertension, and arrhythmogenic right ventricular dysplasia. Figure 7.52 is an example of global right ventricular dysfunction due to acute pulmonary embolus. In contrast, Figure 7.53 demonstrates regional right ventricular free wall akinesis due to infarction as a complication of acute inferior myocardial infarction. As with the left ventricle, regional wall motion can be graded for the extent and severity of dysfunction. Both the free wall and interventricular septum should be evaluated for thickening and endocardial excursion. By assessing regional right ventricular wall motion, a qualitative evaluation of overall right ventricular systolic function can be made. A more quantitative approach involves determination of right ventricular volume at end-diastole and end-systole. From these two volume measurements, the ejection fraction can be derived. A more novel approach involves the quantitative assessment of tricuspid valve anular motion during systole. This can be recorded from the apical four-chamber view using M-mode, two-dimensional, or Doppler tissue imaging techniques (Fig. 7.54). Tricuspid anular velocity is a surrogate for global right ventricular systolic function and has been shown to be affected in several conditions. For example, this value is lower in patients with inferior myocardial infarction, especially if there is evidence of right ventricular involvement. A good correlation between anular velocity and radionuclide ejection fraction also has been reported. More work in this area is needed, but the technique has promise as a simple and reproducible approach to an important problem.

Right Ventricular Overload

Echocardiographic findings characteristic of both right ventricular volume and pressure overload have been described. Pressure overload of the right ventricle results in hypertrophy of both the free wall and interventricular septum. This is often associated with an increase in the trabeculations of the right ventricular walls. By causing septal hypertrophy that is out of proportion to posterior left ventricular free wall hypertrophy, this combination of findings can be misinterpreted as evidence of asymmetric septal hypertrophy, suggesting hypertrophic cardiomyopathy. Because the right ventricle is trabeculated, measurement of right ventricular free wall thickness can be difficult. The medially angulated parasternal long-axis view

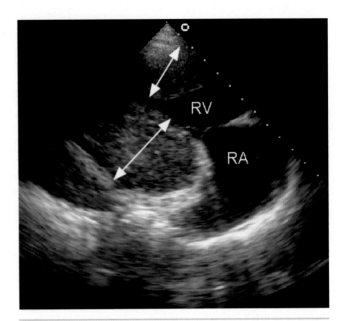

FIGURE 7.55. A parasternal right ventricular inflow view demonstrates severe right ventricular hypertrophy (*arrows*). RA, right atrium; RV, right ventricle.

most often is used for this purpose (Fig. 7.55). It places the right ventricle in the near field with both the endocardial and epicardial surfaces nearly perpendicular to the ultrasound beam. In Figure 7.56, increased right ventricular free wall thickness is apparent from the subcostal four-chamber view. In adults, the normal right ventricular wall thickness has been reported to be 3.4 ± 0.8 mm. A

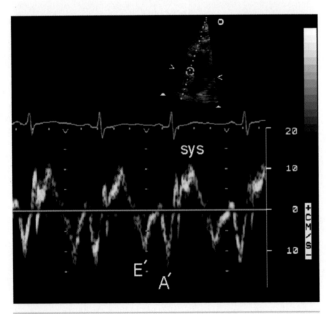

FIGURE 7.54. Doppler tissue imaging can be used to record tricuspid anular velocities. Motion during diastole consists of an early (*E'*) and late (*A'*) component. See text for details. sys, systole.

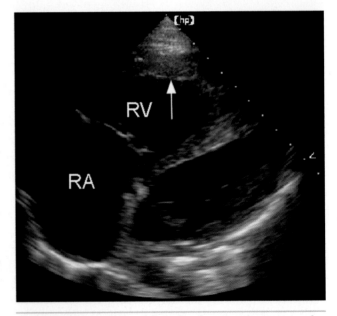

FIGURE 7.56. A subcostal four-chamber view demonstrates hypertrophy of the right ventricular free wall (*arrow*) in a patient with pulmonary hypertension. Both right-sided chambers are dilated. RA, right atrium; RV, right ventricle.

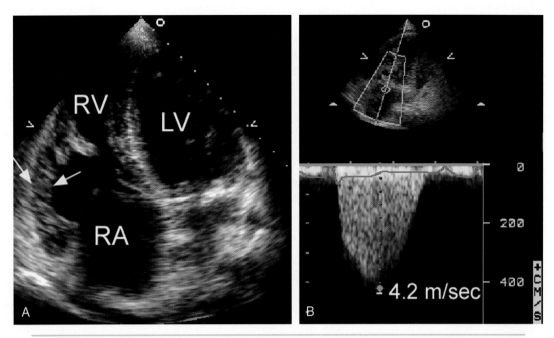

FIGURE 7.57. From a patient with pulmonary hypertension, the apical four-chamber view **(A)** demonstrates a dilated right heart with evidence of right ventricular hypertrophy (*arrows*). Using the tricuspid regurgitation velocity **(B)**, the right ventricular systolic pressure is estimated to be 85 mm Hg. LV, left ventricle; RA, right atrium; RV, right ventricle.

rough correlation exists between the degree of right ventricular hypertrophy and the severity of pulmonary hypertension, although this relationship has obvious limitations (Fig. 7.57).

Right ventricular pressure overload also results in distortion of the shape and motion of the interventricular septum. "Flattening" of the interventricular septum is the result of an abnormal pressure gradient between the left and right ventricles (Fig. 7.58). In the normal heart, the round shape of the left ventricle is maintained throughout the cardiac cycle, a reflection of the higher pressure within the left ventricular cavity (and the instantaneous transseptal pressure gradient). When right ventricular pressure is increased, this normal septal curvature is al-

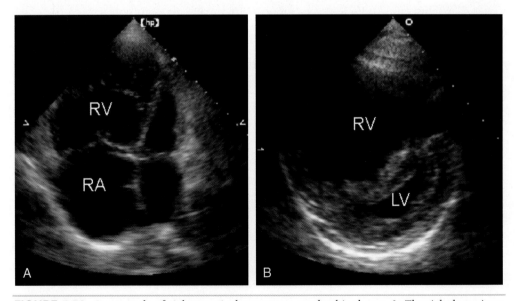

FIGURE 7.58. An example of right ventricular pressure overload is shown. **A:** The right heart is severely dilated, and there is global right ventricular hypocontractility. **B:** The short-axis view demonstrates marked flattening of the septum that was maintained in both systole and diastole. See text for details. RA, right atrium; RV, right ventricle; LV, left ventricle.

tered and the septum appears flattened and displaced toward the left ventricle. The greater the increase in right ventricular systolic pressure, the greater the shift in septal position toward the left ventricular cavity. A characteristic feature of right ventricular pressure overload is the persistence of this septal distortion throughout the cardiac cycle, i.e., in both systole and diastole. As is discussed below, this is in contrast to right ventricular volume overload, which leads to septal flattening predominantly during diastole.

Doppler imaging is very useful to assess right ventricular pressure overload. Both pulmonary valve flow and tricuspid regurgitation velocity should be evaluated (Fig. 7.59). In normal individuals, pulmonary flow has a symmetric contour with a peak velocity occurring in midsystole. As pulmonary pressure increases, peak velocity occurs earlier in systole and late systolic notching is often present (Fig. 7.59C). The acceleration time (time from onset to peak flow velocity) can be measured and provides a rough estimate of the degree of increase in pulmonary artery pressure. The shorter the acceleration time, the higher the pulmonary artery pressure.

A more direct measure of right ventricular pressure is possible by quantifying the tricuspid regurgitation jet velocity. Using the Bernoulli equation to measure the systolic gradient between the right ventricle and atrium,

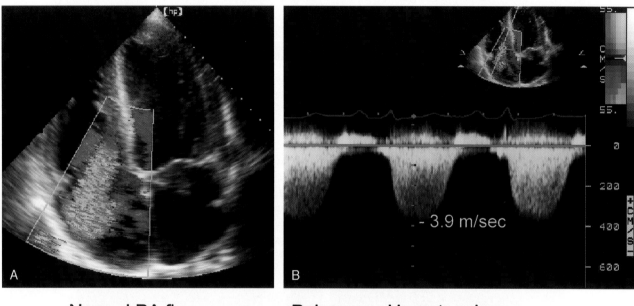

Normal PA flow Pulmonary Hypertension

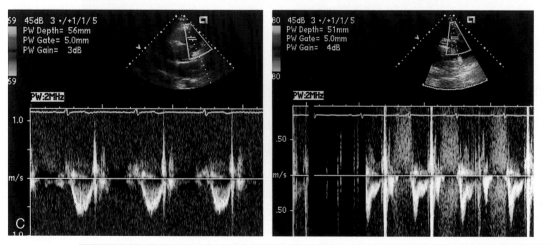

FIGURE 7.59. A: Severe tricuspid regurgitation is demonstrated by color flow imaging. **B:** Continuous wave Doppler imaging demonstrates a pressure gradient of approximately 60 mm Hg consistent with a right ventricular systolic pressure of 70 to 75 mm Hg. **C:** An example of pulmonary flow in the presence of normal (*left*) and elevated (*right*) pulmonary artery pressure is given. Note the shortened acceleration time and late systolic notching in the patient with pulmonary hypertension.

right ventricular systolic pressure (RVSP) is then determined from the following equation:

$$RVSP = 4(TR_{velocity})^2 + P_{RA} \qquad [Eq.\ 7.3]$$

where $TR_{velocity}$ is the maximal velocity of the tricuspid regurgitation jet (in meters per second) and P_{RA} is an estimate of right atrial pressure (guidelines for estimating right atrial pressure are provided in Chapter 8). Because RVSP and pulmonary artery systolic pressure are similar (in the absence of pulmonary stenosis), this approach provides a simple and accurate means of quantifying the presence and severity of pulmonary hypertension.

Pulmonary artery diastolic pressure can be estimated using a similar approach applied to the pulmonary regurgitation flow. In this case, the flow velocity of the regurgitant jet at end-diastole is used in the Bernoulli equation to quantify the pulmonary artery-to-right ventricular gradient. In normal individuals, pulmonary artery diastolic

pressure exceeds right ventricular diastolic pressure by only a few millimeters of mercury, so the regurgitant jet velocity is low. With pulmonary hypertension, pulmonary artery diastolic pressure increases disproportionately, creating a higher pressure gradient and, hence, an increased end-diastolic regurgitant velocity. Thus, in patients with significant pulmonary hypertension, pulmonary regurgitant velocity at end-diastole is often higher than 2 m/sec. These concepts are illustrated in Figure 7.60. In this patient with severe pulmonary hypertension, the right ventricle is dilated and hypokinetic, with septal flattening evident in the short-axis view. Doppler imaging reveals increased tricuspid regurgitation velocity (RVSP = 105 mm Hg). Elevated pulmonary regurgitation velocity (>2 m/sec) is consistent with increased pulmonary artery diastolic pressure.

Right ventricular volume overload typically produces dilation of the right ventricle. In normal subjects, viewed from the apical four-chamber view, right ventricular dia-

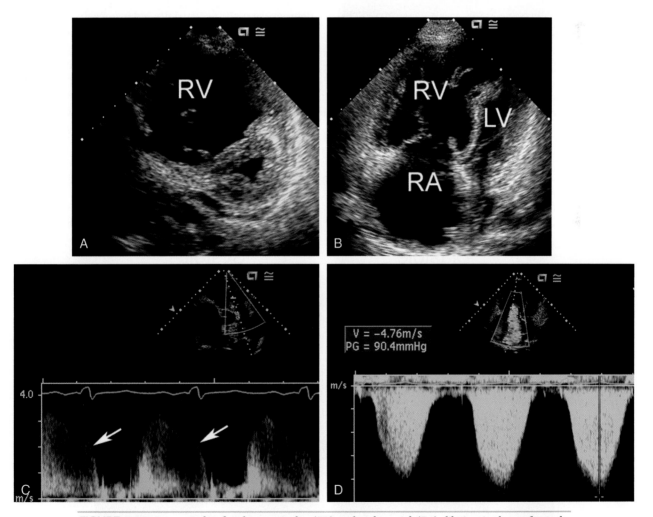

FIGURE 7.60. An example of right ventricular (*RV*) and right atrial (*RA*) dilation is shown from the parasternal short-axis (**A**) and the apical four-chamber (**B**) views. **C:** Pulsed Doppler imaging records pulmonary regurgitation in the right ventricular outflow tract. The end-diastolic velocity is elevated (*arrows*). **D:** High-velocity tricuspid regurgitation is shown and RV systolic pressure is estimated to be 105 mm H, assuming a right atrial pressure of 15 mmHg. See text for details. LV, left ventricle.

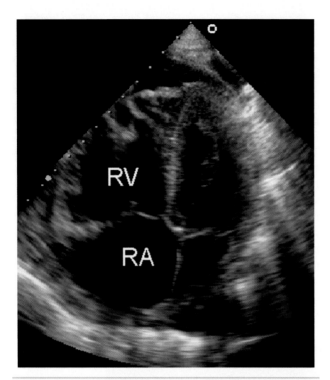

FIGURE 7.61. Severe right ventricular enlargement is demonstrated in this four-chamber view. Note the size of the right ventricle (*RV*) and right atrium (*RA*) relative to their left-sided counterparts. In both cases, the septum is shifted leftward. In addition, the RV free wall is thickened and heavily trabeculated.

stolic area is approximately two-thirds that of the left ventricle. A subjective criterion for right ventricular dilation is a right ventricular diastolic area that appears equal to or greater than that of the left ventricle (Fig. 7.61). Volume overload of the right ventricle also affects septal mo-

tion. During diastole, the increase in right ventricular volume displaces the interventricular septum toward the left ventricular cavity, resulting in flattening of the septum (Fig. 7.62). The normal crescent shape of the right ventricle is replaced by a more spherical appearance. Such abnormalities can be appreciated using both M-mode and two-dimensional imaging techniques. In contrast to right ventricular pressure overload, volume overload of the right ventricle results in septal displacement only during diastole. During systole, because the normal transseptal pressure gradient is maintained, normal septal shape and position are also maintained.

Thus, the degree of septal flattening during systole and diastole can be useful to distinguish volume from pressure overload. This can be qualitatively assessed by deriving an eccentricity index, which is the ratio of two orthogonal minor-axis left ventricular chordae, measured from the short-axis view. A normal round shape would yield a ratio of 1.0, whereas septal flattening would result in an eccentricity index greater than 1.0. Figure 7.63 demonstrates the eccentricity index, measured in diastole and systole, from normal subjects and patients with pressure and volume overload. As can be seen, patients with pure right ventricular volume overload have septal flattening (i.e., a high eccentricity index) confined to diastole. Patients with right ventricular pressure overload maintain septal flattening throughout the cardiac cycle. The degree of septal flattening also roughly correlates with the severity of pulmonary hypertension.

Right Ventricular Dysplasia

Arrhythmogenic right ventricular dysplasia (ARVD) is a rare but important condition in which the normal right

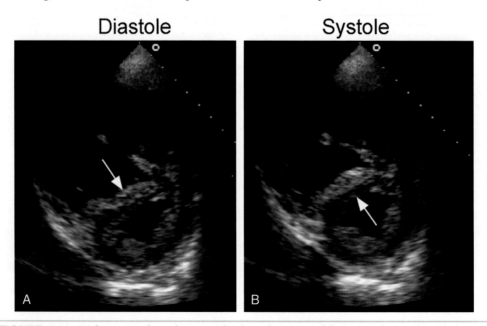

FIGURE 7.62. Right ventricular volume overload results in septal flattening during diastole (*arrow*) (**A**) with restoration of normal septal curvature during systole (*arrow*) (**B**).

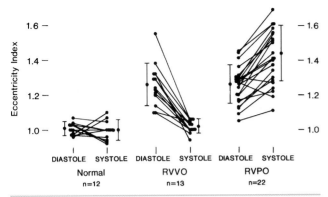

FIGURE 7.63. The eccentricity index reflects the degree of septal flattening resulting in abnormal left ventricular shape from the short-axis view. In normal subjects, the eccentricity index is approximately 1.0 in both diastole and systole. Right ventricular volume overload (*RVVO*) results in an increase in eccentricity index during diastole but near-normal values during systole. With right ventricular pressure overload (*RVPO*), an elevated eccentricity index is maintained throughout the cardiac cycle. (From Ryan T, Petrovic O, Dillon JC, et al. An echocardiographic index for separation of right ventricular volume and pressure overload. J Am Coll Cardiol 1985;5:918—927, with permission.)

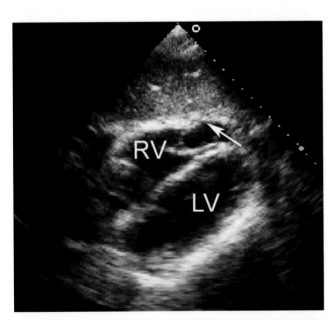

FIGURE 7.64. Arrhythmogenic right ventricular dysplasia (*ARVD*) resulting in aneurysmal dilation of the right ventricular free wall near the apex (*arrow*) is shown from the subcostal four-chamber view. LV, left ventricle; RV, right ventricle. (Illustration courtesy of D. Yoerger, M.D., Massachusetts General Hospital, Boston.)

ventricular free wall myocardium is replaced by adipose and/or collagen-containing tissue. ARVD has a wide range of clinical manifestations, but malignant ventricular arrhythmias and sudden death can occur. Echocardiography has been used extensively for the diagnosis of this abnormality. Right ventricular enlargement, focal right ventricular wall motion abnormalities, and localized

aneurysms of the free wall have been reported. In addition, the affected right ventricular myocardium has a characteristic echogenic appearance, reflecting the presence of fat and/or scar tissue within the free wall. Figure 7.64 is an example of an inferoapical aneurysm in a patient with ARVD. Note also the relative brightness of the right ventricular free wall, possibly indicating fatty tissue within the myocardium. The disease includes a spectrum of abnormalities, from very subtle changes to extensive and obvious involvement of much of the right ventricle (Fig. 7.65). Uhl anomaly, also called parchment right ven-

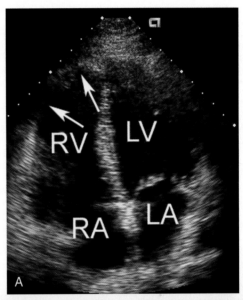

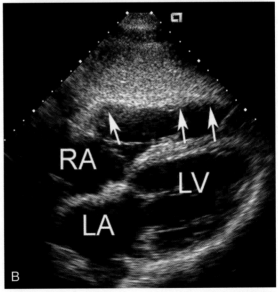

FIGURE 7.65. Extensive right ventricular (*RV*) involvement in a patient with arrhythmogenic right ventricular dysplasia is shown. **A:** The apical four-chamber view demonstrates dilation of the right ventricle and hypokinesis of the RV free wall (*arrows*). **B:** A subcostal view reveals segmental RV dysfunction and aneurysmal dilation near the apex (*arrows*). LA, left atrium; LV, left ventricle; RA, right atrium.

tricle, may be an extreme and generalized manifestation of ARVD. This latter pattern is, however, nonspecific because right ventricular dilation may occur for many reasons. Thus, the sensitivity and specificity of echocardiography to establish the diagnosis depend on the extent of the abnormality and the specific phenotype.

SUGGESTED READINGS

Appleton CP, Jensen JL, Hatle LK, et al. Doppler evaluation of left and right ventricular diastolic function: a technical guide for obtaining optimal flow velocity recordings. J Am Soc Echocardiogr 1997;10:271–292.

Belkin RN, Kisslo J. Atrial septal aneurysm: recognition and clinical relevance. Am.Heart J 1990;120:948–957.

Bommer W, Weinert L, Neumann A, et al. Determination of right atrial and right ventricular size by two-dimensional echocardiography. Circulation 1979;60:91–100.

Cohen GI, Klein AL, Chan KL, et al. Transesophageal echocardiographic diagnosis of right-sided cardiac masses in patients with central lines. Am J Cardiol 1992;70:925–929.

Corboy JR. Patent foramen ovale, atrial septal aneurysm, and recurrent stroke. N Engl J Med 2002;346:1331–1332.

DePace NL, Soulen RL, Kotler MN, et al. Two dimensional echocardiographic detection of intraatrial masses. Am J Cardiol 1981;48:954–960.

Douglas PS. The left atrium: a biomarker of chronic diastolic dysfunction and cardiovascular disease risk. J Am Coll Cardiol 2003;42:1206–1207.

Fujimoto S, Mizuno R, Nakagawa Y, et al. Estimation of the right ventricular volume and ejection fraction by transthoracic three-dimensional echocardiography. A validation study using magnetic resonance imaging. Int J Card Imaging 1998;14:385–390.

Gehl LG, Mintz GS, Kotler MN, et al. Left atrial volume overload in mitral regurgitation: a two dimensional echocardiographic study. Am J Cardiol 1982;49:33–38.

Hirata T, Wolfe SB, Popp RL, et al. Estimation of left atrial size using ultrasound. Am Heart J 1969;78:43–52.

Jiang L, Siu SC, Handschumacher MD, et al. Three-dimensional echocardiography. *In vivo* validation for right ventricular volume and function. Circulation 1994;89:2342–2350.

Keller AM, Gopal AS, King DL. Left and right atrial volume by freehand three-dimensional echocardiography: in vivo validation using magnetic resonance imaging. Eur J Echocardiogr 2000;1:55–65.

Kircher BJ, Himelman RB, Schiller NB. Noninvasive estimation of right atrial pressure from the inspiratory collapse of the inferior vena cava. Am J Cardiol 1990;66:493–496.

Kisslo J. Two-dimensional echocardiography in arrhythmogenic right ventricular dysplasia. Eur Heart J 1989;10(Suppl D):22–26.

Kullo IJ, Edwards WD, Seward JB. Right ventricular dysplasia: the Mayo Clinic experience. Mayo Clin Proc 1995;70:541–548.

LaBarre TR, Stamato NJ, Hwang MH, et al. Left atrial appendage aneurysm with associated anomalous pulmonary venous drainage. Am Heart J 1987;114:1243–1245.

Lemire F, Tajik AJ, Hagler DJ. Asymmetric left atrial enlargement; an echocardiographic observation. Chest 1976;69:779–781.

Levine RA, Gibson TC, Aretz T, et al. Echocardiographic measurement of right ventricular volume. Circulation 1984;69:497–505.

Loperfido F, Pennestri F, Digaetano A, et al. Assessment of left atrial dimensions by cross sectional echocardiography in patients with mitral valve disease. Br Heart J 1983;50:570–578.

Manning WJ, Silverman DI, Katz SE, et al. Atrial ejection force: a noninvasive assessment of atrial systolic function. J Am Coll Cardiol 1993;22:221–225.

Mas JL, Arquizan C, Lamy C, et al. Recurrent cerebrovascular events associated with patent foramen ovale, atrial septal aneurysm, or both. N Engl J Med 2001;345:1740–1746.

Matsukubo H, Matsuura T, Endo N, et al. Echocardiographic measurement of right ventricular wall thickness. A new application of sub xiphoid echocardiography. Circulation 1977;56:278–284.

Mugge A, Daniel WG, Angermann C, et al. Atrial septal aneurysm in adult patients. A multicenter study using transthoracic and transesophageal echocardiography. Circulation 1995;91:2785–2792.

Nagueh SF, Kopelen HA, Zoghbi WA. Relation of mean right atrial pressure to echocardiographic and Doppler parameters of right atrial and right ventricular function. Circulation 1996;93:1160–1169.

Nishimura RA, Abel MD, Hatle LK, et al. Relation of pulmonary vein to mitral flow velocities by transesophageal Doppler echocardiography. Effect of different loading conditions. Circulation 1990;81:1488–1497.

Oh JK, Appleton CP, Hatle LK, et al. The noninvasive assessment of left ventricular diastolic function with two-dimensional and Doppler echocardiography. J Am Soc Echocardiogr 1997;10:246–270.

Oh JK, Hatle LK, Seward JB, et al. Diagnostic role of Doppler echocardiography in constrictive pericarditis. J Am Coll Cardiol 1994;23:154–162.

Panidis IP, Ren JF, Kotler MN, et al. Two-dimensional echocardiographic estimation of right ventricular ejection fraction in patients with coronary artery disease. J Am Coll Cardiol 1983;2:911–918.

Papavassiliou DP, Parks WJ, Hopkins KL, et al. Three-dimensional echocardiographic measurement of right ventricular volume in children with congenital heart disease validated by magnetic resonance imaging. J Am Soc Echocardiogr 1998;11:770–777.

Pearson AC, Labovitz AJ, Tatineni S, et al. Superiority of transesophageal echocardiography in detecting cardiac source of embolism in patients with cerebral ischemia of uncertain etiology. J Am Coll Cardiol 1991;17:66–72.

Pearson AC, Nagelhout D, Castello R, et al. Atrial septal aneurysm and stroke: a transesophageal echocardiographic study. J Am Coll Cardiol 1991;18:1223–1229.

Reynolds T, Appleton CP. Doppler flow velocity patterns of the superior vena cava, inferior vena cava, hepatic vein, coronary sinus, and atrial septal defect: a guide for the echocardiographer. J Am Soc Echocardiogr 1991;4:503–512.

Rossvoll O, Hatle LK. Pulmonary venous flow velocities recorded by transthoracic Doppler ultrasound: relation to left ventricular diastolic pressures. J Am Coll Cardiol 1993;21:1687–1696.

Ryan T, Petrovic O, Dillon JC, et al. An echocardiographic index for separation of right ventricular volume and pressure overload. J Am Coll Cardiol 1985; 5:918–927.

Sakai K, Nakamura K, Satomi G, et al. Hepatic vein blood flow pattern measured by Doppler echocardiography as an evaluation of tricuspid valve insufficiency. J Cardiogr 1983;13:33–43.

Schabelman S, Schiller NB, Silverman NH, et al. Left atrial volume estimation by two-dimensional echocardiography. Cathet Cardiovasc Diagn 1981; 7:165–178.

Schneider B, Hanrath P, Vogel P, et al. Improved morphologic characterization of atrial septal aneurysm by transesophageal echocardiography: relation to cerebrovascular events. J Am Coll Cardiol 1990;16:1000–1009.

Shiota T, Jones M, Chikada M, et al. Real-time three-dimensional echocardiography for determining right ventricular stroke volume in an animal model of chronic right ventricular volume overload. Circulation 1998;97:1897–1900.

Stoddard MF, Dawkins PR, Prince CR, et al. Left atrial appendage thrombus is not uncommon in patients with acute atrial fibrillation and a recent embolic event: a transesophageal echocardiographic study. J Am Coll Cardiol 1995; 25:452–459.

Tomita M, Masuda H, Sumi T, et al. Estimation of right ventricular volume by modified echocardiographic subtraction method. Am Heart J 1992;123:1011–1022.

Tsang TS, Barnes ME, Bailey KR, et al. Left atrial volume: important risk marker of incident atrial fibrillation in 1655 older men and women. Mayo Clin Proc 2001;76:467–475.

Ueti OM, Camargo EE, Ueti Ade A., et al. Assessment of right ventricular function with Doppler echocardiographic indices derived from tricuspid annular motion: comparison with radionuclide angiography. Heart 2002;88:244–248.

Verhorst PM, Kamp O, Visser CA, et al. Left atrial appendage flow velocity assessment using transesophageal echocardiography in nonrheumatic atrial fibrillation and systemic embolism. Am J Cardiol 1993;71:192–196.

Watanabe T, Katsume H, Matsukubo H, et al. Estimation of right ventricular volume with two dimensional echocardiography. Am J Cardiol 1982;49:1946–1953.

Werner JA, Cheitlin MD, Gross BW, et al. Echocardiographic appearance of the Chiari network: differentiation from right-heart pathology. Circulation 1981;63:1104–1109.

Weyman AE, Wann S, Feigenbaum H, et al. Mechanism of abnormal septal motion in patients with right ventricular volume overload: a cross-sectional echocardiographic study. Circulation 1976;54:179–186.

Chapter 8

Hemodynamics

Since its inception, one of the primary goals of echocardiography has been to provide hemodynamic information. This was initially accomplished using M-mode and later two-dimensional imaging, which allowed measurement of dimensions that could be translated into volumetric data. The development of Doppler echocardiography now provides a more direct and quantitative technique from which to derive hemodynamic information. Currently, Doppler imaging, combined with two-dimensional imaging, is the preferred method for the noninvasive measurement of hemodynamics and, in many situations, has supplanted cardiac catheterization for this purpose. The accuracy of the Doppler technique for measuring blood velocity has been validated in numerous ways. Through its ability to quantify blood flow, measure pressure gradients, and estimate intracardiac pressures, the utility of Doppler-derived hemodynamic data is now well established.

USE OF M-MODE AND TWO-DIMENSIONAL ECHOCARDIOGRAPHY

Since the early days of ultrasound, investigators have attempted to extract hemodynamic data from echocardiograms. Such approaches were indirect and qualitative, generally relying on the fact that physiologic changes in blood flow would have predictable effects on the motion of the walls and valves of the heart. One of the earliest applications arose from the recognition that right ventricular pressure and volume overload caused predictable changes in the motion of the interventricular septum. Unfortunately, little quantitative information could be derived from this observation. Thus, once Doppler techniques became available, a more direct quantitative measure of right ventricular pressure was possible, thereby supplanting these more indirect approaches. A more relevant observation involved the early closure of the mitral valve that occurred in patients with acute, severe aortic regurgitation (Fig. 8.1). Here, the high tempo-

ral resolution of the M-mode technique provided a unique approach for timing valvular events. Premature closure of the mitral valve indicated rapidly increasing left ventricular diastolic pressure and became a reliable, if indirect, marker of hemodynamically significant aortic regurgitation before the availability of more direct noninvasive techniques.

A similar example is the B bump of mitral valve closure. This is a particular motion of the mitral valve that occurs in late diastole as the valve drifts shut with increasing left ventricular pressure (Fig. 8.2). The normal rate of mitral valve closure after atrial systole is smooth and of brief duration. In patients with elevated left ven-

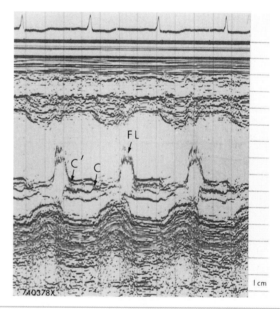

FIGURE 8.1. A mitral valve M-mode echocardiogram is shown from a patient with acute aortic regurgitation. Note partial valve closure (*C'*) in middiastole, significantly earlier than normal. The valve does not reopen with atrial systole and then closes completely with the onset of ventricular contraction (*C*). Fine fluttering (*FL*) of the mitral valve is due to the aortic regurgitant jet.

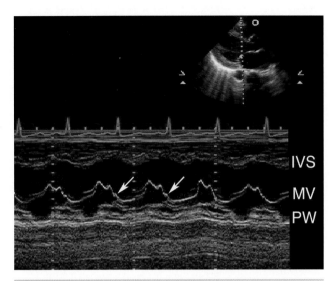

FIGURE 8.2. A mitral valve echocardiogram demonstrating a B bump (*arrows*). See text for details. IVS, interventricular septum; MV, mitral valve; PW, posterior left ventricular wall.

tricular diastolic pressure, the associated increase in left atrial pressure results in an abnormal pattern of mitral valve closure. The onset of mitral valve closure is premature, and mitral valve closure is interrupted because the A point occurs earlier than usual, resulting in a notch between the A point and the C point. The prolongation of the closing phase of the mitral valve has been termed the B bump and has been associated with increased left ventricular end-diastolic (and left atrial) pressure (Fig. 8.3).

Efforts to quantify left ventricular diastolic pressure using this finding have been unreliable. Although the sensitivity of the finding has been debated, the presence of a B bump is consistently associated with a left ventricular diastolic pressure at the time of atrial contraction of at least 20 mm Hg. The application of Doppler techniques to the study of left atrial pressure eventually overshadowed the importance of this finding.

Other M-mode echocardiographic signs of altered hemodynamics also have stood the test of time. Systolic anterior motion of the mitral valve is an important finding in patients with hypertrophic cardiomyopathy and may indicate dynamic outflow tract obstruction. This is demonstrated using either M-mode or two-dimensional techniques. In these patients, partial closure of the aortic valve during mid and late systole, as seen on M-mode echocardiography, is a reliable indicator of significant outflow tract obstruction. Again, however, quantification of the gradient is not possible. One of the most useful echocardiographic indicators of hemodynamic significance is the early diastolic collapse of the right ventricular free wall that occurs when intrapericardial pressure increases in the clinical setting of tamponade (Fig. 8.4). This is discussed in detail in Chapter 9.

A partial listing of M-mode and two-dimensional echocardiographic findings indicating abnormal hemodynamics is provided in Table 8.1. Although most of these

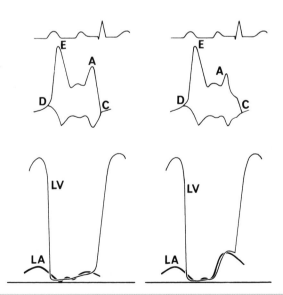

FIGURE 8.3. A schematic demonstrates how the mitral valve echocardiogram reflects changes in left ventricular diastolic pressure. The normal relationship between mitral leaflet motion and intracardiac pressure changes is shown on the left. The genesis of the B bump reflects elevated late diastolic left atrial pressure. See text for details. LA, left atrium; LV, left ventricle.

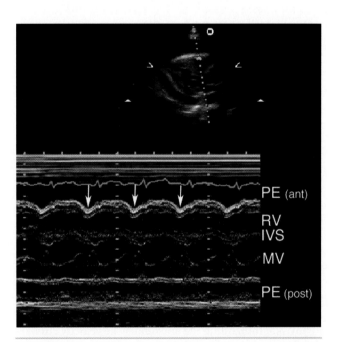

FIGURE 8.4. An M-mode echocardiogram from a patient with pericardial tamponade is demonstrated. The *arrows* indicate early diastolic collapse of the right ventricular (*RV*) free wall. The echo-free space above the RV free wall represents pericardial fluid, which can also been seen posterior to the left ventricle. IVS, interventricular septum; MV, mitral valve; PE, pericardial effusion.

▶ TABLE 8.1 **M-Mode and Two-Dimensional Echocardiographic Findings of Altered Hemodynamics**

Finding	*Hemodynamic Significance*
M-mode	
Early closure of the mitral valve	Acute, severe aortic regurgitation
Delayed closure of the mitral valve (B bump)	Elevated LV end-diastolic pressure
RV free wall early diastolic collapse	Pericardial tamponade
Mid systolic notching of the aortic valve	Dynamic subaortic outflow tract obstruction
Diastolic mitral valve fluttering	Aortic regurgitation
Mid systolic notching of the pulmonary valve	Pulmonary hypertension
Rounding of the opening/closing points of a disk-type prosthetic valve	Mechanical restriction to disc motion
Systolic anterior motion of the mitral valve	Dynamic subaortic outflow track obstruction
Early systolic downward motion (beaking) of the IVS	LBBB
Gradual closure of the aortic valve	Reduced left ventricular stroke volume
Absent pulmonary valve A-wave	Pulmonary hypertension
Two dimensional	
Diastolic flattening of the IVS	RV volume overload
Systolic flattening of the IVS	RV pressure overload (elevated RVSP)
Dilated IVC with abnormal respiratory variation	Elevated RA pressure
Exaggerated IVS bounce, with respiratory variation	Constriction

IVC, inferior vena cava; IVS, interventricular septum; LBBB, left bundle branch block; RA, right atrial; RV, right ventricular; RVSP, right ventricular systolic pressure.

findings have been replaced by more quantitative and direct measurements using the Doppler techniques, they continue to provide useful confirmatory evidence in selected patients.

QUANTIFYING BLOOD FLOW

Doppler echocardiography is able to measure blood flow through its ability to quantify blood velocity. We know that the rate of flow through an orifice is equal to the product of flow velocity and cross-sectional area. Because cross-sectional area can be measured with M-mode or two-dimensional imaging and flow velocity can be determined directly with Doppler imaging, the technique provides a noninvasive measure of flow. If flow were constant (i.e., had a fixed velocity), it would be a simple matter to determine velocity at any point in time and solve the equation accordingly. In the cardiovascular system, however, flow is pulsatile and therefore individual velocities during the ejection phase must be sampled and then integrated to measure flow volume. This sum of velocities is called the time velocity integral (TVI) and is equal to the area enclosed by the Doppler velocity profile during one ejection period. This essential concept is illustrated in Figure 8.5. Integrating the area under the velocity curve is simply measuring the velocities at each point in time and summing all these velocities. It should be noted that when velocity is integrated over time, the units that result from this operation are a measure of distance (in centimeters), hence the term *stroke distance*, which is the linear distance that the blood travels during one flow period. When

TVI and the corresponding cross-sectional area (in centimeters squared) are measured at the same point, such as through one of the four cardiac valves, their product equals stroke volume (in centimeters cubed or milliliters), which is the volume of blood ejected by the heart with each contraction (assuming no valvular regurgitation or cardiac shunt).

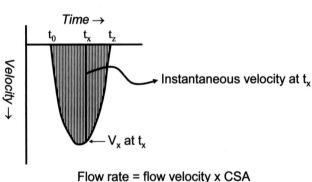

Flow rate = flow velocity x CSA
Flow velocity varies from t_0 to t_z
Sum of all velocities = TVI
TVI = $\Sigma V_{0 \to z}$
Stroke volume = TVI x CSA

FIGURE 8.5. A schematic demonstrates the concept of flow quantification using the Doppler technique. Doppler records instantaneous velocity throughout the cardiac cycle. The area under the Doppler velocity curve represents the time velocity integral (*TVI*). This is the sum of all the individual instantaneous velocities throughout the ejection period. See text for details. CSA, cross-sectional area.

These principles are illustrated in Figure 8.6, which demonstrates how these concepts can be applied to aortic flow to measure stroke volume. Recall from the Doppler equation the importance of the angle θ, that is, the angle between the ultrasound beam and blood flow direction. Because the cosine function varies between 0 and 1 and appears in the numerator of the Doppler equation, errors in θ will have a predictable effect on measured velocities. For example, if θ is between 0 and 20 degrees, the cosine of θ will range between 1.0 and 0.92, leading to a slight underestimation of true velocity. As θ increases to more than 20 degrees, the cosine decreases rapidly and the degree of velocity underestimation increases quickly. Hence, aligning the ultrasound beam as close as possible to the direction of flow is critical if true velocity is to be measured. Equally important, misalignment between the ultrasound beam and flow can only result in underestimation of velocity, never overestimation.

Another factor that will affect the accuracy of the Doppler equation is the pattern of blood flow where velocity is being measured. Normal flow in the heart and great vessels is laminar, meaning that the fluid is traveling at approximately the same velocity and in the same general direction. If a sample volume is placed within such a flow pattern, the Doppler will record a clean signal of uniform velocity. Flow becomes increasingly disturbed or turbulent (i.e., less laminar) as the velocity increases or the cross-sectional area changes (Fig. 8.7A). Viscosity also affects the flow profile. At the edge of the flow pattern, near the vessel wall, flow tends to be slower and more turbulent. The highest velocities and most laminar flow generally occur at the center of the profile. This spatial distribution of velocities across the three-dimensional flow is called the flow velocity profile. In a large, straight vessel,

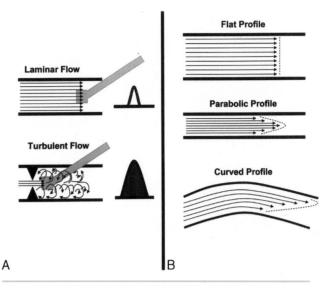

FIGURE 8.7. **A:** The differences between laminar and turbulent flow are demonstrated using pulsed Doppler. Laminar flow is associated with a lower velocity and a thinner flow envelope. **B:** Various flow profiles are provided. See text for details.

with laminar flow, it tends to be flat (Fig. 8.7B), whereas in smaller curved vessels, the profile has a parabolic shape. Velocity will be higher at the center and lower at the margins. Flow patterns through curved vessels, such as the aortic arch, are more complex. Here the distribution of velocities depends on the size of the vessel, the flow profile entering the curve, and the presence and location of branch vessels. If the sample volume is placed within such a flow pattern, the recorded velocity will vary, depending on the exact location.

Fortunately, flow passing through a normal heart valve or the proximal great vessels tends to be laminar with a flat profile and is therefore suitable for quantitative analysis. Because it is easier to determine the average flow velocity with a flat versus a parabolic blood profile, it is not surprising that efforts to measure blood flow attempt to use larger orifices and flow that are close to the origin of vessels. Note also that physiologic blood flow is never perfectly uniform. That is, at any point in time, a distribution of velocities occurs, resulting in a broadening of the Doppler signal. The greater the range of velocities is at any point in time, the broader is the Doppler signal. The darker line through the center of the distribution represents the *modal* frequency, i.e., the velocity at which the largest number of blood cells are traveling (Fig. 8.8). Theoretically, this is the velocity that should be used to determine the TVI. In practice, however, it is common to trace the outer edge of the densest portion of the envelope, and studies have indicated that both techniques provide a reasonably accurate measurement of blood flow. Multiple cycles (usually three to five) should be traced and averaged to minimize error. In patients with atrial fibrillation, between five and 10 beats should be analyzed.

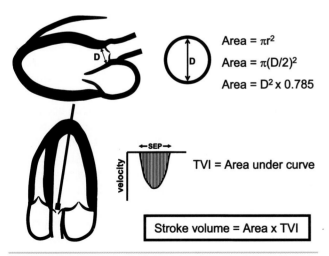

FIGURE 8.6. The method for quantifying stroke volume is demonstrated in the schematic. Two measurements are required: area and time velocity integral. See text for details. D, diameter. SEP, systolic ejection period.

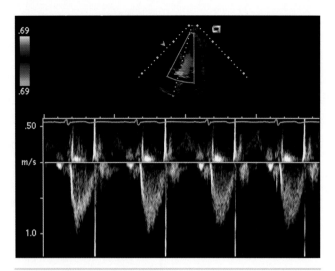

FIGURE 8.8. An example of laminar flow through the aortic valve recorded from the apical view with pulsed Doppler imaging. The vertical velocity spike at end-systole indicates aortic valve closure.

An important potential source of error in the blood flow measurement is the determination of cross-sectional area. It is essential to remember that cross-sectional area must be measured at the same point in space where the Doppler signal is sampled. For example, if blood flow is measured through the aortic valve, both the Doppler signal and the cross-sectional area must be measured at the same level. If the Doppler sample volume is placed at the level of the aortic anulus, then the cross-sectional area of the aortic anulus must be determined. The cross-sectional area can be measured using either M-mode or two-dimensional imaging. In Figure 8.9, three slightly different measurements of the outflow tract diameter are obtained. In most cases, the largest dimension should be used because it most likely corresponds to the true diameter. Another approach to this problem would be to directly measure the cross-sectional area by planimetry of a short-axis image of the orifice. In practice, however, it is common to determine the diameter of the orifice, assume a circular shape, and calculate area using the formula

$$A = \pi r^2 \qquad [\text{Eq. 8.1}]$$

Because $r = \frac{1}{2}D$, and D is what is actually measured, this can be simplified and expressed as

$$A = 0.785 * D^2 \qquad [\text{Eq. 8.2}]$$

Thus, the Doppler equation for stroke volume becomes

$$\text{Stroke volume} = 0.785 * D^2 * \text{TVI} \qquad [\text{Eq. 8.3}]$$

Considering this equation, it is obvious that any error in the measurement of the diameter of the orifice is "squared" and thus contributes greatly to errors in the final determination. For this reason, particular care must be taken to ensure accurate determination of orifice diameter. Multiple measurements should be performed. Generally, the largest dimension is used because it most likely represents the true diameter and smaller measurements represent tangential cuts through the circular outflow tract. The importance of accurately measuring the outflow tract diameter is illustrated in the following example. Assume the "true" diameter is 2.0 cm and the TVI is 20 cm. This would yield a stroke volume of 63 mL. Underestimation of the diameter by just 10%, would have the following effect on stroke volume calculation:

$$\text{Stroke volume} = 0.785 * (1.8 \text{ cm})^2 * 20 = 51 \text{ mL}$$

Thus, a 2-mm (or 10%) underestimation in diameter would lead to a 19% underestimation (51 mL instead of 63 mL) in stroke volume.

Despite these potential sources of error, several investigators have demonstrated the accuracy of this approach for measuring blood flow in a variety of clinical situations. When performed carefully, this noninvasive technique has proven to be an accurate and reproducible way to quantify blood flow within the cardiovascular system. An example of stroke volume calculation from the aortic flow measurement is provided in Figure 8.10.

CLINICAL APPLICATION OF BLOOD FLOW MEASUREMENT

The Doppler approach to measuring blood flow is a general formula that can be applied anywhere that blood passes through an orifice of fixed and measurable dimensions. Thus, it is possible to measure blood flow across all four valves of the heart and in the great vessels. To do so requires pulsed Doppler sampling of flow velocity at a location where cross-sectional area also can be measured. Figure 8.11 illustrates how stroke volume can be measured through each of the four valves. In the absence of valvular regurgitation or intracardiac shunt, flow through all four valves should be equal. The diagram demonstrates how cross-sectional area and TVI vary inversely for the different valves, but the product (cross-sectional area × TVI) is equal at each location. Of course, each site presents its unique set of challenges, and in any given patient, the measurement may or may not be feasible. Accuracy and reproducibility will improve with practice. Thus, performing flow calculation on a routine basis can be expected to increase one's confidence in the results when clinical questions arise.

Although flow can theoretically be measured at any site, in practice, it is customary to measure blood flow through the aortic valve. The Doppler recording is per-

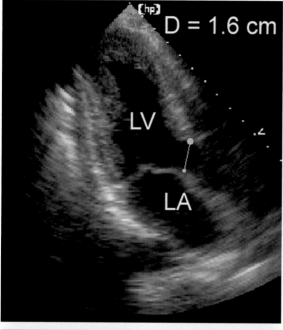
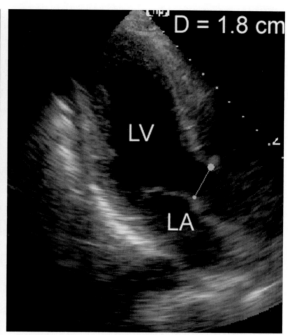
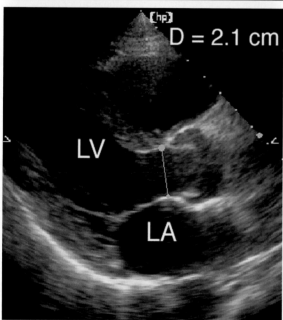

FIGURE 8.9. To measure the cross-sectional area of the left ventricular outflow tract, the diameter (*D*) must be measured carefully. The three examples demonstrate three different values for D obtained from the same patient. In most cases, the correct dimension is the largest, indicating the true diameter. LA, left atrium; LV, left ventricle.

formed using either the apical five-chamber or apical long-axis view and the sample volume is positioned at the level of the aortic anulus, approximately 3 to 5 mm proximal to the valve (Fig. 8.10). At that location, it is usual to record the closing "click" of the aortic valve at end-systole. If the opening click is present in the Doppler recording, the sample volume should be withdrawn slightly into the outflow tract. Cross-sectional area is measured by recording the parasternal long-axis view and determining the diameter of the aortic anulus in systole, assuming a circular shape. Because anular size does not change much over the cardiac cycle, the precise timing of the diameter mea-

surement is not critical. Alternatively, the anulus can be viewed from the short-axis projection and the area measured directly via planimetry. This is theoretically more precise but practically more difficult.

Pulmonary valve flow can be recorded using a similar approach. The sample volume is positioned at the level of the pulmonary valve, usually from the basal short-axis view. Alternatively, especially in children, the subcostal short-axis view can be used. The cross-sectional area is measured as the diameter of the outflow tract at the level of the anulus. An accurate measurement of this diameter is often difficult in adults because of the challenges of vi-

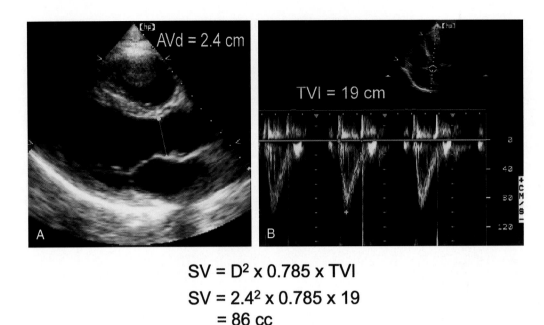

$$SV = D^2 \times 0.785 \times TVI$$
$$SV = 2.4^2 \times 0.785 \times 19$$
$$= 86 \text{ cc}$$

FIGURE 8.10. An example of stroke volume calculation is shown. **A:** The cross-sectional area of the outflow tract (*AVd*) is measured. **B:** The time velocity integral of aortic flow is determined by planimetry. The calculation for stroke volume (*SV*) is shown.

sualizing the lateral border of the right ventricular outflow tract. It is commonly performed in children, however, to quantify right ventricular stroke volume. This can then be compared with stroke volume in the left heart to assess intracardiac shunts and valvular regurgitation. This application is covered later in this section.

Quantitating stroke volume across the mitral valve creates additional challenges. Mitral flow velocity is easily recorded from apical views and consists of two phases: an early diastolic wave (E) and a second wave associated with atrial systole (A). Several studies have demonstrated that Doppler mitral velocity can be used to quantify stroke volume provided that the cross-sectional area of the mitral valve orifice can be determined. This can be performed using a short-axis view to planimeter its cross-sectional area. Next, an M-mode or two-dimensional echocardiographic recording of the mitral valve is used to determine the mitral orifice diameter throughout diastole. From this, the mean mitral diameter is calculated and applied to the Doppler equation. A simplified and more practical approach uses the diameter of the mitral anulus as measured from the apical views as a surrogate for cross-sectional area (Fig. 8.12). The measurement should be performed from the four-chamber view in early diastole. Then, assuming a circular shape, the area is estimated by Equation 8.1, which is $A = \pi r^2$. Alternatively, a second diameter can be measured from the apical two-chamber view and a mean value for cross-sectional area can be obtained. Mitral inflow velocity is then recorded at the level of the anulus, and the TVI is determined by planimetry (Fig. 8.13). The accuracy of quantifying mitral stroke volume is debatable. Recording a clean velocity profile at the anular level (compared with the mitral leaflet tips) can be challenging. It is also more difficult to accurately measure cross-sectional area at the mitral anulus compared with the aortic anulus. For all these reasons, quantifying blood flow across the mitral and tricuspid valves is more cumbersome compared with the aortic and pulmonary valves and is performed infrequently in clinical practice.

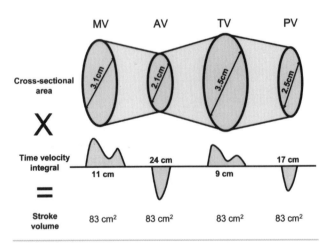

FIGURE 8.11. This schematic demonstrates the principle of conservation of mass. In the absence of valvular regurgitation or intracardiac shunts, the stroke volume through each of the four valves should be equal. See text for details. AV, aortic valve; MV, mitral valve; PV, pulmonic valve; TV, tricuspid valve.

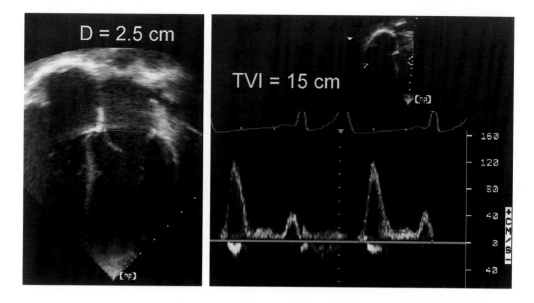

$$SV = 2.5^2 \times 0.785 \times 15$$
$$= 74 \text{ cc}$$

FIGURE 8.12. An example of calculating stroke volume (*SV*) through the mitral valve is demonstrated. **Left:** The cross-sectional area of the mitral anulus is determined. **Right:** Flow velocity at that level is measured using pulsed Doppler imaging. See text for details.

This technique for determining volumetric flow has several practical applications. The noninvasive measurement of stroke volume has obvious value, both as an absolute number and as a relative change. Stroke volume is a fundamental measure of global left ventricular systolic performance and can be readily converted to cardiac output by multiplying by heart rate. In critically ill patients, relative changes in stroke volume may indicate improvement or deterioration or may reflect a response to an intervention. In this case, it is the *relative* change

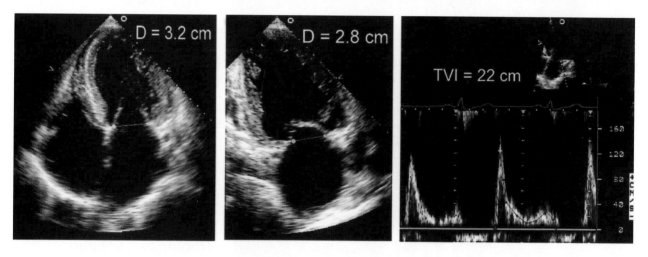

$$SV = (\pi \times r_1 \times r_2) \times 22$$
$$= 152 \text{ cc}$$

FIGURE 8.13. An alternative approach to quantification of flow through the mitral valve assumes an elliptical shape of the mitral anulus. The diameter is measured from the four-chamber **(left)** and two-chamber **(center)** views. The Doppler recording of mitral inflow is shown on the **right.** The equation for the area of an ellipse is $A = \pi \times r_1 \times r_2$. The stroke volume (*SV*) calculation is shown.

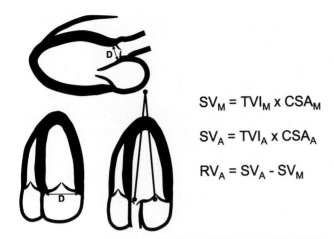

$$SV_M = TVI_M \times CSA_M$$

$$SV_A = TVI_A \times CSA_A$$

$$RV_A = SV_A - SV_M$$

FIGURE 8.14. Differences in stroke volume (*SV*) across the aortic and mitral valves may reflect regurgitation at one of these sites. In this schematic from a patient with aortic regurgitation, regurgitant volume (*RV_A*) is simply the difference between the aortic stroke volume and the mitral stroke volume. D, diameter. See text for details.

tively subtle alterations in cardiac performance can be tracked.

In patients with valvular regurgitation, differences in stroke volume across different valves provide a quantitative assessment of severity. This is illustrated schematically in Figure 8.14. In the absence of regurgitation, stroke volume across all four valves should be equal. In the presence of aortic regurgitation, for example, the difference between aortic flow and mitral flow represents the aortic regurgitant volume as shown in the following formula:

Regurgitant volume = Aortic systolic flow
        − Mitral diastolic flow   [Eq. 8.4]

Regurgitant fraction in aortic regurgitation can also be calculated as

$$\text{Regurgitant fraction (\%)} = \frac{\text{Regurgitant volume}}{\text{Aortic outflow volume}} \times 100\%$$

[Eq. 8.5]

This type of calculation can be performed for any valve of the heart (Fig. 8.15). It assumes that the valve used as the standard for flow is not regurgitant and that a similar degree of accuracy can be achieved at each location. In addition, the calculation is complicated by the presence of valve stenosis.

that matters. If cross-sectional area is assumed to remain constant, changes in the TVI will reflect changes in stroke volume. This has the advantage of avoiding the potential errors that can be introduced when measuring cross-sectional area. By following changes in TVI, relatively

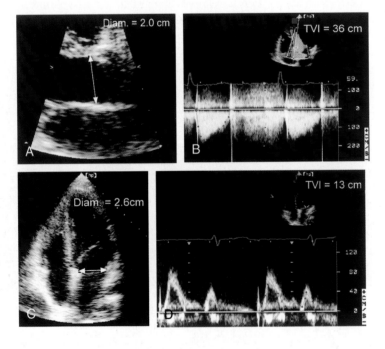

Aortic flow:
CSA_AV = 3.1 cm²
TVI_AV = 36 cm
SV_AV = 112 cc

Mitral flow:
CSA_MV = 5.3 cm²
TVI_MV = 13 cm
SV_MV = 69 cc

Regurgitant volume:
112 − 69 = 43 cc

Regurgitant fraction:
43 / 112 = 38%

FIGURE 8.15. An example of how regurgitant volume (*RV*) and regurgitant fraction (*RF*) can be measured is provided. **A, B:** Stroke volume (*SV*) calculation through the aortic valve. **C, D:** Stroke volume quantification through the mitral valve. The calculations used to determine RV and RF are given on the right. CSA, cross-sectional area; TVI, time velocity integral.

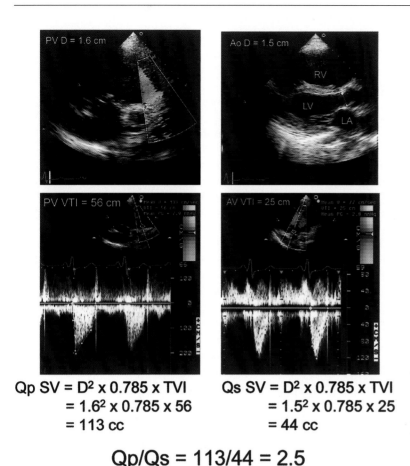

$$Qp\ SV = D^2 \times 0.785 \times TVI$$
$$= 1.6^2 \times 0.785 \times 56$$
$$= 113\ cc$$

$$Qs\ SV = D^2 \times 0.785 \times TVI$$
$$= 1.5^2 \times 0.785 \times 25$$
$$= 44\ cc$$

$$Qp/Qs = 113/44 = 2.5$$

FIGURE 8.16. In the presence of an intracardiac shunt, Q_p/Q_s provides a means to quantify the magnitude of shunting. In this example from a patient with a large secundum atrial septal defect, stroke volume (*SV*) through the pulmonary (**left**) and aortic (**right**) valves are measured and the Q_p/Q_s is determined.

A final application of this principle is the quantitation of intracardiac shunts. Determining the pulmonary-to-systemic flow ratio, or $Q_p:Q_s$, is the principal way to quantitate the size of the shunt (Fig. 8.16). In most cases, the shunt ratio is determined by calculating pulmonary stroke volume and comparing it with aortic stroke volume. The difference equals the net shunt volume in the absence of semilunar valve stenosis or regurgitation. This approach has been used in pediatric echocardiography with success and has been validated against invasive standards.

In summary, calculation of volumetric flow is possible and has been validated in a variety of clinical situations. The formulas are based on sound physiologic principles and, under optimal circumstances, provide an accurate means for quantifying flow. Measurement errors can cause significant mistakes that may or may not be apparent at the time of the calculations. As a consequence, a small and sometimes unrecognized error in measurement can lead to an unacceptable error in the final result. For example, if aortic and mitral stroke volume are derived to calculate regurgitant volume and if each primary calculation is off by 10%, the following scenario is possible. Assume that the correct aortic stroke volume is 90 mL and the mitral stroke volume is 60 mL, yielding a regurgitant volume of 30 mL and a regurgitant fraction of 33%. If the

aortic stroke volume is high by 10% (99 mL) and the mitral stroke volume is low by the same degree (54 mL), the derived regurgitant volume is now 45 mL, and the regurgitant fraction is 45%, a significant difference. To minimize the likelihood of errors, it is essential to do such calculations routinely rather than just on rare occasions. Be aware of the potential sources of error and know when image quality precludes reliable measurements.

MEASURING PRESSURE GRADIENTS

One of the most important applications of the Doppler method is to measure transvalvular pressure gradients. This approach is based on Newton's law of conservation of energy, which states that the total amount of energy within a closed system must remain constant. Thus, as applied to blood flow measurements, the flow velocity through a valve must increase as the valve area decreases. When blood is forced through a stenotic valve, its kinetic energy (which is proportional to the square of velocity) increases, whereas its potential energy must decrease proportionately. In a pulsatile system, some energy may be lost due to inertia as the blood accelerates and decelerates. In addition, a small amount of energy may be lost in the form of heat as a result of viscous friction. These relationships were described mathematically by Bernoulli and expressed as:

$$\Delta P = \tfrac{1}{2}\rho(v_2^2 - v_1^2) + \rho\!\int (dv/dt) * ds + R(\mu) \qquad \text{[Eq. 8.6]}$$

where ΔP is the pressure difference across the stenosis, v_1 and v_2 are the velocities proximal and distal to the stenosis, respectively, ρ is the mass density of blood, R is viscous resistance and μ is viscosity (Fig. 8.17). Essentially, the first term of the equation corresponds to kinetic energy that results from acceleration through the stenosis. The second term accounts for the loss of energy as the blood accelerates and then decelerates. The final term represents the losses due to viscous friction, a function of blood viscosity and velocity. Fortunately, these latter two terms are negligible (under most physiologic conditions) and the Bernoulli equation can be simplified to

$$\Delta P = 4(v_2^2 - v_1^2) \qquad \text{[Eq. 8.7]}$$

Because both velocity terms are squared, if v_2 is significantly greater than v_1, v_1 can be eliminated to a final simplified equation that relates the pressure decrease across a discrete stenosis to the maximal velocity distal to the valve:

$$\Delta P = 4v^2 \qquad \text{[Eq. 8.8]}$$

where v is the maximal velocity of the stenotic jet.

The simplified Bernoulli equation has been validated in numerous clinical situations and correlates well with direct invasive measures of pressure decrease. The technique has had its greatest application in measuring the severity of valve stenosis, a topic that is also covered in several other chapters. This same approach can also be used to estimate intracardiac pressures in patients with valvular regurgitation or intracardiac shunts, such as ventricular septal defects. In essence, wherever velocity can be measured across a discrete stenosis, the Bernoulli equation allows the pressure gradient to be determined.

The accuracy of the Bernoulli equation to predict pressure gradients across stenotic valves is well established. When using the technique clinically, several potential sources of error should be considered and, whenever pos-

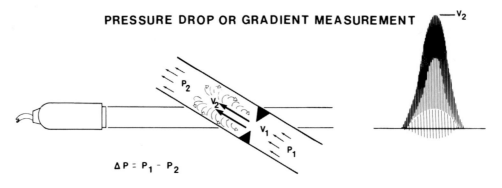

FIGURE 8.17. The principles underlying the modified Bernoulli equation are demonstrated. The complete Bernoulli equation is given. P_2, pressure distal to an obstruction; P_1, pressure proximal to an obstruction; V_2, velocity distal to an obstruction; V_1, velocity proximal to an obstruction; ΔP, difference in pressure across the obstruction.

sible, avoided. As will be apparent, most errors are technical in nature and result in underestimation of the true pressure gradient. The most common example occurs when the ultrasound beam cannot be properly aligned relative to the direction of blood flow. As has been discussed, when the incident angle increases beyond 20 degrees, a significant error is introduced into the Doppler equation that results in underestimation of true velocity. To avoid this problem, color Doppler imaging can be used to visualize the blood flow, thereby facilitating proper alignment. The use of multiple acoustic windows is another way to ensure that the view providing the best alignment is recorded. Two examples of this are shown in Figures 8.18 and 8.19. In Figure 8.18, three different values for tricuspid regurgitation velocity yield three different estimates of right ventricular systolic pressure. The correct value is the highest, in this case recorded from the apical four-chamber view, which affords the best alignment with blood flow. In Figure 8.19, two examples of aortic stenosis are shown. In both cases, the severity of aortic stenosis is underestimated from the apical window but accu-rately assessed from the right parasternal window. Better alignment between the ultrasound beam and the stenotic jet is the explanation for the difference.

Image quality also plays a role in the accuracy of the gradient determination. The signal-to-noise ratio will affect whether the entire Doppler envelope is recorded for analysis. If part of the envelope is "missing" because of an incomplete signal, the peak velocity will be missed and underestimation will occur. In Figure 8.19, notice how the jet envelope is incomplete in some of the beats. Failure to record the entire Doppler envelope will invariably lead to underestimation of velocity. Proper gain setting, optimal beam alignment, and a careful and thorough search for the best image are all necessary to accurately measure pressure gradients. The application of echo contrast agents to boost the signal of the jet is another practical way to avoid underestimation. However, when contrast is used, some noise is inevitably introduced into the signal. Some adjustment of the reject settings may be necessary, and only the densest part of the Doppler contour should be traced. An example of the use of contrast to improve

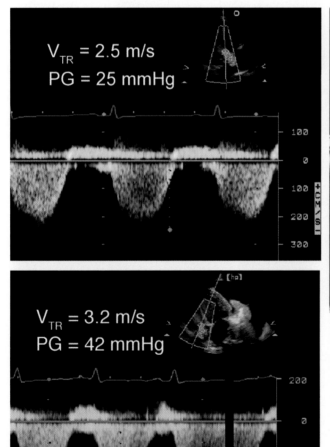

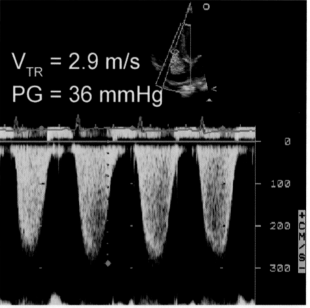

FIGURE 8.18. These three recordings of tricuspid regurgita-tion (*TR*) are taken from one patient. The different panels il-lustrate how various values for velocity (V_{TR}) yield significantly different estimates of pressure gradient (*PG*) and hence right ventricular systolic pressure. The correct value is usually the highest velocity value, in this case recorded from a modified apical four-chamber view. V_{TR}, peak tricuspid regurgitation jet velocity.

Patient A

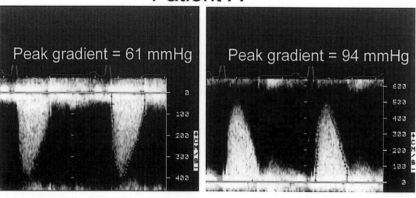

Patient B

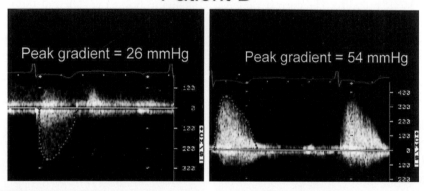

FIGURE 8.19. Two patients with aortic stenosis are included. In both cases, different values for aortic stenosis jet velocity are obtained, yielding different measures of peak gradient. In patient A, the apical view underestimates the true velocity, which is optimally recorded from the right parasternal window. In patient B, the apical window again underestimates true velocity. In this case, the peak gradient was best recorded from the suprasternal notch.

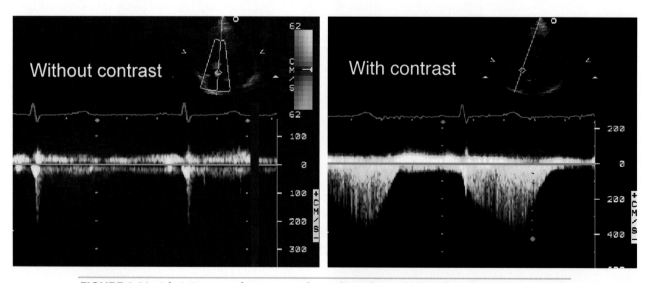

FIGURE 8.20. Administration of contrast can be used to enhance the Doppler signal and improve determination of true velocity. On the left, tricuspid regurgitation is incompletely recorded in a baseline study. After injection of agitated saline through a peripheral vein, the tricuspid regurgitation signal is enhanced and the peak velocity more accurately determined.

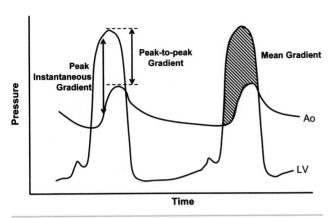

FIGURE 8.21. This schematic demonstrates the relationship between aortic (*Ao*) and left ventricular (*LV*) pressure in the setting of aortic stenosis. The differences between peak instantaneous, peak-to-peak, and mean gradients are demonstrated.

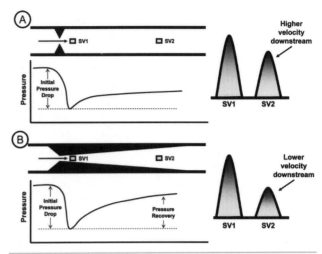

FIGURE 8.22. The concept of pressure recovery is illustrated in this schematic. **Top:** In the absence of pressure recovery, different locations for sample volume (*SV*) measurement yield fairly similar velocities. **Bottom:** Flow through a tapered stenosis results in significant pressure recovery downstream from the obstruction. In this case, sampling within the obstruction (*SV1*) yields a higher velocity compared with a sample site downstream (*SV2*) where pressure recovery has occurred. At this site, the recovery of pressure is associated with a lower velocity. See text for details.

the Doppler signal is provided in Figure 8.20. *It should be emphasized that the maximal velocity should always be sought out and used for the calculation of gradient.*

In most cases, Doppler-derived pressure gradients are compared with cardiac catheterization data. When discrepancies occur, a plausible explanation is often apparent. For example, it is important to remember that Doppler measures peak instantaneous gradient, whereas catheterization data are most often reported as peak to peak, which is usually less. The difference between these two values is illustrated in Figure 8.21. Another potential source of discrepancy is the nonsimultaneous nature of the studies. Valve gradients are dynamic and may vary considerably over time. If the Doppler data and the catheterization data are not recorded at the same time, differences may be expected.

The simplified Bernoulli equation ignores the proximal flow velocity (v_1) and estimates gradient based on the distal, or jet, velocity (v_2). This is an acceptable simplification if v_2 is significantly greater than v_1. However, in cases in which the proximal velocity is relatively high, this simplification may be inappropriate. For example, if antegrade flow is high and/or if the gradient is low, the difference between v_1 and v_2 may be relatively small and a more appropriate version of the Bernoulli equation would be

$$\Delta P = 4(v_2^2 - v_1^2) \qquad \text{[Eq. 8.7]}$$

A potential source of error in some clinical situations involves the concept of *pressure* recovery. Pressure recovery occurs if kinetic energy is not entirely dissipated as turbulent flow distal to the stenosis (Fig. 8.22). Under some conditions, flow may "relaminarize" downstream from the stenosis so that kinetic energy recovers in the form of hydraulic energy. If a measuring catheter is positioned sufficiently far downstream that significant pres-

sure recovery has occurred, it will measure a smaller gradient compared with the Doppler gradient, which measures maximal gradient at the *vena contracta*. In such cases, Doppler imaging will overestimate the catheterization-derived gradient, resulting in a discrepancy, although neither represents an actual error in measurement. Pressure recovery has been demonstrated in some prosthetic valves and may also occur in tapered stenoses, such as supravalvar aortic stenosis and coarctation.

It is apparent that underestimation of the true gradient by the Doppler technique is more common than overestimation. A situation in which overestimation may occur is in the setting of combined aortic stenosis and mitral regurgitation. Because of the proximity of the two jets, as well as their similar timing and appearance, a misplaced Doppler beam may inadvertently record mitral regurgitation instead of aortic stenosis. Because the velocity of mitral regurgitation is invariably high, this can lead to overestimation (Fig. 8.23). To avoid this problem, color flow imaging can be used to ensure spatial orientation. By gradually moving the Doppler beam back and forth from the left atrium to the aortic valve, both jets can be sequentially recorded. This increases the confidence of the interpreter to distinguish one from the other. In addition, the velocity information must "make sense." When anatomic data are incompatible with Doppler data, an explanation must be sought. For example, mitral regurgitation is invariably high velocity, often 5 to 6 m/sec. The jet of aortic stenosis is typically less than that, depending, of

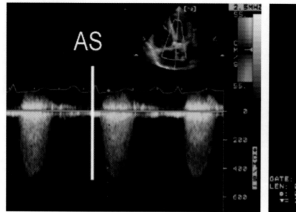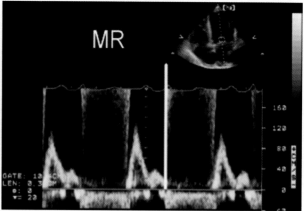

FIGURE 8.23. This illustration demonstrates how the high-velocity systolic jets of mitral regurgitation **(left)** and aortic stenosis **(right)** can be differentiated. Mitral regurgitation begins earlier, during isovolumic contraction, and persists later compared with the aortic stenosis jet. See text for details.

course, on the severity. If, by all other criteria, aortic stenosis appears mild or moderate, but the Doppler velocity is 6 m/sec, the likelihood that the jet represents mitral regurgitation must be considered. It is also helpful to remember that the mitral regurgitation jet will be of greater duration than the systolic ejection period. In Figure 8.23, note the relationship between the onset of flow and the QRS complex; mitral regurgitation begins much earlier than aortic outflow. The onset of mitral regurgitation occurs at the time of mitral valve closure, whereas the jet of aortic stenosis does not begin until after isovolumic contraction. By carefully examining these time intervals within the Doppler signals, the two jets can often be differentiated.

APPLICATIONS OF THE BERNOULLI EQUATION

A list of clinical applications of the Bernoulli equation is provided in Table 8.2. The most common use of the Bernoulli equation is to quantify the severity of valve stenosis. An example of this application is shown in Fig-

ure 8.24. By planimetry of the envelope of the stenotic jet, both maximal and mean gradients are obtained. To determine mean gradient, the instantaneous gradients are measured at multiple points throughout the flow and their sum is divided by the duration of flow. The shape or contour of the Doppler signal also contains relevant information. Two examples of a late-peaking left ventricular outflow tract gradient are shown in Figure 8.25. This pattern is typical of dynamic obstruction, such as occurs with hypertrophic cardiomyopathy. In contrast, valvular stenosis is characterized by rapid acceleration of blood flow in early systole with an earlier peak velocity.

Application of the Bernoulli equation to mitral stenosis has been extensively studied. Although *peak* mitral valve gradient, which occurs in early diastole, can be readily determined, this is of less clinical value than *mean* gradient. By tracing the envelope of the mitral stenosis jet, the mean diastolic gradient across the mitral valve is obtained (Fig. 8.26). In these examples, notice how the presence of an A-wave in the patient with sinus rhythm affects the mean gradient. If the jet velocities are relatively low, the simplified Bernoulli equation will tend to overestimate

▶ **TABLE 8.2 Clinical Applications of the Bernoulli Equation**

Application	*Clinical Utility*
Peak velocity through a stenotic valve	Aortic stenosis maximal gradient
TR jet velocity	RV systolic pressure
LV outflow tract contour and velocity	HOCM gradient
Peak velocity across a VSD	RV systolic pressure
End-diastolic velocity of PR jet	Pulmonary artery diastolic pressure
Velocity through a PDA	Pulmonary artery systolic pressure
MR contour and velocity	Left ventricular dP/dt

HOCM, hypertrophic obstructive cardiomyopathy; LV, left ventricle; MR, mitral regurgitation; PDA, patent ductus arteriosus; PR, pulmonic regurgitation; RV, right ventricular; VSD, ventricular septal defect; TR, tricuspid regurgitation.

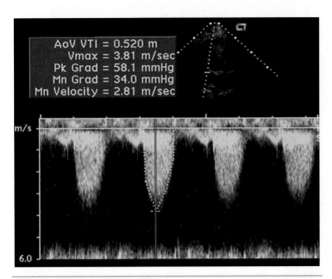

FIGURE 8.24. Continuous wave Doppler can be used to record the aortic stenosis jet. By measuring the maximal velocity of the jet, the peak pressure gradient can be estimated using the Bernoulli equation. In this example, the maximal velocity (V_{max}) is 3.8 m/sec, and the peak and mean gradients are 58 and 34 mm Hg, respectively.

true gradient because the difference between v_2 and v_1 is not great. Under such circumstances, use of the modified Bernoulli equation would be more appropriate:

$$\Delta P = 4(v_2{}^2 - v_1{}^2) \qquad \text{[Eq. 8.8]}$$

This equation is cumbersome when mean (rather than peak) gradient is being measured.

Because the Bernoulli equation provides information on instantaneous pressure gradient, it has several other

applications. The acceleration of blood through a ventricular septal defect in systole is a reflection of the instantaneous pressure difference between the two ventricles (Fig. 8.27). By aligning the Doppler beam parallel to the ventricular septal defect jet, the peak velocity of the shunt can be determined and used to calculate the maximal pressure difference across the ventricular septum. If left ventricular systolic pressure (LV_{SP}) is known, right ventricular systolic pressure (RV_{SP}) can be estimated as the difference between left ventricular pressure and maximal gradient across the defect (PG_{jet}):

$$LV_{SP} - PG_{jet} = RV_{SP} \approx PA_{SP} \qquad \text{[Eq. 8.9]}$$

In the absence of aortic stenosis, cuff-measured systolic blood pressure is an acceptable surrogate for left ventricular pressure, thereby providing a noninvasive means to estimate right ventricular systolic pressure and pulmonary artery systolic pressure (PA_{SP}).

Right ventricular systolic pressure can also be determined by measuring the velocity of tricuspid regurgitation jet. In this case, the tricuspid regurgitation jet is a reflection of the peak pressure difference between the right ventricle and right atrium in systole. If that gradient can be measured using the Bernoulli equation, right ventricular systolic pressure can be estimated, provided right atrial systolic pressure is known. Most patients with elevated right heart pressure will have some degree of tricuspid regurgitation, and obtaining an accurate measure of tricuspid regurgitation jet velocity is possible from multiple views. In some cases, right heart contrast, using agitated saline, is necessary to clearly delineate the jet envelope. The right ventricle-to-right atrial pressure gradi-

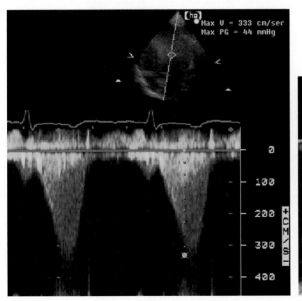

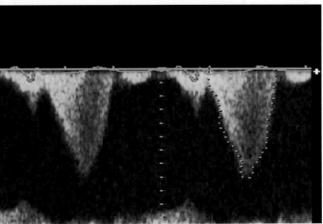

FIGURE 8.25. Two examples of late-peaking left ventricular outflow tract jets are provided. These recordings are taken from patients with hypertrophic obstructive cardiomyopathy.

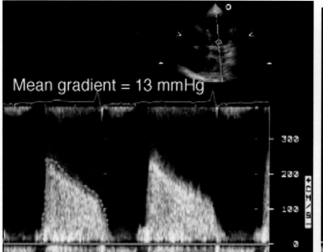

Mean gradient = 13 mmHg

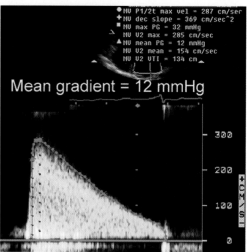

MV P1/2t max vel = 287 cm/sec
MV dec slope = 369 cm/sec^2
MV max PG = 32 mmHg
MV V2 max = 285 cm/sec
MV mean PG = 12 mmHg
MV V2 mean = 154 cm/sec
MV V2 VTI = 134 cm

Mean gradient = 12 mmHg

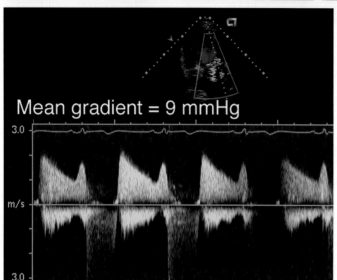

Mean gradient = 9 mmHg

FIGURE 8.26. Three examples of mitral stenosis are provided. **Top:** Images from patients in atrial fibrillation; an online computer system is used to planimeter the mitral jet, thereby providing a measure of the mean pressure gradient. **Bottom:** The same technique is used in a patient in sinus rhythm.

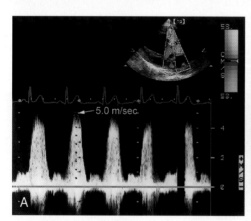

5.0 m/sec.

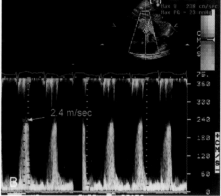

2.4 m/sec

PG = 4v² = 4(5)²
PG = 100 mm Hg
If BP is 130 mm Hg,
RVSP = 130 − 100 = 30 mm Hg

PG = 4v² = 4(2.4)²
PG = 23 mm Hg
If BP is 130 mm Hg,
RVSP = 130 − 23 = 107 mm Hg

FIGURE 8.27. Two examples of ventricular septal defect are provided. Continuous wave Doppler imaging is used to record the maximal velocity through the defects. Using the Bernoulli equation, the left ventricular-to-right ventricular pressure gradients (*PG*) can be calculated. If blood pressure (*BP*) is known, an estimate of right ventricular systolic pressure (*RVSP*) can be derived as shown. **A:** A 5.0 m/sec ventricular septal defect jet predicts an RVSP of 30 mm Hg. **B:** A much lower ventricular septal defect jet velocity (2.4 m/sec) is consistent with significant pulmonary hypertension.

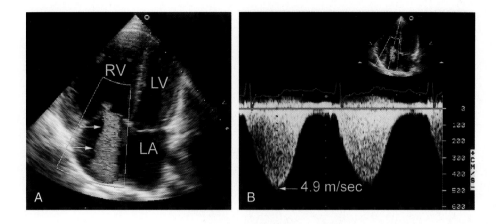

$$RVSP = (4 \times 4.9^2) + 10$$
$$= 96 + 10$$
$$= 106 \text{ mm Hg}$$

FIGURE 8.28. The Bernoulli equation is used to estimate right ventricular systolic pressure. **A:** A significant tricuspid regurgitation (*TR*) jet is demonstrated using color Doppler imaging (*arrow*). **B:** Continuous wave Doppler imaging demonstrates a TR jet velocity of 4.9 m/sec. The calculations used to estimate right ventricular systolic pressure (*RVSP*) are shown. LA, left atrial; LV, left ventricle; RV, right ventricle.

ent may be difficult to estimate in the setting of severe tricuspid regurgitation, when there is a large color flow regurgitant jet. In this case, the peak velocity may not reflect the true pressure gradient.

This approach to determining right ventricular pressure is demonstrated in Figure 8.28. To complete the equation, right atrial pressure can be estimated based on jugular venous pressure or arbitrarily assigned a value, such as 10 or 15 mm Hg. However, in patients with normal or mildly elevated right heart pressure, a reasonable estimate of right atrial pressure is approximately 5 mm Hg. A useful way to estimate right atrial pressure relies on visualization of the inferior vena cava. By observing the degree of dilation and the respiratory variability in inferior vena cava caliber, right atrial pressure can be estimated with reasonable accuracy. If the vessel is normal in size and collapses in response to a "sniff," right atrial pressure is less than 10 mm Hg. Mildly elevated right atrial pressure (10–15 mm Hg) is associated with a normal to mildly dilated inferior vena cava that does not change with sniffing. A dilated inferior vena cava (>2.5 cm), with no response to sniffing, suggests a right atrial pressure greater than 15 mm Hg.

In the setting of pulmonary regurgitation, one can measure the end-diastolic pulmonary regurgitant jet velocity. This measurement provides the pressure gradient between the pulmonary artery and the right ventricle at the end of diastole (Fig. 8.29). Combining this pressure gradient with right ventricular diastolic pressure or right atrial pressure provides a measurement of pulmonary artery diastolic pressure. Specifically, by adding the end-diastolic pressure gradient (from the pulmonary regurgitation velocity) to the right atrial pressure, pulmonary artery diastolic pressure can be estimated. For example, if the end-diastolic pulmonic regurgitation velocity is 2.0 m/sec, this corresponds to a gradient of 16 mm Hg and suggests that the pulmonary artery diastolic pressure is approximately 16 mm Hg *higher* than the mean right atrial (or right ventricular diastolic) pressure.

An estimate of pulmonary vascular resistance can be obtained by dividing the peak TRV (in meters per second) by the TVI of the right ventricular outflow tract (in centimeters). The rationale for this method is based on the recognition that pulmonary vascular resistance is directly related to the change in pressure and inversely related to pulmonary flow (Abbas et al., 2003). The regression equation yielding the best agreement with invasively determined pulmonary vascular resistance was

$$PVR = TRV/TVI_{RVOT} \times 10 + 0.16 \qquad [\text{Eq. 8.10}]$$

This approach may have utility in distinguishing high pulmonary artery pressure due to increased pulmonary flow from pulmonary hypertension due to elevated pulmonary vascular resistance (Fig. 8.30). For example, if the pulmonary artery pressure is high, but the TRV/TVI$_{RVOT}$ is less than 0.2, this most likely indicates low pulmonary vascular resistance, with elevated pressure secondary to increased flow. In the example, the pulmonary artery systolic pressure estimated from the tricuspid regurgitation

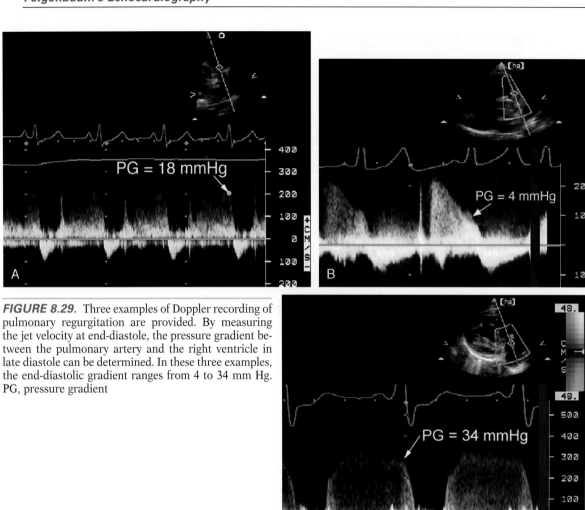

FIGURE 8.29. Three examples of Doppler recording of pulmonary regurgitation are provided. By measuring the jet velocity at end-diastole, the pressure gradient between the pulmonary artery and the right ventricle in late diastole can be determined. In these three examples, the end-diastolic gradient ranges from 4 to 34 mm Hg. PG, pressure gradient

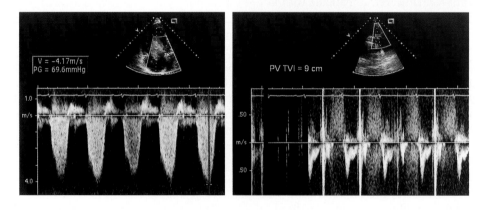

$$PVR = TRV/TVI_{OT} \times 10 + 0.16$$
$$= (4.17/9) \times 10 + 0.16$$
$$= 0.46 \times 10 + 0.16$$
$$= 4.8 \text{ Wood units}$$

FIGURE 8.30. Pulmonary vascular resistance can be estimated by measuring the peak velocity of the tricuspid regurgitation jet (*TRV*) and the time velocity integral (TVI) of the right ventricular outflow tract. See text for details.

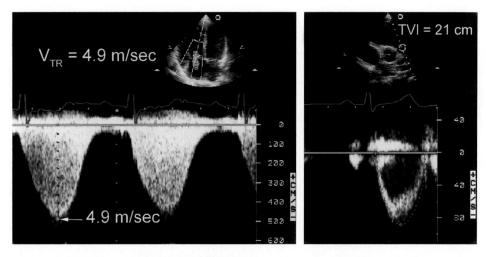

$$PVR = TRV/TVI_{OT} \times 10 + 0.16$$
$$= (4.9/21) \times 10 + 0.16$$
$$= 0.23 \times 10 + 0.16$$
$$= 2.4 \text{ Wood units}$$

FIGURE 8.31. An example of determining pulmonary vascular resistance (*PVR*) is provided. See text for details.

jet would be 70 mm Hg. This high pressure, along with the low pulmonary valve flow, indicated by the TVI_{OT}, is consistent with elevated pulmonary vascular resistance. In contrast, Figure 8.31 demonstrates a high right ventricular pressure but in association with a much higher flow, as indicated by the TVI_{OT}. In this case, despite high pulmonary artery pressure, the pulmonary vascular resistance is significantly lower.

The Bernoulli equation can also be used on the left side of the heart to estimate left ventricular end-diastolic pressure in patients with aortic regurgitation. By measuring the end-diastolic velocity of the aortic regurgitation jet, left ventricular end-diastolic pressure can be determined by subtracting the gradient from the aortic diastolic pressure (Fig. 8.32). The problem with this calculation is that end-diastolic aortic pressure is difficult to estimate non-invasively. It is generally not acceptable to substitute diastolic blood pressure (derived from a cuff measurement) for this value. Also, because left ventricular end-diastolic pressure varies over a relatively narrow range, small errors in the calculation can lead to significant clinical errors in the final estimate.

A final application of the Bernoulli equation involves the use of mitral regurgitation to estimate the rate of left ventricular pressure increase during early systole, also known as dP/dt. Because there is little change in left atrial pressure during the period of isovolumic contraction, the early mitral regurgitation jet velocity reflects dP/dt. By measuring the slope of the mitral regurgitation acceleration velocity, dP/dt can be determined. This is done by

measuring the time interval between 1 m/sec and 3 m/sec on the mitral regurgitation jet, as shown in Figure 8.33. By the Bernoulli equation, this interval corresponds to an increase in pressure difference from 4 to 36 mm Hg, a net change of 32 mm Hg. Thus, dP/dt is calculated as 32 divided by the time interval, expressed in mmHg/sec. Several studies have demonstrated a good correlation be-

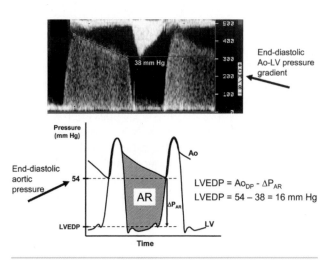

FIGURE 8.32. The Bernoulli equation can be used to estimate left ventricular end-diastolic pressure (*LVEDP*), as shown in this schematic. By measuring the velocity of the aortic regurgitation (*AR*) jet at end-diastole, the aortic-to-left ventricular pressure gradient is estimated. By subtracting this value from the aortic diastolic pressure, LVEDP is determined. See text for details.

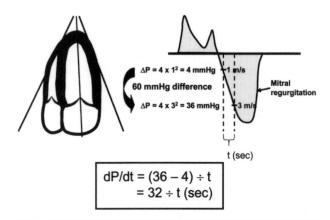

$$\Delta P = 4 \times 1^2 = 4 \text{ mmHg}$$
$$60 \text{ mmHg difference}$$
$$\Delta P = 4 \times 3^2 = 36 \text{ mmHg}$$

Mitral regurgitation

t (sec)

$$dP/dt = (36 - 4) \div t$$
$$= 32 \div t \text{ (sec)}$$

FIGURE 8.33. From a continuous wave recording of the mitral regurgitation jet, dP/dt can be calculated. The schematic demonstrates this approach. See text for details.

tween this Doppler approach and catheter-derived values for dP/dt. Some examples of calculating dP/dt are provided in Figure 8.34.

DETERMINING PRESSURE HALF-TIME

Pressure half-time was originally developed and used in the cardiac catheterization laboratory for evaluating patients with mitral stenosis. By simultaneously plotting left atrial and left ventricular pressure curves, the contour of the diastolic pressure gradient across the mitral valve could be evaluated. Pressure half-time is the time required for the peak pressure gradient to be reduced by one-half (Fig. 8.35). Thus, if the maximal pressure gradient is 14 mm Hg, then the pressure half-time is the time required for the instantaneous gradient to decrease from 14 to 7 mm Hg. With Doppler imaging, we are actually measuring velocity rather than pressure. Because of the quadratic relationship between the two parameters, the Doppler pressure half-time is the time required for the peak velocity to decrease to a value equal to peak velocity divided by $\sqrt{2}$. Because $\sqrt{2}$ equals approximately 1.4, pressure half-time becomes the time required for the initial velocity to decrease to a value of peak velocity divided by 1.4, roughly the same as peak velocity multiplied by 0.7. Thus, the arithmetic involved in deriving pressure half-time from velocity data is summarized as follows:

$$P\tfrac{1}{2}t = \text{time for } P_{max} \text{ to decrease by } \tfrac{1}{2}, \text{ or}$$
$$P\tfrac{1}{2}t = \text{time for } V_{max} \text{ to decrease by } \sqrt{2}, \text{ or}$$
$$P\tfrac{1}{2}t = \text{time when } V = V_{max} \times 0.7 \qquad [\text{Eq. 8.11}]$$

In the setting of mitral stenosis, pressure half-time is a useful measure of severity (Fig. 8.36). As stenosis worsens, pressure half-time increases, i.e., the decrease in ve-

locity during diastole occurs more slowly. It has been empirically shown that mitral valve area is approximately equal to 220 divided by pressure half-time. The advantage of pressure half-time is that it is less dependent on heart rate and flow than other measures of severity, such as gradient. Thus, it is especially useful in patients with atrial fibrillation, in whom variations in the R-R interval alter the diastolic gradient more so than the pressure half-time.

There are several limitations to the pressure half-time approach to mitral stenosis. For example, conditions that alter the diastolic compliance of the left atrium or ventricle (such as left ventricular hypertrophy) will also affect flow velocity and, hence, the pressure half-time. Aortic regurgitation causes the left ventricular pressure to increase more quickly in diastole than would otherwise occur. This can lead to a shortening of the pressure half-time and an underestimation of mitral stenosis severity. Of greater clinical relevance, the temporal changes in atrial and ventricular compliance that accompany balloon mitral valvuloplasty create an unsteady state during which pressure half-time may be inaccurate. This is a temporary problem, lasting between 48 and 72 hours after the procedure. After that, compliance stabilizes and the half-time method can be used to assess the success of the procedure.

The pressure half-time formula has also been applied to aortic regurgitation jets. In this case, the rate of decrease of the jet velocity during diastole is a reflection of the rate of increase of left ventricular diastolic pressure and the rate of decrease of aortic diastolic pressure. The more quickly the left ventricular and aortic pressure curves approach each other during diastole, the steeper the slope of the aortic regurgitation flow profile is and the shorter the pressure half-time (Fig. 8.37). As aortic regurgitation worsens, left ventricular pressure increases more quickly, aortic pressure decreases more quickly, and pressure half-time shortens.

Although there is a general relationship between aortic regurgitation severity and pressure half-time, it must be emphasized that several factors can also affect this value. For example, in the setting of acute aortic regurgitation, left ventricular pressure increases rapidly during diastole as blood fills a normal-size left ventricle from both the aortic root and mitral value. This rapid increase in left ventricular pressure will tend to shorten pressure half-time. In contrast, in the presence of long-standing aortic regurgitation in which the left ventricle is markedly dilated and compliant, a significant amount of aortic regurgitation can occur with a relatively flat left ventricular diastolic pressure curve and a long pressure half-time. These differences are illustrated in Figure 8.37. Thus, pressure half-time is affected by both severity and acuity, and differentiating these factors in an individual patient can be difficult.

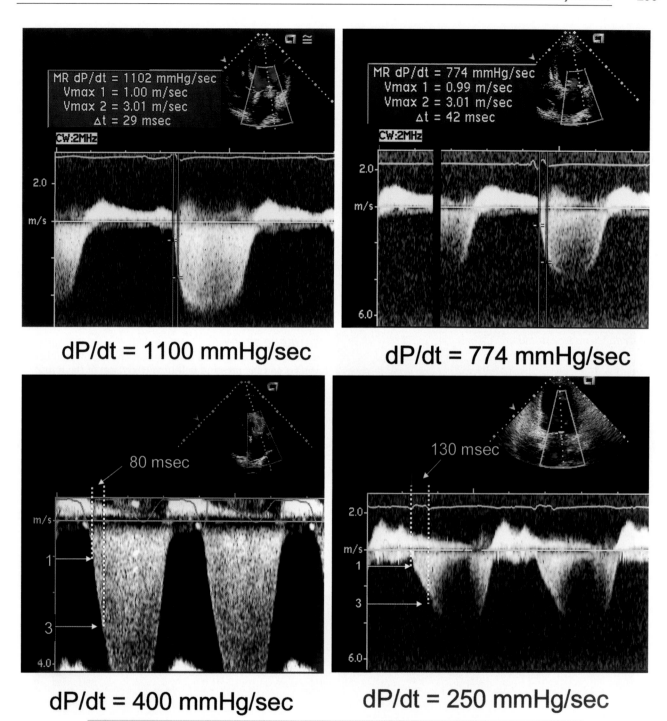

FIGURE 8.34. Four examples of measuring dP/dt from the contour of the mitral regurgitation jet are provided. See text for details.

THE CONTINUITY EQUATION

The continuity equation is based on Newton's second law of thermodynamics, involving the conservation of mass. As it applies to Doppler imaging, this principle states that the volumetric flow rate through the cardiovascular system is constant, assuming that the blood is noncompressible and the conduit is inelastic. Stated differently, the

flow rate (or volume of blood passing through any given point over time) is the same at all points along the circuit. Because flow rate is the product of the TVI and the cross-sectional area, this relationship can be used to solve for the cross-sectional area as follows:

$$\text{flow proximal} = \text{flow distal}$$
$$A_1 \times TVI_1 = A_2 \times TVI_2$$
$$A_2 = A_1 \times TVI_1/TVI_2 \qquad \text{[Eq. 8.12]}$$

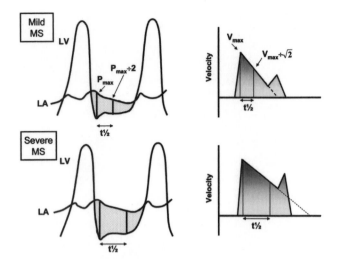

FIGURE 8.35. The determination of pressure half-time of the mitral stenosis jet is demonstrated. **Top:** Pressure tracings and the corresponding Doppler recording are provided in a patient with mild mitral stenosis (*MS*). **Bottom:** More severe stenosis is illustrated. See text for details. LA, left atrium; LV, left ventricle; P_{max}, maximal pressure gradient; V_{max}, maximal velocity; $t^{1/2}$, pressure half-time.

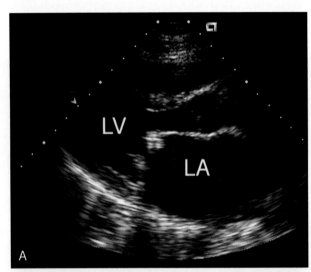

FIGURE 8.36. From a patient with rheumatic mitral stenosis, Doppler is used to calculate the mean gradient (*MnPG*) and the pressure half-time (*P$^{1/2}$ time*) of the mitral valve flow. See text for details. LA, left atrium; LV, left ventricle.

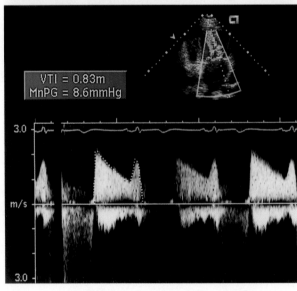

B   **Mean gradient = 9 mmHg**

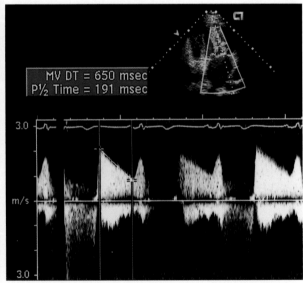

C   **Pressure half-time = 191 msec**

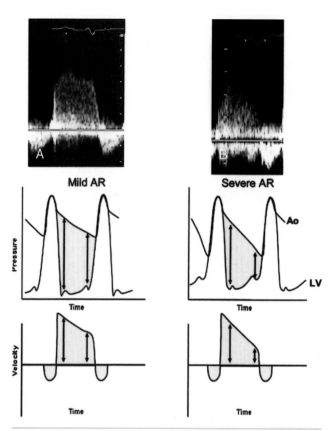

FIGURE 8.37. The contour of the aortic regurgitation (*AR*) jet reflects the instantaneous pressure difference between the aorta (*Ao*) and the left ventricle (*LV*) during diastole. **A:** Mild AR is demonstrated. The relationship between the pressure tracings and the Doppler contour is illustrated. **B:** More severe AR results in a steeper slope of the AR jet. See text for details.

By sampling the TVI at two points and measuring the cross-sectional area at one point, the other cross-sectional area can be determined using this equation (Fig. 8.38). For example, to calculate the cross-sectional area of a stenotic aortic valve, the following three measurements must be made: (1) the TVI of the left ventricular outflow tract, using pulsed Doppler recording just proximal to the stenotic valve, (2) the TVI through the valve, using continuous wave Doppler imaging, and (3) the cross-sectional area of the outflow tract, at the same point where flow was measured.

The advantages of the continuity equation are that it is unaffected by valvular regurgitation and provides quantitative assessment of severity even in the presence of left ventricular dysfunction (when gradient alone may lead to underestimation of severity). Figure 8.39 is a schematic that demonstrates the critical dependence of the Bernoulli equation on stroke volume. The two curves depict the relationship between jet velocity and aortic valve area at different levels of left ventricular function, indicated by different flow rates (the TVI_{OT} values). Beginning at point A,

with a peak gradient of 32 mm Hg and a valve area of 1.3 cm², a worsening of stenosis (at the same flow rate) corresponds to a move to point B, which is a gradient of 74 mm Hg and a valve area of 0.8 cm². This would be typical progression of stenosis with preserved ventricular function. Alternatively, a decrease in flow rate or stroke volume without a change in valve area would imply shifting to the higher curve. On this curve, if the valve area is still 1.3 cm², the corresponding gradient will decrease to 15 mm Hg (point C). At this new stroke volume, a progression of aortic stenosis to a new valve area of 0.8 cm² would return the gradient to the original value of 32 mm Hg (point D). It is apparent that the same gradient can reflect widely different valve areas, depending on the flow rate through the valve. Clearly, in the setting of changing flow states, gradient alone cannot convey adequate diagnostic information about stenosis severity. It is in these situations that the continuity equation can be most helpful.

The continuity equation can be applied to any of the four valves within the heart, although in most instances, the aortic valve is involved. In the setting of left ventricular dysfunction, it can be performed both at baseline and during dobutamine stress to differentiate between severe valvular stenosis and less severe stenosis in the setting of low flow rates. The clinical application of the continuity equation as it applies to the aortic valve is covered in Chapter 10.

PROXIMAL ISOVELOCITY SURFACE AREA

A novel application of the continuity principle involves the proximal isovelocity surface area method. As blood converges toward an orifice, Doppler flow imaging reveals concentric shells or hemispheres, which represent isovelocity surfaces (Fig. 8.40). As the blood accelerates toward the orifice, velocity aliasing occurs and a distinct red-blue interface occurs at the boundary of the shells. At this interface, the velocity is equivalent to the Nyquist limit, which can be read off the velocity color scale. By adjusting the Nyquist limit, the size of the shell can be maximized to allow its surface area to be measured according to the formula:

$$\text{Surface area} = 2\pi r^2 \qquad \text{[Eq. 8.13]}$$

By the continuity equation, we know that flow rate is held constant as blood converges toward the orifice. Thus, flow rate through any given shell will equal the flow rate through the orifice. The rate of flow through any hemispheric shell is the product of the hemisphere area and the flow velocity (i.e., the aliasing velocity). Thus, the following equation can be derived:

$$\text{Flow rate} = 6.28 * r^2 * \text{Aliasing velocity} \quad \text{[Eq. 8.14]}$$

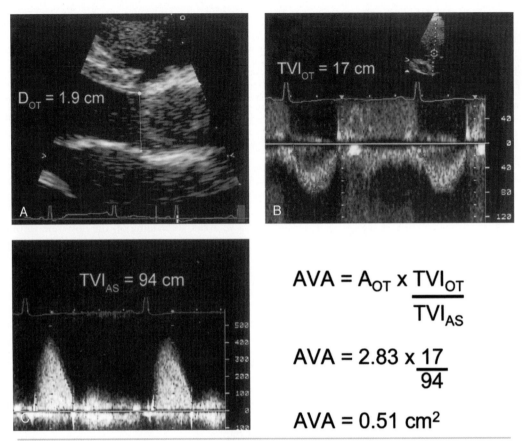

FIGURE 8.38. Calculating aortic valve area (*AVA*) relies on the continuity equation. The three measurements required for this calculation are shown in the illustration. **A:** The cross-sectional area of the outflow tract (A_{OT}) is derived by measuring the diameter (D_{OT}). **B:** The time velocity integral of the outflow tract (TVI_{OT}) is measured using pulsed Doppler imaging. **C:** The TVI_{AS} is measured with continuous wave Doppler imaging. The calculations are shown.

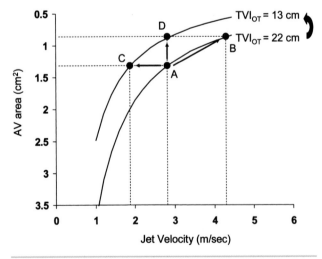

FIGURE 8.39. The relationship among aortic stenosis jet velocity, valve area, and stroke volume is illustrated. See text for details. AV, aortic valve; TVI_{OT}, time velocity integral of the left ventricular outflow tract.

Similarly, the flow rate through a regurgitant orifice is given by the equation:

$$\text{Flow rate} = \text{ERO} * \text{Velocity}_{jet} \qquad [\text{Eq. 8.15}]$$

We can then calculate the effective regurgitant orifice (ERO) according to the formula:

$$\text{ERO} = \text{Flow rate} \div \text{Velocity}_{jet} \qquad [\text{Eq. 8.16}]$$

Regurgitant volume (RV, in milliliters) then becomes

$$\text{RV} = \text{ERO} * \text{FVI}_{MR} \qquad [\text{Eq. 8.17}]$$

Thus,

$$\text{RV} = (2\pi r^2 * \text{Aliasing velocity}) \div (\text{Velocity}_{MR} * \text{TVI}_{MR}) \qquad [\text{Eq. 8.18}]$$

This is illustrated in Figures 8.41 and 8.42.

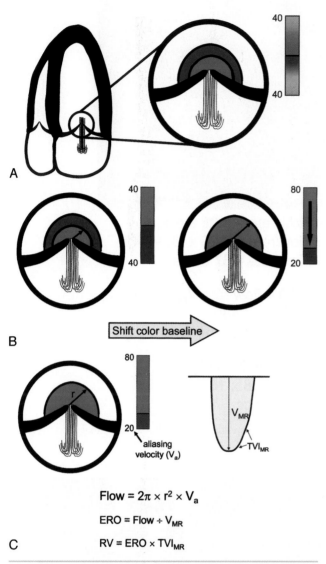

Flow = $2\pi \times r^2 \times V_a$

ERO = Flow ÷ V_{MR}

RV = ERO × TVI_{MR}

C

FIGURE 8.40. Determination of mitral regurgitation (*MR*) severity by the proximal isovelocity surface area method is demonstrated. **A:** The schematic demonstrates how regurgitant flow converges and accelerates in a series of isovelocity shells, indicated by the red and blue patterns. **B:** The radius of the shell is measured, after the baseline has been shifted to maximize its size. From this, the surface area of the shell is determined. **C:** Using the continuity equation, the calculations required to measure flow, effective regurgitant orifice (ERO) area, and regurgitant volume (RV) are demonstrated. See text for details. r, radius; V_a, aliasing velocity; V_{MR}, maximal MR jet velocity.

Although attractive in concept, the routine clinical use of proximal isovelocity surface area has its limitations. Assumptions about the hemispheric shape of the isovelocity shells may be oversimplified. Another assumption states that the shells are converging toward an orifice that lies within a flat plane. In the case of mitral regurgitant flow, this is clearly not the case and some correction is often required. Furthermore, the calculations are cumber-

some and the potential for measurement error must always be considered. This is particularly true with regard to the radius of the isovelocity shells, where precise identification of the center of the regurgitant orifice can be especially challenging. For all these reasons, proximal isovelocity surface area has not yet become a routinely performed measurement. Its application to quantifying mitral regurgitation is covered more in Chapter 11.

MYOCARDIAL PERFORMANCE INDEX

The myocardial performance index (MPI) was developed in the mid-1990s as an expression of global ventricular performance (Tei et al., 1995). It is a simple index that includes both systolic and diastolic parameters and can be applied to either the left or right ventricle. The MPI incorporates three basic time intervals that are readily derived from Doppler recordings: ejection time (ET), isovolumic contraction time (IVCT), and isovolumic relaxation time (IVRT). From these values, the following calculation is performed (Fig. 8.43):

$$MPI = (IVCT + IVRT) \div ET \qquad [Eq. 8.19]$$

Systolic dysfunction is associated with a prolongation of IVCT and a shortening of the ET. Diastolic dysfunction often leads to lengthening of the IVRT. Thus, both systolic and diastolic dysfunction will result in an increase in the MPI (Fig. 8.44). The reported normal range for the MPI is 0.39 ± 0.05. Values greater than 0.50 are considered abnormal. Not surprisingly, this measurement has been shown to be a powerful way to risk stratify patients in a variety of settings. The MPI can also be used to assess right ventricular function. For the right heart, the normal MPI is 0.28 ± 0.04. An increased right ventricular MPI is a sensitive and specific marker of pulmonary hypertension. Thus, the MPI may be of value in patients in whom tricuspid regurgitation is either not present or cannot be quantified to assess for pulmonary hypertension. The MPI also appears to provide powerful prognostic information. Further studies are needed, however, to determine its place among the other Doppler prognostic variables.

ESTIMATION OF LEFT VENTRICULAR FILLING PRESSURE

Left ventricular filling occurs during diastole as left atrial pressure increases, causing mitral valve opening, and creating a pressure gradient between the left atrium and left ventricle. Ventricular filling begins with mitral valve opening and continues throughout diastole, associated with a gradual increase in chamber pressure. One important pa-

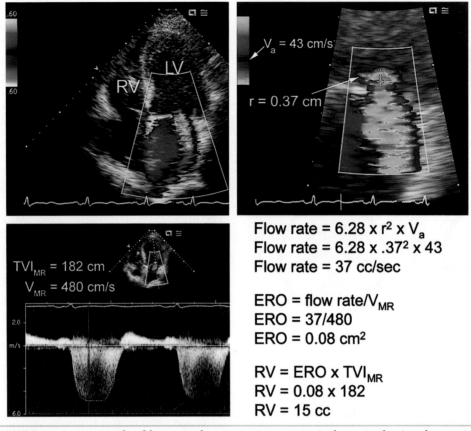

Flow rate = $6.28 \times r^2 \times V_a$
Flow rate = $6.28 \times .37^2 \times 43$
Flow rate = 37 cc/sec

ERO = flow rate/V_{MR}
ERO = 37/480
ERO = 0.08 cm^2

RV = ERO $\times$ TVI$_{MR}$
RV = 0.08 $\times$ 182
RV = 15 cc

FIGURE 8.41. An example of how mitral regurgitation severity is determined using the proximal isovelocity surface area method is provided. The calculations are as described in Figure 8.40.

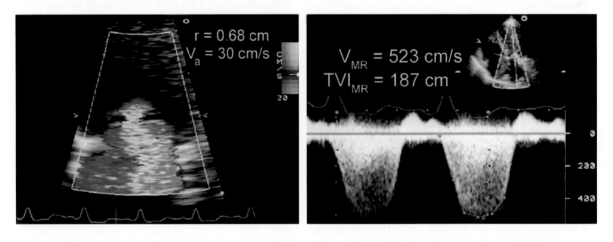

To measure regurgitant flow rate:	To measure effective regurgitant orifice area:	To measure regurgitant volume:
Flow rate = $6.28 \times r^2 \times V_a$	ERO = flow rate/V_{MR}	RV = ERO $\times$ TVI$_{MR}$
Flow rate = $6.28 \times .68^2 \times 30$	ERO = 87/523	RV = 0.17 $\times$ 187
Flow rate = 87 cc	ERO = 0.17 cm^2	RV = 31 cc

FIGURE 8.42. An example of how mitral regurgitation severity is determined using the proximal isovelocity surface area method is provided. The calculations are as described in Figure 8.40. LV, left ventricle; RV, right ventricle.

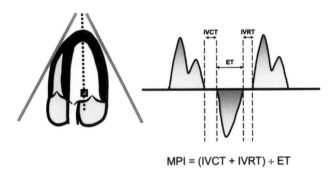

$$MPI = (IVCT + IVRT) \div ET$$

FIGURE 8.43. This schematic demonstrates how the myocardial performance index (*MPI*) is derived. See text for details. ET, ejection time; IVCT, isovolumic contraction time; IVRT, isovolumic relaxation time.

rameter of diastolic function, therefore, is left ventricular filling pressure, which can be expressed as either left ventricular end-diastolic pressure, left atrial mean pressure, or pulmonary capillary wedge pressure. A variety of approaches have been developed to estimate these values, having therapeutic and prognostic implications. Some of these are indirect and qualitative. For example, elevated left atrial pressure is usually associated with dilation of the left atrium. When left atrial size is normal, chronically elevated left atrial pressure is unlikely. However, the correlation between left atrial size and pressure is quite poor due to the myriad of factors that influence this relationship. The mitral E-wave peak velocity is another indirect

measure of left atrial pressure. The E-wave velocity correlates with the difference between left atrial and left ventricular pressure at the time of mitral valve opening (Fig. 8.45). Thus, the higher the left atrial pressure at the time of mitral valve opening, the higher the E-wave velocity. Again, other factors, such as the rate of left ventricular relaxation and atrial contractility, will influence this relationship.

Several other quantitative approaches to measure filling pressure have been tested, primarily using Doppler techniques. For example, mitral E-wave deceleration time is inversely related to mean left atrial pressure. As left atrial pressure increases, the initial pressure gradient between the left atrium and ventricle increases. This leads to a high mitral E-wave and a rapid deceleration of early diastolic flow (Fig. 8.46). Several studies have now shown that deceleration time is inversely and linearly related to filling pressure. This relationship has been demonstrated in patients with dilated cardiomyopathy and those with coronary artery disease and reduced ejection fraction (Fig. 8.47). However, it does not work well in the setting of normal left ventricular function or hypertrophic cardiomyopathy. The confounding effects of age, left ventricular compliance, and left atrial function may account for this lack of correlation. In addition, some "healthy hearts" exhibit relatively high E-wave velocity and rapid deceleration, possibly because the active relaxation process creates a suction effect that accelerates blood flow into the left ventricle during diastole. In such individuals, a high

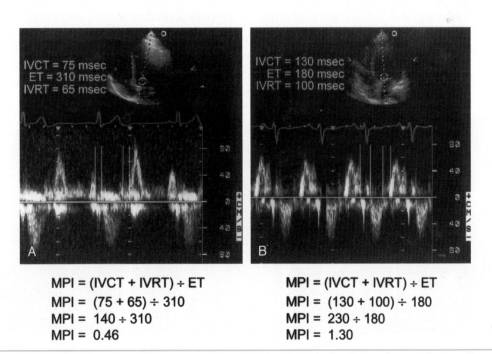

MPI = (IVCT + IVRT) ÷ ET
MPI = (75 + 65) ÷ 310
MPI = 140 ÷ 310
MPI = 0.46

MPI = (IVCT + IVRT) ÷ ET
MPI = (130 + 100) ÷ 180
MPI = 230 ÷ 180
MPI = 1.30

FIGURE 8.44. A: The myocardial performance index (*MPI*) is calculated in a subject with normal systolic and diastolic function, yielding a value of 0.46. **B:** Taken from a patient with acute viral myocarditis, an abnormal MPI is calculated at 1.30. ET, ejection time; IVCT, isovolumic contraction time; IVRT, isovolumic relaxation time.

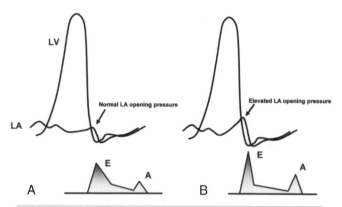

FIGURE 8.45. This schematic demonstrates the relationship between left atrial (*LA*) pressure and E-wave velocity. **A:** In the setting of normal hemodynamics, the left atrial-to-left ventricular pressure gradient at the time of mitral valve opening is relatively low. This pressure difference in part determines the E-wave velocity. **B:** When the LA pressure at the time of mitral valve opening is elevated, a higher driving force is present and the E velocity of mitral flow will be increased as a result.

E-wave velocity and a short deceleration time may occur in the absence of elevated left atrial pressure. Thus, one limitation of the mitral inflow variables is that they are poor predictors of filling pressure in the presence of normal systolic function.

Another approach to left ventricular filling pressure involves a comparison of the time duration of the pulmonary venous A-wave with the mitral A-wave. When the left atrium contracts in late diastole, blood is propelled through the mitral valve and also in a retrograde direction into the pulmonary veins. Normally, the duration of forward flow is greater than that of pulmonary venous retrograde flow. In one study (Rossvoll and Hatle, 1993), the demonstration of a pulmonary venous A-wave that ex-

ceeds the duration of the mitral A-wave predicted a left ventricular end-diastolic pressure of more than 15 mm Hg with a sensitivity of 85% and a specificity of 79% (Fig. 8.48). Furthermore, a modest positive correlation exists between left ventricular end-diastolic pressure and the difference between the pulmonary venous A-wave duration and mitral A-wave duration. Although appealing in concept, a limitation of this method is the technical difficulty in accurately measuring relatively small differences in flow duration. It also appears to be less accurate in the presence of a normal ejection fraction.

The pattern of pulmonary venous flow has also been used to predict mean left atrial pressure. Recall that pulmonary venous flow has two main antegrade components, a systolic wave and a diastolic wave. Normally, the TVI of the systolic wave is greater than that of the diastolic wave. As left atrial pressure increases, the systolic pulmonary venous wave tends to decrease. One group of investigators (Kuecherer et al., 1990), using transesophageal echocardiography, has demonstrated a reasonably strong negative correlation between mean left atrial pressure and systolic fraction, which is the ratio of pulmonary venous systolic TVI divided by the total pulmonary venous TVI. This redistribution of left atrial inflow may reflect the decreased chamber compliance that is associated with elevated left atrial pressure.

More recently, tissue Doppler imaging has been used to estimate left atrial pressure. This approach relies on the Doppler technique to measure the velocity in early diastole of the mitral anulus. This velocity profile appears to be more dependent on left ventricular relaxation and less dependent on the transmitral pressure gradient. Anular velocity can be measured from the apical four-chamber view. Either the medial (i.e., septal) or lateral anulus can be used for this purpose. The sample volume is positioned

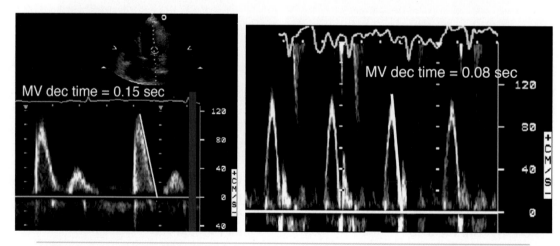

FIGURE 8.46. Two examples of mitral deceleration time are provided. These recordings are taken from patients will elevated filling pressures. In both cases, the deceleration time is shortened. MV dec time, mitral flow deceleration time.

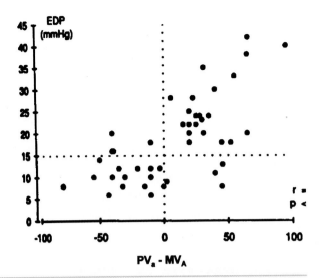

FIGURE 8.47. The inverse linear relationship between mitral flow deceleration time (*DecT*) and pulmonary capillary wedge pressure (*PWP*) is shown. These data are drawn from a clinical study involving 140 patients with a history of myocardial infarction and an ejection fraction less than 35%. (From Giannuzzi P, Imparato A, Temporelli PL, et al. Doppler-derived mitral deceleration time of early filling as a strong predictor of pulmonary capillary wedge pressure in postinfarction patients with left ventricular systolic dysfunction. J Am Coll Cardiol 1994;23:1630–1637, with permission.)

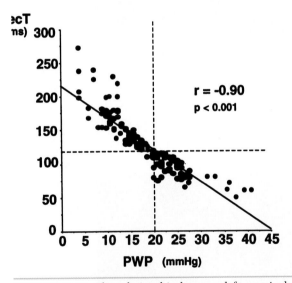

FIGURE 8.48. The relationship between left ventricular end-diastolic pressure (*EDP*) and the difference in duration of the mitral A-wave versus the pulmonary venous a wave is shown ($PV_a - MV_A$). In patients with normal EDP, the duration of forward flow during atrial systole is greater than retrograde flow, as indicated by the negative values. As EDP increases, the relationship reverses, yielding a positive difference. This suggests that with increasing filling pressures, the duration of retrograde flow exceeds forward flow during atrial systole. See text for details. (From Rossvoll O, Hatle LK. Pulmonary venous flow velocities recorded by transthoracic Doppler ultrasound: relation to left ventricular diastolic pressures. J Am Coll Cardiol 1993;21:1687–1696, with permission.)

at the junction of the ventricular myocardium and anulus (Fig. 8.49). A small sample volume should be used, and the gain and filters should be set low. The velocity that coincides with rapid ventricular filling is termed the E_a wave. The ratio of mitral E-wave peak velocity (E) to anular E velocity (E_a) has been shown to correlate well with left atrial pressure (Fig. 8.50). As left atrial pressure increases, E tends to increase (as a function of the opening transmitral pressure gradient) and E_a tends to decrease (due to the compensatory increase in left atrial pressure that accompanies impaired relaxation). Thus, the ratio will increase significantly.

A normal E/E_a is less than 10 (Fig. 8.51). A ratio greater than 15 predicts a left ventricular filling pressure greater than 15 mm Hg (Figs. 8.52 and 8.53). This simple ratio combines the influence of mitral driving pressure and left ventricular relaxation. Thus, including the anular velocity "corrects for" the confounding effects of relaxation on mitral inflow parameters, thereby overcoming some of the limitations of using mitral E velocity alone to predict filling pressures (Fig. 8.54). As such, E/E_a has several advantages. In most studies, it is the most robust of the Doppler indices for reliably predicting left heart filling pressure. Unlike most other markers, it appears to work well in the presence of normal hearts and/or preserved systolic function. Finally, it is a simple, easily derived ratio that discriminates reasonably well between normal and abnormal filling pressures.

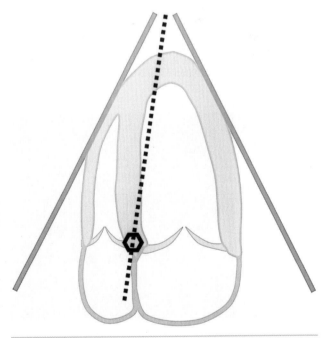

FIGURE 8.49. The technique for measuring the velocity of the mitral anulus is shown. From the apical four-chamber view, the sample volume is positioned on the medial mitral anulus. See text for details.

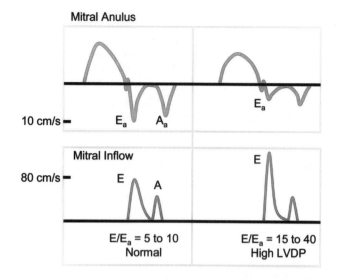

FIGURE 8.50. This schematic demonstrates the relationship between mitral anular velocity and mitral inflow velocity. The corresponding E_a wave of the anulus and mitral E-wave are demonstrated. On the left, in normal individuals, the E/E_a ratio is between 5 and 10. With increasing left ventricular end-diastolic pressure (*LVDP*), the mitral anular E_a wave decreases and the mitral inflow E-wave increases, yielding a ratio of more than 15. See text for details.

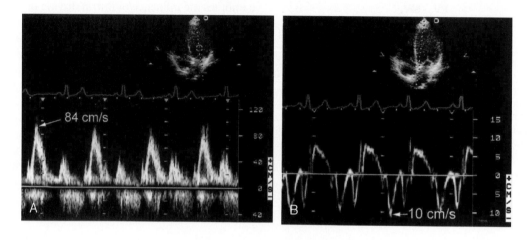

$$E/E_a = 84/10 = 8.4$$

FIGURE 8.51. An example of the derivation of the E/E_a ratio is provided in a patient with normal filling pressure. **A:** Mitral inflow is shown. **B:** Tissue Doppler imaging of mitral anular velocity is shown. The calculated ratio is 8.4.

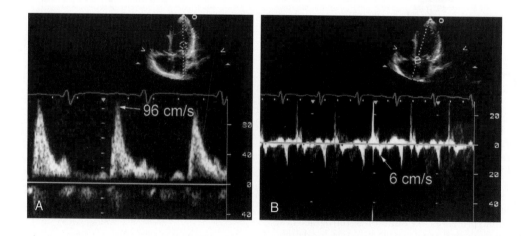

$$E/E_a = 96/6 = 16$$

FIGURE 8.52. Recorded from a patient with mildly elevated left ventricular filling pressure, the E/E_a ratio is derived. A value of 16 is considered mildly elevated.

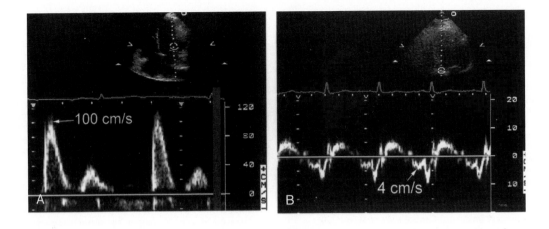

$$E/E_a = 100/4 = 25$$

FIGURE 8.53. From a patient with restrictive cardiomyopathy, an E/E_a ratio of 25 is consistent with elevated left ventricular filling pressure.

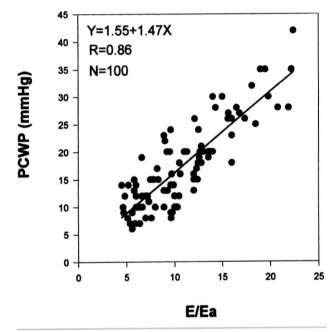

FIGURE 8.54. The relationship between the E/E_a ratio and pulmonary capillary wedge pressure (*PCWP*) is shown. The data were drawn from a study that included 100 patients who underwent simultaneous Doppler imaging and invasive hemodynamic measurements. (From Nagueh SF, Mikati I, Kopelen HA, et al. Doppler estimation of left ventricular filling pressure in sinus tachycardia: a new application of tissue Doppler imaging. Circulation 1998;98:1644–1650, with permission.)

SUGGESTED READINGS

Abbas AE, Fortuin FD, Schiller NB, et al. A simple method for noninvasive estimation of pulmonary vascular resistance. J Am Coll Cardiol 2003;41:1021–1027.

Bargiggia GS, Bertucci C, Recusani F, et al. A new method for estimating left ventricular dP/dt by continuous wave Doppler-echocardiography. Validation studies at cardiac catheterization. Circulation 1989;80:1287–1292.

Baumgartner H, Khan S, DeRobertis M, et al. Discrepancies between Doppler and catheter gradients in aortic prosthetic valves *in vitro*. A manifestation of localized gradients and pressure recovery. Circulation 1990;82:1467–1475.

Botvinick EH, Schiller NB, Wickramasekaran R, et al. Echocardiographic demonstration of early mitral valve closure in severe aortic insufficiency. Its clinical implications. Circulation 1975;51:836–847.

Burstow DJ, Nishimura RA, Bailey KR, et al. Continuous wave Doppler echocardiographic measurement of prosthetic valve gradients. A simultaneous Doppler-catheter correlative study. Circulation 1989;80:504–514.

Callahan MJ, Tajik AJ, Su-Fan Q, et al. Validation of instantaneous pressure gradients measured by continuous-wave Doppler in experimentally induced aortic stenosis. Am J Cardiol 1985;56:989–993.

Chen C, Koschyk D, Brockhoff C, et al. Noninvasive estimation of regurgitant flow rate and volume in patients with mitral regurgitation by Doppler color mapping of accelerating flow field. J Am Coll Cardiol 1993;21:374–383.

Corya BC, Rasmussen S, Phillips JF, et al. Forward stroke volume calculated from aortic valve echograms in normal subjects and patients with mitral regurgitation secondary to left ventricular dysfunction. Am J Cardiol 1981;47:1215–1222.

Currie PJ, Hagler DJ, Seward JB, et al. Instantaneous pressure gradient: a simultaneous Doppler and dual catheter correlative study. J Am Coll Cardiol 1986;7:800–806.

Dubin J, Wallerson DC, Cody RJ, et al. Comparative accuracy of Doppler echocardiographic methods for clinical stroke volume determination. Am Heart J 1990;120:116–123.

Enriquez-Sarano M, Miller FA Jr, Hayes SN, et al. Effective mitral regurgitant orifice area: clinical use and pitfalls of the proximal isovelocity surface area method. J Am Coll Cardiol 1995;25:703–709.

Enriquez-Sarano M, Seward JB, Bailey KR, et al. Effective regurgitant orifice area: a noninvasive Doppler development of an old hemodynamic concept. J Am Coll Cardiol 1994;23:443–451.

Enriquez-Sarano M, Sinak LJ, Tajik AJ, et al. Changes in effective regurgitant orifice throughout systole in patients with mitral valve prolapse. A clinical study using the proximal isovelocity surface area method. Circulation 1995;92:2951–2958.

Fisher DC, Sahn DJ, Friedman MJ, et al. The mitral valve orifice method for noninvasive two-dimensional echo Doppler determinations of cardiac output. Circulation 1983;67:872–877.

Flachskampf FA, Weyman AE, Gillam L, et al. Aortic regurgitation shortens Doppler pressure half-time in mitral stenosis: clinical evidence, *in vitro* simulation and theoretic analysis. J Am Coll Cardiol 1990;16:396–404.

Giannuzzi P, Imparato A, Temporelli PL, et al. Doppler-derived mitral deceleration time of early filling as a strong predictor of pulmonary capillary wedge pressure in postinfarction patients with left ventricular systolic dysfunction. J Am Coll Cardiol 1994;23:1630–1637.

Goldberg SJ, Sahn DJ, Allen HD, et al. Evaluation of pulmonary and systemic blood flow by 2-dimensional Doppler echocardiography using fast Fourier transform spectral analysis. Am J Cardiol 1982;50:1394–1400.

Hatle L, Angelsen B, Tromsdal A. Noninvasive assessment of atrioventricular pressure half-time by Doppler ultrasound. Circulation 1979;60:1096–1104.

Hatle L, Brubakk A, Tromsdal A, et al. Noninvasive assessment of pressure drop in mitral stenosis by Doppler ultrasound. Br Heart J 1978;40:131–140.

Kuecherer HF, Muhiudeen IA, Kusumoto FM, et al. Estimation of mean left atrial pressure from transesophageal pulsed Doppler echocardiography of pulmonary venous flow. Circulation 1990;82:1127–1139.

Lee RT, Lord CP, Plappert T, et al. Prospective Doppler echocardiographic evaluation of pulmonary artery diastolic pressure in the medical intensive care unit. Am J Cardiol 1989;64:1366–1370.

Levine RA, Jimoh A, Cape EG, et al. Pressure recovery distal to a stenosis: potential cause of gradient "overestimation" by Doppler echocardiography. J Am Coll Cardiol 1989;13:706–715.

Meijboom EJ, Horowitz S, Valdes-Cruz LM, et al. A simplified mitral valve method for two-dimensional echo Doppler blood flow calculation: validation in an open-chest canine model and initial clinical studies. Am Heart J 1987;113:335–340.

Meijboom EJ, Rijsterborgh H, Bot H, et al. Limits of reproducibility of blood flow measurements by Doppler echocardiography. Am J Cardiol 1987;59:133–137.

Miller WE, Richards KL, Crawford MH. Accuracy of mitral Doppler echocardiographic cardiac output determinations in adults. Am Heart J 1990;119:905–910.

Moulinier L, Venet T, Schiller NB, et al. Measurement of aortic blood flow by Doppler echocardiography: day to day variability in normal subjects and applicability in clinical research. J Am Coll Cardiol 1991;17:1326–1333.

Nagueh SF, Kopelen HA, Zoghbi WA. Feasibility and accuracy of Doppler echocardiographic estimation of pulmonary artery occlusive pressure in the intensive care unit. Am J Cardiol 1995;75:1256–1262.

Nagueh SF, Middleton KJ, Kopelen HA, et al. Doppler tissue imaging: a noninvasive technique for evaluation of left ventricular relaxation and estimation of filling pressures. J Am Coll Cardiol 1997;30:1527–1533.

Nagueh SF, Mikati I, Kopelen HA, et al. Doppler estimation of left ventricular filling pressure in sinus tachycardia: a new application of tissue Doppler imaging. Circulation 1998;98:1644–1650.

Niederberger J, Schima H, Maurer G, et al. Importance of pressure recovery for the assessment of aortic stenosis by Doppler ultrasound. Role of aortic size, aortic valve area, and direction of the stenotic jet *in vitro*. Circulation 1996;94:1934–1940.

Nishimura RA, Appleton CP, Redfield MM, et al. Noninvasive Doppler echocardiographic evaluation of left ventricular filling pressures in patients with cardiomyopathies: a simultaneous Doppler echocardiographic and cardiac catheterization study. J Am Coll Cardiol 1996;28:1226–1233.

Oh JK, Taliercio CP, Holmes DR Jr, et al. Prediction of the severity of aortic stenosis by Doppler aortic valve area determination: prospective Doppler-catheterization correlation in 100 patients. J Am Coll Cardiol 1988;11:1227–1234.

Ommen SR, Nishimura RA, Appleton CP, et al. Clinical utility of Doppler echocardiography and tissue Doppler imaging in the estimation of left ventricular filling pressures: a comparative simultaneous Doppler-catheterization study. Circulation 2000;102:1788–1794.

Otsuji Y, Toda H, Ishigami T, et al. Mitral regurgitation during B bump of the mitral valve studied by Doppler echocardiography. Am J Cardiol 1991;67:778–780.

Pozzoli M, Capomolla S, Pinna G, et al. Doppler echocardiography reliably predicts pulmonary artery wedge pressure in patients with chronic heart failure with and without mitral regurgitation. J Am Coll Cardiol 1996;27:883–893.

Quinones MA, Otto CM, Stoddard M, et al. Recommendations for quantification of Doppler echocardiography: a report from the Doppler Quantification Task Force of the Nomenclature and Standards Committee of the American Society of Echocardiography. J Am Soc Echocardiogr 2002;15:167–184.

Rasmussen S, Corya BC, Phillips JF, et al. Unreliability of M-mode left ventricular dimensions for calculating stroke volume and cardiac output in patients without heart disease. Chest 1982;81:614–619.

Richards KL, Cannon SR, Miller JF, et al. Calculation of aortic valve area by Doppler echocardiography: a direct application of the continuity equation. Circulation 1986;73:964–969.

Rifkin RD, Harper K, Tighe D. Comparison of proximal isovelocity surface area method with pressure half-time and planimetry in evaluation of mitral stenosis. J Am Coll Cardiol 1995;26:458–465.

Rose JS, Nanna M, Rahimtoola SH, et al. Accuracy of determination of changes in cardiac output by transcutaneous continuous-wave Doppler computer. Am J Cardiol 1984;54:1099–1101.

Rossvoll O, Hatle LK. Pulmonary venous flow velocities recorded by transthoracic Doppler ultrasound: relation to left ventricular diastolic pressures. J Am Coll Cardiol 1993;21:1687–1696.

Ryan T, Petrovic O, Dillon JC, et al. An echocardiographic index for separation of right ventricular volume and pressure overload. J Am Coll Cardiol 1985;5:918–927.

Samstad SO, Hegrenaes L, Skjaerpe T, et al. Half time of the diastolic aortoventricular pressure difference by continuous wave Doppler ultrasound: a measure of the severity of aortic regurgitation? Br Heart J 1989;61:336–343.

Sanders SP, Yeager S, Williams RG. Measurement of systemic and pulmonary blood flow and QP/QS ratio using Doppler and two-dimensional echocardiography. Am J Cardiol 1983;51:952–956.

Segal J, Lerner DJ, Miller DC, et al. When should Doppler-determined valve area be better than the Gorlin formula? Variation in hydraulic constants in low flow states. J Am Coll Cardiol 1987;9:1294–1305.

Silbert DR, Brunson SC, Schiff R, et al. Determination of right ventricular pressure in the presence of a ventricular septal defect using continuous wave Doppler ultrasound. J Am Coll Cardiol 1986;8:379–384.

Stamm RB, Martin RP. Quantification of pressure gradients across stenotic valves by Doppler ultrasound. J Am Coll Cardiol 1983;2:707–718.

Tei C, Ling LH, Hodge DO, et al. New index of combined systolic and diastolic myocardial performance: a simple and reproducible measure of cardiac function—a study in normal and dilated cardiomyopathy. J Cardiol 1995;26:357–366.

Thomas JD, Weyman AE. Fluid dynamics model of mitral valve flow: description with in vitro validation. J Am Coll Cardiol 1989;13:221–233.

Thomas JD, Wilkins GT, Choong CY, et al. Inaccuracy of mitral pressure half-time immediately after percutaneous mitral valvotomy. Dependence on transmitral gradient and left atrial and ventricular compliance. Circulation 1988;78:980–993.

Utsunomiya T, Doshi R, Patel D, et al. Calculation of volume flow rate by the proximal isovelocity surface area method: simplified approach using color Doppler zero baseline shift. J Am Coll Cardiol 1993;22:277–282.

Valdes-Cruz LM, Horowitz S, Mesel E, et al. A pulsed Doppler echocardiographic method for calculating pulmonary and systemic blood flow in atrial level shunts: validation studies in animals and initial human experience. Circulation 1984;69:80–86.

Yock PG, Popp RL. Noninvasive estimation of right ventricular systolic pressure by Doppler ultrasound in patients with tricuspid regurgitation. Circulation 1984;70:657–662.

Yoganathan AP, Cape EG, Sung HW, et al. Review of hydrodynamic principles for the cardiologist: applications to the study of blood flow and jets by imaging techniques. J Am Coll Cardiol 1988;12:1344–1353.

Pericardial Diseases

Anatomically, the pericardium consists of two layers. The visceral pericardium is contiguous with the epicardium, and the parietal pericardium is the thicker fibrous sac surrounding the heart. Although it is often the parietal pericardium that is typically referred to as the pericardium, it should be emphasized that most disease states simultaneously involve both the parietal and visceral pericardia. Normally, there is 5 to 10 mL of normal buffering fluid within the pericardial space. The pericardium encases all four chambers of the heart and extends 1 to 2 cm up the great vessels. The pericardium similarly reflects around the pulmonary veins. The pericardial reflection around the great vessels limits the size of the pericardial space at these junctures.

The pericardium serves to restrain the four cardiac chambers within a relatively confined volume and space within the thorax. Because of pericardial constraint, the total volume of the four cardiac chambers is limited, and alterations in the volume of one chamber must, by necessity, be reflected in a change in volume in the opposite direction of another. This linking of intracardiac volumes is the underlying pathophysiology for development of pulsus paradoxus and other findings seen in tamponade and constriction.

Pericardial disease can present as several different clinical scenarios, and for each of these, echocardiography can play a significant role. Pericardial effusions can accumulate in any infectious or inflammatory process involving the pericardium. Most infectious and inflammatory processes involve both layers of the pericardium. Table 9.1 outlines the diseases that can affect the pericardium. Acute pericarditis of any etiology may result in accumulation of variable amounts of fluid. In the very early phases, inflammation may be present in the absence of any significant accumulation of pericardial fluid. It is important to evaluate left ventricular function in patients presenting with suspected acute pericarditis to exclude a component of myocarditis.

Because the pericardial space is limited in size, accumulation of significant pericardial fluid reduces the total

▶ TABLE 9.1 Etiology of Pericardial Disease

Idiopathic
  Acute idiopathic pericarditis[a]
  Chronic idiopathic effusion
Infectious
  Viral
  Bacterial
    Tuberculosis
    Spread from contiguous infection (e.g., pneumonia)
  Fungal
Inflammatory
  Associated with connective tissue disease
    Rheumatoid arthritis
    Systemic lupus erythematosis
    Other
Post myocardial infarction
  Acute after transmural infarct
  Partial/complete free wall rupture
  Delayed, "Dressler Syndrome"
Associated with systemic disease
  Uremia
  Hypothyroidism
  Pregnancy
  Cirrhosis
Malignancy
  Direct tumor involvement
  Effusion due to lymphatic obstruction
Miscellaneous
  Post trauma
  Post surgical
  Congestive heart failure
  Severe pulmonary hypertension, right heart failure

[a]Many cases of "idiopathic" pericarditis are probably viral or post viral in origin.

volume that the four cardiac chambers can contain and may result in hemodynamic deterioration. It should be recognized that hemodynamic compromise is related to intrapericardial pressure, which in turn is related to the volume of pericardial fluid and the compliance or distensibility of the pericardium. As such, a slowly developing large effusion may be associated with less compromise

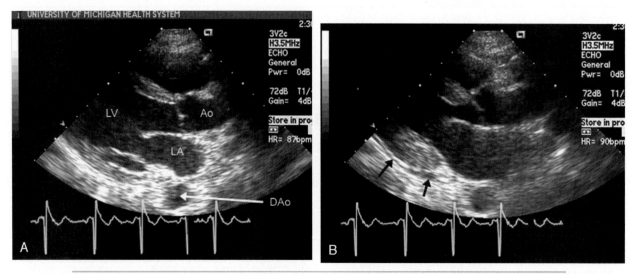

FIGURE 9.1. Parasternal long-axis echocardiogram recorded in a patient with a minimal pericardial effusion. This amount of pericardial fluid represents the normal fluid seen in disease-free individuals. **A:** Recorded at end-diastole. **B:** Recorded at end-systole. Note that at end-diastole, there is no separation between the epicardium and pericardium. At end-systole, the epicardium has lifted off the pericardium revealing a very small pericardial effusion, maximal in the posterior interventricular groove (*arrows*). Ao, aorta; DAo, descending aorta; LA, left atrium; LV, left ventricular.

than a smaller but more rapidly developing effusion. Inflammatory processes of the pericardium typically result in pain and fluid accumulation and more chronically can result in fibrous stranding and stiffening of the pericardium. Thickening of the pericardium eventually can lead to pericardial constriction. Other types of pericardial pathology, such as pericardial cysts and congenital absence of the pericardium, often are noted as incidental findings in asymptomatic individuals or may be associated with atypical and highly variable symptomatology.

ECHOCARDIOGRAPHIC EVALUATION OF THE PERICARDIUM

Anatomically the pericardium can be evaluated with M-mode, two-dimensional, and three-dimensional echocardiography as well as intracardiac ultrasound. Normally, there may be a very small amount of fluid in the pericardial space that typically collects in the dependent areas. It is most often appreciated as a very small echo-free space in the posterior atrioventricular groove. This space may

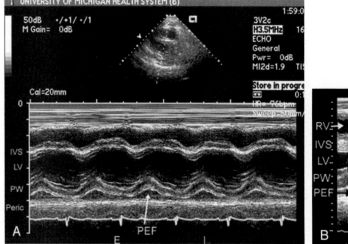

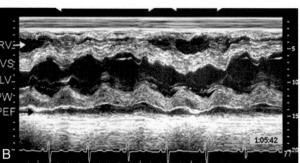

FIGURE 9.2. M-mode echocardiograms recorded in patients with pericardial effusions. **A:** Note the echo-free space (*arrow*) immediately behind the posterior wall of the left ventricle consistent with a small pericardial effusion (*PEF*). Note also that the space is larger in systole than in diastole. **B:** The patient has a larger pericardial effusion with respiratory variation in right ventricular size and septal position.

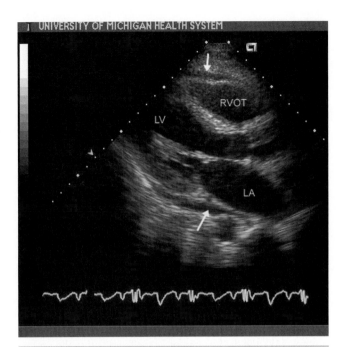

FIGURE 9.3. Parasternal long-axis echocardiogram recorded a patient with a small pericardial effusion. Note the echo-free space, maximal in the posterior interventricular groove (*arrow*) and a smaller anterior echo-free space (*downward-pointing arrow*). In the real-time image, this pericardial effusion can be seen to be present both in diastole and systole. LA, left atrium; LV, left ventricle; RVOT, right ventricular outflow tract.

increase in size during systole (Fig. 9.1). In the absence of a pericardial effusion, dramatic thickening, or calcification, it is unusual to directly visualize the pericardium with either M-mode or two-dimensional echocardiography. Intracardiac ultrasound has been used to directly visualize the pericardium but is infrequently used for this purpose in clinical practice.

Detection and Quantitation of Pericardial Fluid

Pericardial effusion can be detected with all the traditionally used echocardiographic techniques. On M-mode echocardiography, pericardial effusion appears as an echo-free space both anterior and posterior to the heart (Fig. 9.2). The size of the echo-free space is directly proportional to the amount of fluid. There are no accurate M-mode techniques for quantifying the absolute volume of pericardial fluid. It should be emphasized that an isolated anterior free space is not specific for pericardial fluid. An anterior echo-free space may be due to mediastinal fat, fibrosis, thymus, or other tissue.

Most often, two-dimensional echocardiography is used to screen for and quantify pericardial effusion. Most echocardiography laboratories visually quantify pericardial effusion as minimal, small, moderate, or large and further characterize it as either free or loculated. The effusion

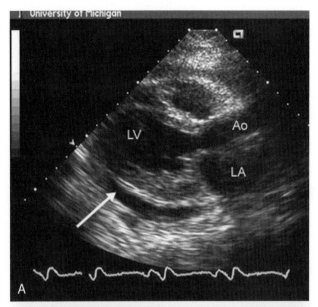

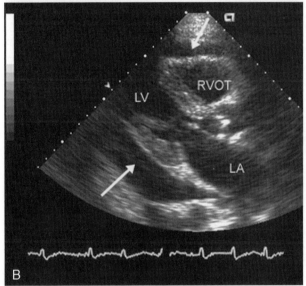

FIGURE 9.4. Parasternal long-axis echocardiograms recorded in patients with a small **(A)** and moderate to large **(B)** pericardial effusion. **A:** There is an approximately 1-cm space between the epicardium and pericardium (*arrow*), consistent with a small pericardial effusion. **B:** A larger pericardial effusion is present both anteriorly and posteriorly (*arrows*). Ao, aorta; LA, left atrium; LV, left ventricle; RVOT, right ventricular outflow tract.

should also be characterized as to the presence or absence of hemodynamic compromise. On two-dimensional echocardiography, pericardial effusion tends to be most prominent in the more dependent (i.e., posterior in a supine patient) area and frequently appears maximal in the posterior atrioventricular groove (Figs. 9.3–9.5). Using additional views including the parasternal short-axis, apical, and subcostal views, the circumferential extent of an effusion can

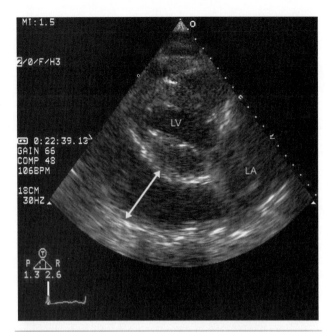

FIGURE 9.5. Parasternal long-axis echocardiogram recorded a patient with a large pericardial effusion, measuring 3 cm in its greatest dimension posteriorly (*arrow*). In a real-time image, there is evidence of a swinging heart within a large pericardial effusion. LA, left atrium; LV, left ventricle.

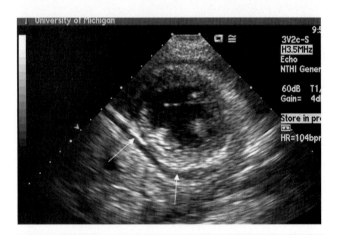

FIGURE 9.6. Parasternal short-axis echocardiogram recorded a patient with a small pericardial effusion. Note the echo-free space between the epicardium and pericardium, which extends from the true posterior wall of the left ventricle past the interventricular groove (*arrows*). In this view, it is also seen behind the right ventricle.

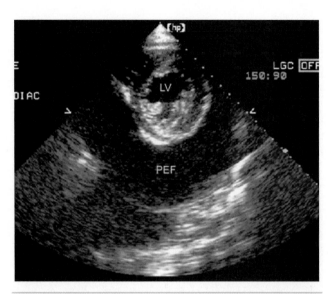

FIGURE 9.7. Parasternal short-axis view recorded a patient with a large pericardial effusion (*PEF*). Note the large echo-free space measuring more than 3 cm surrounding the left ventricle (*LV*) and the free motion of the heart within the pericardial fluid.

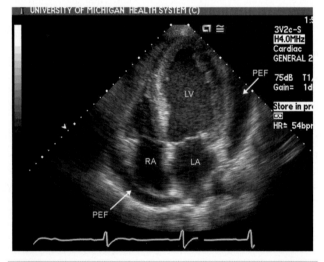

FIGURE 9.8. Apical four-chamber view recorded in a patient with a moderate, predominantly lateral pericardial effusion (*PEF*) (*arrow*). Note also a smaller fluid collection behind the right atrium (*RA*). LA, left atrium; LV, left ventricular.

be reliably determined (Figs. 9.6–9.9). Figures 9.3 through 9.9 were recorded in patients with different amounts of pericardial effusion. Note in Figure 9.7 the circumferential extent of the effusion is confirmed in the short-axis view. This effusion is not constrained by an inflammatory component, and the heart moves freely within the pericardial space buffered by the large pericardial effusion.

Typically, a minimal pericardial effusion represents the normal amount of pericardial fluid in a disease-free state (Fig. 9.1). It is visualized as a small echo-free space in the posterior atrioventricular groove that may be visible only in systole when the heart has pulled away from the pericardium. A small effusion is defined as one resulting in as much as 1 cm of posterior echo-free space, with or without fluid accumulation elsewhere. Moderate effusions have been described as 1 to 2 cm of echo-free space and large effusions as more than 2 cm of maximal separation.

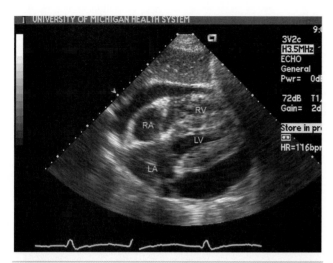

FIGURE 9.9. Subcostal echocardiogram reveals a moderate to large pericardial effusion. Note the effusion surrounding the entire heart, with its greatest dimension lateral to the left ventricular free wall. Fluid is clearly seen surrounding the right atrium (*RA*) and between the pericardium and right ventricle (*RV*). LA, left atrium; LV, left ventricle.

It should be emphasized that these definitions may vary from laboratory to laboratory. In exceptionally large effusions, the heart may swing within the pericardial space (Fig. 9.10). This variable location from beat to beat is the etiology of electric alternans seen on the electrocardiogram.

Effusions may be localized or loculated rather than circumferential. This is not uncommon after cardiac surgery or cardiac trauma in which the inflammatory component of the pericardial effusion has resulted in unequal distribution of fluid in the pericardial space. Figure 9.11 was recorded in an individual with a more localized pericardial effusion, the maximal extent of which is in the area of the lateral wall.

The pericardium reflects around the pulmonary veins and may limit the size of a pericardial effusion behind the left atrium. Previous guidelines had suggested that a fluid collection behind the left atrium was more likely to be plural than pericardial. There are numerous exceptions to this rule, and larger pericardial effusions often collect behind the left atrium as well (Figs. 9.5 and 9.9). Additionally, pericardial fluid may collect in the oblique sinus, which is a potential space bordered by the left atrium and great vessels (Fig. 9.12). In this instance, the pericardial fluid may surround the left atrial appendage and the aorta, left atrium, and pulmonary artery and on occasion has been confused for an abscess cavity.

Several schemes have been used for actual quantitation of the volume of pericardial fluid, none of which have had universal clinical acceptance. Three-dimensional echocardiography may provide the most accurate technique for determining pericardial fluid volume and distri-

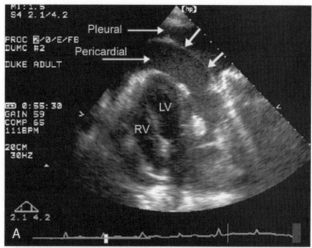

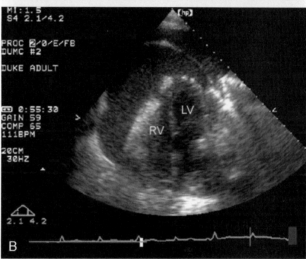

FIGURE 9.10. Apical four-chamber view recorded from a patient with a large pericardial effusion and a swinging heart. A pleural effusion is also present, which allows direct visualization of the pericardial thickness (*arrows*) **(A). A, B:** Recorded from different cardiac cycles. Note the marked change in position of the heart within the pericardial space, which can be appreciated as a swinging heart in the real-time image. This variable position within the thorax is the cause of electrical alternans seen on surface electrocardiography. LV, left ventricle; RV, right ventricle.

bution but is limited in its availability (Fig. 9.13). Using this technique, the three-dimensional volume of the entire pericardial space can be calculated. The overall total volume of the entire heart (all four chambers) is then likewise calculated, and the pericardial fluid volume is calculated as the difference between these two volumes. Although accurate for determining the volume of pericardial fluid, this technique has had little clinical acceptance because of the limited availability of three-dimensional scanning and the lack of a clinical need for determining precise pericardial volume.

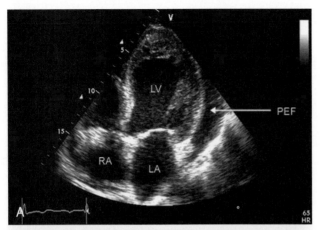

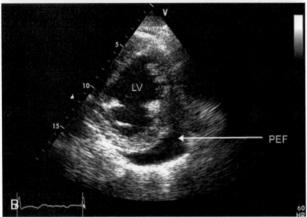

FIGURE 9.11. Apical four-chamber (**A**) and parasternal short-axis (**B**) views recorded in a patient with a small, localized, predominantly lateral pericardial effusion (*PEF*). This echocardiogram was recorded approximately 2 weeks after open-heart surgery. LA, left atrium; LV, left ventricle; RA, right atrium.

Direct Visualization of the Pericardium

In disease-free states, the normal pericardium is rarely visualized with any of the traditional echocardiographic modalities. Intravascular and intracardiac ultrasound may visualize the actual thickness of the pericardium but are obviously invasive techniques. In the absence of a pleural effusion, which creates a fluid layer on either side of the pericardium, the exterior portion of the parietal pericardium abuts the normal intrathoracic structures, and therefore its thickness and character cannot be separated from the surrounding tissues. When both pericardial and pleural effusions are present, the thickness of the pericardium in that area can be ascertained (Figs. 9.10 and 9.14). In instances of marked fibrosis and calcification, it may be possible to infer substantial pericardial thickening, but actual measurement of pericardial thickness will remain problematic. In the presence of calcific pericarditis, there may be marked shadowing seen posterior to the pericardium (Fig. 9.15). It should be empha-

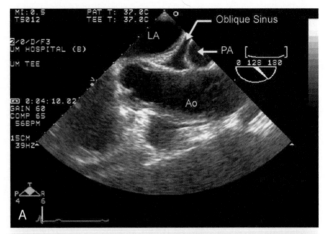

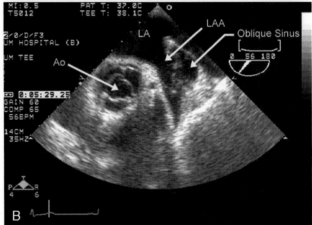

FIGURE 9.12. Transesophageal echocardiogram recorded in a patient with a moderate pericardial effusion and evidence of fluid in the oblique sinus. **A:** Note the echo-free space bounded by the left atrium (*LA*), aorta (*Ao*), and pulmonary artery (*PA*). This represents fluid accumulating in the pericardial reflection around the great vessels. **B:** There is a similar collection of fluid in the pericardial space surrounding the left atrial appendage (*LAA*). In the real-time image (**B**), note the excessive motion of the wall of the left atrial appendage within the pericardial fluid in the oblique sinus. On occasion, the wall of the left atrial appendage can assume a mass-like appearance and be confused with a pathologic mass.

sized that the normal pericardium is a highly reflective structure and that a bright pericardial echo alone should not be used to establish the diagnosis of constrictive pericarditis.

Additionally, in the presence of fluid accumulation, masses and stranding, which occur either on the visceral pericardium or the interior aspect of the parietal pericardium, can be identified with two-dimensional echocardiography. Detection of stranding implies a marked inflammatory or possibly hemorrhagic etiology of the pericardial effusion (Figs. 9.16 and 9.17). It often is seen in uremic or infectious pericarditis due to a bacterial or fungal organism. Masses within the pericardium can be the result of metastatic disease from an intrathoracic ma-

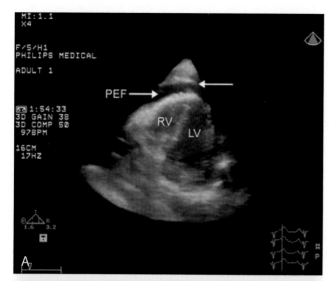

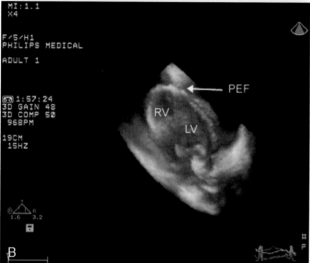

FIGURE 9.13. A, B: Real-time transthoracic three-dimensional echocardiogram recorded in a patient with a moderate pericardial effusion (*PEF*). In these views, the three-dimensional data set was sliced along the plane of a four-chamber view and then the image was rotated and tilted to provide different perspectives. Note that all four chambers of the heart can be clearly visualized, as can the parietal pericardium and the circumferential pericardial fluid within the pericardial space. LV, left ventricle; RV, right ventricle.

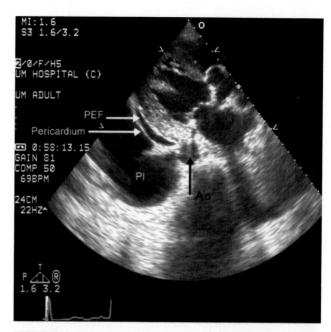

FIGURE 9.14. Parasternal long-axis echocardiogram recorded in a patient with a small pericardial effusion (*PEF*) and a larger pleural effusion (*Pl*). The presence of concurrent pericardial and pleural fluid allows identification of the actual pericardial echo. In this instance, the pericardial thickness can be seen to be approximately 2 mm. Note the position of the two fluid collections with respect to the descending thoracic aorta (*black arrow*).

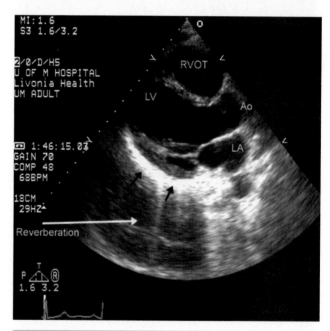

FIGURE 9.15. Parasternal long-axis echocardiogram recorded a patient with a partially calcified posterior pericardium (*arrows*). The posterior pericardium has pathologic echo intensity and appears thickened, although because of reverberation, the actual thickness cannot be reliably determined. Note that the markedly echogenic pericardium has resulted in reverberation artifact, creating a double image of the left ventricular cavity behind the pericardial space. Ao, aorta; LA, left atrium; LV, left ventricle; RVOT, right ventricular outflow tract.

lignancy (Fig. 9.18) but are often in pericardial effusions due to a marked inflammatory process as well.

Using M-mode echocardiography, an indirect assessment of pericardial anatomy can be made. Typically, the heart lifts off the parietal pericardium in systole. By increasing the damping of the M-mode beam to a point at which the myocardium is no longer visualized, the M-mode echocardiogram will visualize only the relatively denser pericardial echoes. A rough assessment of the pericardial thickness and echogenicity can be obtained by this

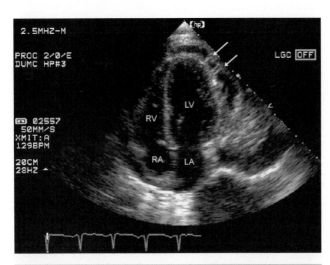

FIGURE 9.16. Apical four-chamber view recorded in a patient with an inflammatory pericardial effusion, maximal at the apical and lateral borders of the heart. Note the strands of tissue connecting the parietal and visceral pericardia (*arrows*), implying an inflammatory process within the pericardium. LA, left atrium; LV, left ventricle; RA, right atrium; RV, right ventricle.

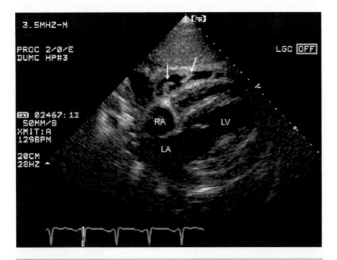

FIGURE 9.17. Subcostal echocardiogram recorded in a patient with a moderate pericardial effusion and stranding arising both from the parietal and visceral pericardia (*arrows*). LA, left atrium; LV, left ventricle; RA, right atrium.

means and has been one of the M-mode signs of pericardial constriction (Fig. 9.19).

Differentiation of Pericardial from Pleural Effusion

A left pleural effusion will result in an echo-free space posterior to the heart in a patient in a supine or left lateral position (Figs. 9.10 and 9.14). Pleural effusion can occasionally be confused for pericardial fluid. There are several echocardiographic clues that help distinguish

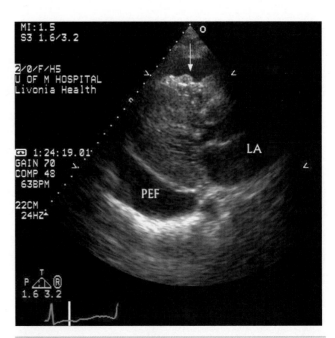

FIGURE 9.18. Parasternal long-axis echocardiogram recorded a patient with a malignant pericardial effusion (*PEF*). Note the nodular densities overlying the visceral aspect of the pericardium anteriorly (*arrow*). Of note, similar densities may be seen in nonmalignant processes as well. LA, left atrium.

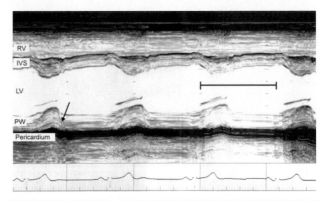

FIGURE 9.19. M-mode echocardiogram recorded in a patient with constrictive pericarditis and thickened posterior pericardial echoes. To the right of this frame, in the area marked by the *black bracket*, damping has been increased to suppress the fainter myocardial echoes. Note the bright pericardial echo has not been suppressed. Also note the flat motion of the posterior wall after the initial rapid posterior motion (*arrow*) of the endocardium. IVS, interventricular septum; LV, left ventricle; PW, posterior wall; RV, right ventricle.

pericardial from pleural fluid. As noted previously, the pericardial reflections surround the pulmonary veins and tend to limit the potential space behind the left atrium. Because of this, fluid appearing exclusively behind the left atrium is more likely to represent pleural than pericardial effusion. One of the more reliable distinguishing features between a pericardial and pleural effusion is the location of the fluid-filled space with respect to the descending thoracic aorta (Fig. 9.14). The pericardial reflection is typically anterior to the descending aorta, and therefore fluid appearing posterior to the descending thoracic aorta is more likely to be pleural, whereas fluid appearing anterior to the aorta is more likely to be pericardial. These observations apply to differentiating pericardial from pleural fluid in the parasternal views. In the apical four-chamber view, separation of a localized lateral pericardial effusion from a pleural effusion can often be problematic. When both pericardial fluid and pleural fluid are present, one can frequently identify the parietal pericardium, which serves as an excellent anatomic landmark to define the extent of each of the two fluid collections (Fig. 9.10).

CARDIAC TAMPONADE

Accumulation of increasing amounts of pericardial fluid results in predictable hemodynamic alterations. Normal intrapericardial pressure ranges between −5 and +5 cm of water and fluctuates with respiration. Because of the previously mentioned constraining effect of the pericardium on the combined volume of the four cardiac chambers, respiratory variation in intrapericardial pressure results in linked variation in filling of the right and left ventricles. With inspiration, intrathoracic and intrapericardial pressures decrease. The result of this is to augment flow into the right heart and reduce flow out of the pulmonary veins. This results in augmented right ventricular filling and stroke volume and, because the total intrapericardial space is limited, also results in a compensatory decrease in left ventricular stroke volume in early inspiration. In expiration, intrathoracic pressure and intrapericardial pressure increase, resulting in a mild decrease in right ventricular diastolic filling and a subsequent increase in left ventricular filling. This cyclic variation of left and right ventricular filling with the respiratory cycle is sufficient to create mild changes in stroke volume and blood pressure with the respiratory cycle (Fig. 9.20). Typically, the normal respiratory variation in stroke volume results in no more than a 10 mm Hg decrease in systemic arterial systolic pressure with inspiration. Any process that results in increasing pressure variation with the respiratory cycle, such as obstructive lung disease, or other states that increase the work of breathing will result in a commensurate increase in intrathoracic pressure swings and subsequently greater reciprocal variation in left and right ventricular filling, stroke volume, and arterial pulse pressure.

With increasing accumulation of pericardial fluid, intrapericardial pressure increases and begins to further affect right heart filling. The overall effect of an increasing volume of pericardial fluid is to limit the total blood volume allowable within the four cardiac chambers and

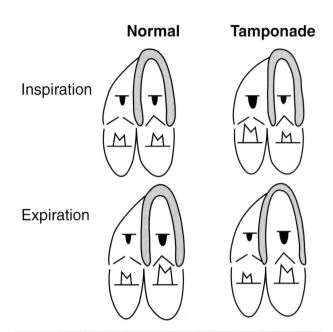

FIGURE 9.20. Schematic depicts the generation of pulsus paradoxus and hemodynamically significant pericardial effusion. Both normal physiology and tamponade physiology are depicted in both inspiration and expiration. In the normal situation, the relative size and geometry of the right and left ventricles are preserved in both inspiration and expiration, and there is little variation of either ventricular outflow or inflow, as depicted by the schematics within the chambers. Exaggerated ventricular interaction in a hemodynamically significant pericardial effusion is shown on the right. Note the relatively greater right ventricular size during inspiration with both augmented inflow and outflow and the concurrent decrease in left ventricular size, outflow tract flow velocity profile, and mitral valve inflow. During expiration (at lower right), left ventricular filling is again augmented as is left ventricular outflow at the expense of reduced right ventricular volume and decreased right ventricular Doppler flow velocities.

to therefore exaggerate the respiration-dependent ventricular volume interaction. Intrapericardial pressure can equal or exceed normal filling pressures of the heart and thus becomes the determining factor for the passive intracardiac pressures. The passively determined intracardiac pressures include right and left atrial pressures, right ventricular diastolic pressure, pulmonary artery diastolic pressure, left ventricular diastolic pressure, and pulmonary capillary wedge pressure. With elevation of intrapericardial pressure above normal filling pressure, the diastolic pressure in all four cardiac chambers becomes equalized and is determined by intrapericardial pressure. This is the hemodynamic hallmark of cardiac tamponade. Because the left ventricle has a stiffer wall and its diastolic pressures are determined by a variety of factors including active relaxation, left ventricular filling is relatively unaffected compared with right ventricular filling.

As a result of increased intrapericardial pressure and the limitation on overall cardiac volume, the interaction between the right and left ventricles becomes exaggerated. Figure 9.20 schematizes the interaction between the right and left ventricles in a large pericardial effusion and outlines the mechanism for pulsus paradoxus. In a large pericardial effusion with pathologic elevation of intrapericardial pressure, inspiration results in a disproportionately greater filling of the right ventricle than in a normal state and subsequently in a disproportionately greater compromise of left ventricular filling. During expiration, the process is reversed and right ventricular filling is impeded to a substantially greater degree. This results in a marked exaggeration in the phasic changes in right and left ventricular stroke volume and subsequently in a substantially greater decrease in systolic arterial blood pressure with inspiration. This is the mechanism of a pathologic pulsus paradoxus as is seen in cardiac tamponade.

Echocardiographic Findings in Cardiac Tamponade

There have been several echocardiographic features described in patients with hemodynamic compromise and frank cardiac tamponade (Table 9.2). It should be empha-

▶ **TABLE 9.2 Echo Doppler Findings in Pericardial Disease**

Anatomic Features
   Pericardial effusion
   Pericardial thickening
   Pericardial standing
Tamponade
   2D echo and M-mode
      Diastolic right ventricular collapse
      Right atrial collapse/inversion
   Doppler
      Exaggerated respiratory variation in inflow velocity
      Phasic variation in right ventricular outflow tract/left
         ventricular outflow tract flow
      Exaggerated respiratory variation in inferior vena cava flow
Constrictive Pericarditis
   Anatomic features
      Thickened pericardium
      Dilated inferior vena cava
      Exaggerated septal shift with inspiration
   M-mode
      Abnormal septal motion
      "Flattened" posterior wall motion
   Doppler
      Exaggerated E/A of mitral inflow
      Exaggerated respiratory variation in E velocity
      Tissue Doppler imaging of anular velocities
      Blunted diastolic inferior vena cava flow with expiration

sized that cardiac tamponade is a clinical diagnosis. Echocardiographic findings may suggest a hemodynamic abnormality that may be the substrate for tamponade, but echocardiographic abnormalities alone do not establish the diagnosis of cardiac tamponade. One of the earliest signs of cardiac tamponade is evidence of a swinging heart, detected on either M-mode or two-dimensional echocardiography (Fig. 9.10). Detection of a swinging heart is simply a marker of a large pericardial effusion in which the four cardiac chambers are free to float within the pericardial space in a phasic manner. A large pericardial effusion is more likely than a small effusion to be associated with intrapericardial pressure elevation, and hence the relationship between a swinging heart and hemodynamic compromise is indirect rather than direct evidence of elevated pressure. Because cardiac position varies within the pericardium from beat to beat, its position in relation to an electrocardiographic lead also varies. This is the mechanism of electrical alternans seen in large pericardial effusions.

More specific signs of hemodynamic compromise have included direct evidence of actual elevation in intrapericardial pressures. Diastolic right ventricular outflow collapse and exaggerated right atrial collapse during atrial systole (ventricular diastole) are well validated as signs of elevated intrapericardial pressure. The earliest description of diastolic right ventricular collapse was obtained using M-mode echocardiography in which a characteristic posterior motion of the anterior right ventricular wall was noted in diastole (Fig. 9.21). This observation was subsequently confirmed using two-dimensional echocardiography. In patients with elevated intrapericardial pressure, intracavitary cardiac pressure may transiently fall below intrapericardial pressure in early diastole, and hydrodynamic compression of these more distensible structures will be seen. Anatomically and experimentally, the right ventricular outflow tract is the more compressible area of the right ventricle and with significantly elevated intrapericardial pressure tends to collapse. In early diastole, immediately after closing of the pulmonary valve, at the time of opening of the tricuspid valve, the right ventricular outflow tract will paradoxically collapse inward (Figs. 9.22 and 9.23). This is indirect evidence that intrapericardial pressure has exceeded right ventricular diastolic pressure at this time point, and hence the underlying substrate for tamponade is likely to be present. Collapse of the right ventricle is often best appreciated in the parasternal long- and short-axis views but occasionally can be appreciated in the apical four-chamber view. When collapse extends from the more compressible outflow tract to the body of the right ventricle, this is evidence that intrapericardial pressure is elevated more substantially.

As a corollary of this, exaggerated right atrial collapse is seen, which is an indication of impeded right atrial fill-

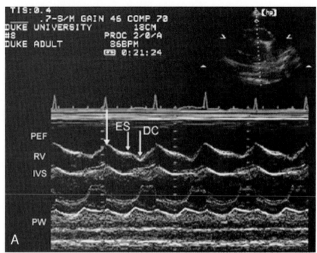

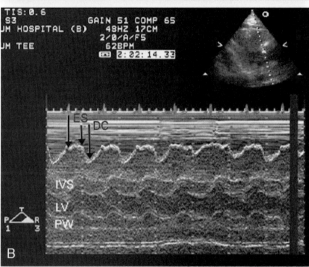

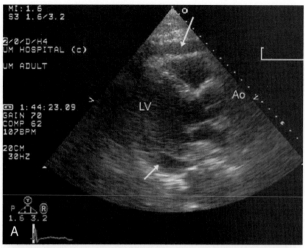

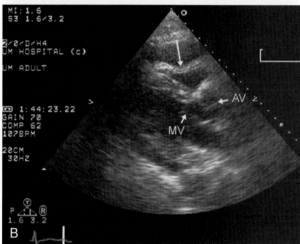

FIGURE 9.21. M-mode echocardiograms **(A, B)** recorded in patients with evidence of hemodynamic compromise and diastolic collapse (*DC*) of the right ventricular free wall. In each example, the *unlabeled arrow* denotes the beginning of systole. The position of the right ventricular free wall at end-systole (*ES*) is also noted. Immediately after end-systole, the right ventricular free wall moves posteriorly, indicative of diastolic collapse. IVS, interventricular septum; LV, left ventricle; PEF, pericardial effusion; PW, posterior wall; RV, right ventricle.

FIGURE 9.22. Parasternal long-axis echocardiogram recorded in a patient with a moderate pericardial effusion (*arrows* in **A**) and evidence of hemodynamic compromise, as manifested by diastolic collapse of the right ventricular free wall. **A:** Recorded at end-diastole. Note the normal shape of the right ventricular outflow tract. **B:** Recorded in early diastole. Note that the aortic valve (*AV*) has closed and that the mitral valve (*MV*) is open. The right ventricular outflow tract has collapsed inward (*arrow*), indicative of elevated intrapericardial pressure, exceeding right ventricular diastolic pressure at this point in the cardiac cycle. In the real-time image, the dynamic nature of this collapse can be appreciated. Ao, aorta; LV, left ventricle.

ing (Fig. 9.24). This occurs with timing opposite that of right ventricular collapse. It is identifiable on two-dimensional echocardiography, typically from the subcostal or apical four-chamber view. Because the right atrium normally contracts in volume with atrial systole, the degree of right atrial collapse must be quantified with respect to either the magnitude of collapse or the duration for which it remains collapsed. Right atrial collapse occurs immediately after normal atrial systolic contraction. In the presence of marked elevation of intrapericardial pressure, the right atrial wall will remain collapsed throughout atrial diastole and buckle inward, reversing the normal wall curvature. In situations in which a local-

ized effusion is resulting in hemodynamic compromise, one may occasionally encounter isolated compression (usually diastolic) of the left atrium or left ventricle.

Doppler Findings in Tamponade

Using Doppler echocardiography, variations in the phasic inflow into the ventricles and in right and left ventricular outflow and stroke volume can be shown. Doppler interrogation can be used to evaluate mitral or tricuspid inflow or aortic or pulmonary outflow and exaggerated phasic variation in flow can be documented. Under normal cir-

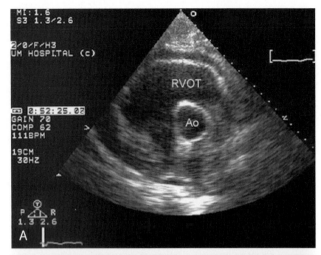

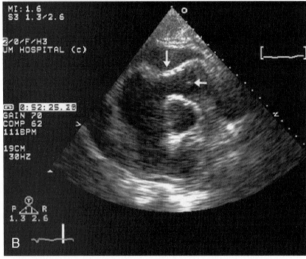

FIGURE 9.23. Parasternal short-axis view recorded at the base of the heart in patient with a hemodynamically significant pericardial effusion and right ventricular outflow tract collapse. **A:** Recorded at end-systole, revealing normal right ventricular outflow tract geometry. **B:** Recorded in early diastole. Note the closed pulmonary valve (*horizontal arrow*). There is definite collapse inward at the right ventricular outflow tract (*RVOT*) free wall (*vertical arrow*), suggesting that pericardial pressure exceeds right ventricular diastolic pressure at that point in the cardiac cycle. Ao, aorta.

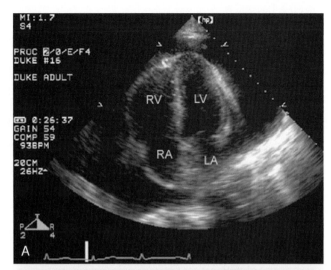

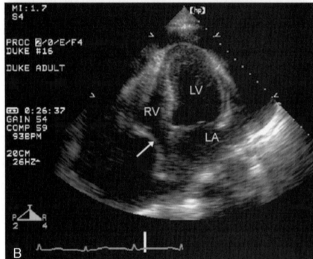

FIGURE 9.24. Apical four-chamber view recorded in a patient with a large pericardial effusion and evidence of right atrial collapse. **A:** Recorded in late diastole. Note the normal contour of the right atrial wall. **B:** Recorded in early ventricular systole, after atrial contraction. Note that, at this point in the cardiac cycle, the right atrial wall has collapsed inward (*arrow*), indicative of elevated pericardial pressure exceeding right atrial pressure. The dynamic nature of the right atrial free wall collapse can be appreciated in this real-time image. LA, left atrium; LV, left ventricle; RA, right atrium; RV, right ventricle.

cumstances, peak velocity of mitral inflow varies by 15% or more with respiration and tricuspid inflow by 25% or more. Variation in peak velocity and time velocity integral of aortic and pulmonary flow profiles typically is less than 10%. In the presence of hemodynamically significant pericardial effusion, respiratory variation in filling is exaggerated above these thresholds, and, as a consequence, respiratory variation in outflow tract velocities and time velocity integral is likewise exaggerated (Figs. 9.25 and 9.26). These Doppler findings are the corollary of a pulsus paradoxus.

Pulsed Doppler imaging of superior vena caval and hepatic vein flows can also reflect the elevated intrapericardial pressure and altered filling patterns. Normally, vena caval flow occurs in both systole and diastole and is nearly continuous. In the presence of elevated intrapericardial pressure, flow during diastole is truncated and the majority of flow into the heart occurs during ventricular systole. The hepatic vein flow pattern may also reflect the exaggerated respiratory phase dependency of right ventricular filling (Fig. 9.27). As a general rule, Doppler flow profiles of vena caval flow are confirmatory of the hemo-

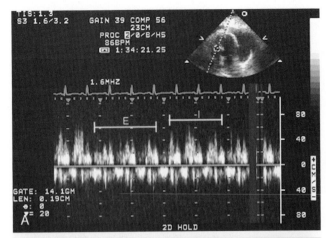

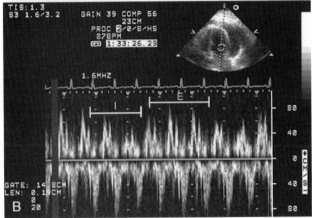

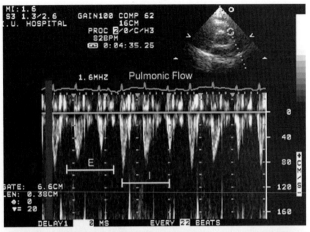

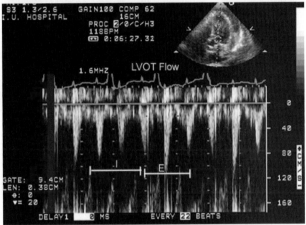

FIGURE 9.25. Doppler recordings of transtricuspid **(A)** and transmitral **(B)** inflow velocities recorded in a patient with a hemodynamically significant pericardial effusion and clinical evidence of cardiac tamponade. The inspiratory (*I*) and expiratory (*E*) phases are as noted in the brackets. For the tricuspid valve, note the augmented inflow during inspiration with diminished inflow during expiration. Note the opposite effect seen on the transmitral inflow velocity.

FIGURE 9.26. Doppler flow profile of the pulmonary outflow tract and left ventricular outflow tract (*LVOT*) recorded in the same patient depicted in Figure 9.25. Again, the phases of the respiratory cycle are as noted in the *brackets*. There are augmented pulmonary flow with inspiration and a reciprocal decrease in left ventricular outflow at the same point in the respiratory cycle. This reciprocal and phasic variation with respiration is physiologic evidence of exaggerated intraventricular interdependence and the underlying phenomenon resulting in pulsus paradoxus. E, expiration.

dynamic abnormality but rarely are necessary as a stand-alone diagnostic finding.

There is a well-defined and predictable hierarchy with which the previously noted findings occur in hemodynamically significant pericardial effusions. These have been well defined experimentally and fit the well-known physiology of the disease states. Typically, the earliest feature to be noted is an exaggerated respiratory variation of tricuspid inflow. Subsequent to this, an exaggeration in mitral inflow patterns can be noted. Abnormal right atrial collapse typically occurs at lower levels of intrapericardial pressure elevation than does right ventricular outflow tract collapse. Right ventricular free wall collapse is seen only later in the development of elevated intrapericardial pressures. It should be noted that with milder elevations in intrapericardial pressure, right ventricular diastolic collapse may be seen in expiration but not in inspiration when right ventricular filling is augmented. This intermittent collapse is

often best documented with M-mode echocardiography (Fig. 9.28). When intrapericardial pressure is elevated and consistently exceeds intravascular pressures, all these findings will be present simultaneously.

There are several instances in which these changes may not be seen. The most common is probably the patient with significant right ventricular hypertrophy, usually due to pulmonary hypertension. In this case, the thick, noncompliant right ventricular wall is not compressed by the relatively modest elevation in pericardial pressure seen in early diastolic with active left ventricular relaxation, and both clinical and echocardiographic signs of compromise may be minimal or absent. Thickening of the ventricular wall due to malignancy, an overlying inflammatory response, or an overlying thrombus in hem-

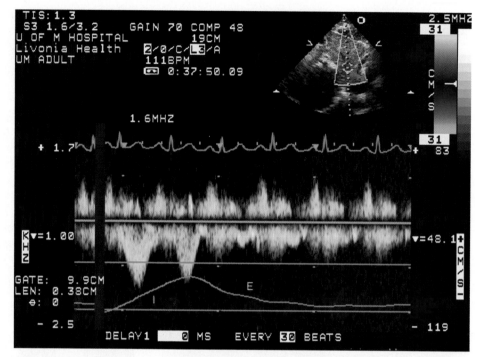

FIGURE 9.27. Pulsed Doppler imaging of the hepatic vein recorded in a patient with a hemodynamically significant pericardial effusion. Note the loss of forward flow in the hepatic veins during the expiratory (*E*) phase of the respiratory cycle. Flow out of the hepatic veins is confined exclusively to the early inspiratory (*I*) phase.

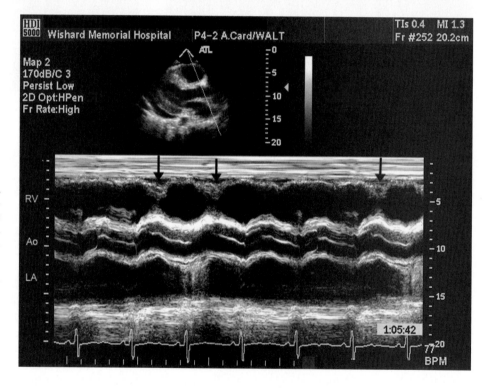

FIGURE 9.28. M-mode echocardiogram recorded through the right ventricular outflow tract in a patient with pericardial effusion and evidence of early hemodynamic compromise. In this instance, right ventricular outflow tract collapse is seen only intermittently (*arrows*) and occurs during expiration, whereas right ventricular filling is less impeded during inspiration. Ao, aorta; LA, left atrium; RV, right ventricle.

orrhagic pericarditis may have the same effect. Similarly, because the magnitude of ventricular interaction is directly related to ventricular volume, these signs may be absent in low-pressure tamponade, as may be seen in hypovolemic patients.

PERICARDIAL CONSTRICTION

Pericardial constriction is a relatively uncommon entity in contemporary practice. The clinical signs and symptoms of pericardial constriction are often vague and may have been present for several years to decades before the diagnosis is finally established. The classic form of pericardial constriction is calcific constriction secondary to tuberculous pericarditis, an entity that obviously has become less and less frequent. Many of the classic physical findings and observations in pericardial constriction were derived from patients with this classic type of calcific constriction. It should be emphasized that other forms of constriction may not share all the classic hemodynamic, physical, and echocardiographic findings or clinical presentations. More commonly in today's practice, constrictive pericarditis may be the result of infectious or inflammatory processes such as connective tissue disease or radiation therapy or develop several years after cardiac surgery. Constrictive pathophysiology can follow virtually any form of pericardial inflammation, and transient constrictive physiology can occasionally occur in the course of otherwise self-limited pericarditis, connective tissue disease or other inflammatory processes, or after cardiac surgery.

Anatomically, constriction occurs when there is stiffening of the pericardium. It is typically the parietal pericardium that becomes the constricting force, although variable degrees of visceral pericardial involvement also occur. This is often seen in association with demonstrable pericardial thickening, again predominantly involving the parietal pericardium but also with inflammation and stiff-

ening of the visceral pericardium. In many instances, the pericardial space between the visceral and parietal pericardium may appear filled with a vague echo-dense substance representing a combination of actual pericardial thickening and organized inflammatory pericardial fluid (Figs. 9.29 and 9.30). In classic calcific constrictive pericarditis, the pericardium forms a rigid shell in which the cardiac chambers are encased and therefore are not affected by changes in intrathoracic pressure. More commonly, an elastic constriction occurs in which there is variable transmission of intrathoracic pressures to the intracardiac chambers, and physical findings and pathophysiology similar to those seen in tamponade may be noted.

Echocardiographic Diagnosis

The diagnosis of constrictive pericarditis requires a combination of clinical and echocardiographic findings. There are no absolutely sensitive and specific echocardiographic or Doppler indicators of constriction; instead, multiple clinical, anatomic, and physiologic observations must be combined to establish the diagnosis. Although pericardial constriction is most often associated with thickening of the pericardium, actual detection of a thickened pericardium is often difficult with transthoracic echocardiography. If an effusion is also present, and especially if pericardial fluid and pleural fluid are both present, the thickness of the pericardium may be directly vi-

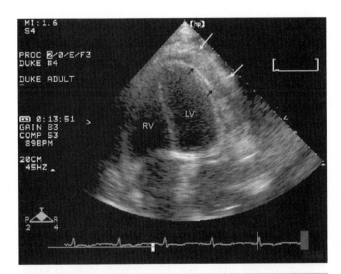

FIGURE 9.29. Apical four-chamber view recorded in a patient with an inflammatory pericardial effusion and an organized pericardial effusion. The *black arrows* represent the margin of the visceral pericardium and the *white arrows* the parietal pericardium. Note that the pericardial space is filled with an echo-dense substance, representing organized pericardial effusion. In this setting, a component of constrictive physiology is often encountered. In the real-time image, note that the cardiac structures appear fixed within the pericardial space rather than moving freely within the mediastinum. LV, left ventricle; RV, right ventricle.

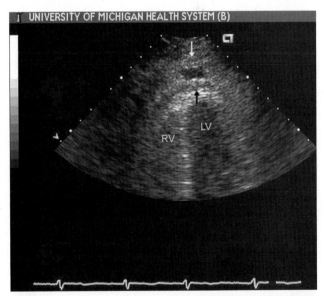

FIGURE 9.30. Apical four-chamber view recorded at a shallow imaging depth. The *black arrow* indicates the external boundary of the left ventricular apex. The *white arrow* denotes the position of the parietal pericardium. Within the pericardial space, there is a combination of free fluid and organized inflammatory material. LV, left ventricle; RV, right ventricle.

sualized by transthoracic or transesophageal echocardiography (Fig. 9.14). When directly visualized, the normal pericardium is no more than 1 to 2 mm in thickness. Additional indicators of a thickened pericardium include its persistence during gradual damping of an M-mode beam through the posterior left ventricular wall (Fig. 9.19). If calcific pericardial disease is present, ultrasound shadowing may occur and again give hints as to the underlying pathology (Fig. 9.15).

One occasionally encounters a patient with signs and symptoms of pericardial constriction in whom there is no direct evidence of pericardial thickening on echocardiography or other imaging techniques such as computed tomography and magnetic resonance imaging. In such cases, if the Doppler evaluation is consistent with constrictive physiology, confirmation of hemodynamics by catheterization is often indicated. Such patients represent a well-defined subset of constrictive pericarditis in which a normal thickness pericardium has become pathologically stiffened and noncompliant, leading to constrictive physiology.

There are several other M-mode abnormalities that have been noted in patients with constrictive pericarditis. These include relatively abrupt relaxation of the posterior wall with subsequent flattening of endocardial motion throughout the remainder of diastole (Fig. 9.19) and abnormal septal motion (Figs. 9.31 and 9.32). Several different septal motion abnormalities have been noted, many of which mimic conduction disturbances and mild right ventricular volume or pressure overload patterns. Typically, early diastolic notching may be seen, followed by paradoxical and then normal motion of the ventricular septum. Septal motion reflects the competitive filling of the two ventricles. With constriction, the ventricles may

fill in an alternative fashion and thus produce a wavy pattern of diastolic septal motion. With atrial systole, there may be an exaggerated motion of the ventricular septum as well.

In elastic constriction (as opposed to classic calcific pericardial constriction), there is exaggerated interaction of the right and left ventricles that manifests as exaggerated septal position shifts with respiration. This can be noted both on M-mode and two-dimensional echocardiography and resembles the type of septal motion abnormality seen in cardiac tamponade (Fig. 9.33). These interventricular septal motion abnormalities are simply a reflection of minor variations in right and left ventricular volume throughout the cardiac and respiratory cycles. They therefore can be seen in any instance in which an abnormal filling relationship exists between the two ventricles. A final indirect sign of constriction is dilation and lack of respiratory variation of the inferior vena caval diameter (Fig. 9.34).

Doppler Echocardiographic Findings in Constriction

Doppler echocardiography has provided substantial insight in to the diagnosis of pericardial constriction and a window on the pathophysiology of intracardiac blood flow in constriction. The classic Doppler findings of pericardial constriction are an exaggerated E/A ratio of mi-

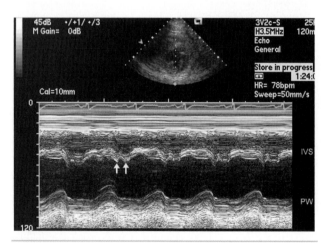

FIGURE 9.31. M-mode echocardiogram recorded in a patient with constrictive pericarditis. Note the flat position of the posterior wall during diastole after initial rapid filling. Also note the abnormal motion of the ventricular septum (*double arrows*). IVS, interventricular septum; PW, posterior wall.

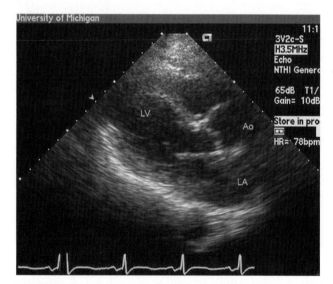

FIGURE 9.32. Parasternal long-axis echocardiogram recorded in a patient with constrictive pericarditis and abnormal motion of the ventricular septum. In this static image, note the normal chamber sizes and configuration of the left ventricle. In the real-time image, note the subtle abnormal motion of the ventricular septum in both diastole and systole. This is a nonspecific septal abnormality, but it is not classic for either left bundle branch block or right ventricular pressure or volume overload. Ao, aorta; LA, left atrium; LV, left ventricle.

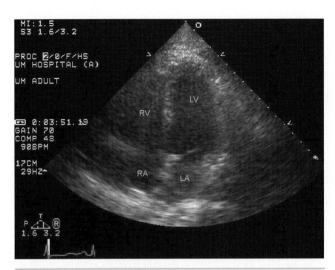

FIGURE 9.33. Apical four-chamber view recorded in a patient with constrictive pericarditis and exaggerated septal position with the respiratory cycle. In this static image, note the normal geometry of all four chambers. In the real-time image, note the exaggerated shift in position of the ventricular septum with the respiratory cycle. During inspiration, there is marked leftward motion of the ventricular septum due to the exaggerated interplay of right ventricular and left ventricular filling during the respiratory cycle. LA, left atrium; LV, left ventricle; RA, right atrium; RV, right ventricle.

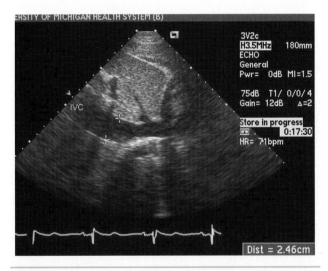

FIGURE 9.34. Subcostal echocardiogram recorded in a patient with constrictive pericarditis revealing a dilated inferior vena cava (*IVC*).

tral valve inflow with a short deceleration time and exaggerated respiratory variation in E-wave velocity (Figs. 9.35–9.38). Although the elevated E/A ratio with a short deceleration time can be seen in any disease state with restrictive or constrictive physiology, exaggerated respiratory variation is a relatively reliable sign of pericardial constriction. In modern practice, it is not uncommon to

see less typical patterns in which there is a normal or reversed E/A ratio with exaggerated respiratory variation or in which only the tricuspid valve inflow reveals classic changes. It should be emphasized, however, that exaggerated respiratory variation in constriction will be seen during normal, quiet, non-labored respiration, whereas an exaggerated respiratory variation in E-wave velocity could be seen in instances of primary respiratory distress as well. Typically, variation of 25% or more in the mitral E-wave velocity between inspiration and expiration has been considered abnormal. The changes noted in atrioventricular valve inflow are maximal with the first several heart beats after inspiration and occur on a reciprocal basis when the mitral and tricuspid flow patterns are compared (Figs. 9.36–9.38). Evaluation of mitral inflow patterns may also reveal exaggerated respiratory variation in the isovolumic relaxation time of the left ventricle.

These classic findings of constriction are usually most prominent when the patient is euvolemic. If absent in a patient in whom constriction is suspected, repeating the Doppler evaluation after volume loading (if volume depleted) or with a head-up tilt (if initially overloaded) may unmask the classic findings.

Doppler interrogation of the hepatic veins often reveals an expiratory increase in diastolic flow reversal (Figs. 9.37 and 9.38). For the more elastic forms of constriction, systolic antegrade flow is increased with inspiration. It should be emphasized that many of these classic findings may not be present in patients with noncalcific pericardial constriction, in patients with localized forms of constriction, and in patients with significant concurrent valvular or myocardial disease.

Effusive Constrictive Pericarditis

Effusive constrictive pericarditis represents a combination of constrictive and tamponade physiology. The most common causes of effusive constrictive pericarditis are malignancy and radiation therapy. Patients with effusive constrictive pericarditis will present with pericardial effusion, often with evidence of marked inflammation. Although hemodynamic embarrassment and tamponade may be present, the thickening of the visceral pericardium may prevent right ventricular or right atrial free wall collapse. This results in a decreased accuracy of individual echocardiographic and Doppler flow patterns for the diagnosis of hemodynamic compromise. From a clinical standpoint, the diagnosis is often established in a patient with hemodynamic compromise and moderate pericardial effusion in whom jugular vein distention and hemodynamic compromise persist after pericardiocentesis. After pericardiocentesis, the effusive component resolves and hemodynamics appear more similar to constriction.

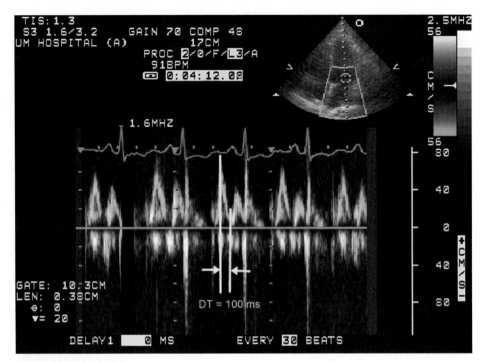

FIGURE 9.35. Pulsed Doppler recording of mitral valve inflow in a 65-year-old patient with constrictive pericarditis. Note the inappropriately elevated E/A ratio and the short deceleration time (*DT*), which averaged 100 milliseconds in this example.

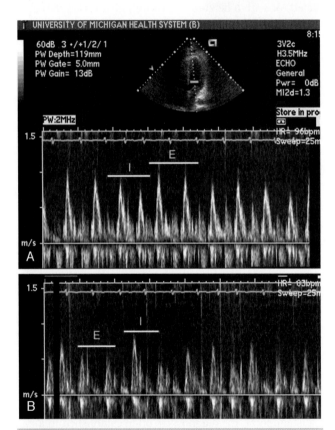

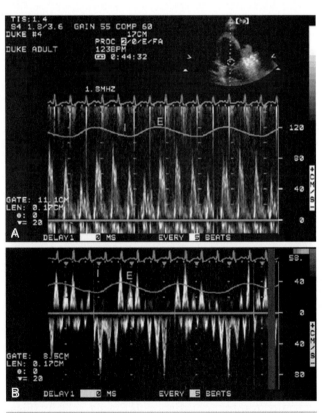

FIGURE 9.36. Pulsed Doppler recording of mitral (**A**) and tricuspid (**B**) inflow in a patient with constrictive pericarditis. Note the exaggerated respiratory variation of the E-wave velocity and the reciprocal relationship between mitral and tricuspid inflow E-wave velocity, dependent on the phase of the respiratory cycle. Note the augmented velocity during inspiration (*I*) and reduced velocity during expiration (*E*) for the tricuspid valve (**B**) compared with the reverse pattern of mitral inflow (**A**).

FIGURE 9.37. Pulsed Doppler recording of mitral inflow and hepatic vein flow recorded in a patient with constrictive pericarditis. **A:** Note the marked respiratory variation in mitral E-wave velocity, similar to that depicted in Figure 9.36. **B:** Note the marked early expiratory (*E*) reversal of flow in the hepatic vein. This results in marked respiratory variation in forward flow in the hepatic vein.

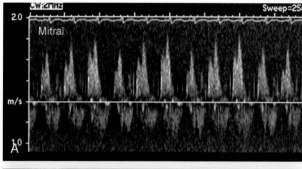

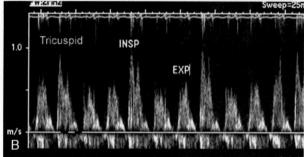

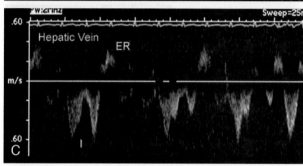

FIGURE 9.38. Pulsed Doppler recording of mitral inflow **(A)**, tricuspid inflow **(B)**, and hepatic vein flow **(C)** from a patient with constrictive pericarditis. In this example from a patient with concurrent diastolic dysfunction, note the reduced E/A ratio of mitral inflow with little respiratory variation. **Middle:** There is definite exaggerated respiratory variation of the tricuspid flow. **Bottom:** Note the respiratory dependency of forward flow in the hepatic vein, with flow confined to inspiration (*INSP*) and the expiratory reversal (*ER*) of flow. EXP, expiration.

Constrictive Pericarditis Versus Restrictive Cardiomyopathy

Both constrictive pericarditis and restrictive cardiomyopathy present as a chronic indolent disease with evidence of volume overload. When classic anatomic abnormalities such as amyloid or other infiltrative cardiomyopathy are noted, the distinction is not difficult. More commonly, the differential diagnosis is between an idiopathic restrictive cardiomyopathy and occult constrictive pericarditis. In these cases, it is important to rely on multiple parameters from a comprehensive Doppler echocardiographic examination to establish the diagnosis. Differentiating features include marked biatrial enlargement in a restrictive cardiomyopathy but relatively normal chamber sizes in con-

striction. In both instances, an elevated E/A ratio may be noted with a shortened deceleration time. Respiratory variation of the E-wave velocity is increased in constriction, whereas it is normal in restrictive cardiomyopathy. Left ventricular isovolumic relaxation time also shows greater respiratory variation in constriction when compared with restrictive cardiomyopathy. Hepatic vein and superior vena caval blood flow patterns also have distinguishing features but are probably less reliable and are substantially more difficult to accurately analyze than are the valve inflow patterns. Typically, in patients with constrictive pericarditis, systolic antegrade flow is enhanced with inspiration, whereas in restriction, there is less respiratory variation and diastolic flow typically exceeds systolic flow.

More recently, Doppler tissue imaging of the mitral anulus has been used to differentiate constrictive pericarditis from restrictive cardiomyopathy. In constriction, there is more rapid early relaxation compared with restriction when diastolic velocities are diminished to below normal (Fig. 9.39). This may be a far more valuable and accurate technique for separating constrictive from restrictive physiology than hepatic or pulmonary view flow analysis.

A final method for differentiating constrictive from restrictive processes is the velocity of propagation (V_p) of mitral inflow determined from mitral color Doppler M-mode imaging (Fig. 9.40). With this technique, the velocity with which the mitral flow moves toward the apex is normal (>55 cm/sec) or frequently exaggerated in constriction, whereas it is pathologically reduced in restriction.

Table 9.3 outlines the expected echocardiographic and Doppler findings in constriction and restriction. It should be

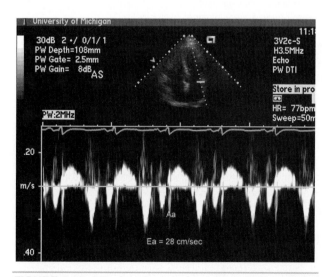

FIGURE 9.39. Mitral anular Doppler tissue imaging recorded in a patient with constrictive pericarditis. Note the E_a and A_a velocities and the E_a velocity of 28 cm/sec, which may be a distinguishing feature when attempting to differentiate constrictive from restrictive physiology.

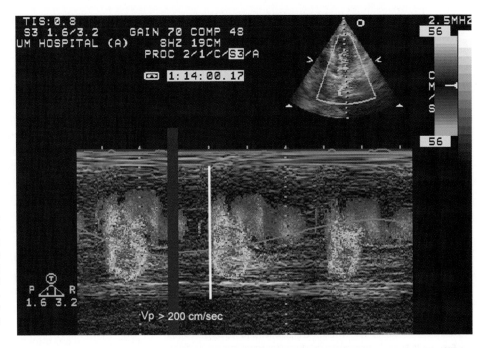

FIGURE 9.40. Color Doppler M-mode recording in a patient with constrictive pericarditis. Note the very steep velocity of propagation (V_p), averaging more than 200 cm/sec in this example. Mitral inflow V_p with this technique may assist in distinguishing constrictive from restrictive physiology.

▶ **TABLE 9.3 Separation of Constrictive Pericarditis from Restrictive Cardiomyopathy**

	Constriction	Restriction
Atrial size	Normal	Dilated
Pericardial appearance	Thick/bright	Normal
Septal motion	Abnormal	Normal
Septal position	Varies with respiration	Normal
Mitral E/A	Increased (≥2.0)	Increased (≥2.0)
Deceleration time	Short (≤160 ms)	Short (≤ 160 ms)
Anular Em	Normal	Reduced (≤10mm/Sec)
Pulmonary hypertension	Rare	Frequent
Left ventricular size/function	Normal	Normal
Mitral/Tricuspid regurgitation	Infrequent	Frequent (TR>MR)
Isovolumic relaxation time	Varies with respiration	Stable with respiration
Respiratory variation of mitral E velocity	Exaggerated (≥25%)	Normal
Color M-mode mitral valve Vp	Increased >55cm/sec	Reduced

The above represents an outline of various parameters which can help in differentiating constrictive pericarditis from restrictive cardiomyopathy. It should be emphasized that in the majority of cases there may be discordant data and that the distinction should be based on the overall appearance and not any single factor. In complex instances such as combined constriction and restriction following radiation or either entity combined with primary valvular heart disease, many exceptions to these guidelines are anticipated.

emphasized that no one finding will be 100% accurate and that a clinical diagnosis of either entity should be based on a combination of clinical and echocardiographic findings combined with other methods (e.g., computed tomography, magnetic resonance imaging) to define pericardial anatomy.

MISCELLANEOUS PERICARDIAL DISORDERS AND OBSERVATIONS

Postoperative Effusions

Pericardial effusion is not uncommon after cardiac surgery and can range from small and self-limited to larger effusions that cause varying degrees of compromise. Postoperative effusions are most commonly localized to the posterior and lateral aspects of the heart and may be loculated (Fig. 9.41 and 9.42). In this location, they can cause isolated, differential compression of one or more chambers, in distinction to a native pericardial effusion, which causes hydrodynamic compression of all cardiac chambers equally. Complicating their assessment is the postoperative status of the patient, which often interferes with transthoracic imaging and for whom transesophageal echocardiography may be necessary. It should also be emphasized that a postoperative pericardial effusion is by definition hemorrhagic and that there

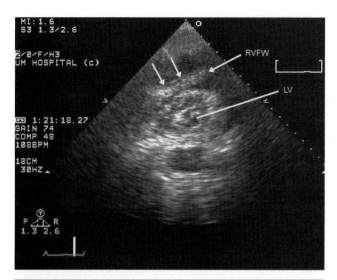

FIGURE 9.41. Parasternal transthoracic echocardiogram recorded in a patient with a compressive pericardial hematoma after bypass surgery. Note the small left ventricular cavity (*LV*) and the abnormal contour of the right ventricular free wall (*RVFW*). In this mid-diastolic frame, the right ventricular free wall is compressed toward the ventricular septum (*arrows*), compromising filling of the right ventricle.

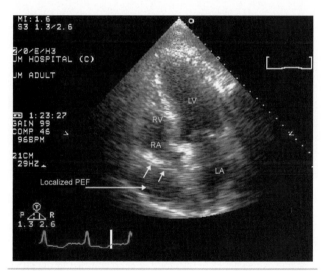

FIGURE 9.42. Apical four-chamber view recorded in a patient after cardiac surgery who had clinical evidence of hemodynamic compromise. Note the normal size and shape of the right ventricle (*RV*), left ventricle (*LV*), and left atrium (*LA*), but the marked compression of the right atrium (*RA*) by a localized pericardial effusion (*arrows*).

will be components of intrapericardial hematoma present as well. The intrapericardial hematoma will have a density similar to that of the myocardium and other mediastinal structures, and a heightened awareness of the possible presence of hematoma within the pericardium is necessary. In evaluating a critically ill patient with a suspected postoperative pericardial effusion or

hematoma, it is important to evaluate the size and geometry of all four cardiac chambers and attempt to identify the inflow from the pulmonary veins and superior inferior vena cava. Loculated effusions and hematoma after cardiac surgery can result in isolated compression of one or more pulmonary veins or of vena caval inflow, either of which can compromise overall cardiac output. Identification of small, underfilled chambers that appear compressed may be indirect evidence of a compressive pericardial hematoma in this setting.

Echocardiography-Guided Pericardiocentesis

Echocardiography plays several valuable roles with respect to therapeutic pericardiocentesis. Obviously, the first role is in determining the presence and distribution of a pericardial effusion and the presence of hemodynamic compromise. If pericardiocentesis is contemplated, multiple echocardiographic imaging windows should be used to determine the distribution of the fluid. Specifically, the distribution and depth from the surface of the chest at which contact with the fluid is anticipated by the pericardiocentesis needle should be determined (Fig. 9.43). Many laboratories perform continuous echocardiographic guidance of pericardiocentesis and attempt to visualize the pericardiocentesis needle as it enters the pericardial cavity (Fig. 9.44). Although this may be helpful to avoid cardiac damage in a relatively small effusion, it plays little incremental role in larger pericardial effu-

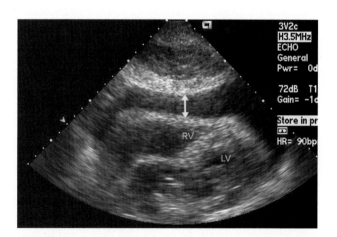

FIGURE 9.43. Echocardiogram recorded from the subcostal position in a patient with a moderate pericardial effusion. Note the approximate 1.5-cm distance between the pericardium and right ventricular free wall (*arrows*), implying a significant distance between the pericardium and heart, which may confer a decreased risk of pericardiocentesis if approached from the subcostal position. LV, left ventricle; RV, right ventricle.

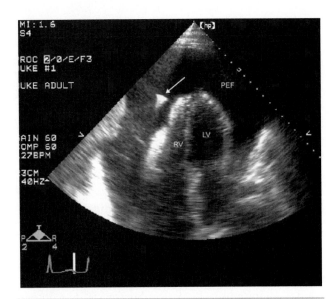

FIGURE 9.44. Apical four-chamber view recorded in a patient with a large pericardial effusion (*PEF*) and cardiac tamponade. Ultrasound guidance is being used as a needle is placed into the pericardial space. The needle is seen as a bright echo density (*arrow*) lateral to the right ventricular free wall. LV, left ventricle; RV, right ventricle.

sions, which are usually the target for a therapeutic pericardiocentesis. If the location of a pericardiocentesis needle is in question, agitated saline can be injected to further define the location of the needle tip (Fig. 9.45). A very reliable indicator that the pericardiocentesis needle is indeed in the pericardial fluid and the procedure can be appropriately continued is when characteristic contrast bubbles are noted in the pericaradial space.

After pericardiocentesis, two-dimensional echocardiography can be used to determine the completeness of fluid removal. In patients with large long-standing pericardial effusions, a syndrome of acute right heart dilation is occasionally seen after large-volume pericardiocentesis. This probably occurs when a large intravascular volume that had been sequestered outside the cardiac chambers is suddenly allowed unlimited entry into the right heart. This can result in acute right heart dilation with clinical evidence of mild right heart failure. This syndrome is typically self-limited.

Congenital absence of the pericardium can occur in either a partial or, less commonly, complete form. It is often asymptomatic; however, in the partial form, the left atrial appendage or, less commonly, the right atrial appendage may herniate through the pericardial defect and become strangulated, resulting in symptoms. Because of the lack of pericardial constraint on cardiac chamber size, there may be an abnormal position of the cardiac silhouette on a chest radiograph and mild degrees of right atrial and right ventricular dilation. Abnormal and frequently paradoxical ventricular septal motion has also been reported.

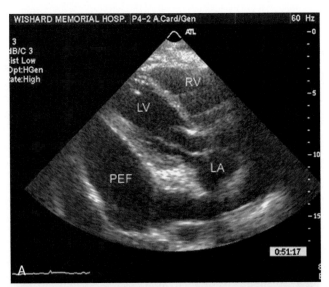

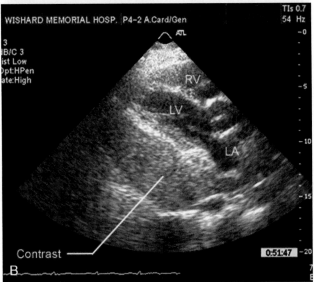

FIGURE 9.45. Parasternal long-axis echocardiogram recorded in a patient with a large posterior pericardial effusion (*PEF*). Pericardiocentesis is being undertaken with echocardiographic guidance. **A:** Note the clear, large posterior pericardial fluid collection. **B:** Agitated saline has been injected via the pericardiocentesis needle. Note the cloud of echo contrast in the previously clear pericardial space confirming that the pericardiocentesis needle is indeed in the pericardium. LA, left atrium; LV, left ventricle, RV, right ventricle.

Pericardial Cysts

Pericardial cysts are benign developmental anomalies that most commonly occur near the costophrenic angle. They appear as a loculated echo-free space adjacent to the cardiac border, most commonly near the right atrium (Fig. 9.46). They frequently distort the normal shape of the atrium. The diagnosis is best confirmed by computed tomography or magnetic resonance imaging. Additional echocardiographic evaluation should include contrast

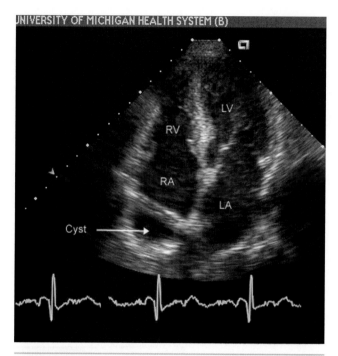

FIGURE 9.46. Apical four-chamber view recorded in a patient with a pericardial cyst. Note the normal geometry of all four cardiac chambers and the echo-free space immediately behind the right atrium (*RA*). Color flow Doppler confirmed that there was no organized flow within the space and no evidence of hemodynamic compromise. This mass was confirmed to be a benign pericardial cyst at the time of thorascopic surgery. LA, left atrium; LV, left ventricle; RV, right ventricle.

echocardiography to exclude an anomalous systemic vein that may also present as an unusually located echo-free structure. Color flow and pulsed Doppler interrogation at low-velocity settings can be used to ensure that there is no phasic flow within the structure.

SUGGESTED READINGS

Applefeld MM, Slawson RG, Hall-Craigs M, et al. Delayed pericardial disease after radiotherapy. Am J Cardiol 1981;47:210–213.

Armstrong WF, Schilt BF, Helper DJ, et al. Diastolic collapse of the right ventricle with cardiac tamponade: an echocardiographic study. Circulation 1982;65:1491–1496.

Armstrong WF, Feigenbaum H, Dillon JC. Acute right ventricular dilation and echocardiographic volume overload following pericardiocentesis for relief of cardiac tamponade. Am Heart J 1984;107:1266–1270.

Byrd BF 3rd, Linden RW. Superior vena cava Doppler flow velocity patterns in pericardial disease. Am J Cardiol 1990;65:1464–1470.

Chandraratna PA. Echocardiography and Doppler ultrasound in the evaluation of pericardial disease. Circulation 1991;84:I303–I310.

Chuttani K, Pandian NG, Mohanty PK, et al. Left ventricular diastolic collapse. An echocardiographic sign of regional cardiac tamponade. Circulation 1991;83:1999–2006.

D'Cruz IA, Cohen HC, Prabhu R, et al. Diagnosis of cardiac tamponade by echocardiography: changes in mitral valve motion and ventricular dimensions, with special reference to paradoxical pulse. Circulation 1975;52:460–465.

Feigenbaum H, Waldhausen JA, Hyde LP. Ultrasound diagnosis of pericardial effusion. JAMA 1965;191:711–714.

Garcia MJ, Rodriguez L, Ares M, et al. Differentiation of constrictive pericarditis from restrictive cardiomyopathy: assessment of left ventricular diastolic velocities in longitudinal axis by Doppler tissue imaging. J Am Coll Cardiol 1996;27:108–114.

Gatzoulis MA, Munk MD, Merchant N, et al. Isolated congenital absence of the pericardium: clinical presentation, diagnosis, and management. Ann Thorac Surg 200;69:1209–1215.

Gibson TC, Grossman W, McLaurin LP, et al. An echocardiographic study of the interventricular septum in constrictive pericarditis. Br Heart J 1976;38:738–743.

Gillam LD, Guyer DE, Gibson TC, et al. Hydrodynamic compression of the right atrium: a new echocardiographic sign of cardiac tamponade. Circulation 1983;68:294–301.

Horowitz MS, Schultz CS, Stinson EB, et al. Sensitivity and specificity of echocardiographic diagnosis of pericardial effusion. Circulation 1974;50:239–247.

Hurrell DG, Nishimura RA, Higano ST, et al. Value of dynamic respiratory changes in left and right ventricular pressures for the diagnosis of constrictive pericarditis. Circulation 1996;93:2007–2013.

King SW, Pandian NG, Gardin JM. Doppler echocardiographic findings in pericardial tamponade and constriction. Echocardiography 1988;5:361–372.

Kronzon I, Cohen ML, Winer HE. Diastolic atrial compression: a sensitive echocardiographic sign of cardiac tamponade. J Am Coll Cardiol 1983;2:770–775.

Ling LH, Oh JK, Schaff HV, et al. Constrictive pericarditis in the modern era: evolving clinical spectrum and impact on outcome after pericardiectomy. Circulation 1999;100:1380–1386.

Mazzoni V, Taiti A, Bartoletti A, et al. The spectrum of pericardial effusion in acute myocardial infarction: an echocardiographic study. Ital Heart J 2000;1:45–49.

Merce J, Sagrista-Sauleda J, Permanyer-Miralda G, et al. Correlation between clinical and Doppler echocardiographic findings in patients with moderate and large pericardial effusion: implications for the diagnosis of cardiac tamponade. Am Heart J 1999;138:759–764.

Miller SW, Feldman L, Palacios I, et al. Compression of the superior vena cava and right atrium in cardiac tamponade. Am J Cardiol 1982;50:1287–1292.

Myers RB, Spodick DH. Constrictive pericarditis: clinical and pathophysiologic characteristics. Am Heart J 2999;138:219–232.

Oh JK, Hatle LK, Mulvagh SL, et al. Transient constrictive pericarditis: diagnosis by two-dimensional Doppler echocardiography. Mayo Clin Proc 1993;68:1158–1164.

Oh JK, Hatle LK, Seward JB, et al. Diagnostic role of Doppler echocardiography in constrictive pericarditis. J Am Coll Cardiol 1994;23:154–162.

Oh JK, Tajik AJ, Appleton CP, et al. Preload reduction to unmask the characteristic Doppler features of constrictive pericarditis. A new observation. Circulation 1997;95:796–799.

Palka P, Lange A, Donnelly J, et al. Differentiation between restrictive cardiomyopathy and constrictive pericarditis by early diastolic Doppler myocardial velocity gradient at the posterior wall. Circulation 2000;102:655–662.

Picard MH, Sanfilippo AJ, Newell JB, et al. Quantitative relation between increased intrapericardial pressure and Doppler flow velocities during experimental cardiac tamponade. J Am Coll Cardiol 1991;18:234–242.

Prakash AM, Sun Y, Chiaramida SA, et al. Quantitative assessment of pericardial effusion volume by two-dimensional echocardiography. J Am Soc Echocardiogr 2003;16:147–153.

Sagrista-Sauleda J, Permanyer-Miralda G, Candell-Riera J, et al. Transient cardiac constriction: an unrecognized pattern of evolution in effusive acute idiopathic pericarditis. Am J Cardiol 1987;59:961–966.

Schiller NB, Botvinick EH. Right ventricular compression as a sign of cardiac tamponade: an analysis of echocardiographic ventricular dimensions and their clinical implications. Circulation 1977;56:774–779.

Senni M, Redfield MM, Ling LH, et al. Left ventricular systolic and diastolic function after pericardiectomy in patients with constrictive pericarditis: Doppler echocardiographic findings and correlation with clinical status. J Am Coll Cardiol 1999;33:1182–1188.

Tabata T, Kabbani SS, Murray RD, et al. Difference in the respiratory variation between pulmonary venous and mitral inflow Doppler velocities in patients with constrictive pericarditis with and without atrial fibrillation. J Am Coll Cardiol 2001;37:1936–1942.

Tsang TS, Barnes ME, Hayes SN, et al. Clinical and echocardiographic characteristics of significant pericardial effusions following cardiothoracic surgery and outcomes of echo-guided pericardiocentesis for management: Mayo Clinic experience, 1979–1998. Chest 1999;116:322–331.

Aortic Valve Disease

The aortic valve is a complex, intricate structure with remarkable durability. It is composed of three cusps of equal size, each of which is surrounded by a sinus. The cusps are separated by three commissures and supported by a fibrous anulus. Each cusp is crescent shaped and capable of opening fully to allow unimpeded forward flow, then closing tightly to prevent regurgitation. The free edge of each cusp curves upward from the commissure and forms a slight thickening at the tip or midpoint, called the Arantius nodule. When the valve closes, the three nodes meet in the center, allowing coaptation to occur along three lines that radiate out from this center point. Overlap of valve tissue along the lines of closure produces a tight seal and prevents backflow during diastole. When viewed from a conventional echocardiographic short-axis projection, these three lines of closure are recorded as a Y shape.

Behind each cusp is its associated Valsalva sinus. The sinuses represent outpouchings in the aortic root directly behind each cusp. They function to support the cusps during systole and provide a reservoir of blood to augment coronary artery flow during diastole. The sinus and its corresponding cusp share the same name. The left and right coronary arteries arise from the left and right sinuses, respectively, and are associated with the left and right aortic cusps. The third, or noncoronary sinus, is posterior and rightward, just above the base of the interatrial septum, and is associated with the noncoronary aortic cusp. At the superior margin of the sinuses, the aortic root narrows at the sinotubular junction.

Diseases of the aortic valve may be either congenital or acquired and may produce either stenosis or regurgitation or a combination of the two. The most common causes of acquired aortic valve disease in adults are degenerative, rheumatic, and infective. Diseases of the aorta may also affect aortic valve function. Subaortic obstruction may also occur. This is due either to hypertrophic cardiomyopathy (see Chapter 17) or membranous and fibromuscular subaortic stenosis (see Chapter 18).

AORTIC STENOSIS

Although obstruction to left ventricular outflow can occur at multiple levels, valvular aortic stenosis is most common. Congenitally abnormal valves may be stenotic at birth or may develop both stenosis and regurgitation over time (Fig. 10.1). Typically, such valves are bicuspid, demonstrate systolic "doming," and tend to become functionally abnormal during adolescence or early adulthood (Fig. 10.2). This form of aortic valve disease is covered more fully in Chapter 18. Most cases of aortic stenosis are acquired, that is, the valves are normal at birth but become gradually dysfunctional over time. The goals of the echocardiographic evaluation of this condition include establishing a diagnosis, quantifying severity, and assessing left ventricular function. A summary of the indications for echocardiography in the setting of valvular stenosis is provided in Table 10.1. The simultaneous assessment of left ventricular function is important because of its prognostic and management implications. In addition, reduced left ventricular function alters the relationship between transvalvular pressure gradient and aortic valve area, thereby complicating the quantitative determination of severity. Other related factors that must be evaluated include the presence and extent of proximal aorta dilation, coexisting mitral valve disease, a measurement of pulmonary artery pressure, and coexisting coronary artery disease.

The *qualitative* diagnosis of aortic stenosis relies heavily on two-dimensional echocardiography. By observing the opening and closing of the valve in systole and diastole, respectively, the presence or absence of valvular stenosis can be determined with confidence. In normal subjects, the aortic valve cusps appear thin and delicate and may be difficult to visualize (Fig. 10.3). In the long-axis view, the cusps open rapidly in systole and appear as linear parallel lines close to the walls of the aorta (Fig. 10.4). With the onset of diastole, they come together and are recorded as a faint linear density within the plane of

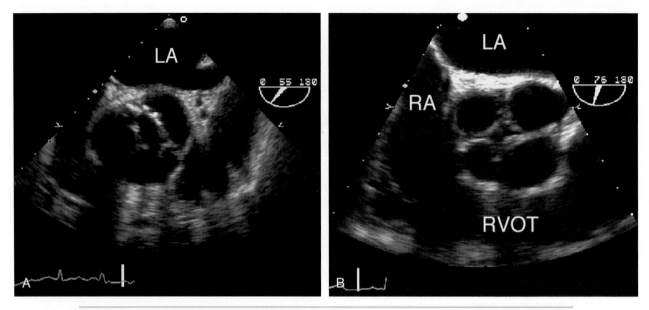

FIGURE 10.1. Examples of congenital forms of aortic valve disease are illustrated. **A:** A short-axis view demonstrates a bicuspid aortic valve. **B:** A quadricuspid aortic valve is shown from transesophageal echocardiography. LA, left atrium; RA, right atrium; RVOT, right ventricular outflow tract.

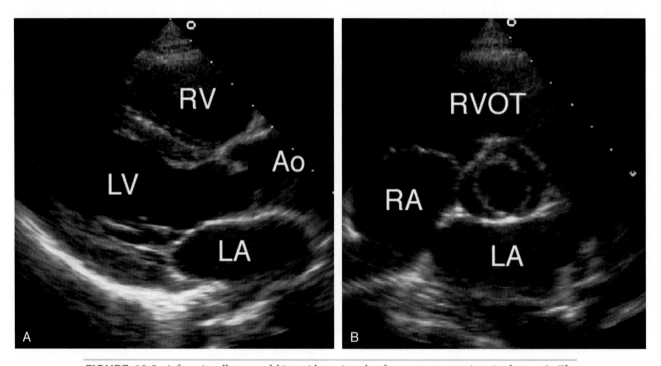

FIGURE 10.2. A functionally normal bicuspid aortic valve from a young patient is shown. **A:** The long-axis view demonstrates doming of the valve in systole. **B:** The basal short-axis view confirms that the valve is bicuspid but with no evidence of stenosis. Ao, aorta; LA, left atrium; RA, right atrium; RV, right ventricle; RVOT, right ventricular outflow tract.

▶ TABLE 10.1 Indications for Echocardiography in Valvular Stenosis

Indication	Class
1. Diagnosis; assessment of hemodynamic severity	I
2. Assessment of left and right ventricular size, function, and/or hemodynamics	I
3. Reevaluation of patients with known valvular stenosis with changing symptoms or signs	I
4. Assessment of changes in hemodynamic severity and ventricular compensation in patients with known valvular stenosis during pregnancy	I
5. Reevaluation of asymptomatic patients with severe stenosis	I
6. Assessment of the hemodynamic significance of mild to moderate valvular stenosis by stress Doppler echocardiography	IIa
7. Reevaluation of patients with mild to moderate aortic stenosis with left ventricular dysfunction hypertrophy even without clinical symptoms	IIa
8. Reevaluation of patients with mild to moderate aortic valvular stenosis with stable signs and symptoms	IIb
9. Dobutamine echocardiography for the evaluation of patients with low-gradient aortic stenosis and ventricular dysfunction	IIb
10. Routine reevaluation of asymptomatic adult patients with mild aortic stenosis having stable physical signs and normal left ventricular size and function	III

Adapted from Cheitlin MD, Alpert JS, Armstrong WF, et al. ACC/AHA Guidelines for the Clinical Application of Echocardiography: A Report of the American College of Cardiology/ American Heart Association Task Force on Practice Guidelines (Committee on Clinical Application of Echocardiography) Developed in Collaboration With the American Society of Echocardiography. Circulation 1997;95:1686–1744, with permission.

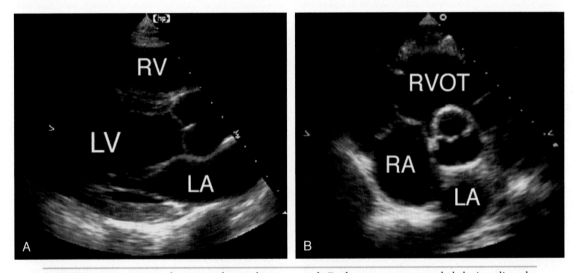

FIGURE 10.3. A normal aortic valve is demonstrated. Both parts were recorded during diastole. **A:** The long-axis view demonstrates the appearance of a typical normal aortic valve in the closed position. **B:** The same valve is demonstrated from the short-axis view. Note that, because of shadowing and lateral resolution, the coaptation line between the left and noncoronary cusps is not visualized. LA, left atrium; LV, left ventricle; RA, right atrium; RV, right ventricle; RVOT, right ventricular outflow tract.

the aortic anulus. Because the velocity of valve motion during opening and closing is high relative to the frame rate of most echocardiographic systems, the normal aortic valve is usually visualized either fully opened or closed but rarely in any intermediate position. In the basal short-axis view, the three aortic cusps can be visualized within the anulus during diastole (Fig. 10.5). The three lines of coaptation can be recorded, normally forming a Y (sometimes referred to as an inverted Mercedes-Benz sign). With the

onset of systole, the cusps open out of the imaging plane, providing a view of the aortic anulus. The short-axis perspective is most helpful to determine the number of cusps and whether fusion of one or more commissures is present. In patients who are difficult to image, normal leaflets are so delicate that they are hard to visualize, generally an indication that they are morphologically normal.

With acquired valvular aortic stenosis, the cusps become thickened and restricted (Fig. 10.6). Their position

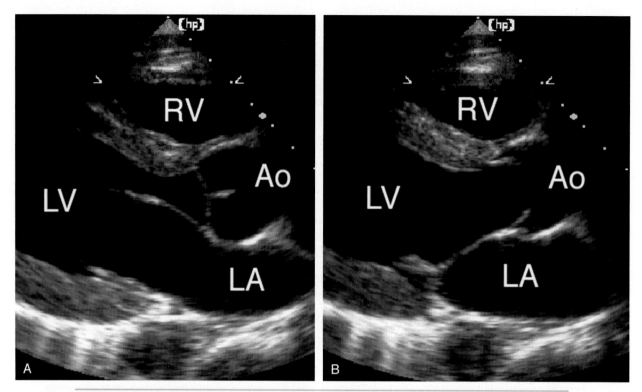

FIGURE 10.4. A normal aortic valve is shown during diastole in the closed position (**A**) and during systole in the open position (**B**). Ao, aorta; LA, left atrium; LV, left ventricle; RV, right ventricle.

during systole is no longer parallel to the aortic walls, and the edges are often seen to point toward the center of the aorta. In severe cases, a nearly total lack of mobility may be present and the anatomy may become so distorted that identification of the individual cusps is impossible. Unfortunately, attempts to quantify the degree of stenosis based on two-dimensional echocardiographic findings have been unsuccessful. However, useful qualitative information is almost always present. For example, if one cusp can be seen to move normally, critical aortic stenosis has been excluded. Figure 10.7 is an example of mild aortic stenosis. Although the diagnosis of aortic stenosis is apparent by two-dimensional imaging, the degree of severity can only be estimated. In the example, the cusps are thickened and exhibit restricted mobility. However, Doppler examination revealed only mild stenosis with a maximal pressure gradient of approximately 28 mm Hg. In this example, based solely on two-dimensional appearance, overestimation of severity would be likely. Figure 10.8 is of a patient with heart failure and moderate left ventricular dysfunction. Note also that the aortic valve is severely calcified with markedly restricted systolic mobility.

One approach to quantitation relies on transesophageal echocardiography. This technique is excellent for determining the morphology of abnormal aortic valves. From a short-axis view at the level of the valve ori-

fice, direct planimetry of the valve area is possible in more than 90% of patients (Fig. 10.9). Limitations of this approach include the three-dimensional nature of the orifice and the shadowing effect of a calcified valve and root. As a result, the technical challenges of this approach are considerable and it is not routinely performed.

Doppler Assessment of Aortic Stenosis

The Doppler assessment of aortic stenosis begins with the determination of the maximal jet velocity through the stenotic valve. From this value, the simplified Bernoulli equation is used to estimate the peak instantaneous gradient. This approach has been validated both in *in vitro* and in clinical situations. It has proved to be a practical, noninvasive method for determining the pressure gradient across the aortic valve, correlating well with simultaneous measurements obtained by invasive means.

An accurate Doppler assessment of aortic stenosis depends on one's ability to record the maximal jet velocity through the stenotic orifice (Fig. 10.10). As blood accelerates through the valve, peak velocity coincides temporally with the maximal pressure gradient. Peak velocity usually occurs in mid systole. As aortic stenosis worsens, velocity tends to peak later in systole, sometimes offering a clue to severity. Late peaking jets are also characteristic of dy-

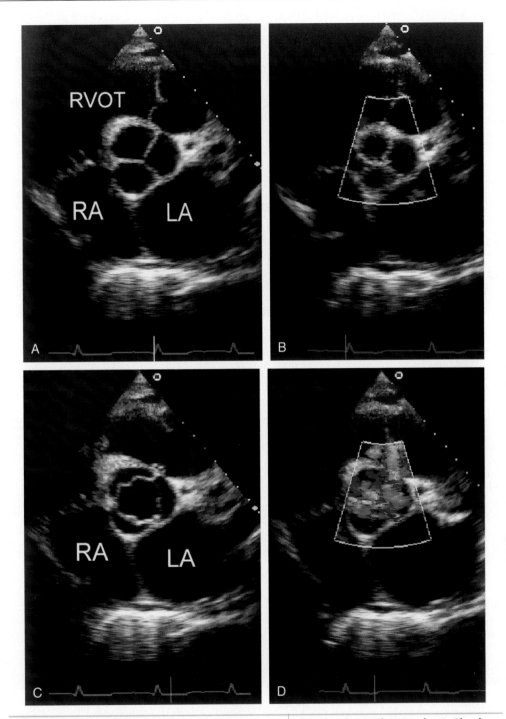

FIGURE 10.5. A normal tricuspid aortic valve is shown with and without color Doppler. **A:** The short-axis view demonstrates the three cusps during diastole. **B:** A diastolic frame with color flow imaging demonstrates trivial aortic regurgitation. **C:** The valve is shown during systole demonstrating the orifice in an open position. **D:** Color flow imaging during systole demonstrates the flow through the valve. LA, left atrium; RA, right atrium; RVOT, right ventricular outflow tract.

namic subaortic stenosis, as occurs in hypertrophic cardiomyopathy (Fig. 10.11). Multiple windows, including the apical five-chamber, suprasternal, and right parasternal, should be used in an attempt to align the Doppler beam with the direction of flow of the stenotic jet. Failure to

achieve parallel alignment will result in underestimation of true velocity (Fig. 10.12). Both imaging and nonimaging continuous wave transducers should be used. Because the direction of jet flow is difficult to predict from two-dimensional imaging, color Doppler imaging may be used to im-

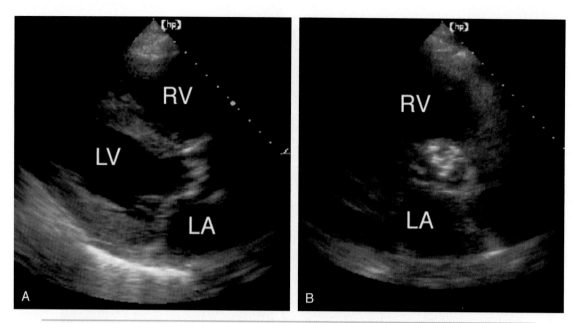

FIGURE 10.6. A two-dimensional echocardiogram from a patient with severe aortic stenosis is shown. **A:** The long-axis view reveals an echogenic and very immobile aortic valve. **B:** The corresponding short-axis view suggests a high degree of calcification of the valve and minimal mobility during systole. LA, left atrium; LV, left ventricle; RV, right ventricle.

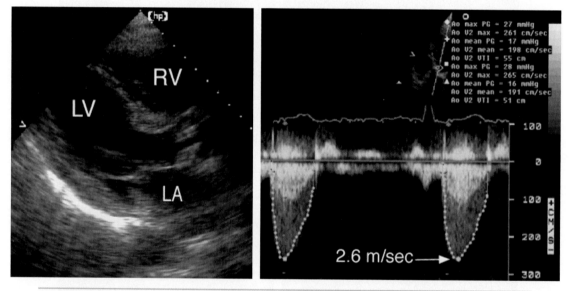

FIGURE 10.7. A patient with mild aortic stenosis is shown. See text for details. LA, left atrium; LV, left ventricle; RV, right ventricle.

prove alignment. In addition, angle correction is available on many ultrasound instruments. This is a simple algorithm that automatically adjusts the displayed gradient or velocity based on a manually defined estimate of angle θ. Although conceptually attractive, this correction is just as likely to introduce error into the gradient calculation, particularly because an accurate three-dimensional determination of θ is so difficult. Thus, in most cases, angle correction should not be used. Instead, careful manipulation

of the transducer position to achieve optimal alignment is recommended. In practice, a thorough and patient interrogation using all available echocardiographic windows is undertaken to record the highest velocity signal possible. By carefully adjusting patient position and instrument gain, both the full envelope and the peak velocity of the stenotic jet can be obtained. In Figure 10.12, the peak gradient would have been underestimated if the echocardiographer had concluded the examination with the apical

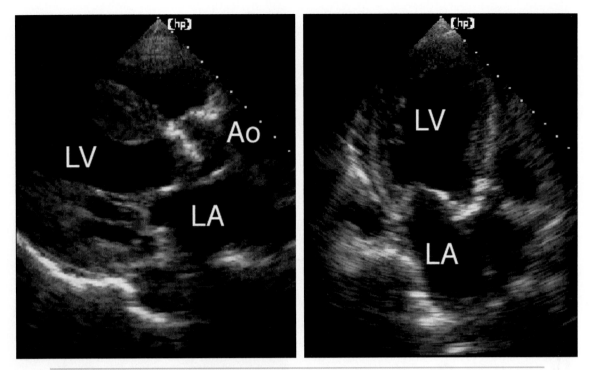

FIGURE 10.8. An example of severe aortic stenosis in the setting of left ventricular dysfunction is provided. The valve is calcified and immobile. A qualitative diagnosis of aortic stenosis is possible, but no quantitative information is available. Ao, aorta; LA, left atrium; LV, left ventricle.

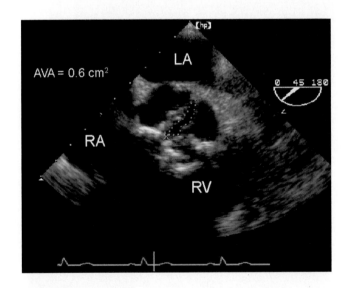

FIGURE 10.9. A transesophageal echocardiogram demonstrates the method of direct planimetry of the aortic valve orifice. By carefully adjusting the level of the short-axis plane, the orifice can be visualized in most patients. In this example, severe stenosis was confirmed. AVA, aortic valve area; LA, left atrium; RA, right atrium; RV, right ventricle.

views rather than moving to the right parasternal window where a higher velocity was recorded.

From the Doppler recording, the peak instantaneous and mean pressure gradient can be determined (Fig. 10.13). The maximal gradient is derived from the equation:

$$\Delta P \text{ (in mm Hg)} = 4v^2 \qquad \text{[Eq. 10.1]}$$

where v equals the maximal jet velocity expressed in meters per second. The mean pressure gradient is most of-

ten obtained by planimetry of the Doppler envelope, which allows the computer to integrate the instantaneous velocity data and provide a mean value. It should be emphasized that mean gradient cannot be obtained by squaring the mean velocity. Because of the nearly linear relationship between mean gradient and maximal gradient, the mean pressure gradient can also be estimated from the formula:

$$\Delta P_{\text{mean}} = \frac{\Delta P_{\text{max}}}{1.45} + 2 \text{ mm Hg} \qquad \text{[Eq. 10.2]}$$

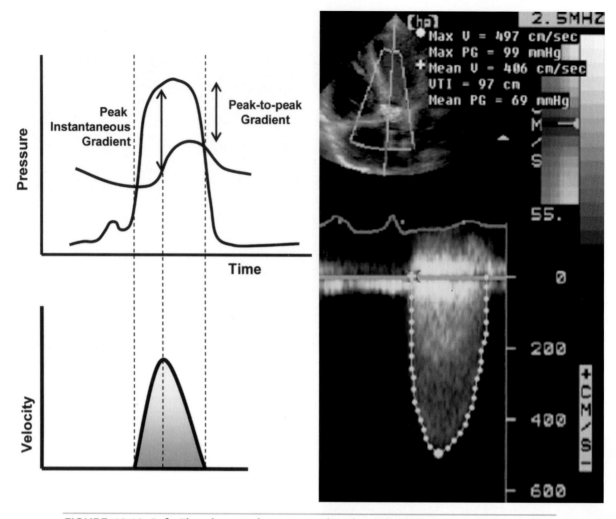

FIGURE 10.10. Left: The schematic demonstrates the relationship between the pressure gradient across a stenotic aortic valve and the velocity tracing obtained by Doppler. The differences between peak-to-peak and peak instantaneous gradients are illustrated. The maximal flow velocity obtained with Doppler imaging corresponds temporally with the peak instantaneous gradient. **Right:** A Doppler recording from a patient with severe aortic stenosis demonstrates a peak instantaneous gradient of approximately 100 mm Hg.

FIGURE 10.11. A late-peaking gradient from a patient with hypertrophic cardiomyopathy is shown. This obstruction occurs at the level of the left ventricular outflow tract and results in a gradient of approximately 50 mm Hg. Note the contour of the jet with acceleration of flow in mid and late systole.

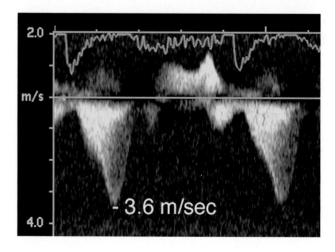

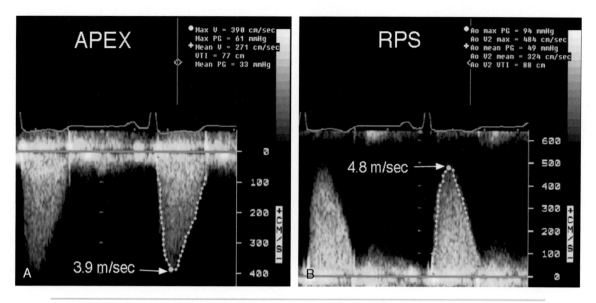

FIGURE 10.12. Aortic stenosis should be quantified using Doppler from multiple windows. **A:** A recording from the apical view is provided. **B:** A higher gradient is obtained from the right parasternal (*RPS*) window. See text for details.

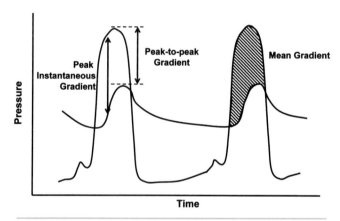

FIGURE 10.13. This schematic demonstrates the differences between peak-to-peak, peak instantaneous, and mean gradients. See text for details.

Stated differently, Equation 10.2 suggests that mean gradient is approximately two-thirds of the peak instantaneous gradient. Both mean and peak gradients should be reported.

The accuracy of the Bernoulli equation to quantify aortic stenosis pressure gradients is well established (Fig. 10.14). Selective studies that have validated the modified Bernoulli equation against invasive hemodynamic measurements are shown in Table 10.2. When discrepancies in measurements occur, several possibilities should be considered. The technical quality of the Doppler data should first be examined. A technically poor recording may fail to display the highest velocity signals, resulting in underestimation of the true gradient. An inability to align the interrogation angle parallel to flow also results

in underestimation. This relationship is demonstrated in Figure 10.15. The various curves plot the relationship between jet velocity and calculated peak gradient (using the Bernoulli equation), assuming different values for angle θ. Note that for low velocity jets (<3 m/sec), the magnitude of the error introduced by angle misalignment is relatively modest. For patients with severe aortic stenosis, errors in alignment cause substantial underestimation of true gradient. Also note that errors less than 20 degrees result in a relatively insignificant degree of underestimation. However, as the intercept angle increases beyond 20 degrees, the magnitude of error increases rapidly.

Because the Doppler technique measures velocity over time, Doppler-derived data always represent *instantaneous* gradients. It is customary in the cardiac catheterization laboratory to report the peak-to-peak gradient, which is often less than the peak instantaneous gradient. This is illustrated in Figure 10.13. It is well known that peak-to-peak gradients are contrived and never exist in time. Failure to recognize the differences in the reported data often leads to miscommunication of clinical information. This can be partially avoided through the use of mean gradients, which correlate better between catheterization and echocardiographic data. Finally, bear in mind that valve gradients are dynamic measurements that vary with heart rate, loading conditions, blood pressure, and inotropic state. Figure 10.16 is an example of varying jet velocities from a patient with an arrhythmia. Note how each recorded beat yields a different peak instantaneous gradient, ranging from approximately 35 to more than 100 mm Hg. If two tests are performed on different days, the results may be expected to vary. It is therefore not surprising that the best correlation between invasive hemo-

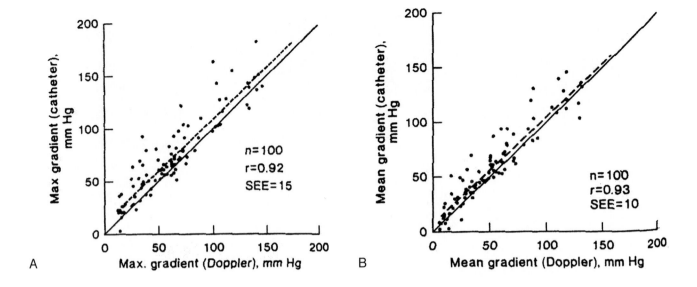

FIGURE 10.14. The correlation between Doppler and cardiac catheterization for measuring peak (**A**) and mean (**B**) gradients are shown. The relationship is linear and a similar degree of correlation is shown for both mean and peak gradient. (From Currie PJ, Seward JB, Reeder GS, et al. Continuous-wave Doppler echocardiographic assessment of severity of calcific aortic stenosis: a simultaneous Doppler-catheter correlative study in 100 adult patients. Circulation 1985;71:1162–1169, with permission.)

dynamics and Doppler is achieved in studies in which the tests are performed simultaneously. When catheterization and Doppler results differ, both tests may be correct but may reflect variations in gradient over time.

Overestimation of the true pressure gradient is less common but can occur. This is usually the result of mistaken identity of the recorded signal. For example, the mitral regurgitation jet has a contour similar to that of a jet of severe aortic stenosis. Because of the similarities in location and direction of the two jets, mistaken identity can occur. To avoid this, the two jets should be recorded by sweeping the transducer back and forth to clearly indicate to the interpreter which jet is which. Another helpful clue involves the timing of the two jets (Fig. 10.17). Mitral regurgitation is longer in duration, beginning during isovolumic contraction and extending into isovolumic relaxation.

▶ TABLE 10.2 **Correlation between Echocardiographic Doppler Techniques and Cardiac Catheterization for Assessing the Severity of Aortic Stenosis**

Ref.	N	Maximal Pressure Gradient		Aortic Valve Area	
		r Value	SSE (mm Hg)	r Value	SSE (cm²)
Stamm and Martin, 1983	35	0.94	12		
Simpson et al., 1985	33	0.92			
Currie et al., 1985	100	0.92	15		
Yeager et al., 1986[a]	52	0.87	11		
Currie et al., 1986	62	0.95	11		
Teirstein et al., 1986[a]	31	0.92	8	0.88	0.17
Zoghbi et al., 1986	39			0.95	0.15
Harrison et al.,1988	58	0.89		0.81	0.16
Oh et al., 1988[a]	100	0.86	10	0.83	0.19
Grayburn et al.,1988[b]	25			0.92	0.26
Tribouilloy et al., 1994[c]	25			0.90	0.12
Cormier et al., 1996	41			0.78	
Kim et al., 1997[c]	81			0.89	0.04

[a]Data are for mean rather than peak gradient.
[b]All patients with severe aortic regurgitation.
[c]Echo valve area by planimetry using transesophageal echocardiography.

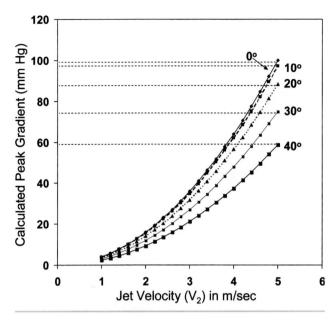

FIGURE 10.15. The effect of incident angle (θ) on recorded velocity is demonstrated. When the angle is 0 degrees (*uppermost curve*), the Bernoulli equation provides an accurate measure of gradient. As θ increases, an increasing degree of underestimation occurs. See text for details.

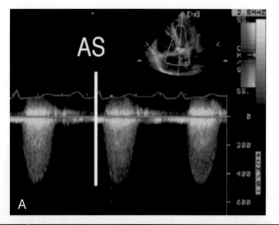

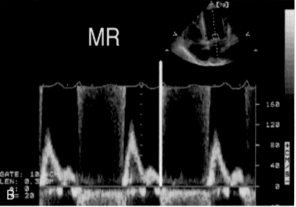

FIGURE 10.17. The jets of aortic stenosis (*AS*) and mitral regurgitation (*MR*) can sometimes be confused. A helpful clue to differentiate between the two involves the timing of flow. **A:** Aortic flow begins after the period of isovolumic contraction. The vertical line provides a reference mark relative to the QRS of the electrocardiogram. Note the gap between the line and the onset of flow. **B:** The same line coincides with the onset of mitral regurgitation. This is because mitral regurgitation occurs during isovolumic contraction. In addition, mitral regurgitation flow extends later in systole compared with aortic stenosis (during isovolumic relaxation).

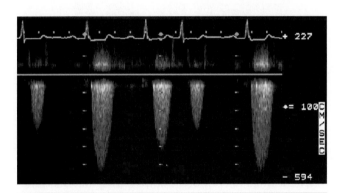

FIGURE 10.16. Doppler recording of aortic stenosis from a patient with an arrhythmia is shown. Note the variability in velocity, depending on the stroke volume and the preceding R-R interval. See text for details.

In most cases, a complete echocardiographic assessment of aortic stenosis includes a determination of aortic valve area using the continuity equation. Based on the principle of conservation of mass, the continuity equation states that the stroke volume proximal to the aortic valve (within the left ventricular outflow tract) must equal the stroke volume *through* the stenotic orifice. Because stroke volume is the product of the cross-sectional area and time velocity integral (TVI), the continuity equation can be arranged to yield:

$$\text{AV area} = \text{CSA}_{OT} * \frac{\text{TVI}_{OT}}{\text{TVI}_{AS}} \qquad \text{[Eq. 10.3]}$$

This is illustrated in Figure 10.18. To calculate aortic valve area, the following three measurements must be performed: (1) the cross-sectional area (CSA) of the left ventricular outflow tract (OT), (2) TVI of the outflow tract, and (3) TVI of the aortic stenosis jet (AS).

To measure the cross-sectional area of the outflow tract, the diameter of the outflow tract is generally measured from the parasternal long-axis view and the shape is assumed to be circular. The equation used is simply

$$\text{Area} = \pi r^2 \qquad \text{[Eq. 10.4]}$$

where *r* is one-half of the measured diameter (in centimeters). The importance of performing this measurement accurately cannot be overemphasized. Because the radius is squared to determine area, small errors in measuring

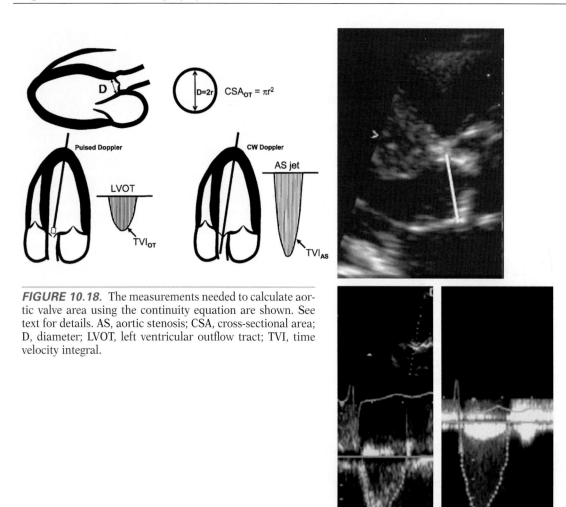

FIGURE 10.18. The measurements needed to calculate aortic valve area using the continuity equation are shown. See text for details. AS, aortic stenosis; CSA, cross-sectional area; D, diameter; LVOT, left ventricular outflow tract; TVI, time velocity integral.

this linear dimension will be compounded in the final formula. The smaller the anulus is, the greater is the percentage error introduced by any given mismeasurement. Potential factors that may contribute to errors include image quality, anular calcification (which obscures the true dimension), a noncircular anulus (which invalidates the formula), and failure to measure the true diameter. In most cases, underestimation of true diameter is much more likely than overestimation. Thus, outflow tract diameter measurement represents an important source of error and must be measured very carefully.

The TVI of the outflow tract is measured from the apical window using pulsed Doppler imaging and positioning the sample volume just proximal to the stenotic valve. In this position, the flow is still laminar and has not yet begun to accelerate through the valve. Then, from the same transducer position, continuous wave Doppler imaging should be used to record the jet velocity envelope. Using planimetry, both envelopes can be traced so that the TVI of each can be derived. If the units used for the measurement of the outflow tract diameter are centimeters,

the value of the aortic valve area will be centimeters squared. A simplified form of the continuity equation, in which maximal velocity of the outflow tract flow and valve jet are used in place of the respective TVIs is possible because flow duration across the two sites is the same. Thus, the simplified continuity equation is

$$\text{AV area} = \text{CSA}_{OT} * \frac{V_{OT}}{V_{AS}} \qquad \text{[Eq. 10.5]}$$

Somewhat technically easier to obtain, this equation yields valve areas that are as accurate as those obtained using the full equation (Equation 10.3).

As with the Bernoulli equation, this approach has also been validated in a variety of clinical and *in vitro* settings. Some of the studies validating the use of the continuity equation to measure aortic valve area are presented in Table 10.2. Thus, the continuity equation provides an accurate and reproducible assessment of the severity of aortic stenosis. It correlates well with invasive data, using the Gorlin equation. However, at very low flow rates, the correlation is not as good, with a consistent overestimation of severity of stenosis by the Gorlin equation. In addition to the challenge of properly measuring the area of the outflow tract, other potential sources of error should also be considered. It is essential that the outflow tract area and flow assessment be measured at the same level. Because the area of the outflow tract is usually measured from the parasternal long-axis view, some conventions are necessary to ensure that this is the case. In practice, the sample volume is positioned in the outflow tract from the apical window and then gradually advanced toward the aortic valve until the flow begins to accelerate. At this point, the peak velocity rises and turbulence is apparent. Then, the sample volume is gradually withdrawn toward the apex until the signal becomes laminar and without evidence of acceleration. This is the point at which the Doppler envelope should be measured.

The continuity equation has two important advantages compared with the Bernoulli equation for the assessment of aortic stenosis. First, coexisting aortic regurgitation may increase the measured transvalvular pressure gradient because of the increase in stroke volume through the valve during systole. The continuity equation, on the other hand, is not affected by the presence of aortic regurgitation. More importantly, left ventricular dysfunction may lead to reduced stroke volume and a low measured gradient even in the presence of severe valve stenosis. Again, the continuity equation is relatively unaffected and will allow an accurate determination of valve area whether the stroke volume is normal or reduced. This concept is demonstrated in Figure 10.19, which is recorded from a patient with aortic stenosis and left ven-

tricular dysfunction. The aortic jet velocity is only 2.9 m/sec, which by the Bernoulli equation yields a peak pressure gradient of approximately 33 mm Hg. However, because the flow is reduced (as evidenced by the left ventricular outflow tract TVI of 11 cm), the calculated aortic valve area is 0.6 cm^2. In this example, the severity of the aortic stenosis would have been significantly underestimated if the peak pressure gradient alone had been reported rather than the aortic valve area. Although an accurate measurement of the pressure gradient is sufficient to make clinical decisions in many cases, a determination of aortic valve area is especially important in patients with significant aortic regurgitation and/or reduced left ventricular function.

The interplay among velocity, stroke volume, and aortic valve area is illustrated graphically in Figure 10.20. The two curves compare the relationship between jet velocity and aortic valve area at different flow rates, indicated by the different outflow tract velocities (1.2 and 0.8 m/sec). Each curve plots the correlation between velocity and valve area for a given level of flow (or stroke volume). At point A, a patient has moderate aortic stenosis, with a peak gradient of 58 mm Hg and a corresponding valve area of 1.0 cm^2. This is in the setting of normal left ventricular function, with a peak left ventricular outflow tract velocity of 1.2 m/sec. Moving from point A to point B is the result of a sudden decrease in stroke volume (e.g., following a myocardial infarction). The associated decline in stroke volume is evident by the change in left ventricular outflow tract velocity to 0.8 m/sec. Because aortic stenosis severity is not affected, the peak gradient

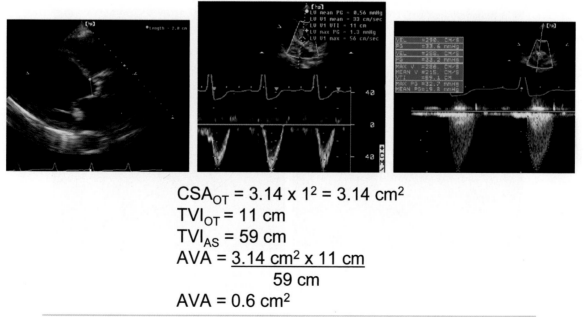

$$CSA_{OT} = 3.14 \times 1^2 = 3.14 \text{ cm}^2$$
$$TVI_{OT} = 11 \text{ cm}$$
$$TVI_{AS} = 59 \text{ cm}$$
$$AVA = \frac{3.14 \text{ cm}^2 \times 11 \text{ cm}}{59 \text{ cm}}$$
$$AVA = 0.6 \text{ cm}^2$$

FIGURE 10.19. Aortic valve area (*AVA*) is calculated in a patient with aortic stenosis and severe left ventricular dysfunction. See text for details.

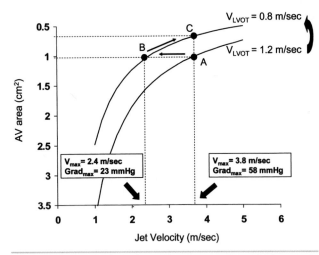

FIGURE 10.20. The relationship among jet velocity, aortic valve area, and stroke volume is demonstrated graphically. See text for details.

decreases to 23 mm Hg and the aortic valve area remains at 1.0 cm². At this level of left ventricular dysfunction, progression of aortic stenosis well into the severe range (point C, a new valve area of 0.7 cm²) would be required to restore the peak gradient back to the original value of 58 mm Hg.

Other Approaches to Quantifying Stenosis

The quantitative approaches described previously, the Bernoulli and the continuity equations, provide sufficient information in most instances. Thus, other parameters,

although available, are used infrequently. Aortic valve resistance is a relatively flow-independent measure of stenosis severity that depends on the ratio of mean pressure gradient and mean flow rate and is calculated as

$$Resistance = (\Delta P_{mean}/Q_{mean}) \times 1333 \quad [Eq. 10.6]$$

The relationship between mean resistance and valve area is given by the formula:

$$Resistance = \frac{28\sqrt{Gradient_{mean}}}{AV\ area} \quad [Eq\ 10.7]$$

Several investigators have demonstrated a close relationship between aortic valve resistance and aortic valve area. The advantages of this method over the continuity equation, however, have not been established.

A novel approach to aortic stenosis severity involves the calculation of left ventricular stroke work loss (SWL). Stroke work loss is calculated as:

$$SWL\ (\%) = (100 * \Delta P_{mean}) \div (\Delta P_{mean} + SBP)$$
$$[Eq.\ 10.8]$$

where SBP is systolic blood pressure, ΔP_{mean} is the mean aortic valve gradient, and stroke work loss is expressed as a percentage. This is based on the concept that the left ventricle expends work during systole to keep the aortic valve open and to eject blood into the aorta. Thus, it accounts for the stiffness of the aortic valve leaflets and is less dependent on flow compared with other parameters. Figure 10.21 is an example of an aortic valve that opens minimally, not because of aortic stenosis but because of

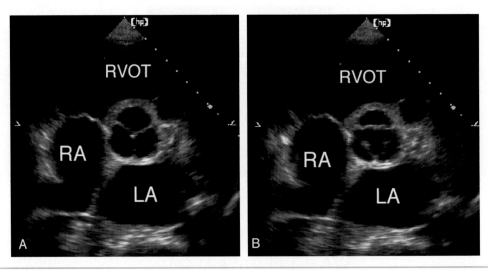

FIGURE 10.21. Short-axis views at the level of the aortic valve illustrate the effect of flow on valve motion. These are taken from a patient with severe left ventricular function and decreased stroke volume. **A:** The aortic valve is shown during diastole in the closed position. **B:** Recorded during mid systole, a minimal degree of cusp opening is the result of decreased flow through the valve. The valve is not stenotic, but the relative immobility is the result of a reduced stroke volume. LA, left atrium; RA, right atrium; RVOT, right ventricular outflow tract.

low stroke volume. The illustration underscores the relationship between flow and valve motion.

A relatively simple calculation, stroke work loss only requires Doppler determination of the mean aortic valve gradient and measurement of systolic blood pressure. With a normal aortic valve, relatively little work is needed to maintain the aortic leaflets in the open position during systole, and the amount of work performed calculated from left ventricular pressures compared with aortic pressures is very similar. In the setting of aortic stenosis, some of the total work performed must be expended on opening the stiff valve leaflets, resulting in a loss or wasting of some amount of total work. Left ventricular stroke work loss is then calculated as the difference between left ventricular work and effective work. One study compared various hemodynamic measures of aortic stenosis severity for their ability to predict symptoms and outcome and concluded that SWL was among the best predictors of symptom status and clinical end points. A cutoff value more than 25% effectively discriminated between patients experiencing a good and poor outcome. Again, although conceptually attractive, the calculation of stroke work loss has limited practical application.

Dobutamine Echocardiography in the Evaluation of Aortic Stenosis

The relationship between valve area and aortic volumetric flow rate has been well studied. These investigations suggest that increases in flow rate are associated with increases in valve area in most patients with aortic stenosis. Conversely, at a very low flow rate, valve opening may be inhibited, perhaps leading to an underestimation of aortic valve area. In practical terms, these phenomena create challenges in the quantitative assessment of aortic stenosis in the presence of significant left ventricular dysfunction.

In such patients, it may be difficult to distinguish true severe valvular stenosis (with low-pressure gradient due to low stroke volume) from mild to moderate stenosis (with reduced aortic valve opening due to low flow). Dobutamine echocardiography may be useful to make this distinction (Fig. 10.22). Using a stepwise infusion of dobutamine from 5 to 30 μg/kg/min (in an effort to increase stroke volume across the stenotic valve) may allow differentiation of the two possibilities. The test assumes that if the leaflets are relatively flexible (mild to moderate stenosis), the valve area will increase in response to an increasing stroke volume. Alternatively, true severe aortic stenosis is associated with a fixed valve area that will not change with dobutamine infusion. In such patients, the dobutamine infusion will increase the maximal velocity of both the outflow tract and the jet proportionally. Thus, the ratio of peak velocity in the outflow tract and of the jet

will remain the same. In milder forms of stenosis, the increase in velocity of the outflow tract will be much greater than that of the jet (due to the functional increase in valve area). In this case, the ratio of outflow tract to jet velocity will increase compared with baseline. Truly severe aortic stenosis is suggested by a critical measure of aortic valve area (<0.6 cm^2) and an outflow tract to jet velocity ratio that does not change during dobutamine infusion (Table 10.3). In the example provided (Fig. 10.22), the initial aortic valve gradient is only 30 mm Hg and the low outflow tract velocity (0.6 m/sec) is consistent with reduced stroke volume. With infusion of dobutamine, both the outflow tract and the jet velocities increase in a stepwise manner. Although stroke volume increases, the ratio between the outflow tract and jet velocity does not change appreciably and the peak gradient rises to approximately 60 mm Hg. These findings support the diagnosis of severe aortic stenosis. This method has proven to be safe and clinically useful for many patients. One limitation is that the study results cannot be interpreted if the ventricle does not respond to dobutamine with an increase in contractility, as might occur in the setting of concurrent coronary artery disease.

Natural History of Aortic Stenosis

In addition to its pivotal role in diagnosis, echocardiography has contributed significantly to an understanding of the natural history of valvular aortic stenosis and its rate of progression. Because of the relatively long asymptomatic period, predicting the rate of progression to severe aortic stenosis is helpful in the timing of follow-up evaluation and the planning for surgical intervention. The definition of severe aortic stenosis varies, but echocardiographic criteria have been established. When the maximal aortic valve velocity exceeds 4.5 m/sec, indicating a peak pressure gradient of greater than 80 mm Hg, the stenosis is considered severe. Some investigators have argued that the mean pressure gradient is a better predictor of severity, often using a cutoff of 50 mm Hg as the criterion for severe.

As can be seen in Figure 10.23, a precise correlation between maximal velocity or mean gradient and the aortic valve area is lacking and considerable overlap exists. Using an aortic valve area less than 0.75 cm^2 as the standard definition of severe stenosis, patients with mean Doppler gradients between 10 and 110 mm Hg would be included (Fig. 10.23B). Much of this range is accounted for on the basis of left ventricular dysfunction. Furthermore, significant overlap occurs in measured severity between symptomatic and asymptomatic individuals.

Recent studies have shed new light on our understanding of the rate of disease progression in adult patients with aortic stenosis. Despite individual variability, most patients demonstrate an average increase in mean

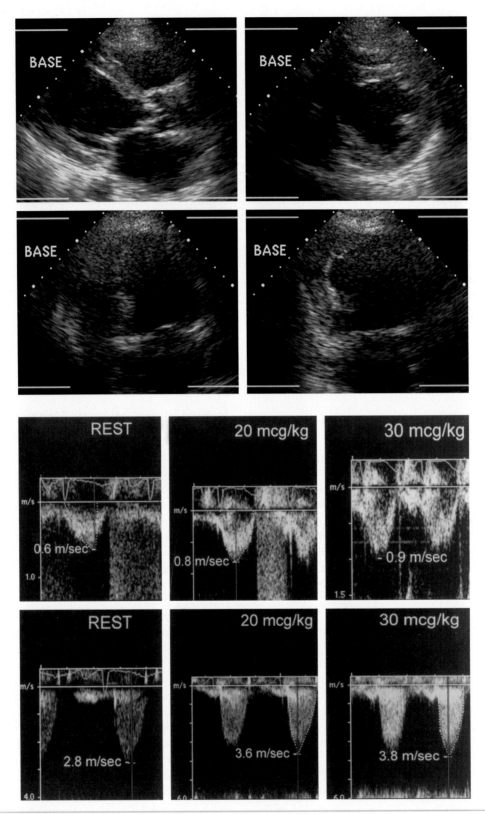

FIGURE 10.22. Dobutamine stress echocardiography can be used to assess the severity of aortic stenosis in patients with left ventricular dysfunction. **Top:** Baseline two-dimensional echocardiogram demonstrating significant left ventricular dysfunction. **Bottom:** Doppler recordings of left ventricular outflow tract velocity (above) and aortic jet velocity (below) at rest, 20, and 30 mcg/kg/min. See text for details.

▶ **TABLE 10.3 Dobutamine Echocardiographic Responses in Patients with Aortic Stenosis and Left Ventricular Dysfunction**

Baseline			Low Dose			Mid Dose			Interpretation
LVOT Velocity	Jet Velocity	Maximal Gradient	LVOT Velocity	Jet Velocity	Maximal Gradient	LVOT Velocity	Jet Velocity	Maximal Gradient	
0.6	3.0	36	0.8	4.0	64	1.0	5.0	100	Severe AS with LV dysfunction
0.6	3.0	36	0.8	3.2	41	1.0	3.4	46	Moderate AS with LV dysfunction
0.6	3.0	36	0.6	3.0	36	0.6	3.0	36	AS with LV dysfunction and no evidence of myocardial viability

Values for velocity are in meters per second; for gradient, in millimeters of mercury.
AS, aortic stenosis; LV; left ventricular; LVOT, left ventricular outflow tract.

pressure gradient of 0 to 10 mm Hg per year (mean, 7 mm Hg) with a corresponding decrease in aortic valve area of 0.12 ± 0.19 cm² per year. Figure 10.24 illustrates progression of aortic stenosis over a 2-year period. In this example, the peak aortic gradient increases from 49 to 69 mm Hg. To date, attempts to predict the determinants of more rapid progression have been largely unsuccessful. Progression can also occur in the absence of an increase in jet velocity if left ventricular function declines (Fig. 10.20).

Clinical Decision Making

The management of patients with aortic stenosis must take into account the presence or absence of symptoms, the severity of the stenosis, the status of the left ventricle, and the existence of any comorbidities. Most asymptomatic adults with significant aortic stenosis are managed

medically, and thus the role of echocardiography in this group focuses on measuring severity, rate of progression, and assessment of left ventricular function. The indications for echocardiography in patients being considered for aortic valve replacement are listed in Table 10.4. Based on these recommendations, it is clear that echocardiography plays a role before, during, and after such interventions. Among symptomatic patients, Otto and colleagues have devised an algorithm that incorporates a measure of jet velocity, valve area, and the severity of aortic regurgitation (Fig. 10.25). The scheme relates the hierarchy of Doppler echocardiographic data to clinical outcome. At the extremes, maximal velocity (V_{max}) alone is sufficient. For patients with a V_{max} between 3.0 and 4.0 m/sec, calculation of aortic valve area provides further discrimination. Then, for those patients with borderline valve areas, the presence and severity of aortic regurgitation (A1) were useful to discriminate between patients who might be

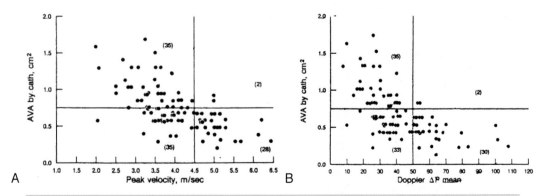

FIGURE 10.23. A: The correlation between jet velocity by Doppler imaging and aortic valve area (*AVA*) obtained by cardiac catheterization is demonstrated. **B:** Doppler mean gradient is plotted against aortic valve area obtained by cardiac catheterization. Note the degree of scatter of the data. See text for details. (From Oh JK, Taliercio CP, Holmes DR Jr, et al. Prediction of the severity of aortic stenosis by Doppler aortic valve area determination: prospective Doppler-catheterization correlation in 100 patients. J Am Coll Cardiol 1988;11:1227–1234, with permission.)

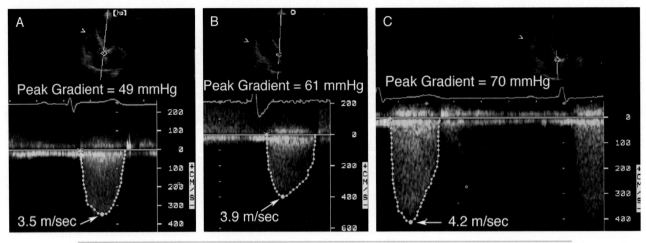

FIGURE 10.24. Doppler imaging is useful to document the rate of progression of aortic stenosis. **A:** A baseline study; **B**, **C:** recorded at 1- and 2-year intervals, respectively. The series demonstrates a gradual increase in peak gradient across the valve.

treated medically and those for whom aortic valve replacement is recommended. Although the confounding factor of severe left ventricular dysfunction is not directly addressed, this diagnostic approach is a useful guideline for most clinicians and underscores the importance of echocardiography in diagnosis and follow-up. These same investigators have also demonstrated the power and simplicity of using maximal jet velocity to predict event-free survival, as shown in Figure 10.26. Although attractive in its simplicity, it should be emphasized that progression can occur in the absence of a change in velocity due to a reduction in the volume flow rate. Thus, an assessment of

left ventricular function is always a key component in the evaluation of patients with aortic stenosis.

AORTIC REGURGITATION

Aortic regurgitation may be congenital or acquired and may be caused by either abnormalities of the aortic root or the valve itself. Some of the more common causes of aortic regurgitation are listed in Table 10.5. Long-standing hypertension may result in dilation of the aortic root and anulus, leading to valvular regurgitation. Other dis-

▶ **TABLE 10.4** **Indications for Echocardiography in Interventions for Valvular Heart Disease and Prosthetic Valves**

	Class
1. Assessment of the timing of valvular intervention based on ventricular compensation, function, and/or severity of primary and secondary lesions	I
2. Use of echocardiography (especially transesophageal echocardiography) in performing interventional techniques (e.g., balloon valvotomy) for valvular disease	I
3. Postintervention baseline studies for valve function (early) and ventricular remodeling (late)	I
4. Reevaluation of patients with valve replacement with changing clinical signs and symptoms; suspected prosthetic dysfunction (stenosis, regurgitation) or thrombosis[a]	I
5. Routine reevaluation study after baseline studies of patients with valve replacements with mild to moderate ventricular dysfunction without changing clinical signs or symptoms	IIa
6. Routine reevaluation at the time of increased failure rate of a bioprosthesis without clinical evidence of prosthetic dysfunction	IIb
7. Routine reevaluation of patients with valve replacements without suspicion of valvular dysfunction and unchanged clinical signs and symptoms	III
8. Patients whose clinical status precludes therapeutic interventions	III

[a]Transesophageal echocardiography may provide incremental value in addition to information obtained by transthoracic echocardiography. From Cheitlin MD, Alpert JS, Armstrong WF, et al. ACC/AHA Guidelines for the Clinical Application of Echocardiography: A Report of the American College of Cardiology/ American Heart Association Task Force on Practice Guidelines (Committee on Clinical Application of Echocardiography) Developed in Collaboration With the American Society of Echocardiography. Circulation 1997;95:1686–1744, with permission.

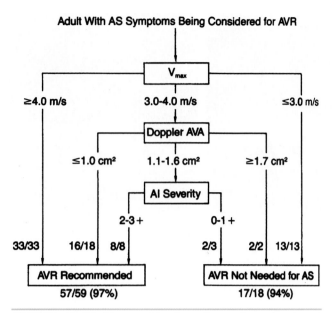

Adult With AS Symptoms Being Considered for AVR

FIGURE 10.25. The combination of two-dimensional and Doppler echocardiography is useful for clinical decision making in patients with aortic stenosis (*AS*) who have symptoms and are being considered for aortic valve replacement. See text for details. (From Otto CM, Pearlman AS. Doppler echocardiography in adults with symptomatic aortic stenosis. Diagnostic utility and cost-effectiveness. Arch Intern Med 1988;148:2553–2560, with permission.)

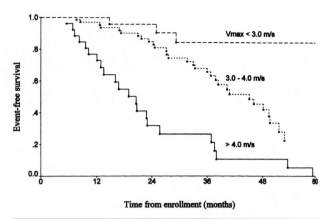

FIGURE 10.26. The simple parameter of maximal jet velocity (V_{max}) is a powerful determinant of outcome in patients with aortic stenosis. Event-free survival curves for three groups of patients defined based on V_{max} are plotted. A highly significant difference in survival is demonstrated. (From Otto CM, Burwash IG, Legget ME, et al. Prospective study of asymptomatic valvular aortic stenosis. Clinical, echocardiographic, and exercise predictors of outcome. Circulation 1997;95:2262–2270, with permission.)

▶ **TABLE 10.5 Causes of Aortic Regurgitation**

Congenital aortic valve disease (usually bicuspid)
Other congenital causes, e.g., prolapse from a ventricular septal defect
Hypertension
Rheumatic
Infective endocarditis
Marfan syndrome
Ankylosing spondylitis
Degenerative
Trauma
Rheumatoid arthritis
Syphilis
Aortic dissection
Membranous subaortic stenosis

eases of the aortic root often associated with aortic regurgitation include Marfan syndrome, syphilitic aortitis, cystic medial necrosis, and aortic dissection. Often, dilation of the sinotubular junction is the underlying mechanism for these causes of aortic regurgitation. More commonly, aortic regurgitation is due to defects in the valve leaflets, including bicuspid aortic valve, rheumatic heart disease, endocarditis, and degenerative calcific aortic valve disease. An unusual cause of aortic regurgitation is membranous subaortic stenosis. In these patients, the impact of the jet through the stenotic membrane damages the valve, leading to regurgitation (Fig. 10.27). Recently, the anorexigens fenfluramine and dexfenfluramine have been implicated as causes of aortic regurgitation. Regardless of etiology, aortic regurgitation imposes a volume overload on the left ventricle and, eventually, a reduced forward stroke volume. Thus, the echocardiographic assessment of this condition includes establishing a diagnosis, determining an etiology, evaluating the effects of volume overload on the left ventricle, and a careful assessment of the aortic root. Indications for echocardiography in patients with valvular regurgitation are summarized in Table 10.6.

M-Mode and Two-Dimensional Imaging

As the aortic jet cascades across the anterior mitral leaflet, it creates a high-frequency fluttering that requires the rapid sampling rate of M-mode echocardiography for de-

tection. This was one of the earliest examples of the use of the M-mode technique to indirectly assess valve disease (Fig. 10.28). In acute aortic regurgitation, premature closure of the mitral valve (due to rapidly increasing left ventricular diastolic pressure) was also initially detected with this technique (Fig. 10.29). As with other forms of valve disease, however, the development of two-dimensional imaging and Doppler techniques largely supplanted the M-mode technique in this setting.

Two-dimensional echocardiographic imaging focuses on a detailed evaluation of the aortic valve and root and an assessment of left ventricular size and function. Many of the causes of aortic regurgitation, including rheumatic, degenerative, and congenital, are established based on two-dimensional echocardiographic findings. Very impor-

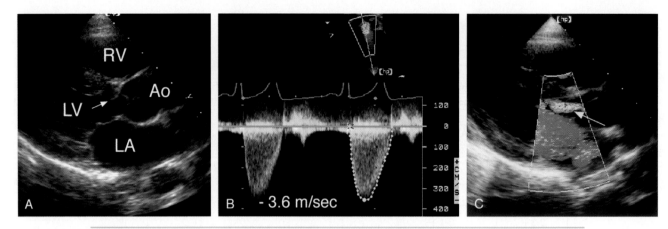

FIGURE 10.27. An unusual cause of aortic regurgitation is the presence of a subaortic membrane. **A:** A parasternal long-axis view demonstrates narrowing just below the aortic valve (*arrow*) due to the membrane. **B:** Doppler imaging demonstrates a peak gradient of approximately 50 mm Hg, at the level of the subaortic membrane. **C:** A mild degree of aortic regurgitation (*arrow*) recorded using color flow imaging is shown. Ao, aorta; LA, left atrium; LV, left ventricle; RV, right ventricle.

tantly, manifestations of endocarditis are accurately assessed with a combination of transthoracic and transesophageal echocardiography. Figure 10.30 is an example of abnormal mitral valve motion due to impingement on the anterior leaflet by a posteriorly directed aortic regurgitation jet. Note how the mid portion of the leaflet is deformed during diastole.

Diseases that affect the aortic root can cause regurgitation by altering the geometry of aortic leaflet coapta-tion, primarily through dilation at the level of the sinotubular junction. Conditions such as hypertension, Marfan syndrome, and cystic medial necrosis typically result in the combination of a dilated aortic root and some degree of aortic regurgitation (Fig. 10.31). In such conditions, the aortic regurgitation jet arises centrally and may vary over the full range of severity. Causes of *acute* aortic regurgitation that can be identified using two-dimensional echocardiography include endocarditis and aortic

▶ **TABLE 10.6 Indications for Echocardiography in Native Valvular Regurgitation**

	Class
1. Diagnosis; assessment of hemodynamic severity	I
2. Initial assessment and reevaluation (when indicated) of left and right ventricular size, function, and/or hemodynamics	I
3. Reevaluation of patients with mild to moderate valvular regurgitation with changing symptoms	I
4. Reevaluation of asymptomatic patients with severe regurgitation	I
5. Assessment of changes in hemodynamic severity and ventricular compensation in patients with known valvular regurgitation during pregnancy	I
6. Reevaluation of patients with mild to moderate regurgitation with ventricular dilation without clinical symptoms	I
7. Assessment of the effects of medical therapy on the severity of regurgitation and ventricular compensation and function when it might change medical management	I
8. Assessment of valvular morphology and regurgitation in patients with a history of anorectic drug use or the use of any drug or agent known to be associated with valvular heart disease, who are symptomatic, have cardiac murmurs, or have a technically inadequate auscultatory examination	I
9. Reevaluation of patients with moderate aortic regurgitation without chamber dilation and without clinical symptoms	IIb
10. Routine reevaluation in asymptomatic patients with mild valvular regurgitation having stable physical signs and normal left ventricular size and function	III
11. Routine repetition of echocardiography in past users of anorectic drugs with normal previous studies or known trivial valvular regurgitation	III

From Cheitlin MD, Alpert JS, Armstrong WF, et al. ACC/AHA Guidelines for the Clinical Application of Echocardiography: A Report of the American College of Cardiology/American Heart Association Task Force on Practice Guidelines (Committee on Clinical Application of Echocardiography) Developed in Collaboration with the American Society of Echocardiography. Circulation 1997;95:1686–1744, with permission.

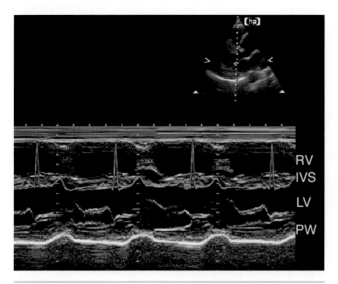

FIGURE 10.28. An M-mode echocardiogram from a patient with aortic regurgitation demonstrates fine fluttering of the anterior mitral leaflet as a result of the jet. IVS, interventricular septum; LV, left ventricle; PW, posterior wall; RV, right ventricle.

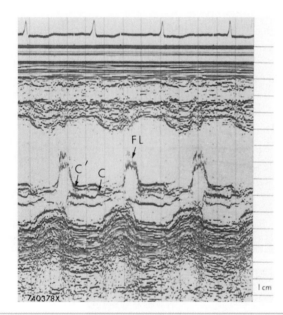

FIGURE 10.29. An M-mode recording from a patient with acute and severe aortic regurgitation demonstrates both fluttering (*FL*) of the anterior mitral leaflet and premature closure (*C'*) of the mitral valve, the result of rapidly increasing diastolic left ventricular pressure.

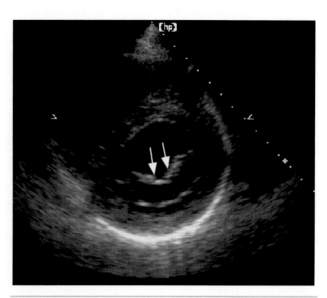

FIGURE 10.30. A two-dimensional short-axis echocardiogram is shown from a patient with significant aortic regurgitation and a posteriorly directed jet. The *arrows* indicate the effect of the jet on the anterior mitral leaflet. The mid portion of the leaflet is deformed during diastole as a result.

dissection (Figs. 10.32 and 10.33). Figure 10.34 is an example of perivalvular regurgitation occurring as a result of abscess formation in a patient with a stentless aortic prosthesis.

Two-dimensional echocardiography is critically important in patients with aortic regurgitation to evaluate the left ventricle's response to volume overload. Over an extended period, chronic aortic regurgitation leads to dila-

tion of the left ventricle and a characteristic change to a more spherical shape. Left ventricular systolic function is typically preserved and left ventricular mass increases, although the increase in wall thickness is often quite modest. Hyperdynamic interventricular septal motion occurs as a result of left ventricular volume overload due to unequal filling and stroke volume of the ventricles. This abnormal septal motion is best appreciated with M-mode imaging, which often reveals an exaggeration of the normal early diastolic septal dip and an overall increase in the amplitude of septal motion compared with the posterior left ventricular wall.

The enlarging left ventricle remains compliant and is able to accept the simultaneous filling through the mitral and aortic valves throughout diastole without a significant increase in pressure. Eventually, left ventricular function begins to deteriorate, although this generally does not occur until a significant increase in end-systolic volume is present. Figure 10.35 is taken from a patient with long-standing aortic regurgitation. The left ventricular end-diastolic dimension was 6.2 cm. Note also the globular shape of the chamber. The reduction in left ventricular function should be viewed as a late and sometimes irreversible change in the natural history of the disease. The implications of these changes on clinical decision making will be discussed later.

Establishing a Diagnosis

By directly visualizing the aortic valve, two-dimensional echocardiography can frequently identify an anatomic

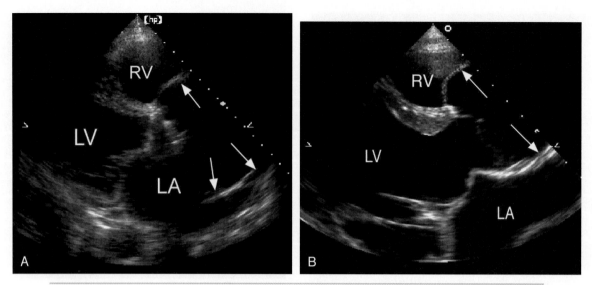

FIGURE 10.31. Aortic regurgitation can result from dilation of the aortic root. **A:** A severely dilated aortic root in a patient with a prosthetic aortic valve is shown. **B:** A similar degree of dilation is demonstrated from a patient with Marfan syndrome. In both cases, significant aortic regurgitation was present. LA, left atrium; LV, left ventricle; RV, right ventricle.

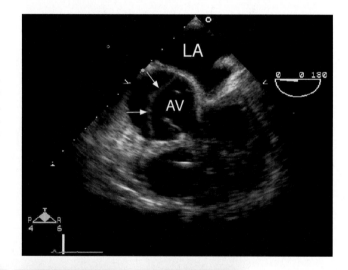

FIGURE 10.32. A transesophageal echocardiogram at the base of the heart is shown from a patient with aortic dissection involving the proximal aorta. The aortic valve (*AV*) is seen in an off-axis plane. The *arrows* point to the dissection flap within the aortic root. The location of the dissection flap affected the ability of the valve to close in diastole, thereby causing aortic regurgitation. LA, left atrium.

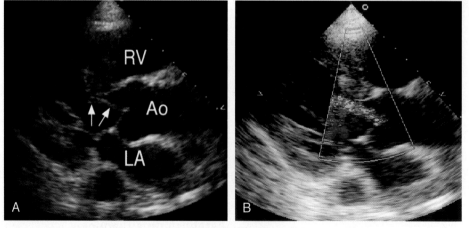

FIGURE 10.33. Endocarditis can cause aortic regurgitation through a variety of mechanisms. **A:** A long-axis view demonstrates a long, thin mass attached to the aortic valve, extending into the outflow tract (*arrows*). **B:** Color Doppler imaging demonstrates mild aortic regurgitation. Ao, aorta; LA, left atrium; RV, right ventricle.

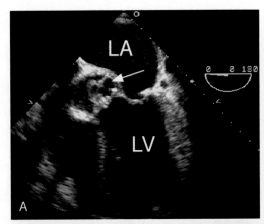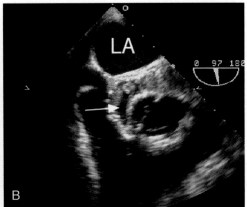

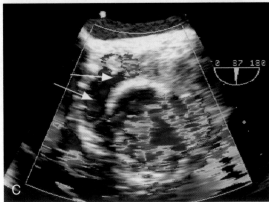

FIGURE 10.34. Images were recorded from a patient with a Medtronic Freestyle aortic prosthesis who developed an aortic root abscess. **A:** The transesophageal echocardiogram demonstrates a complex echo-free space (*arrow*) surrounding the aortic valve. **B:** The same abnormality is demonstrated from the short-axis view (*arrow*). **C:** Color Doppler imaging demonstrates flow within the abscess cavity and evidence of perivalvular regurgitation (*arrows*). LA, left atrium; LV, left ventricle.

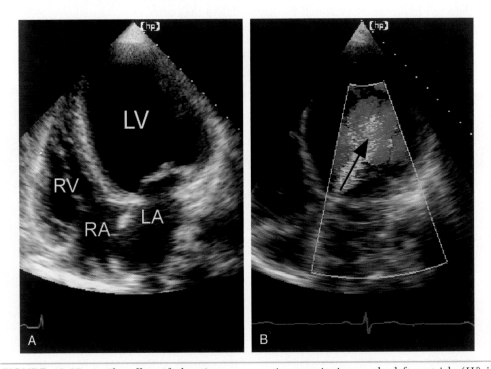

FIGURE 10.35. **A:** The effect of chronic, severe aortic regurgitation on the left ventricle (*LV*) is demonstrated. The volume overload imposed by the regurgitation eventually results in left ventricular enlargement and dysfunction. The chamber assumes a more spherical shape. **B:** Color Doppler imaging demonstrates the aortic regurgitation jet. See text for details. LA, left atrium, LV, left ventricle; RA, right atrium; RV, right ventricle.

condition that would predispose to the development of aortic regurgitation. Although such indirect indicators may provide a clue to the presence of aortic regurgitation, the specific diagnosis requires Doppler techniques. In some cases, even when aortic regurgitation is severe, two-dimensional imaging will be surprisingly unremarkable, even suggesting that the valve is "anatomically" normal. In such cases, Doppler imaging will be the most important, and sometimes the only, clue to a diagnosis.

The jet of aortic regurgitation can be recorded with pulsed, continuous wave, or color flow Doppler imaging. All three methods are highly sensitive for the detection of regurgitation and should be viewed as complementary in the evaluation of individual patients (Figs. 10.36 and 10.37). Pulsed Doppler echocardiography relies on the demonstration of turbulent flow during diastole in the left ventricular outflow tract on the ventricular side of the aortic valve (Fig. 10.38). Because the velocity of the aortic regurgitation jet is high, aliasing occurs inevitably, but simply the presence of turbulence will usually establish the diagnosis. The method is highly sensitive but requires a methodical and careful search for the regurgitant jet, using multiple views and echocardiographic windows. There can be false-positive findings, sometimes in the setting of mitral stenosis or a prosthetic mitral valve, where turbulent diastolic flow may be mistaken for aortic regurgitation. Early attempts to "map" the aortic regurgitation jet using pulsed Doppler techniques provided the first approach to estimating severity using Doppler imaging. Once the jet was detected immediately proximal to the aortic valve, the sample volume was gradually withdrawn toward the apex to track the length of the regurgitant jet.

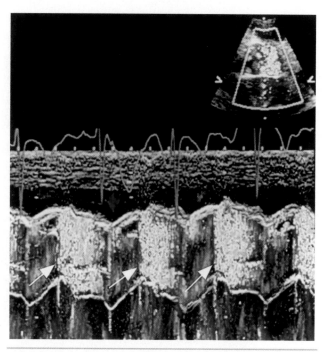

FIGURE 10.37. A color M-mode imaging example of aortic regurgitation is provided. The mosaic flow signal during diastole (*arrows*) identifies the aortic regurgitation jet.

Although simplistic in concept, this approach proved reasonably accurate to distinguish among mild, moderate, and severe degrees of regurgitation. One obvious limitation of the pulsed Doppler mapping technique was the assumption that the regurgitant jet is centrally directed and can be tracked back toward the apex. Figure 10.39 is an

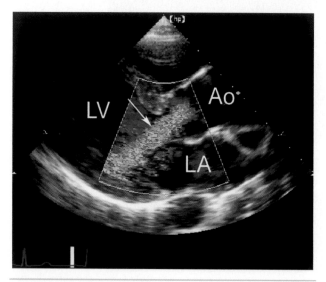

FIGURE 10.36. An example of severe aortic regurgitation recorded using color flow imaging is shown. The jet is indicated by the *arrow*. Note the width and length of the regurgitant jet. Ao, aorta; LA, left atrium; LV, left ventricle.

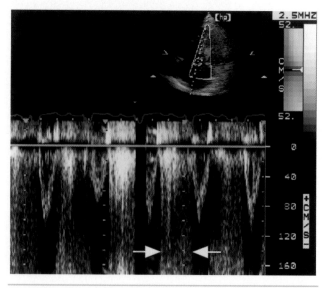

FIGURE 10.38. Pulsed Doppler echocardiography can detect aortic regurgitation as turbulent flow within the left ventricular outflow tract during diastole. In this example, aliasing of the high-velocity regurgitant jet is evident (*arrows*).

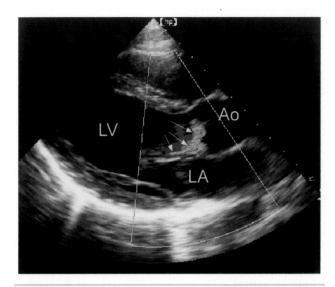

FIGURE 10.39. An example of an eccentric aortic regurgitant jet (*arrows*) is demonstrated. Note the impingement of the jet on the anterior mitral valve leaflet. Ao, aorta; LA, left atrium; LV, left ventricle.

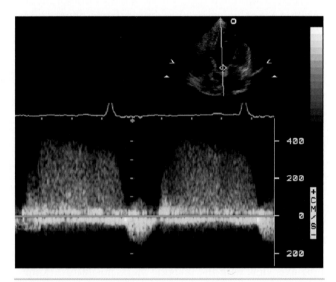

FIGURE 10.40. Continuous wave Doppler recording of an aortic regurgitant jet from the apical window is provided. The velocity and contour of the jet are best appreciated using this technique.

example of a very eccentric aortic regurgitant jet that is directed posteriorly toward the anterior mitral leaflet. Pulsed Doppler mapping of such a jet could significantly underestimate its severity.

Because the aortic regurgitation jet is invariably high-velocity, continuous wave Doppler imaging is necessary for the contour of the envelope to be recorded (Fig. 10.40). The density of the jet, a qualitative indication of the volume of regurgitation, can also be assessed. Density is a function of the number of blood cells being sampled and will generally increase as the regurgitant volume in-

creases. The velocity of the regurgitation jet and particularly the rate of deceleration of retrograde flow can be measured (Fig. 10.41). Continuous wave Doppler imaging is especially helpful when there is confusion about whether a flow disturbance is due to aortic regurgitation or mitral stenosis (Fig. 10.42). The velocity and contour of the jet will generally allow this distinction to be established.

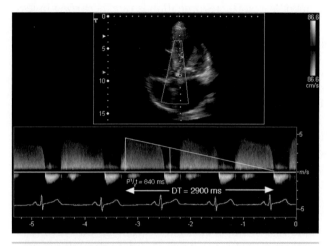

FIGURE 10.41. The slope, or rate of deceleration, of the aortic regurgitation jet provides information about severity. In this example, the deceleration slope is plotted to permit calculation of the pressure half-time (840 milliseconds). The deceleration time is 2,900 milliseconds. These findings are consistent with mild regurgitation.

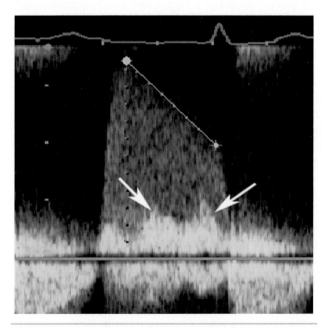

FIGURE 10.42. Because of the proximity of the aortic regurgitant jet to mitral inflow, the two flow patterns can sometimes be recorded simultaneously. In this example, severe aortic regurgitation is superimposed on the mitral inflow pattern (*arrows*).

By far the most commonly used technique to assess aortic regurgitation is color flow imaging. This technique has a reported sensitivity of greater than 95% and a specificity of nearly 100% for establishing the diagnosis. In fact, minor degrees of aortic regurgitation may be detected using color flow imaging in a percentage of otherwise normal individuals. Most cases involve "trivial" or "mild" regurgitation, and the prevalence increases with advancing age. Among normal subjects younger than 40 years of age, aortic regurgitation is rare, occurring in less than 1%. The reported frequency in older individuals is much higher, however, occurring in between 10% and 20% of subjects older than 60 years of age. In very elderly individuals, e.g., those older than 80 years of age, some degree of aortic regurgitation can be detected using color Doppler imaging in the vast majority.

Color flow imaging will demonstrate a turbulent jet in the left ventricular outflow tract of nearly all patients with clinical evidence of aortic regurgitation. The jet usually persists throughout diastole, and its dimensions provide useful information regarding severity. False-negative findings are rare but may occur in the setting of very high heart rate, in which diastole is short in duration and the frame rate of the ultrasound instrument only permits a few diastolic frames to be displayed. In this setting, continuous wave Doppler, by virtue of its higher sampling rate, is often useful.

Evaluating the Severity of Aortic Regurgitation

The severity of aortic regurgitation can be judged using several different criteria. The size or extent of the regurgitant jet within the left ventricle, the effective regurgitant orifice area, and the volume or fraction of regurgitant flow are distinct, but obviously interrelated, measures of severity. Although the effective regurgitant orifice area may be the most hemodynamically important parameter, it is quite challenging to derive in patients with aortic regurgitation. By far the most commonly used approach relies on the relationship between the size of the regurgitant jet, visualized by color flow imaging, and the regurgitant volume. The jet should be recorded in multiple imaging planes to provide a three-dimensional assessment of its dimensions. It is now generally believed that the length of the jet conveys unreliable information about overall severity. In any given plane, the area of the jet can be estimated or measured by planimetry. Figure 10.43 is recorded from a patient with mild regurgitation. The jet originates posteriorly and is narrow at the orifice. Both the area and length of the color jet are small. Figure 10.44 shows three examples of aortic regurgitation recorded with color flow imaging, demonstrating the differences in appearance of the regurgitant jet in mild, moderate, and severe disease. Again, this approach has several limita-

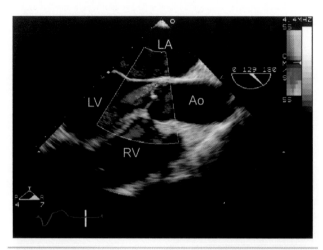

FIGURE 10.43. A transesophageal echocardiogram demonstrates mild aortic regurgitation. The jet originates posteriorly. Ao, aorta; LA, left atrium; LV, left ventricle; RV, right ventricle.

tions and correlates only modestly with other measures of severity.

A related approach relies on the visualization of the regurgitant jet at its origin (i.e., immediately downstream from the valve) as an indicator of regurgitant orifice size (Fig. 10.45). From the parasternal long-axis view, the "height" of the jet just below the valve can be measured using electronic calipers. This dimension can also be expressed as a percentage of left ventricular outflow tract dimension to provide an estimate of severity. In the three examples in Figure 10.44, note the differences in jet height/outflow tract dimension ratio. Figure 10.45 illustrates a jet height that occupies more than 70% of the left ventricular outflow tract dimension. The greater the percentage is of the left ventricular outflow tract that is filled by the jet at its origin, the more severe the regurgitation. A jet that occupies more than 60% of the left ventricular outflow tract (either height or area) usually indicates severe aortic regurgitation. A similar approach uses the short-axis view with the imaging plane positioned immediately proximal to the aortic valve (Fig. 10.46). The outflow tract is directly visualized as a circular space, and the regurgitant jet is visualized as a two-dimensional shape within this circle.

There are several limitations to the use of color flow mapping as a direct indicator of severity. Eccentric jets may become entrained along a wall of the left ventricle, which tends to alter their appearance and hence the perception of severity (Fig. 10.47). It must be remembered that the jet is inherently three-dimensional so that no one imaging plane conveys complete information about its shape and extent. The apparent size of the jet is very instrument dependent. Changes in gain, color scale, transducer frequency, and wall filters will affect the jet appearance, independent of severity. For example, the width of

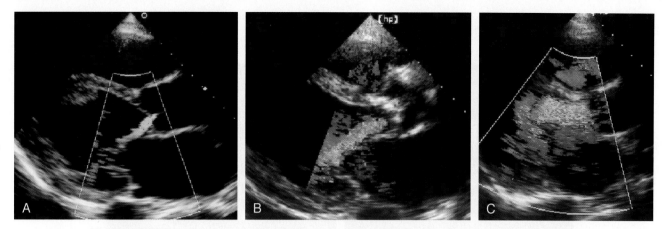

FIGURE 10.44. Three examples of aortic regurgitation are provided, all taken from the parasternal long-axis view using color Doppler. Mild **(A)**, moderate **(B)**, and severe **(C)** aortic regurgitation are illustrated.

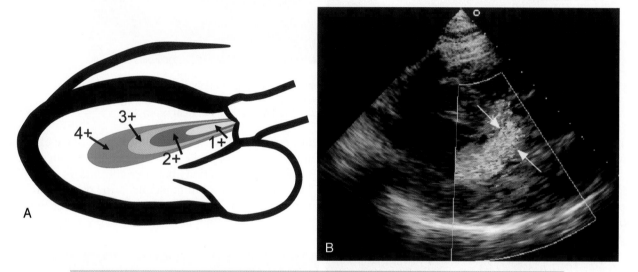

FIGURE 10.45. **A:** The schematic demonstrates how the dimensions of the color jet of aortic regurgitation can be used to estimate severity. **B:** The jet height just below the aortic valve (*arrows*) can be measured and compared with the dimension of the left ventricular outflow tract. This is a useful measure of severity. See text for details.

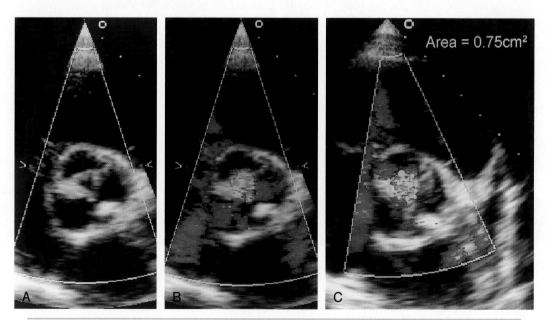

FIGURE 10.46. Using transesophageal echocardiography, the jet can be visualized from the short-axis view, just below the aortic valve. **A:** The regurgitant orifice is visualized with two-dimensional imaging. **B:** Color Doppler is used to demonstrate flow within the regurgitant orifice. **C:** The regurgitant orifice area is measured by planimetry (0.75 cm²).

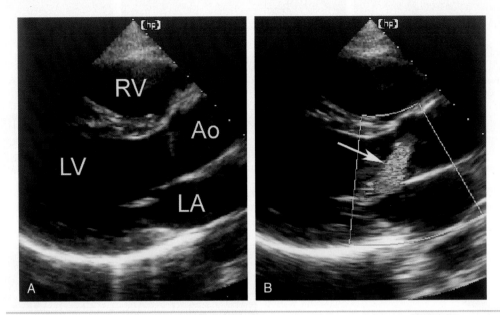

FIGURE 10.47. A bicuspid aortic valve and moderate aortic regurgitation in a patient is shown. **A:** The long-axis view is shown. **B:** An eccentric jet is indicated by the *arrow* and is directed toward the anterior mitral valve leaflet. Ao, aorta; LA, left atrium; LV, left ventricle; RV, right ventricle.

an aortic regurgitant jet is often greater from an apical view compared with a parasternal view. This is because the jet's width recorded from a parasternal projection depends on axial resolution, whereas the same dimension recorded apically will rely more on lateral resolution, resulting in the appearance of a wider jet. Alternatively, im-age quality and/or the three-dimensional shape of the jet may create the opposite effect. Figure 10.48 is an example of aortic regurgitation that appears mild in the apical four-chamber view but moderate in the parasternal long-axis projection. The example merely points out the limi-tations of color flow imaging in assessing regurgitation

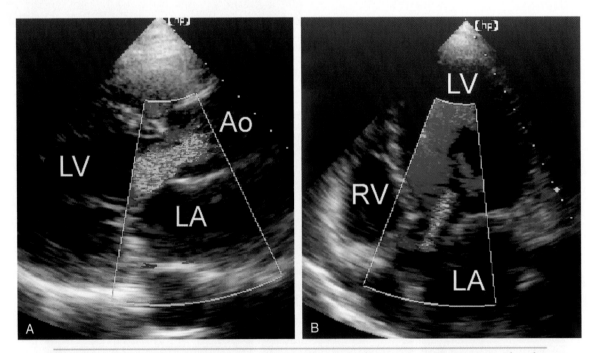

FIGURE 10.48. A: The parasternal long-axis view records the aortic regurgitant jet with color Doppler imaging. The height of the jet relative to the dimension of the left ventricular outflow tract suggests that the regurgitation is moderate. **B:** Taken from the same patient, the apical four-chamber view suggests mild aortic regurgitation. See text for details. Ao, aorta; LA, left atrium; LV, left ventricle; RV, right ventricle.

severity and underscores the fact that no single view conveys all the necessary information for measuring severity. Finally, there is evidence that the regurgitant orifice area in patients with chronic aortic regurgitation changes (and usually decreases) during diastole. This finding has implications for techniques such as color Doppler and may explain the temporal variability in jet size in many patients. A gradual decrease in regurgitant orifice area would also account for the tendency of color Doppler to overestimate severity because the visualized jet area would reflect peak rather than mean orifice area.

Continuous wave Doppler imaging can also be used to estimate severity. The simplest approach compares the density or darkness of the envelope of the antegrade aortic flow and the regurgitant jet. The larger the regurgitant volume is, the darker the regurgitant jet is on continuous wave imaging. The shape of the envelope also contains information. The velocity of the jet is simply a reflection of the pressure gradient between the aorta and left ventricle throughout diastole (Fig. 10.49). This can be thought of as the driving force for the regurgitant flow. In early diastole, the gradient is highest and the velocity will be in the range of 4 to 6 m/sec, depending on the blood pressure. As diastole progresses, the gradient diminishes as aortic pressure decreases and left ventricular pressure increases.

With mild aortic regurgitation, a compliant left ventricle allows a slow and modest increase in left ventricular pressure and aortic diastolic pressure is maintained throughout. Thus, the velocity of the regurgitant jet remains relatively high and the envelope appears flat. With more severe aortic regurgitation, the combination of increasing left ventricular pressure and more rapidly decreasing aortic pressure leads to a more rapid deceleration of the regurgitant jet velocity resulting in a steeper slope of the Doppler envelope (Fig. 10.50). The deceleration of jet velocity can be described as either the slope or the pressure half-time of the jet. These parameters have been correlated with other measures of severity, and a reasonable agreement has been demonstrated. A pressure half-time less than 250 milliseconds or a slope greater than 400 cm/sec^2 are indicators of severe aortic regurgitation. However, other factors, including aortic compliance, blood pressure, and left ventricular size and compliance will also affect these measures. As is discussed later, a rapid rate of deceleration of the aortic regurgitation jet is more an indicator of acuity rather than severity.

A final nonquantitative approach using pulsed Doppler imaging assesses diastolic flow reversal in the descending aorta. This is illustrated in Figure 10.51. As aortic regurgitation becomes worse, a greater degree of flow reversal occurs and retrograde velocities can be recorded throughout diastole. Again, this parameter is dependent on vessel compliance and the location of the sample volume but does provide a simple and practical marker of severity. The presence of holodiastolic flow reversal in the de-

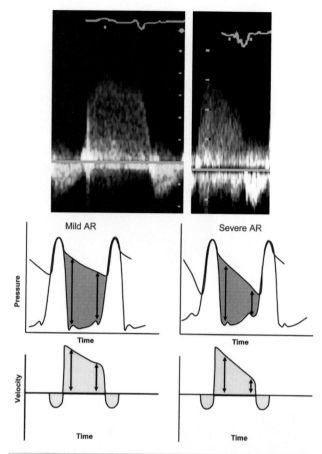

FIGURE 10.49. This schematic illustrates how hemodynamic changes are reflected in the Doppler velocity tracing. **Left:** Mild aortic regurgitation (*AR*) is associated with a fairly flat contour of the regurgitant jet. **Right:** As severity increases, the slope of the jet becomes steeper. These changes are the result of the instantaneous pressure gradient between the aorta and left ventricle during diastole. See text for details.

scending aorta has been correlated with severe aortic regurgitation.

Several more quantitative approaches are also available to assess aortic regurgitation. Because the four valves of the heart exist in series, the flow or stroke volume at any point must be equal. In the setting of aortic regurgitation, the total stroke volume through the aortic valve in systole must equal the forward stroke volume (which can be determined at another nonregurgitant valve) plus the regurgitant volume (Fig. 10.52). As described previously, stroke volume is simply the product of the cross-sectional area and TVI. If the mitral valve is competent, *forward* stroke volume is typically measured at this location. Then, *total* stroke volume across the aortic valve is determined. This value will include both forward and regurgitant volumes. Hence, the regurgitant volume is the difference between the forward flow across the aortic and mitral valves (Fig. 10.53). This approach has been validated in several laboratories. Both the regurgitant stroke volume and the

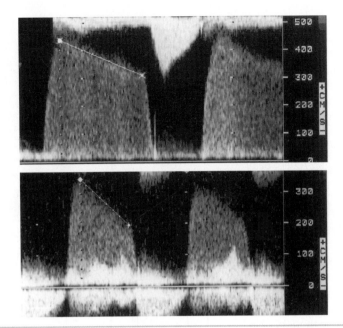

FIGURE 10.50. Continuous wave Doppler imaging of the aortic regurgitation (*AR*) jet permits quantitation of both slope and pressure half-time (P$^1/_2$t). **Top:** An example of mild aortic regurgitation is demonstrated. The slope is relatively flat and the P$^1/_2$t is long. **Bottom:** An example of severe aortic regurgitation demonstrates a much steeper slope and shorter P$^1/_2$t.

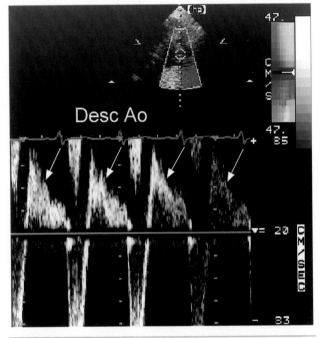

FIGURE 10.51. A pulsed Doppler recording within the descending aorta (*Desc Ao*) from a patient with severe aortic regurgitation demonstrates flow reversal throughout diastole (*arrows*). See text for details.

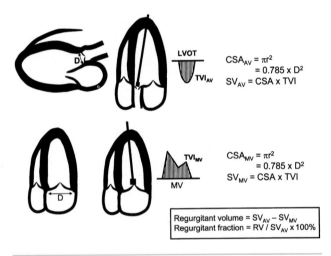

FIGURE 10.52. Stroke volume can be measured through any valve within the heart. This schematic demonstrates how stroke volume can be calculated at the level of the aortic valve (*#1*) and mitral valve (*#2*). The difference in stroke volume represents the regurgitant volume. In addition, the regurgitant fraction can be calculated. See text for details.

regurgitant fraction can be quantified. As a reference, a regurgitant fraction greater than 50% or a regurgitant volume greater than 60 mL indicates severe aortic regurgitation. In the example provided in Figure 10.53, stroke volume is calculated as 112 cc across the aortic valve and 69 cc across the mitral valve. The difference is the result of significant aortic regurgitation. Based on these values, the regurgitant volume is approximately 43 cc and the regurgitant fraction is 38%.

Proximal isovelocity surface area, in theory, can be applied to any regurgitant valve to measure regurgitant area and volume. However, because of the technical challenges

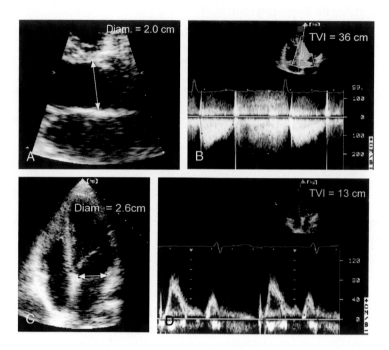

Aortic flow:
$CSA_{AV} = 3.1 \text{ cm}^2$
$TVI_{AV} = 36 \text{ cm}$
$SV_{AV} = 112 \text{ cc}$

Mitral flow:
$CSA_{MV} = 5.3 \text{ cm}^2$
$TVI_{MV} = 13 \text{ cm}$
$SV_{MV} = 69 \text{ cc}$

Regurgitant volume:
$112 - 69 = 43 \text{ cc}$

Regurgitant fraction:
$43 / 112 = 38\%$

FIGURE 10.53. An example of how regurgitant volume and regurgitant fraction can be quantified is provided. See text for details.

of visualizing the isovelocity shells that converge on the aortic regurgitant orifice, this technique has limited application to the aortic valve. Finally, an interesting approach to the quantification of severity of aortic regurgitation involves the concept of conservation of momentum. Momentum, the product of volumetric flow rate and velocity, is constant at any point within the regurgitant jet. Thus, as the jet expands in diastole to include a greater volume of blood, the velocity must decrease proportionately. Because flow is the product of the cross-sectional area and velocity, through substitution,

$$\text{Momentum} = \text{Flow}(Q) * v \text{ or} \quad [\text{Eq. 10.9}]$$

$$\text{Momentum} = \text{Area} * v^2 \quad [\text{Eq. 10.10}].$$

To measure the regurgitant orifice area (ROA), momentum is determined at two points, one of which is at the regurgitant orifice. Because momentum is conserved, just like mass, a form of the continuity equation is employed to yield

$$\text{ROA} = (\text{Jet area} * v^2_{\text{jet}}) \div v^2_{\text{ROA}} \quad [\text{Eq. 10.11}].$$

This is an attractive concept based on sound theoretical principles. By measuring the jet area and velocity at two points (one of which is within the regurgitant orifice), the regurgitant orifice area can be determined. The measurements are reasonably straightforward and reproducible, and *in vitro* studies have demonstrated the accuracy of this approach. However, jet momentum calculation remains a research tool and is difficult to apply clinically. A summary of the various approaches to measuring the severity of aortic regurgitation is provided in Table 10.7. It should be evident that no single measure of regurgitation severity is sufficient for clinical decision making. Each provides clues to severity but is imperfect and cannot be relied on in isolation. Instead, the clinician/echocardiographer must take into account all available data so that a comprehensive assessment of severity can be obtained.

Acute Versus Chronic Aortic Regurgitation

Several important differences exist between acute and chronic aortic regurgitation. Acute regurgitation is usually caused by endocarditis, leading to disruption or destruction of the aortic leaflets, aortic dissection, leading to anular and/or aortic root dilation, or by impingement of the dissection flap on the valve itself. Less commonly, chest trauma can result in this condition.

▶ **TABLE 10.7 Estimating the Severity of Aortic Regurgitation**

Modality	Parameter	Criteria for Severe	Example of Limitations
Color flow	Jet area	>60% LVOT area	Instrument (gain) dependent, eccentric jet, temporal variability
	Jet height	>60% LVOT height	
	PISA	Effective regurgitation orifice >0.3 cm²	Multiple measurements, technically challenging
CW Doppler imaging	Signal density	Nonquantitative	Affected by other factors, e.g., blood pressure, LV compliance, acuity
	P½t	<250 ms	
	Slope	>400 cm/s²	
Pulsed Doppler imaging	Regurgitant volume	>60 mL	Requires multiple measurements, assumes no regurgitation at reference valve;
	Regurgitant fraction	>50%	
	Descending aortic flow reversal	Holodiastolic retrograde flow	limited quantitative information; affected by sample volume location
2D echocardiography	LV end-diastolic dimension	>7 cm	Nonspecific, affected by multiple factors
	LV end-systolic dimension	>4.5 cm	

CW, continuous wave; LV, left ventricular; LVOT, left ventricular outflow tract; PISA, proximal isovelocity surface area; P½t; 2D, two-dimensional.

A primary difference between acute and chronic aortic regurgitation involves the response of the left ventricle. Over time, the left ventricle has a remarkable capacity to dilate, remaining compliant and accommodating even a large regurgitant volume while maintaining nearly normal diastolic filling pressures. This is not possible with acute aortic regurgitation in which the volume overload is poorly tolerated (due to the normal left ventricular size and the constraining effects of the pericardium) so that left ventricular diastolic pressure increases rapidly. The shape of the regurgitant jet envelope on continuous wave Doppler imaging and especially the rate of deceleration of flow are perhaps the most useful hemodynamic markers to distinguish between the two (Fig. 10.54). In this example, the aortic regurgitation was the result of leaflet de-

struction from staphylococcal endocarditis. In acute aortic regurgitation, the rapid increase in left ventricular diastolic pressure may also lead to premature closure of the mitral valve, which can be recorded using M-mode imaging (Fig. 10.29). Thus, echocardiography is critical to establish the cause of aortic regurgitation and to distinguish acute from chronic disease.

Assessing the Left Ventricle

In most patients, chronic aortic regurgitation is slowly progressive and is associated with a long asymptomatic period. Because left ventricular dysfunction may precede the onset of symptoms, the longitudinal evaluation of patients with chronic significant aortic regurgitation

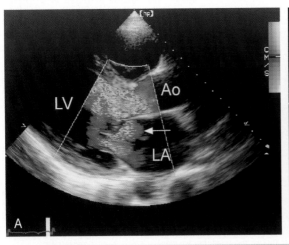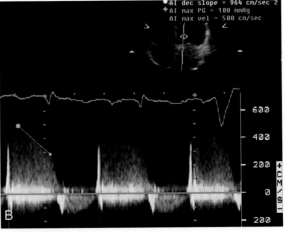

FIGURE 10.54. An example of acute aortic regurgitation is provided in a patient with endocarditis involving the aortic valve. **A:** Color Doppler imaging demonstrates severe aortic regurgitation. There is also evidence of diastolic mitral regurgitation (*arrow*), due to high diastolic left ventricular pressure. **B:** Continuous wave Doppler imaging is consistent with severe regurgitation, based on the slope of the jet. Ao, aorta; LA, left atrium; LV, left ventricle.

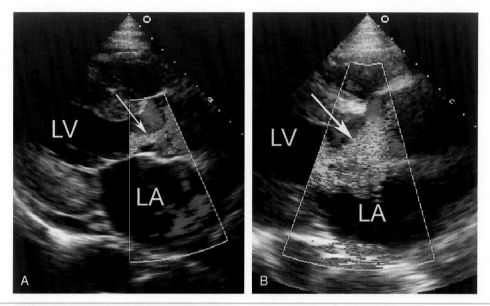

FIGURE 10.55. Progression of severity of aortic regurgitation can be assessed using echocardiography. **A:** Mild aortic regurgitation (*arrow*) is demonstrated. **B:** The same patient is evaluated 2 years later. During the interim, the severity of regurgitation (*arrow*) has increased dramatically. See text for details. LA, left atrium; LV, left ventricle.

focuses on the left ventricle. Several clinical studies, initially using M-mode echocardiography and later two-dimensional imaging, have demonstrated the value of serial studies in detecting the earliest signs of left ventricular decompensation in asymptomatic patients. Recent studies have also explored the rate of progression of chronic aortic regurgitation. These longitudinal series have confirmed that chronic aortic regurgitation is a slowly progressive condition and that patients with more severe disease progress more rapidly than those with mild or moderate regurgitation. However, more rapid and unexpected progression is possible. In Figure 10.55, a patient with mixed connective tissue disease is shown. In the first study, mild aortic regurgitation is present. Two years later, the regurgitation has become severe. The role of echocardiography in selecting patients for surgery and in the timing of intervention is well established (Table 10.4).

A variety of measures have been proposed to aid in clinical decision making. End-diastolic and end-systolic minor-axis left ventricular dimensions, ejection fraction, fractional shortening, and end-systolic wall stress have all been shown to predict outcome in patients with severe aortic regurgitation. When patients are initially evaluated, left ventricular systolic dysfunction thought secondary to aortic regurgitation is often an indication for surgical intervention. Among patients with preserved systolic function, an increase in chamber size, particularly the end-systolic dimension or volume, is generally regarded as an early manifestation of decompensation

and frequently an indication for aortic valve replacement. Thus, the echocardiographic evaluation of these patients must pay particular attention to evidence of systolic dysfunction or progressive chamber enlargement. These parameters, together with the symptom status of the patient and his or her exercise capacity, provide most of the information needed for management decisions in aortic regurgitation.

MISCELLANEOUS ABNORMALITIES OF THE AORTIC VALVE

Lambl's excrescences are thin, delicate filamentous strands that arise from the ventricular edge of aortic cusps. Considered normal variants, these structures are seen increasingly with advancing age and improved image quality (Fig. 10.56). As such, they may represent a form of degenerative change of the valve that occurs over time. They can occasionally be multiple. An important goal in the evaluation of such structures is to distinguish a Lambl's excrescence from pathologic entities, especially vegetations. This can be difficult and generally requires some consideration of the clinical setting. For example, if a patient has fever and positive blood cultures, a small aortic valve mass likely represents a vegetation. If the patient is afebrile and asymptomatic, the possibility of a Lambl's excrescence should be strongly considered. Tumors affecting the aortic valve, such as fibroelastoma, are rare and are discussed in Chapter 21.

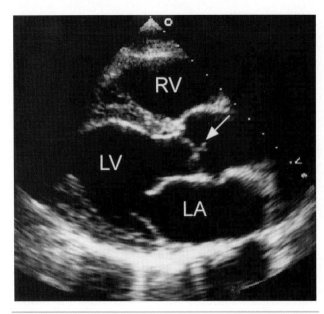

FIGURE 10.56. A parasternal long-axis view demonstrates an example of Lambl's excrescence (*arrow*). LA, left atrium; LV, left ventricle; RV, right ventricle.

SUGGEST READINGS

Akasaka T, Yoshikawa J, Yoshida K, et al. Age-related valvular regurgitation: a study by pulsed Doppler echocardiography. Circulation 1987;76:262–265.

Bermejo J, Odreman R, Feijoo J, et al. Clinical efficacy of Doppler-echocardiographic indices of aortic valve stenosis: a comparative test-based analysis of outcome. J Am Coll Cardiol 2003;41:142–151.

Bernard Y, Meneveau N, Vuillemenot A, et al. Planimetry of aortic valve area using multiplane transoesophageal echocardiography is not a reliable method for assessing severity of aortic stenosis. Heart 1997;78:68–73.

Bonow RO, Epstein SE. Is preoperative left ventricular function predictive of survival and functional results after aortic valve replacement for chronic aortic regurgitation? J Am Coll Cardiol 1987;10:713–716.

Bouchard A, Yock P, Schiller NB, et al. Value of color Doppler estimation of regurgitant volume in patients with chronic aortic insufficiency. Am Heart J 1989;117:1099–1105.

Burwash IG, Dickinson A, Teskey RJ, et al. Aortic valve area discrepancy by Gorlin equation and Doppler echocardiography continuity equation: relationship to flow in patients with valvular aortic stenosis. Can J Cardiol 2000;16:985–992.

Burwash IG, Thomas DD, Sadahiro M, et al. Dependence of Gorlin formula and continuity equation valve areas on transvalvular volume flow rate in valvular aortic stenosis. Circulation 1994;89:827–835.

Cannon JD Jr, Zile MR, Crawford FA Jr, et al. Aortic valve resistance as an adjunct to the Gorlin formula in assessing the severity of aortic stenosis in symptomatic patients. J Am Coll Cardiol 1992;20:1517–1523.

Cape EG, Skoufis EG, Weyman AE, et al. A new method for noninvasive quantification of valvular regurgitation based on conservation of momentum. *In vitro* validation. Circulation 1989;79:1343–1353.

Choong CY, Abascal VM, Weyman J, et al. Prevalence of valvular regurgitation by Doppler echocardiography in patients with structurally normal hearts by two-dimensional echocardiography. Am Heart J 1989;117:636–642.

Ciobanu M, Abbasi AS, Allen M, et al. Pulsed Doppler echocardiography in the diagnosis and estimation of severity of aortic insufficiency. Am J Cardiol 1982;49:339–343.

Connolly HM, Crary JL, McGoon MD, et al. V. Valvular heart disease associated with fenfluramine-phentermine. N Engl J Med 1997;337:581–588.

Cormier B, Iung B, Porte JM, et al. Value of multiplane transesophageal echocardiography in determining aortic valve area in aortic stenosis. Am J Cardiol 1996;77:882–885.

Currie PJ, Hagler DJ, Seward JB, et al. Instantaneous pressure gradient: a simultaneous Doppler and dual catheter correlative study. J Am Coll Cardiol 1986;7:800–806.

Currie PJ, Seward JB, Reeder GS, et al. Continuous-wave Doppler echocardiographic assessment of severity of calcific aortic stenosis: a simultaneous Doppler-catheter correlative study in 100 adult patients. Circulation 1985;71:1162–1169.

deFilippi CR, Willett DL, Brickner ME, et al. Usefulness of dobutamine echocardiography in distinguishing severe from nonsevere valvular aortic stenosis in patients with depressed left ventricular function and low transvalvular gradients. Am J Cardiol 1995;75:191–194.

Esper RJ. Detection of mild aortic regurgitation by range-gated pulsed Doppler echocardiography. Am J Cardiol 1982;50:1037–1043.

Espinal M, Fuisz AR, Nanda NC, et al. Sensitivity and specificity of transesophageal echocardiography for determination of aortic valve morphology. Am Heart J 2000;139:1071–1076.

Godley RW, Green D, Dillon JC, et al. Reliability of two-dimensional echocardiography in assessing the severity of valvular aortic stenosis. Chest 1981;79:657–662.

Grayburn PA, Smith MD, Harrison MR, et al. Pivotal role of aortic valve area calculation by the continuity equation for Doppler assessment of aortic stenosis in patients with combined aortic stenosis and regurgitation. Am J Cardiol 1988;61:376–381.

Grayburn PA, Handshoe R, Smith MD, et al. Quantitative assessment of the hemodynamic consequences of aortic regurgitation by means of continuous wave Doppler recordings. J Am Coll Cardiol 1987;10:135–141.

Harrison MR, Gurley JC, Smith MD, et al. A practical application of Doppler echocardiography for the assessment of severity of aortic stenosis. Am Heart J 1988;115:622–628.

Henry WL, Bonow RO, Rosing DR, et al. Observations on the optimum time for operative intervention for aortic regurgitation. II. Serial echocardiographic evaluation of asymptomatic patients. Circulation 1980;61:484–492.

Kim KS, Maxted W, Nanda NC, et al. Comparison of multiplane and biplane transesophageal echocardiography in the assessment of aortic stenosis. Am J Cardiol 1997;79:436–441.

Labovitz AJ, Ferrara RP, Kern MJ, et al. Quantitative evaluation of aortic insufficiency by continuous wave Doppler echocardiography. J Am Coll Cardiol 1986;8:1341–1347.

Lin SS, Roger VL, Pascoe R, et al. Dobutamine stress Doppler hemodynamics in patients with aortic stenosis: feasibility, safety, and surgical correlations. Am Heart J 1998;136:1010–1016.

Nishimura RA, Tajik AJ. Determination of left-sided pressure gradients by utilizing Doppler aortic and mitral regurgitant signals: validation by simultaneous dual catheter and Doppler studies. J Am Coll Cardiol 1988;11:317–321.

Oh JK, Taliercio CP, Holmes DR Jr, et al. Prediction of the severity of aortic stenosis by Doppler aortic valve area determination: prospective Doppler-catheterization correlation in 100 patients. J Am Coll Cardiol 1988;11:1227–1234.

Otto CM, Pearlman AS. Doppler echocardiography in adults with symptomatic aortic stenosis. Diagnostic utility and cost-effectiveness. Arch Intern Med 1988;148:2553–2560.

Otto CM. The difficulties in assessing patients with moderate aortic stenosis. Heart 1999;82:5–6.

Otto CM. Valvular aortic stenosis: which measure of severity is best? Am Heart J 1998;136:940–942.

Otto CM, Burwash IG, Legget ME, et al. Prospective study of asymptomatic valvular aortic stenosis. Clinical, echocardiographic, and exercise predictors of outcome. Circulation 1997;95:2262–2270.

Otto CM, Pearlman AS, Gardner CL, et al. Simplification of the Doppler continuity equation for calculating stenotic aortic valve area. J Am Soc Echocardiogr 1988;1:155–157.

Padial LR, Oliver A, Vivaldi M, et al. Doppler echocardiographic assessment of progression of aortic regurgitation. Am J Cardiol 1997;80:306–314.

Perry GJ, Helmcke F, Nanda NC, et al. Evaluation of aortic insufficiency by Doppler color flow mapping. J Am Coll Cardiol 1987;9:952–959.

Reimold SC, Maier SE, Aggarwal K, et al. Aortic flow velocity patterns in chronic aortic regurgitation: implications for Doppler echocardiography. J Am Soc Echocardiogr 1996;9:675–683.

Reimold SC, Maier SE, Fleischmann KE, et al. Dynamic nature of the aortic regurgitant orifice area during diastole in patients with chronic aortic regurgitation. Circulation 1994;89:2085–2092.

Reimold SC, Thomas JD, Lee RT. Relation between Doppler color flow variables and invasively determined jet variables in patients with aortic regurgitation. J Am Coll Cardiol 1992;20:1143–1148.

Richards KL. Assessment of aortic and pulmonic stenosis by echocardiography. Circulation 1991;84:I182–I187.

Richards KL, Cannon SR, Miller JF, et al. Calculation of aortic valve area by Doppler echocardiography: a direct application of the continuity equation. Circulation 1986;73:964–969.

Roberts WC. Valvular, subvalvular and supravalvular aortic stenosis: morphologic features. Cardiovasc Clin 1973;5:97–126.

Roger VL, Seward JB, Bailey KR, et al. Aortic valve resistance in aortic stenosis: Doppler echocardiographic study and surgical correlation. Am Heart J 1997;134:924–929.

Roger VL, Tajik AJ, Bailey KR, et al. Progression of aortic stenosis in adults: new appraisal using Doppler echocardiography. Am Heart J 1990;119:331–338.

Rokey R, Sterling LL, Zoghbi WA, et al. Determination of regurgitant fraction in isolated mitral or aortic regurgitation by pulsed Doppler two-dimensional echocardiography. J Am Coll Cardiol 1986;7: 1273–1278.

Rosenhek R, Binder T, Porenta G, et al. Predictors of outcome in severe, asymptomatic aortic stenosis. N Engl J Med 2000;343:611–617.

Simpson IA, Houston AB, Sheldon CD, et al. Clinical value of Doppler echocardiography in the assessment of adults with aortic stenosis. Br Heart J 1985;53:636–639.

Smith MD, Grayburn PA, Spain MG, et al. Observer variability in the quantitation of Doppler color flow jet areas for mitral and aortic regurgitation. J Am Coll Cardiol 1988;11:579–584.

Springings DC, Chambers JB, Cochrane T, et al. Ventricular stroke work loss: validation of a method of quantifying the severity of aortic stenosis and derivation of an orifice formula. J Am Coll Cardiol 1990;16:1608–1614.

Stamm RB, Martin RP. Quantification of pressure gradients across stenotic valves by Doppler ultrasound. J Am Coll Cardiol 1983;2: 707–718.

Stoddard MF, Hammons RT, Longaker RA. Doppler transesophageal echocardiographic determination of aortic valve area in adults with aortic stenosis. Am Heart J 1996;132:337–342.

Taylor R. Evolution of the continuity equation in the Doppler echocardiographic assessment of the severity of valvular aortic stenosis. J Am Soc Echocardiogr 1990;3:326–330.

Teague SM, Heinsimer JA, Anderson JL, et al. Quantification of aortic regurgitation utilizing continuous wave Doppler ultrasound. J Am Coll Cardiol 1986;8:592–599.

Teirstein P, Yeager M, Yock PG, et al. Doppler echocardiographic measurement of aortic valve area in aortic stenosis: a noninvasive application of the Gorlin formula. J Am Coll Cardiol 1986;8:1059–1065.

Tribouilloy C, Shen WF, Peltier M, et al. Quantitation of aortic valve area in aortic stenosis with multiplane transesophageal echocardiography: comparison with monoplane transesophageal approach. Am Heart J 1994;128:526–532.

Vandenbossche JL, Massie BM, Schiller NB, et al. Relation of left ventricular shape to volume and mass in patients with minimally symptomatic chronic aortic regurgitation. Am Heart J 1988;116: 1022–1027.

Yeager M, Yock PG, Popp RL. Comparison of Doppler-derived pressure gradient to that determined at cardiac catheterization in adults with aortic valve stenosis: implications for management. Am J Cardiol 1986;57:644–648.

Zoghbi WA, Farmer KL, Soto JG, et al. Accurate noninvasive quantification of stenotic aortic valve area by Doppler echocardiography. Circulation 1986;73:452–459.

Mitral Valve Disease

The mitral valve was the first of the four cardiac valves to be evaluated with echocardiography. In large part, this was due to the relatively high prevalence of rheumatic heart disease and the relatively large excursion of the mitral valve leaflets, which made them an easier target for early M-mode techniques. M-mode echocardiography was instrumental in providing early clues to the severity of mitral stenosis and documenting changes after open mitral commissurotomy. Modern two-dimensional and Doppler techniques have made echocardiography an instrumental tool in the management of patients with known and suspected mitral valve disease of any etiology.

Primary mitral valve disease can be the major contributor to cardiovascular symptoms. In addition, the mitral valve often is affected in a secondary manner in other cardiac diseases. Table 11.1 outlines the primary and secondary causes of mitral valve disease. These include congenital lesions such as congenital mitral stenosis and acquired valve disease such as rheumatic heart disease. Other forms of acquired disease, typically presenting later in life, include ischemic papillary muscle dysfunction and degenerative diseases.

ANATOMY OF THE MITRAL VALVE

It is important to recognize that the leaflets of the mitral valve constitute only a portion of the mitral valve apparatus and that diseases resulting in mitral dysfunction often are caused by abnormalities in the overall apparatus rather than in the actual leaflets. The components of the mitral valve apparatus are schematized in Figure 11.1. The components of the mitral apparatus include the mitral anulus, the leaflets, chordae tendineae papillary muscles, and the underlying ventricular wall. Pathologic changes in any of these components of the mitral valve apparatus can result in mitral valve dysfunction. The classic form of mitral valve disease is rheumatic heart disease, which involves predominantly the leaflets and chordae. Other forms of mitral valve disease involve the different aspects of mitral apparatus. Table 11.2 outlines the impact of different disease states on the different components of the mitral apparatus and the degree to which they result in mitral regurgitation or stenosis.

The mitral anulus is a more complex structure then previously recognized. The initial concept of the mitral anulus was that of a planar structure (Fig. 11.2A). The mitral anulus is part of the fibrous skeleton of the heart, which also includes the aortic anulus, the junction of the anterior mitral valve leaflet and aorta (anuloaortic fibrosa), and the tricuspid anulus. The mitral anulus itself is a complex three-dimensional structure. Three-dimensional echocardiography has been instrumental in demonstrating the nonplanar nature of the mitral anulus and the implications of this complex geometry for the diagnosis of mitral valve prolapse as well as for the design of therapeutic interventions such as mitral anuloplasty

▶ **TABLE 11.1 Etiology of Mitral Valve Disease**

Diseases directly affecting the mitral apparatus
Rheumatic heart disease
Congenital mitral stenosis
Congenital cleft mitral valve
Infectious endocarditis
Marantic endocarditis
Libman-Sacks endocarditis
Hypereosinophilic heart disease
Coronary artery disease
Diet drug valvulopathy
Mitral anular calcification
Degenerative
Infiltrative
Carcinoid
Indirect effect on mitral valve function
Dilated cardiomyopathy
Hypertrophic cardiomyopathy
Left atrial myxoma
Myocardial ischemia or infarction

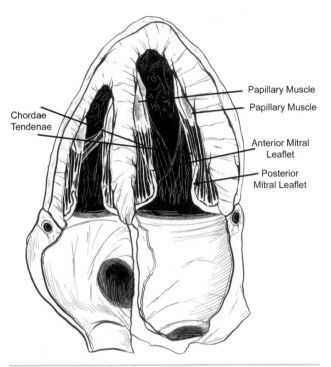

Chordae
Tendenae

Papillary Muscle

Papillary Muscle

Anterior Mitral
Leaflet

Posterior
Mitral Leaflet

FIGURE 11.1. Anatomic rendering of the normal mitral valve and mitral valve apparatus in the open position. Note that the chordae are attached not only to the tips of the mitral valve leaflets but also to the mid portion of the leaflets as well. (Artwork by Amanda Almon and Travis Vermilye.)

rings. Figure 11.2B depicts the normal nonplanar anatomy of the mitral anulus and its relationship to mitral leaflet closure patterns.

There are two mitral valve leaflets, typically referred to as anterior and posterior. (An alternate nomenclature uses

the terms septal and mural respectively.) Inspection of Figure 11.3, which details mitral valve leaflet anatomy further, reveals that the mitral leaflet should be viewed not as a two-leaflet structure but as a six-scallop structure. (Some investigators have proposed an even more complex description of mitral valve anatomy including as many as eight separate coaptation points.) This figure also depicts the perspective with which the mitral valve is viewed anatomically (from the left atrium) and with transthoracic and transesophageal echocardiography. Clinically, the most easily understood and clinically useful description of mitral valve anatomy involves dividing it into six scallops, three each for the anterior and posterior leaflet, designated as scallop 1, 2, and 3. Scallop 1 is most lateral and scallop 3 is most medial. Chordae attach throughout the entire length of the coaptation line of each of the mitral valve leaflets and insert into the tips of the papillary muscles.

Anatomically, there are two major papillary muscles, each of which may have several heads. The anterolateral papillary muscle provides chordae to the anterolateral half of both mitral leaflets. The posteromedial papillary muscle provides chordae to the posteromedial aspect of both leaflets. There is substantial variability from patient to patient in the exact number of chordae and the percentage of chords that are devoted to the anterior and posterior leaflets, but in general both papillary muscles provide chordal attachments to a portion of each of the leaflets. The posteromedial papillary muscle typically is perfused by the right coronary artery, and the anterior lateral papillary muscle has a dual blood supply. Because of the dual blood supply of the anterior lateral papillary muscle, it is less susceptible to ischemic injury than the posteromedial papillary muscle.

▶ **TABLE 11.2 Physiologic and Anatomic Effect of Disease on the Mitral Valve**

	MS	*MR*	*Anulus*	*Leaflets*	*Chordae*	*Papillary Muscles*	*Left Ventricular Wall*
Rheumatic heart disease	✓	✓		✓	✓		
Congenital mitral stenosis	✓			✓	✓	✓	
Cleft mitral valve		✓		✓			
Bacterial endocarditis		✓	*	✓	✓	*	
Coronary artery disease—myocardial infarction		✓				✓	✓
Diet drug valvulopathy		✓		✓	✓		
Mitral anular calcium	±	✓	✓	±			
Dilated cardiomyopathy		✓	✓			✓	✓
Hypertrophic cardiomyopathy		✓		✓		✓	✓
Myxoma	✓	✓		±			
Radiation	±	✓		✓	✓		
Infiltrative		✓		✓			✓
Carcinoid	✓	✓		✓	✓		
Papilloma		±		✓	✓		
Metastatic disease		±		±	±	±	±

MS, mitral stenosis; MR, mitral regurgitation; ✓, common and primary involvement; ±, infrequent or late-stage involvement; *, rare abscess formation.

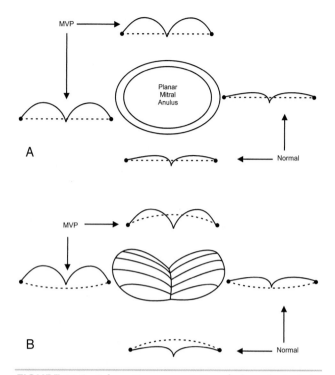

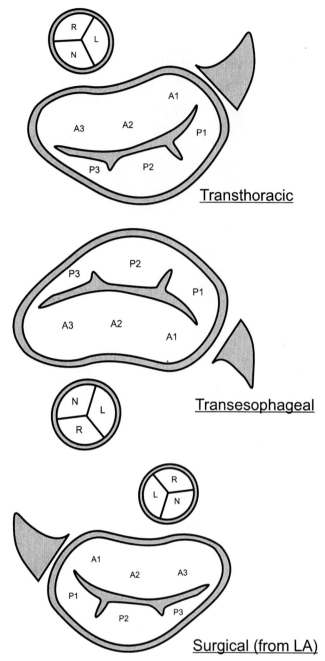

FIGURE 11.2. Schematic representation of a hypothetical planar mitral valve anulus **(A)** and the more accurate three-dimensional geometry of the anulus **(B)**. In each set of schematics, the plane of the anulus is depicted as a *dotted line* and either a normal mitral valve or a mitral valve with mitral valve prolapse, depicted as viewed from orthogonal planes. **A:** Note that a planar anulus results in the same appearance of the mitral valve when viewed from two perspectives 90 degrees apart. Normal mitral closure is noted on the right and the bottom of each schematic and mitral valve prolapse at the top and left. Note that the normal valve closes with the belly of the leaflet slightly behind the plane of the anulus, irrespective of the viewing perspective, and that the prolapse valve bows to a substantially greater degree. **B:** The three-dimensional saddle-shape geometry of the mitral anulus as described by Levine et al. Because of the saddle shape, the anulus may be either concave or convex toward the apex of the left ventricle depending on the viewing perspective. With a normal closure pattern in the lower anular schematic, note that the leaflet does not protrude above the plane of the anulus. The schematic to the right represents the identical closing geometry of the mitral valve, which now appears to prolapse behind the plane of the anulus because of its geometry in that perspective. The upper and leftward schematics depict the appearance of mitral valve prolapse as it relates to the saddle-shape geometry. In each instance, the geometry of the prolapse schematic is identical. Note the substantially greater degree to which prolapse is apparent on the left in **B** versus **A**, which is related to the different contour of the anulus when viewed from the orthogonal views.

FIGURE 11.3. Schematic representation of the mitral valve from multiple perspectives. **Bottom:** The view of the mitral valve in a surgical approach from inside the left atrium (*LA*). **Top:** The mitral valve as viewed from a traditional transthoracic parasternal short-axis view. **Middle:** The mitral valve is seen from a transesophageal approach at the mid gastric level. In each instance, the proximal aorta is as noted in the schematic, as is the left atrial appendage. The three distinct scallops of the anterior and posterior leaflets (*A1, A2, A3, P1, P2, P3*) are also schematized. L, left coronary sinus; N, non-coronary sinus; R, right coronary sinus.

Figure 11.4 schematizes the relationship between the anterior and posterior leaflets and their scallops to transesophageal echocardiographic planes. Figures 11.5 through 11.8 depict normal transthoracic and transesophageal echocardiographic images recorded in various imaging planes outlining the relationship of the echocar-

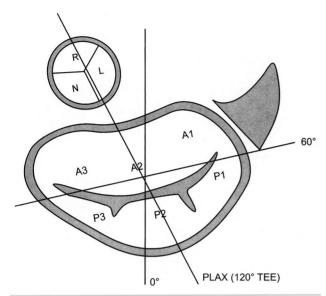

FIGURE 11.4. Expanded view of the mitral valve as seen from a transthoracic echocardiographic (*TEE*) approach. This image corresponds to the middle image of Figure 11.3. The imaging plane of a traditional transverse (0-degree) plane and parasternal long-axis view (or 120-degree transesophageal echocardiographic view) are as noted. Note that when imaged from a 60-degree imaging plane (commissural view) with a transesophageal echocardiographic probe, the imaging plane will intersect the P1, A2, P3 intersection. A1, A2, A3, anterior scallops 1 through 3; P1, P2, P3, posterior scallops 1 through 3; L, left coronary sinus; N, non-coronary sinus; PLAX, transthoracic parasternal long-axis plane; R, right coronary sinus.

diographic image to the anatomic mitral valve. Because of the curved C shape of the closed mitral valve, confusion often arises when dealing with a flail mitral valve leaflet. The C-shaped coaptation results in image planes in which alternating portions of the anterior and posterior leaflets may be visualized simultaneously (see the 60-degree plane in Figs. 11.4 and 11.8). It is not uncommon to detect multiple regurgitation jets in this view. This is discussed further in the section on flail mitral valve leaflets and in Chapter 19.

Coaptation of the mitral valve is complex and involves overlap of mitral valve tissue over a variable length of the mitral valve leaflet. Coaptation is not isolated to the mitral valve tips but rather is the result of overlap of several millimeters of tissue (the *zona coapta*) (Figs. 11.7 and 11.9). Because of this, the closing force of the mitral valve in systole actually increases with systolic pressure as the leaflets are forced to coapt along a longer portion of their terminal length. Any disease process that reduces the ability of the mitral valve to coapt along a several-millimeter length will result in inefficient or possibly incomplete coaptation and subsequent mitral regurgitation. Figure 11.10 schematizes abnormal coaptation patterns seen in a variety of disease states. It should be emphasized that disease processes occurring

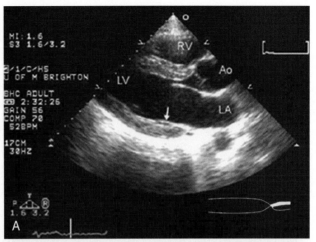

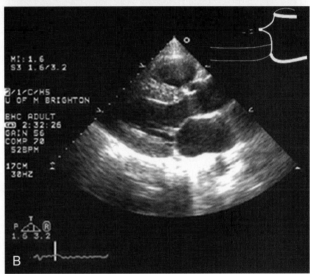

FIGURE 11.5. Parasternal long-axis view recorded in diastole **(A)** and systole **(B)** in a patient with a normal mitral valve. **A:** Note the anterior and posterior mitral valve leaflets. The posterior leaflet lies against the inferoposterior wall of the left ventricle (*LV*) (*arrow*) and may not be clearly seen when fully open. **B:** Both leaflets have moved toward the center of the left ventricular cavity and have closed with a 2- to 3-mm zone of overlap (the *zona coapta*). This is schematized in the middle to the right. Ao, aorta; LA, left atrium, RV, right ventricle.

anywhere along the length of the mitral apparatus (from the anulus to the base of the papillary muscle) can result in malfunction of the mitral valve.

PHYSIOLOGY OF MITRAL VALVE DISEASE

Physiologic abnormalities of mitral valve disease can be classified as stenosis, regurgitation, and combinations of the two. The classic form of mitral valve disease is rheumatic mitral stenosis in which the leaflet tips and chordae are involved and a transvalvular gradient develops, obstructing flow from the left atrium to the left ventricle.

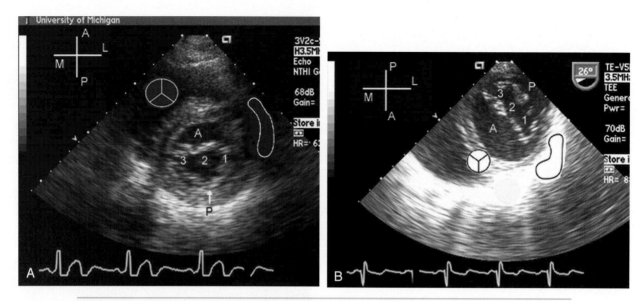

FIGURE 11.6. Parasternal short-axis view **(A)** and transesophageal short-axis view from a transgastric position **(B)** recorded in normal patients. The positions of the aorta and left atrial appendage are as noted by the schematics superimposed on the echocardiographic images. In each of these examples, recorded in diastole, the anterior (*A*) and posterior (*P*) leaflets of the mitral valve are clearly visualized and the three distinct regions (*1–3*) can be seen. For each imaging format, notice that the A1/P1 coaptation point is closest to the left atrial appendage and the A3/P3 coaptation closest to the ventricular septum. M, medial; L, lateral.

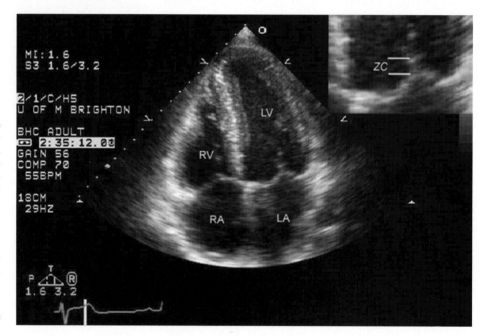

FIGURE 11.7. Apical four-chamber view recorded in systole in a normal patient. In this image, the normal closure pattern of the anterior and posterior leaflets of the mitral valve is clearly demonstrated. At the upper right, the closure pattern has been expanded. Note that the anterior and posterior mitral valve leaflets do not close tip to tip but rather along a 4-mm length [the *zona coapta* (*ZC*)]. LA, left atrium; LV, left ventricle, RA, right atrium; RV, right ventricle.

This has the effect of increasing the left atrial pressure throughout the entire cardiac cycle. Increased left atrial pressure is transmitted retrogradely to the pulmonary veins and pulmonary capillary bed. This elevated pressure then translates to an increased driving force for transudation of fluid into the alveoli and development of pulmonary congestion. Typically, with normal plasma on-cotic pressure, fluid extravasation into the alveoli occurs at a pulmonary capillary pressure of approximately 24 mm Hg. With reduced plasma oncotic pressure, extravasation of fluid will occur at lower hydrostatic pressures. Extravasation of fluid into the alveoli interrupts pulmonary gas exchange and results in dyspnea, initially with exercise but subsequently at rest, and to a variable

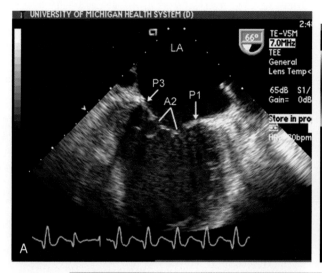
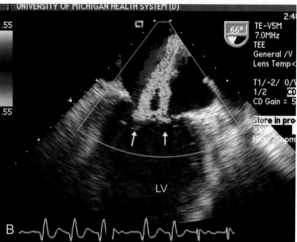

FIGURE 11.8. Transesophageal echocardiogram recorded at 66 degrees. In this view, the P1, A2, and P3 scallops are clearly visualized **(A)**. **B:** Note the two separate mitral regurgitation jets (*arrows*) arising from the P1-A2 and P3-A2 commissures. A1, A2, A3, anterior scallops 1 through 3; P1, P2, P3, posterior scallops 1 through 3. LA, left atrium; LV, left ventricle.

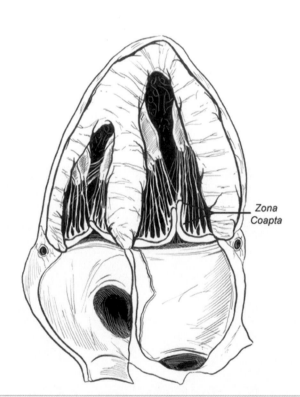

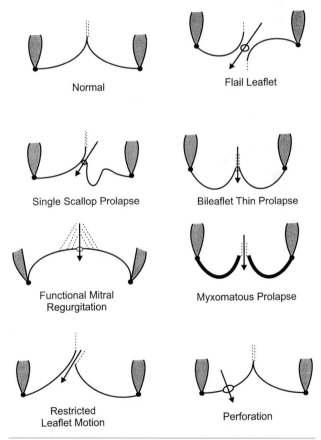

FIGURE 11.9. Anatomic rendering of the normal mitral valve in a closed position. Again note the chordae that attach not only to the leaflet tips but to the belly of the leaflet as well. Also note that the normal mitral valve does not close in a tip-to-tip manner but that there is an overlap of the leaflets as they close (the *zona coapta*). (Artwork by Amanda Almon and Travis Vermilye.)

FIGURE 11.10. Schematic drawings demonstrate a normal mitral valve closure pattern (*upper left*) and multiple different pathologic closure patterns. In each example, the anulus (*small black dot*) and proximal ventricular wall are denoted. At the point of the intended coaptation, the *open circle* denotes the regurgitant orifice and the *arrow* denotes the direction of the regurgitant flow. The *dotted lines* denote the mitral valve chordae.

degree may lead to secondary pulmonary hypertension. Development of pulmonary hypertension in the presence of increased pulmonary venous pressure is initially due to increased pulmonary vasoreactivity, but in chronic cases, fixed anatomic changes occur in the pulmonary vascular bed leading to both fixed and reactive pulmonary hypertension.

Chronically elevated left atrial pressure, due to obstruction at the mitral valve level, results in secondary dilation of the left atrium. Over time, this results in progressive fibrosis in the atrial myocardium with a subsequent decrease in atrial contractility, stasis of the blood, and the potential for atrial fibrillation and thrombus formation.

MITRAL STENOSIS

In adult populations, the etiology of mitral stenosis is overwhelmingly rheumatic heart disease. Because of the decreased incidence of recognized rheumatic heart disease in many developed countries, many patients with classic rheumatic involvement of the mitral valve have no known history of rheumatic fever. A far less common etiology of mitral stenosis is congenital mitral stenosis. Infrequently, mitral anular calcification develops to the point that it obstructs mitral valve inflow and mimics mitral stenosis. Tumors such as left atrial myxoma classically have been described as mimicking mitral stenosis, but presentation as occult mitral stenosis by a myxoma is exceptionally rare in contemporary practice.

Two-Dimensional Echocardiography in Rheumatic Mitral Stenosis

The classic findings of rheumatic mitral stenosis involve thickening and fusion of the mitral valve commissural edges and chordae. This results in characteristic abnormalities of the mitral leaflet opening motion. Normally, the anterior and posterior leaflets open with a motion pattern that involves maximal excursion at the leaflet tips. In mitral stenosis, due to commissural fusion, the leaflets open with a "doming" motion. In rheumatic heart disease, the open anterior leaflet has also been described as having a "hockey stick" appearance. Initially, this results in reduction of the orifice and conversion of the mitral leaflet–chordal apparatus from a tubular channel to a funnel-shaped orifice. It should be recognized that the limiting factor in flow from the left atrium to the left ventricle will be the orifice of the mitral valve and chordae at their junction. The degree of chordal thickening and mitral valve commissural fusion is highly variable. Over time, there is progressive fibrosis at the initial site of fusion as well as throughout the more distal chordae and more proximal leaflets. Eventually, this

results in stiffening and calcification of these structures. Figures 11.11 through 11.16 were recorded in patients with varying degrees of rheumatic mitral valve involvement. Note in Figures 11.11 and 11.12 the relatively pliable belly of the mitral valve leaflets with the disease

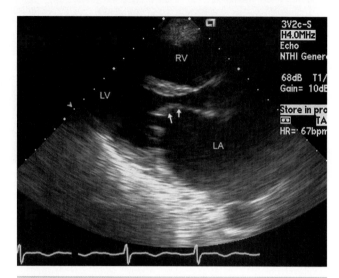

FIGURE 11.11. Transthoracic parasternal long-axis view echocardiogram recorded in a patient with rheumatic heart disease and mitral stenosis. In this image, recorded in early diastole, note the doming motion of the anterior mitral valve leaflet with restriction of motion at the tips. The belly of the leaflet (*arrows*) is pliable, and there is little or no fibrosis, calcification, or thickening of the leaflets. Also note the secondary dilation of the left atrium (*LA*). In the real-time image, note the relatively fixed position of the leaflet tips with all motion of the leaflet occurring at the mid and proximal portions of the leaflets. LV, left ventricle; RV, right ventricle.

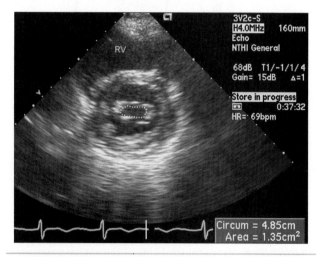

FIGURE 11.12. Parasternal short-axis view recorded in a patient with rheumatic heart disease and mitral stenosis. This image has been recorded at the level of the tips of the mitral valve and reveals the actual restrictive orifice. In this instance, the actual mitral valve area can be measured as 1.35 cm². RV, right ventricle.

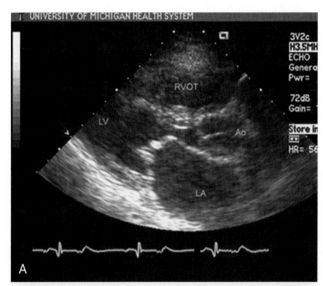

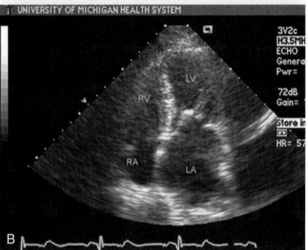

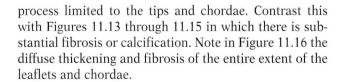

FIGURE 11.13. Parasternal long-axis view **(A)** and apical four-chamber view **(B)** recorded in a patient with mitral stenosis. **A:** Note the marked doming nature of the mitral valve opening in diastole with focal thickening at the tips of both the anterior and posterior leaflets. In the real-time image, note that pliability of the mid portion of the mitral valve is preserved. **B:** Apical four-chamber view reveals a similar phenomenon with doming of the mitral valve in diastole toward the apex. Ao, aorta; LA, left atrium; LV, left ventricle; RA, right atrium; RV, right ventricle; RVOT, right ventricular outflow tract.

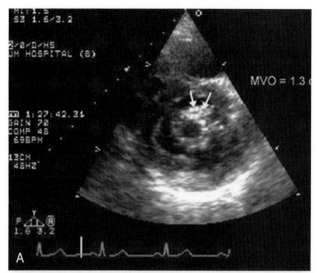

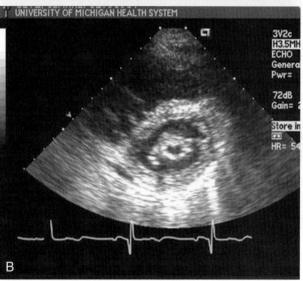

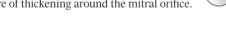

FIGURE 11.14. Parasternal short-axis views recorded in patients with rheumatic mitral stenosis. In each instance, note the restricted mitral valve orifice. **A:** The orifice can be planimetered as 1.3 cm². In this example, note the localized thickening of the chordae at the anterolateral border of the mitral orifice (*arrows*). **B:** Recorded in a patient with more severe stenosis. The mitral orifice has been planimetered at 0.7 cm². Also note the diffuse nature of thickening around the mitral orifice.

process limited to the tips and chordae. Contrast this with Figures 11.13 through 11.15 in which there is substantial fibrosis or calcification. Note in Figure 11.16 the diffuse thickening and fibrosis of the entire extent of the leaflets and chordae.

Congenital Mitral Stenosis

Congenital mitral stenosis is infrequently encountered in contemporary adult practice. There are two forms of con-

genital mitral stenosis. The first is "parachute" mitral valve. It typically occurs in conjunction with a single papillary muscle to which all chordae of an otherwise normal valve attach. This limits the mobility of the leaflets and results in restriction of inflow to a variable degree. The second type of congenital mitral stenosis is due to an anatomic abnormality of the valve and chordae resulting in a combination of reduced mobility and an intrinsic reduction in the anatomic orifice due to abnormal leaflet morphology (Fig. 11.17). This is discussed further in Chapter 18, Congenital Heart Diseases.

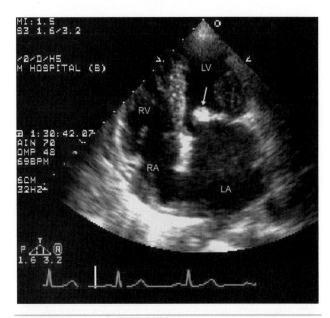

FIGURE 11.15. Apical four-chamber view recorded in a patient with rheumatic mitral stenosis. Note the marked dilation of the left atrium (*LA*). In this example, there is substantial but focal calcification of the anterior mitral valve leaflet (*arrow*). Note also the relatively restricted motion of both leaflets along their full length. LV, left ventricle; RA, right atrium; RV, right ventricle.

M-Mode Echocardiographic Appearance

M-mode echocardiography was one of the early tools used for evaluation of rheumatic mitral valve disease. The hallmark of rheumatic heart disease on M-mode echocardiography was increased echogenicity of the leaflets with decreased excursion and reduced separation of the anterior and posterior leaflets. This was accompanied by a reduced diastolic E-F slope of the mitral closure (Fig. 11.18). The E-F slope could be measured in millimeters per second and followed after intervention (the only intervention available at the time that this measurement was commonly undertaken was open mitral commissurotomy). The E-F slope was inversely correlated with the severity of mitral stenosis and improved (i.e., became steeper) after successful commissurotomy. The E-F slope ultimately proved to be nonspecific and was noted in any situation in which left ventricular filling was impaired such as in diastolic dysfunction. Thus, the E-F slope is of more historical than clinical value today. Additional features of mitral stenosis noted on M-mode echocardiography included "paradoxical" anterior diastolic motion of the posterior mitral valve leaflet. This occurred because tethering at the tips resulted in an obligatory anterior motion of the posterior mitral valve leaflet tips that, due to commissural fusion, were tethered to the larger anterior leaflet. Because M-mode echocardiography provided only a qualitative assessment of the presence of mitral steno-

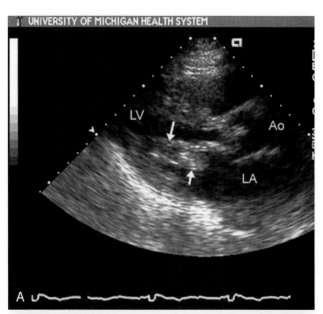

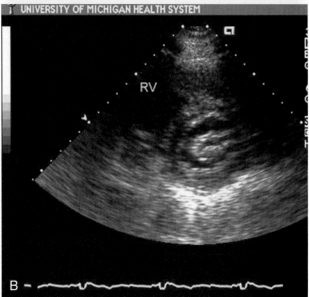

FIGURE 11.16. Parasternal long-axis (**A**) and short-axis (**B**) transthoracic echocardiograms recorded in a patient with rheumatic mitral stenosis. **A:** Note the marked thickening of the chordae throughout their entire length, from the mitral leaflet tips to the papillary muscles. In the short-axis view (**B**), the slit-like orifice of the mitral valve can be visualized. Ao, aorta, LA, left atrium; LV, left ventricle; RV, right ventricle.

sis, it has almost been completely replaced by two-dimensional echocardiography and Doppler techniques.

Transesophageal Echocardiography

Transesophageal echocardiography can provide additional information on patients with rheumatic mitral stenosis. It should be emphasized, however, that for diag-

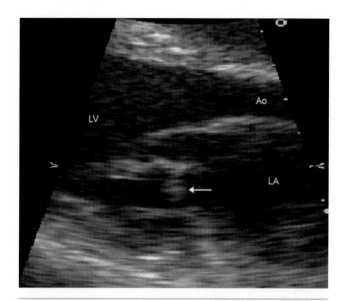

FIGURE 11.17. Expanded parasternal long-axis view recorded in a young patient with congenital mitral stenosis. Note the abnormal position of chordae to the posterior mitral leaflet (*arrow*), which restricts its motion, resulting in mitral stenosis. Ao, aorta; LA, left atrium; LV, left ventricle.

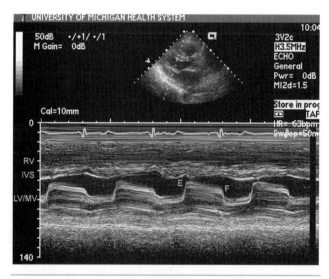

FIGURE 11.18. M-mode echocardiogram recorded in a patient with rheumatic mitral stenosis. Note the marked thickening of the mitral valve leaflets and the flat E-F slope during diastole. The posterior leaflet appears to move anteriorly in diastole as well.

nosis and quantification, there is little incremental yield afforded by transesophageal echocardiography in patients in whom a high-quality, high-resolution two-dimensional echocardiogram can be obtained. There is incremental value of the transesophageal echocardiogram with respect to some secondary findings such as left atrial appendage thrombus. Although transesophageal echocar-

diography provides a higher resolution view of the mitral valve apparatus, it may understate the severity of mitral anular and chordal involvement when the mitral valve is viewed from the left atrial aspect. Use of transgastric planes in 90- to 120-degree views can provide highly detailed visualization of the chordal apparatus (Figs. 11.19 and 11.20).

Three-Dimensional Echocardiography

Using the latest generation scanners, three-dimensional imaging of the entire mitral apparatus can be obtained

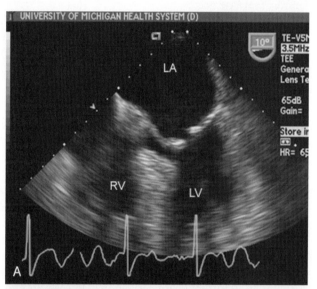

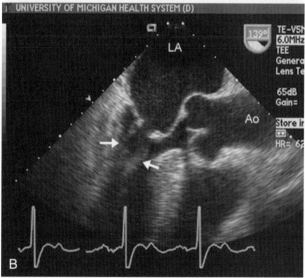

FIGURE 11.19. Transesophageal echocardiogram recorded in transverse and longitudinal views in a patient with mitral stenosis. **A, B:** In both images, note the diffuse thickening of the mitral leaflets with the doming motion in diastole. **B:** Also note the diffuse thickening of the chordae (*arrows*). Ao, aorta; LA, left atrium; LV, left ventricle; RV, right ventricle.

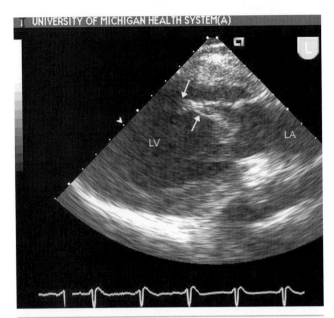

FIGURE 11.20. Transesophageal echocardiogram recorded in a longitudinal view in a patient with rheumatic mitral stenosis. Note the diffuse thickening of the chordae and fibrosis of the papillary muscle tip (*arrows*). LA, left atrium; LV, left ventricle.

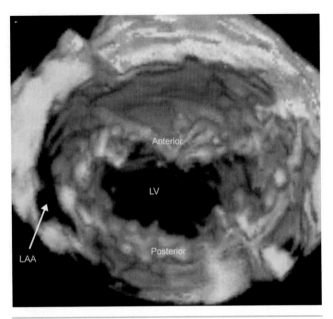

FIGURE 11.21. Three-dimensional echocardiographic reconstruction of the mitral orifice in a normal patient. The viewing perspective is from the cavity of the left atrium looking distally into the left ventricle. Note the echo lucency at the left, which represents the mouth of the left atrial appendage (*LAA*). LV, left ventricle.

from the transthoracic or transesophageal approach. Currently (2004) available scanners rely on reconstruction techniques from the transesophageal approach or real-time acquisition of a true three-dimensional data set from the transthoracic approach. This technique improves the reliability for determination of involvement of chordal structures and further characterization of fibrosis and calcification (Figs. 11.21 and 11.22). At this time, it is limited by its availability and technical complexity of offline reconstruction required in some systems.

Anatomic Determination of Severity

M-mode, two-dimensional, and three-dimensional echocardiography have all been used for the anatomic determination of severity of mitral stenosis. As noted previously, M-mode echocardiography relied on determination of leaflet thickness and the E-F slope as indirect measures of leaflet restriction. Although previously useful for serial follow-up, M-mode echocardiography provided no quantitative data regarding the actual restrictive orifice.

Using two-dimensional echocardiography, it is possible to visualize the actual restrictive orifice of the stenotic mitral valve at its limiting orifice (Figs. 11.12, 11.14, and 11.16). In patients with relatively symmetric involvement, the orifice area can accurately be planimetered and correlates well with that determined from hemodynamic data. There are several technical factors that must be accounted for in determining anatomic orifice size from this approach. First, one should recognize that, in mitral

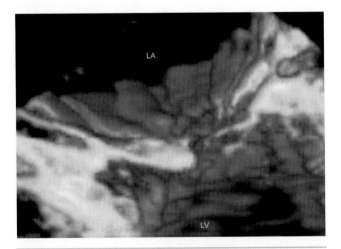

FIGURE 11.22. Three-dimensional reconstruction of a stenotic mitral valve in a patient with rheumatic heart disease. Note the diffusely thickened leaflets with restricted motion in the real-time image. LA, left atrium; LV, left ventricle.

stenosis, the mitral valve represents a funnel-shaped structure that tapers to its limiting orifice at the tips. Therefore, the actual limiting orifice is located at the tips, and careful scanning must be performed to ensure that the image is frozen and planimetered at the mitral valve tips and not more proximally where the orifice area would be overstated (Fig. 11.23). Second, instrumentation settings such as gain, reject, and transmission power all af-

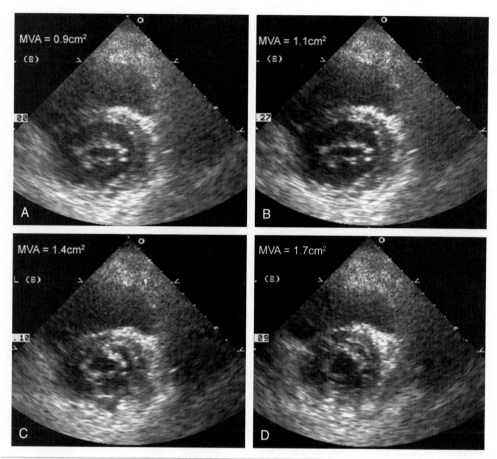

FIGURE 11.23. Series of parasternal short-axis views recorded in a patient with rheumatic mitral stenosis. **A:** Recorded at the actual restrictive orifice, and the mitral valve area (*MVA*) can be planimetered at 0.9 cm². **B–D:** The three additional views were recorded progressively closer to the anulus and show a progressive increase in the planimetered mitral orifice depending on the position at which the "orifice" is planimetered.

fect the ability to accurately visualize the limiting orifice. Increased gain will result in a "blooming" of the echoes, which then overstates their boundary and thereby diminishes the visualized orifice. When appropriately recorded, the measured orifice area correlates very well with that determined by hemodynamics. After commissurotomy, the orifice often becomes more irregular and the area of the commissural opening may be difficult to accurately planimeter.

Doppler Echocardiographic Determination of Severity

There are several methods for assessing the severity of mitral stenosis that can be derived from the Doppler mitral inflow pattern (Fig. 11.24). Doppler echocardiography can be used to determine the transvalvular gradient from the left atrium to the left ventricle. Determination of this gradient may be the single most important factor in determining the severity of mitral stenosis and the relationship to the patient's symptomatic and functional status. If

one understands the hemodynamic and physiologic principles noted previously and can provide an estimate of left ventricular diastolic pressure, then the overall hemodynamic effect of mitral stenosis can be derived from the transthoracic echocardiogram. It should be recognized that the transmitral gradient plus the anticipated left ventricular diastolic pressure equals the left atrial pressure. As noted previously, left atrial, pulmonary venous, and pulmonary capillary pressures are all similar and represent the hydrostatic driving pressure leading to pulmonary congestion. The pressure gradient is dependent on both volume status and heart rate, which affect filling time. Determination of the pressure gradient and its overall relevance to left atrial pressure should play an equal role in management to determination of a mitral valve area alone.

Determination of the mitral pressure gradient is easily accomplished from the transthoracic echocardiogram recorded from the apical approach in most patients. It often can be recorded in individuals in whom two-dimensional scanning provides suboptimal anatomic definition

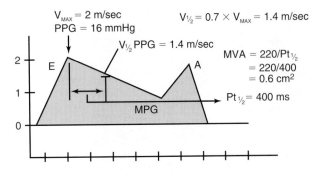

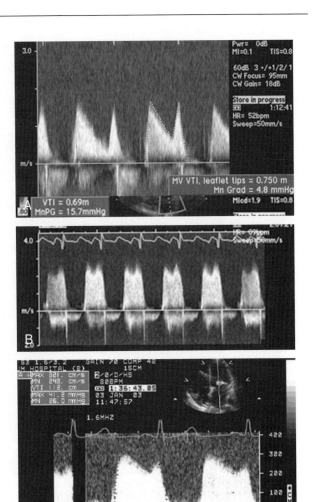

FIGURE 11.24. Schematic representation of mitral valve inflow depicting different parameters that can be extracted for determination of the severity of mitral stenosis. In the schematic, note the relatively flat decay of pressure from the E point. Parameters that can be measured include integration of the overall pressure gradient beneath the spectral display to calculate the mean pressure gradient (*MPG*) as well as calculation of mitral valve area (*MVA*) from the pressure half-time method. For the pressure half-time method, the time required for the pressure to decay from its peak value (16 mm Hg in this example) to one-half of that value (8 mm Hg) is determined. The velocity at which the gradient has declined to one-half its peak can be calculated as 0.7 × V$_{MAX}$. This value (400 milliseconds in this example) is then entered into the equation MVA = 220/Pt$_{1/2}$. In the schematic, the mitral valve area calculates to 0.6 cm². PPG, peak pressure gradient.

of mitral valve disease. The transmitral gradient should be recorded using continuous wave Doppler imaging aligned as parallel as possible to the anticipated flow. If pulsed wave Doppler imaging is used, it is essential that the sample volume be placed at the level of the restrictive orifice and not further back near the anulus. Placement of the sample volume near the anulus will result in systematic underestimation of the transmitral gradient. In general, rheumatic mitral stenosis results in a central stenotic orifice with flow directed from the center of the left atrium toward the apex of the left ventricle. As such, traditional two- and four-chamber viewing planes usually suffice for measurement. If necessary, color flow imaging can be used to determine the direction of flow and further refine this assessment. The peak and mean pressure gradient can be obtained online by electronic planimetry of the spectral profile at the time of examination or offline on a review station (Fig. 11.25). It should be emphasized that this mean gradient represents the mean of multiple instantaneous pressure gradients (each determined by the equation: $\Delta P = 4V^2$) and is not calculated from the calculated mean velocity.

Atrial fibrillation with an irregular heart rate poses additional problems. Depending on the diastolic filling time, there may be a dramatic variation in the mean transvalvular gradient (Fig. 11.26).

Examination of the spectral profile in Figures 11.24 and 11.27 suggests that there are several additional parameters of this pressure relationship that may be re-

FIGURE 11.25. Transmitral Doppler tracings recorded in patients with varying degrees of mitral stenosis. **A:** Recorded in a patient with very mild mitral stenosis. Note the relatively brisk pressure gradient decay and a mean gradient of 4.8 mm Hg. **B:** Recorded in a patient with more severe mitral stenosis and a mean gradient of 15.7 mm Hg. **C:** Recorded in a patient with severe mitral stenosis and a mean pressure gradient of 26 mm Hg. Also note the flat slope of pressure decay in this instance.

lated to mitral stenosis. The issue of the mean gradient was noted previously. An additional feature of the pressure gradient is the rapidity with which the instantaneous pressure gradient decays over time. It was recognized relatively early in the hemodynamic laboratory that individuals in whom the pressure gradient persisted to the end of diastole had more severe stenosis than those individuals in whom the pressure gradient declined to near zero at end-diastole. A measure of the rate of decay of the mitral valve gradient can be calculated as the pressure half-time ($Pt_{1/2}$) or the time in milliseconds at which the initial instantaneous pressure gradient declines to one-half its peak value. The mathe-

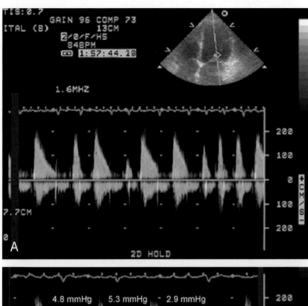

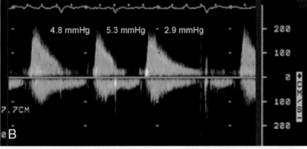

FIGURE 11.26. Transmitral continuous wave Doppler image recorded in a patient with mitral stenosis in atrial fibrillation with an irregular ventricular response. **A:** Note the marked variation in diastolic filling time and the obvious variation in the spectral profile. **B:** Recorded in the same patient, revealing three different diastolic filling profiles. Note the marked variation in the mean pressure gradient, dependent on diastolic filling time. MVA, mitral valve area.

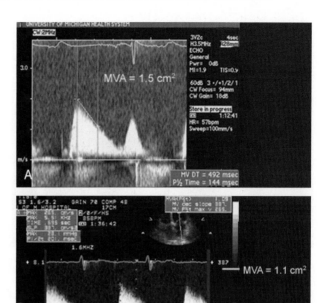

FIGURE 11.27. Transmitral spectral Doppler image recorded in patients with mitral stenosis. Images recorded in a patient with relatively mild stenosis **(A)** and in a patient with more severe mitral stenosis **(B)**. In each example, the pressure half-time has been used to calculate the mitral valve area, which is as noted on the figure. At the top, note the relatively steep decay of the pressure curve compared with the relatively flat pressure decay at the bottom.

matical calculation of $Pt_{1/2}$ is depicted in Figure 11.24. Empirically, $Pt_{1/2}$ is related to the mitral valve area by the formula: mitral valve area = $220/Pt_{1/2}$ (Fig. 11.24). There are several technical factors that affect this calculation. First, from a methodologic standpoint, the initial validation was done in a very small number of patients with hemodynamic rather than Doppler correlations. Second, the $P_{1/2}t$ calculation represents the "pressure decay" between the left atrium and left ventricle and as such will be affected by any factor that changes either left atrial driving pressure or left ventricular compliance and pressure. Situations in which the latter can be altered include severe left ventricular hypertrophy with reduced relaxation or concurrent aortic insufficiency, in which there is additional competitive filling of the left ventricle and an additional cause for an increase in left ventricular pressure. In many instances, the mitral stenosis signal is not a uniform slope but may have an early rapid decay followed by a more gradual decay,

giving a "ski slope" appearance to the spectral signal. In this instance, caution is advised, but the more accurate reflector of area will be derived from the flatter portion of the spectral envelope. In general, the derived anatomic area from the pressure half-time calculation is often less valuable for patient management than determination of pressure gradients and anatomically measured valve areas.

Although the mean pressure gradient is directly related to the average area of the restricted orifice and cardiac output, the peak instantaneous early pressure gradient between the left atrium and left ventricle is related to the early transmitral flow volume. Early flow volume is dependent on cardiac output and also affected by high early left atrial volumes, as may be seen with mitral regurgitation or high-output states. In the presence of mitral regurgitation or high cardiac output, there is a disproportionate increase in the early transvalvular velocity and gradient compared with the mean mitral valve gradient (Fig. 11.28). On occasion, this exaggerated early pressure gradient, compared with the mean pressure gradient, can be a clue to the presence of concurrent mitral regurgitation in situations in which the mitral regurgitation may not be directly visualized.

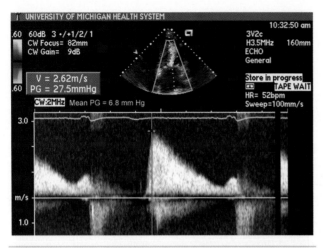

FIGURE 11.28. Transmitral Doppler image recorded in a patient with concurrent mitral stenosis and mitral regurgitation. Note the high peak early gradient (27.5 mm Hg) but the rapid decay and a negligible pressure gradient at end-diastole. Compare the peak early gradient of 27.5 mm Hg with the mean gradient of only 6.8 mm Hg. This discrepancy between peak and mean pressure gradient is often seen in patients with concurrent mitral regurgitation.

Exercise Gradients

By remeasuring the transmitral gradient with exercise, valuable information can be obtained regarding the physiologic impact of mitral stenosis. Although it is uncommon for there to be a clinical dilemma as to the severity of mitral stenosis and its link to symptoms when high transmitral gradients are measured at rest, occasional patients are encountered in whom there is a moderate resting gradient of 6 to 8 mm Hg but who have substantial clinical impairment. As noted previously in the section on physiology of mitral stenosis, the transmitral gradient is related to the volume of flow as well as the anatomic degree of obstruction. Increasing cardiac output and increasing heart rate result in an increasing volume of flow and a decrease in diastolic filling time. This has the effect of increasing pressure gradients for any degree of anatomic obstruction. Limited exercise such as 30 to 60 seconds of leg lifts frequently increases the heart rate and, in a supine position, allows registration of transmitral gradients that can then be compared with resting values. Figure 11.29 is an example in which transmitral gradients were recorded at rest and again after 30 seconds of leg lifts. The resting gradient is relatively unimpressive but increased dramatically with limited exercise. Keeping in mind the physiologic principals and relationship between this transvalvular gradient and pulmonary capillary pressures, one can then surmise valuable information regarding the physiologic abnormalities present in these patients after limited exercise.

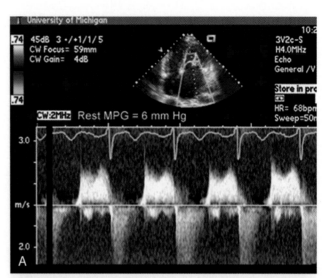

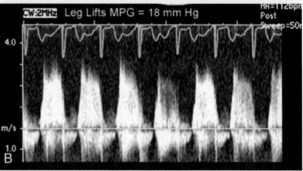

FIGURE 11.29. Transmitral pressure gradient recorded at rest **(A)** and after 30 seconds of leg lifts **(B)**. Note that the resting gradient is 6 mm Hg, and with minimal exercise, this gradient increases to 18 mm Hg. MPG, mean pressure gradient.

Secondary Features of Mitral Stenosis

Chronic mitral stenosis results in several common and easily recognized secondary features, the overwhelming majority of which are related to an increase in left atrial pressure. Chronic elevation in left atrial pressure results in left atrial dilation and eventual fibrosis of the atrial myocardium. Over time, fibrosis of the atrial myocardium results in decreased atrial contraction and serves as a substrate for development of atrial fibrillation. Dilation of the left atrium occurs both in the atrial body and left atrial appendage. The combination of atrial and atrial appendage dilation with decreasing mechanical function results in stasis of the blood with an enhanced propensity to thrombus formation, most commonly in the left atrial appendage. The tendency to develop stasis and clot is markedly increased in the presence of atrial fibrillation. Using either high-resolution transthoracic imaging or more often transesophageal imaging, it is not uncommon to see varying degrees of stasis of the blood flow in the atrium of patients with mitral stenosis. This typically appears as a swirling mass of echoes in the body of the left atrium, referred to as spontaneous echo contrast, and is often maximal in the left atrial appendage. Figures 11.30 through 11.34 were recorded in patients with rheumatic mitral stenosis and varying degrees of spontaneous echo contrast and thrombus formation within the left atrium and left atrial appendage. Current opinion suggests that spontaneous echo contrast and stasis of the blood are precursors to thrombus formation in the left atrium that carry a nearly equivalent risk of thromboembolic disease, especially if seen in the presence of atrial fibrillation. This issue is discussed further in Chapters 21 and 22.

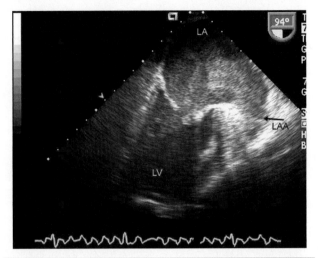

FIGURE 11.30. Transesophageal echocardiogram recorded in a patient with rheumatic mitral stenosis, left atrial dilation, and marked stasis of the blood within the left atrium and left atrial appendage. In the real-time image, the stasis of the blood appears as a dense swirling cloud of "smoke" filling the left atrium (*LA*) and left atrial appendage (*LAA*). LV, left ventricle.

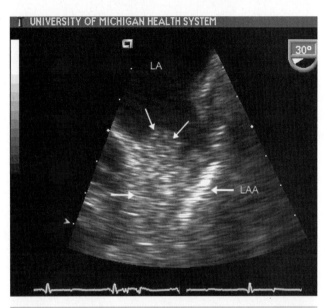

FIGURE 11.32. Transesophageal echocardiographic image of the left atrial appendage (*LAA*) in a patient with rheumatic mitral stenosis and a left atrial appendage thrombus. Note the irregular echo density mass filling the left atrial appendage (*thin arrows*). The boundary of the wall of the left atrial appendage is as noted by the *heavier arrows*. LA, left atrium.

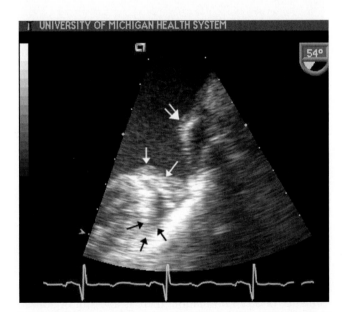

FIGURE 11.31. Transesophageal echocardiogram recorded in a patient with mitral stenosis who was in sinus rhythm. The *black arrows* denote the boundary of the left atrial appendage, which is filled with a relatively solid immobile mass of echoes consistent with left atrial appendage thrombus (*white arrows*). Additionally, there is a highly mobile, vague echo density (*double arrow*), which in the real-time image can be seen to have the characteristics of spontaneous echo contrast.

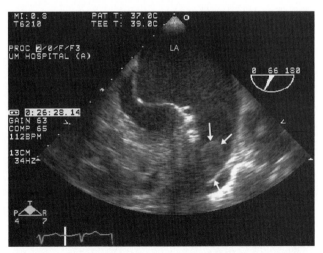

FIGURE 11.33. Transesophageal echocardiogram recorded in a patient with rheumatic mitral stenosis and atrial fibrillation. Note the oval-shaped small echo density in the apex of the left atrial appendage (*arrows*), which is consistent with left atrial appendage thrombus. LA, left atrium.

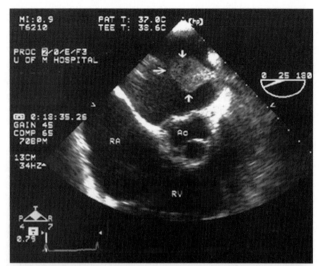

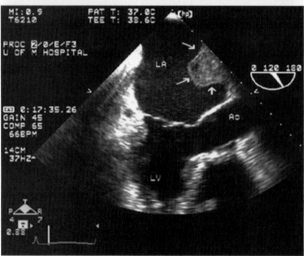

FIGURE 11.34. Transesophageal echocardiogram recorded in two views in a patient with mitral stenosis and a large left atrial thrombus. This thrombus arose from the left atrial appendage but protruded into the body of the left atrium (*LA*) (*arrows*). Ao, aorta; LV, left ventricle; RA, right atrium; RV, right ventricle.

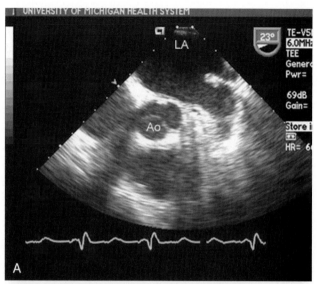

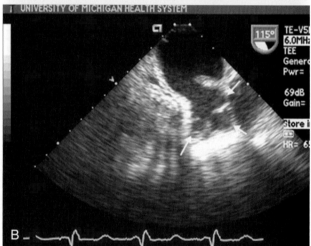

FIGURE 11.35. Transesophageal echocardiogram recorded from two different imaging planes in a patient with complex left atrial appendage anatomy. **A:** Note the relatively normal geometry of the left atrial appendage, which appears as a "dog ear"–shaped space immediately adjacent to the aorta (*Ao*). **B:** Recorded in a view orthogonal to that in **A.** Note the three distinct lobes of the left atrial appendage (*arrows*). LA, left atrium.

When evaluating a patient for a possible left atrial appendage thrombus, it is important to recognize the range in anatomic variability of the atrial appendage. Traditionally, the left atrial appendage has been considered a single-lobe structure with varying degrees of trabeculation due to pectinate muscles. It is now well recognized that the left atrial appendage has multiple lobes in a substantial percentage (>30%) of patients (Fig. 11.35). This raises several concerns when evaluating patients for a left atrial appendage thrombus. The first is that all lobes of the appendage must be identified and examined. The second issue is the need to recognize the septation tissue between appendage lobes as normal tissue and not as protruding thrombus.

Atrial Fibrillation

A frequent sequela of left atrial dilation is atrial fibrillation, which can be either intermittent or persistent. In the presence of atrial fibrillation, there is a loss of organized mechanical activity of the left atrium. This intensifies the tendency to form spontaneous echo contrast and thrombus. The fibrillatory mechanical activity of the atrium can be appreciated by either two-dimensional visualization or M-mode echocardiography of the left atrial wall. Additionally, Doppler echocardiography at the mouth of the atrial appendage reveals indirect evidence of the reduction in mechanical force due to atrial fibrillation. In Figure 11.36, note the high-frequency but low-velocity signals recorded by pulsed Doppler imaging at the mouth of the left atrial appendage. This represents a marked reduction in velocity and volume of flow out of the left atrial appendage compared with velocities seen in normal sinus rhythm and is the anatomic/physiologic basis for stasis and formation of clot. Patients with atrial fibrillation and relatively intact atrial appendage transport function as documented by preserved emptying velocities (>50 cm/sec) are less likely to have spontaneous contrast (and presumably thrombosis) than are those with reduced atrial appendage velocities.

Secondary Pulmonary Hypertension

An additional sequela of long-standing severe mitral stenosis is secondary pulmonary hypertension. In the early phases, this is due in large part to reactive changes in pulmonary vascular resistance and is reversible with correction of mitral stenosis. In long-standing severe mitral stenosis, a fixed component occurs, and in this instance, pulmonary artery systolic hypertension may be only partially reversible.

Echocardiographic manifestations of secondary pulmonary hypertension in mitral stenosis are similar to those seen in pulmonary hypertension of any cause. Concurrent tricuspid regurgitation is present in the majority of these patients, usually due to right ventricular dilation and less often due to direct involvement of the tricuspid valve by the rheumatic process.

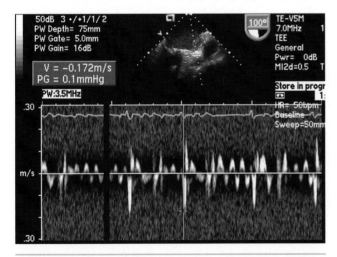

FIGURE 11.36. Pulsed Doppler image recorded from the left atrial appendage in a patient with mitral stenosis and atrial fibrillation. Note the high-frequency, low-velocity signals (<20 cm/sec), indicative of reduced mechanical transport in the left atrial appendage.

Decision Making Regarding Intervention

Medical management plays only a minor role in alleviating symptoms in moderate and severe mitral stenosis. Therapy is predominantly directed at increasing the effective mitral orifice area, by open surgical commissurotomy, percutaneous balloon valvotomy, or mitral valve replacement.

Once a decision has been made that the severity of mitral stenosis warrants intervention, two-dimensional echocardiography plays a valuable role in determining the most appropriate interventional or surgical technique. As a general rule, valves with heavy degrees of calcification, chordal shortening and fibrosis, and prominent subvalvar involvement, are not good candidates for either surgical or interventional correction. Figures 11.11 and 11.12 were recorded in a patient with relatively mild fibrosis of the valve for which either surgical or balloon intervention would be feasible. Compare these figures with Figures 11.13 through 11.16, in which there are varying degrees of diffuse fibrosis and calcification of the mitral valve apparatus.

A mitral valve score has been proposed to further characterize and stratify the degree to which the valve is anatomically compromised. The components of this mitral valve score are schematized in Figure 11.37. The components of the score are leaflet thickening, leaflet mobility, calcification, and subvalvular involvement. Each of these is then graded numerically as 0 (none or absent) to 4 (severe or extensive), depending on severity of none to severe. There is a direct relationship between the score and the likelihood of successful balloon valvotomy, with higher scores mitigating against successful intervention. In general, calcification and subvalvular involvement represent a disproportionate contribution to the likelihood of technical failure at the time of balloon valvotomy. Individuals with a mitral valve score of ≤8 typically are excellent candidates for balloon valvotomy, and those with scores greater than 12 are less likely to have a satisfactory result. The issue of balloon valvotomy and intraprocedural monitoring success of this procedure with transesophageal echo is discussed further in Chapter 19, which deals with monitoring of operative and interventional procedures.

MITRAL REGURGITATION

Mitral regurgitation is a commonly encountered hemodynamic lesion. It can occur due to primary disease of the mitral leaflets or can occur secondary to other abnormalities of the mitral apparatus. Etiologies of mitral regurgitation are outlined in Tables 11.1 and 11.2. Mitral regurgitation represents a pathologic leak of blood typically under systolic pressure, from the left ventricle

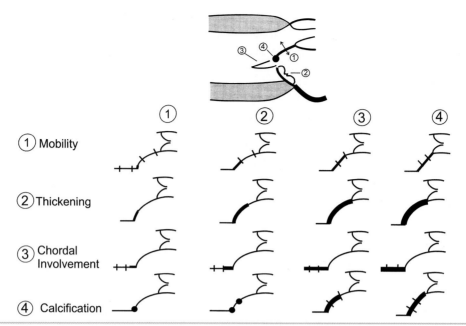

FIGURE 11.37. Schematic demonstration of the calculation of the mitral stenosis score. This figure is adapted from the work of Wilkins et al. The large schematic at top denotes the four components for calculation of the score, which included leaflet mobility (*1*); leaflet thickening (*2*); chordal involvement (*3*), and calcification (*4*). For each characteristic, involvement is graded with respect to its extension from the proximal to mid to distal one-third of the leaflet. To calculate the total mitral stenosis score, involvement for each characteristic is summed. (See text for details).

into the left atrium. Acute severe mitral regurgitation often results in acute pulmonary congestion, whereas chronic mitral regurgitation may be tolerated for decades. By definition, mitral regurgitation occurs during systole, which, at normal resting heart rates, constitutes approximately one-third of the cardiac cycle. As such, the left atrial pressure elevation is not present consistently but only transiently. The transient nature of the pressure increase seen in mitral regurgitation represents less of a drive to development of pulmonary congestion and secondary pulmonary hypertension than does the chronic (although lower intensity) pressure elevation seen in mitral stenosis. Additionally, mitral regurgitation is a volume overload of the left ventricle. This volume overload may be well tolerated for relatively long periods of time but eventually results in a reduction in left ventricular myocardial contractile force, which may not be reversible even with correction of the mitral regurgitation.

Doppler Evaluation of Mitral Regurgitation

The full range of echocardiographic techniques should be used for complete evaluation of mitral regurgitation (Table 11.3). Currently, color Doppler imaging is the primary echocardiographic tool for detection and quantitation of mitral regurgitation. It should be emphasized that not all color Doppler signals appearing within the left atrium represent mitral regurgitation. There are several potential sources of color Doppler flow signal in the left atrium. These include normal posterior motion of the blood pool caused by mitral valve closure (Fig. 11.38), reverberation from aortic flow (Fig. 11.39), normal pulmonary vein inflow (Fig. 11.40) (which occurs in systole and diastole), and low velocity overall atrial motion augmented by inappropriate gain and Nyquist limits. Any of these can result in the appearance of a color Doppler signal in the left atrium in systole. On occasion, these spurious signals have been erroneously attributed to mitral regurgitation and either a false diagnosis of regurgitation has been made or the extent of true regurgitation overstated. The characteristics of a true mitral regurgitation jet are as follows: (1) there is evidence of proximal flow acceleration [proximal isovelocity surface area (PISA)], (2) the flow conforms to the appearance of a true "jet" or ejection flow with a *vena contracta*, (3) the downstream (left atrial) appearance is consistent with a volume of blood being ejected through a relatively constraining orifice, (4) the flow signal is appropriately confined to systole, and (5) the color Doppler signals are appropriate in color for the anticipated direction and/or reveal the appropriate variance or turbulence encoding. Finally, in equivocal cases pulsed and/or continuous wave Doppler should be used to confirm the origin, timing, and direction of flow (Figs. 11.41 and 11.42).

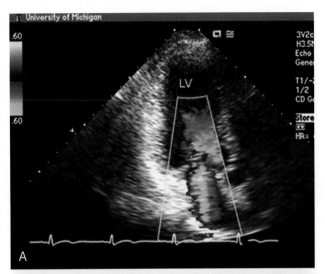

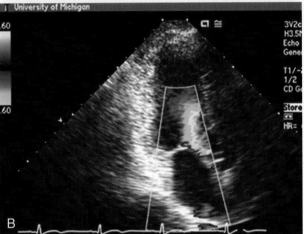

FIGURE 11.38. Apical view recorded in a patient with faint, early systolic blue color Doppler encoding within the left atrium. This color signal represents overall posterior motion of the pre-existing blood pool in the left atrium, combined with backwash of flow forced to motion by the closing mitral valve leaflets. Note that it is present only in **A,** recorded in very early systole, immediately after mitral closure and is not present in the subsequent image (**B**) recorded 50 milliseconds later. Also note the lack of any convergence zone, *vena contracta* or high velocity color coding. This signal should not be mistaken for true mitral regurgitation. LV, left ventricle.

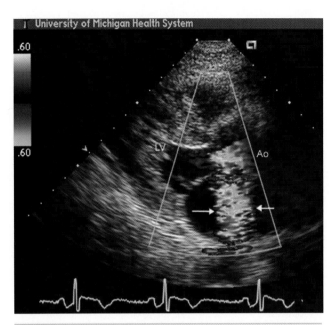

FIGURE 11.39. Parasternal long-axis view recorded in a patient with color reverberation in the left atrium (*between the arrows*). This signal is a color artifact arising from the aorta (*Ao*) and should not be confused for mitral regurgitation. Note that it is a direct extension of the turbulent flow in the proximal aorta and that it does not arise from any area of mitral valve closure. In the real-time image, note the very brief duration of this signal. LV, left ventricle.

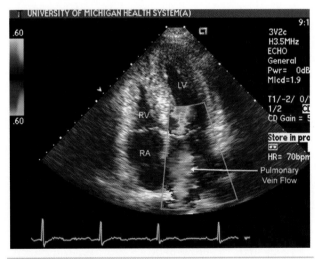

FIGURE 11.40. Apical four-chamber view recorded in a patient with prominent pulmonary vein flow in the left atrium in systole. Note that although this signal extends from the plane of the mitral valve to the wall of the left atrium, it is encoded in red, indicative of flow toward the transducer and that there is no evidence of high-velocity turbulent flow, *vena contracta*, or flow convergence. LV, left ventricle, RA, right atrium; RV, right ventricle.

Although color flow Doppler imaging has largely replaced the use of spectral recordings for detection and quantification of mitral regurgitation, these modalities can be useful for confirmation. Because of the high gradient between the left ventricle and left atrium, the velocity of a mitral regurgitation jet will virtually always exceed the Nyquist limit and aliasing will occur (Fig. 11.43). Inspection of the spectral signal can provide clues as to the severity and timing of mitral regurgitation as well as downstream (left atrial) pressure.

By definition, hemodynamically significant mitral regurgitation results in a volume overload of the left ventricle with subsequent left ventricular and left atrial dilation. As a consequence, there is elevation of left atrial pressure, which is transmitted to the pulmonary venous vasculature resulting in pulmonary congestion. The physiology of

▶ TABLE 11.3 **Echo-Doppler Parameters of Mitral Regurgitation**

Anatomic
  Chambers
    Left ventricular dimensions/size
    Left atrial dilation
    Left ventricle volume and stroke volume
    Valve Perforation
Doppler
  Color flow
    Jet area
    Jet area indexed to left atrium
    Central vs. eccentric jets
    Vena contracta width
    Proximal isovelocity surface area
      Size/qualitative
      Volumetric flow/regurgitant volume
      Effective regurgitant orifice
  Pulmonary vein flow reversal
  Spectral
    Forward flow calculation at the mitral anulus
    Signal density
    Elevated E/A ratio (with normal left ventricular function)

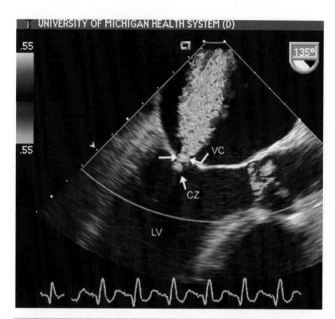

FIGURE 11.42. Transesophageal echocardiogram in a patient with moderate mitral regurgitation demonstrates the components of true mitral regurgitation as schematized in Figure 11.41. Note the flow acceleration convergence zone (*CZ*), the relatively narrow *vena contracta* (*VC*), and a high-velocity turbulent downstream jet. LV, left ventricle.

acute severe mitral regurgitation is substantially different from chronic mitral regurgitation. In the acute setting, there is insufficient time for chamber dilation to occur and for left atrial compliance to increase. As such, acute severe mitral regurgitation is associated with dramatic

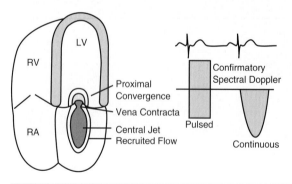

FIGURE 11.41. Schematic demonstrates the principal features of true mitral regurgitation. The various components of the true regurgitant signal are outlined on the schematic, including the proximal flow acceleration zone, the *vena contracta*, and a central high-velocity jet surrounded by lower velocity recruited flow. The figure also schematizes a confirmatory spectral Doppler image recorded in both continuous wave and pulsed wave modes. Note the aliasing phenomenon with pulsed wave Doppler imaging. LV, left ventricle; RA, right atrium; RV, right ventricle.

and substantial elevation of left atrial pressure acutely, which results in the instantaneous onset of symptoms. With chronic mitral regurgitation, the left atrium dilates and compliance increases. Because of this, left atrial pressure is lower in the chronic than in the acute setting for any given degree of mitral regurgitation.

The jet of mitral regurgitation may be either central, peripheral, single or multiple and may be eccentric within the left atrium and impinge on a wall. Figure 11.10 schematizes the mitral closure pattern and jet direction in a number of disease states. Figures 11.44 through 11.52 were recorded in patients with mitral regurgitation of varying severity and regurgitation jet morphology. The direction taken by the mitral regurgitation jet provides valuable clues as to the etiology of mitral regurgitation. In general, an eccentric jet suggests an anatomic abnormality resulting in flail or partial flail of one leaflet. The initial observation was made in patients with flail leaflets in which the jet direction was opposite to that of the involved leaflet. As such, a posterior flail leaflet generally results in an anteriorly directed jet, whereas the converse is true for an anterior flail leaflet. The mechanism by which this occurs is schematized in Figure 11.53.

It should be emphasized that mechanisms other than a flail leaflet can result in an eccentric mitral regurgitation jet. Ischemic disease commonly results in retraction of one mitral leaflet with subsequent malcoaptation. A fairly

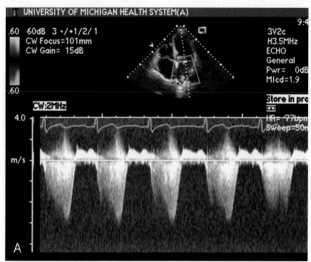

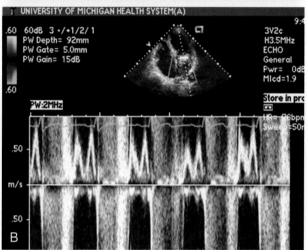

FIGURE 11.43. Spectral Doppler image recorded in a patient with mitral regurgitation using continuous wave Doppler **(A)** and pulsed Doppler **(B)** imaging. Note the aliasing phenomenon with pulsed Doppler imaging in which the signal directed away from the transducer is paradoxically recorded above the zero crossing line after exceeding the Nyquist limit (1.0 m/sec in this example). In the continuous wave signal, note the ability to record the full maximal velocity of the mitral regurgitation jet (6 m/sec).

common scenario is restriction of motion of the posterior mitral valve leaflet due to inferior ischemia or infarction and tethering of the normal motion. This results in the anterior leaflet tip coapting behind the restricted posterior leaflet (Fig. 11.54). This has the result of directing the regurgitant jet in a posterior direction, thus mimicking a partial flail of the anterior leaflet (Fig. 11.55).

In patients with dilated cardiomyopathy, the papillary muscles are apically displaced, which tethers the valve apically and limits normal coaptation (Fig. 11.56). When both leaflets are equally affected, the regurgitant jet is typ-

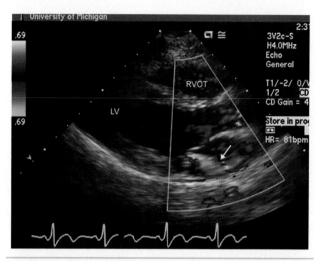

FIGURE 11.44. Parasternal long-axis view recorded in a patient with mild mitral regurgitation (*arrow*). Note the relatively small color flow area when compared with the total left atrial area. LV, left ventricle; RVOT, right ventricular outflow tract.

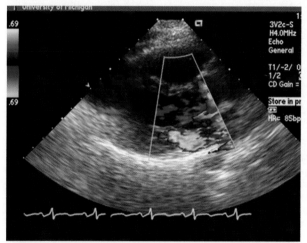

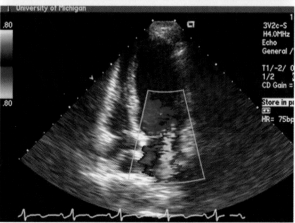

FIGURE 11.45. Parasternal long-axis and apical four-chamber views recorded in a patient with moderate mitral regurgitation. In each instance, note the intermediate-sized jet encompassing approximately 25% of the left atrial area.

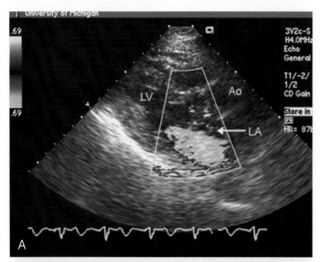

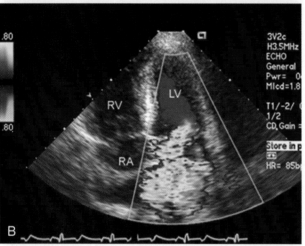

FIGURE 11.46. Transthoracic echocardiograms recorded in patients with severe mitral regurgitation. Recorded in the parasternal long-axis view **(A)** and in the apical four-chamber view **(B)**. In each instance, note the large color flow Doppler signal filling greater than 50% of the left atrial area. Ao, aorta; LA, left atrium; LV, left ventricle; RA, right atrium; RV, right ventricle.

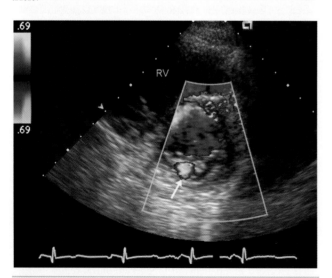

FIGURE 11.47. Parasternal short-axis transthoracic echocardiogram recorded in a patient with mitral regurgitation. This image was recorded at the level of the mitral valve tips and allows direct visualization of the short-axis area of the mitral regurgitation jet, which can be seen to arise from an area slightly medial to midline (*arrow*). RV, right ventricle.

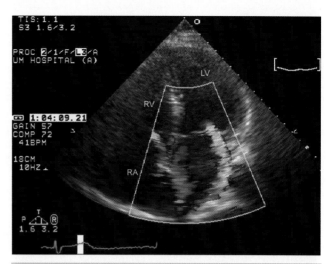

FIGURE 11.48. Apical four-chamber view recorded in a patient with a highly eccentric mitral regurgitation jet. In both the static and real-time images, note that the jet originates at the lateral margin of the mitral valve and then courses laterally along the left atrial wall. The actual color Doppler area of an eccentric jet such as this understates the true severity of mitral regurgitation (see text for details). LV, left ventricle; RA, right atrium; RV, right ventricle.

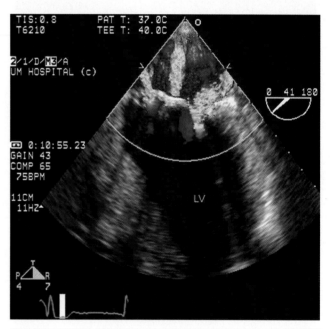

FIGURE 11.49. Transesophageal echocardiogram recorded from a patient with three separate mitral regurgitation jets. Inspection of Figure 11.4 reveals that in this imaging plane, these jets are likely to be arising from the coaptation of different anterior and posterior scallops. LV, left ventricle.

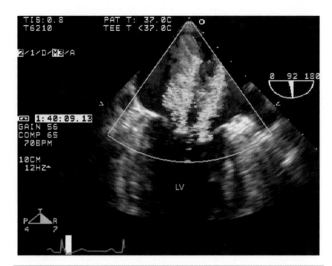

FIGURE 11.50. Transesophageal echocardiogram recorded in a patient with two distinct mitral regurgitation jets. In this instance, the two relatively limited jets combined probably represent moderate mitral regurgitation. LV, left ventricle.

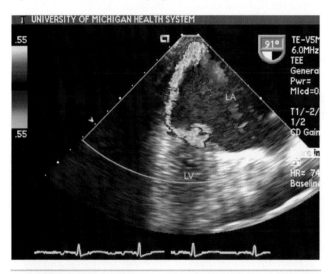

FIGURE 11.51. Transesophageal echocardiogram recorded in a patient with a highly eccentric mitral regurgitation jet. Note the origin of the jet near the midpoint of mitral valve closure but its highly eccentric nature as it courses along the posterior wall of the left atrium (*LA*). Note also that the jet does not appear in a traditional echocardiographic view, the transducer position has been optimized for the left atrium and mitral regurgitation jet, and the left ventricle (*LV*) has been markedly foreshortened.

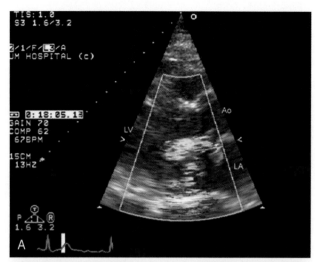

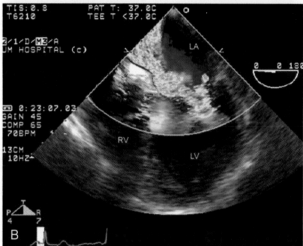

FIGURE 11.52. Transthoracic (**A**) and transesophageal echocardiograms (**B**), both recorded in a patient with mitral regurgitation due to a flail leaflet. In both instances, note the highly eccentric mitral regurgitation jet. **A:** An organized jet is not visualized, but rather there is a disorganized color signal appearing immediately below the anterior mitral leaflet. Note in the real-time image that this jet does not appear to fill a significant portion of the left atrium (*LA*). **B:** Recorded in the same patient, note the obvious convergence zone on the left ventricular side of the mitral valve and the substantial size of the eccentric mitral regurgitation jet, which is directed along the aorta (*Ao*) and atrial wall. LV, left ventricle; RV, right ventricle.

ically central (Fig. 11.57). See Chapter 17 for further discussion of this phenomenon.

Determination of Mitral Regurgitation Severity

Determination of the severity of mitral regurgitation relies heavily on color flow Doppler imaging. There are numerous limitations to using this methodology for assessing regurgitation jets which were discussed in Chapter 2. Initial validation studies were done with contrast left ven-

triculography as the standard in relatively small cohorts. These all suggested a rough correlation between the angiographic grade of regurgitation and the color flow area within the left atrium. Instrumentation used in earlier studies probably did not have the sensitivity of current-generation scanners. Over time, these advantages may have resulted in systematic overestimation of regurgitation severity when assessed with color flow imaging. In general, the severity of mitral regurgitation is directly proportional to the area of the regurgitation jet in the left

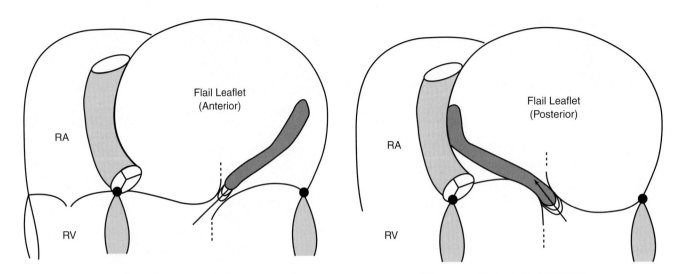

FIGURE 11.53. Schematic representation of jet direction in the presence of a flail anterior **(left)** or posterior **(right)** leaflet. In each instance, note that the tip of the flail leaflet is located behind the belly of the intact leaflet. This results in eccentric orientation of the regurgitant orifice, with the direction of the regurgitant jet opposite that of the flail leaflet. Note that the flail posterior leaflet results in a jet directed along the left atrial wall and the posterior wall of the aorta. This may result in a mitral regurgitation jet, which on auscultation is heard in the typical aortic area. The more laterally directed jet, attributable to the anterior flail leaflet, will result in a jet directed toward the lateral wall of the left atrium and a murmur heard best laterally rather than anteriorly. RA, right atrium; RV, right ventricle.

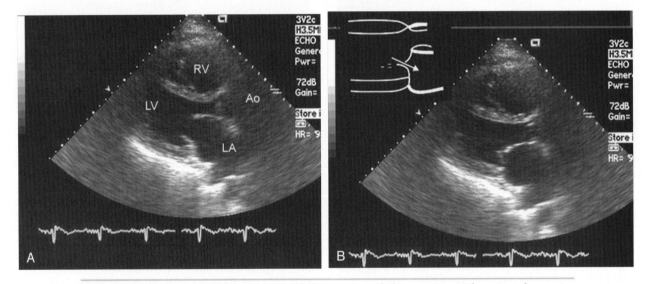

FIGURE 11.54. Parasternal long-axis echocardiogram recorded in a patient with restricted posterior mitral leaflet motion. **A:** Recorded in diastole. Note the relatively normal-appearing mitral leaflets. **B:** Recorded at end-systole. Note the relative immobility of the posterior leaflet, which has remained tethered toward the left ventricular apex. The tip of the anterior leaflet coapts behind the tip of the posterior leaflet. This closure pattern is schematized to the left. In this instance (Fig. 11.55), the restricted posterior leaflet has resulted in a posteriorly directed mitral regurgitation jet. Ao, aorta; LA, left atrium; LV, left ventricle; RV, right ventricle.

atrium. When assessing regurgitation jet size, it is imperative to adjust Doppler gains appropriately to avoid "blooming," which will increase the apparent jet size. Additionally, an inappropriately low Nyquist limit will result in low-velocity pulmonary vein flow and recruited flow being encoded as turbulence and systematically overstate the severity of regurgitation (Fig. 11.58). It should be emphasized that jet size will vary over the systolic cycle. While the eye rapidly integrates this change in size over time to estimate overall jet size, any given still frame may either dramatically over- or underestimate the jet size and hence mischaracterize severity.

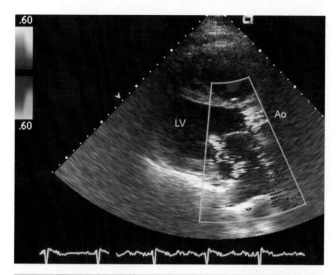

FIGURE 11.55. Parasternal long-axis view with color flow Doppler imaging recorded in the same patient depicted in Figure 11.54. Note the posteriorly directed mitral regurgitation jet, which in many instances would imply pathology of the anterior leaflet but in this instance is due to restricted motion of the posterior leaflet. Ao, aorta; LV, left ventricle.

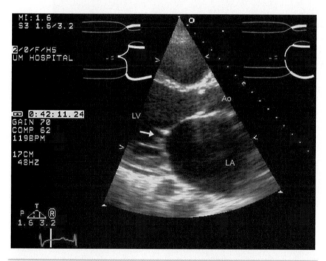

FIGURE 11.56. Parasternal long-axis view recorded in a patient with a dilated cardiomyopathy and apical displacement of the papillary muscles, leading to functional mitral regurgitation. Note the dilation of the left ventricle (*LV*) and left atrium (*LA*). This frame was recorded in mid-systole. Because of the displacement of the papillary muscles, the mitral leaflets are tethered apically and cannot coapt along a normal zone. The mitral valve is attempting to coapt in a tip-to-tip manner. In this example, the actual regurgitant orifice (*arrow*) can be visualized. In the upper left, the normal mitral closure along a 2 to 3 mm distance is schematized. In the upper right, the abnormal closure pattern with incomplete coaptation is schematized. Ao, aorta.

The assessment of mitral regurgitation severity can be enhanced by indexing the regurgitation jet area to left atrial size (Figs. 11.59 and 11.60). Several relatively small studies have confirmed the correlation between this type of assessment of mitral regurgitation severity and a stan-

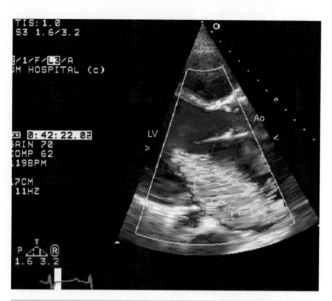

FIGURE 11.57. Parasternal long-axis echocardiogram with color flow Doppler recorded in the same patient depicted in Figure 11.56. Note the large color flow Doppler jet filling more than 50% of the left atrial cavity, consistent with severe mitral regurgitation. Note also that the origin of the jet is in the area identified by the *arrow* in Figure 11.56 as non-coaptation of the mitral leaflets. Ao, aorta; LV, left ventricle.

dard such as contrast ventriculography. Figures 11.44 through 11.46 were recorded in patients with different grades of severity of mitral regurgitation. Additionally, the width of the regurgitant jet at its origin (the *vena contracta*) can be measured from the color Doppler image and has been correlated with regurgitation severity as well.

Most schemes for determining the severity of mitral regurgitation were developed in the presence of central jets where the regurgitant jet recruits into motion left atrial blood adjacent along all its surfaces. As such, the overall Doppler encoded size of the "jet" in the left atrium overstates the true volume of flow from the left ventricle by the amount of preexisting left atrial blood recruited into motion. If a similar volume of regurgitant flow arises from an eccentric jet, so that the regurgitant jet impinges on a wall, then recruitment of left atrial blood into motion occurs only over the portion of the jet surface area that is not constrained by a wall. This results in a relatively smaller amount of recruitment for an impinging jet than for a central jet. This effect results in underestimation of regurgitation severity when an impinging jet is compared with an identical regurgitant volume due to a central jet. This phenomenon is schematized in Figure 11.61. In general, color flow Doppler imaging of a highly eccentric jet impinging on the left atrial wall will understate the regurgitation volume by approximately 40% when compared with an identical regurgitant volume that is centrally located.

An additional parameter that relates to the severity of regurgitation is the density of the spectral Doppler signal. Spectral density is directly proportional to the number of

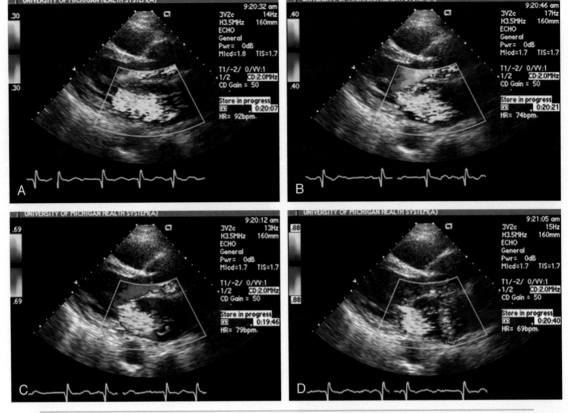

FIGURE 11.58. Impact of Nyquist limit on apparent regurgitation jet size. All four images were recorded in the same patient with moderate mitral regurgitation. C, D: Recorded at Nyquist limits of 0.69 m/sec and 0.88 m/sec, resulting in a smaller apparent jet than A, B, recorded at inappropriately low Nyquist limits of 0.3 m/sec and 0.4 m/sec. Note that at the low Nyquist limit of 0.3 m/sec, even normal pulmonary vein inflow has been encoded as turbulent flow, thus resulting in a substantially larger area of turbulence in the left atrium and overstating the severity of mitral regurgitation.

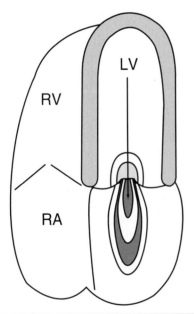

FIGURE 11.59. Schematic representation demonstrates the methodology by which jet area is used to determine jet severity. A series of centrally located, not eccentric, jets are demonstrated, which encompass approximately 15%, 25%, 35%, and 60% of the left atrial area, representing grades 1 through 4 (mild to severe) mitral regurgitation. LV, left ventricle; RA, right atrium; RV, right ventricle.

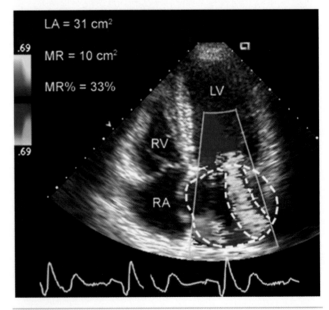

FIGURE 11.60. Apical four-chamber view recorded in a patient with mitral regurgitation. In this example, the left atrial area (LA) is 31 cm² and the area of the mitral regurgitation (MR) jet is 10 cm², which results in a jet-to-left atrial area ratio of 33%. LV, left ventricle; RA, right atrium; RV, right ventricle.

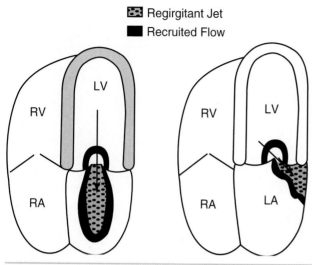

Legend:
- ⊞ Regirgitant Jet
- ■ Recruited Flow

FIGURE 11.61. Schematic representation of the effect of an impinging wall jet versus a centrally located wall jet on overall jet size detected with color Doppler flow imaging. **Left:** A centrally located "free" jet within the body of the left atrium, which is not constrained by a solid boundary such as the atrial wall. The darker central jet represents the actual volume of regurgitant blood, which originated in the left ventricle (*LV*) and has been ejected into the left atrium (*LA*). The fainter outer signal represents the blood that has been recruited into motion and is also detected by color flow Doppler imaging. Note that the total amount of blood in motion exceeds the actual regurgitant volume by approximately 40%. **Right:** The effect on jet size for a jet directed along a constraining surface, such as the left atrial wall. The dark area represents the blood ejected from the left ventricle into the left atrium and is the same area as the dark regurgitant jet on the left. Note that the blood is recruited into motion only along one surface of the jet, hence making the total area of the jet (regurgitant blood plus recruited blood) smaller than the free jet, even though the total true regurgitant volume is identical. RA, right atrium; RV, right ventricle.

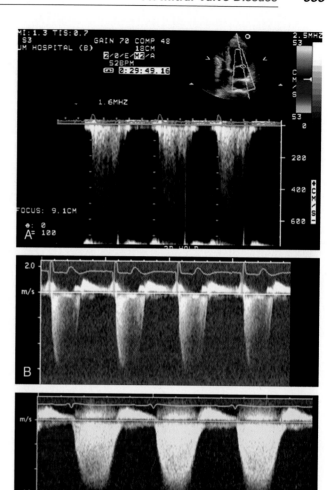

FIGURE 11.62. Continuous wave Doppler spectral recordings from patients with mild **(A)**, moderate **(B)**, and severe **(C)** mitral regurgitation. Note the progressive increase in signal density with increasing severity of mitral regurgitation due to interrogation of the larger volume of red blood cells with greater degrees of mitral regurgitation.

red cells being interrogated by the Doppler beam. If only a few cells are in motion, the spectral signal will be relatively faint, whereas with severe regurgitation, more cells are in motion and the spectral signal is substantially more robust (Fig. 11.62).

In addition to the assessment of mitral regurgitation severity by color flow Doppler imaging, there are other physiologically related measurements that can be made for determination of mitral regurgitation severity. These include determination of volumetric flow by the PISA method and determination of regurgitant volume and regurgitant fraction based on calculation of ventricular volumes and forward stroke volume. Using the volumetric analyses described in Chapters 2 and 8, one can determine the diastolic and systolic volumes of the left ventricle from which total stroke volume can then be calculated. Using principles elucidated in Chapter 8 to determine volumetric flow in the left ventricular outflow tract, one can then calculate the forward stroke volume. The difference between the total left ventricular stroke

volume and forward stroke volume in the left ventricular outflow tract then equals the mitral valve regurgitant volume (Figs. 11.63 and 11.64). This calculation assumes the absence of aortic regurgitation. A major limitation of this technique is the number of different measurements that must be made, each of which introduces a quantitative error. Alternatively, one can use the mitral valve inflow time velocity integral and an assumed mitral orifice to determine forward-going mitral flow in diastole. This volume of flow is then equal to the regurgitant mitral volume plus the forward stroke volume and can provide a different route for determination of mitral regurgitation volume. In general, this later methodology has seen little acceptance because of the difficulty in determining the true mitral anular area.

Finally, by inspection of the isovelocity curves in the proximal convergence zone (Figs. 11.65 and 11.66), the

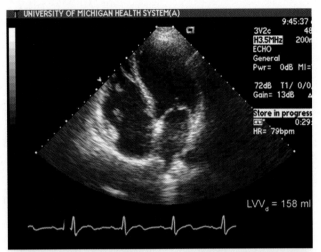

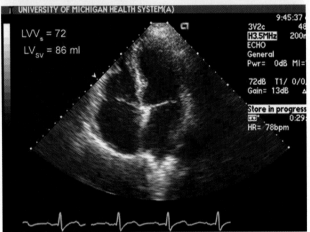

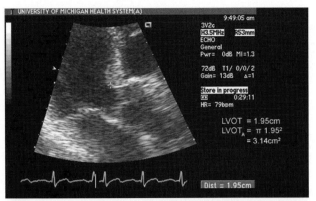

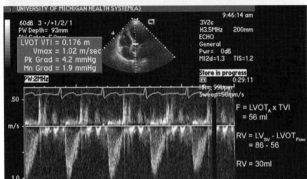

FIGURE 11.63. Method for determining mitral regurgitation volume using left ventricular volume. An apical four-chamber view was recorded in diastole **(Top)** and in systole **(Bottom)** from which diastolic and systolic volumes are determined. The difference between the diastolic and systolic volumes is the total left ventricular stroke volume (LV_{SV}), which represents the sum of forward flow in the left ventricular outflow tract and the regurgitant volume. Alternatively, this view can also be used to determine the diastolic transmitral flow by determining the diameter of the anulus from which anular area can be calculated. The product of anular area and the time velocity integral of mitral flow equals forward flow from the left atrium into the left ventricle in diastole, which in turn equals the sum of regurgitant flow and forward flow. This total left ventricular stroke volume is used to calculate regurgitant volume as seen in Figure 11.64. LVV_d, left ventricular volume in diastole; LVV_s, left ventricular volume in systole.

FIGURE 11.64. Example of calculating forward flow in the left ventricular outflow tract (*LVOT*). A parasternal long-axis view is recorded from which the diameter of the left ventricular outflow tract is measured and then the outflow tract area ($LVOT_A$) determined as demonstrated. The time velocity integral (*TVI*) in the left ventricular outflow tract is recorded from an apical view and the product of left ventricular outflow tract area times time velocity integral equals forward stroke volume (*F*). This forward stroke volume can then be subtracted from the total transmitral volume or from the total left ventricular stroke volume (LV_{SV}) calculated in Figure 11.63 to determine the regurgitant volume. RV, right ventricle.

regurgitant volume and several derived indices can be calculated. The general use of PISA for determining volumetric flow is discussed in Chapter 8. With this technique, one maximizes the dimension of the proximal velocity hemisphere by using a relatively low Nyquist limit and by shifting the baseline toward the direction of regurgitant flow. One can then determine the velocity of flow in the hemispherical flow zone at its aliasing line as well as the radius of any given hemisphere of flow. If one then as-

sumes a hemispherical flow profile toward the regurgitant orifice, the surface area of this hemisphere of flow can be calculated by the formula: surface area = $2\pi r^2$. The product of the hemisphere area and the velocity determined from the aliasing limit of the color flow display equals the flow rate. Limitations of this technique include the fact that flow convergence toward a regurgitant orifice is seldom truly hemispherical. In this instance, the surface area of flow may be either greater or larger than that calculated, resulting in an expected measurement error.

Once the volumetric regurgitant flow (RF) has been determined, the effective regurgitant orifice (ERO) can be calculated. This is calculated as regurgitant flow (calculated as previously noted from PISA) divided by the peak velocity of the mitral regurgitation jet (MR_{max}), from the continuous wave spectral profile (ERO = RF/MR_{max}). The effective regurgitant orifice area thus determined can be related to the regurgitant volume by the formula: RV = ERO $\times$ TVI_{MR}, where TVI_{MR} is the time velocity integral of

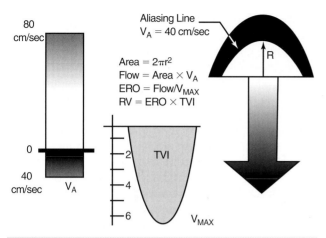

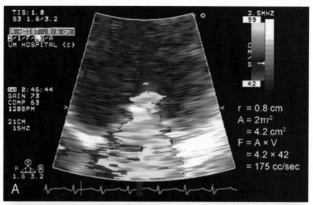

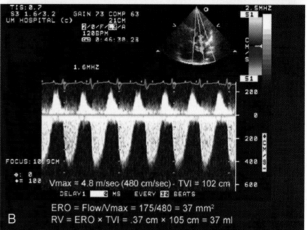

FIGURE 11.65. Schematic demonstration of the principle involved in calculating mitral regurgitation severity from the proximal isovelocity surface area method. In this schematic, mitral regurgitation has been visualized from the apical four-chamber view. The color Doppler scale has been shifted downward so that the mitral regurgitation aliasing velocity has been reduced to 40 cm/sec, thus maximizing resolution for measuring the aliasing radius. The area of hemispherical flow through the regurgitant orifice can be calculated as $2\pi r^2$. Instantaneous flow can be calculated as area $\times$ flow velocity at the aliasing boundary (V_A). The effective regurgitant orifice (*ERO*) is calculated as flow/V_{MAX}. The regurgitant volume (*RV*) can be calculated as the product of ERO $\times$ TVI (where TVI is the time velocity integral of the mitral regurgitation flow as measured by continuous wave Doppler imaging).

FIGURE 11.66. Example of using the proximal isovelocity surface area method for determining mitral regurgitation severity. **A:** An expanded view of the mitral regurgitation convergence zone, from which a radius of 0.8 cm can be determined. The area of the proximal convergence zone can be calculated as 4.2 cm² and the flow as 175 mL/sec. **B:** A continuous wave Doppler image of the mitral regurgitation jet has been recorded. The V_{max} is 4.8 m/sec (480 cm/sec) and the time velocity integral (*TVI*) is 102 cm. Calculations of effective regurgitant orifice (*ERO*) and regurgitant volume (*RV*) are as noted in the schematic. These values are consistent with moderate to severe mitral regurgitation.

the mitral regurgitation jet (Fig. 11.65). There are several limitations to the PISA method, the most important of which is the fact that flow convergence may not conform to a true hemispherical shape. If convergence toward the regurgitant orifice occurs over a surface less than 180 degrees, the flow volume will be overstated by the PISA method. Correction for nonhemispherical shapes is technically possible but rarely employed in clinical practice.

Another common source of error with the PISA method is a mitral regurgitation jet, which occurs along a variable length of the leaflet commissure. In this case, the surface area of the regurgitation flow volume does not conform to a hemisphere but rather to a half cylinder. Inspection of the PISA shape in an orthogonal plane should help avoid this source of underestimation by this method (Fig. 11.67). In many instances, the geometry of the proximal regurgitant jet may preclude accurate use of the PISA method, and severity assessment should be based on other factors.

Other Considerations in Assessing Mitral Regurgitation

The majority of schemes for quantifying mitral regurgitation have assumed holosystolic regurgitation flow. In many instances, such as mitral valve prolapse, regurgita-

tion may be confined to only a portion of systole. As such, the volume of flow either estimated from a color flow image area or calculated by the PISA technique should be reduced by the fraction of systole over which flow occurs. One occasionally encounters the situation of apparent moderate or severe mitral regurgitation on color flow Doppler imaging, which is known to be of long-standing duration but which is not associated with secondary left atrial dilation. This situation is often encountered in individuals in whom mitral regurgitation was incidentally detected and who have few or no symptoms suggesting congestive heart failure. Careful attention to the timing of mitral regurgitation in these instances often reveals that the mitral regurgitation jet, although encompassing a substantial area of the left atrium, is present only for 30%

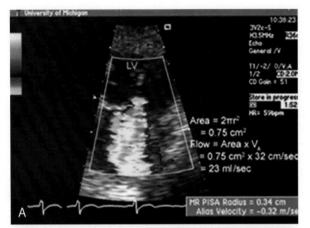

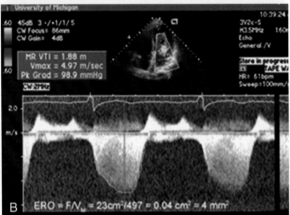

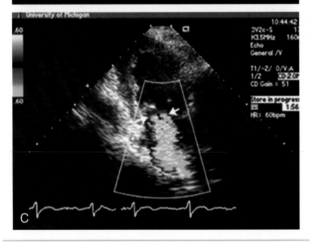

FIGURE 11.67. This is an example of a patient in whom the proximal isovelocity surface area method for calculation of mitral regurgitation characteristics is inaccurate. **A:** Note the very small convergence zone with a radius of 0.3 cm. Using this value, regurgitant flow is calculated as 23 mL/sec and the regurgitant orifice as 4 mm². Inspection of the color flow signal (**A**) suggests that mitral regurgitation is substantially more severe than would be suggested by these calculations. **B:** Recorded in the same patient with an orthogonal view. Note that the convergence zone no longer appears hemispherical but extends along a substantial length of the commissural closure of the mitral valve (*arrows*). This is an example in which the mitral regurgitation jet does not adhere to the principles for which a simple proximal isovelocity surface area calculation can be employed. ERO, effective regurgitant orifice; LV, left ventricle.

to 50% of systole. This typically is occurring toward end-systole when overall volumes are relatively smaller as well. Thus, mitral regurgitation confined to late systole is overestimated by simple assessment of maximal jet area and is a not infrequent finding in patients with functional mitral regurgitation or mitral valve prolapse. Figure 11.68 illustrates an example in which the color jet area fills approximately 60% of the left atrium but has not resulted in chamber dilation in spite of the known chronicity of the mitral regurgitation. Figure 11.69 is a color M-mode image of a similar mitral regurgitation jet demonstrating that it is confined to the later 40% of systole, and hence the jet area method will overstate the actual severity of regurgitation. Similar observations regarding the timing of mitral regurgitation can be made from a spectral Doppler profile (Fig. 11.43).

An additional characteristic of severe mitral regurgitation is retrograde flow in the pulmonary veins during systole. This can be directly attributed to the increasing left atrial pressure and regurgitant volume in the left atrium. Typically, this is thought to be a marker of moderate to severe mitral regurgitation and is not seen in mild regurgitation. It occasionally can be absent in the presence of a highly eccentric jet, which is directed away from the pulmonary veins. Although its presence is a reliable marker of

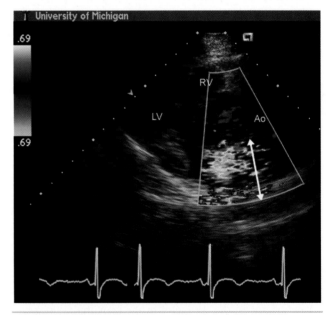

FIGURE 11.68. Example of a patient with apparent hemodynamically significant mitral regurgitation but normal left ventricular size and only mild left atrial dilation. When one encounters this discrepancy between the apparent severity of mitral regurgitation and downstream effects (i.e., atrial dilation), one should consider either acute onset of mitral regurgitation or nonholosystolic mitral regurgitation. Note in the real-time image, the mitral regurgitation is present for less than 50% of systole, thus explaining the discrepancy between apparent jet size in a single frozen image and left atrial size. Ao, aorta; LV, left ventricle; RV, right ventricle.

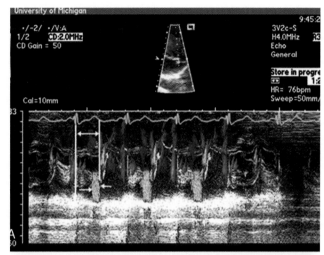

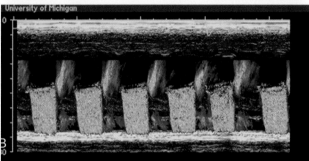

FIGURE 11.69. Color Doppler M-mode images recorded in patients with mitral regurgitation. Both tracings were recorded from the left ventricular apex. **A:** Recorded in a patient with mitral valve prolapse and regurgitation confined to the latter 40% of systole. The *two vertical lines* indicate the duration of mechanical systole (*double-headed arrow*). **B:** Recorded in a patient with holosystolic mitral regurgitation.

moderate and severe mitral regurgitation, its absence should not be used to exclude significant mitral regurgitation in the presence of other echocardiographic and Doppler features suggesting that it is present. Figure 11.70 presents examples of mitral regurgitation associated with retrograde flow in a pulmonary vein.

Table 11.4 outlines various findings seen in mitral regurgitation and their relationship to determining the severity of regurgitation. It should be emphasized that no single parameter is completely accurate for determining severity and that assessment of the severity of mitral regurgitation should be based on a combination of findings. Many of those observations are valid only at the extremes, i.e., in accurately identifying mild and severe regurgitation but having suboptimal accuracy with substantial overlap in the moderate range. In many instances, one or more of these findings may not correlate with other findings. In this instance, severity should be based on the overall findings and not one isolated feature.

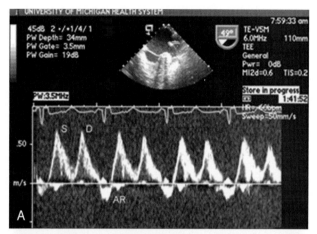

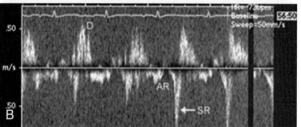

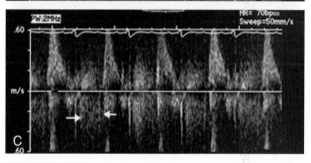

FIGURE 11.70. A: The normal flow pattern from the pulmonary vein (recorded from a transesophageal echocardiogram). Note the systolic predominance of flow out of the pulmonary vein and the relatively brief atrial reversal (*AR*). **B:** Recorded from an apical view (transthoracic) in a patient with moderate mitral insufficiency. Note the loss of systolic forward flow in most cardiac cycles with only a very brief systolic reversal (*SR*). **C:** Recorded (transthoracic apical view) in a patient with severe mitral regurgitation. Note the holosystolic retrograde flow in the pulmonary vein (flow between the *arrows*). D, diastole; S, systole.

MITRAL VALVE PROLAPSE

The diagnosis of mitral valve prolapse is a commonly encountered dilemma in clinical cardiology and echocardiography. Early studies suggesting a prevalence of mitral valve prolapse of 6% to 21% in otherwise healthy female patients were clearly erroneous and dramatically overestimated the true prevalence of this entity. Using modern criteria for diagnosis, mitral valve prolapse can be expected to be found in 2% to 4% of the population. There are two basic forms of mitral valve prolapse that repre-

▶ TABLE 11.4 Mitral Regurgitation Severity

	I (Mild)	II	III	IV (Severe)
Left ventricular size	N	N	↑	↑↑
Left atrial size	N	N	↑	↑↑
MR jet (% LA)	<15	15–30	35–50	>50
Spectral Doppler density	Faint	—	—	Dense
Vena contracta	<3 mm	—	—	>6 mm
Pulmonary vein flow	S > D	—	—	Systolic reversal
RV (ml)	<30	30–44	45–59	≥60
ERO (cm²)	<0.2	0.2–0.29	0.3–0.39	>0.40
PISA	Small	—	—	Large

For some parameters, the observation is valid at the extremes of mitral regurgitation severity and there may be marked overlap in intermediate (grades II and III) mitral regurgitation. In these instances, no value is presented.
MR, mitral regurgitation; % LA, percentage of left atrial area encompassed by the mitral regurgitation jet with color flow Doppler imaging; S, antegrade flow in systole (pulmonary vein flow); D, antegrade flow in diastole (pulmonary vein flow); RV, regurgitant volume determined either by proximal isovelocity surface area or volume method; ERO, effective regurgitant orifice; PISA, proximal isovelocity surface area. N, normal; ↑, increased; ↑↑, markedly increased.

sent the two ends of a spectrum of abnormality. It should be emphasized that in clinical practice many patients will fall between these two extremes. The first, which represents a true form of organic heart disease, is mitral valve prolapse associated with myxomatous thickening of the mitral valve leaflets. The second form of mitral valve prolapse represents mild buckling of an otherwise anatomically normal valve. It was inclusion of individuals with the latter type of mitral valve "prolapse" that inflated the apparent prevalence of the disease. From a clinical outcome standpoint, it is individuals with thickening of the leaflets in association with prolapse who are most prone to complications such as progressive mitral regurgitation, spontaneous chordal rupture, neurologic events, and endocarditis. Individuals with prolapse but with otherwise anatomically normal leaflets and no mitral regurgitation are at substantially lower risk of complications.

Multiple criteria have been proposed for the diagnosis of mitral valve prolapse. With M-mode echocardiography (Fig. 11.71), mitral valve prolapse was diagnosed in the presence of leaflet thickening with posterior bowing of the mitral valve apparatus during systole. This bowing could be present either throughout entire systole or confined to late systole. From a technique standpoint, it is important to recognize that the M-mode interrogation beam should be aligned in a manner to encompass the area just behind the mitral anulus if one is to document buckling of the mitral valve leaflet into the left atrium.

Two-dimensional echocardiography is a more commonly employed technique for screening for mitral valve prolapse. Several quantitative techniques have been recommended including determining the angle in systole between the posterior aortic wall and the proximal anterior mitral valve leaflet. In general, quantitative techniques for separating mitral valve prolapse from normal closure patterns have not seen clinical acceptance. In the past, there has been much debate regarding the sensitivity and speci-

ficity of mitral valve bowing when seen in a parasternal versus apical view. It is more important to appreciate the presence or absence of valve thickening and the symmetry versus asymmetry with which the valve "prolapses." Because the mitral anulus is not a planar structure, gradual bowing of both leaflets is to be anticipated in the apical four-chamber view but is less common in the apical two-chamber view (Fig. 11.2). As a general rule, the four-chamber view will be less specific for the diagnosis of mitral valve prolapse than detection of buckling in either a

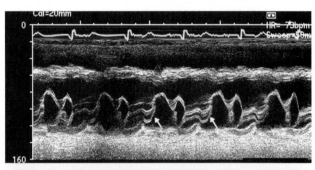

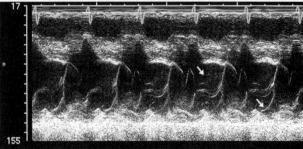

FIGURE 11.71. **Top and Bottom:** M-mode echocardiograms recorded in two patients with mitral valve prolapse. In each instance, note the distinct posterior motion of the mitral valve (*arrow*). **Bottom:** Note the chordal systolic anterior motion (*upper arrow*), which may also be seen in mitral valve prolapse.

parasternal long-axis view or apical two-chamber view. Recognizing that the mitral anulus is a complex three-dimensional structure and that the mitral valve has multiple scallops, one should recognize that the view in which mitral valve prolapse is best appreciated will depend on which anatomic portion of the mitral valve is involved in the prolapse process. The diagnosis of mitral valve prolapse should be made when one or both leaflets breaks the plane of the mitral anulus in a nonsymmetric manner, typically taking on a buckling appearance. As noted previously, the leaflet should be described as thickened or anatomically normal as well. Figures 11.72 through 11.78 depict patients with varying degrees of mitral valve prolapse. Figure 11.72 represents classic myxomatous mitral

valve disease with diffuse leaflet thickening and bileaflet prolapse. Figure 11.75 is from an individual with normal mitral valve thickness and definite prolapse of the posterior leaflet. Occasionally, a patient is encountered in whom there is very marked myxomatous degeneration, leaflet thickening, and redundancy. On occasion, this may result in a mass-like appearance on the valve, which could be confused with vegetation or tumor (Fig. 11.77). Similarly, a markedly redundant valve may buckle back on itself and result in the appearance of a cystic structure on the valve (Fig. 11.78).

Several sequelae and complications of mitral valve prolapse can be identified from the echocardiogram. These include mitral regurgitation, ruptured chordae, and flail leaflets as well as endocarditis. Figure 11.76 was recorded in an individual with mitral valve prolapse and mitral regurgitation. Note the eccentric mitral regurgitation jet due to eccentric coaptation secondary to prolapse. Figure 11.79 was also recorded in a patient with mitral valve prolapse and a flail scallop. Note the highly disorganized regurgitation jet in the left atrium. Figure 11.80 was recorded in an individual with prolapse and flail. Note the small highly mobile filamentous echoes protruding into the left atrium, which represent the proximal end of the ruptured chordae.

Once the diagnosis of mitral valve prolapse has been established, it is important to further characterize other areas of the cardiovascular system that may also be involved. Mitral valve prolapse can be an integral part of Marfan syndrome, in which case aortic pathology may be encountered and should be evaluated. As such, detailed attention to the

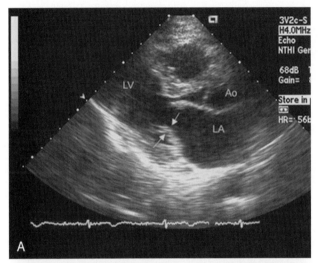

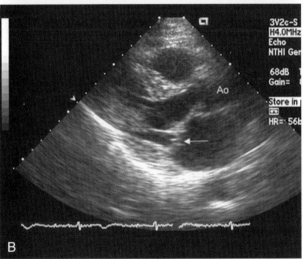

FIGURE 11.72. Parasternal long-axis echocardiogram recorded in diastole **(A)** and end-systole **(B)** in a patient with mitral valve prolapse. **A:** Note the pathologic thickening of the posterior leaflet (*arrows*). **B:** Note the prolapse of the posterior leaflet behind the plane of the mitral valve anulus (*arrow*). In the real-time image, note the distinct abnormal buckling motion of the posterior mitral valve leaflet in systole.

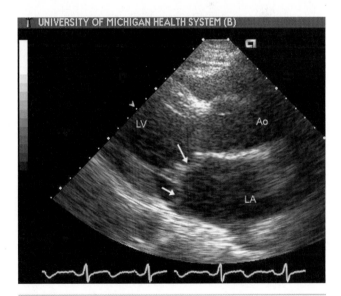

FIGURE 11.73. Parasternal long-axis echocardiogram recorded in a patient with bileaflet mitral valve prolapse and myxomatous thickening of the leaflets. This frame was recorded in systole. Note distinct prolapse of both the anterior and posterior leaflets behind the plane of the mitral anulus (*arrows*). Ao, aorta, LA, left atrium; LV, left ventricle.

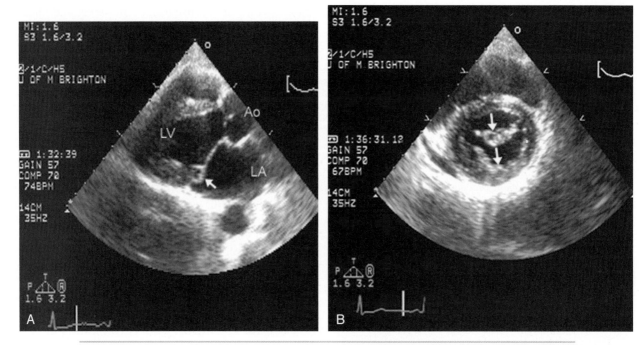

FIGURE 11.74. Parasternal long-axis **(A)** and short-axis **(B)** views recorded in a patient with posterior mitral valve prolapse. **A:** Recorded at end-systole. Note distinct prolapse of the posterior leaflet (*arrow*), well behind the plane of the mitral anulus. **B:** Note the diffuse thickening of both the anterior and posterior mitral valve leaflets (*arrows*). Ao, aorta; LA, left atrium; LV, left ventricle.

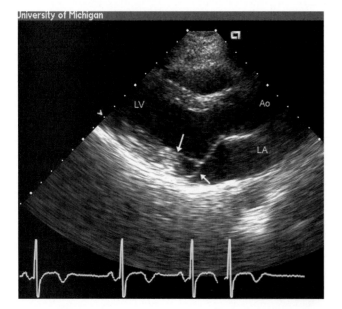

FIGURE 11.75. Parasternal long-axis echocardiogram recorded in a patient with mitral valve prolapse and thin mitral valve leaflets. This frame was recorded at end-systole. Note the normal thickness of both mitral leaflets but the distinct prolapse of the posterior leaflet (*upward-pointing arrow*) behind the mitral anulus into the body of the left atrium (*LA*). The *downward-pointing arrow* denotes the position of the mitral anulus for reference. Ao, aorta; LV, left ventricle.

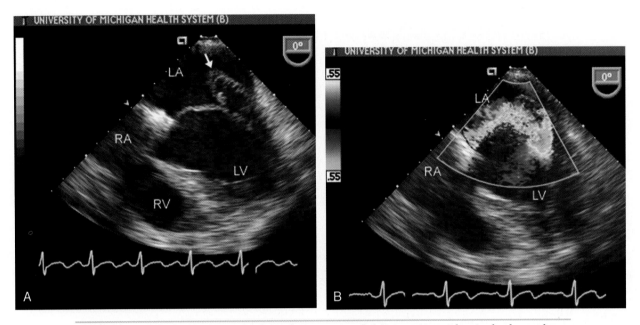

FIGURE 11.76. Transesophageal echocardiogram recorded in a patient with mitral valve prolapse. Both panels were recorded in systole. **A:** Note the marked prolapse of the posterior leaflet into the body of the left atrium (*LA*) (*arrow*). **B:** A color Doppler image also recorded in systole. Note the relatively large convergence zone and the highly eccentric mitral regurgitation jet directed toward the atrial septum. LV, left ventricle; RA, right atrium; RV, right ventricle.

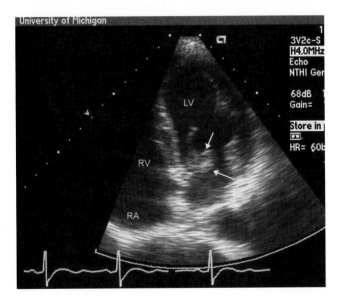

FIGURE 11.77. Apical four-chamber view recorded in a patient with myxomatous mitral valve disease and pronounced mitral valve prolapse. In this example, the combination of myxomatous thickening and exaggerated buckling of the leaflet results in the appearance of a mass on the left atrial side of the mitral leaflet. Transesophageal echocardiography confirmed the absence of a mass and that this effect was due to the pronounced myxomatous thickening and prolapse alone. LV, left ventricle; RA, right atrium; RV, right ventricle.

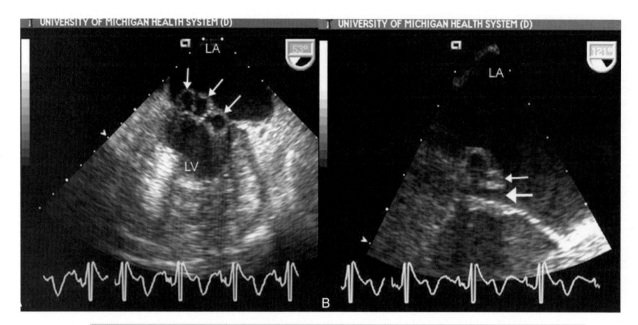

FIGURE 11.78. A: Transesophageal echocardiogram recorded in a patient with marked mitral valve prolapse of multiple scallops, resulting in the appearance of cystic masses (*arrows*) on the mitral valve. **B:** An expanded view of a different portion of the mitral valve revealing a partial flail of one scallop (*small arrow*) and direct visualization of the regurgitant channel (*large arrow*). LA, left atrium; LV, left ventricle.

FIGURE 11.79. Parasternal long-axis view echocardiogram with color flow Doppler imaging recorded in a patient with mitral valve prolapse and a partial flail leaflet. There is a highly eccentric and disorganized mitral regurgitation jet, with one component confined behind the anterior mitral leaflet and the second component directed immediately posteriorly (*arrow*). Ao, aorta; LV, left ventricle.

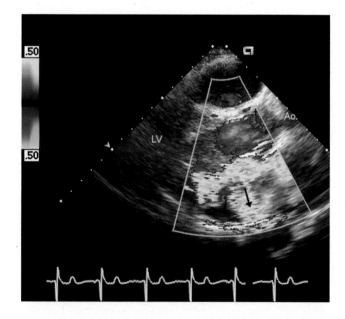

aortic valve and proximal aorta should be undertaken in patients in whom prolapse has been diagnosed.

FLAIL LEAFLETS

Any portion of the mitral apparatus can become anatomically disrupted and result in a portion of the mitral valve becoming flail (Figs. 11.80–11.83). As noted previously, this is a not uncommon sequela of a myxomatous

mitral valve. The degree of resultant regurgitation is directly related to the extent of anatomic disruption. Rupture of several isolated chordae may not result in disruption of normal coaptation and hence can be seen in the absence of mitral regurgitation. Rupture of an entire papillary muscle or papillary muscle head typically results in acute severe mitral regurgitation. Between these two extremes, a wide range of anatomic disruption with varying degrees of mitral regurgitation can be noted. As

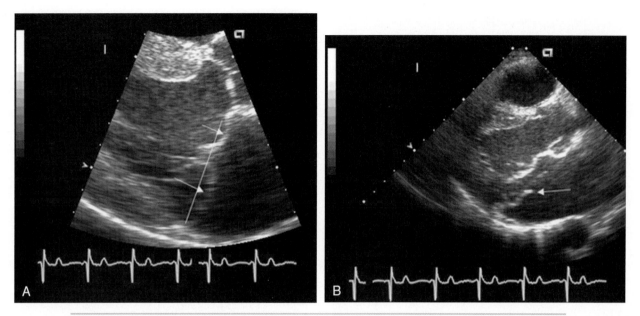

FIGURE 11.80. Parasternal long-axis view recorded in a patient with mitral valve prolapse. **A:** Note the prolapse of both the anterior and posterior leaflets behind the plane of the mitral anulus (*white line*). **B:** With a slightly different angulation, note the evidence of flail chordae, with a portion of the posterior leaflet seen well behind the anterior leaflet in systole (*arrow*).

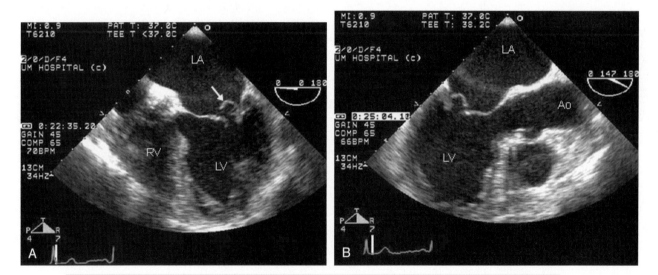

FIGURE 11.81. Transesophageal echocardiogram recorded in a transverse plane **(A)** and longitudinal plane **(B)** in a patient with a flail posterior scallop (P2) of the mitral valve. **A:** Note the portion of the posterior leaflet of the mitral valve curling behind the anterior leaflet in systole (*arrow*). **B:** A similar phenomenon is noted recorded at 147 degrees. In both of these planes, the posterior scallop (P2) is at the mid portion of the mitral valve (Fig. 11.4). RV, right ventricle; Ao, aorta; LA, left atrium; LV, left ventricle.

previously described, anatomic disruption of a portion of the mitral apparatus results in an eccentric direction of the regurgitation jet with an orientation opposite in direction to the leaflet with the anatomic defect.

The recognition and complete description of flail mitral valve leaflet can play a critical role in patient man-

agement. Figure 11.3 depicts the detailed anatomy of the anterior and posterior mitral valve leaflets and the different viewing perspectives. As noted earlier, both leaflets can be described as having three separate scallops termed anterior 1 through 3 (A1, A2, A3) and posterior 1 through 3 (P1, P2, P3). By definition, the A1 and P1 scallops are

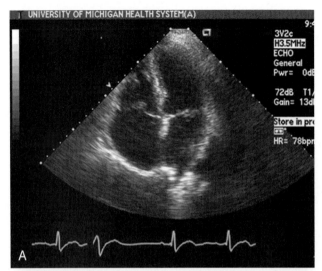

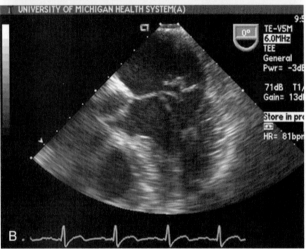

FIGURE 11.82. Transthoracic (**A**) and transesophageal (**B**) echocardiograms recorded in a patient with a flail posterior mitral valve leaflet. **A:** Note the distinct buckling of the posterior leaflet, the tip of which points away from the left ventricular apex. **B:** This phenomenon is more clearly demonstrated when recorded from the transesophageal approach in the same patient.

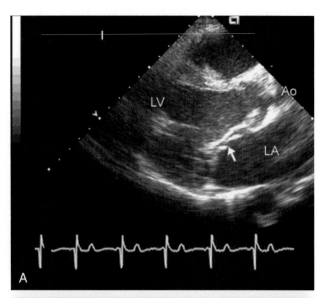

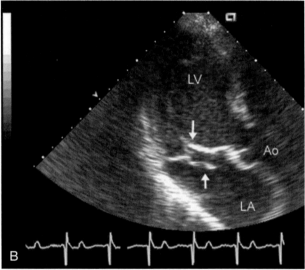

FIGURE 11.83. Transthoracic echocardiogram recorded in parasternal long-axis and apical views in a patient with a flail posterior leaflet. **A:** Note that the posterior leaflet and attached chordae are positioned behind the anterior leaflet (*arrow*), indicative of disruption of the anatomic attachment of the posterior leaflet. **B:** Recorded from apical transducer position, this phenomenon is better visualized. The *downward-pointing arrow* denotes the normally closed anterior leaflet and the *upward-pointing arrow* indicates the flail posterior leaflet. Ao, aorta; LA, left atrium; LV, left ventricle.

most anterolaterally located, nearest the left atrial appendage. The A3 and P3 scallops are more inferomedial in location. A common source of confusion arises when describing the location of a flail scallop. It should be recognized that when viewed surgically from within the left atrium, the A1 and P1 scallops will be at the left of the surgeon's field of view, whereas when viewed in an echocardiographic imaging plane, they will be to the right and inferior when viewed by transesophageal echocardiography. Figure 11.3 depicts this difference in viewing perspective. Depending on the depth of the probe insertion and the angle of rotation, imaging planes can be obtained that will simultaneously view two or three scallops. Typically, when viewing the left ventricle in a longitudinal plane (120 degrees), the imaging plane intersects the A2/P2 boundary.

Confusion may arise when imaging the mitral valve in a view orthogonal to this (60 degrees). In this view, the P1, A2, and A3 scallops may be simultaneously visualized. Because of this imaging plane, confusion may arise between a flail P3 and A3 scallop in this view. Substantial experience is necessary to accurately identify the precise scallop. This may have particular relevance with respect to patient management because, in general, repair of a posterior flail is technically easier than that of an anterior flail, or it may have relevance for feasibility of repair de-

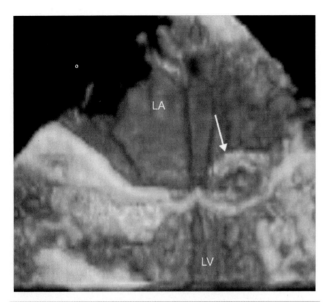

FIGURE 11.84. Three-dimensional reconstruction recorded from the transesophageal echocardiographic approach in a patient with a flail posterior mitral valve leaflet. Note the distinct buckling of a portion of the posterior leaflet (*arrow*) into the left atrium (*LA*). In the real-time image, note that this pathologic buckling occurs over only a portion of the systolic cycle. LV, left ventricle.

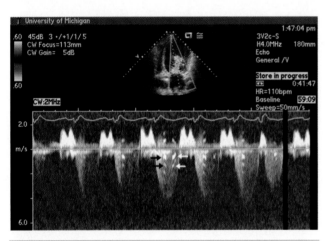

FIGURE 11.85. Continuous wave spectral Doppler image recorded in a patient with a partial flail leaflet. In the spectral signal, note the bright tissue signatures (*arrows*) within the mitral regurgitation jet. This signal arises from oscillating tissue density structures in the regurgitant jet. This spectral image corresponds to a "whistling" or "cooing" character to the mitral regurgitation murmur.

pending on surgical expertise and experience. Three-dimensional echocardiography (Fig. 11.84) has shown tremendous promise for localization of the specific area of anatomic description.

In the presence of a flail leaflet, the mitral regurgitation spectral signal may have an atypical appearance. The interrogation beam may intersect the jet either tangentially

or partially for part of the cycle. This may result in varying density and velocity of the signal, mimicking a less than holosystolic jet (Fig. 11.85). Additionally, if there are flail portions of the mitral apparatus that oscillate in the regurgitation flow stream, they result in a "tiger stripe" appearance of the spectral signal associated with a "whistling" sound on the audible signal (Fig. 11.85).

Surgical repair of a partial mitral flail typically involves placing an anuloplasty ring and resection of the flail portion of the leaflet. Other surgical techniques include placement of prosthetic chordae, chordal shortening procedures, and translocation of chordae from one leaflet to another. After repair, the anuloplasty ring typically appears as an echo density most easily seen in the posterior anulus area (Fig. 11.86). Because the most common re-

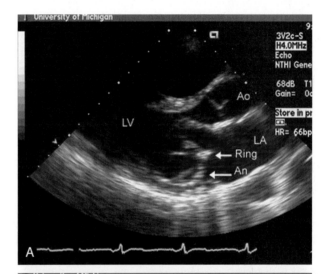

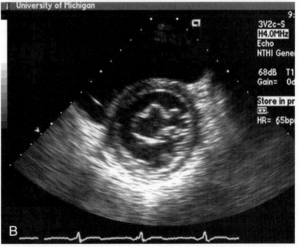

FIGURE 11.86. Parasternal long-axis (**A**) and short-axis (**B**) echocardiograms recorded in a patient after mitral valve repair with an anular ring. The ring is noted as an echo density at the base of the posterior mitral leaflet. In both the long- and short-axis views in real-time, note that most of the mitral valve leaflet motion occurs with the anterior rather than the posterior leaflet. An, mitral anulus; Ao, aorta; LA, left atrium; LV, left ventricle.

pair is of the posterior leaflet, this leaflet often appears foreshortened with the majority of valve function being controlled by the anterior leaflet. This topic is discussed in greater detail in Chapters 14 and 19.

MISCELLANEOUS MITRAL VALVE ABNORMALITIES
Calcification of the Mitral Anulus

Fibrosis and calcification of the fibrous skeleton of the heart are common sequelae of aging. This is most often appreciated in the posterior mitral valve anulus and can range from limited degrees of focal deposits to nearly circumferential heavy calcification. Figures 11.87 through 11.89 are echocardiographic examples of anular calcium. In addition to age, other conditions that accelerate the rate at which anular calcium occurs include hypertension and chronic renal insufficiency. In patients with chronic renal insufficiency, the degree of anular calcium can be substantial and take on a mass-like effect that on occasion has been confused with tumor.

Mild degrees of mitral regurgitation are not uncommon; however, the presence of severe mitral regurgitation is unlikely in uncomplicated anular calcification. If the fibrotic and calcific process extends throughout the entire anulus and into the valve leaflets, secondary leaflet dysfunction can occur and result in substantially greater degrees of mitral regurgitation. Other rare associated abnormalities include superimposed thrombus formation or vegetation. An additional complication of heavy mitral anular calcification is the potential difficulty in seating a prosthetic valve in patients in whom mitral valve replacement is necessary. Patients with heavy mitral anular cal-

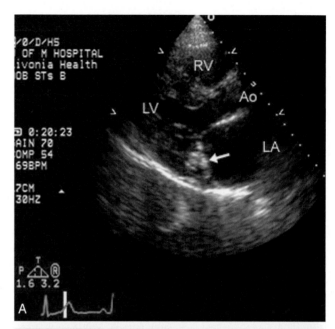

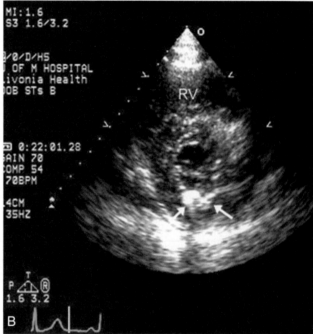

FIGURE 11.88. Parasternal long-axis **(A)** and short-axis **(B)** echocardiograms recorded in a patient with mitral anular calcification. **A:** Note the irregular echo densities within the anulus (*arrow*). This is also visualized in the short-axis view at the base of the heart (*arrows*). Ao, aorta; LA, left atrium; LV, left ventricle, RV, right ventricle.

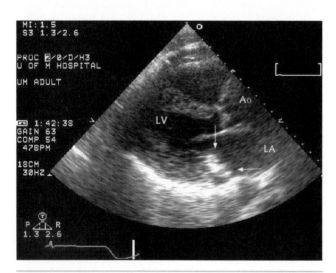

FIGURE 11.87. Parasternal long-axis echocardiogram recorded in a patient with mitral anular calcification. Note the bright echo densities in the mitral anulus (*arrows*) that protrude into the body of the left atrium (*LA*) (*horizontal arrow*). Ao, aorta; LV, left ventricle.

cification are more likely to have subsequent paravalvular regurgitation than are patients without calcification.

Although mild degrees of mitral regurgitation are common with a calcified mitral anulus, calcification rarely progresses to the point of causing clinically relevant obstruction to flow. In advanced cases, invasion of the prox-

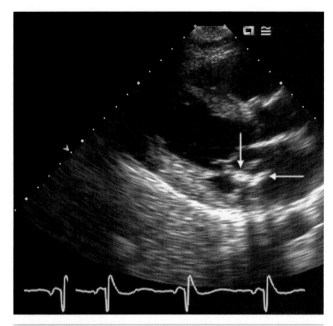

FIGURE 11.89. Parasternal long-axis echocardiogram recorded in a patient with irregular calcification of the mitral anulus. In this example, note that the anular calcium has taken on an irregular configuration that protrudes into the body of the left atrium (*arrows*). In the real-time image, note that the marked echo density of the anular calcification results in a beam width artifact, which can mimic a mobile mass in the left atrial cavity.

imal leaflet portions by the fibrotic and calcific process can reduce the mitral orifice and result in functional mitral stenosis (Fig. 11.90). This type of mitral stenosis is not amenable to balloon valvuloplasty.

Tumors of the Mitral Valve

On occasion, cardiac myxomas arise from the mitral valve rather than from the atrial septum (Fig. 11.91). They present as a relatively large, bulky tissue density mass moving with the mitral valve tissue. Not infrequently, a typically located atrial myxoma on a relatively long stalk will move in such close conjunction with the mitral valve leaflets that it appears to be physically attached to the leaflet. Transesophageal echocardiography often can identify the true location of the tumor attachment and confirm the separation of the tumor from the left atrial side of the mitral leaflet.

Other mitral valve tumors include the papilloma or fibroelastoma. These typically present as smooth, spherical masses 2 to 10 mm in diameter, attached to the distal mitral valve or to the chordae tendineae. Their characteristic regular spherical shape and location on the chordae should allow definitive diagnosis with an echocardiogram (Fig. 11.92). Occasionally, fibroelastoma may appear as a highly mobile, strand-like mass as well.

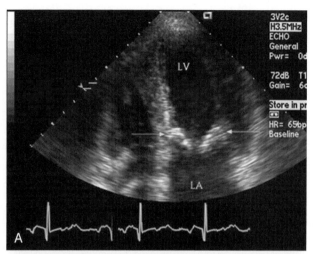

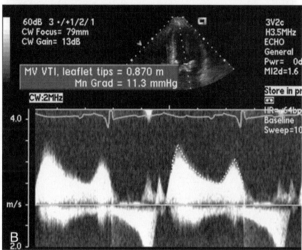

FIGURE 11.90. Apical four-chamber view **(A)** recorded in a patient with advanced anular calcification. In this example, note that the anular calcification extends onto the proximal mitral valve leaflets. This has resulted in functional mitral stenosis, as can be documented by the transmitral Doppler flow gradient of 11.3 mm Hg recorded **(B)**. LA, left atrium; LV, left ventricle.

A final, rare mass to be noted on a mitral valve is the mitral blood cyst. This is a developmental cystic structure that is more commonly encountered in pediatric populations. Cysts can range in size from 2 to 3 mm to 1 cm and appear as smooth, usually spherical or ovoid cystic structures. Single or multiple cysts can be encountered on the mitral valve. Figure 11.93 was recorded in an asymptomatic woman with multiple mitral valve blood cysts. Because of the cyst bulk, they can interfere with appropriate mitral valve coaptation and result in secondary mitral regurgitation.

Aneurysms of the Mitral Valve

On occasion, one encounters a discrete aneurysmal outpouching of the mitral leaflet, most commonly at the base

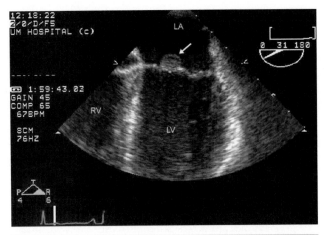

FIGURE 11.91. Transesophageal echocardiogram recorded in a patient with a myxoma of the mitral valve leaflet. Note the smooth, homogeneous, nearly spherical mass attached to the mitral leaflet (*arrow*), which was demonstrated at the time of surgical excision to be an atypically located myxoma. LA, left atrium; LV, left ventricle; RV, right ventricle.

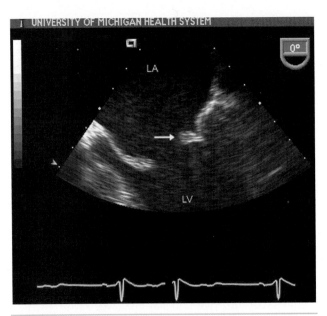

FIGURE 11.92. Transesophageal echocardiogram recorded in a patient with a mitral fibroelastoma. Note the small, nearly spherical mass attached to the tip of the mitral leaflet (*arrow*). LA, left atrium; LV, left ventricle.

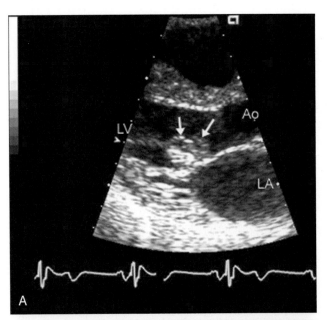

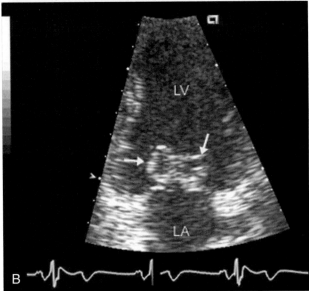

FIGURE 11.93. Transthoracic echocardiogram recorded in the parasternal long-axis (**A**) and apical two-chamber (**B**) views in a patient with mitral valve blood cysts. In both views (*arrows*), note the nearly spherical, cystic echo masses that are attached to the tips of the mitral leaflets. Ao, aorta, LA, left atrium; LV, left ventricle.

of the anterior leaflet and protruding into the left atrium. In many instances, this is the sequela of endocarditis, in which case the aneurysm may be thick walled or irregular in contour and associated with perforation into the left atrium. More rarely, a similar aneurysm is seen with thin walls and without evidence of endocarditis. The etiology of these aneurysms is unknown but assumed to be a congenital developmental anomaly.

Mitral Valve Perforation

An additional etiology of mitral regurgitation is perforation of one or both leaflets. This typically is the sequela of infective endocarditis, which has eroded through the leaflet but in which there has been resolution of the vegetation (Fig. 11.94). The degree of mitral regurgitation is obviously directly proportional to the size of the perforation.

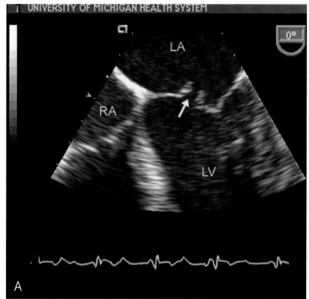

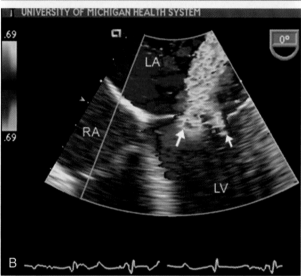

FIGURE 11.94. Transesophageal echocardiogram recording a transverse view in a patient with mitral valve endocarditis and a perforation of the anterior leaflet. **A:** Note the distinct break in the continuity of the anterior leaflet (*arrow*), with remnants of mitral valve tissue protruding into the left atrium (*LA*). **B:** Note the distinct convergence zone directed through the defect in the anterior leaflet (*left arrow*) and a lesser degree of mitral regurgitation through the mitral coaptation point (*right arrow*). LV, left ventricle; RA, right atrium.

Anular Abscess

Abscess of the mitral valve anulus is an uncommon sequela of endocarditis and typically is confined to the posterior anulus. Further discussion of anular abscess and other sequelae of endocarditis can be found in Chapter 13.

Anular Dehiscence

Anular dehiscence is a very infrequent sequela of blunt chest trauma. The presumed mechanism is a sudden dramatic increase in intracardiac pressure against a closed mitral valve resulting in tearing of the posterior leaflet from the mitral valve anulus or less commonly of a portion of the anulus from the adjoining wall. Anular dehiscence results in substantial mitral regurgitation with an eccentrically directed mitral regurgitation jet. Transesophageal echocardiography is essential to confirm the diagnosis. Anatomically, the defect is similar to that seen in an anular abscess and the diagnosis of dehiscence requires both the echocardiographic appearance and a history of chest trauma sufficient to have caused the injury.

Radiation Damage

Because of the degree to which radiation therapy is anatomically targeted and the cardiovascular system shielded, it is increasingly uncommon to encounter radiation-induced mitral valve disease. When present, it may be the sequela of radiation therapy occurring 10 to 15 years before presentation. The degree and location of damage are highly variable and dependent on the direction of the radiation beam. Because most radiation portals are anterior, it is the more anterior cardiac structures that are most prone to injury, including the anterior mitral valve leaflet (Fig. 11.95). Although the nature of radiation damage can be highly variable, the most common finding is fibrosis and stiffening of the proximal portions of the anterior leaflet.

Carcinoid and Diet Drug Valvulopathy

There are several metabolic and toxic syndromes that can affect the mitral valve. The first to be described was carcinoid heart disease, which most often involves the tricuspid and pulmonary valves. The lesions are similar to those seen in ergotamine heart disease and consist of diffuse thickening of the valve tissue and chordae with a combination of stenosis and regurgitation, predominantly of the tricuspid valve. Because the biologically active serotonin-related metabolites are deactivated in the lung, left-sided structures are typically spared. In instances of pulmonary metastases or a right-to-left shunt, the mitral or aortic valves may also be involved. More recently, a nearly identical appearance, both pathologically and echocardiographically, of valve pathology has been noted in patients taking anorexic agents, typically a combination of phentermine and fenfluramine. Substantial controversy exists regarding the true prevalence of diet drug valvulopathy. The majority of well-done, case-controlled trials suggest a prevalence of significant (moderate or greater) mitral in-

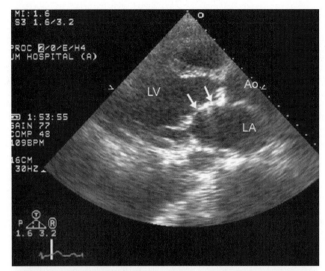

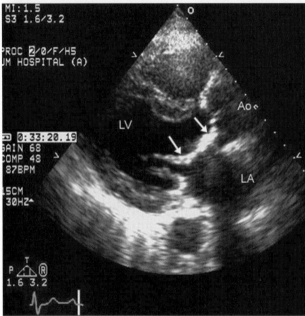

FIGURE 11.95. Parasternal long-axis view echocardiograms recorded in two patients with radiation-induced heart disease. In both instances, note the pathologic echo density of the anterior mitral leaflet (*arrows*) and reduced mobility of the proximal portion of the mitral valve, appreciable in the real-time image. Also note the increased echo densities in the aortic valve, which is also a consequence of radiation therapy in these two relatively young patients.

sufficiency due to diet drugs substantially less than suggested in initial reports. More recent studies have suggested that diet drug valvulopathy often regresses after withdrawal of the agents.

SUGGESTED READINGS

Abascal VM, Moreno PR, Rodriguez L, et al. Comparison of the usefulness of Doppler pressure half-time in mitral stenosis in patients < 65 and > or = 65 years of age. Am J Cardiol 1996;78:1390–1393.

Abascal VM, Wilkins GT, O'Shea JP, et al. Prediction of successful outcome in 130 patients undergoing percutaneous balloon mitral valvotomy. Circulation 1990;82:448–456.

Ascah KJ, Stewart WJ, Jiang L, et al. A Doppler-two-dimensional echocardiographic method for quantitation of mitral regurgitation. Circulation 1985;72:377–383.

Blumlein S, Bouchard A, Schiller NB, et al. Quantitation of mitral regurgitation by Doppler echocardiography. Circulation 1986;74: 306–314.

Bryg RJ, Williams GA, Labovitz AJ, et al. Effect of atrial fibrillation and mitral regurgitation on calculated mitral valve area in mitral stenosis. Am J Cardiol 1986;57:634–638.

Cape EG, Skoufis EG, Weyman AE, et al. A new method for noninvasive quantification of valvular regurgitation based on conservation of momentum. *In vitro* validation. Circulation 1989;79:1343–1353.

Cape EG, Yoganathan AP, Weyman AE, et al. Adjacent solid boundaries alter the size of regurgitant jets on Doppler color flow maps. J Am Coll Cardiol 1991;17:1094–1102.

Castello R, Pearson AC, Lenzen P, et al. Effect of mitral regurgitation on pulmonary venous velocities derived from transesophageal echocardiography color-guided pulsed Doppler imaging. J Am Coll Cardiol 1991;17:1499–1506.

Chao K, Moises VA, Shandas R, et al. Influence of the Coanda effect on color Doppler jet area and color encoding. *In vitro* studies using color Doppler flow mapping. Circulation 1992;85:333–341.

De Simone R, Glombitza G, Vahl CF, et al. Three-dimensional color Doppler: a new approach for quantitative assessment of mitral regurgitant jets. J Am Soc Echocardiogr 1999;12:173–185.

Enriquez-Sarano M, Dujardin KS, Tribouilloy CM, et al. Determinants of pulmonary venous flow reversal in mitral regurgitation and its usefulness in determining the severity of regurgitation. Am J Cardiol 1999;83:535–541.

Foster GP, Isselbacher EM, Rose GA, et al. Accurate localization of mitral regurgitant defects using multiplane transesophageal echocardiography. Ann Thorac Surg 1998;65:1025–1031.

Freed LA, Levy D, Levine RA, et al. Prevalence and clinical outcome of mitral-valve prolapse. N Engl J Med 1999;341:1–7.

Gilon D, Buonanno FS, Joffe MM, et al. Lack of evidence of an association between mitral-valve prolapse and stroke in young patients. N Engl J Med 1999;341:8–13.

Gonzalez-Torrecilla E, Garcia-Fernandez MA, Perez-David E, et al. Predictors of left atrial spontaneous echo contrast and thrombi in patients with mitral stenosis and atrial fibrillation. Am J Cardiol 2000;86:529–534.

Grigioni F, Enriquez-Sarano M, Zehr KJ, et al. Ischemic mitral regurgitation: long-term outcome and prognostic implications with quantitative Doppler assessment. Circulation 2001;103:1759–1764.

Hernandez R, Banuelos C, Alfonso F, et al. Long-term clinical and echocardiographic follow-up after percutaneous mitral valvuloplasty with the Inoue balloon. Circulation 1999;99:1580–1586.

Himelman RB, Kusumoto F, Oken K, et al. The flail mitral valve: echocardiographic findings by precordial and transesophageal imaging and Doppler color flow mapping. J Am Coll Cardiol 1991;17:272–279.

Karp K, Teien D, Bjerle P, et al. Reassessment of valve area determinations in mitral stenosis by the pressure half-time method: impact of left ventricular stiffness and peak diastolic pressure difference. J Am Coll Cardiol 1989;13:594–599.

Klein AL, Obarski TP, Stewart WJ, et al. Transesophageal Doppler echocardiography of pulmonary venous flow: a new marker of mitral regurgitation severity. J Am Coll Cardiol 1991;18:518–526.

Levine RA, Handschumacher MD, Sanfilippo AJ, et al. Three-dimensional echocardiographic reconstruction of the mitral valve, with implications for the diagnosis of mitral valve prolapse. Circulation 1989;80:589–598.

Loperfido F, Laurenzi F, Gimigliano F, et al. A comparison of the assessment of mitral valve area by continuous wave Doppler and by cross sectional echocardiography. Br Heart J 1987;57:348–355.

Marks AR, Choong CY, Sanfilippo AJ, et al. Identification of high-risk and low-risk subgroups of patients with mitral-valve prolapse. N Engl J Med 1989;320:1031–1036.

Martin RP, Rakowski H, Kleiman JH, et al. Reliability and reproducibility of two dimensional echocardiograph measurement of the stenotic mitral valve orifice area. Am J Cardiol 1979;43:560–568.

Nishimura RA, McGoon MD, Shub C, et al. Echocardiographically documented mitral-valve prolapse. Long-term follow-up of 237 patients. N Engl J Med 1985;313:1305–1309.

Otsuji Y, Handschumacher MD, Liel-Cohen N, et al. Mechanism of ischemic mitral regurgitation with segmental left ventricular dysfunction: three-dimensional echocardiographic studies in models of acute and chronic progressive regurgitation. J Am Coll Cardiol 2001;37:641–648.

Padial LR, Abascal VM, Moreno PR, et al. Echocardiography can predict the development of severe mitral regurgitation after percutaneous mitral valvuloplasty by the Inoue technique. Am J Cardiol 1999;83:1210–1213.

Palacios IF, Sanchez PL, Harrell LC, et al. Which patients benefit from percutaneous mitral balloon valvuloplasty? Prevalvuloplasty and postvalvuloplasty variables that predict long-term outcome. Circulation 2002;105:1465–1471.

Pearson AC, St Vrain J, Mrosek D, et al. Color Doppler echocardiographic evaluation of patients with a flail mitral leaflet. J Am Coll Cardiol 1990;16:232–239.

Pu M, Thomas JD, Vandervoort PM, et al. Comparison of quantitative and semiquantitative methods for assessing mitral regurgitation by transesophageal echocardiography. Am J Cardiol 2001;87:66–70.

Pu M, Vandervoort PM, Greenberg NL, et al. Impact of wall constraint on velocity distribution in proximal flow convergence zone. Implications for color Doppler quantification of mitral regurgitation. J Am Coll Cardiol 1996;27:706–713.

Recusani F, Bargiggia GS, Yoganathan AP, et al. A new method for quantification of regurgitant flow rate using color Doppler flow imaging of the flow convergence region proximal to a discrete orifice. An in vitro study. Circulation 1991;83:594–604.

Salgo IS, Gorman JH 3rd, Gorman RC, et al. Effect of annular shape on leaflet curvature in reducing mitral leaflet stress. Circulation 2002;106:711–717.

Smallhorn J, Tommasini G, Deanfield J, et al. Congenital mitral stenosis. Anatomical and functional assessment by echocardiography. Br Heart J 1981;45:527–534.

Smith MD, Wisenbaugh T, Grayburn PA, et al. Value and limitations of Doppler pressure half-time in quantifying mitral stenosis: a comparison with micromanometer catheter recordings. Am Heart J 1991;121:480–488.

Spain MG, Smith MD, Grayburn PA, et al. Quantitative assessment of mitral regurgitation by Doppler color flow imaging: angiographic and hemodynamic correlations. J Am Coll Cardiol 1989;13:585–590.

Stamm RB, Martin RP. Quantification of pressure gradients across stenotic valves by Doppler ultrasound. J Am Coll Cardiol 1983;2:707–718.

Stevenson JG. Two-dimensional color Doppler estimation of the severity of atrioventricular valve regurgitation: important effects of instrument gain setting, pulse repetition frequency, and carrier frequency. J Am Soc Echocardiogr 1989;2:1–10.

Sun JP, Asher CR, Yang XS, et al. Clinical and echocardiographic characteristics of papillary fibroelastomas: a retrospective and prospective study in 162 patients. Circulation 2001;103:2687–2693.

Thomas JD, Weyman AE. Doppler mitral pressure half-time: a clinical tool in search of theoretical justification. J Am Coll Cardiol 1987;10:923–929.

Thomas JD, Wilkins GT, Choong CY, et al. Inaccuracy of mitral pressure half-time immediately after percutaneous mitral valvotomy. Dependence on transmitral gradient and left atrial and ventricular compliance. Circulation 1988;78:980–993.

Thomas L, Foster E, Hoffman JI, et al. The Mitral Regurgitation Index: an echocardiographic guide to severity. J Am Coll Cardiol 1999;33:2016–2022.

Van Camp G, Carlier S, Cosyns B, et al. Quantification of mitral regurgitation by the automated cardiac output method: an in vitro and in vivo study. J Am Soc Echocardiogr 1998;11:643–651.

Voelker W, Jacksch R, Dittmann H, et al. Validation of continuous-wave Doppler measurements of mitral valve gradients during exercise—a simultaneous Doppler-catheter study. Eur Heart J 1989;10:737–746.

Wang A, Krasuski RA, Warner JJ, et al. Serial echocardiographic evaluation of restenosis after successful percutaneous mitral commissurotomy. J Am Coll Cardiol 2002;39:328–334.

Wang A, Ryan T, Kisslo KB, et al. Assessing the severity of mitral stenosis: variability between noninvasive and invasive measurements in patients with symptomatic mitral valve stenosis. Am Heart J 1999;138:777–784.

Wann LS, Weyman AE, Feigenbaum H, et al. Determination of mitral valve area by cross-sectional echocardiography. Ann Intern Med 1978;88:337–341.

Wilkins GT, Weyman AE, Abascal VM, Block PC, Palacios IF. Percutaneous balloon dilatation of the mitral valve: an analysis of echocardiographic variables related to outcome and the mechanism of dilation. British Heart Journal 1988;60, 299–308.

Yiu SF, Enriquez-Sarano M, Tribouilloy C, et al. Determinants of the degree of functional mitral regurgitation in patients with systolic left ventricular dysfunction: a quantitative clinical study. Circulation 2000;102:1400–1406.

Yoshida K, Yoshikawa J, Yamaura Y, et al. Assessment of mitral regurgitation by biplane transesophageal color Doppler flow mapping. Circulation 1990;82:1121–1126.

Tricuspid and Pulmonary Valves

CLINICAL OVERVIEW

Primary pathology of the tricuspid and pulmonary valve is relatively infrequent in adult populations. Secondary or functional abnormalities due to disease of the ventricle or pulmonary hypertension are more common in adult populations. Clinical entities resulting in detectable pulmonary and tricuspid valvular disease are listed in Table 12.1. Congenital pulmonary and tricuspid valve lesions are discussed in Chapter 18. Disease of the tricuspid valve can be divided into primary and secondary anatomic abnormalities. Primary abnormalities include congenital diseases such as Ebstein anomaly as well as acquired abnormalities such as endocarditis and carcinoid valve disease. The most common form of tricuspid valvular pathology encountered in adults is secondary tricuspid

regurgitation due to anular dilation and malcoaptation of the leaflets. This is a common secondary finding in pulmonary hypertension or any other disease resulting in right ventricular dilation. In general, detection of tricuspid regurgitation with a dilated anulus should lead to a search for an underlying cause such as pulmonary hypertension, primary left heart disease, or disease of the right ventricular myocardium such as infarction or cardiomyopathy.

PULMONARY VALVE

The normal pulmonary valve is a three-leaflet structure, anatomically similar to the aortic valve. It is inserted into the pulmonary artery anulus distal to the right ventricular outflow tract. Developmentally, the aorta and pulmonary arteries arise in a parallel fashion. The two arteries then rotate such that the right ventricular outflow tract, pulmonary valve, and proximal pulmonary artery effectively wrap around the aortic valve and ascending aorta.

When viewed with two-dimensional echocardiography, typically only one or two leaflets are simultaneously visualized. On occasion, unusual imaging planes allow visualization of the pulmonary valve in its short axis; however, the relatively thin, highly pliable leaflets are infrequently directly visualized in their entirety. Visualization of the pulmonary valve in adults typically is optimal from a parasternal short-axis transducer position at the base of the heart, at which time the aortic valve and/or proximal aorta are simultaneously visualized (Fig. 12.1). The bifurcation of the pulmonary artery is also visualized from this view (Fig. 12.2). Anatomically, the pulmonary valve should be described in conjunction with the right ventricular outflow tract, including an assessment of the degree of hypertrophy in the outflow tract. In addition to the parasternal short-axis view, a long-axis projection of the right ventricular outflow tract and pulmonary valve can be obtained by rotation of the transducer approximately 90 degrees while angulating the transducer toward the

▶ **TABLE 12.1 Diseases of the Tricuspid and Pulmonary Valves**

Disease	Stenosis	Regurgitation
Rheumatic heart disease	✓	✓
Carcinoid heart disease	✓	✓
Obstructive tumors	✓	—
Congenital pulmonary stenosis	✓	±
Endocarditis	±	✓
Ebstein anomaly	—	✓
Endocardial fibroelastosis	±	✓
Tricuspid valve prolapse	—	✓
Traumatic rupture	—	✓
Right ventricular infarction	—	✓
Ischemic papillary muscle dysfunction	—	✓
Pulmonary hypertension[a]	—	✓
Left-to-right shunt with dilation[a]	—	✓
Right ventricular cardiomyopathy[a]	—	✓
Pacemaker leads, right heart catheter	—	✓

[a]Tricuspid disease is secondary to right ventricular dilation. The leaflets are anatomically normal.

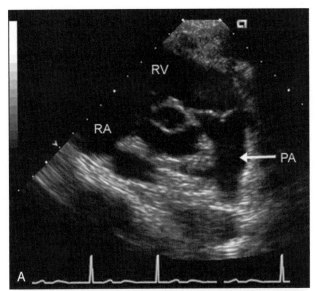

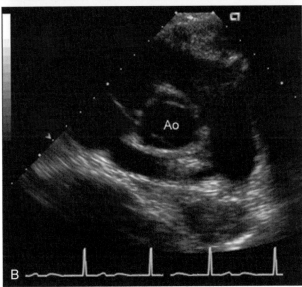

FIGURE 12.1. Transthoracic parasternal short-axis view at the base of the heart visualizes the pulmonary valve. Notice the central closure point in diastole **(A)** and the inability to visualize the normal leaflets that are fully open in systole **(B).** Ao, aorta; PA, pulmonary artery; RA, right atrium; RV, right ventricle.

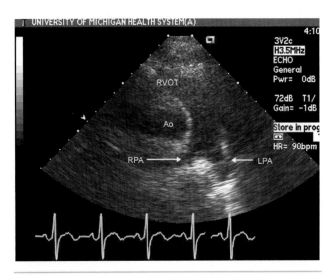

FIGURE 12.2. Parasternal short-axis view at the base of the heart with a slightly different angulation than presented in Figure 12.1. In this view, the bifurcation of the pulmonary artery into right and left pulmonary arteries (*RPA, LPA*) can be visualized. Ao, aorta, RVOT, right ventricular outflow tract.

right shoulder (Fig. 12.3). This visualization plane is often problematic in large-stature adults but is often available in adolescents and smaller stature individuals. A final imaging plane for transthoracic visualization of the pulmonary valve is the subcostal view in which, with anterior angulation, the entire sweep of the right ventricular outflow tract can often be visualized including the pulmonary valve leaflets (Fig. 12.4).

The pulmonary valve can also be visualized with transesophageal echocardiography. The views that maximize visualization of the pulmonary valve include horizontal (0 degrees) plane imaging at relatively shallow depths (typi-

cally 25–30 cm from the incisors) with clockwise rotation of the probe. In this view, the bifurcation of the pulmonary artery is typically seen and the pulmonary valve can be likewise visualized (Fig. 12.5). An additional transesophageal echocardiographic window providing visualization of the pulmonary valve is often obtained from a deep gastric view in a longitudinal or 120-degree imaging plane. With clockwise rotation of the transducer, the entire sweep of the right ventricular inflow and outflow tracts can often be obtained and simultaneous visualization of the right atrium, tricuspid valve, right ventricular outflow tract, pulmonary valve, and proximal pulmonary artery often accomplished.

Using M-mode echocardiography from a parasternal approach, motion of the pulmonary valve can be recorded. Only one leaflet will be intersected by the M-mode interrogation beam. The likelihood of visualizing pulmonary valve motion on M-mode is maximized by using two-dimensional echocardiography-guided M-mode imaging. Characterization of pulmonary valve motion provided one of the earlier clues to the presence of pulmonary hypertension and indirect evidence of other right heart pathology. There are several components to normal pulmonary valve motion (Fig. 12.6). The first is presystolic A-wave motion away from the transducer, which is due to relatively low-amplitude excursion (<6 mm) of the pulmonary valve with atrial systole. This phenomenon is dependent on mechanical atrial systole and is not present in atrial fibrillation. It is also dependent on relatively low pulmonary artery diastolic pressures, so that atrial contraction creates the driving force for partial opening of the pulmonary valve. The pulmonary valve leaflet then moves posteriorly (in a supine patient), i.e., away from

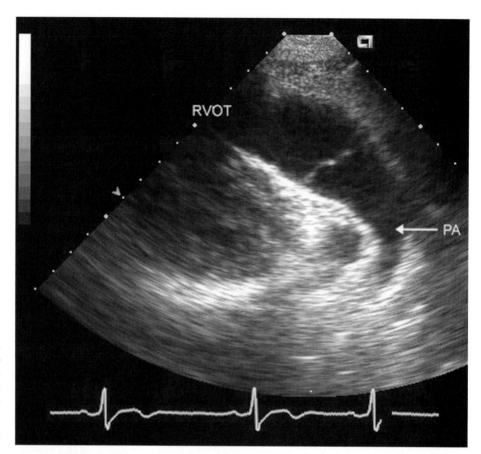

FIGURE 12.3. Parasternal long-axis view of the right ventricular outflow tract (*RVOT*), pulmonary artery (*PA*), and pulmonary valve recorded in diastole. In the real-time image, note the full motion of the valve to the margins of the arterial wall.

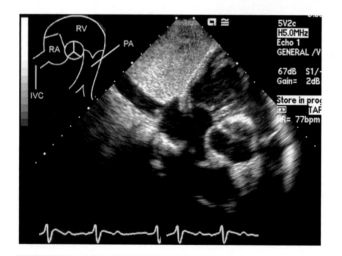

FIGURE 12.4. Subcostal short-axis view of the base of the heart shows a portion of the right atrium (*RA*), tricuspid valve, right ventricle (*RV*) and outflow tract, pulmonary valve, and pulmonary artery (*PA*). Structures are as noted on the schematic in the upper left of the figure. IVC, inferior vena cava.

the transducer during systole. It is not uncommon for visualization to be incomplete throughout the entire cardiac cycle and for only the A-wave and opening slope of the pulmonary valve to be detectable. With excellent acoustic windows, the full opening of the pulmonary valve and the degree to which it remains in a fully open position during systole can occasionally be appreciated (Fig. 12.7) and its subsequent closure in diastole also noted.

Pulsed and continuous wave Doppler imaging can also be recorded at the level of the pulmonary valve. The data derived from this interrogation can provide information on the status of pulmonary vasculature. Typically, the pulmonary valve flow profile is recorded from a parasternal short-axis view along an interrogation line identical to that used for M-mode echocardiography. Figure 12.8 schematizes the appropriate sample volume position and provides an example of a normal pulsed Doppler imaging of pulmonary flow. It should be emphasized that many of the indirect parameters of right heart hemodynamics that can be derived from the pulmonary outflow tract spectral profile are dependent on optimal imaging planes, including the central position of the sample volume within the pulmonary artery (as opposed to recording it along the periphery of the wall) and recording at a level just distal to the tips of the pulmonary valve. The normal pulmonary outflow tract velocity ranges from 1 to 1.5 msec. As with other valves, the time velocity integral of this valve can be determined and in combination with the outflow tract dimension

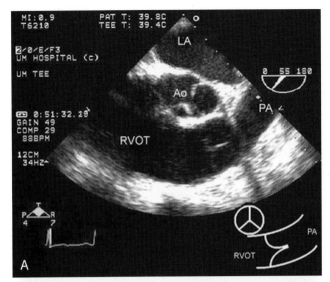

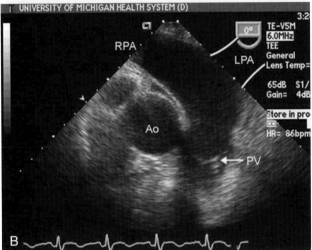

FIGURE 12.5. Transesophageal echocardiogram recorded in a 55-degree view at the base of the heart. **A:** The right ventricular outflow tract (*RVOT*) and pulmonary artery (*PA*) are clearly visualized as is the pulmonary valve (*PV*). **B:** The pulmonary valve and a larger portion of the main pulmonary artery and right pulmonary artery (*RPA*) are shown. In this view, it is often difficult to visualize simultaneously the right (*RPA*) and left (*LPA*) pulmonary arteries. Ao, aorta; LA, left atrium.

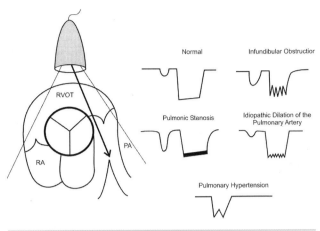

FIGURE 12.6. Schematic representation of M-mode echocardiograms of normal and abnormal pulmonary valves. In the normal schematic, note the normal A-wave and box-like opening of the valve. Various disease states are also schematized.

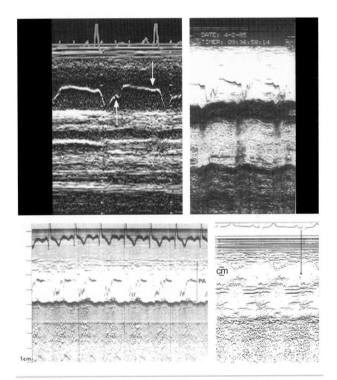

FIGURE 12.7. M-mode echocardiograms recorded in patients with different abnormalities. **Top left:** Recorded in a patient with pulmonary hypertension. Note the loss of the pulmonic valve A-wave (*downward-pointing arrow*) and mid systolic notching (*upward-pointing arrow*) of the valve. **Top right:** Note the low-amplitude biphasic A-wave. **Bottom left:** Image recorded in a patient with infundibular obstruction shows coarse fluttering of the valve in systole. **Bottom right:** Recorded in a patient with pulmonary valve stenosis. Note the accentuated A-wave (1 cm). PA, pulmonary artery.

can be used to calculate volumetric flow (Fig. 12.8). Other parameters of the pulmonary outflow tract velocity include acceleration time. Acceleration time is defined as the time in milliseconds from the onset of ejection to peak systolic velocity. In normal individuals, acceleration time exceeds 140 milliseconds and progressively shortens with increasing degrees of pulmonary hypertension (Fig. 12.9).

The inverse relationship between pulmonary acceleration time and pulmonary artery systolic, diastolic, and mean pressures has been demonstrated in numerous studies. Most have suggested that at an acceleration time

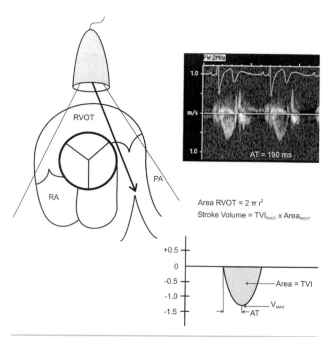

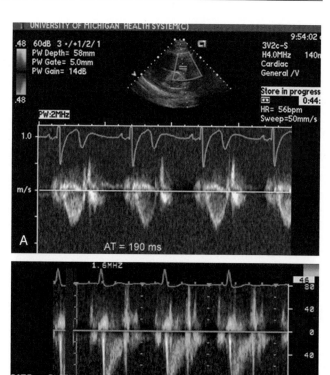

FIGURE 12.8. Schematic representation of the methods for recording pulmonary/right ventricular outflow tract (*RVOT*) velocities. The parasternal short-axis view is used with the interrogating beam aimed posteriorly along the long axis of the right ventricular outflow tract and proximal pulmonary artery (*PA*). The spectral display is schematized at the lower right, including its various components such as time velocity ventricle (*TVI*) and acceleration time (*AT*). In the upper right is an example of a normal flow profile. The method for calculating stroke volume from these parameters is also displayed. RA, right atrium.

FIGURE 12.9. Spectral flow profiles recorded in a normal individual (**A**) with an acceleration time (*AT*) of 190 milliseconds and a patient with significant pulmonary hypertension in whom the acceleration time is 80 milliseconds (**B**).

of less than 70 to 90 milliseconds, pulmonary artery systolic pressures will exceed 70 mm Hg. This assessment has been largely replaced by the more direct Doppler assessment of right ventricular systolic pressure from the tricuspid regurgitation signal. On occasion, in a patient without a measurable tricuspid regurgitation velocity, shortening of the pulmonary acceleration time may be the only evidence of pulmonary hypertension.

Color flow imaging can be accomplished in the vast majority of patients and often, when using high-resolution, high-sensitivity imaging platforms, results in detection of inconsequential degrees of pulmonary regurgitation (Fig. 12.10). As minor degrees of pulmonary regurgitation are detected in the majority of adults when using modern imaging platforms, they should be considered a normal variant.

Pulmonary Valve Stenosis

Pulmonary valve stenosis is a congenital cardiac lesion and is discussed in detail in Chapter 18. The classic anatomic abnormality is fusion of the commissures such that the pulmonary valve is effectively converted to a unicuspid or bicuspid funnel-shaped valve. This results in restriction of the orifice at the distal portion of the valve, and the resultant stenosis ranges in severity from mild and inconsequential to severe and life-threatening in infancy.

Pulmonary valve stenosis is easily detected and quantified using two-dimensional echocardiographic and Doppler techniques. On two-dimensional echocardiography, thickening and doming of the pulmonary valve are often appreciated (Fig. 12.11) and continuous wave Doppler imaging can be used to accurately determine the peak instantaneous and mean gradients (Fig. 12.12). Because the orientation of the right ventricular outflow tract and pulmonary artery flow is directed posteriorly, there is a natural alignment of the interrogating beam with the direction of flow, and off-angle interrogation is less of a problem than with aortic stenosis. The same techniques for determining mean and peak instantaneous gradients were discussed previously for the aortic valve, and there is an excellent correlation between catheterization and Doppler hemodynamics for pulmonary valve stenosis as well.

M-mode echocardiography can provide clues to the presence of pulmonary valve stenosis, although it is rarely

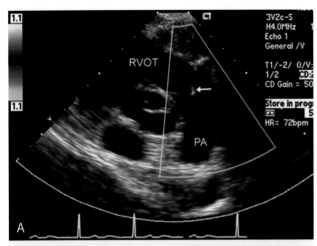

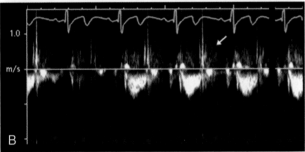

FIGURE 12.10. Parasternal short-axis view at the base of the heart in a normal individual reveals trivial central pulmonary valve insufficiency. **A:** Note the very small central regurgitant jet (*arrow*). **B:** Note the faint early diastolic retrograde Doppler spectral signal consistent with minimal pulmonary insufficiency. PA, pulmonary artery; RVOT, right ventricular outflow tract.

necessary in contemporary practice in which Doppler techniques predominate for detection and quantification of pulmonary valve stenosis. On M-mode echocardiography (Fig. 12.7), the hallmark findings of pulmonary valve stenosis are an accentuated A-wave amplitude (>6 mm) with thickening of the leaflets. The accentuated A-wave occurs only in patients in sinus rhythm and in individuals with right ventricular hypertrophy. It does not allow quantitation of severity, but the presence of an accentuated A-wave is indirect evidence of pulmonary valve stenosis. The origin of the accentuated A-wave is the relatively elevated right ventricular diastolic pressure in comparison with the pulmonary artery diastolic pressure. Atrial contraction generates a greater than usual amount of hemodynamic force, and this pressure is transmitted by the hypertrophied noncompliant right ventricle to the pulmonary valve and pulmonary artery. With atrial contraction, the right ventricular outflow tract pressure exceeds pulmonary artery diastolic pressure, and there is accentuated presystolic opening of the pulmonary valve. As noted previously, this is a qualitative descriptor imply-

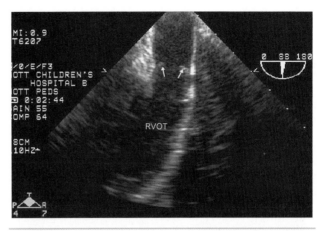

FIGURE 12.11. Transesophageal echocardiogram recorded in an adolescent with congenital pulmonary valve stenosis. This image was recorded in mid-systole. Note the thickening of the pulmonary valve leaflets and the doming motion (*arrows*) characteristic of valvar pulmonary stenosis. RVOT, right ventricular outflow tract. (Courtesy of Gregory Ensing, M.D.)

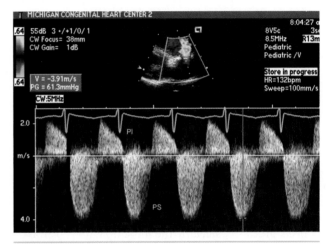

FIGURE 12.12. Continuous wave Doppler imaging through the right ventricular outflow tract and pulmonary valve in a patient with pulmonary valve stenosis. Note the peak pressure gradient of 61 mm Hg and the presence of concurrent pulmonary valve insufficiency. PI, pulmonary valve insufficiency; PS, pulmonary valve stenosis.

ing the presence of pulmonary valve stenosis but provides no further quantitative information.

Pulmonary Valve Regurgitation

Minor degrees of pulmonary valve regurgitation are commonly encountered in the normal disease-free population and do not necessarily imply anatomic disease of the pulmonary valve, pulmonary artery, or elevated pulmonary artery pressures (Figs. 12.10 and Fig. 12.13). There are several pathologic causes of pulmonary valve regurgitation, including its association with pulmonary valve stenosis. Dilation of the pulmonary anulus, which can be

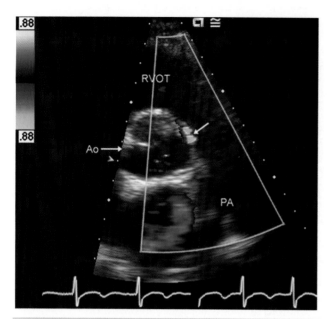

FIGURE 12.13. Parasternal short-axis view recorded at the base of the heart in a patient with minimal pulmonary valve insufficiency originating at the lateral aspect of the cusp commissure. Because this jet originates immediately adjacent to the aorta (*Ao*), it could be confused for an aorta-pulmonary fistula. Note, however, the exclusively diastolic flow, which would not be expected in the presence of the true shunt. PA, pulmonary artery; RVOT, right ventricular outflow tract.

idiopathic or due to pulmonary artery dilation, which in turn is a consequence of pulmonary hypertension, also results in pulmonary valve regurgitation. Occasionally, one encounters congenital absence of one or more pulmonary valve cusps, which results in substantial degrees of pulmonary valve regurgitation (Fig. 12.15).

Detection of pulmonary valve regurgitation relies almost exclusively on color flow imaging and spectral Doppler profile analysis. Using color Doppler imaging, typically from a parasternal short-axis view at the base of the heart, one detects a diastolic retrograde jet. The location of the jet can be highly variable and often occurs at the margins of commissural fusion, immediately adjacent to the wall of the pulmonary artery (Fig. 12.13). On occasion, this could be confused with an aorta-pulmonary communication; however, its exclusive diastolic flow profile should allow exclusion of an aorta-pulmonary window in which flow would occur throughout the entire cardiac cycle. Using pulsed Doppler imaging, one can detect a retrograde spectral profile directed toward the transducer similar to that seen in aortic pulmonary regurgitation. Because mild degrees of pulmonary valve regurgitation can be highly eccentric, blind scanning with spectral Doppler can often miss the pulmonary valve regurgitation jet, whereas they are easily detected by color flow Doppler imaging.

Determination of the severity of pulmonary valve regurgitation has been less well validated than determina-

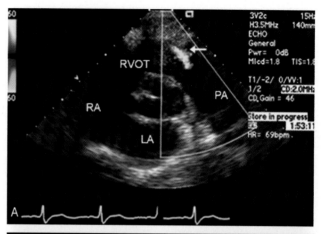

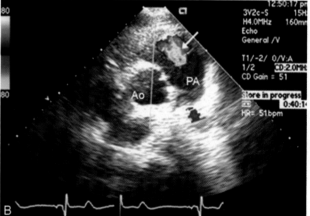

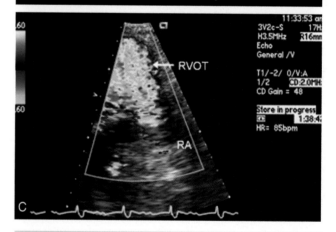

FIGURE 12.14. Parasternal short-axis view color Doppler flow images recorded in patients with mild **(A)**, moderate **(B)**, and severe **(C)** pulmonary valve insufficiency. Ao, aorta; LA, left atrium; PA, pulmonary artery; RA, right atrium; RVOT, right ventricular outflow tract.

tion of aortic regurgitation, in large part due to the lack of reliable standards for comparison. In general, similar guidelines are clinically used for determining the severity of pulmonary valve regurgitation, including determination of overall jet size, depth of penetration into the right

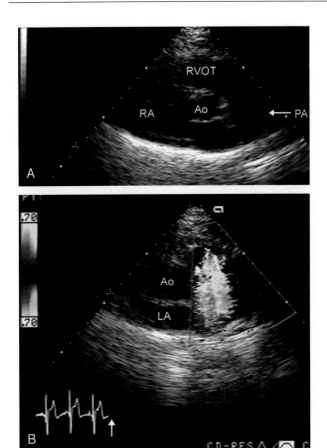

FIGURE 12.15. Parasternal short-axis view images recorded in a patient with wide-open pulmonary insufficiency due to congenital absence of pulmonary valve leaflets. Notice the absence of any pulmonary valve tissue **(A)** and the "free" insufficiency that fills the entire right ventricular outflow tract **(B)**. Note the absence of any high-velocity or organized jet, which is attributable to the absence of any constraining valve tissue. Ao, aorta; LA, left atrium; PA, pulmonary artery; RA, right atrium; RVOT, right ventricular outflow tract.

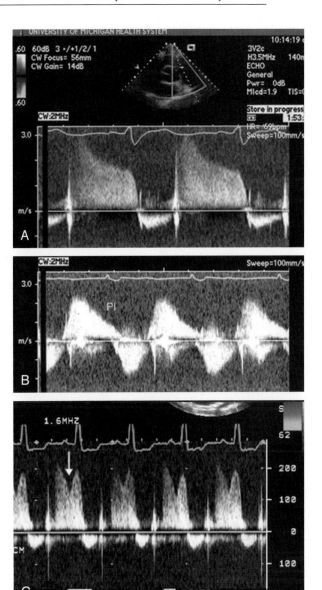

FIGURE 12.16. Continuous wave spectral recording of patients with pulmonary valve insufficiency. **A:** Note the relatively faint signal and slow diastolic decay consistent with relatively mild insufficiency. Compare this with the denser signal with a steeper decay slope **(B)**, which was recorded in a patient with severe pulmonary valve insufficiency. **C:** Image recorded in a patient with moderate pulmonary valve insufficiency and a hypertrophied noncompliant right ventricle. Note the late systolic interruption of regurgitant flow coincidental with atrial systole *(arrow)*. This phenomenon occurs when the atrium contracts, ejecting blood into a noncompliant right ventricle. This results in pre-systolic flow into the right ventricular outflow tract, which interrupts the diastolic insufficiency flow. PI, pulmonary valve insufficiency.

ventricle *vena contracta* width, and its overall width in relation to the right ventricular outflow tract (Figs. 12.14 and 12.15). One should also rely heavily on indirect evidence of a hemodynamic effect from the pulmonary valve regurgitation such as right ventricular dilation and the presence of a right ventricular volume overload. The latter, in the absence of other causes of right ventricular overload, is evidence of at least moderate pulmonary valve regurgitation.

As with other valvular lesions, inspection of the quality of the retrograde spectral signal also provides indirect clues to the severity of pulmonary valve regurgitation, with relatively dense signals suggesting a higher volume of regurgitant blood flow than faint signals and short deceleration times having the same implication as for aortic regurgitation (Fig. 12.16).

The diastolic flow velocities of pulmonary valve regurgitation can be used to calculate pulmonary artery diastolic pressure using the modified Bernoulli equation. In this setting, one calculates the end-diastolic gradient between the pulmonary artery and right ventricular outflow tract from the velocity of the pulmonary regurgitation jet (Fig. 12.17). If one then adds an assumed right

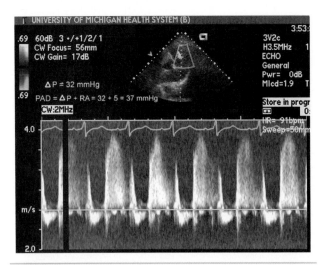

FIGURE 12.17. Continuous wave Doppler image recorded in a patient with pulmonary hypertension illustrates the manner in which pulmonary artery diastolic pressure can be calculated from the diastolic flow velocity and an assumed right atrial pressure of 5 mm Hg.

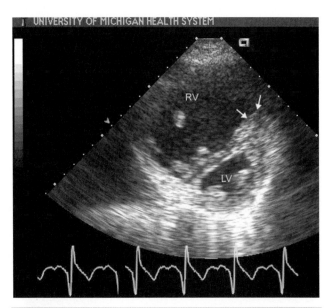

FIGURE 12.18. Parasternal short-axis view recorded at the papillary muscle level in a patient with significant pulmonary hypertension and secondary infundibular hypertrophy. Note the massively dilated right ventricle (*RV*) and hypertrophied muscle bundles, the flattened ventricular septum with a small left ventricular cavity, and marked hypertrophy of the right ventricular infundibulum (*arrows*). LV, left ventricle.

ventricular diastolic pressure (in turn assumed to equal right atrial pressure), the equation PADP = RVEDP + ΔP_{pv} can be applied, where ΔP_{pv} equals the pressure gradient between the pulmonary artery and right ventricular outflow tract from the spectral profile. This calculation of pulmonary artery diastolic pressure has had substantial use in congenital heart disease. When combined with the determination of right ventricular systolic pressure from the tricuspid regurgitation jet, it allows calculation of both systolic and diastolic pulmonary artery pressures. Using the combination of pulmonary artery diastolic and systolic pressures, one can then calculate mean pulmonary artery pressure as $PA_{mean} = (PA_{systolic} + 2PA_{diastolic})/3$.

Evaluation of the Right Ventricular Outflow Tract

The right ventricular outflow tract is defined as the portion of the right ventricle extending from the crista terminalis to the pulmonary artery anulus. It is a relatively trabeculated area of the right ventricle. Because of its muscular nature, diseases that elevate right ventricular pressure, such as pulmonary hypertension and pulmonary valve stenosis, result in compensatory hypertrophy in the right ventricular outflow tract. Because of its proximity to the anterior chest wall, the right ventricular outflow tract is usually easily evaluated from a parasternal short-axis view, where its dimension and degree of trabeculation and hypertrophy can frequently be easily ascertained (Fig. 12.18). Obstruction can occur in the right ventricular outflow tract as a primary abnormality such as discrete outflow tract obstruction or more commonly

due to physiologic hypertrophy. Physiologic hypertrophy often has a dynamic component. Obstruction in the right ventricular outflow tract can result in characteristic abnormalities of pulmonary valve motion, which are often best appreciated on M-mode echocardiography. In a manner similar to the abnormalities seen on the aortic valve in discrete subvalvar stenosis, coarse fluttering of the pulmonary valve can be seen (Fig. 12.6). Other instances in which specific abnormalities of the right ventricular outflow tract can be noted include patients in whom corrective surgery has been undertaken, in which case, either a patch or aneurysmal dilation of the outflow tract can be noted.

Miscellaneous Abnormalities of the Pulmonary Valve

There are rare tumors and masses that can be seen on the pulmonary valve. As with any of the four cardiac valves, infectious endocarditis can involve the pulmonary valve, although it is substantially less frequent than involvement of any of the other three cardiac valves. When present, vegetations take on a similar oscillating appearance to that noted in other valve involvement. Occasionally, a fibroma or papilloma can be seen on the pulmonary valve, in which case, it takes on the typical appearance of a small spherical mass, usually attached to the leaflet by a thin stalk.

There is a clinically described phenomenon of idiopathic dilation of the pulmonary artery typically seen in elderly female patients. This can result in marked dilation of the proximal pulmonary artery, occasionally involving both major branches, and frequently results in secondary pulmonary valve regurgitation. An additional finding noted in idiopathic dilation of the pulmonary artery is high-frequency oscillation of the pulmonary valve leaflets.

TRICUSPID VALVE

Anatomically, the tricuspid valve is the most complex of the four cardiac valves. The three tricuspid valve leaflets are attached around the tricuspid anulus, which has a more variable geometry than does the mitral valve anulus. The three leaflets are not equally sized, with the anterior (or lateral) leaflet typically being substantially larger than the septal and posterior leaflets. Typically, the septal leaflet is smaller than the other two and inserts in a more apical position compared with the anterior leaflet of the mitral valve. This relatively apical position is one of the key discriminators between the tricuspid and mitral valves and is a reliable means of identifying the anatomic right ventricle in complex congenital heart disease. Coaptation of the tricuspid valve involves interaction of all three leaflets with a variable degree of overlap of leaflet tissue at the coaptation line. Chordal attachments are to three papillary muscles arising from the ventricular septum and free wall of the right ventricle. Because of the variable size of each of the three tricuspid leaflets, it is often difficult to ascertain the independent location, size, and motion of any given tricuspid leaflet in systole. Similarly, chordal attachments connect each of the three leaflets to one or more heads of each of the papillary muscles. Figure 12.19 schematizes the different echocardiographic views from which the tricuspid valve is visualized.

As noted in Figure 12.19, the tricuspid valve can be visualized from multiple transthoracic and transesophageal imaging planes. From the parasternal transducer position, the tricuspid valve is very well visualized from the right ventricular inflow tract view, obtained by medial angulation of the transducer such that the ultrasound beam is directed beneath the sternum. In this view, the right atrium and right ventricle as well as the coronary sinus and occasionally the inferior vena cava with an associated eustachian valve are clearly visualized (Fig. 12.20A). From this view, the posterior and anterior leaflets of the tricuspid valve can be clearly seen. In a parasternal short-axis view at the base of the heart, the tricuspid valve can be seen at the 9-o'clock position in relation to the aorta (Fig. 12.20B). In this view, the septal and anterior leaflets are

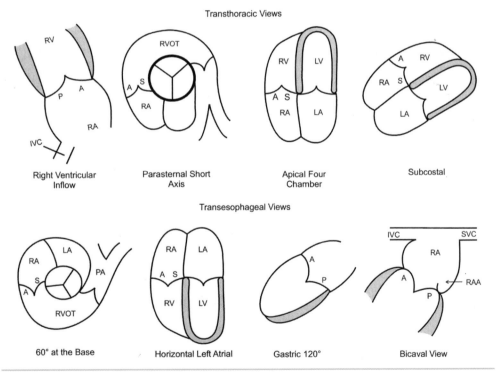

FIGURE 12.19. Schematic representation of transthoracic and transesophageal echocardiographic views illustrates the position of the tricuspid valve leaflets in each. Visualization of the anterior (*A*), posterior (*P*), and septal (*S*) leaflets are as noted in each figure. IVC, inferior vena cava; LA, left atrium; LV, left ventricle; PA, pulmonary artery; RA, right atrium; RAA, right atrial appendage; RV, right ventricle; RVOT, right ventricular outflow tract; SVC, superior vena cava.

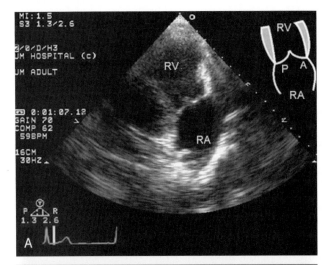

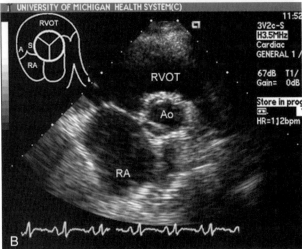

FIGURE 12.20. Parasternal views of the normal tricuspid valve in the right ventricular inflow tract view **(A)** and parasternal short-axis view **(B)**. Ao, aorta; RA, right atrium; RV, right ventricle; RVOT, right ventricular outflow tract.

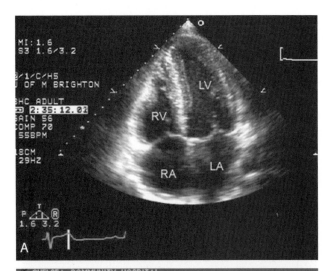

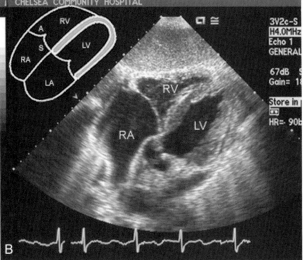

FIGURE 12.21. Apical four-chamber view **(A)** and subcostal view **(B)** recorded in a patient with a normal tricuspid valve. A, anterior leaflet; S, septal leaflet; LA, left atrium; LV, left ventricle; RA, right atrium; RV, right ventricle.

visualized. From an apical four-chamber view, the tricuspid valve can be visualized and its position relative to the mitral valve ascertained (Fig. 12.21). As discussed in Chapter 18, the tricuspid anulus is more apically positioned than is the mitral anulus. From an apical four-chamber view, the septal and anterior leaflets of the tricuspid valve are clearly visualized. Because the tricuspid valve is complex both in its anatomy and motion, M-mode echocardiography plays little role in identification of tricuspid valve pathology. When employed, it can demonstrate a two-phase opening pattern of the tricuspid valve, similar to that seen for the mitral valve (Fig. 12.22).

Using transesophageal echocardiography, the tricuspid valve can be imaged in multiple imaging planes as well. In general, the incremental yield of transesophageal echocardiography is less for the tricuspid valve than for imaging the mitral valve. This is particularly true if only mono- or biplane transesophageal probes are used. An experienced operator using a multiplane probe can often provide a detailed and comprehensive visualization of the tricuspid valve. The tricuspid valve can be visualized in the four-chamber equivalent view from behind the left atrium (Fig. 12.23), in which case its appearance is similar to that noted for a transthoracic apical four-chamber view. It is also well visualized at the base of the heart in a 60-degree view (Fig. 12.24). The deeper gastric views in a longitudinal plane often provide superb visualization of the tricuspid valve as well (Fig. 12.25).

Doppler Evaluation of the Tricuspid Valve

Both tricuspid valve inflow and tricuspid regurgitation can be evaluated from multiple echocardiographic windows, including the parasternal inflow tract view, short-

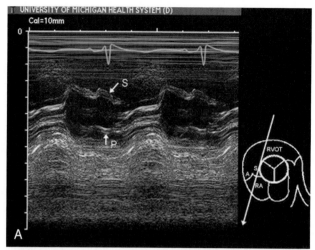

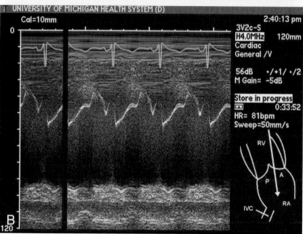

FIGURE 12.22. M-mode echocardiograms recorded in the parasternal short-axis **(A)** and right ventricular inflow tract **(B)** views demonstrate normal tricuspid valve motion. A, anterior leaflet; IVC, inferior vena cava; P, posterior leaflet; RA, right atrium; RV, right ventricle; RVOT, right ventricular outflow tract; S, septal leaflet.

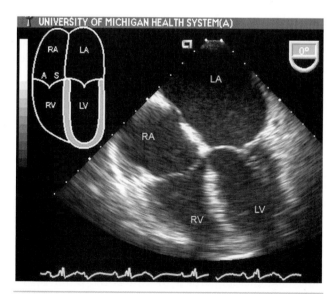

FIGURE 12.23. Transesophageal echocardiogram recorded in a horizontal (0-degree) view from behind the left atrium. Note the slight apical positioning of the tricuspid valve septal leaflet (S) compared with the anterior leaflet (A) of the mitral valve. See Figure 12.19 for leaflet anatomy.

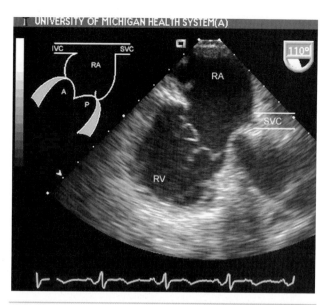

FIGURE 12.24. Transesophageal echocardiogram recorded in a 110-degree view at the base of the heart. See Figure 12.19 for leaflet anatomy. A, anterior leaflet; P, posterior leaflet; IVC, inferior vena cava; RA, right atrium; RV, right ventricle; SVC, superior vena cava.

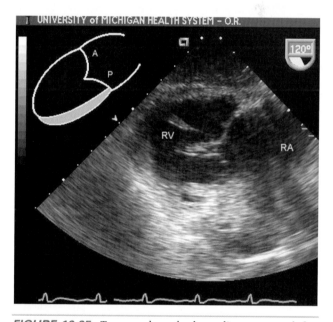

FIGURE 12.25. Transesophageal echocardiogram recorded at 120 degrees from the gastric probe position. The apex of the right ventricle (RV), tricuspid valve, and a portion of the right atrium (RA) are clearly visualized. This view gives excellent visualization of the tricuspid valve chordae and papillary muscles.

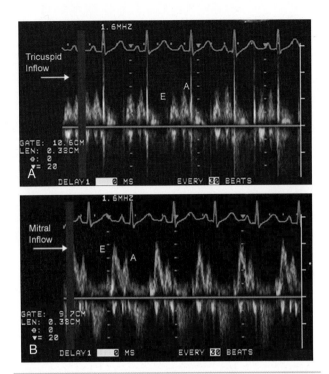

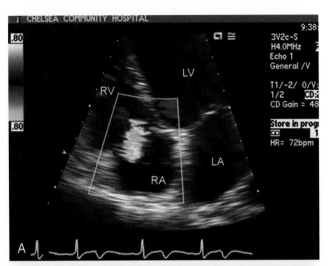

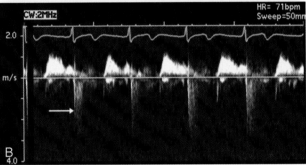

FIGURE 12.26. Pulsed spectral Doppler recording of tricuspid inflow (**A**) and mitral inflow for comparison (**B**). Note the relatively lower absolute velocity of the tricuspid inflow due to the larger effective orifice area of the tricuspid valve compared with the mitral valve.

FIGURE 12.27. A: Apical four-chamber view recorded in an individual with mild pulmonary hypertension and mild tricuspid regurgitation. **B:** Note the very faint spectral signal confined to early systole. LA, left atrium; LV, left ventricle; RA, right atrium; RV, right ventricle.

axis view at the base of the heart, and apical four-chamber view. Because the effective orifice area of the tricuspid valve is substantially greater than that of the mitral valve, the inflow velocities are lower than for the mitral valve. As for the mitral valve, however, the normal pattern consists of relatively higher early inflow (E-wave) and a lower velocity flow concordant with atrial systole (A-wave). In the absence of significant pathology, the tricuspid valve E/A ratio typically exceeds 1.0 (Fig. 12.26). Color flow imaging can be used to document the presence of tricuspid regurgitation. It should be emphasized that in the normal disease-free state, the tricuspid valve, because of its complex closure pattern, often exhibits mild degrees of valvular regurgitation, which may be confined to early systole (Fig. 12.27). The prevalence of regurgitation increases with patient age. When noted, the normal physiologic degrees of regurgitation typically are associated with relatively low tricuspid regurgitation velocities, implying right ventricular systolic pressures in the normal range.

Tricuspid Stenosis

Tricuspid stenosis is infrequently encountered in both adults and children. The etiologies of tricuspid stenosis include exceptionally rare cases of congenital stenosis, tricuspid stenosis due to rheumatic heart disease, in which

case mitral stenosis will invariably be present, and milder degrees of stenosis in the carcinoid syndrome (see below). The stenotic tricuspid valve has thickened leaflets with restricted motion at the level of the tips and chordae (Fig. 12.28); with the mitral valve, the transvalvular gradient can be determined from any of the available imaging planes.

Tricuspid Regurgitation

Unlike tricuspid stenosis, tricuspid regurgitation is common and can be due to primary disease of the tricuspid valve or secondary to anular dilation. As noted previously, small physiologic degrees of tricuspid regurgitation are often encountered in the normal disease-free individual. Etiologies of tricuspid regurgitation are listed in Table 12.1. Probably the most common cause of tricuspid regurgitation is functional valvular regurgitation secondary to anular dilation, which in turn is the result of pulmonary hypertension of any cause. The severity of functional tricuspid regurgitation can range from mild to se-

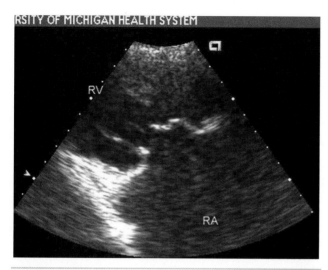

FIGURE 12.28. Right ventricular inflow tract view recorded in a patient with rheumatic tricuspid stenosis. Note the thickening of the leaflets, which is maximal at the tips and chordae, and the preserved mobility of the mid portion of the leaflets in the real-time image. Compare this with the rigidity of the entire leaflet seen in Figure 12.41, which was recorded in a patient with carcinoid syndrome. RA, right atrium; RV, right ventricle.

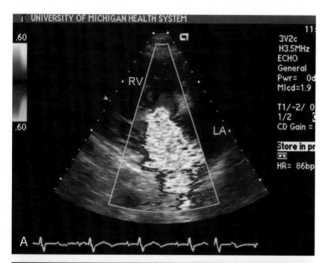

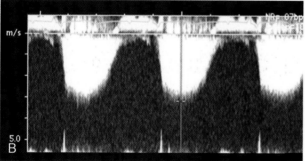

FIGURE 12.29. Right ventricular inflow tract view recorded in a patient with severe tricuspid regurgitation. In the color Doppler image, note the turbulent jet filling the majority of the right atrial cavity **(A)** and the very dense spectral profile **(B)**. LA, left atrium; RV, right ventricle.

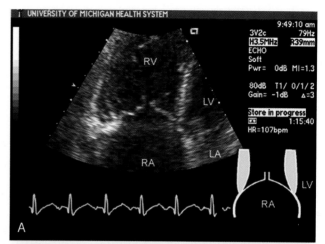

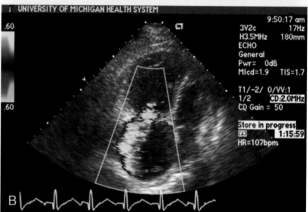

FIGURE 12.30. **A:** Recorded from an apical transducer position is an expanded view of the right ventricle (*RV*) and right atrium (*RA*) demonstrating a dilated tricuspid anulus with tethering of the tricuspid leaflets due to right ventricular dilation and dysfunction. **A:** Recorded in early systole, note that the tricuspid leaflets fail to coapt. **B:** Note the somewhat eccentric tricuspid regurgitation jet filling approximately 30% of the right atrium. Because this jet impinges on a wall, the jet size will understate the true severity of tricuspid regurgitation. LA, left atrium; LV, left ventricle.

vere. Figures 12.29 and 12.30 are examples of functional tricuspid regurgitation due to anular dilation. Additional causes of tricuspid regurgitation include ruptured chordae, which can occur as a sequela of endocarditis, spontaneously, or on occasion as a result of blunt chest trauma. Figure 12.31 was recorded in a patient after a motor vehicle accident. There is a partial flail of the tricuspid valve secondary to chordal rupture, which presumably was the result of blunt chest trauma.

As with any of the other cardiac valves, involvement by endocarditis can lead to tricuspid regurgitation. A final cause of tricuspid regurgitation is tricuspid valve prolapse seen in myxomatous valve syndrome (Fig. 12.32). In most instances, this will be seen in conjunction with mitral valve prolapse. Because of the variable anatomy of the tricuspid valve leaflets, its motion both in diastole and sys-

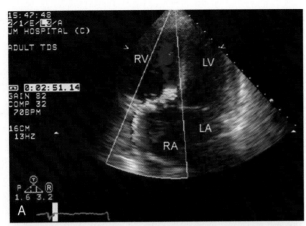

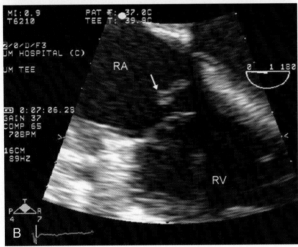

FIGURE 12.31. A: A transthoracic echocardiogram recorded in an apical four-chamber view revealing highly eccentric tricuspid regurgitation. **B:** A transesophageal echocardiogram recorded in a horizontal imaging plane from behind the left atrium. Note the disruption of the septal tricuspid leaflet (*arrow*), which protrudes behind the plane of the anulus in systole. These images were recorded in an individual with a traumatic rupture of the tricuspid valve due to a motor vehicle accident. LA, left atrium; LV, left ventricle; RA, right atrium; RV, right ventricle.

tole is far less predictable than that of the mitral valve, and in one or more views, the normal tricuspid valve may appear to prolapse behind the plane of its anulus.

Quantitation of tricuspid regurgitation relies heavily on color flow Doppler imaging. These standards have in large part been extrapolated from recommendations for quantification of mitral regurgitation. There are several anatomic findings in the presence of significant tricuspid regurgitation including right atrial and right ventricular dilation and detection of a right ventricular volume overload. Figure 12.33 was recorded in a patient with moderate tricuspid regurgitation in whom there is marked right heart enlargement, and a right ventricular volume overload is apparent when scanning in the parasternal short-axis view. Evidence of right heart dilation with a right

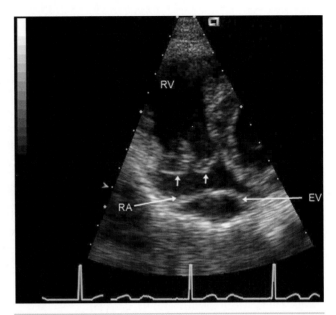

FIGURE 12.32. Transthoracic echocardiogram recorded in a patient with the Marfan syndrome. Note the myxomatous changes in the tricuspid valve with pronounced bileaflet prolapse (*small arrows*). Incidental note is made of a prominent eustachian valve (*EV*) as well. RA, right atrium; RV, right ventricle.

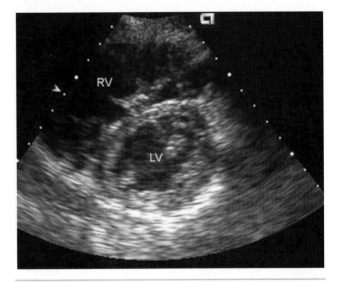

FIGURE 12.33. Parasternal short-axis view recorded in a patient with moderately severe tricuspid regurgitation. Note the secondary effects on the heart from the right-side volume overload, which include a dilated right ventricle and diastolic flattening of the ventricular septum consistent with a right ventricular volume overload. LV, left ventricle; RV, right ventricle.

ventricular volume overload is not specific for tricuspid regurgitation but can be noted in left-to-right atrial level shunts, pulmonary valve regurgitation, and anomalous pulmonary venous return as well. When due to tricuspid regurgitation, it implies at least moderate tricuspid regurgitation.

Color Doppler flow imaging is used to quantify tricuspid regurgitation in a manner analogous to that for the mitral valve. Because standards for determining the severity of tricuspid regurgitation are less robust than for mitral regurgitation, the algorithms for relating jet area to severity of tricuspid regurgitation are less well developed. In clinical practice, most echocardiography laboratories rely on a qualitative assessment of tricuspid regurgitation as being minimal (within normal limits), mild, moderate, or severe. Generally, the same thresholds of jet area, indexed to the right atrial area as used for mitral regurgitation, are used for tricuspid regurgitation. Figures 12.27, 12.29 through 12.31, 12.34, and 12.35 are examples of color flow Doppler imaging in tricuspid regurgitation demonstrating varying severity. The same limitations and cautions that were discussed with respect to color Doppler evaluation of mitral regurgitation also apply to the evaluation of tricuspid regurgitation.

An additional indirect marker of tricuspid regurgitation is dilation and systolic pulsation of the inferior vena cava. With persistent elevation of right heart pressure, the inferior vena cava will become dilated and lose its normal respiratory variation in size (Fig. 12.36). In some patients

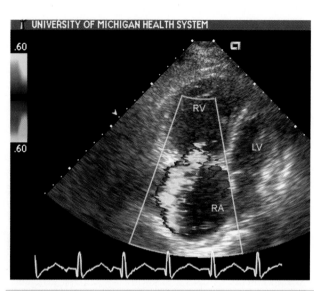

FIGURE 12.35. Apical four-chamber view recorded with color flow imaging revealing moderate tricuspid regurgitation with an eccentric jet. LV, left ventricle; RA, right atrium; RV, right ventricle.

with significant tricuspid regurgitation, systolic pulsations may be noted. Additionally, retrograde systolic flow can also be seen with either color flow or pulsed Doppler imaging in patients with significant tricuspid regurgitation (Fig. 12.37).

A final marker of tricuspid regurgitation that is infrequently used and has been largely replaced by color Doppler flow imaging is the use of contrast echocardiography. When agitated saline is injected into an arm vein, the contrast effect typically remains confined to the right atrium. Because non–contrast-enhanced blood is flowing into the atrium from the inferior vena cava, contrast is rarely present in the more inferior portion of the atrium and is not present in the inferior vena cava. Phasic (systolic) appearance of contrast in the inferior vena cava is another indirect marker of tricuspid regurgitation. As for other valve regurgitation, assessment of severity requires integrating multiple observations. Table 12.2 presents one recommended matrix for determining the severity of tricuspid regurgitation.

Determination of Right Ventricular Systolic Pressure

As noted in Chapter 8, the tricuspid regurgitation jet can be used to determine right ventricular systolic pressure. This is done by calculating the right ventricle to right atrial pressure gradient using the modified Bernoulli equation and then adding an assumed right atrial pressure. Figure 12.38 schematizes this approach, and Figure 12.39 is an example of this application. The relationship between the gradient determined by Doppler and the gra-

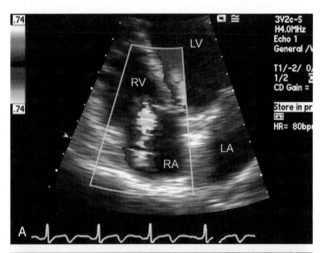

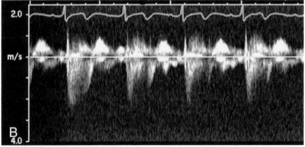

FIGURE 12.34. Apical four-chamber view recorded in a patient with mild to moderate tricuspid regurgitation. **A:** Note the color Doppler signal filling approximately 25% of the right atrium (*RA*). **B:** Note the holosystolic nature of the flow confirmed by spectral Doppler imaging. LA, left atrium; LV, left ventricle; RV, right ventricle.

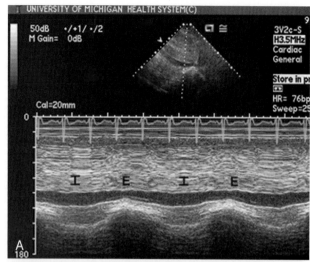

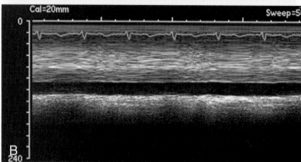

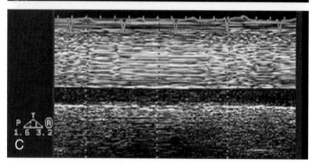

FIGURE 12.36. M-mode echocardiograms from the subcostal transducer position of the inferior vena cava (IVC). **A:** Recorded in a normal patient. Note the respiration-dependent phasic variation in IVC size. A normal IVC size but a loss of respiratory variation is shown **(B)**, and a dilated IVC also without respiratory variation **(C)**.

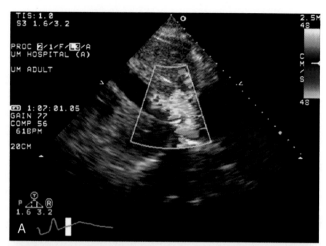

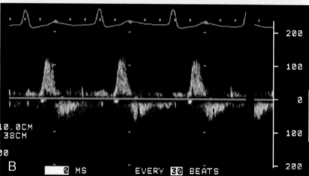

FIGURE 12.37. Subcostal echocardiogram recorded in a patient with severe tricuspid regurgitation. **A:** The color Doppler flow confirms retrograde flow into the inferior vena cava and hepatic veins in systole consistent with significant tricuspid regurgitation. **B:** A spectral Doppler recording from a hepatic vein, also confirming the systolic retrograde flow.

dient determined invasively in the catheterization laboratory has been demonstrated to be quite good. The major variable in determining the right ventricular systolic pressure is the method by which a right atrial pressure is either assumed or calculated. Multiple algorithms have been proposed, each of which has provided a relatively good correlation over a broad range of pulmonary artery pressures (Fig. 12.40). Some of the potential methods for determining right atrial pressure are listed in Table 12.3. Many laboratories use a floating constant of 5, 10, or 15 mm Hg, based on size of the right atrium and the severity

of tricuspid regurgitation. Using this qualitative approach, when tricuspid regurgitation is mild and the right atrial size is normal, an assumed right atrial pressure of 5 mm Hg is used. For moderate degrees of tricuspid regurgitation with mild or no right atrial enlargement, an assumed constant of 10 mm Hg can be used. If tricuspid regurgitation is severe and noted in the presence of a dilated right atrium, an assumed constant of 15 mm Hg can be used. An alternate approach is to use an assumed fixed constant in all patients. Typically, either 10 or 14 mm Hg has been used. Although this approach provides excellent correlation over a broad range of right ventricular systolic pressures, it will systematically overestimate the right ventricular systolic pressure in the low ranges and potentially underestimate it in the high ranges in which the right atrial pressure could exceed 20 mm Hg. Table 12.4 outlines one scheme used to determine right atrial pressure based on a combination of echocardiographic features. It should be emphasized that this is one of many proposed schemes, and multiple different algorithms can be used with similar success.

▶ TABLE 12.2 Echocardiographic and Doppler Parameters Used in Grading Tricuspid Regurgitation Severity

Parameter	Mild	Moderate	Severe
Tricuspid valve	Usually normal	Normal or abnormal	Abnormal/flail leaflet/poor coaptation
RV/RA/IVC size	Normal[a]	Normal or dilated	Usually dilated[b]
Jet area-central jets (cm^2)[c]	<5	5–10	>10
VC width (cm)[d]	Not defined	Not defined, but <0.7	>0.7
PISA radius (cm)[e]	≤0.5	0.6–0.9	>0.9
Jet density and contour CW	Soft and parabolic	Dense, variable contour	Dense, triangular with early peaking
Hepatic vein flow[f]	Systolic dominance	Systolic blunting	Systolic reversal

[a]Unless there are other reasons for right atrial or right ventricular dilation. Normal two-dimensional measurements from the apical four-chamber view: right ventricular mediolateral end-diastolic dimension: ≤4.3 cm, right ventricular end-diastolic area ≤35.5 cm^2; normal right atrial mediolateral and superoinferior dimensions: ≤4.6 cm and 4.9 cm, respectively, maximal RA volume ≤33 mL/m^2.

[b]The exception is acute tricuspid regurgitation.

[c]At a Nyquist limit of 50 to 60 cm/sec. Not valid in eccentric jets. Jet area is not recommended as the sole parameter of tricuspid regurgitation severity due to its dependence on hemodynamics and technical factors.

[d]At a Nyquist limit of 50 to 60 cm/sec.

[e]Baseline shift with Nyquist limit of 28 cm/sec.

[f]Other conditions may cause systolic blunting (e.g., atrial fibrillation, elevated right atrial pressure).

CW, continuous wave Doppler imaging; IVC, inferior vena cava; PISA, proximal isovelocity surface area; RA, right atrium; RV, right ventricle; VC, *vena contracta*.

Modified from Zoghbi WA, et al. Recommendations for evaluation of the severity of native valvular regurgitation with two-dimensional and Doppler echocardiography. J Am Soc Echocardiogr 2003;16:777–802, with permission.

ESTIMATION OF RIGHT VENTRICULAR PRESSURE

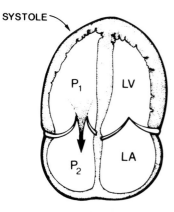

SYSTOLE

$$P_1 - P_2 = 4v^2$$

$$P_1 = 4v^2 + P^2$$

$$RVSP = 4v^2 + P_{RA}$$

v = Peak velocity of TR jet

P_{RA} = Jugular venous pulse

FIGURE 12.38. Schematic representation of the method by which right ventricular systolic pressure (*RVSP*) can be calculated from the tricuspid regurgitation jet velocity. Using the Bernoulli equation, the pressure gradient (Δ*P*) between the right ventricle and right atrium is calculated as noted. Solving the equation for RVSP requires adding an assumed right atrial (*RA*) pressure, which can be calculated using a variety of methods (see text for details). LA, left atrium; LV, left ventricle.

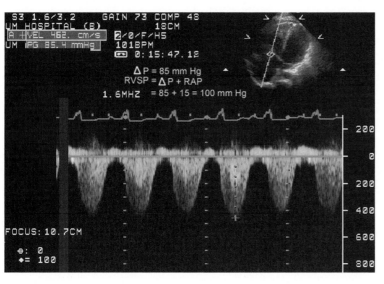

FIGURE 12.39. Demonstration of calculation of right ventricular systolic pressure (*RVSP*) from the continuous wave Doppler recording of tricuspid regurgitation in a patient with severe pulmonary hypertension. In this example, a right atrial pressure (*RAP*) of 15 mm Hg has been assumed based on the severity of tricuspid regurgitation, right atrial size, appearance of the inferior vena cava, and the tricuspid regurgitation jet velocity.

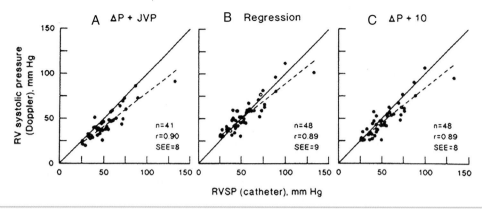

FIGURE 12.40. Doppler imaging– versus catheterization-derived right ventricular systolic pressures (RVSP). For each graph, the same ΔP has been used in combination with a different method for estimating right atrial pressure. **A:** Right atrial pressure has been estimated from the jugular venous pressure (*JVP*). An empiric constant of 10 mm Hg **(C)** and a regression equation **(B)** have been used. Note the relatively linear relationship of Doppler versus catheterization RVSP, irrespective of the method for calculating right atrial pressure. (From Currie PJ, et al. Continuous wave Doppler determination of right ventricular pressure: a simultaneous Doppler-catheterization study in 127 patients. J Am Coll Cardiol 1985;6:750–756, with permission.)

▶ **TABLE 12.3** **Methods for Determining Right Atrial Pressure**

Jugular vein height
Inferior vena caval appearance
   Dilated vs. normal
   Sniff plesmography
   Respiratory variation in size
Empiric constant value (i.e., 10 or 14 mm Hg)
Floating constant (5, 10, 15, 20 mm Hg)
Percentage constant (10% of ΔP)

ΔP, right ventricular–right atrial pressure gradient from the tricuspid regurgitation jet.

▶ **TABLE 12.4** **Estimation of Right Atrial Pressure**

RAP (mm Hg)	RA Size	TR	TR V_{max}	IVC
5	Normal	≤Mild	≤2.5 m/s	Normal
10	↑	Moderate	2.6–4 m/s	Dilated
15	↑↑	Severe	>4 m/s	Dilated, no respiratory variation

IVC, inferior vena cava; RA, right atrium; RAP, estimated right atrial pressure; TR, severity of tricuspid regurgitation; TR V_{max}, Doppler determined peak velocity of the tricuspid regurgitation jet.

MISCELLANEOUS CONDITIONS

Carcinoid Heart Disease

Carcinoid heart disease occurs when an endocrine-secreting tumor releases high levels of serotonin and its metabolites such as 5-hydroxytryptophan into the bloodstream. This results in an inflammatory reaction on the endothelial surface of valves and the endocardium, with a particular predilection to involve the tricuspid valve with lesser involvement of the pulmonary valve. The active metabolite is deactivated in the lungs. As such, pulmonary vein blood does not contain the active metabolites, thus sparing the left-side heart structures. There are two exceptions in which the left-side valves can be involved as well. If a left-to-right shunt exists so that the active compound is not deactivated in the pulmonary bed, then left-sided involvement can occur. Similarly, if pulmonary metastases have occurred, then there will be direct release of metabolically active metabolites into the left-side bloodstream and the mitral and aortic valves may be involved as well.

Figure 12.41 is an example of carcinoid heart disease in which the tricuspid valve has been heavily involved. Typically, the entire length of the leaflets are involved and have a rigid stiffened appearance. There is some retraction of overall leaflet length resulting in failure of coaptation and tricuspid regurgitation on this basis, resulting in noncoaptation of the leaflets. Typically, pulmonary hypertension is not present, and thus the tricuspid regurgitation jet occurs at a relatively low velocity.

Endocardial Fibroelastosis

Endocardial fibrosis can occur due to a variety of diseases including the hypereosinophilia syndrome and tropical forms of endocardial fibroelastosis. The underlying pathology is a marked inflammatory response in the endocardium that extends to the chordae and subsequently interferes with normal valve coaptation. Typically, the leaflets will appear to be restricted and bound down toward the ventricular wall. This is often seen in association

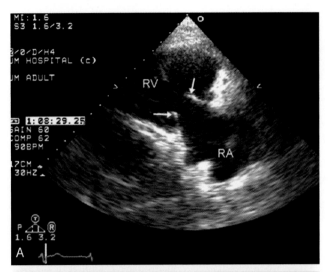

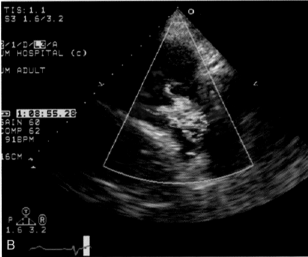

FIGURE 12.41. Transthoracic echocardiogram recorded in a patient with carcinoid syndrome and tricuspid valve involvement. **A:** A right ventricular inflow tract view reveals diffusely thickened and immobile tricuspid valve leaflets (*arrows*). This image was recorded in early systole. Note the complete failure of coaptation of the leaflets, which results in severe tricuspid regurgitation, confirmed in an apical four-chamber view with color flow Doppler imaging **(B)**. In the real-time image, note that the tricuspid leaflets lack mobility along their entire length, which is classic for carcinoid involvement. RA, right atrium; RV, right ventricle.

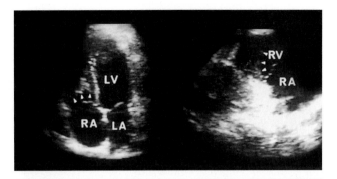

FIGURE 12.42. Echocardiogram recorded in a patient with a hypereosinophilic syndrome and involvement of the right ventricle (*RV*) and tricuspid valve. An apical four chamber view is presented on the left and a right ventricular inflow view on the right. Note the involvement and obliteration of the right ventricular apex (*arrowheads*). LA, left atrium; LV, left ventricle; RA, right atrium. (From Presti C, Ryan T, and Armstrong WF. Two-dimensional and Doppler echocardiographic findings in hypereosinophilic syndrome. Am Heart J 114:173, 1987.)

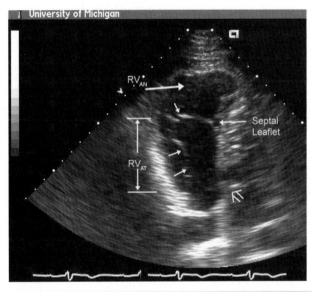

FIGURE 12.43. Apical view recorded in a patient with the Ebstein anomaly of the tricuspid valve. Note the marked distortion of right ventricular and right atrial geometry. The approximate position of the mitral anulus is noted by the *broad arrow* at the lower right. Note that the septal leaflet of the tricuspid valve is apically displaced from the anulus by approximately 3 cm and that the lateral leaflet is tethered to the right ventricular wall along much of its length (*small arrows*). It is also pathologically elongated. The tricuspid valve closes at a markedly apical position, resulting in a small anatomic right ventricle (RV_{AN}) and a larger atrialized portion of the right ventricle (RV_{AT}).

with obliteration of the right ventricular apex due to inflammatory tissue and secondary thrombosis. Figure 12.42 was recorded in a patient with hypereosinophilia and obliteration of the right ventricular apex with restriction and involvement of the tricuspid chordae.

Ebstein Anomaly

Ebstein anomaly is a congenital abnormality of the tricuspid valve in which there is apical displacement of the septal leaflet and tethering of the lateral leaflet to the ventricular wall. This results in atrialization of a portion of the right ventricle. Tricuspid regurgitation is invariably present. Figures 12.43 and 12.44 are examples of patients with Ebstein anomaly. This entity is discussed further in Chapter 18.

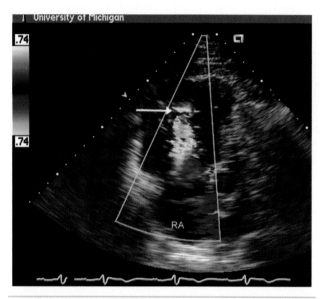

FIGURE 12.44. Color Doppler image recorded in a patient with the Ebstein anomaly of the tricuspid valve. Note the presence of significant tricuspid regurgitation with a convergence zone and *vena contracta* present near the apex (*arrow*). On occasion, in marginal quality studies, noting the abnormal origin of the tricuspid regurgitation jet may be an early valuable clue to the presence of the Ebstein anomaly. RA, right atrium.

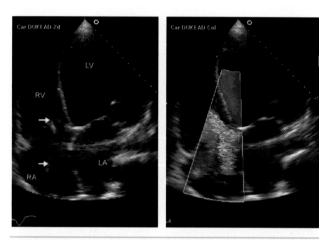

FIGURE 12.45. Transthoracic echocardiogram recorded in a patient with a chronic ventricular pacemaker (*arrows*). In this instance, the pacemaker wire has restricted motion of the tricuspid valve and resulted in moderate tricuspid regurgitation. LA, left atrium; LV, left ventricle; RA, right atrium; RV, right ventricle.

Pacemakers and Catheters

On occasion, a transvenous pacemaker wire or catheter interferes with tricuspid valve function. The stiffer, larger diameter leads used for implantable defibrillators may interrupt normal coaptation to a greater degree. Typically, because of the redundancy of the tricuspid valve, coaptation occurs around catheters or pacemaker wires and does not result in significant tricuspid regurgitation. On rare occasions, placement of a catheter can be such that normal coaptation is prevented and variable degrees of tricuspid regurgitation ensue. More chronically, fibrosis of a leaflet can occur due to contact with a catheter, resulting in regurgitation as well. Figure 12.45 is an example of a pacemaker catheter traversing the right ventricular inflow tract, resulting in moderate tricuspid regurgitation.

Tricuspid Valve Resection

As a treatment for bacterial endocarditis, a number of patients in the late 1970s and early 1980s underwent removal of a tricuspid valve leaflet. This obviously results in free tricuspid regurgitation. Many of these patients have presented 15 to 20 years later with evidence of significant right heart failure. Figure 12.46 was recorded in a patient who had undergone resection of a tricuspid valve leaflet for bacterial endocarditis approximately 15 years before this echocardiogram. Note the absence of any tricuspid valve tissue. By definition, wide-open tricuspid regurgitation is present. Because of the complete absence of tricuspid valve tissue, there is no organized flow from the right ventricle to the right atrium and no increase in velocity or organized jet. This results in the absence of a convergence zone, which is usually seen with organized regurgitant flow, and in low velocities of the regurgitant jet (Fig. 12.46). On occasion, this entity is encountered, and because of the absence of typical findings of regurgitation, the severity of tricuspid regurgitation is not appreciated. Recognition of the marked dilation of the right heart and absence of tricuspid valve tissue should alert the sonographer and clinician to the presence of this situation.

Cardiac Biopsy

In patients who have undergone cardiac transplantation, repeated right ventricular myocardial biopsy often results in significant tricuspid regurgitation. This is presumably due to trauma to the tricuspid valve and/or chordae tendineae. Typically, other features of a post-transplantation heart are noted including biatrial enlargement and prominent suture lines. Figure 12.47 was recorded in a patient 3 years status postcardiac transplantation who had undergone numerous endomyocardial biopsies. Note the moderate tricuspid regurgitation and the apparent mild thickening of the tricuspid valve leaflets.

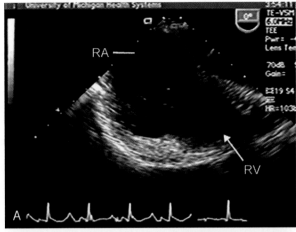

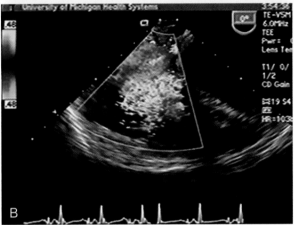

FIGURE 12.46. Transesophageal echocardiogram recorded in a horizontal view from behind the left atrium in a patient who previously had undergone resection of a tricuspid leaflet for bacterial endocarditis. **A:** Note the marked dilation of the right atrium (*RA*) and right ventricle (*RV*) and the absence of visible tricuspid valve tissue. **B:** In the color Doppler image, note the free tricuspid regurgitation with the absence of any organized jet. On occasion, the absence of a true jet with a *vena contracta* and convergence zone may result in the true severity of the tricuspid regurgitation not being appreciated.

Tumors and Other Masses

Rarely, a primary tumor can arise on the tricuspid valve. Tumors that have been reported on the tricuspid valve have included very infrequent myxomas and occasional fibroelastoma. When present, they have the same appearance as these atypical tumors do on the mitral valve.

Ischemic Heart Disease

Both right ventricle and papillary muscle apparatus can become involved secondary to ischemic heart disease. Tricuspid regurgitation is the usual sequela.

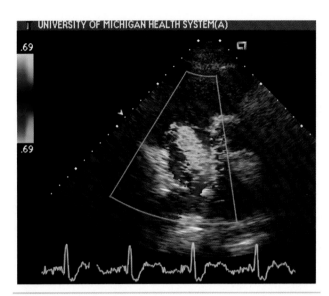

FIGURE 12.47. Parasternal short-axis view recorded in a patient several years after cardiac transplantation. As a consequence of multiple transvenous right ventricular biopsies, there has been trauma to the tricuspid valve apparatus, which has resulted in moderate tricuspid regurgitation

SUGGESTED READINGS

ACC/AHA guidelines for the management of patients with valvular heart disease. A report of the American College of Cardiology/American Heart Association. Task Force on Practice Guidelines (Committee on Management of Patients with Valvular Heart Disease). J Am Coll Cardiol 1998;32:1486–1588.

Aessopos A, Farmakis D, Taktikou H, et al. Doppler-determined peak systolic tricuspid pressure gradient in persons with normal pulmonary function and tricuspid regurgitation. J Am Soc Echocardiogr 2000;13:645–649.

Bossone E, Rubenfire M, Bach DS, et al. Range of tricuspid regurgitation velocity at rest and during exercise in normal adult men: implications for the diagnosis of pulmonary hypertension. J Am Coll Cardiol 1999;33:1662–1666.

Chan KL, Currie PJ, Seward JB, et al. Comparison of three Doppler ultrasound methods in the prediction of pulmonary artery pressure. J Am Coll Cardiol 1987;9:549–554.

Chopra HK, Nanda NC, Fan P, et al. Can two-dimensional echocardiography and Doppler color flow mapping identify the need for tricuspid valve repair? J Am Coll Cardiol 1989;14:1266–1274.

Currie PJ, Seward JB, Chan KL, et al. Continuous wave Doppler determination of right ventricular pressure: a simultaneous Doppler-catheterization study in 127 patients. J Am Coll Cardiol 1985;6:750–756.

Dabestani A, Mahan G, Gardin JM, et al. Evaluation of pulmonary artery pressure and resistance by pulsed Doppler echocardiography. Am J Cardiol 1987;59:662–668.

Dib JC, Abergel E, Rovani C, et al. The age of the patient should be taken into account when interpreting Doppler assessed pulmonary artery pressures. J Am Soc Echocardiogr 1997;10:72–73.

Ehrsam RE, Perruchoud A, Oberholzer M, et al. Influence of age on pulmonary haemodynamics at rest and during supine exercise. Clin Sci (Lond) 1983;65:653–660.

Graettinger WF, Greene ER, Voyles WF. Doppler predictions of pulmonary artery pressure, flow, and resistance in adults. Am Heart J 1987;113:1426–1437.

Herrera CJ, Mehlman DJ, Hartz RS, et al. Comparison of transesophageal and transthoracic echocardiography for diagnosis of right-sided cardiac lesions. Am J Cardiol 1992;70:964–966.

Himelman RB, Schiller NB. Clinical and echocardiographic comparison of patients with the carcinoid syndrome with and without carcinoid heart disease. Am J Cardiol 1989;63:347–352.

McQuillan BM, Picard MH, Leavitt M, et al. Clinical correlates and reference intervals for pulmonary artery systolic pressure among echocardiographically normal subjects. Circulation 2001;104:2797–2802.

Pellikka PA, Tajik AJ, Khandheria BK, et al. Carcinoid heart disease. Clinical and echocardiographic spectrum in 74 patients. Circulation 1993;87:1188–1196.

Robiolio PA, Rigolin VH, Wilson JS, et al. Carcinoid heart disease. Correlation of high serotonin levels with valvular abnormalities detected by cardiac catheterization and echocardiography. Circulation 1995;92:790–795.

Tribouilloy CM, Enriquez-Sarano M, Bailey KR, et al. Quantification of tricuspid regurgitation by measuring the width of the vena contracta with Doppler color flow imaging: a clinical study. J Am Coll Cardiol 2000;36:472–478.

Weyman AE. Pulmonary valve echo motion in clinical practice. Am J Med 1977;62:843–855.

Weyman AE, Hurwitz RA, Girod DA, et al. Cross-sectional echocardiographic visualization of the stenotic pulmonary valve. Circulation 1977;56:769–774.

Zoghbi WA, Enriquez-Sarano M, Foster E, et al. Recommendations for evaluation of the severity of native valvular regurgitation with two-dimensional and Doppler echocardiography. J Am Soc Echocardiogr 2003;16:777–802.

Infective Endocarditis

Despite advances in antibiotic therapy and surgical options, infective endocarditis remains a challenging and often fatal condition. One reason for this is the difficulty of establishing an accurate diagnosis, particularly early in the course of the disease when proper management can be lifesaving. As therapeutic approaches have become more successful, the importance of early and accurate diagnosis is self-evident. Unfortunately, no single test or finding establishes the diagnosis in all cases. Instead, a constellation of findings that constitutes the diagnostic criteria continue to evolve.

The central role that echocardiography plays in the diagnosis of endocarditis began in the early 1970s with the echocardiographic demonstration of a valvular vegetation by the M-mode technique. With the advent of two-dimensional and Doppler modalities, echocardiography has become virtually indispensable in the diagnosis and management of these patients. Today, echocardiographic findings are a central part of the diagnostic criteria for infective endocarditis.

CLINICAL PERSPECTIVE

Infective endocarditis is defined as a localized infection anywhere on the endocardium, including the chamber walls, vessels, and within congenital defects. The vast majority of vegetations, however, occur on valve leaflets. Infection may also develop on any implanted or prosthetic material such as prosthetic valves, conduits, pacing electrodes, and catheters. In recent years, the importance of intracardiac devices as a risk factor for the development of endocarditis has increased. As the proliferation of such devices increases, especially in older and sicker patients, the incidence of infection in this setting will further rise. The process of developing endocarditis occurs in the setting of bacteremia or fungemia. The initiating event usually requires the presence of a high-velocity jet, which may be due to a congenital anomaly such as a ventricular septal defect, a regurgitant valve, or a prosthetic valve. It

is thought that the jet interferes with the protective endothelial surface, allowing the blood-borne pathogens to adhere and coalesce. As the nidus of infection organizes, masses of microorganisms attract platelets, fibrin, and other material and become adherent to the endothelial surface to form a vegetation. The vegetation will grow in size, either as a sessile clump or a highly mobile and even pedunculated mass with the potential for embolization. As the hallmark of endocarditis, the ability to detect the vegetation is the focal point of diagnosis. This sequence of events offers a mechanism for development of endocarditis in patients with underlying heart disease. However, since as many as 50% of patients who get endocarditis do not have lesions associated with a high-velocity jet, some other set of conditions must be operational in these patients to explain the link between bacteremia and cardiac involvement.

Thus, the classic approach to the diagnosis of endocarditis, developed by von Reyn and colleagues in the early 1980s, focused on pathologic evidence of infection within the heart and relied heavily on the presence of positive blood cultures for an appropriate organism in association with clinical evidence suggesting endocarditis (Table 13.1). This initial series included 123 cases diagnosed using strict clinical criteria (von Reyn et al, 1981). The von Reyn criteria quickly became the standard by which the diagnosis of endocarditis was established. Because "probable" endocarditis required confirmatory clinical evidence, early or less severe forms of the disease were not included. Importantly, the von Reyn definitions did not include echocardiographic findings as part of the criteria.

ECHOCARDIOGRAPHIC CHARACTERISTICS OF A VEGETATION

The versatility of echocardiography in the evaluation of endocarditis is illustrated in Table 13.2. Among its important functions is the identification of underlying heart dis-

▶ TABLE 13.1 von Reyn Criteria for Establishing a Diagnosis of Infective Endocarditis

Definite
Direct evidence based on histology from surgery or autopsy or on bacteriology of valvular vegetation or peripheral embolus
Probable
A. Persistently positive blood cultures plus one of the following:
   1. New regurgitant murmur
   2. Predisposing heart disease and vascular phenomena
B. Negative or intermittently positive blood cultures plus all 3 of the following:
   1. Fever
   2. New regurgitant murmur
   3. Vascular phenomena
Possible
A. Persistently positive blood cultures plus one of the following:
   1. Predisposing heart disease
   2. Vascular phenomena
B. Negative or intermittently positive blood cultures plus all three of the following:
   1. Fever
   2. Predisposing heart disease
   3. Vascular phenomena
C. For *Streptococcus viridans* cases only: at least two positive blood cultures without an extracardiac source, and fever
Rejected
A. Endocarditis unlikely, alternate diagnosis generally apparent
B. Endocarditis likely, empiric antibiotic therapy warranted
C. Culture negative endocarditis diagnosed clinically, but excluded by postmortem

Adapted from von Reyn CF, Levy BS, Arbeit RD, et al. Infective endocarditis: an analysis based on strict case definitions. Ann Intern Med 1981;194:505–518, with permission.

▶ TABLE 13.2 Role of Echocardiography in Patients with Endocarditis

Identifies predisposing heart disease
Pivotal role in diagnosis
Detects complications
Assesses hemodynamic consequences
Serial evaluation (assesses efficacy of therapy)
Prognosis (risk of complications)

▶ TABLE 13.3 Echocardiographic Criteria for Defining a Vegetation

Positive Feature	Negative Feature
Low reflectance	High echogenicity
Attached to valve, upstream side	Nonvalvular location
Irregular shape, amorphous	Smooth surface or fibrillar
Mobile, oscillating	Nonmobile
Associated tissue changes, valvular regurgitation	Absence of regurgitation

the valve, i.e., the ventricular side of the aortic valve and the atrial side of the mitral valve (Fig. 13.1). They may be sessile or pedunculated but usually have motion that is independent of the valve itself. Because they often occur in the path of a high-velocity jet, their motion is frequently described as oscillating or fluttering. The presence of sig-

ease known to increase a patient's risk of infection. Although the absence of underlying disease does not confer protection against endocarditis, particular conditions, such as congenital heart disease and a myxomatous mitral valve, are known risk factors. At the same time, these conditions often confound the diagnosis of endocarditis by creating abnormalities that mimic or conceal echocardiographic evidence of infection.

An essential first step in the echocardiographic evaluation is to search for evidence of acute ongoing infection. Although there are several manifestations of endocarditis, including abscesses and fistulae, the most common and direct evidence of infective endocarditis is the vegetation. Because a vegetation begins as a microscopic focus of infection and gradually grows into a conspicuous mass, its presence may or may not be evident on an imaging study. Thus, echocardiography must be sensitive enough to detect the vegetation and specific enough to distinguish it from other echocardiographic abnormalities or artifacts. A vegetation is typically an irregularly shaped, highly mobile mass attached to the free edge of a valve leaflet (Table 13.3). Vegetations tend to develop on the upstream side of

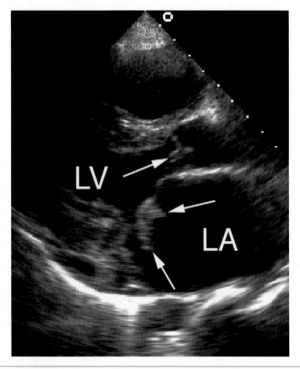

FIGURE 13.1. An example of vegetations involving the mitral and aortic valves is shown. The vegetations are indicated by the *arrows*. LA, left atrium; LV, left ventricle.

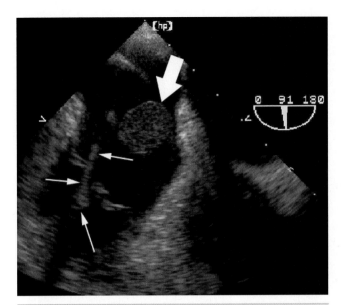

FIGURE 13.2. Transesophageal echocardiography shows a large mass (*large arrow*) attached to a pacemaker lead (*small arrows*) in the right atrium. This mass most likely represents an infected thrombus.

Although typically attached to a valve, vegetations may also attach to chordae, chamber walls, or any foreign body, such as a pacemaker lead, indwelling catheter, and prosthetic valve sewing ring (Fig. 13.2). The mass itself is typically homogeneous with echogenicity similar to that of the myocardium. However, vegetations can occasionally be cystic or appear more dense and calcified. The infectious process often alters valve structure and function. As a result, some degree of regurgitation is associated with most cases of acute endocarditis. In Figure 13.3, a patient with a mitral valve vegetation is shown. The involvement is extensive, and the valve appears partially flail. There is severe mitral regurgitation. A patient with significant aortic regurgitation associated with an aortic valve vegetation is shown in Figure 13.4. Although the vegetation does not appear to be large, its effect on valve function is evident. If the process results in destruction of underlying tissue leading to a flail or perforated valve structure, the degree of regurgitation will be severe. For example, if the infection leads to mitral chordal rupture, severe mitral regurgitation will ensue. This is demonstrated in Figure 13.5, taken from a patient with a flail mitral valve in the setting of staphylococcal endocarditis. Figure 13.6 is an example of a small perforation of the noncoronary cusp of the aortic valve due to infection. Mild aortic regurgitation was present, but no definite vegetation was identified. Much less often, a large vegetation will obstruct the valve orifice, leading to a functional form of valve stenosis (Fig. 13.7). Although most vegetations involve the valves, in severe cases the infection may extend to other structures, such as the wall of the chambers. An example of this is shown in Figure 13.8. In this case, the vegetation adhered to the wall of the left atrium and the posterior mitral valve anulus.

nificant mobility, or oscillating motion, is a typical feature of most vegetations. In fact, the absence of mobility argues against the diagnosis and should suggest the possibility of an alternative diagnosis. The shape and size of vegetations are quite variable and may either increase (due to progression of disease) or decrease (due to healing or embolization) over time. Fungal vegetations tend to be larger than those caused by bacterial infections, and those involving the tricuspid valve tend to be larger compared with vegetations that affect the aortic or mitral valve.

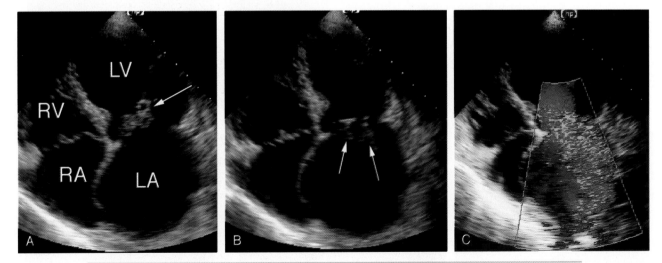

FIGURE 13.3. A large vegetation involving the anterior mitral leaflet is shown. **A:** The size and location of the mass is evident (*arrow*). **B:** During systole, the vegetation can be seen on the left atrial side of the mitral valve (*arrows*). **C:** Color Doppler imaging reveals severe mitral regurgitation. LA, left atrium; LV, left ventricle; RA, right atrium; RV, right ventricle.

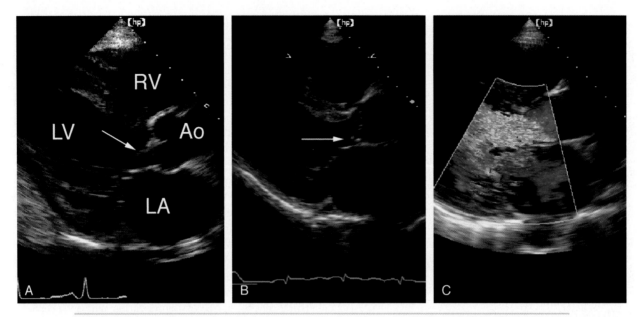

FIGURE 13.4. A small aortic valve vegetation (*arrow*) is shown during diastole **(A)** and systole **(B)**. **C:** Color Doppler demonstrates severe aortic regurgitation. Ao, aorta; LA, left atrium; LV, left ventricle; RV, right ventricle.

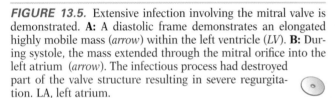

FIGURE 13.5. Extensive infection involving the mitral valve is demonstrated. **A:** A diastolic frame demonstrates an elongated highly mobile mass (*arrow*) within the left ventricle (*LV*). **B:** During systole, the mass extended through the mitral orifice into the left atrium (*arrow*). The infectious process had destroyed part of the valve structure resulting in severe regurgitation. LA, left atrium.

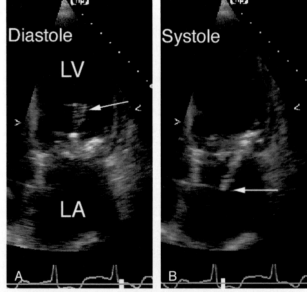

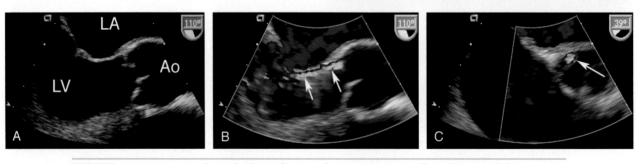

FIGURE 13.6. A transesophageal echocardiogram demonstrates a small perforation of the noncoronary cusp of the aortic valve. **A:** Focal thickening is seen but no definite vegetation. **B:** Color Doppler imaging demonstrates the jet extending through the cusp (*arrows*). **C:** A short-axis view confirms the location of the perforation (*arrow*). Ao, aorta; LV, left ventricle; LA, left atrium.

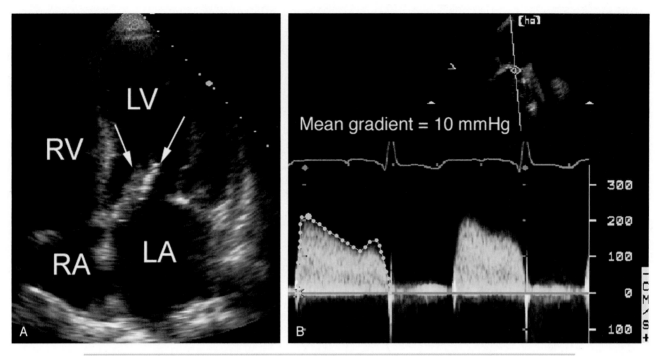

FIGURE 13.7. A: A large vegetation involving the anterior mitral leaflet is demonstrated (*arrows*). **B:** Spectral Doppler imaging recorded a 10 mm Hg mean gradient across the mitral valve. LA, left atrium; LV, left ventricle; RA, right atrium; RV, right ventricle.

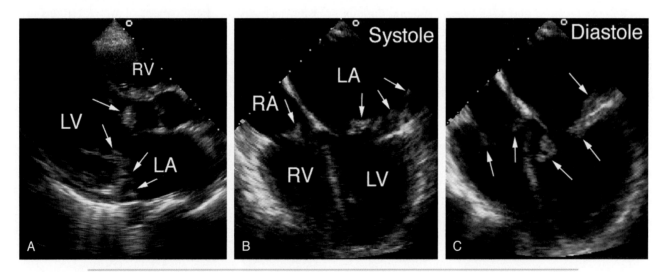

FIGURE 13.8. A: The *arrows* indicate multiple masses within the left ventricle (*LV*) and left atrium (*LA*), consistent with vegetations. Transesophageal echocardiography confirmed these findings and also revealed involvement of the tricuspid valve (*arrows*). **B:** Note the location of the mass within the left atrium, extending from the base of the mitral leaflet along the wall of the left atrium (*arrows*). **C:** A diastolic frame demonstrates the highly mobile nature of the vegetations (*arrows*). RA, right atrium; RV, right ventricle.

It should be emphasized that there is no single characteristic on the echocardiogram that will conclusively identify a mass as a vegetation. The ability to detect a vegetation, when one is present, depends on several factors including vegetation size, location, the presence of underlying heart disease, image quality, and instrument settings. All available echocardiographic windows should be used, and Doppler flow mapping should be performed to identify any associated valvular regurgitation. Although masses as small as 2 mm have been reported, in most cases, a vegetation must be at least 3 to 6 mm in size to be reliably seen. Image quality will also influence our ability to visualize small structures. As is discussed later, these are areas in which the advantages of transesophageal echocardiography have been demonstrated.

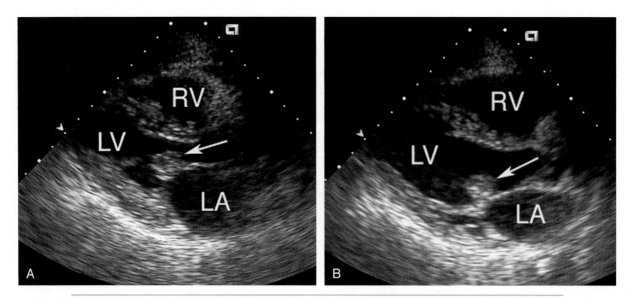

FIGURE 13.9. An example of a blood cyst (arrow) is demonstrated within the mitral valve. Diastolic **(A)** and systolic **(B)** frames are shown. Such an appearance could easily be confused with vegetation. LA, left atrium; LV, left ventricle; RV, right ventricle.

To avoid false-positive results, vegetations must be differentiated from other echo-producing abnormalities, such as myxomatous processes, degenerative changes (including Lambl's excrescences and calcification), tumors, thrombi, and imaging artifacts. Figure 13.9 is taken from a patient who was asymptomatic. The large mitral valve mass could easily be mistaken for a vegetation. However, the absence of clinical signs of infection suggests an alternative diagnosis. In this case, the mass was a blood cyst. Underlying heart disease both obscures the presence of a vegetation

and increases the likelihood of false-positive findings through misinterpretation (Fig. 13.10). Thus, the accuracy of echocardiography is greater in patients without underlying valve disease. Furthermore, active vegetations must be differentiated from old or healed vegetations. Some studies have suggested that vegetations tend to become smaller and more circumscribed and echogenic over time as part of the healing process. Although this is generally true, a reduction in vegetation size might also suggest embolization. Thus, distinguishing active from healed vegeta-

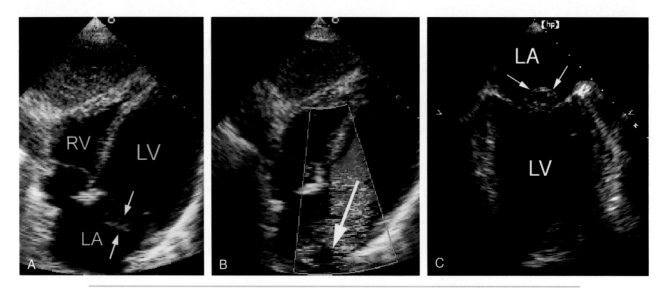

FIGURE 13.10. This echocardiogram was recorded from a patient with mitral valve prolapse and significant mitral regurgitation. The mitral valve was myxomatous and partially flail. **A:** The prolapsing valve is indicated by the *arrows*. **B:** Severe mitral regurgitation is demonstrated (*arrow*). **C:** A transesophageal echocardiogram demonstrates the prolapsing scallop (*arrows*). This could easily be mistaken for a vegetation. LA, left atrium; LV, left ventricle; RV, right ventricle.

tions can never rely on echocardiography alone but must take into account clinical factors.

DIAGNOSTIC ACCURACY OF ECHOCARDIOGRAPHY

Over the past 30 years, numerous clinical studies have been performed to test the accuracy of echocardiography to detect vegetations and other manifestations of acute endocarditis. A limitation of all these studies is the difficulty in defining the standard by which the diagnosis is established. In most series, a clinical standard for diagnosis was used that incorporated clinical findings, blood culture results, response to therapy, and outcome measures. Although practical, this approach has obvious limitations and very likely permitted the inclusion of some patients who had bacteremia but never had endocarditis. More rigorous diagnostic standards that required pathologic and/or surgical confirmation must, by definition, exclude patients who have endocarditis but never come to either surgery or autopsy. As a result, only the "sickest of the sick" would be included in such series. Finally, the recognition over time of the fundamental involvement of echocardiography in establishing a diagnosis made it increasingly difficult to "test the test." That is, it becomes impossible to establish the accuracy of a test (in this case, echocardiography) that is fundamentally involved in the definition of disease. For all these reasons, the exact sensitivity and specificity of the various echocardiographic techniques must be interpreted in context. Despite these limitations, the overall utility of echocardiography as an integral part of the diagnostic algorithm is well established.

A summary of the studies examining transthoracic echocardiography for the diagnosis of endocarditis is presented in Table 13.4. The sensitivity of the transthoracic technique to detect vegetations is approximately 60% to 70%. Size and image quality are clear determinants of the ability of echocardiography to detect a vegetation when one is present. Using the transthoracic approach, sensitivity for the detection of endocarditis in patients with prosthetic valves is significantly lower, as is discussed later. It should be recognized that some patients with endocarditis may not have vegetations, thereby accounting for some false-negative results. Establishing the specificity of the technique is more difficult. Although the reported false-positive rate is quite low in most series, specificity will vary widely depending on the population being studied. As previously discussed, distinguishing active vegetations from healed vegetations, myxomatous change, or tumors in the absence of clinical information is nearly impossible. In most cases, echocardiography is interpreted in context, thereby avoiding most false-positive results.

Beginning in the mid-1980s, the potential advantages of transesophageal echocardiography in assessing pa-

▶ **TABLE 13.4** Diagnostic Accuracy of Echocardiography for Detecting Endocarditis

| | | Sensitivity (%) | |
Reference	N	TTE	TEE
Erbel et al., 1988	166	63	100
Mugge et al., 1989	91	58	90
Shively et al., 1991	66	44	94
Birmingham et al., 1992	63	30	88
Shapiro et al., 1994	64	68	91
Lowry et al., 1994	93	36	93
Werner et al., 1996	104	60	93

TEE, transesophageal echocardiography; TTE, transthoracic echocardiography

tients with suspected endocarditis were first recognized. As is apparent in Table 13.4, the sensitivity of transesophageal echocardiography is consistently higher than that of the transthoracic technique. The improved image quality and the closer proximity between transducer and valves account for much of this difference. Smaller vegetations, those associated with prosthetic valves, and those in locations that would be shadowed or obscured during transthoracic scanning are some of the areas in which the transesophageal approach is superior.

When the two echocardiographic techniques are compared in the same patient population, the superior sensitivity of transesophageal imaging has been a consistent finding (Fig. 13.11). At the same time, many of these contemporary series have reported a sensitivity of transthoracic echocardiography that is lower than would be oth-

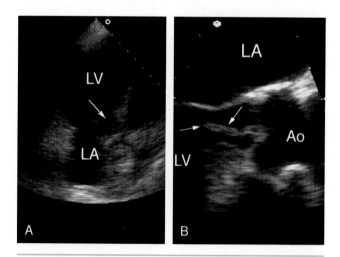

FIGURE 13.11. This aortic valve vegetation was not detected on transthoracic imaging **(A)**. The *arrow* points toward the aortic valve, but the mass was not visualized. **B:** The transesophageal echocardiogram clearly demonstrates the vegetation. Ao, aorta; LA, left atrium; LV, left ventricle.

erwise expected. This may be partly explained by the mere availability of transesophageal imaging. If the transthoracic examination is approached with less determination and rigor, small lesions may be missed, thereby contributing to the wide difference in sensitivity between the two tests. Although the superiority of the transesophageal approach is beyond question, the magnitude of the difference (i.e., the surprisingly low sensitivity of transthoracic echocardiography) is noteworthy. Some of this may be explained based on patient selection that included a greater percentage of individuals with a relatively low pretest likelihood of disease. Alternatively, the availability of transesophageal echocardiography may have indirectly contributed to the performance of a more cursory and less rigorous transthoracic study, followed by a thorough and complete transesophageal examination.

An additional advantage of transesophageal echocardiography lies in its ability to identify other manifestations of endocarditis, such as ring abscesses and fistulae (Fig. 13.12). Despite the relatively modest sensitivity of transthoracic echocardiography, a normal study in the presence of excellent image quality is strong evidence against endocarditis.

EVOLUTION OF THE DIAGNOSTIC CRITERIA

The clinical diagnosis of infective endocarditis has always been challenging. Before the routine use of echocardiography, establishing the diagnosis of endocarditis focused on evidence of ongoing infection within the blood coupled with clinical evidence of cardiac involvement. In 1994, the Duke Endocarditis Service published new criteria for the diagnosis of endocarditis that relied heavily on echocardiographic findings. In this original study, 405 cases were retrospectively reviewed and classified as either definite, possible, or rejected based on the presence or absence of major and minor criteria (Table 13.5). When compared with previously used criteria, the newly proposed Duke criteria classified significantly more cases as definite endocarditis. Among pathologically proven cases, the Duke criteria were significantly more sensitive (80%) compared with the von Reyn criteria (51%) (Table 13.6).

Since this original report, the higher sensitivity of the Duke criteria has been validated in multiple series involving diverse patient groups. In one study (Habib et al., 1999) that compared the two diagnostic approaches in 93 consecutive pathologically proven cases, the sensitivity of the Duke criteria was 76% compared with 56% for the von Reyn criteria. Most of the false-negative results were due

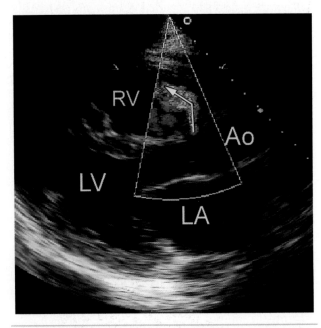

FIGURE 13.12. A fistula between the left ventricular outflow tract and the right ventricle (*RV*) (*arrow*) is demonstrated from this transthoracic echocardiogram using color Doppler imaging. This developed as a complication of an aortic ring abscess. Ao, aorta; LA, left atrium; LV, left ventricle.

▶ **TABLE 13.5 Duke Criteria for Diagnosing Endocarditis**

Major criteria
Two or more separate positive blood cultures, appropriate organisms[a]
Positive echocardiographic findings: oscillating mass, abscess, prosthetic valve dehiscence
New valvular regurgitation
Minor criteria
Predisposing factors (underlying heart disease or intravenous drug use)
Fever
Vascular phenomena
Immunologic phenomena
Microbiologic evidence

Definite infective endocarditis: two major + one minor, or three minor criteria

Possible infective endocarditis: one major + one minor, or findings consistent with infective endocarditis, but neither definite nor rejected

Recent modifications of the criteria
1. Possible endocarditis defined as:
   one major + one minor criterion; or
   three minor criteria
2. New major criteria:
   Positive Q-fever serology
   Staphylococcus aureus bacteremia
      Whether community-acquired or nosocomial
      Regardless of whether source of bacteremia is apparent
3. Eliminates echocardiographic minor criteria

[a]For example, *Streptococcus viridans, Streptococcus bovis, Staphylococcus aureus, Enterococcus* species, HACEK.
From Durack DT, Lukes AS, Bright DK. New criteria for diagnosis of infective endocarditis: utilization of specific echocardiographic findings. Am J Med 1994;96:200–209 and Li JS, Sexton DJ, Mide N, et al. Proposed modifications to the Duke criteria for the diagnosis of infective endocarditis. Clin Infect Dis 2000;30:633–638, with permission.

▶ **TABLE 13.6** Comparison of von Reyn and Duke Criteria for Diagnosing Endocarditis

Duke Definitions	von Reyn Definitions			
	Probable	**Possible**	**Rejected**	**Total**
Definite	65	59	11	40%
Possible	6	56	87	44%
Rejected	0	0	52	15%
Total	21%	34%	45%	100%

From Durack DT, Lukes AS, Bright DK. New criteria for diagnosis of infective endocarditis: utilization of specific echocardiographic findings. Am J Med 1994;96:200–209, with permission.

▶ **TABLE 13.7** Complications of Endocarditis

Structural	Hemodynamic
Leaflet rupture	Acute valvular regurgitation
Flail leaflet	Valve obstruction
Leaflet perforation	Heart failure
Abscess	Intracardiac shunt
Aneurysm	Tamponade
Fistula	Perivalvular regurgitation
Prosthetic valve dehiscence	
Embolization	
Pericardial effusion	

to negative blood cultures. These were attributed to either previous antibiotic therapy or Q-fever endocarditis. The subsequent revision of the Duke criteria to include Q-fever serology as a major criterion has addressed the latter issue. However, the widespread use of antibiotics in the community remains a source of false-negative blood cultures and will therefore continue to be a challenge in the diagnosis of endocarditis. The enhancement in sensitivity provided by the Duke criteria is achieved without a significant loss in specificity. Although more difficult to test, most series have concluded that specificity is maintained and has been reported to be as high as 99%. This is primarily attributable to the inclusion of specific echocardiographic findings.

The value of this approach is now well established. In addition to providing a more sensitive means to establish the diagnosis of endocarditis, the Duke criteria have emphasized the essential relationship between clinical and echocardiographic findings. Despite the well-recognized importance of echocardiography in the evaluation of these patients, both false-positive and false-negative results may occur, underscoring the need to incorporate other (i.e., clinical) criteria. Furthermore, the inclusion of echocardiographic criteria has provided an impetus to standardize the various criteria used to define the essential pathologic processes, including vegetations and abscesses. These will be discussed subsequently. Finally, recent modifications in the Duke criteria have been proposed and are now being used in clinical practice. These are reflected in Table 13.5.

COMPLICATIONS OF ENDOCARDITIS

A variety of complications may occur in the setting of active endocarditis that may affect outcome and alter management (Table 13.7). The vegetation itself is an important source of possible complications in the setting of endocarditis. Infection of the valve can lead to tissue destruction or perforation that results in acute,

severe regurgitation (Fig. 13.13). This may lead to hemodynamic instability and heart failure. Two-dimensional echocardiography is useful to detect such structural changes in the valve, confirm the hemodynamic sequelae using Doppler imaging, and to measure the overall impact on cardiac function. It is important to recognize that, in the setting of active endocarditis, such changes in valve function often occur suddenly and lead to dramatic changes in clinical status. The availability and appropriate use of echocardiography in such situations may be lifesaving. Figure 13.14 includes two examples of anterior mitral leaflet perforation due to the destructive effects of the infectious process. Note the difference in the severity of regurgitation between the two cases.

An abscess is a localized pocket of infection (most often caused by staphylococci or enterococci bacteria) that appears on ultrasound as either an echo dense or echo lucent mass within the tissue. The most common location for an abscess is near the anulus of the aortic or mitral valve where it can affect valve function and/or the conducting system of the heart. An example of an aortic anulus (or ring) abscess is shown in Figure 13.15. This form of infection will sometimes develop in the absence of an associated vegetation. Abscesses may extend locally to affect adjacent structures. For example, an abscess of the aortic anulus may involve the anterior mitral valve leaflet (Fig. 13.16) or the sinus of Valsalva.

An abscess may rupture to allow communication with one of the cardiac chambers. Echocardiographically, this can be detected as a fistulous connection between two chambers of the heart (such as the right and left ventricles) or between the aortic root and a chamber (i.e., between a sinus of Valsalva and the left or right atrium). An example of this is provided in Figure 13.17. When rupture does occur, color flow imaging may demonstrate flow within the abscess cavity. Doppler is essential to document flow within the fistula and to demonstrate its connection to another chamber or space. Depending on the coronary sinus involved, the location of the fistula varies

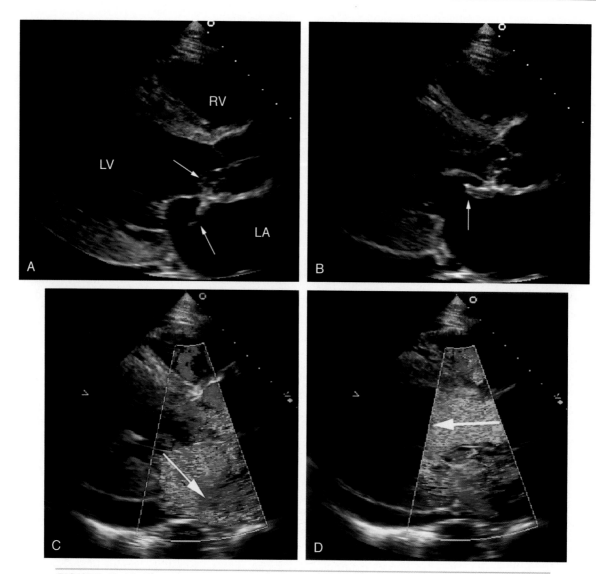

FIGURE 13.13. These images were recorded from a patient undergoing treatment for staphylococcal bacteremia. **A:** Masses (*arrows*) can be seen at the base of the aortic valve, extending through the anulus into the left atrium (*LA*). **B:** A diastolic frame confirms the extent of tissue involvement (*arrow*). **C:** Severe mitral regurgitation is evident (*arrow*). **D:** Severe aortic regurgitation (*arrow*) is demonstrated. Note the presence of a pericardial effusion. LA, left atrium; LV, left ventricle; RV, right ventricle.

widely and may communicate with any of the cardiac chambers.

Detecting abscess formation is difficult on clinical grounds. Aside from the development of atrioventricular conduction abnormalities, there are few clinical clues that suggest abscess development. Echocardiography therefore plays a critically important role in diagnosis. Although it is well established that transthoracic imaging has low sensitivity to detect abscesses, transesophageal echocardiography is an excellent technique for this purpose. Areas, particularly in the region of the aortic anulus, with abnormal thickening (Fig. 13.18), either echo dense

or echo lucent, should raise the suspicion of abscess formation in the appropriate clinical setting.

Mycotic aneurysms of the heart usually involve the aortic root and are similar in many ways to abscesses. A mycotic aneurysm is defined as an echo lucent outpouching of the vessel wall or, in the case of the aortic root, the coronary sinuses. It is usually connected through a single channel with the vessel from which it arises. As such, it can be either filled with infectious material or contain free-flowing blood. Such aneurysms may rupture to produce an intracardiac shunt or may undermine the function of the aortic valve. Figure 13.19 is taken from a pa-

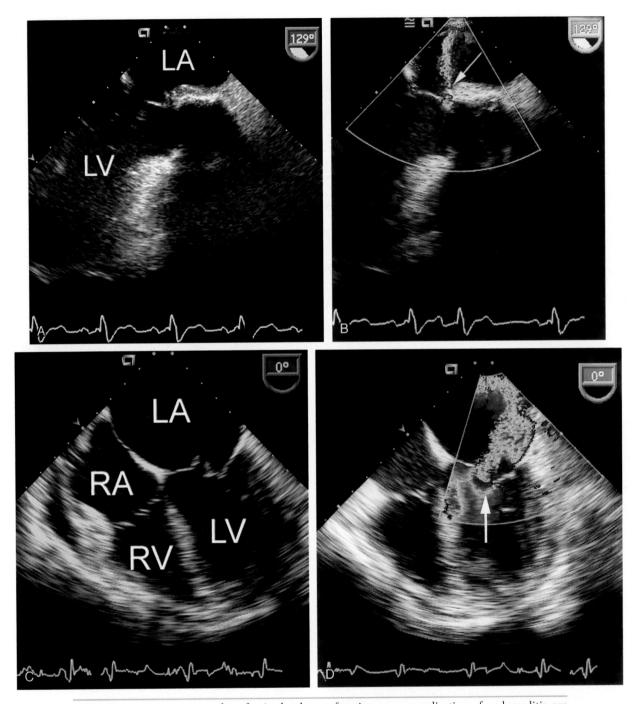

FIGURE 13.14. Two examples of mitral valve perforation as a complication of endocarditis are shown. **A, B:** Images are from a patient with a small perforation studied with transesophageal echocardiography. **A:** Thickening at the base of the anterior leaflet, involving the aortic anulus is evident. **B:** Color Doppler imaging during systole demonstrates a jet into the left atrium (*arrow*). A larger perforation involving the anterior mitral leaflet is demonstrated **(C, D)**. **C:** The defect within the mid portion of the leaflet is apparent. **D:** Color Doppler imaging reveals a severe degree of regurgitation through the perforation (*arrow*). LA, left atrium; LV, left ventricle; RA, right atrium; RV, right ventricle.

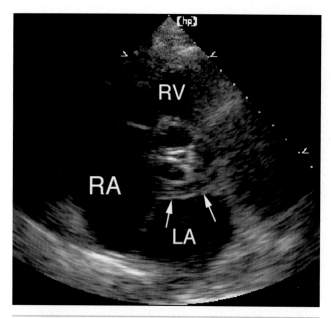

FIGURE 13.15. An aortic ring abscess (*arrows*) is seen from a transthoracic echocardiogram. Thickening in the posterior portion of the anulus adjacent to the left atrium (*LA*) is apparent. RA, right atrium; RV, right ventricle.

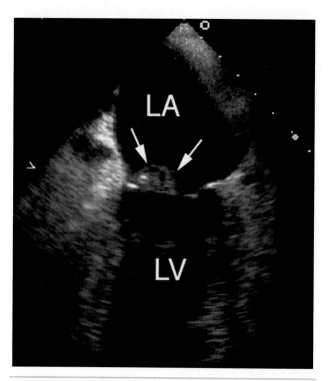

FIGURE 13.16. A transesophageal echocardiogram demonstrates an abscess (*arrows*) involving the anterior mitral leaflet. This patient also had an aortic ring abscess. LA, left atrium; LV, left ventricle.

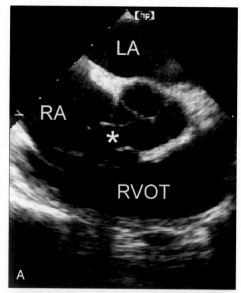

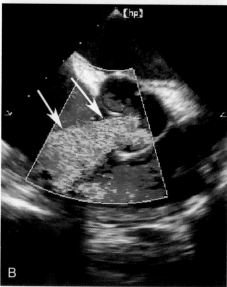

FIGURE 13.17. As a complication of aortic valve endocarditis, this patient demonstrated a ruptured sinus of Valsalva aneurysm (*). In this case, the noncoronary sinus was involved **(A)**. When rupture occurred, a shunt developed between the aortic root and right atrium (*arrows*) **(B)**. LA, left atrium; RA, right atrium; RVOT, right ventricular outflow tract.

tient who underwent aortic valve replacement and then presented 1 month later with fever. The aneurysm was evident just below the sewing ring and had partially ruptured into the right ventricle.

Complications such as abscess or aneurysm formation may result in spread of infection into the pericardial space producing purulent pericarditis. Clinical evidence of pericarditis in an acutely ill patient, coupled with echocardiographic evidence of a pericardial effusion, should suggest the possibility of purulent pericarditis,

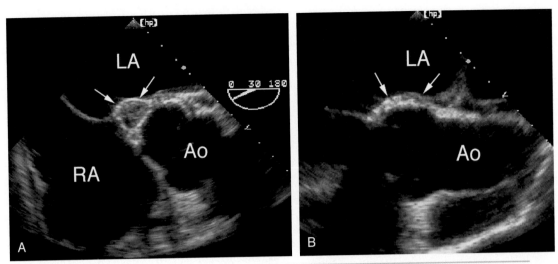

FIGURE 13.18. An abscess of the aortic root is demonstrated by transesophageal echocardiography. **A:** The location of the abscess is indicated by the *arrows* in the region of the noncoronary cusp. **B:** A long-axis view of the proximal aorta (*Ao*) demonstrates thickening in the posterior wall of the aortic root (*arrows*). LA, left atrium; RA, right atrium.

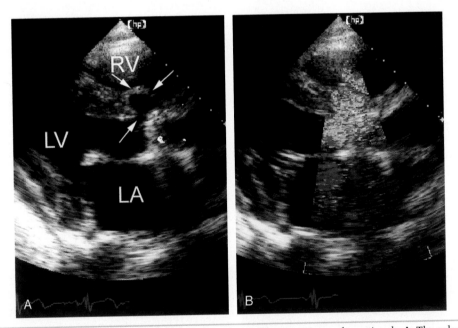

FIGURE 13.19. This patient underwent aortic valve replacement 1 month previously. **A:** The valve became infected, which led to the development of a mycotic aneurysm (*arrows*). **B:** Color Doppler imaging demonstrates a fistulous connection through the aneurysm and into the right ventricle. LA, left atrium; LV, left ventricle; RV, right ventricle.

usually a surgical emergency. Such effusions are rarely large in volume. Effusions due to purulent pericarditis may be difficult to differentiate from other causes of effusion, and the diagnosis is generally established on clinical grounds.

Among the most devastating of complications of endocarditis is an embolic event. Vegetations in the left side of the heart can embolize to cause stroke, distal infection, or ischemia. Figure 13.20 is taken from a patient who pre-

sented with signs of an embolic stroke. In this case, the vegetation was small, but its high mobility was a clue to the embolic risk. Figure 13.21 demonstrates a similar appearance involving the mitral valve. A thin and very mobile mitral valve vegetation is present. Right-sided endocarditis can lead to pulmonary emboli and pneumonia. In some cases, an embolic event is the first manifestation of endocarditis. More often, patients undergoing antibiotic therapy are suddenly affected, usually without warning.

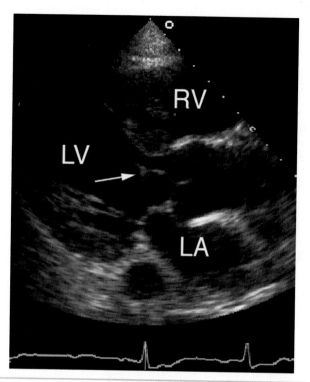

FIGURE 13.20. A highly mobile but small aortic valve vegetation (*arrow*) was visualized in this patient who presented with a stroke. LA, left atrium; LV, left ventricle; RV, right ventricle.

After such an event, echocardiography will sometimes show a reduction in size or a change in appearance of the vegetation (Fig. 13.22). The most important role of echocardiography in this setting is to predict patients at risk of these devastating events, a topic that is covered in the next section.

PROGNOSIS AND PREDICTING RISK

For most patients with acute endocarditis, outcome is largely dependent on the likelihood of developing a complication that can occur in as many as 40% of patients being treated for active endocarditis. Such complications are invariably associated with a worsening prognosis. Thus, identifying patients at risk of developing complications before they occur is an important goal. Several investigations have attempted to stratify patients into low- and high-risk subsets and to identify those at risk of complications based on clinical and echocardiographic findings. Most of the parameters that determine high- and low-risk status are clinical, including age, type of organism, and development of heart failure. In addition, stroke occurrence consistently has been a strong negative determinant of outcome in patients with endocarditis. Echocardiography, if it could predict the likelihood of embolization, would be very useful to predict high-risk status before complications developed.

The only echocardiographic parameter that has been consistently associated with an increased risk of complications is vegetation size. In one study (Sanfilippo et al., 1991), there was a strong and nearly linear relationship between vegetation size and the risk of complications. For example, vegetations less than 7 mm in size accounted for less than 10% of all complications, whereas those that were greater than 11 mm accounted for more than half of the complications. In a meta-analysis by Tischler and Vaitkus (1997) involving 10 studies and 738 cases, the risk of an embolic event in patients with a vegetation greater than 10 mm was threefold higher than in patients with smaller vegetations (Fig. 13.23). It is clear that a direct relationship exists between vegetation size and risk. The

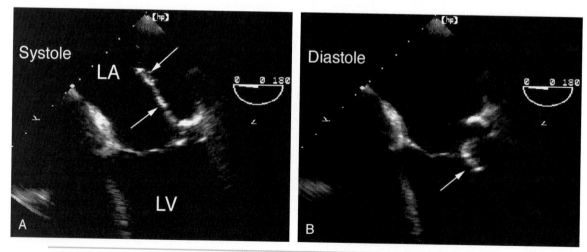

FIGURE 13.21. An elongated and highly mobile vegetation is demonstrated. **A:** During systole, the mass (*arrows*) extends into the left atrium (*LA*). **B:** During diastole, the vegetation was carried through the mitral valve into the left ventricle (*arrow*). LV, left ventricle.

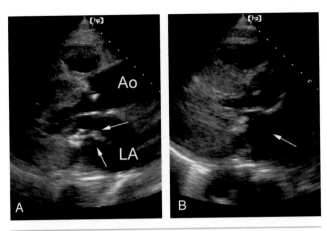

FIGURE 13.22. The appearance of a vegetation may change as a result of embolization. **A:** A large and mobile vegetation (*arrows*) can be seen attached to the left atrial (*LA*) side of the posterior mitral leaflet. **B:** An echocardiogram recorded 1 week later, after a stroke. Note that the vegetation (*arrow*) is much smaller, most likely the result of embolization. Ao, aorta.

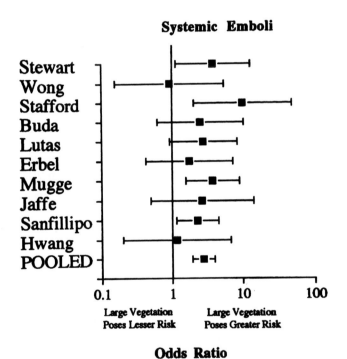

Systemic Emboli

Stewart
Wong
Stafford
Buda
Lutas
Erbel
Mugge
Jaffe
Sanfillipo
Hwang
POOLED

0.1   1   10   100

Large Vegetation Poses Lesser Risk   Large Vegetation Poses Greater Risk

Odds Ratio

FIGURE 13.23. A meta-analysis of studies that examine whether vegetation size could predict the risk of systemic emboli. The pooled odds ratio for increased risk associated with large vegetation was 2.80 (95% confidence interval 1.95 to 4.02, *p* <0.01). (From Tischler MD, Vaitkus PT. The ability of vegetation size on echocardiography to predict clinical complications: a meta-analysis. J Am Soc Echocardiogr 1997;10:562–568, with permission.)

larger the vegetation is, the greater the likelihood of complications, particularly embolic events (Fig. 13.24). Furthermore, an increase in vegetation size after 4 weeks of antibiotic therapy is additional evidence of high-risk sta-

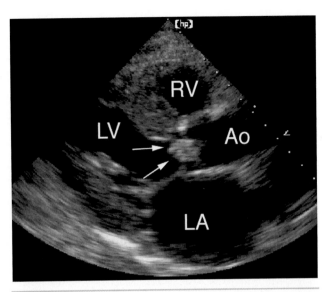

FIGURE 13.24. An example of a large vegetation (*arrows*) involving the aortic valve is shown. Ao, aorta; LA, left atrium; LV, left ventricle; RV, right ventricle.

tus and should prompt consideration for surgical intervention. Other parameters that have been implicated as increasing the risk of complications include high mobility of the vegetation, multiple sites of involvement, and extension to extravalvular structures.

More recently, vegetation location has also been associated with risk. In one study by Cabell and colleagues (2001), patients with mitral valve involvement were three times more likely to develop embolic complications compared with patients with aortic valve vegetations. However, mitral valve vegetations also tended to be larger, so it may be that size, rather than location, was the factor that predicted embolic potential. In this same study, vegetation location was not predictive of overall mortality at 1 year. In the future, it is very likely that refinement in risk stratification will involve a multivariate approach that combines clinical, bacteriologic, and echocardiographic measures.

PROSTHETIC VALVE ENDOCARDITIS

Endocarditis involving a prosthetic valve is challenging, both from a diagnostic and a management standpoint. On echocardiography, the highly reflective nature of prosthetic material, the shadowing created by the prosthesis, and the effect of the device being implanted on the underlying tissue combine to make diagnosis difficult. Vegetations on prosthetic valves most often occur on the base or sewing ring of the structure (Fig. 13.25). Distinguishing small vegetations from the prosthetic material (and especially from the sutures used to secure the valve in place) can be extremely difficult. Therefore, diagnosis of endocarditis in this setting requires a thorough echocardio-

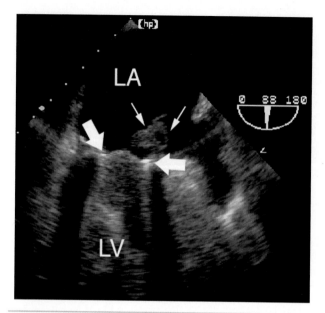

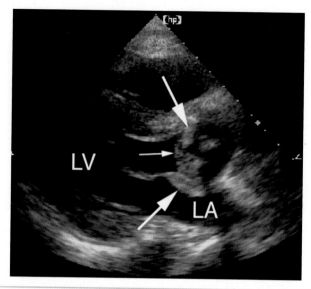

FIGURE 13.25. From a patient with a St. Jude mitral prosthesis, a large vegetation (*small arrows*) can be seen in the left atrium (*LA*) attached to the sewing ring (*large arrows*). LV, left ventricle.

FIGURE 13.26. A porcine aortic prosthesis is shown. The leaflets are severely infected, and multiple vegetations are present (*small arrow*). In addition, thickening of the aortic anulus adjacent to the sewing ring (*large arrows*) indicates ring abscess formation. LA, left atrium; LV, left ventricle.

graphic assessment from all available windows. Transthoracic echocardiography is limited in its ability to secure the diagnosis of prosthetic valve endocarditis. When extensive infection is present, as is shown in Figure 13.26, chest wall imaging may be adequate. However, transthoracic echocardiography is rarely sufficient to exclude the diagnosis of endocarditis in patients with prosthetic valves in whom there is a high index of suspicion. For example, in a patient with a mitral valve prosthesis, visualizing that portion of the left atrium immediately behind the prosthesis may be impossible from any transthoracic window. In such cases, the perspective available from transesophageal imaging is most helpful (Fig. 13.27). Conversely, the ventricular aspect of a tricuspid valve prosthesis may be more readily imaged from the chest wall as opposed to the esophagus. Thus, a combination of the two techniques may be necessary for a complete interrogation. Figure 13.26 illustrates an extensive infection in a patient with a bioprosthetic aortic valve. The valve itself is completely obscured by the vegetation, and the aortic root is diffusely thickened due to a ring abscess. Another example of obstruction due to a prosthetic valve vegetation is shown in Figure 13.28. In this case, a porcine mitral prosthesis is involved and the large vegetation results in a significant diastolic pressure gradient, which was recorded both on transthoracic and transesophageal imaging.

Multiplane transesophageal echocardiography has increased the accuracy of detecting endocarditis in this setting. Investigators have consistently demonstrated a much higher sensitivity for transesophageal echocardiog-

raphy in the presence of prosthetic valves. The improvement in accuracy is so great that many echocardiographers view transesophageal echocardiography as the initial procedure of choice when prosthetic valve endocarditis is suspected. In addition, complications associated with prosthetic valve endocarditis (especially anular abscesses) are more consistently visualized from the transesophageal approach (Fig. 13.29).

INFECTED INTRACARDIAC DEVICES

In addition to prosthetic valves, other types of prosthetic material within the heart or vasculature can become infected. As with prosthetic valves, infection can occur early or later after implantation. When infection occurs early after implantation, it is usually due to the presence of preexisting infection or as a complication of the procedure itself. Late infection is most often the result of seeding of the prosthetic material by hematogenously borne organisms. In either case, infected prosthetic devices are difficult to treat without removal and are associated with a poor prognosis. An example of an infected pacemaker lead is shown in Figure 13.30. In most cases, detection of evidence of infection requires transesophageal echocardiography. Distinguishing vegetations from thrombus is virtually impossible on echocardiographic grounds alone and invariably requires clinical correlation. With the growing use of these devices, the incidence of this type of endocarditis will certainly increase.

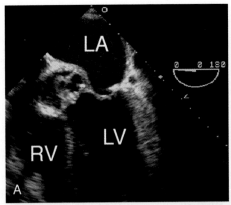

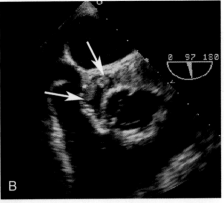

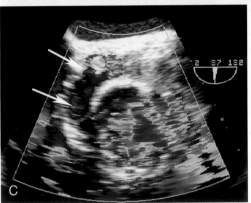

FIGURE 13.27. A stentless aortic valve is recorded with transesophageal echocardiography. **A:** The aortic root is thickened and echogenic. **B:** A short-axis view demonstrates abscess formation posteriorly (*arrows*). **C:** Color Doppler imaging reveals flow within the abscess cavity (*arrows*). LA, left atrium; LV, left ventricle; RV, right ventricle.

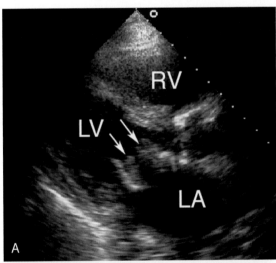

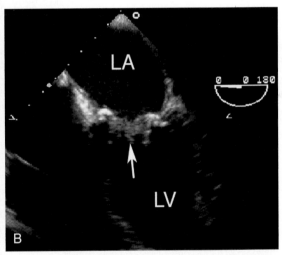

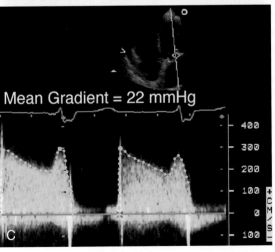

Mean Gradient = 22 mmHg

FIGURE 13.28. An infected porcine mitral prosthesis is shown. The valve leaflets are thickened and relatively immobile (*arrows*) **(A)**. **B:** On the transesophageal echocardiogram, thickening and decreased motion (*arrow*) were apparent. **C:** Doppler demonstrates a mean gradient of 22 mm Hg across the prosthesis. LA, left atrium; LV, left ventricle; RV, right ventricle.

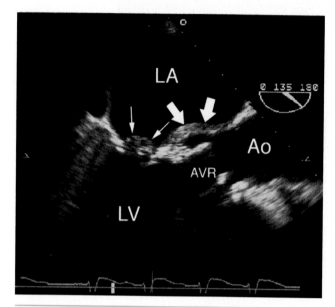

FIGURE 13.29. Endocarditis in a patient with a porcine aortic prosthesis is demonstrated on this transesophageal echocardiogram. The aortic prosthesis itself was spared. However, thickening of the aortic root, consistent with abscess formation, is indicated by the *large arrows*. A mitral valve vegetation is demonstrated by the *small arrows*. Ao, aorta; LA, left atrium; LV, left ventricle; AVR, aortic valve replacement.

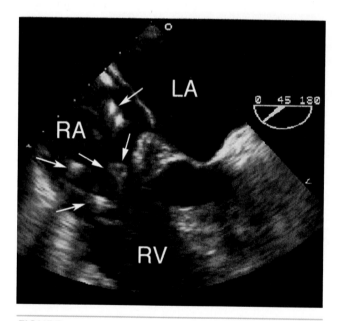

FIGURE 13.30. A transesophageal echocardiogram recorded from a patient with multiple pacemaker leads in the right heart is shown. The *arrows* indicate mobile masses attached to the leads, consistent with vegetations. LA, left atrium; RA, right atrium; RV, right ventricle.

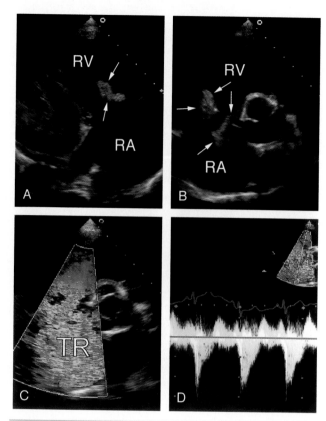

FIGURE 13.31. A large and highly mobile tricuspid valve vegetation is demonstrated. **A:** During diastole, a vegetation could be seen attached to the tricuspid valve (*arrows*). The short-axis view (**B**) was recorded during systole indicating the highly mobile nature of the mass (*arrows*). **C:** Color Doppler imaging reveals severe tricuspid regurgitation (*TR*). **D:** The spectral Doppler tracing is shown. RA, right atrium; RV, right ventricle.

RIGHT-SIDED ENDOCARDITIS

Endocarditis involving the tricuspid valve is most commonly seen in the setting of intravenous drug use (Fig. 13.31). In one series by Hecht et al. (1992) involving 121 intravenous drug users, a tricuspid valve vegetation was seen in all cases, whereas the pulmonary valve was involved in only four. Vegetation size tends to be greater in right-sided endocarditis, and some degree of tricuspid regurgitation is generally present. Pulmonary valve vegetations are less common and can be difficult to visualize. They may develop in patients as a complication of pulmonary artery catheterization. Figure 13.32 is an example of a small vegetation affecting the pulmonary valve in an immunocompromised patient. In this case, a tricuspid valve vegetation was also present.

The advantages of transesophageal echocardiography are less well established in right-sided endocarditis, and both echocardiographic techniques have demonstrated high sensitivity for this diagnosis. Even after successful

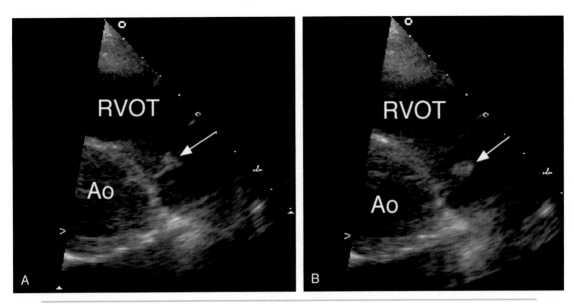

FIGURE 13.32. A small vegetation involving the pulmonary valve is shown. This occurred in the setting of tricuspid valve endocarditis. Two diastolic frames are provided, showing the small mass (*arrow*) on the right ventricular aspect of the valve leaflet. Ao, aorta; RVOT, right ventricular outflow tract.

antibiotic therapy, when infection is no longer clinically active, masses on the tricuspid valve often remain. Thus, differentiating active from healed endocarditis in this situation is often difficult.

APPROACH TO THE PATIENT WITH ENDOCARDITIS

Although it is clear that echocardiography is indispensable in the evaluation of patients with suspected endocarditis, the decisions about when and how often the test should be performed must still be made. Some guidelines for the use of echocardiography in patients with known or suspected endocarditis are provided in Table 13.8. In most patients in whom there is a clinical suspicion of endocarditis, echocardiography is helpful whether the results are positive or negative. The results help to establish or exclude the diagnosis and also provide prognostic information, establish a baseline for comparison, and may even identify patients in whom prompt surgical intervention is recommended.

An inevitable consequence of the utility of echocardiography in endocarditis is the potential for overuse. This is particularly true among patients in whom the pretest likelihood of endocarditis is extremely low and no additional testing, including echocardiography, is likely to yield important new information. Thus, the rationale to perform echocardiography must depend on clinical findings that increase the pretest likelihood of disease, such as fever, an abnormal physical examination, or blood culture results for an appropriate organism.

Once the decision is made to perform an echocardiogram, the choice between transthoracic and transesophageal echocardiography must be made. Given the well-documented superior sensitivity of transesophageal imaging, it is tempting to conclude that this should be the test of choice. However, in a study by Lindner and colleagues (1996), the relative value of transthoracic echocardiography was demonstrated and the advantages of transesophageal imaging were shown to be confined to specific situations (Fig. 13.33). This series compared the yield of echocardiography in different cohorts of patients grouped based on the clinical probability of endocarditis. Not surprisingly, among patients who were categorized as having either a low or high likelihood of endocarditis, based on clinical grounds, neither echocardiographic technique added much to the ultimate classification of the patient. However, among patients with a medium pretest probability of disease, both tests were helpful to reclassify most patients as having either a low or high probability, and transesophageal echocardiography was superior for this purpose.

Thus, because of its greater cost and invasiveness, the higher sensitivity of transesophageal echocardiography must be weighed against these factors. As a result, a transthoracic echocardiogram is the initial test of choice for many situations. The negative predictive value of the test is high, and, if image quality if acceptable, the absence of positive findings is often sufficient to avoid the need for further testing. Situations in which transesophageal echocardiography should be considered as the initial test of choice include (1) those patients in whom image quality on chest wall imaging is unacceptable, (2)

TABLE 13.8 Indications for Echocardiography in Infective Endocarditis: Native Valves

Indication	Class
1. Detection and characterization of valvular lesions, their hemodynamic severity, and/or ventricular compensation[a]	I
2. Detection of vegetations and characterization of lesions in patients with congenital heart disease suspected of having infective endocarditis	I
3. Detection of associated abnormalities (e.g., abscesses, shunts)[a]	I
4. Reevaluation studies in complex endocarditis (e.g., virulent organism, severe hemodynamic lesion, aortic valve involvement, persistent fever or bacteremia, clinical change, or symptomatic deterioration)	I
5. Evaluation of patients with high clinical suspicion of culture-negative endocarditis[a]	I
6. If transthoracic echocardiography is equivocal, transesophageal echocardiography evaluation of staphylococcus bacteremia without a known source	I
7. Evaluation of persistent nonstaphylococcus bacteremia without a known source[a]	IIa
8. Risk stratification in established endocarditis[a]	IIa
9. Routine reevaluation in uncomplicated endocarditis during antibiotic therapy	IIb
10. Evaluation of transient fever without evidence of bacteremia or a new murmur	III

[a]Transesophageal echocardiography may provide incremental value in addition to information obtained by transthoracic echocardiography. The role of transesophageal echocardiography in first-line examination awaits further study.

Adapted with permission from Cheitlin MD, Alpert JS, Armstrong WF, et al. ACC/AHA Guidelines for the Clinical Application of Echocardiography: a report of the American College of Cardiology/American Heart Association Task Force on Practice Guidelines (Committee on Application of Echocardiography) developed in collaboration with the American Society of Echocardiography. Circulation 1997;95:1686–1744, with permission.

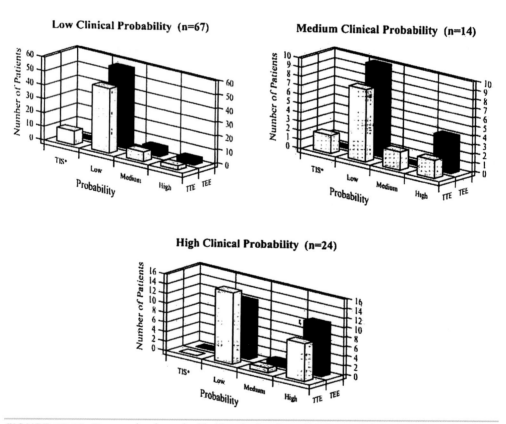

FIGURE 13.33. Bar graphs show the likelihood of endocarditis by transthoracic echocardiography (TTE) and transesophageal echocardiography (TEE) in patients with low, medium, and high clinical probability of disease. See text for details. TIS, technically inadequate study. (From Lindner JR, Case RA, Dent JM, et al. Diagnostic value of echocardiography in suspected endocarditis. An evaluation based on the pretest probability of disease. Circulation 1996;93:730–736, with permission.)

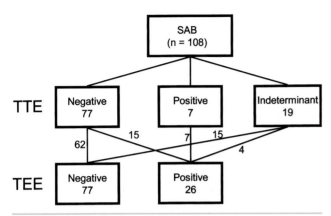

FIGURE 13.34. Block diagram demonstrates the yield of transthoracic (TTE) and transesophageal (TEE) echocardiography in patients with *Staphylococcus aureus* bacteremia (SAB). See text for details. (From Fowler VG Jr, Li J, Corey GR, et al. Role of echocardiography in evaluation of patients with *Staphylococcus aureus* bacteremia: experience in 103 patients. J Am Coll Cardiol 1997;30:1072–1078, with permission).

clinical setting, the advantages of transesophageal imaging were clearly demonstrated, perhaps because the imaging was performed so early in the course of the disease, when vegetations are likely to be relatively small (Fig. 13.35).

The choice between transthoracic and transesophageal echocardiography can also be addressed from the perspective of cost-effectiveness. Heidenreich and colleagues (1999) used a decision-analysis technique to compare the two tests in patients with a high pretest probability (4%–60%) of having endocarditis. These investigators assessed the health and economic outcomes of various groups using six different strategies: (1) empiric treatment of bacteremia (short-course therapy), (2) empiric treatment of endocarditis (long-course therapy), (3) treatment based on transthoracic echocardiographic results, (4) treatment based on transesophageal echocardiographic results, (5) treatment based on transesophageal echocardiography after negative transthoracic study, and (6) treatment based on transthoracic echocardiographic results (unless the study was negative and image quality was poor, in which case, a transesophageal echocardiogram was obtained). Their results confirmed that the pretest probability of endocarditis, based on the history and physical and laboratory data, was essential in deciding which strategy was most effective. Their model suggested that transesophageal echocardiography alone increased the quality-adjusted life days and reduced the cost of diagnosis compared with transthoracic echocardiography for a wide range of relative costs for the two tests

those with prosthetic valves, and (3) those in whom complications such as abscess formation are suspected on clinical grounds. In one study (Fowler et al., 1997), the yields of transthoracic and that of transesophageal echocardiography were compared in a series of 103 patients with staphylococcal bacteremia who were evaluated relatively early in the course of their illness. Both forms of echocardiography were performed, and the results were interpreted independently (Fig. 13.34). In this

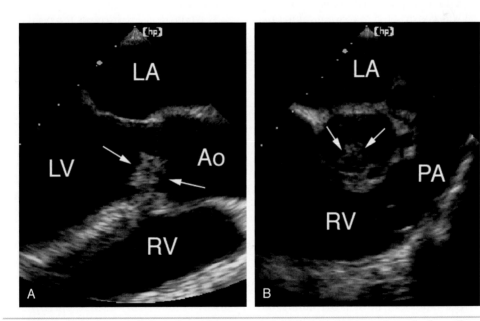

FIGURE 13.35. An aortic valve vegetation is demonstrated on this transesophageal echocardiogram (*arrows*). The mass was clearly seen from the long-axis **(A)** and short-axis **(B)** views. The mass was not detected on transthoracic imaging. Ao, aorta; LA, left atrium; LV, left ventricle; RV, right ventricle; PA, pulmonary artery.

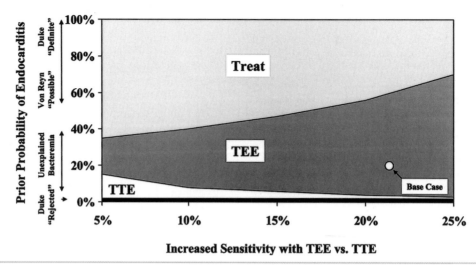

FIGURE 13.36. Using a decision tree and Markov model of published data, this graph shows the relationship between the prior probability of endocarditis, the incremental sensitivity provided by transesophageal echocardiography (TEE), and the appropriate diagnostic strategy. TTE, transthoracic echocardiography. See text for details. (From Heidenreich PA, Masoudi FA, Maini B, et al. Echocardiography in patients with suspected endocarditis: a cost-effectiveness analysis. Am J Med 1999;107:198–208, with permission.)

(Fig. 13.36). Although the limitations of this approach are evident, the results do support a prominent role for transesophageal echocardiography in many patients with suspected endocarditis.

A related question is whether echocardiography can be used to guide duration of antibiotic therapy. This issue has been addressed in the subset of patients with catheter-associated *Staphylococcus aureus* bacteremia (Rosen et al., 1999). A model was constructed to test the value (and cost-effectiveness) of transesophageal echocardiography in deciding the optimal duration of therapy. The model compared empiric short-course therapy (2 weeks), long-course therapy (4 weeks), and echocardiography-guided therapy (long-course if there was evidence of endocarditis and short-course otherwise). The study tested whether the incremental cost of transesophageal echocardiography could be justified based on superior outcomes and/or reduced duration of therapy. The results suggested that the echocardiography-guided strategy offered improved life expectancy compared with empiric short-course therapy and was more cost-effective compared with long-course therapy. Over a wide range of costs and levels of accuracy, echocardiography was found to be cost-effective in this clinical setting.

The decision to proceed with surgery is a complex one that must rely on clinical criteria as well as echocardiographic findings. The development of heart failure, an embolic event, stroke, or extension of the infection are some indications for surgical intervention. Some echocardiographic findings are also considered in this decision-making process. For example, an aortic ring abscess and valve tissue destruction leading to severe regurgitation are often considered surgical indications. Other less dramatic signs should also be sought. Evidence of disease progression might include increase in vegetation size, worsening regurgitation, chamber enlargement, ventricular dysfunction, or extension of infection to other sites. These changes may occur during therapy in the absence of clinical deterioration and often affect management plans.

The final decision involves the need for repeat echocardiographic analysis in a patient with an established diagnosis. There are no firm data to support the use of serial echocardiograms in this setting. In most cases, the decision to perform subsequent echocardiograms depends on the clinical course. Figure 13.37 shows echocardiograms from a patient with a repaired mitral valve. In the first study, the patient had clinical evidence of endocarditis, but no vegetations were apparent on the study and the patient was clinically stable. The prosthetic ring is seen and the leaflets appear normal. Seven months later, the second study shows marked progression of disease, despite a prolonged course of antibiotics. In patients who demonstrate clinical deterioration, repeat testing can be valuable in establishing a cause and guiding subsequent decision making. Alternatively, patients who demonstrate a good response to antibiotic therapy based on subsequent blood culture results as well as history and physical examination are unlikely to benefit from any form of additional testing. Some high-risk subsets of patients, such as those with staphylococcal endocarditis involving the aortic valve, may benefit from a second echocardiogram 7 to 10 days after initiation of therapy to exclude complications such as abscess formation.

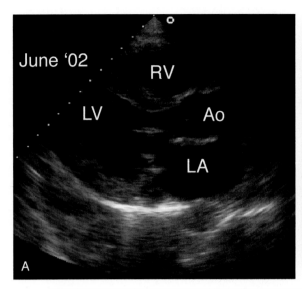 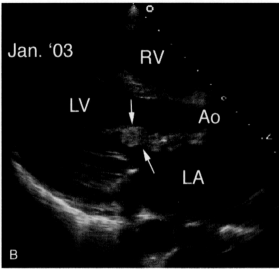

FIGURE 13.37. Serial changes can be detected echocardiographically. This patient had undergone mitral valve repair and a mitral anular ring was present. **A:** No evidence of endocarditis was detected, despite clinical signs suggesting infection. **B:** Seven months later, marked progression of disease is apparent, despite antibiotic therapy. A large vegetation involving the anterior mitral leaflet (*arrows*) is present. Ao, aorta; LA, left atrium; LV, left ventricle; RV, right ventricle.

SUGGESTED READINGS

Alam M, Rosman HS, Sun I. Transesophageal echocardiographic evaluation of St. Jude Medical and bioprosthetic valve endocarditis. Am Heart J 1992;123:236–239.

Alton ME, Pasierski TJ, Orsinelli DA, et al. Comparison of transthoracic and transesophageal echocardiography in evaluation of 47 Starr-Edwards prosthetic valves. J Am Coll Cardiol 1992;20:1503–1511.

Bayer AS. Diagnostic criteria for identifying cases of endocarditis—revisiting the Duke criteria two years later. Clin Infect Dis 1996;23:303–304.

Birmingham GD, Rahko PS, Ballantyne F. Improved detection of infective endocarditis with transesophageal echocardiography. Am Heart J 1992;123:774–781.

Blumberg EA, Karalis DA, Chandrasekaran K, et al. Endocarditis-associated paravalvular abscesses. Do clinical parameters predict the presence of abscess? Chest 1995;107:898–903.

Cabell CH, Jollis JG, Peterson GE, et al. Changing patient characteristics and the effect on mortality in endocarditis. Arch Intern Med 2002;162:90–94.

Cabell CH, Pond KK, Peterson GE, et al. The risk of stroke and death in patients with aortic and mitral valve endocarditis. Am Heart J 2001;142:75–80.

Chamis AL, Peterson GE, Cabell CH, et al. *Staphylococcus aureus* bacteremia in patients with permanent pacemakers or implantable cardioverter-defibrillators. Circulation 2001;104:1029–1033.

Cheitlin MD, Alpert JS, Armstrong WF, et al. ACC/AHA Guidelines for the Clinical Application of Echocardiography: a report of the American College of Cardiology/American Heart Association Task Force on Practice Guidelines (Committee on Clinical Application of Echocardiography) developed in collaboration with the American Society of Echocardiography. Circulation 1997;95:1686–1744.

Daniel WG, Mugge A, Grote J, et al. Comparison of transthoracic and transesophageal echocardiography for detection of abnormalities of prosthetic and bioprosthetic valves in the mitral and aortic positions. Am J Cardiol 1993;71:210–215.

Daniel WG, Mugge A, Martin RP, et al. Improvement in the diagnosis of abscesses associated with endocarditis by transesophageal echocardiography. N Engl J Med 1991;324:795–800.

Dodds GA, Sexton DJ, Durack DT, et al. Negative predictive value of the Duke criteria for infective endocarditis. Am J Cardiol 1996;77:403–407.

Durack DT, Lukes AS, Bright DK. New criteria for diagnosis of infective endocarditis: utilization of specific echocardiographic findings. Am J Med 1994;96:200–209.

Erbel R, Rohmann S, Drexler M, et al. Improved diagnostic value of echocardiography in patients with infective endocarditis by transoesophageal approach. A prospective study. Eur Heart J 1988;9:43–53.

Fowler VG Jr, Li J, Corey GR, et al. Role of echocardiography in evaluation of patients with *Staphylococcus aureus* bacteremia: experience in 103 patients. J Am Coll Cardiol 1997;30:1072–1078.

Habib G, Derumeaux G, Avierinos JF, et al. Value and limitations of the Duke criteria for the diagnosis of infective endocarditis. J Am Coll Cardiol 1999;33:2023–2029.

Hecht SR, Berger M. Right-sided endocarditis in intravenous drug users. Prognostic features in 102 episodes. Ann Intern Med 1992;117:560–566.

Heidenreich PA, Masoudi FA, Maini B, et al. Echocardiography in patients with suspected endocarditis: a cost-effectiveness analysis. Am J Med 1999;107:198–208.

Jaffe WM, Morgan DE, Pearlman AS, et al. Infective endocarditis, 1983–1988: echocardiographic findings and factors influencing morbidity and mortality. J Am Coll Cardiol 1990;15:1227–1233.

Joffe II, Jacobs LE, Owen AN, et al. Noninfective valvular masses: review of the literature with emphasis on imaging techniques and management. Am Heart J 1996;131:1175–1183.

Karalis DG, Bansal RC, Hauck AJ, et al. Transesophageal echocardiographic recognition of subaortic complications in aortic valve endocarditis. Clinical and surgical implications. Circulation 1992;86:353–362.

Khandheria BK. Suspected bacterial endocarditis: to TEE or not to TEE. J Am Coll Cardiol 1993;21:222–224.

Leung DY, Cranney GB, Hopkins AP, et al. Role of transoesophageal echocardiography in the diagnosis and management of aortic root abscess. Br Heart J 1994;72:175–181.

Li JS, Sexton DJ, Mick N, et al. Proposed modifications to the Duke criteria for the diagnosis of infective endocarditis. Clin Infect Dis 2000;30:633–638.

Lindner JR, Case RA, Dent JM, et al. Diagnostic value of echocardiography in suspected endocarditis. An evaluation based on the pretest probability of disease. Circulation 1996;93:730–736.

Lowry RW, Zoghbi WA, Baker WB, et al. Clinical impact of transesophageal echocardiography in the diagnosis and management of infective endocarditis. Am J Cardiol 1994;73:1089–1091.

Mohr-Kahaly S, Kupferwasser I, Erbel R, et al. Value and limitations of transesophageal echocardiography in the evaluation of aortic prostheses. J Am Soc Echocardiogr 1993;6:12–20.

Mugge A, Daniel WG, Frank G, et al. Echocardiography in infective endocarditis: reassessment of prognostic implications of vegetation size determined by the transthoracic and the transesophageal approach. J Am Coll Cardiol 1989;14:631–638.

O'Brien JT, Geiser EA. Infective endocarditis and echocardiography. Am Heart J 1984;108:386–394.

Rodbard S. Blood velocity and endocarditis. Circulation 1963;27:18–28.

Rohmann S, Erbel R, Darius H, et al. Prediction of rapid versus prolonged healing of infective endocarditis by monitoring vegetation size. J Am Soc Echocardiogr 1991;4:465–474.

Rosen AB, Fowler VG Jr, Corey GR, et al. Cost-effectiveness of transesophageal echocardiography to determine the duration of therapy for intravascular catheter-associated *Staphylococcus aureus* bacteremia. Ann Intern Med 1999;130:810–820.

Roy P, Tajik AJ, Giuliani ER, et al. Spectrum of echocardiographic findings in bacterial endocarditis. Circulation 1976;53:474–482.

San Roman JA, Vilacosta I, Zamorano JL, et al. Transesophageal echocardiography in right-sided endocarditis. J Am Coll Cardiol 1993;21:1226–1230.

Sanfilippo AJ, Picard MH, Newell JB, et al. Echocardiographic assessment of patients with infectious endocarditis: prediction of risk for complications. J Am Coll Cardiol 1991;18:1191–1199.

Schulz R, Werner GS, Fuchs JB, et al. Clinical outcome and echocardiographic findings of native and prosthetic valve endocarditis in the 1990's. Eur Heart J 1996;17:281–288.

Shapiro SM, Young E, De Guzman S, et al. Transesophageal echocardiography in diagnosis of infective endocarditis. Chest 1994;105:377–382.

Shively BK, Gurule FT, Roldan CA, et al. Diagnostic value of transesophageal compared with transthoracic echocardiography in infective endocarditis. J Am Coll Cardiol 1991;18:391–397.

Strom BL, Abrutyn E, Berlin JA, et al. Dental and cardiac risk factors for infective endocarditis. A population-based, case-control study. Ann Intern Med 1998;129:761–769.

Tak T, Rahimtoola SH, Kumar A, et al. Value of digital image processing of two-dimensional echocardiograms in differentiating active from chronic vegetations of infective endocarditis. Circulation 1988;78:116–123.

Tischler MD, Vaitkus PT. The ability of vegetation size on echocardiography to predict clinical complications: a meta-analysis. J Am Soc Echocardiogr 1997;10:562–568.

von Reyn CF, Levy BS, Arbeit RD, et al. Infective endocarditis: an analysis based on strict case definitions. Ann Intern Med 1981;94:505–518.

Vuille C, Nidorf M, Weyman AE, et al. Natural history of vegetations during successful medical treatment of endocarditis. Am Heart J 1994;128:1200–1209.

Werner GS, Schulz R, Fuchs JB, et al. Infective endocarditis in the elderly in the era of transesophageal echocardiography: clinical features and prognosis compared with younger patients. Am J Med 1996;100:90–96.

Zabalgoitia M, Herrera CJ, Chaudhry FA, et al. Improvement in the diagnosis of bioprosthetic valve dysfunction by transesophageal echocardiography. J Heart Valve Dis 1993;2:595–603.

Chapter 14

Prosthetic Valves

The era of valve surgery preceded the development of echocardiography by only a few years. It is therefore not surprising that one of the earliest applications of echocardiography was the study of prosthetic valve function. With the tremendous advances in surgical techniques over the past four decades, the role of echocardiography has evolved and broadened in this important field. Because neither the perfect valve repair nor the perfect prosthesis yet exists, ongoing assessment of valve function is a key aspect of the management of patients after valve surgery. Echocardiography, with its noninvasive ability to evaluate both anatomy and function, has become the diagnostic modality of choice for this purpose.

The echocardiographic assessment of prosthetic valves is complex. Flow dynamics are different through prosthetic compared with native valves. Both the size and type of the prosthesis influence the range of expected flow velocities and thus the definition of normal versus abnormal function. The echocardiographer must determine the specific type of prosthetic valve and whether the structural and functional parameters exceed the limits of normal for a given size and type. Despite these challenges, the combination of echocardiography and Doppler imaging techniques is ideally suited to assessing prosthetic valves. Whether monitoring valve function over time or detecting the specific cause of prosthesis dysfunction, echocardiographic techniques have become indispensable in this important clinical area.

TYPES OF PROSTHETIC VALVES

The two major categories of prosthetic valves include mechanical valves and tissue valves or bioprostheses. These are listed in Table 14.1. The mechanical prosthetic valves can be further divided into caged ball and tilting disk designs. The caged ball prosthesis was the first type of artificial heart valve and the Starr-Edwards valve is by far the most common (Fig. 14.1). It consists of a circular sewing ring on which is mounted a U-shaped cage that contains a silastic ball occluder. To open, the ball moves forward into the cage, allowing blood flow around the entire circumference. To occlude, the ball is driven back into the sewing ring to prevent backflow.

Several tilting disk prostheses are currently in use (Fig. 14.2). The single disk prosthesis consists of a round sewing ring and a circular disk fixed eccentrically to the ring via a hinge. The disk moves through an arc of less than 90 degrees (usually 55–70 degrees), thereby allowing antegrade flow in the open position and seating within the

▌TABLE 14.1 Types of Prosthetic Valves

Mechanical
  Caged ball
    Starr-Edwards
  Single disc
    Björk-Shiley
    Medtronic-Hall
    Omnicarbon
    Lillehei-Kaster
  Bileaflet disc
    St. Jude Medical
    CarboMedics
    Duramedics Jyros
Tissue
  Porcine
    Carpentier-Edwards
    Hancock
  Bovine
    Hancock
  Pericardial
    Carpentier-Edwards
    Ionescu-Shiley
    Hancock
  Stentless
    St. Jude Toronto
    Medtronic Freestyle
    Biocor
    Edwards Prima
  Homografts

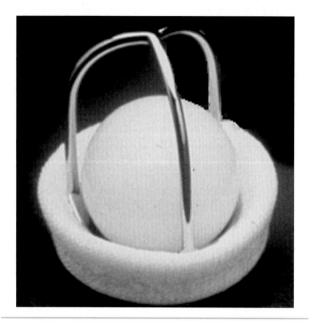

FIGURE 14.1. A Starr-Edwards prosthesis is shown.

sewing ring to prevent backflow in the closed position. The Björk-Shiley and Medtronic-Hall are examples of single tilting disk prostheses. Because the hinge is eccentrically positioned within the sewing ring and the disk opens less than 90 degrees, major and minor orifices are created and some stagnation of flow occurs behind the disk. Bileaflet tilting disk valves consist of two semicircular disks that open and close on a hinge mechanism within the sewing ring. The opening angle is generally more vertical (approximately 80 degrees) than the single disk prosthesis and results in three distinct orifices: two larger ones

on either side and a smaller central rectangular-shaped orifice. Examples of bileaflet titling disks include the St. Jude Medical and CarboMedics valves.

Unlike mechanical valves, bioprostheses are constructed from either human or animal tissue (Fig. 14.3). Among the most commonly used are the porcine bioprostheses, including the Hancock and Carpentier-Edwards valves. These are porcine aortic valves that have been preserved and fixed within a polypropylene mount attached to a Dacron sewing ring. Pericardial prostheses are also in use today. Because the tissue has been preserved, it is less pliable than native valve tissue. The leaflets themselves are supported by stents, which vary in number and design and arise vertically from the sewing ring. More recently, "stentless" bioprostheses have been developed for use in the aortic position. This design is characterized by leaflet support via a flexible cuff and the absence of rigid stents. Freestyle valves are porcine aortic valves that include the anulus, valve, and root preserved intact. They are customized by the surgeon in the operating room at the time of implantation.

Homograft valves are derived from human aortic or pulmonary valve tissue that has undergone cryopreservation and may be either stented or unstented. Such prosthetic valves have several advantages, and the Ross procedure is an example of their use. Homografts are also used in valved conduits but are rarely used to replace a mitral or tricuspid valve.

NORMAL PROSTHETIC VALVE FUNCTION

The indications for echocardiography in patients with prosthetic valves are summarized in Table 14.2. Visualization of prosthetic valves often requires a combination of transthoracic and transesophageal imaging. Two-dimensional echocardiography is used to determine the type of valve and to evaluate its structure and function. Using this modality, the stability of the sewing ring is assessed. Rocking or independent motion of the prosthesis is often an indication of dehiscence. The presence of abnormal

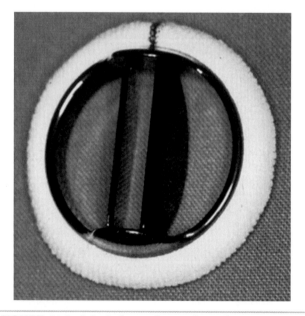

FIGURE 14.2. A St. Jude prosthetic valve is shown.

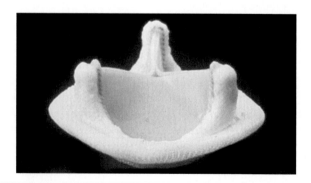

FIGURE 14.3. A porcine bioprosthetic valve is shown.

▶ **TABLE 14.2 Indications for Echocardiography in Interventions for Valvular Heart Disease and Prosthetic Valves**

Indications	Class
1. Assessment of the timing of valvular intervention based on ventricular compensation, function, and/or severity of primary and secondary lesions	I
2. Selection of alternative therapies for mitral valve disease (such as balloon valvuloplasty, operative valve repair, valve replacement)[a]	I
3. Use of echocardiography (especially TEE) in guiding the performance of interventional techniques and surgery (eg, balloon valvotomy and valve repair) for valvular disease	I
4. Postintervention baseline studies for valve function (early) and ventricular remodeling (late)	I
5. Reevaluation of patients with valve replacement with changing clinical signs and symptoms; suspected prosthetic dysfunction (stenosis, regurgitation) or thrombosis[a]	I
6. Routine reevaluation study after baseline studies of patients with valve replacements with mild to moderate ventricular dysfunction without changing clinical signs or symptoms	IIa
7. Routine reevaluation at the time of increased failure rate of a bioprosthesis without clinical evidence of prosthetic dysfunction	IIb
8. Routine reevaluation of patients with valve replacements without suspicion of valvular dysfunction and unchanged clinical signs and symptoms	III
9. Patients whose clinical status precludes therapeutic interventions	III

[a]TEE may provide incremental value in addition to information obtained by TTE.
Adapted with permission from Cheitlin MD, Alpert JS, Armstrong WF, et al. ACC/AHA Guidelines for the Clinical Application of Echocardiography: a report of the American College of Cardiology/American Heart Association Task Force on Practice Guidelines (Committee on Application of Echocardiography) developed in collaboration with the American Society of Echocardiography. Circulation 1997;95:1686-1744, with permission.
TEE, transesophageal echocardiography; TTE, transthoracic echocardiography.

masses, such as thrombi or vegetations, should be determined. Bear in mind that shadowing from the prosthesis may obscure such pathology and multiple imaging windows may be required for a complete evaluation. Motion of the leaflets, disks, or occluder mechanism should also be assessed from the two-dimensional study. An important early step in the echocardiographic assessment of prosthetic valves is recognizing the range of normal find-

ings. Figure 14.4 is a normally functioning porcine aortic prosthesis. Leaflet opening during systole resembles that of a normal native valve. The overall appearance is so similar, in fact, that normally functioning aortic bioprostheses are occasionally mistaken for "normal" aortic valves when historical information is not available. When examined carefully, however, the sewing ring and struts are more echogenic than normal and tend to shadow the leaflets, a clue to the presence of prosthetic material.

Figure 14.5 shows a Starr-Edwards valve in the mitral position. The protruding, high-profile cage in the left ventricle is diagnostic. When examined in real-time, the poppet can be seen moving forward and backward in the cage. These valves are highly echogenic, and small thrombi or vegetations can be easily hidden or overlooked. A normally functioning St. Jude mitral prosthesis is presented in Figure 14.6. The two hemidisks open and close in synchrony, although it is often difficult to distinguish both on transthoracic imaging. Significant shadowing occurs, and the left atrium is not well seen in most cases. Figure 14.7 is a stable aortic St. Jude valve. In this example, the disks are obscured by the walls of the aorta. A distinct shadow from the sewing ring is apparent, extending into the left atrium. Stentless aortic valves are the most recent option in prostheses and are being implanted with increasing frequency. An example of a normal Medtronic Freestyle valve is provided in Figure 14.8. Distinguishing a normally functioning stentless valve from a native aortic valve can be impossible.

Blood flow through normally functioning prosthetic valves differs from flow through native valves in several important ways. First, artificial heart valves are inher-

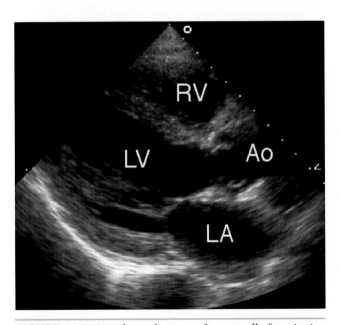

FIGURE 14.4. An echocardiogram of a normally functioning porcine bioprosthetic aortic valve is demonstrated. Ao, aorta; LA, left atrium; LV, left ventricle; RV, right ventricle.

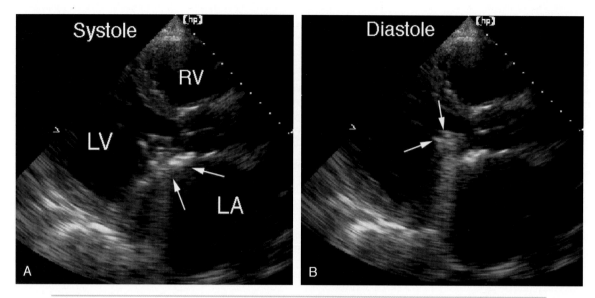

FIGURE 14.5. A normally functioning Starr-Edwards mitral prosthesis is shown. **A:** During systole, the poppet is seated within the sewing ring (*arrows*). **B:** During diastole, the poppet moves forward into the cage (*arrows*), allowing blood flow around the occluder. LA, left atrium; LV, left ventricle; RV, right ventricle.

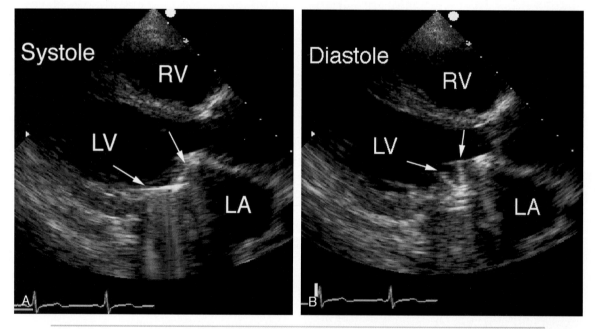

FIGURE 14.6. A normally functioning St. Jude mitral prosthesis is demonstrated. **A:** During systole, the hemidisks are shown in the closed position (*arrows*). **B:** During diastole, the two disks are recorded in the open position (*arrows*). LA, left atrium; LV, left ventricle; RV, right ventricle.

ently stenotic. There is a variety of explanations for this consistent observation. The sewing ring of the valve may be too small relative to the flow. In young patients, what passes for an adequately sized valve in childhood may become increasingly stenotic as the patient grows. More importantly, the effective orifice area is significantly smaller than the area of the sewing ring because the valve assembly (i.e., the occluder mechanism) occupies some of the central space. Leaflets of bioprostheses, by virtue of the preservation process, are stiffer and therefore these valves have a higher resistance to forward flow compared with equivalently sized native valves. Thus, flow velocity through a normally functioning artificial valve is generally higher than would occur through a normal native valve. However, the range of velocities through a normally functioning bioprosthesis is consid-

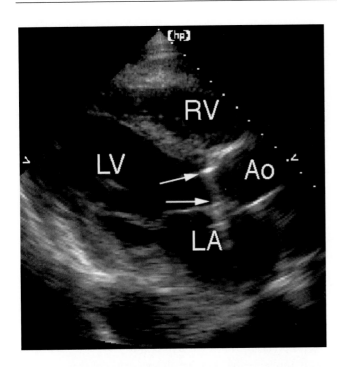

FIGURE 14.7. A normally functioning St. Jude aortic prosthesis is demonstrated. The sewing ring is indicated by the *arrows*. The walls of the aortic root (*Ao*) often obscure the motion of the disks. LA, left atrium; LV, left ventricle; RV, right ventricle.

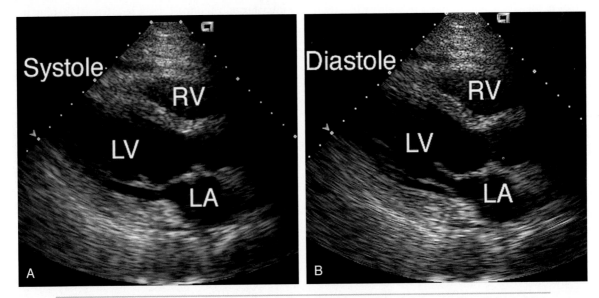

FIGURE 14.8. A normally functioning Medtronic Freestyle valve is shown in the aortic position. **A:** During systole, the valve is shown in the opened position. **B:** During diastole, the cusps are barely visible. Normally functioning stentless valves appear very similar to normal native valves. LA, left atrium; LV, left ventricle; RV, right ventricle.

erable. Both valve size and type determine the pressure gradient that one can expect in the absence of dysfunction. For example, stented bioprosthetic valves may have slightly higher gradients than mechanical valves of similar size, which tend to have higher gradients than stentless valves. For all these reasons, the range of velocities that must be considered normal varies widely among prosthetic valves. This is illustrated in Figure 14.9. In Figure 14.9A, a newly implanted St. Jude aortic prosthesis is shown. Although functioning normally by clinical criteria, the Doppler study demonstrates a maximal velocity of 290 cm/sec and a mean gradient of 20 mm Hg. Also note the distinctive "clicks" that correspond to the opening and closing of the disks. In contrast, Figure 14.9B illustrates flow through a normally functioning bioprosthetic aortic valve. In this case, no significant increase in velocity is present. Prosthetic valve clicks are not typically seen in normally functioning bioprostheses.

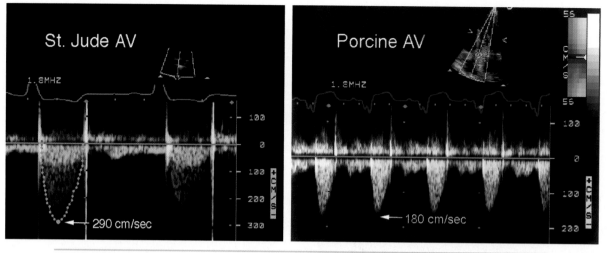

FIGURE 14.9. Doppler evaluations of a normally functioning St. Jude bileaflet prosthesis **(left)** and a porcine prosthesis **(right)** are provided. In both cases, contour of the flow signal and maximal velocity are within the expected range. Note the opening and closing valve clicks that are associated with the mechanical but not the tissue prosthesis.

Another important difference between native and prosthetic valves is the shape and number of orifices through which forward flow occurs. As noted previously, a bileaflet tilting disk valve has three separate orifices, a rectangular-shaped central orifice surrounded by two larger semicircular orifices (Fig. 14.10). Flow velocity is highest through the central orifice, and if this flow is sampled with continuous wave Doppler imaging, an overestimation of the true gradient can occur. This is because flow through all three orifices contributes to net gradient. By only sampling the highest velocity through the central orifice and ignoring lower velocity flow through the other two, an overestimation of true gradient occurs. Flow through a caged ball valve does not go through a well-defined orifice but rather goes around the periphery of the spherical occluder (Fig. 14.11). The variability and orientation of the flow complicate the Doppler interrogation of these valves. Flow through bioprostheses is often triangular in shape and may occur through an area that is significantly smaller than the sewing ring itself. Note in Figure 14.12 the position of the three struts and how they effectively form a triangular orifice, the area of which is considerably smaller than the surrounding sewing ring. All these factors contribute to the challenges inherent to assessing prosthetic valve function by any technique.

A potentially important phenomenon affecting flow through prosthetic valves involves *pressure recovery*. This occurs when a portion of the kinetic energy released as blood crosses the valve is recovered in the form of pressure downstream. The amount of energy that is recovered depends on how smoothly the transition of flow occurs between the valve and the downstream conduit. For this

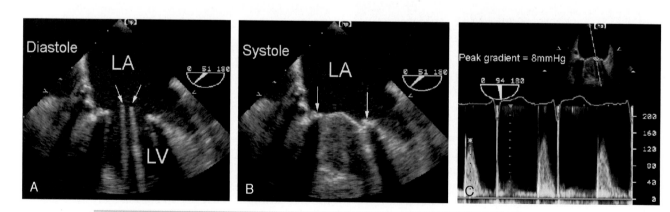

FIGURE 14.10. A transesophageal echocardiogram from a patient with a St. Jude mitral prosthesis demonstrates the appearance of the discs during diastole **(A)** and systole **(B)**. This technique is ideal to record opening and closing of the hemidisks. **C:** Flow through one of the larger semicircular orifices is recorded using transthoracic Doppler imaging. LA, left atrium; LV, left ventricle.

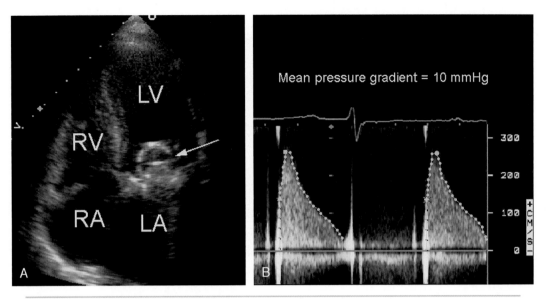

FIGURE 14.11. A: A Starr-Edwards mitral prosthesis is shown (*arrow*). **B:** Doppler imaging demonstrates flow through the valve. The mean pressure gradient is approximately 10 mm Hg. LA, left atrium; LV, left ventricle; RA, right atrium; RV, right ventricle.

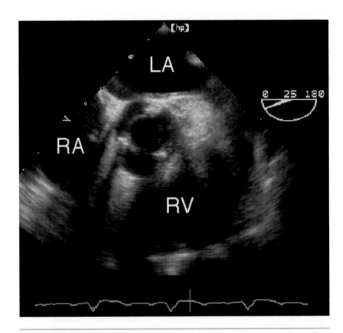

FIGURE 14.12. A short-axis view of a porcine aortic prosthesis from transesophageal echocardiography is demonstrated. The three struts are visualized, forming a triangular-shaped orifice. LA, left atrium; RA, right atrium; RV, right ventricle.

reason, pressure recovery is most clinically relevant at the aortic position in the presence of a St. Jude prosthesis. The net effect is the development of a high, but very localized, gradient through the central orifice of the prosthesis immediately distal to the disks (Fig. 14.13). Then, as pressure recovers (or increases) downstream, the net pressure gradient diminishes. It should be emphasized

that this overestimation is a real phenomenon, although less physiologically relevant than the net gradient between the left ventricle and the aorta.

Another unique aspect of prosthetic valve function is the presence of normal, or physiologic, regurgitation. This occurs with virtually all types of mechanical prostheses and is actually part of the design of the valve. Physiologic regurgitation can be divided into two types: closure backflow and leakage. Closure backflow occurs due to the flow reversal required to close the occluding mechanism. This results in a small amount of regurgitation that ends once the occluder mechanism is seated in the sewing ring (Fig. 14.14). Leakage backflow occurs after the prosthesis has closed and is the result of a small amount of retrograde flow between and around the occluding mechanism. It is often part of the design of the prosthesis to provide a washing mechanism and prevent thrombus formation on its upstream side. Because leakage backflow may be holosystolic (or holodiastolic, depending on valve location), it must be distinguished from pathologic regurgitation. This depends on the severity and the pattern of regurgitation. For example, leakage through a bileaflet valve often results in two symmetric narrow jets directed obliquely from the edges of the valve. This type of physiologic regurgitation is illustrated in Figure 14.15.

Despite these differences in flow characteristics, the basic Doppler principles applied to native valves are also relevant to the study of prosthetic valves. For example, Doppler imaging can be used to measure both the maximal and mean pressure gradient across prostheses (Fig. 14.16). The assumptions that are critical to the modified

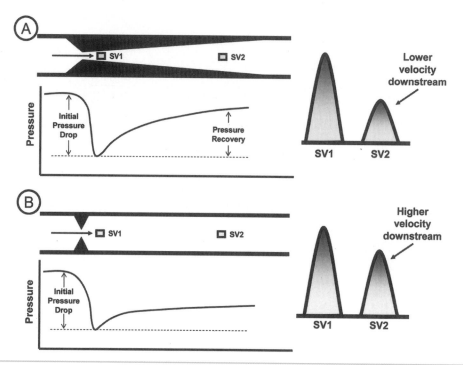

FIGURE 14.13. The concept of pressure recovery is illustrated in this schematic. In the top panel, in the absence of pressure recovery, different locations for sample volume (SV) measurement yield fairly similar velocities. In panel B, flow through a tapered stenosis results in significant pressure recovery downstream from the obstruction. In this case, sampling within the obstruction (SV1) yields a higher velocity compared to a sample site downstream (SV2) where pressure recovery has occurred. At this site, the recovery of pressure is associated with a lower velocity. See text for details.

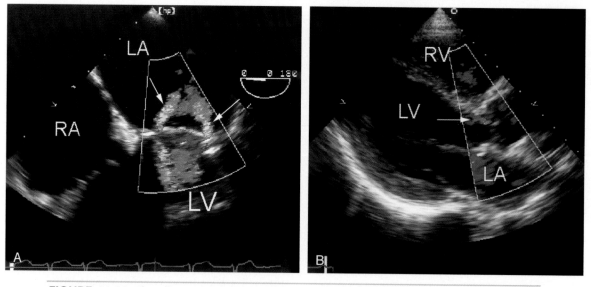

FIGURE 14.14. Physiologic regurgitation is demonstrated through a normally functioning St. Jude mitral prosthesis (*arrows*) **(A)** and a porcine aortic prosthesis (*arrow*) **(B)**. LA, left atrium; RA, right atrium; RV, right ventricle; LV, left ventricle.

Bernoulli equation apply to prosthetic valves as well. Thus, the correlation between pressure gradients obtained by the Doppler technique compared with cardiac catheterization is generally very good. However, because of the existence of multiple jets through many types of prosthetic valves, more than one velocity pattern can often be recorded. As noted previously, the phenomenon of pressure recovery may also lead to overestimation of the pressure gradient. Figure 14.17 illustrates flow through different types of mitral prostheses. Note the variability in the contour and velocity among the four examples. Gradients across "normal" prosthetic valves vary across a wider range compared with native valves. For this reason, it is often helpful to obtain a baseline Doppler imaging

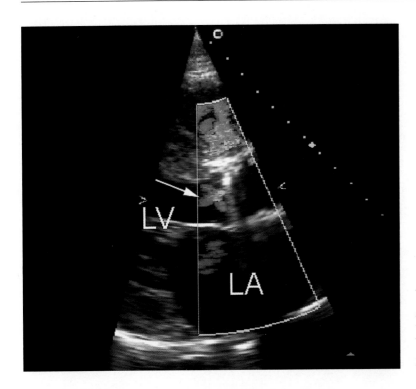

FIGURE 14.15. Physiologic regurgitation through a St. Jude aortic valve is shown. The jets originate at the periphery and appear to cross just below the valve (*arrow*). The occurrence of this type of regurgitation is part of the design of many prosthetic valves. LA, left atrium; LV, left ventricle.

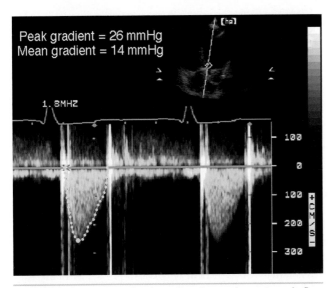

FIGURE 14.16. Doppler imaging is used to record flow through an aortic prosthesis. The peak and mean gradients are indicated. Note the presence of valve clicks at the time of opening and closing.

study in all patients at a time when the valve is known to be functioning normally, such as during the first postoperative clinic visit. This can then be used as a reference for future evaluations to help determine whether a given pressure gradient is normal or abnormal for the individual. In addition, tables have been published providing a range of normal values for different types of valves in the various positions.

The continuity equation can also be used to measure the effective orifice area of prosthetic valves. The value of this measurement has the same limitations just described for pressure gradients. Finally, for prosthetic mitral and tricuspid valves, the pressure half-time technique is useful to quantify the severity of stenosis. However, pressure half-time generally overestimates the valve area in the presence of a mitral prosthesis. Again, having a baseline study and using the patient as his or her own control is essential for future management.

GENERAL APPROACH TO IMAGING

Transthoracic two-dimensional imaging is generally adequate to distinguish among the various types of prosthetic valves. However, the high reflectance of the prosthetic material creates challenges for the echocardiographer. Because the speed of sound changes as it passes through prosthetic materials, size and appearance can be distorted. Some decrease in gain setting is generally necessary to compensate for these differences. The high reflectance also leads to shadowing behind the prostheses. Reverberations frequently appear behind the prosthetic structures, which may obscure targets of interest. To overcome these problems, multiple echocardiographic windows must be used to fully interrogate the areas around prosthetic valves. In many cases, transesophageal echocardiography is necessary to provide a thorough examination.

The two-dimensional echocardiographic appearance of bioprostheses more closely approximates that of native

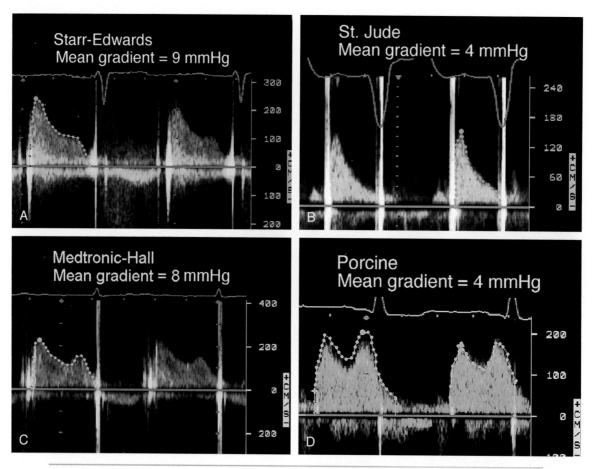

FIGURE 14.17. A–D: Doppler recording of flow through four different mitral prosthetic valves is demonstrated. The mean gradient across each prosthesis is indicated.

valves. In fact, newer stentless aortic prostheses can be nearly indistinguishable from a normal native aortic valve. For stented valves, imaging is ideally performed with the ultrasound beam aligned parallel to flow to avoid the shadowing effects of the stents and sewing ring. The leaflets themselves are quite similar to native valve tissue, both in texture and excursion. Over time, bioprostheses tend to thicken and become more fibrotic, leading to increased echogenicity and reduced excursion on two-dimensional imaging (Fig. 14.18). Such valves can become stenotic and/or regurgitant. This illustration demonstrates a brittle, fibrotic porcine mitral valve with partial rupture of one cusp leading to severe mitral regurgitation. In all cases, a combination of two-dimensional and Doppler imaging is required to thoroughly assess bioprosthetic valves (Fig. 14.19).

For the reasons noted above, mechanical valves can be quite difficult to assess with two-dimensional echocardiography. Although gross abnormalities can be detected, more subtle changes are often missed, especially with transthoracic imaging. The primary goals of two-dimensional echocardiography in this setting are to confirm stability of the sewing ring, determine the specific type of prosthesis, confirm the opening and closing motion of the occluding mechanism, and evaluate for gross structural abnormalities such as vegetations and thrombi. Assessing the mobility of the occluding mechanism can be difficult. However, through careful interrogation, the rapid motion of the leading edge of the disk or ball generally can be recorded. In normal prostheses, the motion is brisk and consistent with each beat (Figs. 14.5–14.8). M-mode imaging can be useful in this case to more precisely define the brisk opening and closing and the degree of excursion of the occluder (Fig. 14.20). For bileaflet prostheses, it is important to search for both hemidisks, which often have slightly out of phase motion as they open and close in close proximity (Figs. 14.6 and 14.10).

As with two-dimensional imaging, the Doppler examination also faces unique challenges in the setting of a prosthetic valve. Because of the variability of flow through and around the different prostheses, color flow imaging is often helpful to define the location and direction of the various flow patterns. Some prosthetic valves have more than one orifice and, consequently, a complex

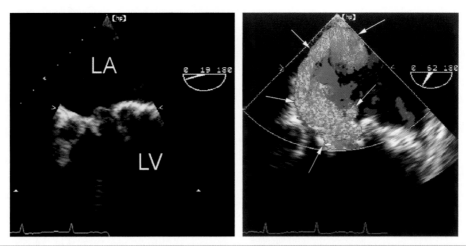

FIGURE 14.18. An example of primary tissue degeneration involving a porcine mitral valve is provided. The leaflets are thickened and fibrotic with decreased mobility **(left)**. **Right:** Color Doppler imaging demonstrates severe mitral regurgitation with an eccentric jet (*arrows*). LA, left atrium; LV, left ventricle.

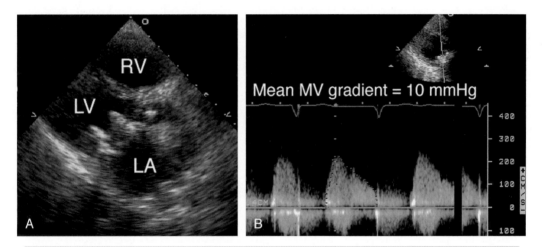

FIGURE 14.19. **A:** An example of a mildly thickened porcine mitral prosthesis is shown. The structure and motion of the leaflets are often obscured by the struts. **B:** Doppler imaging demonstrates a mean gradient of 10 mm Hg. LA, left atrium; LV, left ventricle; RV, right ventricle.

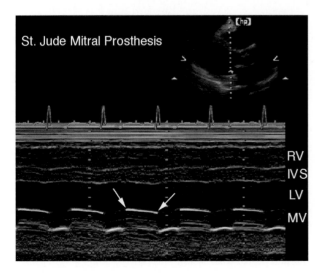

FIGURE 14.20. M-mode echocardiogram of a St. Jude mitral prosthetic valve. M-mode echocardiography is ideal to record the brisk opening and closing of the disks (*arrows*). IVS, interventricular septum; LV, left ventricle; MV, mitral valve; RV, right ventricle.

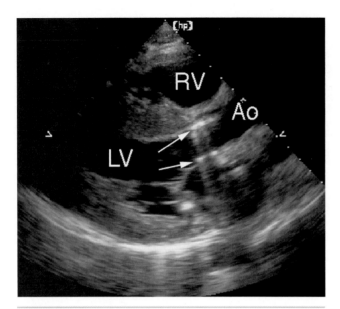

FIGURE 14.21. The presence of a St. Jude aortic prosthesis (*arrows*) creates a pattern of reverberations that extends into the left atrium. This creates a shadowing effect and can obscure the presence of mitral regurgitation. Ao, aorta; LV, left ventricle; RV, right ventricle.

flow profile. Once the desired flow patterns are localized with color flow imaging, pulsed and continuous wave Doppler imaging can be oriented to quantify flow velocity. As already noted, velocities will always tend to be higher through prosthetic valves, depending in part on the size of the specific prosthesis. Whenever velocity is higher than expected, consider the possibility of pressure recovery, as discussed previously.

Assessing valvular regurgitation is primarily limited by the shadowing effect of the prosthetic valve itself. Because the signal-to-noise ratio for Doppler imaging is lower compared with two-dimensional echocardiographic imaging, the shadowing effect is even more pronounced and the ability to record a Doppler signal "behind" a prosthetic valve is very limited. Multiple views must be used to fully interrogate the regurgitant signal. Figure 14.21 demonstrates how the shadowing effect of an aortic prosthesis obscures the left atrium from the parasternal window. It is also important to distinguish transvalvular from perivalvular regurgitation. This is best accomplished using color flow imaging to interrogate the circumference of the sewing ring on the upstream side of the valve (Fig. 14.22). With the increased sensitivity of modern equipment, particularly using the transesophageal approach, a small amount of perivalvular regurgitation may be recorded in the immediate postoperative period that will often disappear or diminish over time (Fig. 14.23). Spectral Doppler recordings of prosthetic valve flow will also include brief, high-velocity signals referred to as "clicks." These are intense recordings associated with both the opening and closing of the occluder mechanism. They provide useful information on timing and are particularly helpful to identify the various phases of filling and ejection. In Figure 14.24, both normal and an abnormal St. Jude aortic prostheses are shown. In Figure 14.24A, note the valve clicks marking opening and closing of the normal valve. Figure 14.24B is taken from a patient with a prosthesis that is partially obstructed by a thrombus on the sewing ring. Note that the opening valve click is absent, and the closing click is very faint. The high velocity is evidence of the increased pressure gradient across the partially obstructed valve.

PROSTHETIC AORTIC VALVES

Transthoracic M-mode and two-dimensional echocardiography have relatively low sensitivity for detecting dysfunction of aortic prostheses. Gross abnormalities, such

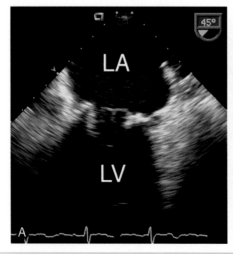
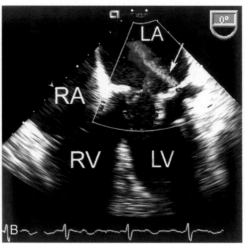

FIGURE 14.22. **A:** A porcine mitral prosthesis is visualized using transesophageal echocardiography. **B:** Color Doppler imaging demonstrates both transvalvular and perivalvular (*arrow*) mitral regurgitation. LA, left atrium; LV, left ventricle; RA, right atrium; RV, right ventricle.

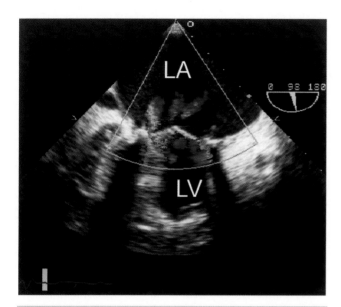

FIGURE 14.23. This St. Jude mitral prosthesis was evaluated in the operating room immediately after implantation when a mild degree of perivalvular regurgitation may be present. In most cases, this resolves over time. Color Doppler imaging indicates both central and peripheral jets, consistent with mild mitral regurgitation. LA, left atrium; LV, left ventricle.

as valve dehiscence or large thrombi or vegetations, can be identified using two-dimensional echocardiography from the apical window. Thickened and fibrocalcific leaflets of bioprostheses can also be visualized, but assessing the functional significance of such changes is difficult. Thus, most of the diagnostic information related to aortic prostheses depends on a thorough and quantitative Doppler study. Both the peak instantaneous and mean pressure gradients across the prosthesis should be

recorded from multiple views. The correlation between Doppler gradients and values obtained with cardiac catheterization is quite high, especially when the tests are performed simultaneously. Agreement between Doppler imaging and catheterization tends to be highest for mean gradient and the inherent differences between peak instantaneous and peak-to-peak gradients should be considered.

The range of normal values depends primarily on the size of the prosthesis (Table 14.3). For example, a 29 mm St. Jude aortic prosthesis will generally have a maximal velocity of less than 2.5 m/sec, whereas a normally functioning 19 mm St. Jude prosthesis may have a maximal velocity of as high as 4 to 4.5 m/sec. Consequently, the mean gradient across a 19 mm valve is roughly twice the mean gradient across a corresponding 29 mm prosthesis. Differences among the various types of prosthetic valves (assuming a similar size) are much less. The exceptions to this are aortic homografts and stentless valves, which consistently have lower gradients and exhibit hemodynamics that more closely approximate the native valve.

When the continuity equation is used to estimate the effective orifice area of a prosthetic valve, it should be remembered that this area corresponds to the *vena contracta* of flow rather than the actual orifice. The equation itself is identical to the one used in the setting of native valve stenosis (Fig. 14.25). If the outflow tract dimension cannot be accurately measured, some investigators suggest substituting the sewing ring outer diameter for this value. Again, the most important point is that the Doppler recording and the diameter measurement be obtained at the same level. The Doppler velocity index (DVI) is a simple and useful alternative for evaluating stenosis. DVI is dimensionless and is calculated as the ratio between the

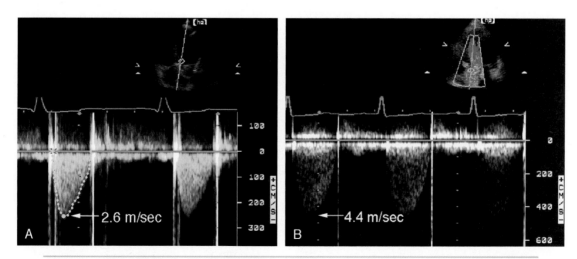

FIGURE 14.24. Examples of flow through two different St. Jude aortic prosthetic valves are provided. **A:** Flow velocity is normal and crisp valve clicks are present. **B:** Jet velocity is increased, indicating a peak pressure gradient of approximately 77 mm Hg. Valve clicks, especially at the time of valve opening, are diminished.

▶ TABLE 14.3 **Range of Normal Values for Doppler Evaluation of Aortic Prostheses**

Category	Specific Type	Size (mm)	Gradient (mm Hg) Maximum	Gradient (mm Hg) Mean	Peak Velocity (m/sec)
Stentless					
	Biocor stentless	21	36±4	18±4	
		23	29±8	19±7	3.0±0.6
		25	29±7	18±7	2.8±0.5
		27	26±3	18±3	2.7±0.2
	Edwards Prima stentless	21	31±17	16±11	
		23	23±10	12±5	2.8±0.4
		25	20±10	11±9	2.7±0.3
		27	16±7	7±4	
		29	11±9	5±4	
	Toronto porcine	21	19±12	8±4	
		23	23	7±4	
		25	12±6	6±3	
		27	10±5	5±2	
		29	8±4	4±2	
Bioprosthetic stented					
	Carpentier-Edwards	19	43±13	26±8	
		21	28±8	17±6	2.4±0.5
		23	29±7	16±6	2.8±0.4
		25	24±7	13±4	2.4±0.5
		27	22±8	12±5	2.3±0.4
		29	22±6	10±3	2.4±0.4
	Hancock II	21	20±4	15±4	
		23	25±6	17±7	
		25	20±2	11±3	
		27	14±3		
		29	15±3		
	Medtronic intact	19	39±15	24±9	
		21	34±13	19±8	2.7±0.4
		23	31±10	19±6	2.7±0.4
		25	27±11	16±6	2.6±0.4
		27	25±8	15±4	2.5±0.4
		29	31±12	16±2	2.8
Tilting disk					
	Björk-Shiley monostrut	19	46	27±8	3.3±0.6
		21	32±10	19±6	2.9±0.4
		23	27±10	15±6	2.7±0.5
		25	22±7	13±5	2.5±0.4
		27	18±8	10±4	2.1±0.4
		29	12±8	8±4	1.9±0.2
	Medtronic-Hall	20	34±13	17±5	2.9±0.4
		21	27±11	14±6	2.4±0.4
		23	27±9	14±5	2.4±0.6
		25	17±7	10±4	2.3±0.5
		27	19±10	9±6	2.1±0.5
Bileaflet					
	CarboMedics	19	33±11	12±5	3.1±0.4
		21	26±10	13±4	2.6±0.5
		23	25±7	11±4	2.4±0.4
		25	20±9	9±5	2.3±0.3
		27	19±7	8±3	2.2±0.4
		29	13±5	6±3	1.9±0.3

▶ TABLE 14.3 Range of Normal Values for Doppler Evaluation of Aortic Prostheses (continued)

Category	Specific Type	Size (mm)	Gradient (mm Hg) Maximum	Mean	Peak Velocity (m/sec)
Bileaflet *(cont.)*					
	St. Jude Medical	19	35±11	19±6	2.9±0.5
		21	28±10	16±6	2.6±0.5
		23	25±8	14±5	2.6±0.4
		25	23±8	13±5	2.4±0.5
		27	20±8	11±5	2.2±0.4
		29	18±6	10±3	2.0±0.1
Caged ball					
	Starr-Edwards	23	33±13	22±9	3.5±0.5
		24	34±10	22±8	3.4±0.5
		26	32±9	20±6	3.2±0.4
		27	31±6	19±4	
		29	29±9	16±6	

Modified from Rosenhek R, Binder T, Maurer G, Baumgartner H. Normal values for Doppler echocardiographic assessment of heart valve prostheses. J Am Soc Echocardiogr 2003;16:1116–1127, with permission.

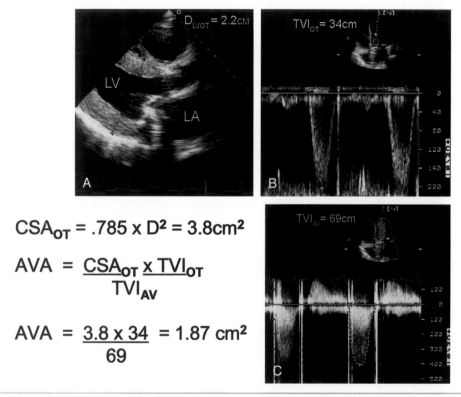

$$CSA_{OT} = .785 \times D^2 = 3.8 cm^2$$

$$AVA = \frac{CSA_{OT} \times TVI_{OT}}{TVI_{AV}}$$

$$AVA = \frac{3.8 \times 34}{69} = 1.87 cm^2$$

FIGURE 14.25. The continuity equation can be used to calculate the effective valve area across prostheses. **A:** The diameter of the left ventricular outflow tract is measured. **B:** Time velocity integral (TVI) of the outflow tract is calculated using planimetry. **C:** Using continuous wave Doppler imaging, flow through the prosthetic valve is recorded. Because of a hyperdynamic left ventricle (LV), the TVI$_{OT}$ and the maximal pressure gradient are quite high. Despite the maximal gradient of 65 mm Hg, the aortic valve area is approximately 1.9 cm². The calculations used to measure valve area are provided. CSA, cross-sectional area; D$_{LVOT}$, outflow tract diameter; LA, left atrium.

outflow tract velocity and the maximal velocity through the prosthesis. In the absence of any gradient, the two velocities will be the same, yielding a ratio of one. Because all prostheses are somewhat stenotic, a DVI of less than 1 is consistently obtained. The expected range for normally functioning aortic prostheses is 0.35 to 0.5. Although this dimensionless number has limited utility in isolation, it can be obtained reproducibly and provides a useful parameter to detect changes over time. In addition, it avoids the challenges of measuring the outflow tract diameter, as described above.

Assessing regurgitation is similar in prosthetic and native aortic valves with two exceptions. First, it must be remembered that some degree of regurgitation is a normal finding for most prostheses. Distinguishing physiologic from pathologic regurgitation is generally a matter of degree. Second, shadowing from the prosthesis can obscure significant regurgitant jets, mandating the use of multiple windows (and often transesophageal echocardiography) to completely interrogate the left ventricular outflow tract. Distinguishing valvular from perivalvular regurgitation is also important. Using either the transthoracic or transesophageal approach, a short-axis view at and immediately below the level of the sewing ring often allows this distinction to be made (Figs. 14.26 and 14.27). For many patients, however, transesophageal imaging is a more accurate way of detecting the presence and extent of perivalvular regurgitation. Figure 14.28 is an example of mild perivalvular regurgitation associated with a stentless aortic prosthesis.

PROSTHETIC MITRAL VALVES

Visualizing mitral prostheses with transthoracic echocardiography is somewhat easier than visualizing aortic prostheses. This is because the prosthetic mitral valve is seated within the mitral anulus and can be easily visualized from both the parasternal and apical windows. In contrast, aortic prostheses may be partially obscured by the walls of the

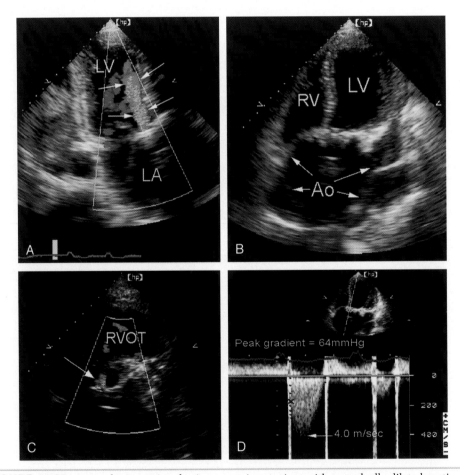

FIGURE 14.26. A prosthetic aortic valve is present in a patient with a markedly dilated aortic root. **A:** The presence of aortic regurgitation is detected using color Doppler imaging (*arrows*). **B:** The dilated aortic root (*Ao*) is demonstrated from the apical window. **C:** The short-axis view identifies the origin of the regurgitant jet (*arrow*). **D:** The gradient across the prosthesis is demonstrated. LA, left atrium; LV, left ventricle; RV, right ventricle; RVOT, right ventricular outflow tract.

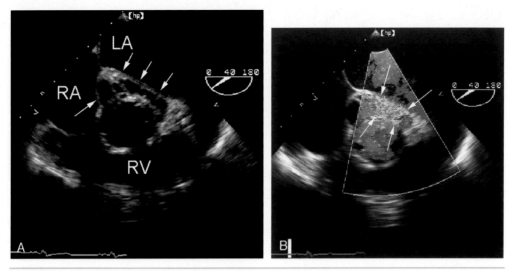

FIGURE 14.27. An example of an aortic root abscess is demonstrated. **A:** In the short-axis view, an echo-free space is seen posterior to the aortic root (*arrows*). **B:** Color Doppler imaging demonstrates flow within the abscess cavity (*arrows*) and associated perivalvular regurgitation. LA, left atrium; RA, right atrium; RV, right ventricle.

aorta (from the parasternal view) and by the prostheses itself from the apical view. Evaluating the stability of the mitral prosthesis, excluding dehiscence, and visualizing the motion of leaflets or the occluding mechanism are generally possible with transthoracic imaging.

Using Doppler imaging, the antegrade flow through the prosthesis can be accurately recorded (Fig. 14.29). Normal values for the various types and sizes of mitral prosthetic valves are provided in Table 14.4. The mean mitral pressure gradient is derived by planimetry of the mitral envelope, taking care to align the Doppler beam as close as possible to the direction of inflow (Figs. 14.19 and 14.30). Because of the orientation of the prosthesis and

the resulting transprosthesis flow direction, nonstandard views may be necessary for optimal alignment of the Doppler beam. Note in Figure 14.30 that the mitral flow recording is obtained from the parasternal long-axis view. The pressure half-time method can also be performed in the setting of prosthetic valves. With native valves, it was empirically determined that mitral valve area was approximated by the equation

$$\text{MV area} = 220 \div P_{1/2}t \qquad \text{[Eq. 14.1]}$$

When the same approach is applied to prosthetic valves, the formula tends to overestimate the effective ori-

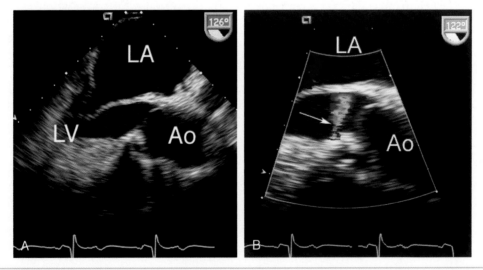

FIGURE 14.28. **A:** A transesophageal echocardiogram from a patient with a stentless aortic prosthesis is provided. **B:** A mild degree of perivalvular aortic regurgitation (*arrow*) is demonstrated using color Doppler imaging. Ao, aorta; LA, left atrium; LV, left ventricle.

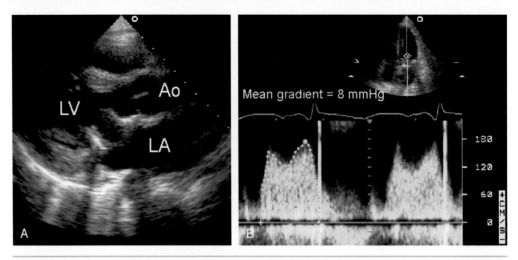

FIGURE 14.29. A normally functioning porcine mitral prosthesis is shown. **A:** The long-axis view records the struts. The leaflet themselves were not visualized. **B:** Doppler imaging demonstrates a mean pressure gradient of 8 mm Hg across the prosthesis. Ao, aorta; LA, left atrium; LV, left ventricle.

▶ TABLE 14.4 **Range of Normal Values for Doppler Evaluation of Mitral Prostheses**

Category	Specific Type	Size (mm)	Gradient (mm Hg) Maximum	Gradient (mm Hg) Mean	Peak Velocity (m/sec)
Stentless					
	Biocor	27	13±1		
		29	14±2		
		31	12±1		
		33	12±1		
Bioprosthetic stented					
	Carpentier-Edwards	27		6±2	98±28
		29		5±2	92±14
		31		4±2	92±19
		33		6±3	93±12
	Hancock I	27	10±4	5±2	
		29	7±3	2±1	115±20
		31	4±1	5±2	95±17
		33	3±2	4±2	90±12
	Ionescu-Shiley	25		5±1	93±11
		27		3±1	100±28
		29		3±1	85±8
		31		4±1	100±36
Tilting disk					
	Omnicarbon	25		6±2	102±16
		27		5±2	105±33
		29		5±2	120±40
		31		4±1	134±31
	Björk-Shiley	25	12±4	6±2	99±27
		27	10±4	5±2	89±28
		29	8±3	3±1	79±17
		31	6±3	2±2	70±14
Bileaflet					
	St. Jude Medical	25		3±1	75±4
		27		5±2	75±10
		29		4±2	85±10
		31		4±2	74±13
	CarboMedics	25	10±2	4±1	93±8
		27	9±3	3±1	89±20
		29	9±3	3±1	88±17
		31	9±2	3±1	92±24
		33	9±2	5±3	93±12
Caged ball					
	Starr-Edwards	28		7±3	
		30	12±5	7±3	125±25
		32	12±4	5±3	110±25

Modified from Rosenhek R, Binder T, Maurer G, Baumgartner H. Normal values for Doppler echocardiographic assessment of heart valve prostheses. J Am Soc Echocardiogr 2003;16:1116–1127, with permission.

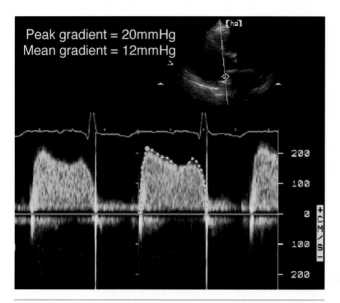

Peak gradient = 20mmHg
Mean gradient = 12mmHg

FIGURE 14.30. Doppler recording of flow through a porcine mitral valve is shown. Both the peak and mean gradient are derived by planimetry. Note that the recording was obtained from the parasternal window. In this case, this view provided optimal alignment with mitral inflow.

fice area. Despite this limitation, prolongation of the pressure half-time, especially when a baseline has been established, is a reliable marker of obstruction across the prosthesis and is less flow-dependent than gradient alone. In most patients, both mean gradient and pressure half-time should be assessed to determine whether prosthetic valve stenosis is present. Alternatively, the continuity equation can be applied (in the absence of mitral regurgitation) according to the formula, in which MV is the mitral valve, LVOT is the left ventricular outflow tract, and TVI is the time velocity integral:

$$\text{MV area} = \text{Area}_{\text{LVOT}} * \left(\frac{\text{TVI}_{\text{LVOT}}}{\text{TVI}_{\text{MV}}} \right) \quad [\text{Eq. 14.2}]$$

Detecting regurgitation through or around a mitral prosthesis using transthoracic echocardiography is limited by the shadowing effect of the prosthetic material. Whether imaging is performed from the parasternal or the apical view, the prosthetic valve will always obscure a portion of the left atrium so the sensitivity of this method is reduced (Figs. 14.31 and 14.32). In the presence of both aortic and mitral prostheses, most of the left atrium is shadowed and the detection of mitral regurgitation in such patients is very limited. In contrast, the transesophageal approach offers an excellent opportunity to assess the entire left atrium in the presence of prosthetic valves (Fig. 14.33). Differentiating between physiologic and pathologic mitral regurgitation is based on a variety of factors. Using the transesophageal approach, some degree of regurgitation is detected in as many as 90% of normally functioning mitral prostheses. Characteristics of "normal" prosthetic regurgitation include a jet area less than 2 cm^2 and a jet length less than 2.5 cm. In addition, the patterns of regurgitant flow are typical for each individual prosthesis. For example, a St. Jude mitral prosthesis often displays one central and two peripheral small jets, whereas a Medtronic-Hall valve typically has a single central regurgitant jet. Transesophageal echocardiography is also well suited for distinguishing valvular from perivalvular regurgitation.

SPECIFIC CAUSES OF DYSFUNCTION

Obstruction

Obstruction to antegrade flow through a prosthetic valve has several possible causes. As has been mentioned previously, all prostheses are inherently stenotic, demonstrating a wide range of pressure gradients that depend on prosthesis size and stroke volume. Thus, a common cause of obstruction results from a mismatch between the valve

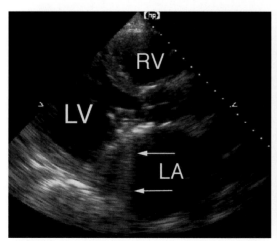
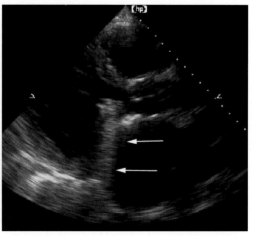

FIGURE 14.31. Detecting the presence of mitral regurgitation in patients with mechanical mitral prostheses can be difficult. In this example, a portion of the left atrium is obscured by the shadowing effect of the prosthesis, as indicated by the arrows during both systole **(left)** and diastole **(right)**. LA, left atrium; LV, left ventricle; RV, right ventricle.

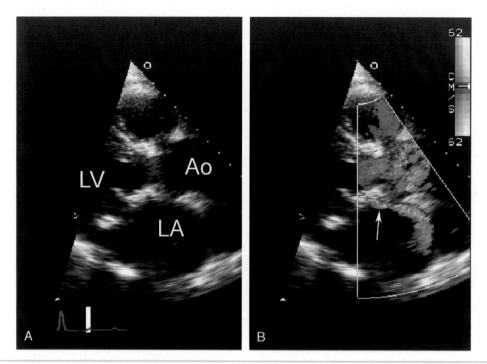

FIGURE 14.32. **A:** Despite the presence of a prosthetic mitral valve, the presence of perivalvular mitral regurgitation was recorded on this transthoracic study. **B:** The eccentric regurgitant jet (*arrow*) can be seen along the anterior wall of the left atrium (*LA*). Ao, aorta; LV, left ventricle.

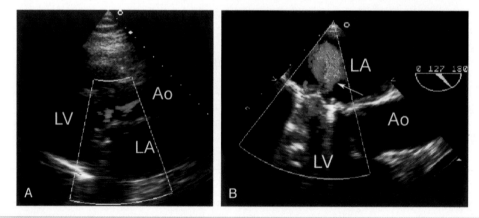

FIGURE 14.33. Transesophageal echocardiography is superior to transthoracic imaging to detect prosthetic mitral regurgitation. **A:** Poor image quality and the shadowing effect of the St. Jude prosthesis prevent mitral regurgitation from being detected on this transthoracic study. **B:** The proximity of the left atrium (*LA*) to the transesophageal probe facilitates diagnosis of mitral regurgitation (*arrow*). Ao, aorta; LV, left ventricle.

and the patient. In this situation, the prosthesis functions as intended but is too small to accommodate the necessary flow. When the effective orifice area is small relative to the patient's body surface area, hemodynamic abnormalities occur. This results in the generation of a significant pressure gradient across the valve. A common reason for prosthesis-patient mismatch occurs in young patients who outgrow their prosthetic valve. In other words, the prosthesis is properly sized for a child but becomes gradually stenotic over time as the child outgrows it. Small patients, especially women, are prone to this condition be-

cause of the necessity to implant small prostheses that result in suboptimal hemodynamics. Figure 14.34 is taken from a 24-year-old patient who had had a disk-type aortic prosthesis implanted at 9 years of age. Over time, the pressure gradient had gradually increased as he "outgrew" the valve. Although asymptomatic and clinically stable, the peak gradient had increased to approximately 64 mm Hg.

In other cases, for technical reasons, a prosthetic valve that is too small is implanted and the patient is left with a significant transvalvular gradient. A form of prosthesis-

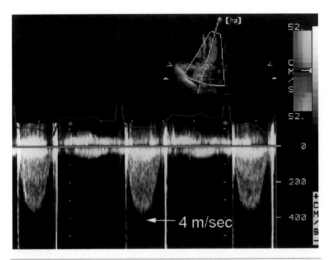

FIGURE 14.34. An example of patient-prosthesis mismatch is shown. This prosthetic valve had been implanted when the patient was young. Over time, the patient outgrew the prosthesis. The result is a 64 mm Hg peak gradient across the valve, as indicated by the Doppler recording.

patient mismatch involves a prosthetic valve that functions adequately at rest but is unable to accommodate the hemodynamic demands of exercise. Distinguishing mismatch dysfunction from other causes of acquired prosthesis obstruction can be difficult. The diagnosis depends

on a careful assessment of prosthesis function, knowledge of the prosthesis size relative to the patient, a quantitative evaluation of stroke volume, and a careful search to exclude other causes of prosthesis dysfunction. It should be pointed out that a high flow velocity alone is not proof of an obstructed prosthesis. A high cardiac output or severe regurgitation are additional causes of increased velocity without obstruction.

Obstruction can occur as a result of technical difficulties encountered while implanting the prosthesis. Figure 14.35 is an example an intraoperative transesophageal echocardiogram that demonstrates immobility of one hemidisk. The hemidisk was stuck in the closed position, resulting in both stenosis and regurgitation. Thrombotic interference is the most common cause of obstruction of mechanical prostheses. It may develop gradually over time or occur suddenly with catastrophic consequences. A relatively small thrombus in a location that interferes with opening of the ball or disk can result in a substantial increase in the pressure gradient across the prosthetic valve (Fig. 14.36). The abnormality may be either permanent or intermittent and may or may not be associated with regurgitation. Transthoracic echocardiography has low sensitivity for visualizing obstructive thrombi affecting mechanical prostheses. Most often, prosthesis dysfunction is suspected when transthoracic Doppler imaging reveals evidence of an

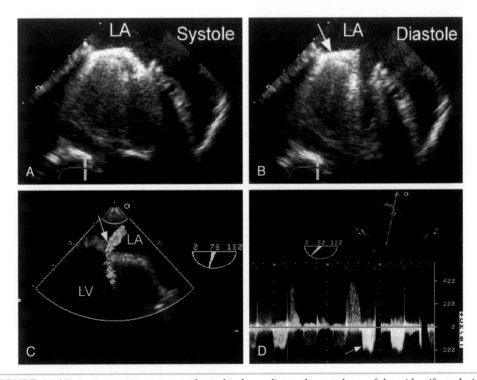

FIGURE 14.35. Intraoperative transesophageal echocardiography can be useful to identify technical problems related to prosthesis insertion. In this example, one of the hemidisks of a St. Jude mitral valve was stuck in the closed position. **A, B:** Lack of motion of the hemidisk was apparent (*arrow*). **C:** Mild mitral regurgitation was detected (*arrow*) using color Doppler imaging. **D:** Continuous wave Doppler imaging confirms both an increased gradient (*arrow*) and regurgitation through the valve. The problem was rectified before leaving the operating room. LA, left atrium; LV, left ventricle.

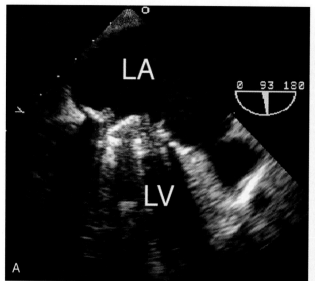

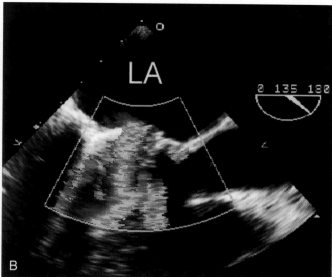

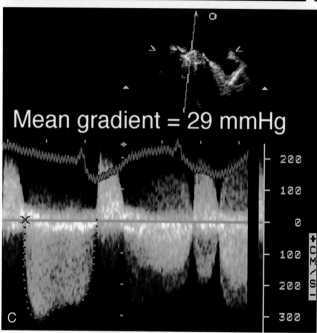

FIGURE 14.36. The most common cause of prosthesis obstruction is the presence of a thrombus. In this example, a small thrombus was barely visible on transesophageal imaging **(A)**. **B:** Color Doppler imaging demonstrates increased turbulence but no significant mitral regurgitation. **C:** Doppler imaging confirms obstruction by demonstrating a very high mean pressure gradient of 29 mm Hg. LA, left atrium; LV, left ventricle.

increased pressure gradient. Then, the precise cause of the gradient is determined with transesophageal imaging. Occasionally, a larger thrombus can be seen with the transthoracic approach (Fig. 14.37). Careful scrutiny of the motion of the occluder is a key to diagnosis. The range of occluder motion should be assessed from multiple planes. M-mode echocardiography can be helpful in this setting, particularly if the abnormality is intermittent with varying occluder motion from beat to beat. Two-dimensional echocardiography can sometimes demonstrate the absence of motion of one hemidisk of a bileaflet prosthesis. Frequently, a combination of transthoracic and transesophageal imaging is necessary for a complete diagnosis. Figure 14.38 is an example of a thrombus within the left

atrium affecting the function of a St. Jude mitral valve. In this example, the location of the thrombus prevented one of the hemidisks from opening, thereby resulting in a moderate diastolic gradient.

Sometimes the obstruction is not apparent from two-dimensional imaging, but Doppler imaging reveals a significant increase in gradient. Figure 14.39 is taken from a patient who developed heart failure 4 months after insertion of a St. Jude aortic prosthesis. Although a thrombus could not be visualized, significant regurgitation and stenosis were demonstrated. The patient had discontinued his warfarin 3 weeks before presentation. Figure 14.40 shows a case of obstruction suspected on transthoracic imaging and then confirmed using transesophageal

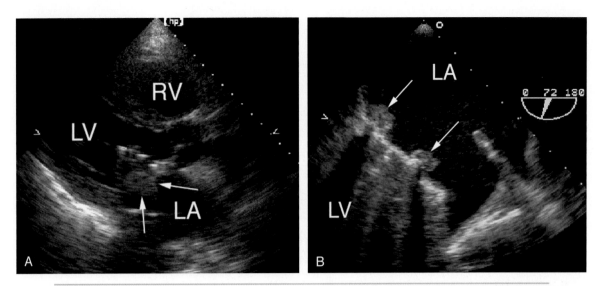

FIGURE 14.37. In this example, a large thrombus was visualized on transthoracic **(A)** and transesophageal **(B)** imaging. The thrombus can be seen on the left atrial (*LA*) aspect of the mitral prosthesis (*arrows*). **B:** Multiple thrombi were demonstrated (*arrows*) adjacent to the sewing ring. LV, left ventricle; RV, right ventricle.

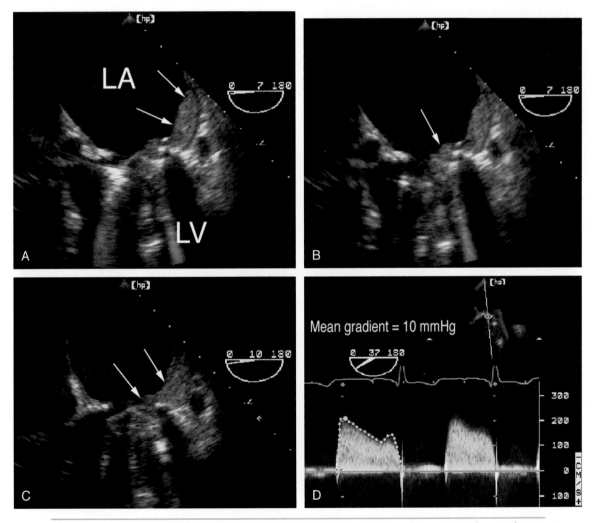

FIGURE 14.38. An extensive thrombus within the left atrium (*LA*) involving a St. Jude mitral prosthesis is demonstrated. **A–C:** The extent of the size and location of the thrombus are demonstrated (*arrows*). Reduced motion of one of the hemidisks resulted. **D:** Doppler imaging demonstrates a mean pressure gradient of 10 mm Hg. Ao, aorta; LV, left ventricle.

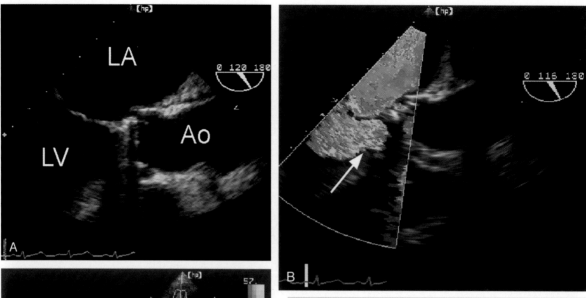

FIGURE 14.39. Even a small thrombus, if properly located, can result in obstruction. **A:** A St. Jude aortic prosthesis is shown. A thrombus was not visualized. **B:** Color Doppler imaging demonstrates increased turbulence and significant aortic regurgitation (*arrow*). **C:** From the transthoracic study, a peak pressure gradient of 95 mm Hg confirms the presence of significant obstruction. Ao, aorta; LA, left atrium, LV, left ventricle.

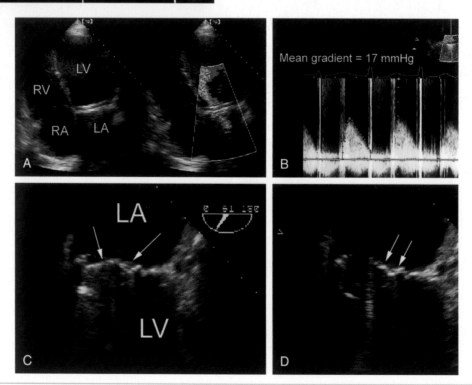

FIGURE 14.40. Thrombus formation leading to partial obstruction of mitral inflow in a patient with a St. Jude mitral prosthesis is demonstrated. **A:** Abnormal function of the prosthesis is suggested based on the direction of the mitral inflow jet. **B:** An increased gradient confirms partial obstruction. **C:** Transesophageal echocardiography demonstrated abnormal motion of the disks (*arrows*). **D:** Failure of one hemidisk to open properly is shown (*arrows*). LA, left atrium; LV, left ventricle; RA, right atrium; RV, right ventricle.

echocardiography. In this case, the unusual pattern and direction of the mitral inflow jet, recorded from the apical four-chamber view, was the first indication of abnormal prosthetic valve function. Pulsed Doppler imaging confirmed a significant diastolic gradient, but transesophageal imaging was required to fully demonstrate the obstructed hemidisk. Less often, obstruction is due to the presence of a vegetation within the sewing ring, restricting antegrade flow through the prosthesis. An example of this is provided in Figure 14.41.

Echocardiography may also play a role in selecting patients for thrombolytic therapy, which is sometimes used to treat prosthetic valve thrombosis, and in assessing its success (Fig. 14.42). This therapy has an overall success rate of 80% to 90% but carries a 20% risk of serious complications. Selecting candidates for thrombolytic therapy must take into account several factors. Poor overall clinical status, previous stroke, extension of thrombus beyond the valve, and large thrombus size are risk factors for complications. In one large multicenter registry (Tong et al., 2004), a thrombus area (measured using transesophageal echocardiography) more than 0.8 cm² and his-

tory of stroke were the most powerful predictors of poor outcome after thrombolytic therapy. Because the decision to proceed with thrombolysis depends in part on the size and location of the thrombus, echocardiography plays a key role in decision making. In addition, serial studies are helpful to evaluate the progress of therapy and determine whether prosthesis function has improved.

Bioprosthetic valves may become obstructed through the process of fibrocalcific degeneration, a primary degenerative process that occurs slowly and leads to prosthesis obstruction, almost always with a component of regurgitation (Figs. 14.18, 14.30, and 14.43). Two-dimensional imaging demonstrates increased echogenicity and decreased mobility of the leaflets and Doppler imaging can be used to confirm an abnormally high pressure gradient across the valve. Acute rupture or fracture of a calcified leaflet can lead to sudden and severe regurgitation, often a medical emergency. This can often be visualized with two-dimensional imaging from a window that records the bioprosthesis from the upstream side. Typically, this results in an unusual flow pattern on pulsed Doppler interrogation, illustrated in Figure 14.44. This striated signal generally in-

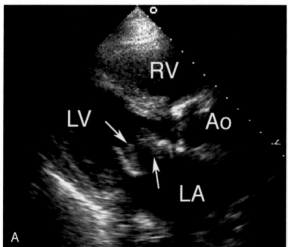

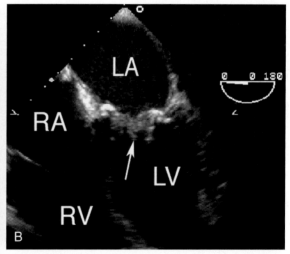

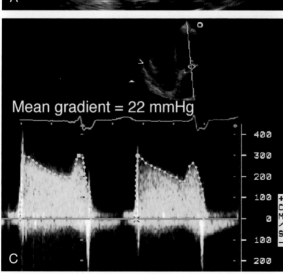

FIGURE 14.41. An example of prosthesis obstruction from a vegetation is provided. The mass effect of the vegetation (*arrows*) partially obstructs mitral inflow. This is demonstrated with transthoracic (**A**) and transesophageal (**B**) imaging. **C:** Doppler imaging demonstrates a mean pressure gradient of 22 mm Hg. Ao, aorta; LA, left atrium; LV, left ventricle; RA, right atrium; RV, right ventricle.

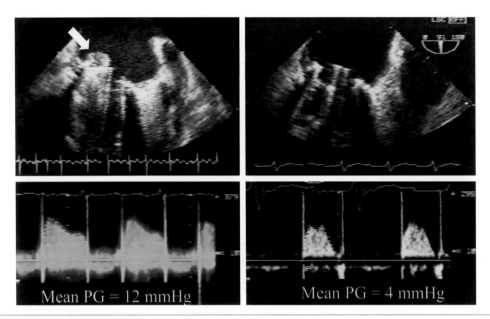

FIGURE 14.42. In the left panels, a St. Jude mitral prosthesis with thrombotic obstruction is shown. The thrombus is evident on transesophageal echocardiography (*arrow*) and Doppler demonstrates a mean gradient of 12 mm Hg. Note how the thrombus prevents opening of one hemidisc in this diastolic frame. In the right panels, following thrombolytic therapy using streptokinase, normal opening motion of both hemidiscs is restored and the mean gradient is reduced to 4 mm Hg. PG, pressure gradient. (Courtesy of W. Zoghbi, MD)

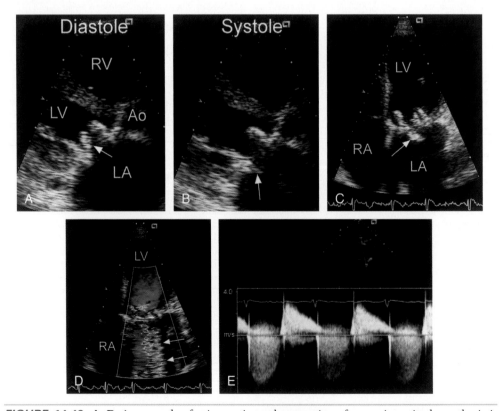

FIGURE 14.43. **A, B:** An example of primary tissue degeneration of a porcine mitral prosthesis is provided. **C:** The leaflets are markedly thickened and partially flail (*arrows*). **D:** Color Doppler imaging confirms severe mitral regurgitation (*arrows*). **E:** Continuous wave Doppler imaging demonstrates both stenosis and regurgitation. Ao, aorta; LA, left atrium; LV, left ventricle; RA, right atrium; RV, right ventricle.

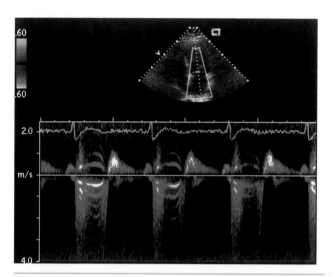

FIGURE 14.44. This particular signal may be recorded in the presence of a flail bioprosthetic valve. The unusual Doppler pattern may be the result of coarse fluttering of the flail leaflets.

dicates the presence of a torn or perforated leaflet. Figure 14.45 is an example of primary tissue degeneration resulting predominantly in regurgitation. In Figure 14.45A, thickened leaflets are apparent, but no significant regurgitation is detected. However, in Figure 14.45B, spectral Doppler imaging reveals a high inflow velocity without prolongation of the $P_{1/2}t$, suggesting increased antegrade flow. A high peak gradient with a relatively low mean gradient suggests the possibility of significant mitral regurgitation. This is confirmed in Figure 14.45C, which demonstrates severe mitral regurgitation. The absence of regurgitation in Figure 14.45A was the result of shadowing by the fibrotic leaflets and sewing ring.

Infective Endocarditis

Infective endocarditis is a potentially catastrophic complication of prosthetic valves. As with native valves, an early and accurate diagnosis is essential to a favorable outcome. In contrast to native valve endocarditis, infec-

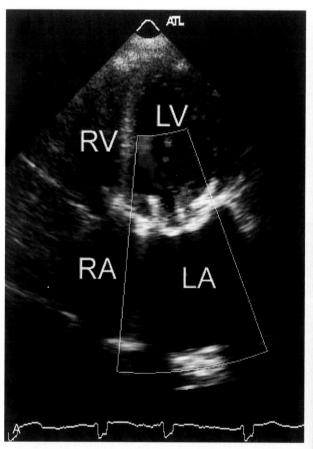

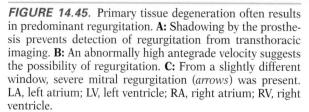

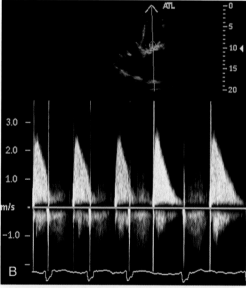

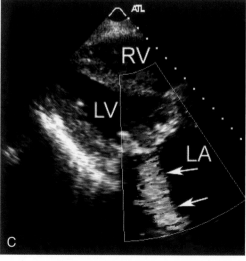

FIGURE 14.45. Primary tissue degeneration often results in predominant regurgitation. **A:** Shadowing by the prosthesis prevents detection of regurgitation from transthoracic imaging. **B:** An abnormally high antegrade velocity suggests the possibility of regurgitation. **C:** From a slightly different window, severe mitral regurgitation (*arrows*) was present. LA, left atrium; LV, left ventricle; RA, right atrium; RV, right ventricle.

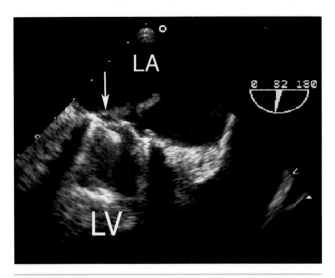

FIGURE 14.46. In patients with prosthetic valves, the most common site for attachment of a vegetation is the sewing ring. In this case, a large vegetation can be seen in the left atrium (*LA*) (*arrow*), attached to the sewing ring of a St. Jude mitral prosthesis. LV, left ventricle.

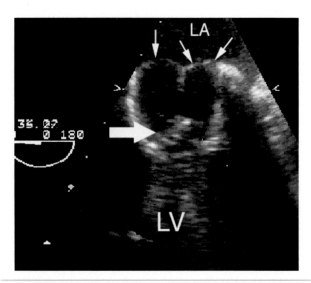

FIGURE 14.48. An atypical location for a vegetation is shown. The vegetation is attached to the distal edge of the stents of a bioprosthetic mitral valve. The valve leaflets (*small arrows*) and the vegetation (*large arrow*) are shown. The leaflets themselves appeared free of infection. LA, left atrium; LV, left ventricle.

tion involving prostheses is more variable and more difficult to diagnose. Due to the reflectance of the prosthetic material, as well as its shadowing effect, detecting vegetations is challenging. Like thrombi, they are easily obscured and require imaging from multiple windows to detect. The most common site for attachment of a vegetation is at the base or sewing ring of the prosthetic valve (Fig. 14.46). Small vegetations can be missed. Pannus or loose suture material can be confused with small vegetations and are sources of false-positive findings. Fur-

thermore, distinguishing vegetation from thrombus is nearly impossible from echocardiographic criteria alone. The distinction relies heavily on the clinical situation, i.e., the presence of fever and the results of blood cultures. Figure 14.47 is an example of a large vegetation attached to mitral ring. In this case, the appearance and location of the mass are most consistent with a vegetation. Figure 14.48 shows an atypical location for a vegetation, attached to the stents of a porcine mitral prosthesis. The unusual location of this mass suggests other possible diagnoses, such as thrombus. In this case, the diagnosis was established based on clinical grounds and then confirmed at surgery. In patients with prosthetic valves in whom endocarditis is being considered, transesophageal echocardiography is recommended in the majority of cases (Fig. 14.49). A combination of transthoracic and transesophageal imaging provides the most complete interrogation of the prosthesis, taking advantage of all available windows to secure a diagnosis.

A common complication of prosthetic valve endocarditis is the development of an abscess. As is the case with native valves, transesophageal echocardiography is significantly more sensitive for detecting abscesses. However, because of the reflectance of the sewing ring and the tissue changes that occur after valve surgery, this diagnosis can be difficult even when transesophageal imaging is performed. A careful interrogation that focuses on a distortion of the tissue subjacent to the sewing ring is critical. Abscesses may be either echo dense or echo lucent, and color flow imaging may reveal evidence of flow within the abscess cavity (Fig. 14.50). Rupture of the abscess into an adjacent chamber or space may occur and is best detected with color Doppler imaging. Perivalvular regurgi-

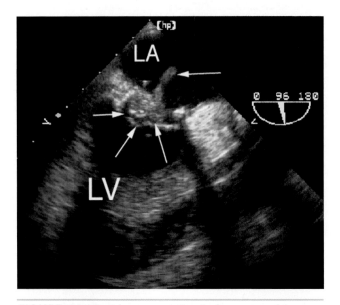

FIGURE 14.47. A large vegetation is demonstrated in a patient with a repaired mitral valve and mitral ring. The vegetation can be seen filling the mitral orifice (*arrows*). LA, left atrium; LV, left ventricle.

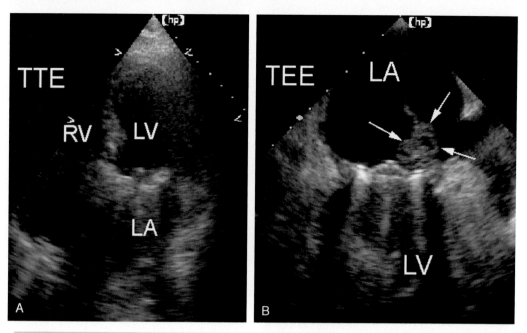

FIGURE 14.49. In patients with prosthetic valves, the combination of transthoracic and transesophageal imaging is often necessary. In this example, transthoracic echocardiography (*TTE*) **(A)** was unable to identify the large vegetation present on this St. Jude mitral prosthesis. **B:** The large mass (*arrows*) was recorded in the left atrium (*LA*) using transesophageal echocardiography (*TEE*). LV, left ventricle; RV, right ventricle.

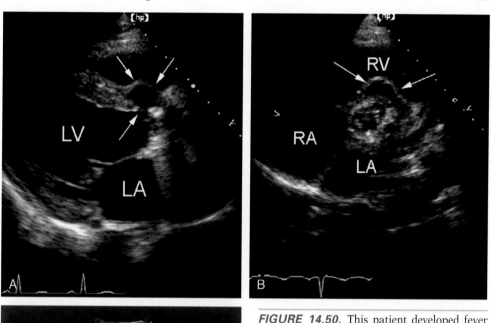

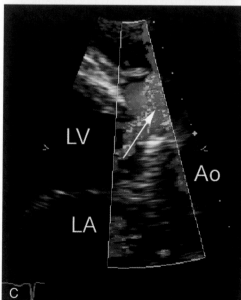

FIGURE 14.50. This patient developed fever approximately 1 month after aortic valve replacement. **A:** A mycotic aneurysm (*arrows*) developed as the result of abscess formation adjacent to the sewing ring. **B:** The aneurysm (*arrows*) is further demonstrated from the short-axis view. **C:** Flow through the aneurysm into the right ventricle (*arrow*) is shown. LA, left atrium; LV, left ventricle; RA, right atrium; Ao, aorta.

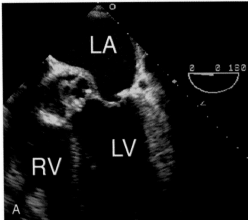

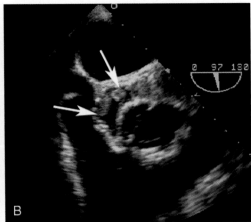

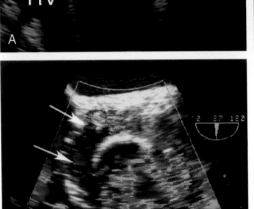

FIGURE 14.51. A ring abscess occurring in a patient with a stentless aortic prosthesis is shown. The abscess (*arrows*) is clearly visualized in both long-axis **(A)** and short-axis **(B)** views. **C:** Color Doppler imaging reveals flow within the abscess cavity (*arrows*). LA, left atrium; LV, left ventricle; RV, right ventricle.

tation is commonly associated with abscess formation. Although perivalvular regurgitation may occur simply as a technical complication after implantation, its development late after valve surgery suggests an infectious etiology (Fig. 14.51). If the degree of destabilization of the sewing ring reaches a certain point, dehiscence of the prosthesis may occur (Fig. 14.52). This leads to a characteristic rocking of the sewing ring within the implantation site. Dehiscence is a serious complication of prosthetic valve endocarditis, almost always associated with significant perivalvular regurgitation. It is, in fact, one of the major factors of the Duke diagnostic criteria. Establishing the diagnosis of dehiscence is relatively straightforward in the mitral position where rocking of the prosthesis relative to the mitral anulus is easy to detect. Dehiscence of an aortic prosthesis may be more difficult to establish because of the shadowing effect of the aortic root (Fig. 14.53). In this example, dilation of the aortic root makes the diagnosis of dehiscence easier to establish.

Although transesophageal echocardiography is very accurate for detection of abscess formation in the presence of a prosthetic valve, errors in diagnosis may occur. Figure 14.54 is an example of a recently placed stentless aortic valve that was implanted using an inclusion technique. In this type of implantation, the porcine aortic valve and root are inserted inside the native aortic root,

creating a double-density appearance of the two walls. With time, the walls become adherent, but until that happens, the presence of two walls separated by an echo-free space can easily be confused with a root abscess.

Mechanical Failure

Primary mechanical failure or defects in manufacturing are increasingly rare causes of prosthesis dysfunction. In the past, several recognized defects occasionally developed in some specific types of prostheses. For example, a gradual change in the shape of the occluder of Starr-Edwards prosthesis, termed ball variance, sometimes resulted in dysfunction as the ball intermittently became stuck within the cage. Older models of the Björk-Shiley valve occasionally developed fractured struts that resulted in embolization of the disk. Disk fracture has also been reported, although it is quite rare. Each of these types of abnormality can be assessed with echocardiography. Fortunately, improvements in design and manufacture have made such catastrophic failures exceedingly uncommon.

RIGHT-SIDED PROSTHETIC VALVES

Most prosthetic valves inserted in the tricuspid position are bioprosthetic. Doppler echocardiographic evaluation

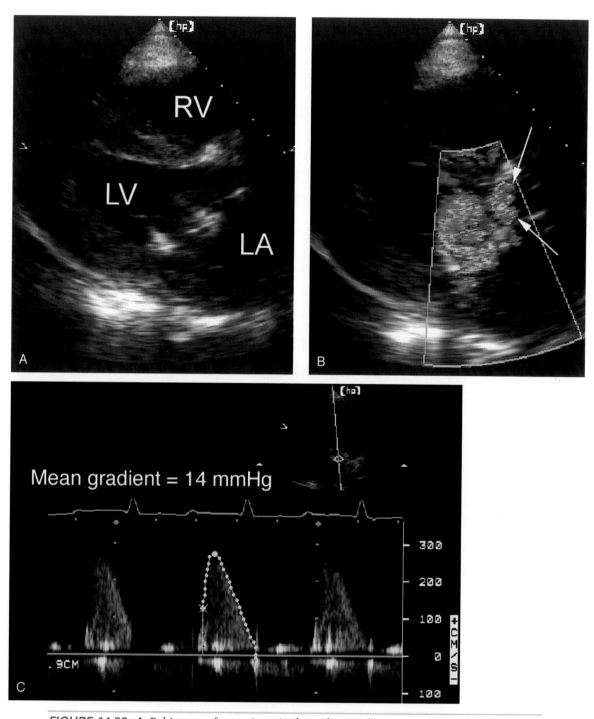

FIGURE 14.52. A: Dehiscence of a porcine mitral prosthesis is demonstrated. In real time, excessive motion of the prosthetic valve was evident. **B:** Color flow imaging revealed significant perivalvular regurgitation (*arrows*). **C:** Abnormally high peak flow velocity (2.8 cm/sec) and an increased gradient (14 mm Hg) are demonstrated by Doppler imaging. LA, left atrium; LV, left ventricle; RV, right ventricle.

of prosthetic tricuspid valves follows an approach similar to that of mitral prostheses. Using a combination of the medially angulated parasternal view and the apical four-chamber view, prosthetic tricuspid valves can be adequately interrogated from the transthoracic approach (Fig.

14.55). Experience with right-sided prosthetic valves is significantly less compared with left-sided valves so published data regarding range of normal function are limited. Flow through right-sided prosthetic valves normally occurs at low velocities, thereby increasing the risk of

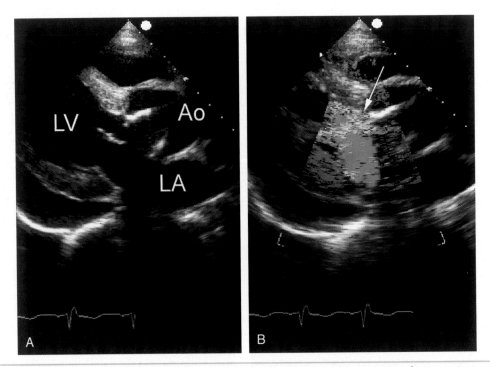

FIGURE 14.53. Severe dehiscence of a porcine aortic prosthesis is shown. **A:** Prosthesis motion was evident, independent of motion of the aortic root. **B:** Significant perivalvular regurgitation (*arrow*) is demonstrated. Ao, aorta; LA, left atrium; LV, left ventricle.

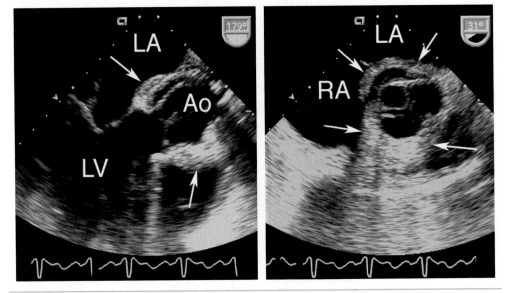

FIGURE 14.54. A recently implanted stentless aortic valve (*Ao*) is evaluated with transesophageal echocardiography. The valve is shown in the long-axis **(left)** and short-axis **(right)** views. Thickening of the aortic root and an echo-free space (*arrows*) are the result of inclusion of the porcine aortic root within the patient's aortic root, creating the appearance of a double-walled aorta. See text for details. LA, left atrium; LV, left ventricle; RA, right atrium.

thrombus formation. In assessing tricuspid prostheses, the normal respiratory variation that characterizes right heart flow must be taken into account. More commonly, repair of the tricuspid valve is undertaken and an anuloplasty ring is implanted. On two-dimensional echocardiography, these rings appear as dense echogenic structures within the anulus. Echocardiographic evaluation focuses on documenting stable positioning of the ring, excluding functional stenosis from an improperly placed ring and assessing residual tricuspid regurgitation that might be present.

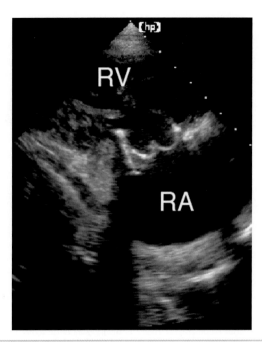

FIGURE 14.55. A normally functioning porcine valve in the tricuspid position is shown. RA, right atrium; RV, right ventricle.

Prosthetic valves in the pulmonary position are even less common. The parasternal short-axis view at the base of the heart and subcostal views are most helpful in their assessment. A form of aortic valve surgery, the Ross procedure, involves replacement of a dysfunctional aortic valve with the patient's own pulmonary valve (autograft) followed by implantation of a homograft in the pulmonary position. Both the valve and the proximal pulmonary artery are replaced. After a successful Ross procedure, a mild pressure gradient across the pulmonary valve is often present, sometimes associated with a minor degree of pulmonary regurgitation. Progressive stenosis, often due to degeneration of the proximal pulmonary artery, has been reported and may lead to a significant pulmonary artery gradient that is readily detected with Doppler imaging (Fig. 14.56).

VALVED CONDUITS

Valved conduits are also part of the repair of some forms of complex congenital heart disease. Not all conduits contain valves and those that do may use either bioprosthetic or mechanical prostheses. The conduit material itself often has a characteristic echocardiographic appearance due to the conduit material and the ribbed design. An example is provided in Figure 14.57. Visualizing the valve within such conduits may be difficult. However, Doppler imaging is critical to assess the function of such valves and to exclude stenosis and regurgitation. Stenosis within a valved conduit may be the result of either prosthetic valve dysfunction or neointimal proliferation along the

entire length of the tubing. Color flow imaging may allow this distinction to be made and continuous wave Doppler imaging should be used to assess its severity. This topic is covered more fully in Chapter 18.

MITRAL VALVE REPAIR

Repairing, rather than replacing, a dysfunctional mitral valve has several advantages and is being performed with increasing frequency. Selecting patients for mitral valve repair depends heavily on etiology, morphology, and severity of the valve disease as well as on the status of the left ventricle. For all these reasons, echocardiography is critical to patient management and is generally the primary factor in the decision to attempt valve repair. Because the surgical approach must be individualized, clinicians rely on a precise and thorough assessment of valve anatomy and function to plan the procedure. The success rate of repair in patients with myxomatous degeneration and mitral valve prolapse is linked to factors that are assessed echocardiographically before and during surgery. For example, posterior leaflet prolapse carries a greater likelihood of successful repair than anterior or bileaflet prolapse. The location and extent of leaflet excision and the decision to shorten the chordae and/or perform a ring anuloplasty also rely on echocardiographic guidance. Figure 14.58 illustrates an excellent result of repair of mitral valve prolapse with a Carpentier ring. The ring is well positioned and effectively improves the coaptation of the leaflets during systole. At the same time, mobility of the leaflets is maintained with adequate excursion during diastole to allow unimpeded left ventricular filling. Figure 14.59 is another example of successful mitral valve repair. Mild mitral regurgitation is present, but normal mitral inflow is preserved. Figure 14.60 illustrates an unsuccessful attempt to repair a regurgitation mitral valve. The mitral ring has become dislodged and appears partially detached within the left atrium. Severe mitral regurgitation is present. This topic is discussed further in Chapter 11.

Mitral valve repair can also be accomplished using a newer technique referred to as an Alfieri, or edge-to-edge, repair. This method involves suturing together the free edges of the mitral leaflets at the site of regurgitation. Thus, spatial localization of the regurgitant orifice is a key part of patient evaluation. The suturing results in a localized area of fixed "stenosis" around which mitral inflow occurs. An example of this is provided in Figure 14.61. In this case, regurgitation involved the middle scallops, so the Alfieri stitches are placed centrally, creating the appearance of a double-orifice mitral valve. The potential for creating a degree of mitral stenosis exists and part of the echocardiographic examination should address this possibility. In the example shown, mild residual mitral regurgitation was documented with color Doppler imaging.

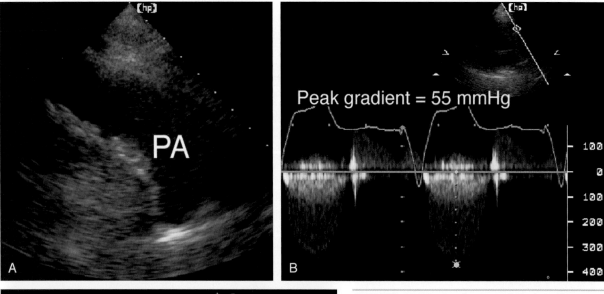

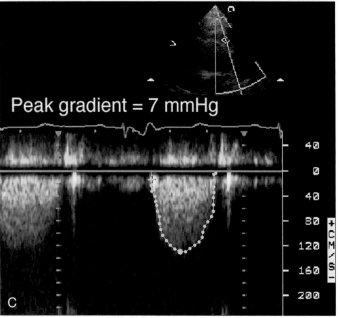

FIGURE 14.56. **A:** A homograft in the pulmonary position is recorded from a patient after a Ross procedure. With two-dimensional imaging, evidence of narrowing was not apparent. **B:** Stenosis within the homograft is demonstrated with continuous wave Doppler imaging. **C:** After surgical revision, the pressure gradient was no longer present. PA, pulmonary artery.

FIGURE 14.57. A Bentall repair of the aortic root is shown. **A:** The long-axis of the conduit is shown, and the highly echogenic walls of the prosthetic material are apparent. A disk-type mechanical prosthetic valve is shown. **B:** A short-axis view demonstrates the origin of the left coronary artery (*arrow*) just below the left atrial appendage. Ao, aorta; LA, left atrium.

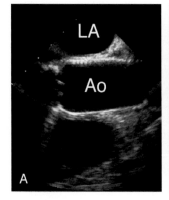

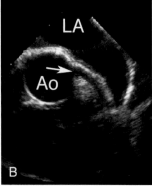

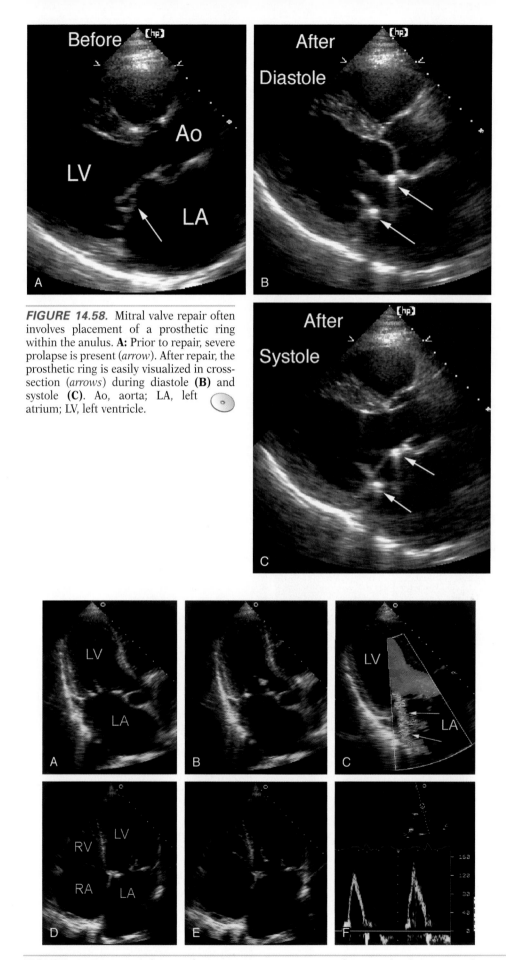

FIGURE 14.58. Mitral valve repair often involves placement of a prosthetic ring within the anulus. **A:** Prior to repair, severe prolapse is present (*arrow*). After repair, the prosthetic ring is easily visualized in cross-section (*arrows*) during diastole **(B)** and systole **(C)**. Ao, aorta; LA, left atrium; LV, left ventricle.

FIGURE 14.59. Some degree of regurgitation may remain after mitral valve repair. This study demonstrates a stable ring in the mitral position during systole **(A, D)** with well-preserved leaflet excursion during diastole **(B, E)**. **C:** Mitral regurgitation (*arrows*) is present. **F:** Doppler imaging demonstrates no evidence of obstruction across the repaired mitral valve. LA, left atrium; LV, left ventricle; RA, right atrium; RV, right ventricle.

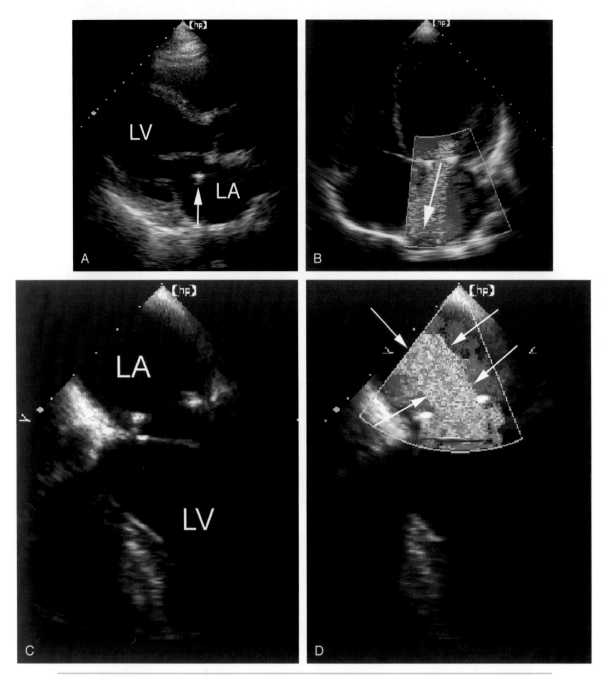

FIGURE 14.60. Unsuccessful mitral valve repair is demonstrated. **A:** The ring has become detached from the anulus and appears to float within the left atrial (*LA*) cavity (*arrow*). **B:** Color Doppler imaging demonstrates severe mitral regurgitation. These findings were confirmed using transesophageal echocardiography **(C)** and severe mitral regurgitation was documented (**D**, *arrows*). LV, left ventricle.

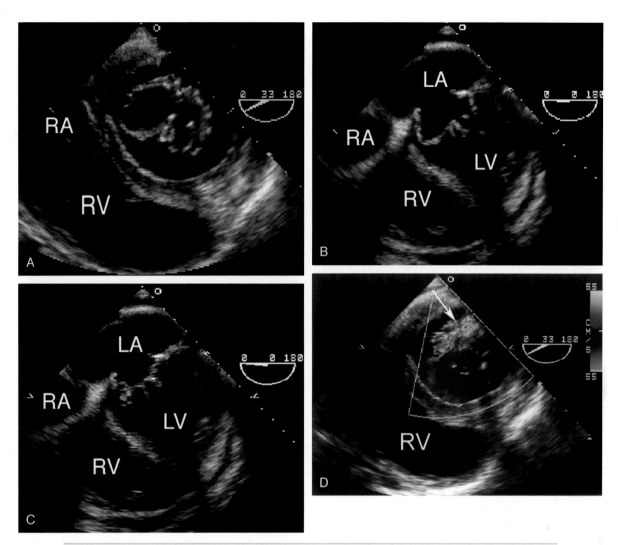

FIGURE 14.61. Mitral valve repair using the Alfieri stitch, or edge-to-edge repair, is demonstrated. In this case, a patient with mitral valve prolapse had severe mitral regurgitation. Scallops A2 and P2 were sewn together creating a double-orifice appearance to the mitral valve **(A–C)**. See text for details. In **D,** mild residual mitral regurgitation (*arrow*) is demonstrated. LA, left atrium; LV, left ventricle; RA, right atrium; RV, right ventricle.

SUGGESTED READINGS

Alam M, Madrazo AC, Magilligan DJ, et al. M-mode and two dimensional echocardiographic features of porcine valve dysfunction. Am J Cardiol 1979;43:502–509.

Alam M, Rosman HS, Polanco GA, et al. Transesophageal echocardiographic features of stenotic bioprosthetic valves in the mitral and tricuspid valve positions. Am J Cardiol 1991;68:689–690.

Alton ME, Pasierski TJ, Orsinelli DA, et al. Comparison of transthoracic and transesophageal echocardiography in evaluation of 47 Starr-Edwards prosthetic valves. J Am Coll Cardiol 1992;20:1503–1511.

Baumgartner H, Khan S, DeRobertis M, et al. Discrepancies between Doppler and catheter gradients in aortic prosthetic valves *in vitro*. A manifestation of localized gradients and pressure recovery. Circulation 1990;82:1467–1475.

Blot WJ, Omar RZ, Kallewaard M, et al. Risks of fracture of Björk-Shiley 60 degree convexo-concave prosthetic heart valves: long-term cohort follow up in the UK, Netherlands and USA. J Heart Valve Dis 2001;10:202–209.

Burstow DJ, Nishimura RA, Bailey KR, et al. Continuous wave Doppler echocardiographic measurement of prosthetic valve gradients. A simultaneous Doppler-catheter correlative study. Circulation 1989;80:504–514.

Chafizadeh ER, Zoghbi WA. Doppler echocardiographic assessment of the St. Jude Medical prosthetic valve in the aortic position using the continuity equation. Circulation 1991;83:213–223.

Chambers J, McLoughlin N, Rapson A, et al. Effect of changes in heart rate on pressure half time in normally functioning mitral valve prostheses. Br Heart J 1988;60:502–506.

Daniel WG, Mugge A, Martin RP, et al. Improvement in the diagnosis of abscesses associated with endocarditis by transesophageal echocardiography. N Engl J Med 1991;324:795–800.

Dismukes WE, Karchmer AW, Buckley MJ, et al. Prosthetic valve endocarditis. Analysis of 38 cases. Circulation 1973;48:365–377.

Effron MK, Popp RL. Two-dimensional echocardiographic assessment of bioprosthetic valve dysfunction and infective endocarditis. J Am Coll Cardiol 1983;2:597–606.

Grunkemeier GL, Starr A. Late ball variance with the Model 1000 Starr-Edwards aortic valve prosthesis. Risk analysis and strategy of operative management. J Thorac Cardiovasc Surg 1986;91:918–923.

Heinle S, Wilderman N, Harrison JK, et al. Value of transthoracic echocardiography in predicting embolic events in active infective endocarditis. Duke Endocarditis Service. Am J Cardiol 1994;74:799–801.

Hixson CS, Smith MD, Mattson MD, et al. Comparison of transesophageal color flow Doppler imaging of normal mitral regurgitant jets in St. Jude Medical and Medtronic Hall cardiac prostheses. J Am Soc Echocardiogr 1992;5:57–62.

Ledain LD, Ohayon JP, Colle JP, et al. Acute thrombotic obstruction with disc valve prostheses: diagnostic considerations and fibrinolytic treatment. J Am Coll Cardiol 1986;7:743–751.

Levine RA, Jimoh A, Cape EG, et al. Pressure recovery distal to a stenosis: potential cause of gradient "overestimation" by Doppler echocardiography. J Am Coll Cardiol 1989;13:706–715.

Linden PA, Cohn LH. Medium-term follow up of pulmonary autograft aortic valve replacement: technical advances and echocardiographic follow up. J Heart Valve Dis 2001;10:35–42.

McHenry MM, Smeloff EA, Fong WY, et al. Critical obstruction of prosthetic heart valves due to lipid absorption by Silastic. J Thorac Cardiovasc Surg 1970;59:413–425.

Mohr-Kahaly S, Kupferwasser I, Erbel R, et al. Regurgitant flow in apparently normal valve prostheses: improved detection and semiquantitative analysis by transesophageal two-dimensional color-coded Doppler echocardiography. J Am Soc Echocardiogr 1990;3:187–195.

Morguet AJ, Werner GS, Andreas S, et al. Diagnostic value of transesophageal compared with transthoracic echocardiography in suspected prosthetic valve endocarditis. Herz 1995;20:390–398.

Nellessen U, Masuyama T, Appleton CP, et al. Mitral prosthesis malfunction. Comparative Doppler echocardiographic studies of mitral prostheses before and after replacement. Circulation 1989;79:330–336.

Nettles RE, McCarty DE, Corey GR, et al. An evaluation of the Duke criteria in 25 pathologically confirmed cases of prosthetic valve endocarditis. Clin Infect Dis 1997;25:1401–1403.

Onoda K, Yasuda F, Takao M, et al. Long-term follow-up after Carpentier-Edwards ring annuloplasty for tricuspid regurgitation. Ann Thorac Surg 2000;70:796–799.

Otto CM, Yoganathan AP, Brandon T. Fluid dynamics of prosthetic valves. In: Otto CM, ed. The Practice of Clinical Echocardiography. 2nd Ed. Philadelphia: WB Saunders, 2002:514–518.

Panidis IP, Ross J, Mintz GS. Normal and abnormal prosthetic valve function as assessed by Doppler echocardiography. J Am Coll Cardiol 1986;8:317–326.

Rahimtoola SH. The problem of valve prosthesis-patient mismatch. Circulation 1978;58:20–24.

Rosenhek R, Binder T, Maurer G, Baumgartner H. Normal values for Doppler echocardiographic assessment of heart valve prostheses. J Am Soc Echocardiogr 2003;16:1116–1127.

Ross DN. Replacement of aortic and mitral valves with a pulmonary autograft. Lancet 1967;2:956–958.

Rothbart RM, Castriz JL, Harding LV, et al. Determination of aortic valve area by two-dimensional and Doppler echocardiography in patients with normal and stenotic bioprosthetic valves. J Am Coll Cardiol 1990;15:817–824.

Ryan T, Armstrong WF, Dillon JC, et al. Doppler echocardiographic evaluation of patients with porcine mitral valves. Am Heart J 1986;111:237–244.

Saad RM, Barbetseas J, Olmos L, et al. Application of the continuity equation and valve resistance to the evaluation of St. Jude Medical prosthetic aortic valve dysfunction. Am J Cardiol 1977;80:1239–1242.

Shively BK, Gurule FT, Roldan CA, et al. Diagnostic value of transesophageal compared with transthoracic echocardiography in infective endocarditis. J Am Coll Cardiol 1991;18:391–397.

Tischler MD, Cooper KA, Rowen M, et al. Mitral valve replacement versus mitral valve repair. A Doppler and quantitative stress echocardiographic study. Circulation 1994;89:132–137.

Tong AT, Roudaut R, Ozkan M, et al. Transesophageal echocardiography improves risk assessment of thrombolysis of prosthetic valve thrombosis: results of the international PRO-TEE registry. J Am Coll Cardiol 2004;43:77–84.

Vandervoort PM, Greenberg NL, Powell KA, et al. Pressure recovery in bileaflet heart valve prostheses. Localized high velocities and gradients in central and side orifices with implications for Doppler-catheter gradient relation in aortic and mitral position. Circulation 1995;92:3464–3472.

Watarida S, Shiraishi S, Nishi T, et al. Strut fracture of Björk-Shiley convexo-concave valve in Japan—risk of small valve size. Ann Thorac Cardiovasc Surg 2001;7:246–249.

Wilkes HS, Berger M, Gallerstein PE, et al. Left ventricular outflow obstruction after aortic valve replacement: detection with continuous wave Doppler ultrasound recording. J Am Coll Cardiol 1983;1:550–553.

Wilkins GT, Gillam LD, Kritzer GL, et al. Validation of continuous-wave Doppler echocardiographic measurements of mitral and tricuspid prosthetic valve gradients: a simultaneous Doppler-catheter study. Circulation 1986;4:786–795.

Xie GY, Bhakta D, Smith MD. Echocardiographic follow-up study of the Ross procedure in older versus younger patients. Am Heart J 2001;142:331–335.

Yoganathan AP. Flow characteristics of prosthetic heart valves. Int J Cardiovasc Imaging 1989;4:5–8.

Young E, Shapiro SM, French WJ, et al. Use of transesophageal echocardiography during thrombolysis with tissue plasminogen activator of a thrombosed prosthetic mitral valve. J Am Soc Echocardiogr 1992;5:153–158.

Zoghbi WA, Desir RM, Rosen L, et al. Doppler echocardiography: application to the assessment of successful thrombolysis of prosthetic valve thrombosis. J Am Soc Echocardiogr 1989;2:98–101.

Coronary Artery Disease

CLINICAL OVERVIEW

Coronary artery disease is the most common form of organic heart disease encountered in adults. Its clinical syndromes are the result of atherosclerotic disease of the coronary arteries and include syndromes of stable and unstable angina, acute myocardial infarction, ischemic cardiomyopathy with congestive heart failure, and sudden cardiac death. The use of echocardiography in patients with known or suspected ischemic heart disease is broad ranging and includes playing a role in diagnosis, detecting complications, and assessing prognosis. The current American College of Cardiology/American Heart Association Guidelines for Clinical Application of Echocardiography have established areas for which echocardiography is an appropriate diagnostic tool in patients with coronary artery disease (Tables 15.1 and 15.2).

▶ **TABLE 15.1 Recommendations for Echocardiography in the Diagnosis of Acute Myocardial Ischemic Syndromes**

Class I
1. Diagnosis of suspected acute ischemia or infarction not evident by standard means
2. Measurement of baseline left ventricular function
3. Evaluation of patients with inferior myocardial infarction and clinical evidence suggesting possible right ventricular infarction
4. Assessment of mechanical complications and mural thrombus[a]

Class IIa
Identification of location/severity of disease in patients with ongoing ischemia

Class III
Diagnosis of acute myocardial infarction already evident by standard means

[a]Transesophageal echocardiography is indicated when transthoracic echocardiographic studies are not diagnostic.
From Cheitlin MD, et al. ACC/AHA/ASE 2003 Guideline Update for the Clinical Application of Echocardiography: summary article. A report of the American College of Cardiology/American Heart Association Task Force on Practice Guidelines (ACC/AHA/ASE Committee to Update the 1997 Guidelines for the Clinical Application of Echocardiography). J Am Soc Echocardiogr 2003;16:1091–1110, with permission.

▶ **TABLE 15.2 Recommendations for Echocardiography in Risk Assessment, Prognosis, and Assessment of Therapy in Acute Myocardial Ischemic Syndromes**

Class I
1. Assessment of infarct size and/or extent of jeopardized myocardium
2. In-hospital assessment of ventricular function when the results are used to guide therapy
3. In-hospital or early postdischarge assessment of the presence/extent of inducible ischemia whenever baseline abnormalities are expected to compromise electrocardiographic interpretation[a]
4. Assessment of myocardial viability when required to define potential efficacy of revascularization[b]

Class IIa
1. In-hospital or early postdischarge assessment of the presence/extent of inducible ischemia in the absence of baseline abnormalities expected to compromise electrocardiographic interpretation[a]
2. Reevaluation of ventricular function during recovery when results are used to guide therapy
3. Assessment of ventricular function after revascularization

Class IIb
Assessment of late prognosis (≥2 years after acute myocardial infarction)

Class III
Routine reevaluation in the absence of any change in clinical status

[a]Exercise or pharmacologic stress echocardiogram.
[b]Dobutamine stress echocardiogram.
From Cheitlin MD, et al. ACC/AHA/ASE 2003 Guideline Update for the Clinical Application of Echocardiography: summary article. A report of the American College of Cardiology/American Heart Association Task Force on Practice Guidelines (ACC/AHA/ASE Committee to Update the 1997 Guidelines for the Clinical Application of Echocardiography). J Am Soc Echocardiogr 2003;16:1091–1110, with permission.

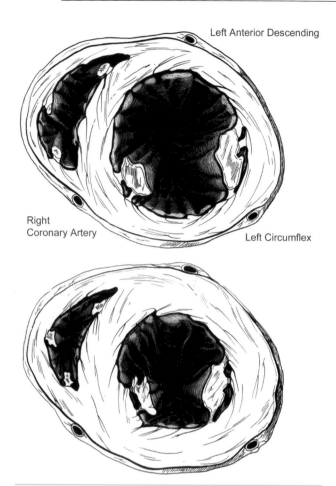

Left Anterior Descending

Right
Coronary Artery

Left Circumflex

FIGURE 15.1. Anatomic rendering of a short-axis view of the left ventricle in diastole **(top)** and systole **(bottom)**. Note the circular geometry of the left ventricle in both diastole and systole and the crescent-shaped geometry of the right ventricle. In the real-time image, note the symmetric wall thickening and inward endocardial excursion. The location of the major epicardial coronary arteries is also shown.

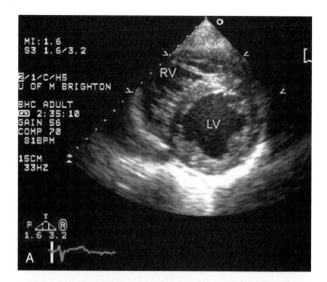

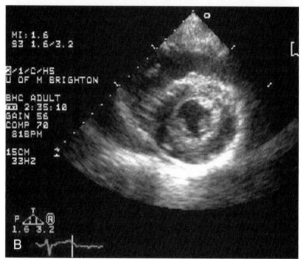

FIGURE 15.2. Parasternal short-axis view of the left ventricle (*LV*) at the papillary muscle level. As with the accompanying schematic (Fig. 15.1), note the circular geometry of the left ventricle and the symmetric endocardial inward motion and wall thickening from diastole **(A)** to systole **(B)**. RV, right ventricle.

Pathophysiology of Coronary Syndromes

Normal left ventricular wall motion consists of simultaneous wall thickening and endocardial excursion so that the cavity decreases in size in a relatively symmetric manner (Figs. 15.1–15.3). Interruption of contraction, due to ischemia, infarction, or other process, results in regional abnormalities of motion.

There is a well-defined hierarchy of functional abnormalities that occur as a consequence of interruption in coronary blood flow. This has been termed the ischemic cascade and is schematized in Figure 15.4. Resting blood flow to the myocardium is preserved until a coronary artery stenosis approaches 90% diameter narrowing. It should be emphasized that simple diameter narrowing is only one component of the anatomic abnormality that results in reduced coronary flow, and lesion eccentricity, length, and number of sequential lesions all play crucial roles. At lesser degrees of stenosis, rest flow is preserved,

but coronary flow reserve may be reduced, and at times of increasing demand such as exercise, a supply-demand mismatch occurs. Creation and detection of a supply-demand mismatch in the presence of an otherwise nonflow obstructive lesion are the underlying principles of stress echocardiography and other stress-testing techniques designed to unmask occult coronary artery stenoses.

With the above hierarchy of functional abnormalities in mind, one can then appreciate the predictable sequence of events that can be detected with echocardiographic imaging in the presence of a coronary stenosis. Experimentally, immediately after coronary artery occlusion, abnormalities in diastolic function occur and can be detected with echocardiographic and Doppler techniques (Fig. 15.5). The easiest and most commonly identified ab-

Diastole & Systole

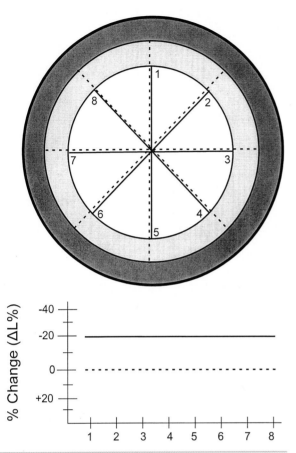

FIGURE 15.3. Schematic diagram of normal endocardial wall motion. The *outer dark circle* represents the diastolic thickness of the left ventricle and the *inner lighter shaded circle* represents the extent of systolic contraction. Eight radians from the center of mass have been drawn for both the diastolic (*dashed line*) and systolic (*solid line*) endocardial boundaries. At bottom, the percentage of change in length from diastole to systole is schematized. The *dashed line* represents zero change in length and the *solid line* represents the actual percentage of change in length for the normally contracting ventricle, which, in this example, is a 20% reduction in length. This diagram will be subsequently repeated for demonstration of wall motion abnormalities and algorithms for correction of translation and rotational motion (see Chapter 6). In each subsequent similar figure, the darker outer circle will represent the normal diastolic contour and a solid circle will represent the systolic endocardial contour demonstrating a wall motion abnormality.

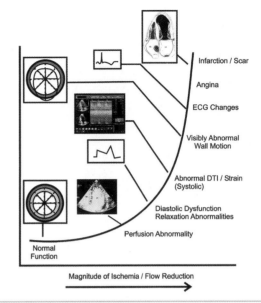

FIGURE 15.4. Demonstration of the ischemic cascade outlining the sequence of events as the magnitude of ischemia or coronary flow reduction progresses from none to severe. ECG, electrocardiographic; DTI, Doppler tissue imaging.

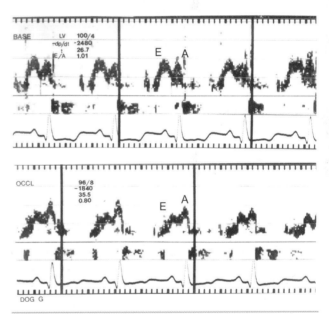

FIGURE 15.5. Pulsed Doppler recording of mitral inflow in an experimental model of myocardial ischemia. **Top:** Note the normal E/A ratio and the reversal of the E/A ratio within seconds of coronary occlusion in the bottom panel.

normality is abnormal mitral valve inflow, with reduction in E-wave velocity and an increase in A-wave velocity occurring within seconds of total coronary occlusion. Additionally, there may be a visibly abnormal relaxation pattern to the wall, mimicking a conduction abnormality. Detailed analysis methods such as strain or strain rate imaging have demonstrated that, in many instances, this abnormality is the result of postsystolic contraction. This is followed almost immediately by loss of systolic wall thick-

ening and decreased endocardial excursion in the region perfused by the obstructed coronary artery (Figs. 15.6 and 15.7). If the coronary artery obstruction persists for a threshold period (typically defined as ≥4 hours), myocardial necrosis ensues and a persistent wall motion abnormality will develop.

Depending on the presence or absence of collaterals and the duration of occlusion, a series of identifiable wall

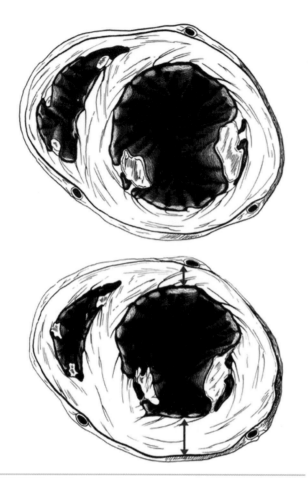

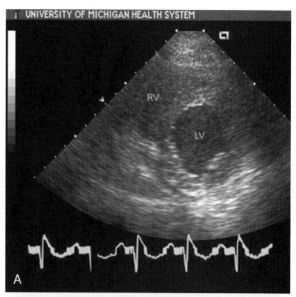

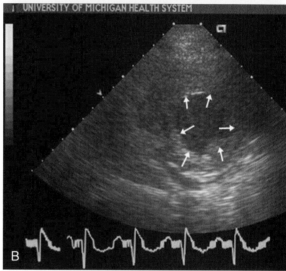

FIGURE 15.6. Anatomic rendering in diastole **(top)** and systole **(bottom)** of ischemia or myocardial infarction in the distribution of the left anterior descending coronary artery. When comparing diastole and systole, note the lack of thickening in the anterior wall and anterior septum compared with normal hyperdynamic motion in the uninvolved segments.

FIGURE 15.7. Parasternal short-axis view recorded in diastole **(A)** and in systole **(B)** in a patient with acute left anterior descending coronary artery occlusion and myocardial infarction. **B:** Note the lack of wall thickening and the dyskinesis of the anterior septum (*outward-pointing arrows*) and the normal motion of the posterior wall (*inward-pointing arrows*). LV, left ventricle; RV, right ventricle.

motion abnormalities can be noted. Obviously, if flow is not restored, myocardial necrosis occurs and a wall motion abnormality persists as a permanent feature of ventricular function. If flow is restored before the onset of myocardial necrosis, variable degrees of recovery of function can be expected. In most instances, a total occlusion of 4 to 6 hours will result in irreversible loss of transmural myocardium. Total interruption for less than 60 minutes will result in lesser degrees of loss of myocardium. In between these two extremes of flow interruption, varying degrees of nontransmural necrosis occur. This predominantly involves the subendocardial layers of the myocardium. As is discussed subsequently, the severity, nature, and extent of wall motion abnormalities depend on the amount of transmural versus nontransmural infarction present in a given segment.

If a substantial period of ischemia has occurred, as may be seen in transient occlusion of 40 to 120 minutes, recovery of function may not be immediate but rather de-

layed due to myocardial stunning. Myocardial stunning is a phenomenon easily demonstrated on echocardiography and represents persistent wall motion abnormalities after restitution of coronary blood flow. These abnormalities recover over a variable time period. Typically, with brief occlusions of 5 minutes or less, recovery of function occurs within 60–120 seconds. With coronary occlusions of 30 to 120 minutes, there may be a 48- to 72-hour delay in recovery of function. There is a substantial degree of variability in the time course over which stunning recovers, and in clinical practice, recovery of function occasionally is delayed for weeks to months.

A phenomenon of repetitive stunning has also been well described. In this scenario, the myocardium is subject to repetitive, brief episodes of ischemia. No single episode of ischemia is sufficient to result in postischemic dysfunction; however, the combined effect of multiple episodes over time may result in prolonged postischemic dysfunction that mimics myocardial hibernation.

After complete coronary occlusion and transmural infarction, a series of events known as remodeling occurs. Over a period of roughly 6 weeks, the necrotic myocardium is replaced by fibrosis and scar tissue, which is thinner and denser than normal myocardium but which has similar tensile strength, rendering it unlikely to rupture. There may be regional dilation in the area of the scar that results in a ventricular aneurysm (Figs. 15.8 and 15.9). An aneurysm is defined as a regional area of akinesis or dyskinesis and scar that has abnormal geometry in both diastole and systole. This is in contrast to a regional wall motion abnormality that has normal geometry in diastole and the distortion occurs exclusively in systole.

On occasion, there can be acute remodeling in an infarct segment that results in expansion of the myocardium in that area. Myocardial expansion occurs typically in the first 48 hours after extensive transmural myocardial infarction and represents acute thinning of the infarcted myocardium. Because expansion occurs acutely, there is no time for scar formation or gradual re-

modeling, and, as such, the wall in the area of myocardial expansion consists of relatively thin necrotic myocardium with reduced tensile strength. Myocardial infarct expansion typically is heralded by new electrocardiographic changes and pain but without enzymatic evidence of further necrosis. It is the anatomic substrate for free-wall rupture, ventricular septal defect, and other mechanical complications of myocardial infarction.

Although the location of a wall motion abnormality is an accurate marker for the site of ischemia or infarction, the extent of the wall motion abnormality often overestimates the anatomic extent of ischemia or infarction. This is in large part due to tethering. Myocardial tethering refers to the impact that an abnormal segment has on a normal adjacent border segment. Tethering occurs both on a horizontal and vertical basis. Horizontal tethering occurs when there is akinesis or dyskinesis of a segment that then results in the reduction in endocardial excursion in the adjacent functionally normal boundary tissue. The effect of horizontal or lateral tethering is for the extent of a wall motion abnormality to overrepresent the anatomic circumferential extent of myocardial necrosis because the detected wall motion abnormality includes not only the infarcted tissue but also a variable percentage of the immediately adjacent boundary tissue. Generally, the wall motion abnormality will overestimate the anatomic extent of a myocardial infarction by approximately 15% due

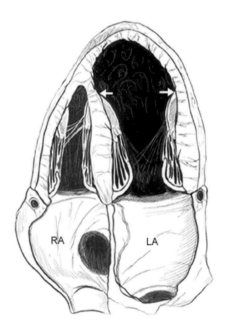 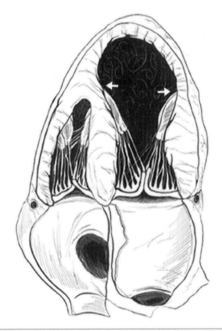

FIGURE 15.8. Anatomic rendering in the four-chamber view depicts a left ventricular apical aneurysm. **Left:** Diastole. **Right:** Systole. Note in diastole the abnormal geometry of the apex with localized apical and septal dilation and the relative thinning of the wall compared with the thickness in the proximal walls. **Right:** The preserved thickening of the proximal walls and a lack of thickening in the aneurysmal segment in all segments distal to the *arrows* are shown. This abnormal geometry in both diastole and systole with wall thinning is the hallmark of true ventricular aneurysm. LA, left atrium; RA, right atrium.

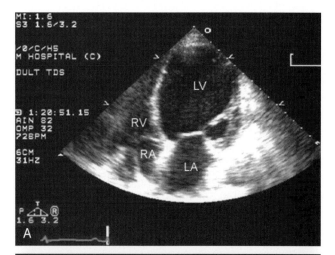

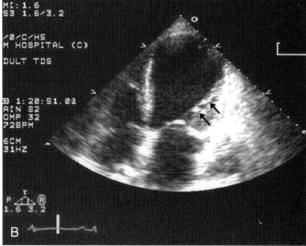

FIGURE 15.9. Apical four-chamber view recorded in a patient with a large apical and septal aneurysm. This two-dimensional echocardiogram corresponds to the anatomic rendering in Figure 15.8. As with the anatomic rendering, note the abnormal geometry of the left ventricle in both diastole **(A)** and systole **(B)** with dilation in the apical segments. In systole, only the proximal lateral wall (*arrows*) has preserved contraction. LA, left atrium; LV, left ventricle; RA, right atrium; RV, right ventricle.

to this phenomenon. The impact that tethering has on quantification of infarct size is demonstrated subsequently.

Normal contraction is heavily dependent on endocardial rather than epicardial contraction. Both the velocity and magnitude of contraction are greater in the subendocardial than in the subepicardial layers. As such, a contraction abnormality in the subendocardium has a disproportionate impact on overall wall thickening. This phenomenon is known as vertical tethering. Vertical tethering has been demonstrated both experimentally and clinically and has relevance for the determination of myocardial infarction size, based on wall motion abnormalities. In general, ischemia or infarction of the inner 20% of the myocardial wall will result in frank akinesis or dyski-

nesis of that segment. As such, nontransmural involvement (either infarction or ischemia) results in malfunction of the entire wall thickness, and thus the wall motion abnormality is indistinguishable from that seen with full transmural myocardial infarction or ischemia.

DETECTION AND QUANTITATION OF WALL MOTION ABNORMALITIES

Regional left ventricular wall motion and global ventricular function can be analyzed and quantified using a number of schemes. These can be classified as purely qualitative, semiquantitative, and quantitative assessments. Table 15.3 outlines many of the schemes that are either commonly used today or have been proposed in the past for evaluation of regional wall motion abnormalities. Although detailed quantitative schemes, which measure regional or global function as a percentage of anticipated normal, may be useful for serial studies and investigational protocols, they are not necessary for detection and localization of an ischemic event for clinical diagnosis. A

▶ **TABLE 15.3 Wall Motion Analysis Methods**

Regional
Qualitative
  "Eyeball" assessment
  Normal vs. abnormal
  Normal–hypokinetic–akinetic–dyskinetic
  Presence of scar/aneurysm
Semiquantitative
  Wall motion score/score index
Quantitative
  Fractional shortening
  Radial shortening
  Cavity/fractional cavity area change
  Chordal centerline analysis
  Doppler tissue based
    Wall velocity
    Myocardial displacement
    Myocardial gradient
    Strain
    Strain rate
Global
Ventricular geometry
Short-axis area change
Left ventricular volumes
  Diastole
  Systole
Ejection fraction
Doppler forward flow (TVI$_{LVOT}$)
Anular displacement (DTI)
Myocardial performance index
Left ventricular dP/dt (from mitral regurgitation)

DTI, Doppler tissue imaging; TVI$_{LVOT}$, Doppler time velocity integral in the left ventricular outflow tract.

compromise that allows semiquantitation and that can be employed easily is the generation of a wall motion score. The wall motion score is a unitless hierarchical number directly proportional to the severity and magnitude of wall motion abnormalities.

M-mode left ventricular measurements provide only limited information on patients with coronary artery disease, not only because of the regional nature of the left ventricular function but also because the M-mode dimensions are not true minor axis measurements (Fig. 15.10). On the other hand, linear two-dimensional measurements still can be very valuable. The linear minor-axis dimension between the posterior left ventricular endocardium and the septum at the level of the mitral chordae provides an assessment of left ventricular systolic function at the base of the heart. The proximal septum is perfused by the first septal perforator; thus, this measurement in systole and diastole and resultant fractional shortening is a good indication of whether a left anterior descending coronary obstruction is proximal or distal to the first septal perforator.

Determination of global ventricular function can provide both diagnostic and prognostic information on patients with ischemic syndromes. Many of the algorithms for determining global function are discussed in Chapter 6. The most commonly used assessment of left ventricular systolic function is the ejection fraction. As a matter of convenience, many echocardiographic laboratories give an "eyeball" or visually estimated qualitative assessment of the ejection fraction. Although there are data supporting this approach, it is a subjective assessment that is highly observer dependent. One can quantitatively measure left ventricular diastolic and systolic volumes, from which the ejection fraction is then calculated. The volumes are frequently indexed to body surface area to allow normalization of data for investigational purposes. Because coronary artery disease results in regional abnormalities, precise calculation of the ejection fraction typically requires a biplane approach to volume determination.

Two-dimensional imaging has replaced M-mode echocardiography for evaluation of global and regional wall motion. The most commonly used method for volume determination is the Simpson rule or the rule of disks, in which the endocardial border in diastole and systole is outlined, and then mathematically a series of disks of identical height, each of which corresponds to one of the minor-axis dimensions of the ventricle, is generated (Fig. 15.11). The volume of each individual disk is then summed to provide a volume. In any given view, a circular disk is assumed at each level along the ventricle. Obviously, if a regional wall motion abnormality is not visualized in the plane of examination, this technique will overestimate the ejection fraction. For this reason, when dealing with patients with coronary disease in whom regional abnormalities are anticipated, biplane methodology is necessary if precise measurements are required. Because of the regional nature of coronary disease, other methods, such as area length calculations, have had less acceptance in evaluating patients with coronary disease.

A two-dimensional area measurement of the short axis at the papillary muscle level has some of the same limitations as M-mode dimensions. The advantage of the short-axis area is that there is less myocardial dropout than with the apical views, and all three coronary artery territories contribute to the measurement. Thus, the resultant fractional area change is a reasonable global assessment, unless there is isolated apical dysfunction.

Evaluation of regional left ventricular function is substantially more complex. There are multiple schemes for

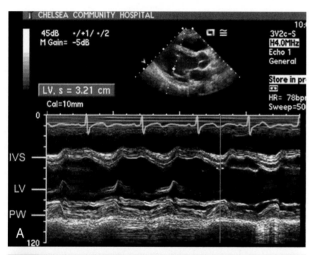

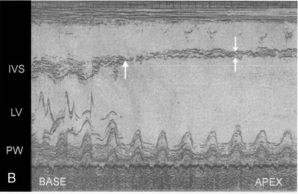

FIGURE 15.10. A: A two-dimensionally guided M-mode echocardiogram through the mid left ventricular level in a normal subject. Note the symmetric contraction of both the anterior septum and posterior wall (*PW*). **B:** Recorded in a patient with an anteroseptal myocardial infarction and extensive areas of scar. Note the normal contraction of the posterior wall from the base (on left) to the apex (on right). At the base, the anterior septum has normal contraction but at the level of the mitral valve (*upward-pointing arrow*), there is an abrupt loss of wall thickness and endocardial motion (*rightward arrows*) of the anterior septum. IVS, interventricular septum; LV left ventricle.

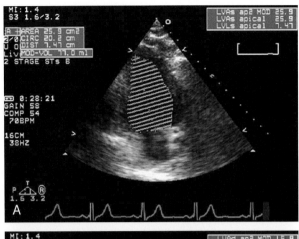

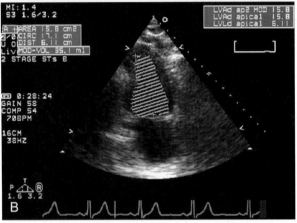

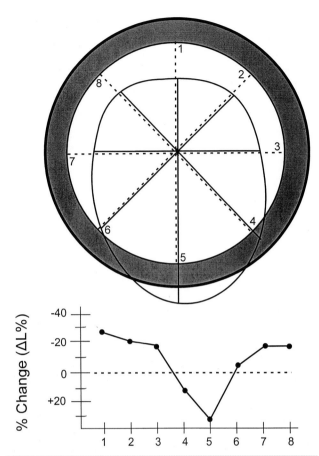

FIGURE 15.11. Apical two-chamber view recorded in a patient with normal ventricular function using automatic endocardial border detection to automatically outline the diastolic **(A)** and systolic **(B)** contours, from which the left ventricular diastolic and systolic volumes are calculated using the rule of disks (Simpson rule). From these volumes, the ejection fraction can be calculated.

FIGURE 15.12. Schematic demonstrates posterior dyskinesis with no translational or rotational motion. The *dark outer circle* represents the contour of the ventricle in diastole and the *inner circle* represents the endocardial contour in systole. Note the maximal area of dyskinesis at segment 5 with less dyskinesis at segment 4 and essential akinesis at segment 6. At bottom, the graph illustrates the change in radian length from diastole to systole. Note the hyperkinesis of the noninvolved segments with increased radian shortening compared with normal contraction in Figure 15.3.

regional wall motion assessment (Table 15.3). The assessment can be undertaken on purely qualitative terms such as an "eyeball" assessment of wall motion as being normal or abnormal or further characterized as hypokinetic, akinetic, or dyskinetic, or undertaken in detailed quantitative schemes in which shortening of multiple endocardial chords around the circumference of the ventricular cavity is undertaken (Figs. 15.3 and 15.12). Figure 15.12 schematizes the simplest, truly quantitative analysis of wall motion using a radian shrinkage analysis and assuming no overall translational or rotational motion of the heart from diastole to systole. Each of the schemes outlined in Table 15.3 can introduce error into a quantitative assessment of regional wall motion. (See Chapter 6 for a more detailed discussion of quantitative techniques.)

It is important to recognize that normal myocardial motion in systole consists of two closely related events. The first is myocardial thickening during which all layers of the wall contract, resulting in augmentation of the thickness of the myocardium from its normal 9 to 11 mm to 14 to 16 mm. This typically represents a 35% to 40% change in wall thickness. There are several layers of myocardial fibers, some of which contract circumferentially in a "wringing" fashion and others that contract in an apex-to-base direction. Because of the electrical activation of the heart, not all regions contract at the identical rate or time. In addition to there being substantial temporal and mechanical heterogeneity of contraction in the normal setting, ischemia results in further temporal and mechanical heterogeneity. Although abnormal wall motion is typically described as being akinetic or dyskinetic, detailed analysis of the temporal sequence of contraction often reveals variations of these contraction abnormalities. One is early systolic contraction followed by dyskinetic motion rather than dyskinesis throughout the entire duration of systole. A second is marked delay in onset of contraction

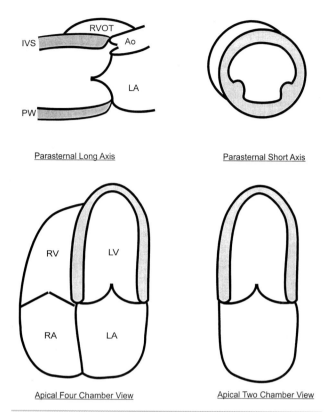

on an apical echocardiogram means that the transducer is not over the true apex. Apical motion with other imaging methods is also due to artifact. This bullet-shaped geometry is noted in the apical four- and two-chamber views as well as in the subcostal view. In the short-axis view, normal left ventricular geometry is circular. In the parasternal long-axis view, normal geometry involves a slight concave curvature of both the ventricular septum and inferoposterior wall, with the direction of concavity for each wall pointing toward the center of the ventricle. Normal geometry is schematized in Figure 15.13 and further illustrated in Figure 15.14. Abnormal geometry is often most apparent in the apical four-chamber view and may involve rounding of the apex or asymmetry of apical

FIGURE 15.13. Schematic representation of normal left ventricular geometry in parasternal **(top)** and apical views **(bottom)**. In the parasternal long-axis view, note the slight concavity of the septum and the posterior wall (*PW*) toward the center of the cavity. Note in the parasternal short-axis view the circular geometry of the left ventricle and the crescent-shaped right ventricle. In the apical views, note the tapering of the apex with the apical segment being thinner than the other walls. In the apical view, the left ventricular geometry has been referred to as bullet shaped or as representing a cone on top of a cylinder. Ao, aorta, IVS, interventricular septum; LA, left atrium; LV, left ventricle; RA, right atrium; RV, right ventricle; RVOT, right ventricular outflow tract.

but with nearly normal excursion (tardokinesis). The implications of these latter two wall motion abnormalities vary with the clinical setting. Either can be seen as a normal variant, as a manifestation of ischemia, or in the postischemia period. As a general rule, if the wall motion abnormality is very brief (50–100 milliseconds), it is more likely to be a normal variant than a manifestation of myocardial ischemia.

An additional qualitative indicator of abnormal ventricular function involves assessment of ventricular geometry. The normal left ventricle is best described as a cylinder with an apical cone. The geometry is therefore "bullet" shaped with gradual tapering of the diameter toward the apex. It should be pointed out that the apex has very limited, if any, motion during the ejection and filling phases of the left ventricle. The apex only moves briefly during the isovolumic periods. Significant apical motion

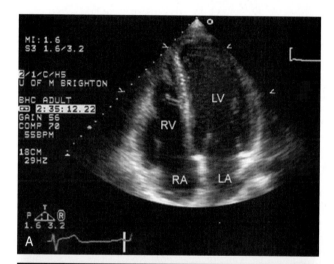

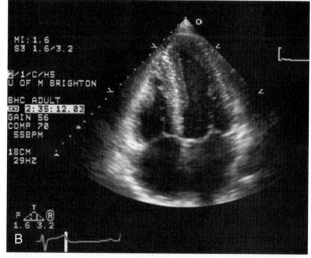

FIGURE 15.14. Apical four-chamber views recorded in a normal ventricle in diastole **(A)** and systole **(B)**. Note the normal bullet-shaped geometry of the left ventricle that tapers at the apex and the symmetric contraction of all visualized walls. Note also the stable position of the apex in the real-time image, indicating that the transducer is at the true apex. LA, left atrium; LV, left ventricle; RA, right atrium; RV, right ventricle.

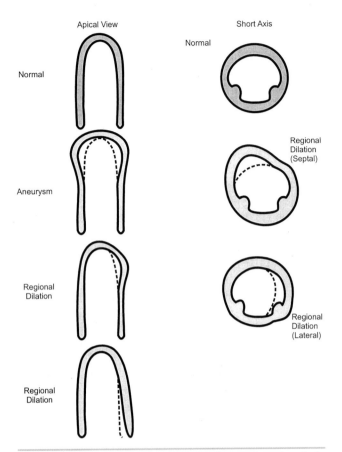

FIGURE 15.15. Schematic representation of normal and abnormal left ventricular geometry shows varying degrees of regional dilation, including a classic apical aneurysm and less typical regional dilation, which also may be a manifestation of myocardial ischemia or infarction. Note that in the schematic depicting lateral wall regional dilation that the posterolateral papillary muscle has been laterally displaced as well. This may result in mitral valve malcoaptation and functional mitral regurgitation. In each schematic, the *dotted line* represents the normal geometry.

shape as opposed to smooth bullet-like tapering (Fig. 15.15). When evaluating echocardiograms for an ischemic wall motion abnormality, it is important to quickly assess the left ventricular geometry because it often provides a very rapid clue to the presence of abnormal regional function.

With the complex nature of myocardial contraction and wall motion abnormalities in mind, one can then employ several different algorithms for quantitation of wall motion abnormalities. These were outlined in Table 15.3. Many of these are further discussed in Chapter 6. When dealing with coronary disease, it is imperative to adopt a regional approach to the description of wall motion abnormalities, whether that description is a highly detailed quantitative scheme or a simple "eyeball" approach. Figure 15.16 schematizes the standard segments of the left ventricle that are commonly employed for analysis as well as the coronary arteries that usually perfuse those seg-

ments. Previous schemes employed a 16-segment model. More recently, a 17-segment approach has been recommended in which the 17th segment represents the true apex. This approach allows a more precise correlation with the segments visualized and analyzed by competing imaging techniques. The new segmentation schematic renames the segments, dropping the term posterior (Table 15.4). In general, the anterior septum and anterior wall are perfused by the left anterior descending coronary artery and its branches, and the inferior wall in the area of the posterior interventricular groove by the right coronary artery. Figure 15.16 outlines the most likely distribution of coronary arteries to the various segments. There can be substantial overlap in the inferior, lateral, and an-

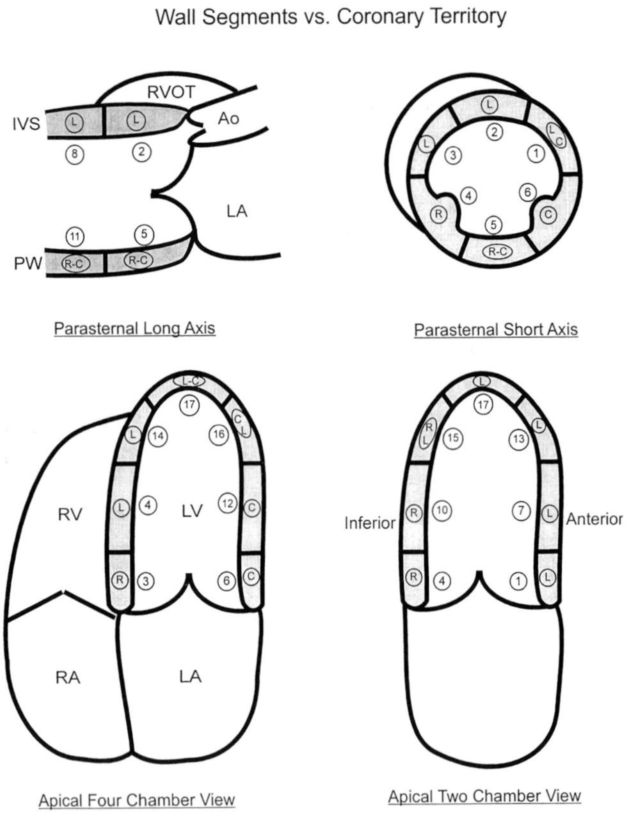

Wall Segments vs. Coronary Territory

Parasternal Long Axis

Parasternal Short Axis

Apical Four Chamber View

Apical Two Chamber View

FIGURE 15.16. Schematic representation of the currently recommended 17-segment model of the left ventricle (*LV*). The parasternal and apical views are depicted. The circled numbers correspond to the current segment numbers recommended by the American Society of Echocardiography (Table 15.4). For each segment, the coronary distribution most likely responsible for the wall motion abnormality in that area is noted. When more than one coronary territory is listed, overlap between coronary distributions is anticipated in that segment. The true apex is most often perfused by the left anterior descending coronary artery (*L*); however, in the presence of a dominant right coronary artery (*R*) or circumflex coronary artery (*C*), it may also be perfused by that artery. Ao, aorta; IVS, interventricular septum; LA, left atrium; PW, posterior wall; RA, right atrium; RV, right ventricle; RVOT, right ventricular outflow tract.

▶ TABLE 15.4 Comparison of Current (17 Segment) and Former (16 Segment) Nomenclature for Left Ventricular Segmentation

New Segment No.	New Nomenclature	Views	Old Nomenclature
1	Basal anterior	PSx, 2C	Same
2	Basal anterior septal	PSx, PLAX	Same
	Dropped		Basal septal
3	Basal inferior septal	PSx, 4C	$\frac{1}{2}$ basal inferior + $\frac{1}{2}$ basal septal
4	Basal inferior	PSx, 2C	$\frac{1}{2}$ basal inferior + $\frac{1}{2}$ basal post
	Dropped		Basal posterior
5	Basal inferior lateral	PSx, PLAX	Basal lateral
6	Basal anterior lateral	PSx, 4C	Basal lateral
7	Mid anterior	PSx, 2C	Same
8	Mid anterior septal	PSx, PLAX	Same
9	Mid inferior septal	PSx, 4C	$\frac{1}{2}$ mid septal + $\frac{1}{2}$ mid inferior
	Dropped		Mid posterior
10	Mid inferior	PSx, 2C	$\frac{1}{2}$ mid inferior + $\frac{1}{2}$ mid posterior
11	Mid inferior lateral	PSx, PLAX	Mid lateral
12	Mid anterior lateral	PSx, 4C	Mid lateral
13	Apical anterior	2C	Same
14	Apical septal	4C	Same
15	Apical inferior	2C	Same
16	Apical lateral	4C	Same
17	True apex	4C/2C	N/A

PLAX, parasternal long-axis view; PSx, parasternal short-axis view; 4C, apical four-chamber view; 2C, apical two-chamber view; N/A, not available.

terolateral segments, depending on the dominance of the right and left circumflex coronary arteries. The inferoapical segment represents an overlap zone between the distal left anterior descending coronary artery and the distal right coronary artery, and the apical lateral wall represents an overlap between the circumflex and left anterior descending coronary arteries. This type of scheme that attributes the coronary artery territories to different regions can be superimposed on any of these semiquantitative or quantitative schemes to assist in linking regional wall motion abnormalities to the coronary artery responsible for wall motion abnormality.

The simplest assessment of wall motion consists of description of wall motion as being normal or abnormal, typically further characterized as hypokinetic, akinetic, and dyskinetic in each region of the myocardium. This assessment suffices for the immediate detection of an ischemic event but does not provide information that can be readily communicated with respect to the size of myocardial infarction or the size of an area in jeopardy.

The next level of complexity for quantitation of wall motion abnormalities involves generation of a wall motion score or score index. This methodology involves describing the wall motion characteristics of each of the predefined segments as being normal, hypokinetic, akinetic, dyskinetic, or aneurysmal. A numerical score, typically 1 to 5, is then applied to each of these segments (Table 15.5), and the total score is divided by the number of segments evaluated to create a wall motion score index. A ventricle with completely normal wall motion would have a score index of 1.0 (total score divided by the number of segments), with higher scores representing progressively greater degrees of ventricular dysfunction. This global score, representing overall left ventricular wall motion, can then be subdivided into an anterior score, representing the distribution of the left anterior descending coronary artery, and a posterior score, representing the right plus circumflex coronary artery territories. Often, because of the tremendous overlap in the posterior circulation, an effort is not made to separate the independent contribution of the right coronary artery and the circumflex coronary artery. It is often helpful to also calculate the percentage of seg-

▶ TABLE 15.5 Wall Motion Score

Standard Scores		Optional Scores
	0	Hyperdynamic
Normal	1	
	1.5	Mildly hypokinetic
Hypokinetic	2	
	2.5	Severely hypokinetic
Akinetic	3	
Dyskinetic	4	
Aneurysm	5	
	6	Akinetic with scar[a]
	7	Dyskinetic with scar[a]

[a]Descriptive numbers only. The actual numeric value added to the global score is that corresponding to the motion pattern (i.e., 0–5).

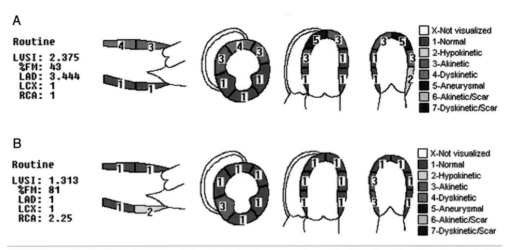

FIGURE 15.17. Wall motion score index recorded in two patients. **A:** A wall motion score recorded in a patient with extensive anteroapical myocardial infarction. **B:** A wall motion score from a patient with a more limited inferior wall myocardial infarction. In each instance, note the global left ventricular score index and the ability to separate the score for each of the three major coronary territories. LAD, left anterior descending coronary artery; LCX, circumflex coronary artery; %FM, percent of segments with normal wall motion; LVSI, left ventricular wall motion score index; RCA, right coronary artery.

ments with normal motion. Figure 15.17 presents examples of wall motion score indexes generated in patients with varying size wall motion abnormalities. It is often beneficial to subdivide the wall motion score into an anterior or posterior score or a separate score for each coronary territory. In Figure 15.17A, note that the global score of 2.375 is made up entirely of a wall motion abnormality in the left anterior descending coronary territory, whereas the posterior territories are normal.

Additional modifications of the wall motion score index have included an additional descriptive score for scar that allows a numeric designation that can then be tabulated. Typically, the number assigned for scar is used only for descriptive purposes and the numeric value corresponding to the wall motion abnormality is used to calculate the score and score index. For example, a scarred segment that is akinetic will receive a descriptive value of 6, but when calculating the wall motion score index, it is given a value of 3 because it is akinetic. The same is true for a scarred dyskinetic segment. Although allowing for the description of the scar and its extent, it avoids attributing a greater than usual functional deficit to a wall that is essentially akinetic or dyskinetic.

Other modifications have included using a score of 0 for hyperdynamic. As with the aneurysm score, this allows description and tabulation of walls with compensatory hyperkinesis; however, it results in a relative underestimation of the deficit attributable to the infarct because the global numeric score now allows the compensatory hyperkinesis to reduce the numeric impact of the wall motion abnormality. In this instance, the regional wall motion score, reflecting either anterior or posterior territories or individual coronary arteries, will remain abnormal even if overall left ventricular function is normal

due to compensatory hyperkinesis. Further modifications of a wall motion score scheme have included intermediate scores of 1.5 and 2.5 for mildly and severely hypokinetic, respectively, which provides additional quantitative information when evaluating patients during cardiovascular stress for viable myocardium or in following recovery of function after myocardial infarction.

More quantitative methods for regional wall motion analysis include radian or area shrinkage analysis (Figs. 15.3 and 15.12) and centerline chordal shortening, which are discussed in Chapter 6. For any of the quantitative or semiquantitative methods, tethering will result in a predictable overestimation of actual infarct or ischemic zone size. The impact of horizontal tethering is schematized in Figure 15.18.

A different approach to quantitation of regional wall motion in ischemic syndromes can be obtained by application of Doppler tissue imaging. This technique is described in Chapter 3 and Chapter 6. Doppler tissue imaging can be used for both global and regional assessment of wall motion. For a global assessment, the entire left ventricular area is superimposed with a Doppler tissue imaging region of interest. The myocardium is then color encoded to reflect direction and velocity of wall motion. There are several limitations to this methodology including a slow frame rate and the inability to adequately saturate the entire ventricular myocardium with returning Doppler signal.

Doppler tissue imaging can also be used in a targeted fashion to quantitatively determine myocardial velocities in specific regions and has been shown to provide evidence of very early diastolic and systolic dysfunction in acutely ischemic myocardium. The major limitation of the technique is that the quantitative aspects can only be employed

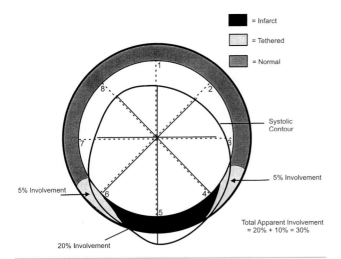

FIGURE 15.18. Schematic representation of horizontal tethering. This diagram represents posterior dyskinesis without translational motion. Note that the true extent of the infarct is as noted in the *darkly shaded area* encompassing radian 5 and parts of radians 6 and 4. Note that there is a border zone (*lightly shaded areas*) adjacent to the infarct area that is anatomically normal but has abnormal motion due to the tethering effect of posterior dyskinesis. In the schematic, the true anatomic defect represents 20% of the circumference of the left ventricle, with the tethered border zone giving an apparent total extent of 30%.

in one region of interest. Technology is under development to extract multiple Doppler velocities simultaneously.

Further advancements on determination of Doppler tissue velocities have included calculation of the endocardial to epicardial velocity gradient. By using Doppler tissue imaging to determine the velocity and magnitude of motion in the subendocardial and subepicardial layers along the same chord of shortening, a description of the difference in the two velocities can be determined. Subendocardial velocity and magnitude of motion exceeds subepicardial velocity and motion. In early ischemia, there may be a selective decrease in subendocardial function. This may be reflected as a change in the endocardial to epicardial gradient. Because the velocities of the two regions are each measured in relation to the transducer, there is little angle dependence on the measurement when expressed as a ratio of velocities. Calculation of this gradient requires specialized instrumentation that is not widely available at this time.

Myocardial Strain and Strain Rate Imaging

Myocardial strain rate imaging is a recently developed technique based on Doppler principles for evaluating regional wall motion. This technique relies on continuous determination of myocardial velocities in two segments of the ventricular myocardium separated by a known distance. Strain rate is defined as the rate of change in velocity between these two points. Experimental data have suggested that calculation of the strain rate is a more sensitive and early indicator of myocardial dysfunction than is mere determination of velocity from Doppler tissue imaging (Fig. 15.19).

Other Methods for Evaluating Ischemic Myocardium

There are several other technologies that can be brought to bear in evaluating patients with acute ischemic syndromes. Tissue characterization has shown promise for

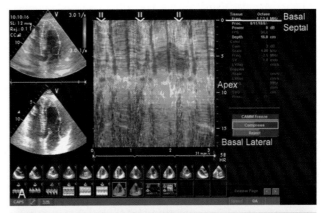

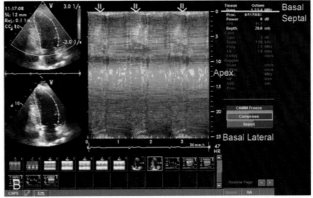

FIGURE 15.19. Strain rate imaging recorded in an apical four-chamber view in a patient with normal systolic function (**A**) and a patient with apical and septal wall motion abnormality (**B**). The color image in the middle of each panel represents the strain rate image. On the horizontal axis is time over three cardiac cycles and on the vertical axis is location along the perimeter of the left ventricle. The basal septal wall is at the top of each image (point 0), the apex at the middle, and the basal lateral wall at the bottom (point 17). In the normally contracting ventricle, note the phasic coloration in systole for both the lateral wall and septum (*arrows at the top of the image*). The lateral wall signal has areas of nonhomogeneous color due to echo dropout. In the image depicting septal and apical wall motion abnormality, note the early yellow coloration in the septum indicating hypokinesis with late systolic contraction. The lateral wall signal is compromised by echo dropout.

providing incremental information regarding the status of myocardial contractility in both experimental and clinical models of acute myocardial infarction. This technique relies on evaluating the cyclic variation in backscatter (returning signals from the myocardium). In the absence of myocardial ischemia, the overall intensity of returning signals within the myocardium varies in a cyclic manner timed with the phase of the cardiac cycle. The presence of even mild myocardial ischemia results in a reduction in this cyclic variation. (See Chapter 3 for a further discussion of tissue characterization.)

Recently, contrast echocardiography using new perfluorocarbon- or nitrogen-based agents has shown tremendous promise for evaluating the integrity of capillary level flow in the myocardium. Detection of preserved microvascular perfusion with myocardial contrast echocardiography has correlated with myocardial viability and subsequent recovery of function in both animal experimental models and clinical myocardial infarction. This topic is discussed further in Chapter 4.

ECHOCARDIOGRAPHIC EVALUATION OF CLINICAL SYNDROMES

Angina Pectoris

Resting echocardiography alone plays little role in the evaluation of patients with exertional angina pectoris. For patients with transient exertional chest pain, stress echocardiography can play an instrumental role in establishing the diagnosis of occult coronary artery disease. This is discussed in detail in Chapter 16.

For patients with clinical angina pectoris, a resting echocardiogram occasionally can provide information of both exclusionary and confirmatory nature. In rare instances, a patient may experience an episode of spontaneous chest pain while imaging is taking place or in a situation in which imaging can be undertaken immediately. If this fortuitous timing occurs, detection of a regional wall motion abnormality during ongoing pain is excellent evidence that the pain is due to myocardial ischemia. The specificity of this observation is obviously greatest if the wall motion abnormality is transient and resolves simultaneously with resolution of chest pain or electrocardiographic changes.

Similarly in a patient with chest pain and a moderate or high likelihood of underlying coronary disease, detection of a resting wall motion abnormality can provide excellent confirmatory evidence that underlying coronary artery disease is present. It should be emphasized that the resting abnormality may represent results of occult myocardial infarction or be the residua of repetitive episodes of myocardial ischemia. Some studies have suggested that as many as 40% of patients with chronic coronary artery disease, but without documented myocardial infarction, may have regional wall motion abnormalities on a resting echocardiogram. The potential mechanisms are repetitive stunning due to recurrent ischemia myocardial hibernation in the presence of severe coronary stenosis, or clinically unrecognized previous nontransmural infarction. Detection of a resting regional wall motion abnormality, persistent or otherwise, in a patient with clinical suspicion of coronary disease is excellent confirmatory evidence that significant underlying coronary artery disease is present and is a likely cause for the chest pain syndrome.

Conversely, by detecting other forms of organic heart disease, echocardiography can play an exclusionary role in evaluating patients with chest pain. When the resting echocardiogram reveals evidence of severe valvular heart disease such as aortic stenosis or of other diseases such as pulmonary hypertension and dilated or hypertrophic cardiomyopathy, this may provide a definitive diagnosis and a plausible explanation for the presenting symptoms. In this instance, the echocardiogram is used to establish an alternative diagnosis, and coronary artery disease may become a less likely alternative.

Acute Myocardial Infarction

Urgent transthoracic two-dimensional echocardiography can play a crucial role in establishing the diagnosis of acute myocardial infarction and determining its location, extent, and prognosis. As noted in Chapter 6 and in the previous sections on pathophysiology and evaluation of wall motion abnormalities, a regional wall motion abnormality is the hallmark of an acute ischemic syndrome. In the presence of chest pain with electrocardiographic changes, detection of a regional wall motion abnormality is direct evidence of myocardial ischemia, and the extent of the wall motion abnormality is directly related to the volume of myocardium in jeopardy. Based on the fundamentals previously noted, including the disproportionate impact of subendocardial ischemia, one should appreciate the independence of the wall motion abnormality from electrocardiographic changes because wall motion abnormalities will be seen in the absence of traditional Q-wave infarct.

Classic inferior myocardial infarction with ST-segment elevation and/or Q-waves in leads II, III, and AVF typically involves segments bordering the posterior interventricular groove with variable amounts of involvement of the inferoposterior wall. Classic anterior and anterolateral myocardial infarction with ST-segment elevation and/or Q-waves in the anterior precordial leads involves the anterior septum, anterior wall, and apex. Circumflex coronary artery occlusions represent a diverse combination of electrocardiographic changes, often presenting as an inferior myocardial infarction with exaggerated R-waves in the anterior precordium (leads V_1 and V_2) combined with changes in the inferior leads. The location of wall motion abnormalities in this instance is predominantly in the inferior and inferolateral walls. Apical involvement on echocardiography can be seen in virtually any of the classic electrocardiographic distributions of myocardial infarction and is not limited to the classic anterior infarct pattern. As such, detection of an apical abnormality in the presence of an inferior or posterolateral wall motion abnormality does not necessarily imply multivessel coronary disease or concurrent anterior myocardial infarction, but rather can be the effect of a single posterior dominant coronary territory. Figures 15.20 through 15.27 were recorded in patients presenting with classic Q-wave myocardial infarction in different territories. Figure 15.28 was recorded in patients with remote myocardial infarction and reveal variable degrees of wall thinning and scar formation.

The presence of a left bundle branch block pattern, either antecedent or occurring as a complication of myocardial infarction, confounds wall motion analysis. There are several guidelines that one can use to separate the bundle branch block wall motion abnormality from superimposed ischemia or myocardial infarction. These are listed in Table 15.6. In general, wall motion abnormalities due exclusively to left bundle branch block are most prominent in the proximal and mid anterior septum and are less often manifest in the anterior wall or apex. They typically do not result in alteration of left ventricular geometry or regional dilation. By using M-mode echocar-

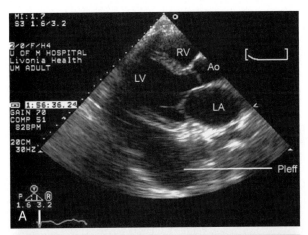

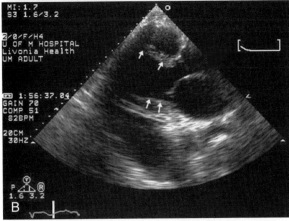

FIGURE 15.20. Parasternal long-axis echocardiogram recorded in a patient with extensive anteroapical and anterior wall myocardial infarction. Figures 15.20 through 15.23 are recorded in the same patient. **A:** In the parasternal long-axis view, note the normal geometry of the left ventricle (*LV*) in diastole. **B:** In systole, note the normal motion of the proximal inferior wall and a lack of thickening and akinesis of the entire anterior septum (*arrows*). Incidental note is made of a pleural effusion (*Pleff*). Ao, aorta; LA, left atrium; LV, left ventricle.

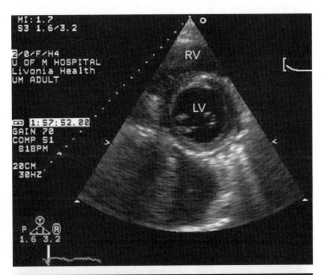

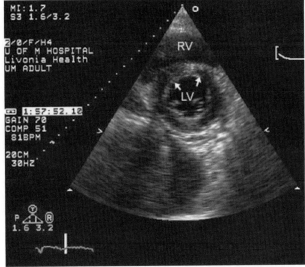

FIGURE 15.21. Parasternal short-axis view recorded in the same patient depicted in Figure 15.20. Note preserved circular geometry of the left ventricle (*LV*) in diastole (**A**) and the normal myocardial thickening and endocardial excursion of the posterior wall. **B:** Recorded in systole, the anterior and mid septum are both full thickness but dyskinetic (*arrows*). RV, right ventricle.

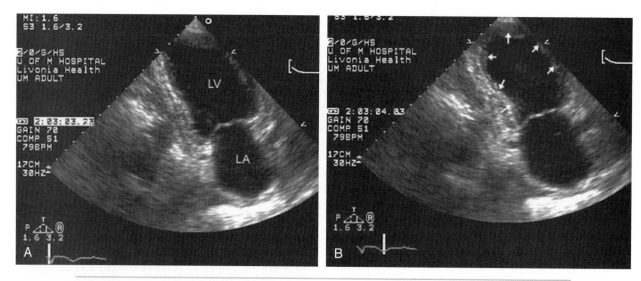

FIGURE 15.22. Apical two-chamber view recorded in diastole **(A)** and systole **(B)** in the patient previously presented with extensive left anterior descending coronary artery territory myocardial infarction. In the two-chamber view, note the preserved function of the proximal 50% of the inferior wall and the akinesis or dyskinesis of the distal inferior wall, apex, and anterior wall (*arrows*). In this example, the involvement of the distal inferior wall is due to a wraparound left anterior descending coronary artery and not the result of concurrent ischemia in the right coronary artery. LA, left atrium; LV, left ventricle.

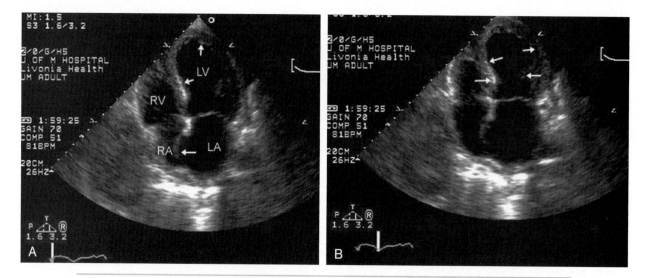

FIGURE 15.23. Apical four-chamber view recorded in the same patient depicted in the three previous figures. In the four-chamber view, note the abnormal geometry of the distal septum (*area between the two arrows*) present in diastole **(A)**. **B:** In systole, function is preserved at the base of the heart (*inward-pointing arrows*) with akinesis or dyskinesis in the distal half of the left ventricle (*outward-pointing arrows*). Incidental note is also made of an atrial septal aneurysm [*arrow in the left atrium (LA)*]. Note the bowing of the atrial septum from left to right, implying elevated left atrial pressure, presumably secondary to left ventricular dysfunction. LV, left ventricle, RA, right atrium; RV, right ventricle.

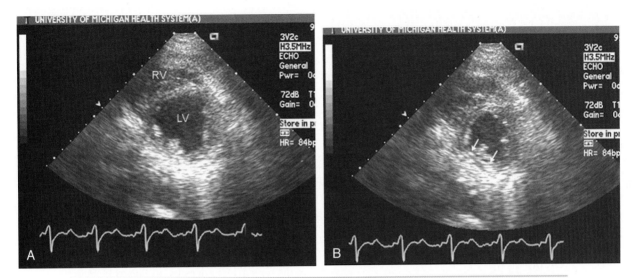

FIGURE 15.24. Parasternal short-axis view recorded in a patient with a classic inferior wall myocardial infarction. **A:** Recorded in diastole. Note the normal shape of the left ventricle (*LV*) in diastole. In systole **(B)**, the true inferior wall is thin and frankly dyskinetic (*arrows*), whereas the remaining walls contract normally. RV right ventricle.

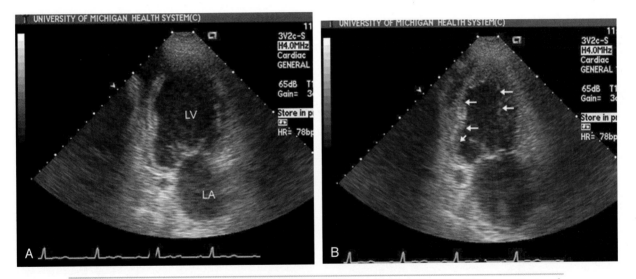

FIGURE 15.25. Apical two-chamber view recorded in diastole **(A)** and systole **(B)** in a patient with an inferior myocardial infarction. In systole **(B)**, note the normal motion of the anterior wall and the frank dyskinesis of the proximal two-thirds of the inferior wall (*arrows*). LA, left atrium; LV, left ventricle.

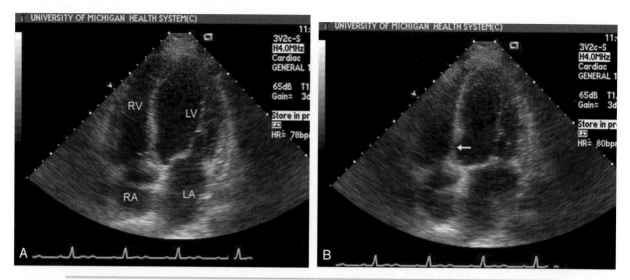

FIGURE 15.26. Apical four-chamber view recorded in the same patient depicted in Figure 15.25 in diastole **(A)** and systole **(B)**. Note the dyskinesis of the proximal 25% of the ventricular septum, which in this instance is attributable to septal involvement by the inferior myocardial infarction. Caution is advised when interpreting a wall motion abnormality in this location. The proximal ventricular septum in the apical four-chamber view often has abnormal motion. Only when the abnormality is seen in association with concurrent inferior wall myocardial infarction should it be presumed to be infarct as well. LA, left atrium; LV, left ventricle; RA, right atrium; RV, right ventricle.

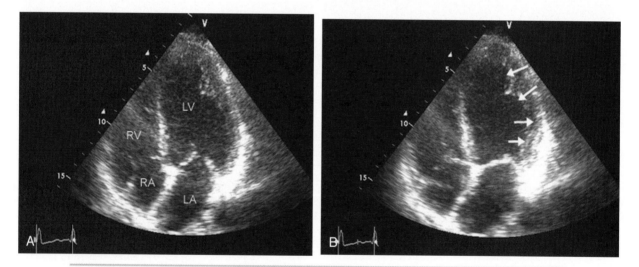

FIGURE 15.27. Apical four-chamber view recorded in a patient with a lateral wall myocardial infarction. The four-chamber view in diastole **(A)** and systole **(B)** is presented. Note the normal geometry of the left ventricle **(A)** but the dyskinesis of the proximal half of the lateral wall in systole (*rightward-pointing arrows*) with preserved function in the distal lateral wall (*leftward pointing arrows*) **(B)**. LA, left atrium; LV, left ventricle; RA, right atrium; RV, right ventricle.

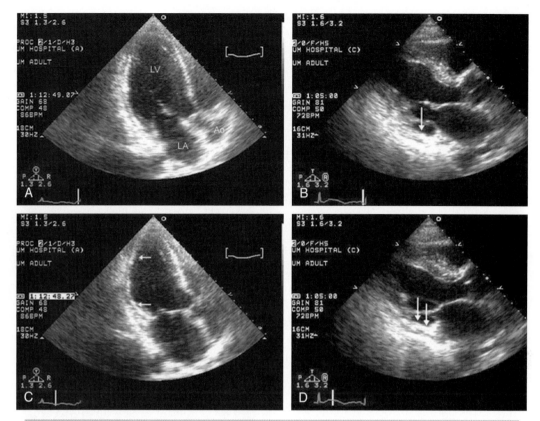

FIGURE 15.28. Echocardiograms recorded in two patients with remote myocardial infarctions. **Left:** Apical long-axis views recorded in diastole **(A)** and systole **(C)** in a patient with an inferior myocardial infarction attributed to disease of the left circumflex coronary artery. Note in systole that the proximal two-thirds of the inferoposterior wall are dyskinetic and there is normal contraction of the anterior septum and apex. **Right:** Parasternal long-axis views recorded in a patient with a remote inferior/inferolateral myocardial infarction. Image at the top **(B)** was recorded in diastole; note that the proximal one-third of the inferior wall is pathologically thinned with a dense echo signature consistent with scar. In the image at the bottom **(D)**, there is normal contraction of the anterior septum and more distal portions of the inferoposterior wall with akinesis of the infarct area (*downward-pointing arrows*). LA, left atrium; LV, left ventricle.

diography or careful attention to frame-by-frame analysis of two-dimensional echocardiography, wall thickening can be seen to be preserved and there is often multiphasic motion of the septum (Fig. 15.29). M-mode echocardiography is the more definitive method for demonstrating the mechanical effects of the left bundle branch block. With this technique, a classic early downward "beak" is noted with the onset of ventricular depolarization followed by concurrent anterior motion of the septum and myocardial thickening. In contrast, an ischemic abnormality in the left anterior descending territory results in loss of systolic thickening of the myocardium in the ventricular septum and wall motion abnormalities that often extend to the anterior wall and apex (Fig. 15.30). These are not infrequently associated with abnormal geometry of the left ventricular cavity. Finally, because the wall motion in left bundle branch block is due to electric delay, there is often marked mechanical dyssynchrony between the onset of motion (normal or abnormal) in the noninvolved walls

compared with a normal time frame for onset of motion in ischemia. These guidelines generally suffice for separation of ischemic from nonischemic abnormalities in the presence of a left bundle branch block in the majority of patients. It should be emphasized that there are numerous exceptions to these guidelines, and the diagnostic accuracy for detecting ischemia in the presence of a left bundle branch block is diminished to less than that seen for the other coronary territories, even for the most experienced echocardiographer.

As noted previously in the section on pathophysiology, it is not necessary to render the entire transmural thickness of the myocardium ischemic to result in a wall motion abnormality. Ischemia involving more than 20% of the wall thickness will result in akinesis or dyskinesis of the entire wall. This is in large part due to vertical tethering. As such, nontransmural myocardial infarction, typified by the non–Q-wave or non–ST-segment elevation myocardial infarction, can result in wall motion abnor-

▶ TABLE 15.6 **Left Bundle Branch Block Versus Ischemic Wall Motion Abnormality**

	Ischemic WMA	*LBBB*	*RV Paced*
Maximal location	Distal septum, apex, and anterior wall	Proximal/mid anterior septum	Distal septum, often inferior septum
Thickening	Absent or thinning	Partially preserved	Partially preserved
Duration	Usually monophasic	Multiphasic	Multiphasic
Abnormal geometry	Common	Uncommon	Uncommon
Temporal dyssynchrony	No	Yes	Yes

LBBB, left bundle branch block; RV, right ventricle; WMA, wall motion abnormality.

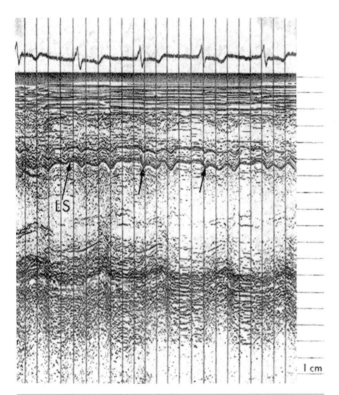

FIGURE 15.29. M-mode echocardiogram recorded in a patient with a left bundle branch block. Note the early systolic beak of the left septum (LS) occurring immediately after the QRS (*arrows*), followed by subsequent thickening of the ventricular septum.

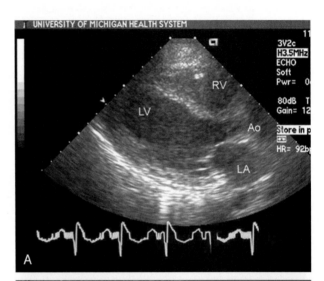

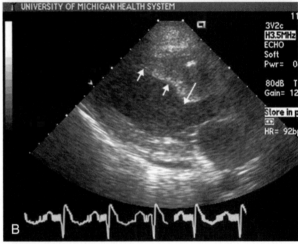

FIGURE 15.30. Parasternal long-axis echocardiogram recorded in a patient presenting with an acute myocardial infarction and left bundle branch block. Note from diastole (**A**) to systole (**B**), only the very proximal portion of the anterior septum has moved downward (*long arrow*) and the more distal portions of the septum are dyskinetic (*upward-pointing arrows*). This pattern should be easily distinguished from the wall motion abnormality seen in left bundle branch block. Ao, aorta; LA, left atrium; LV, left ventricle; RV, right ventricle.

malities virtually identical to those seen in Q-wave or transmural myocardial infarction. Because the extent of the wall motion abnormality reflects the distribution of the ischemic territory, two-dimensional echocardiography provides incremental information compared with electrocardiography for determining the amount of myocardium in jeopardy that in turn is related to prognosis and the likelihood of complications. Figure 15.31 was recorded in a patient with non–Q-wave myocardial infarction whose electrocardiogram revealed only isolated T-wave inversion and ST-segment depression. Note the extent of wall motion abnormalities in this patient similar to that seen in ST-segment or Q-wave infarction. A not un-

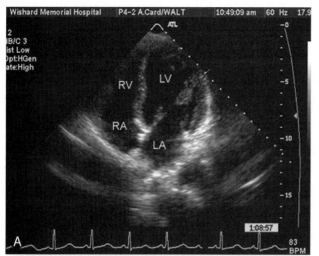

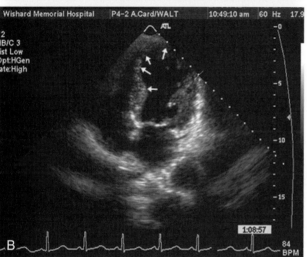

FIGURE 15.31. Apical four-chamber view recorded in a patient presenting with a non–ST-segment elevation myocardial infarction. In this instance, only ST-segment depression with T-wave inversion was noted on the electrocardiogram, maximally in the anterior precordium. **A** was recorded in diastole. **B:** Note the fairly extensive area of dyskinesis in the distal septum and apex *(arrows)*. The wall motion abnormality noted here is virtually identical to that seen with typical ST-segment elevation or Q-wave myocardial infarction. LA, left atrium; LV, left ventricle, RA, right atrium; RV, right ventricle.

common clinical scenario is the presentation of a patient with known coronary artery disease and previous myocardial infarction who now has an acute chest pain syndrome suggesting myocardial ischemia. In this situation, it can be problematic to identify additional wall motion abnormalities in the background of a preexisting wall motion abnormality, especially if the preexisting abnormality is large.

Numerous studies have evaluated the clinical utility of transthoracic two-dimensional echocardiography for detecting wall motion abnormalities in suspected acute

myocardial infarction. Many of the published studies are outlined in Table 15.7. In general, 80% to 95% of patients with documented myocardial infarction will have detectable wall motion abnormalities. Experimentally, there is a threshold of myocardium required to produce a wall motion abnormality. The transmural threshold was discussed previously. It also appears that there is a total myocardial burden that must be rendered ischemic before a wall motion abnormality develops. Animal models have suggested that involvement of 1.0 g of myocardium or more is necessary before a wall motion abnormality is expected to be detectable with standard echocardiography. For this reason, myocardial infarction or ischemia involving exceptionally small territories may not result in a detectable wall motion abnormality and, as such, may be missed with echocardiographic techniques. In contemporary practice, resting transthoracic echocardiography is rarely used as a stand-alone technique in patients presenting with chest pain syndromes. Many aggressive centers have adopted an approach of early stress echocardiography in patients with normal resting wall motion who have presented with chest pain suggesting an acute coronary syndrome. The safety of this approach has been demonstrated in numerous studies, and the accuracy of combined rest and stress echocardiography for detecting underlying coronary artery disease likewise has been demonstrated and appears equivalent to the capability of competing radionuclide techniques. The use of stress echocardiography is discussed in Chapter 16.

Natural History of Wall Motion Abnormalities

Once the diagnosis of acute myocardial infarction has been established, transthoracic echocardiography can be used to follow the progression of remodeling or regression of wall motion abnormalities. In contemporary practice, if successful reperfusion is obtained either by mechanical or pharmacologic strategies, wall motion can be expected to recover substantially or in part in most patients. Because reperfusion strategies often are not completed within the critical time window to avoid all myocardial necrosis, many patients are left with varying degrees of nontransmural myocardial fibrosis. Because of the residual fibrosis, wall motion abnormalities may persist, even in the presence of relatively full-thickness myocardium. Figures 15.32 and 15.33 were recorded in patients in whom serial follow-up echocardiograms were available after myocardial infarction. Notice in Figure 15.32 that there has been complete recovery of wall motion after successful early reperfusion. In Figure 15.33, the magnitude of the wall motion abnormality is dramatically less, but the apex remains akinetic. This would be a typical pattern seen after less optimal reperfusion, in which nontransmural infarction

TABLE 15.7 Diagnosis of Acute Myocardial Infarction in Patients with Chest Pain

Ref.	Population	Total No. of Patients	Abnormal Test	Sens (%)	Spec (%)	PPV (%)	NPV (%)	Overall Accuracy (%)
Patients with documented AMI								
Heger et al., 1980	Consec AMI	44	Seg WMA	100	—	—	—	—
Parisi et al., 1981	Prior AMI	20	Seg WMA	95	—	—	—	—
Visser et al., 1981	Consec AMI	66	Seg WMA	98	—	—	—	—
Stamm et al., 1983	Prior AMI	51	Seg WMA	100	—	—	—	—
Nishimura et al., 1984	Consec AMI	61		93	—	—	—	—
Lundgren et al., 1990	Consec AMI	20	Seg WMA	83	—	—	—	—
Patents with chest pain, suspected AMI								
Horowitz et al., 1982	No prior MI	65	Seg WMA	94	84	86	93	89
Sasaki et al., 1986	No prior MI, During CP	18	Seg WMA	86	82	75	90	83
Sasaki et al., 1986	No prior MI, After CP	28	Seg WMA	100	90	80	100	93
Peels et al., 1990	No prior MI	43	Seg WMA	92	53	46	94	65
Sabia et al., 1991	Consec	169	Seg WMA	93	57	31	98	63
Saeian et al., 1994	No prior MI	60	Seg WMA	88	94	91	92	92
Gibler et al., 1995	Consec	901	Any WMA	47	99	50	99	98

AMI, acute myocardial infarction; Consec, consecutive patients; NPV, negative predictive value; PPV, positive predictive value; Seg, segmental; CP, chest pain; Sens, sensitivity; Spec, specificity; WMA, wall motion abnormality.
From Cheitlin MD, et al. ACC/AHA/ASE 2003 Guideline Update for the Clinical Application of Echocardiography: summary article. A report of the American College of Cardiology/American Heart Association Task Force on Practice Guidelines (ACC/AHA/ASE Committee to Update the 1997 Guidelines for the Clinical Application of Echocardiography). J Am Soc Echocardiogr 2003;16:1091–1110, with permission.

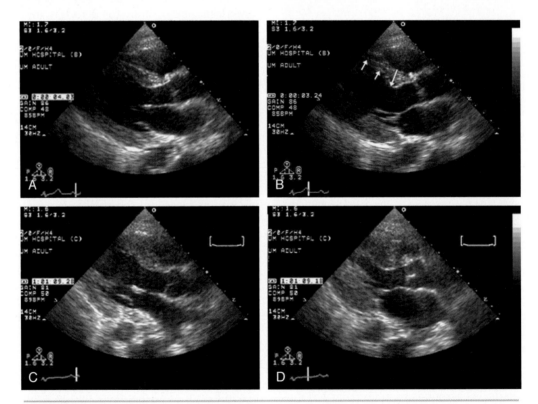

FIGURE 15.32. Parasternal long-axis echocardiogram recorded in a patient at the time of presentation with an impending anterior ST-segment elevation myocardial infarction (**A, B**). **C,D:** The same patient on a follow-up echocardiogram recorded several days after successful reperfusion therapy. For each set of images, the end-diastolic frames are on the left and end-systolic on the right. At the time of acute presentation, note preserved motion of the proximal anterior septum (*downward-pointing arrow*) with dyskinesis of the distal septum (*upward-pointing arrows*). **D:** Recorded in systole after reperfusion therapy and recovery of function; note the normal motion of both the anterior septum and inferoposterior walls.

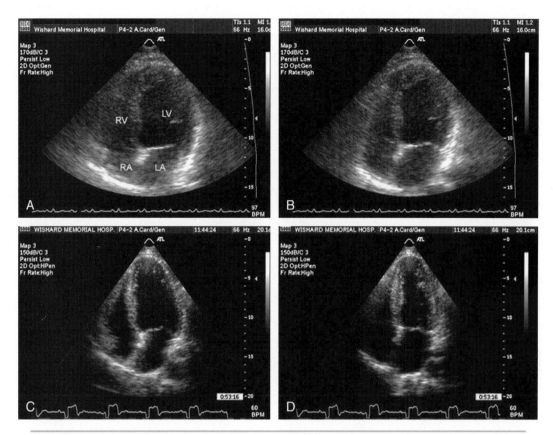

FIGURE 15.33. Apical four-chamber views recorded in a patient presenting with extensive LAD distribution myocardial infarction. **A, B:** Recorded at the time of presentation; **C, D:** recorded approximately 3 months later after successful reperfusion therapy. For each set of images, diastole is on the left and systole on the right. Note the extensive wall motion abnormalities at the time of presentation with the acute event and near complete recovery of function 3 months later, with only a limited residual apical wall motion abnormality. LA, left atrium; LV, left ventricle; RA, right atrium; RV, right ventricle.

and fibrosis occurred after delayed reperfusion. It is important to distinguish between the persistent dysfunction attributable to relatively successful reperfusion and nontransmural infarction from failed reperfusion with hibernating myocardium.

Without successful restoration of flow, the natural course of acute myocardial infarction is for transmural necrosis to occur. In this instance, there will be no recovery of function in the infarct zone. The border zones that may have compromised myocardial perfusion acutely and hence have abnormal wall motion may show recovery of function; however, the central transmural infarct zone will remain akinetic. Over approximately a 6-week period, myocardial necrosis is replaced by fibrosis and scar. Both pathologically and echocardiographically, the wall becomes thinner and denser. Figures 15.9 and 15.28 were recorded in patients with nonintervened myocardial infarction in which thinning of the wall and frank akinesis can be seen. More chronically, aneurysm formation and remodeling may occur that can have deleterious effects

on ventricular performance. These issues are discussed further in the section on chronic coronary artery disease.

Several investigators have evaluated recovery of function after myocardial infarction on a serial basis. More recently, several large clinical trials have evaluated the impact of pharmacologic therapy with either beta-blockers or angiotensin-converting enzyme inhibitors for preventing adverse remodeling. Depending on the size of the initial infarction, degree of success of reperfusion, and, in some instances, presence or absence of active treatment, adverse remodeling can be minimized. Long-term prognostic studies have demonstrated that patients with adverse ventricular remodeling are more likely to develop ventricular arrhythmias, congestive heart failure, evidence of diastolic dysfunction and, in general, have a substantially worse prognosis than patients in whom adverse remodeling has not occurred. Remodeling has been quantified by a number of techniques including assessment of endocardial surface area and calculation of diastolic and systolic volumes.

▶ **TABLE 15.8** Prognostic Value of Wall Motion Abnormalities in Patients with Acute Myocardial Infarction

Ref.	Population	Total No. of Patients	Adverse Outcomes	Criteria	Prediction of Adverse Outcomes (%)				
					Sensitivity (%)	Specificity (%)	PPV (%)	NPV (%)	Overall Accuracy (%)
Horowitz et al, 1982	No prior AMI	65	D, PumF, MaligAR, RecAP	SWMA	100	53	28	100	60
Gibson et al., 1982	Consec AMI	68	D, PumF, MI	Remote WMA	81	81	78	83	81
Horowitz et al., 1982	Proved AMI	43	D, PumF, MaligAr	WSM >7	85	83	69	93	84
Nishimura et al., 1984	Consec AMI	61	D, PumF,	WSM index >2	80	90	89	82	85
Jaarsma et al., 1984	AMI; Killip	77	MaligAR Progression to PumF	WMS >7	88	57	35	95	64
Sabia et al., 1984	Consec AMI	29	PumF, MaligAR, RecAP	SWMA	100	13	48	100	52
Sabia et al., 1984	Consec CP (ED)	171	D, MI, MaligAR RecAP < 48 h	LV dysfx	94	48	28	97	54
Sabia et al., 1984	Consec CP (ED)	139	D, MI	LV dysfx MaligAr, RecAP >48 h	83	50	25	94	55

CP (ED), chest pain in the emergency department;
D, death; LV dysfx, left ventricular dysfunction; MaligAr, malignant arrhythmias; MI, myocardial infarction; PumF, pump failure; RecAP, recurrent angina pectoris; SWMA, segmental wall motion abnormality; WMA, wall motion abnormality; WMS, wall motion score.
Other abbreviations as in Table 15.7.
From Cheitlin MD, et al. ACC/AHA/ASE 2003 Guideline Update for the Clinical Application of Echocardiography: summary article. A report of the American College of Cardiology/American Heart Association Task Force on Practice Guidelines (ACC/AHA/ASE Committee to Update the 1997 Guidelines for the Clinical Application of Echocardiography). J Am Soc Echocardiogr 2003;16:1091–1110, with permission.

Prognostic Implications

Several studies have demonstrated the adverse prognosis of wall motion abnormalities in patients presenting with acute myocardial infarction (Table 15.8). In general, the more extensive the wall motion abnormality is, whether determined by a wall motion score index, ejection fraction, or more detailed quantitative techniques, the greater is the likelihood of complications such as congestive heart failure, arrhythmia, and death. The extent of regional wall motion abnormalities as well as parameters of global ventricular dysfunction such as end-diastolic and end-systolic volume index and ejection fraction all correlate with the likelihood of an adverse outcome in both the short and long term.

Several other echocardiographic observations have direct relevance to prognosis. In the presence of isolated, single-vessel coronary artery disease, resulting in an acute ischemic syndrome, normally there is compensatory hyperkinesis of the remaining segments. This mitigates against the overall adverse impact of the ischemic regional wall motion abnormality and serves to protect global function. Failure to develop compensatory hyperkinesis has been noted as a marker of underlying multivessel coronary artery disease and carries a worse prognosis compared with the finding of hyperkinesis in noninvolved segments. There are several Doppler parameters that also correlate with prognosis.

Doppler Evaluation of Systolic and Diastolic Function in Acute Myocardial Infarction

As discussed in Chapter 6, Doppler techniques can be used to determine left ventricular systolic function. This has had little use in routine clinical practice because assessment of the location and magnitude of regional wall motion abnormalities generally provides more clinically relevant information. Interrogation of the left ventricular outflow tract or ascending aorta can be used to record a time velocity integral that is directly proportional to left ventricular stroke volume. This can be successfully tracked during the course of acute myocardial infarction to determine the degree of impairment, degree of recovery, and effect of interventions. This is infrequently used in contemporary clinical practice.

More recently, Doppler interrogation of the mitral valve has been undertaken to assess left ventricular diastolic function at the time of acute myocardial infarction. Assuming normal diastolic properties of the left ventricle before myocardial infarction, there is an immediate reduction in left ventricular compliance at the time of acute ischemia or myocardial infarction. This typically results in a reduced E/A ratio with a prolonged deceleration time (Figs. 15.5 and 15.34A). Several clinical studies have demonstrated that the presence of a restrictive pattern (Fig. 15.34C) or even a normal pattern of mitral valve inflow at the time of acute myocardial infarction represents a high-risk subset with a substantially worse prognosis than patients with delayed relaxation. The fact that the "normal" mitral valve inflow pattern confers a poor prognosis suggests that this represents a pseudonormal pattern rather than truly normal diastolic properties. The pseudonormal pattern is seen in patients with poor ventricular compliance and elevated left ventricular filling pressure. As anticipated, this hemodynamic situation is the result of more extensive myocardial infarction or ischemia. Clinical studies have suggested an adverse outcome in 21% to 65% of individuals with restrictive filling (or pseudonormal) patterns in the presence of acute myocardial infarction compared with adverse outcomes of 13% to 24% in patients with delayed relaxation patterns (Table 15.9). Confounding the evaluation of mitral valve inflow patterns is the wide range of inflow patterns that may exist immediately before myocardial infarction in any given patient. Although normal diastolic properties can be assumed in an otherwise healthy younger patient before myocardial infarction, in the elderly population with coexistent left ventricular hypertrophy or other disease (including previous myocardial infarction), one cannot assume that the patient began with a normal baseline diastolic function. This represents a confounding variable in the assessment of diastolic properties at the time of acute myocardial infarction. Nevertheless, detection of a classic restrictive inflow pattern does convey an adverse prognosis irrespective of the presence, nature, and degree of previously existing underlying abnormalities.

COMPLICATIONS OF ACUTE MYOCARDIAL INFARCTION

Virtually all mechanical complications of acute myocardial infarction can be visualized and diagnosed using two-dimensional echocardiography. In most instances, routine transthoracic scanning suffices for this assessment.

Obviously, color Doppler flow imaging is an integral part of the comprehensive examination in patients with acute myocardial infarction and is crucial for detection and quantitation of lesions such as mitral and tricuspid regurgitation and ventricular septal defect.

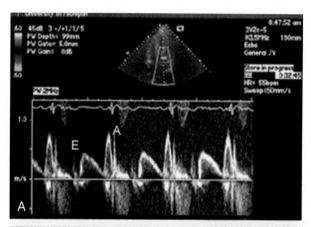

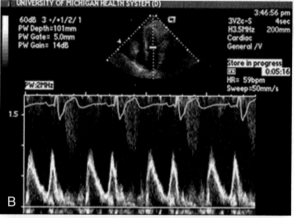

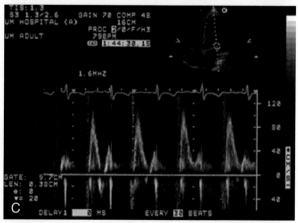

FIGURE 15.34. Mitral valve inflow recorded in three patients presenting with acute myocardial infarction. Classic delayed relaxation **(A)** and a restrictive pattern **(C)** are shown. **B:** An apparently normal mitral inflow pattern is recorded. However, in the presence of acute myocardial infarction in which abnormal diastolic dysfunction would be expected, this most likely represents a pseudonormal inflow pattern.

▶ **TABLE 15.9** **Prognostic Features in Acute Myocardial Infarction**

Ref.	No.	follow-up (mo)	Parameter	Outcome	% with Adverse Event	% without Adverse Event
Barzilai et al., 1990	849	48	On admission MR murmur	Death	36	15
Feinberg et al., 2000	417	12	≥Mild MR	Death	16	4.8
Grigioni et al., 2001	303	60	MR at ≥16 d S/P MI	Death	62 ± 5	39 ± 6
Møller et al., 2000	125	12 ± 7	Normal	Death	0	
			DR		13	
			PN		48	
			RFP		65	
Cerisano et al., 2001	104	32 ± 10	DT≤130 ms	Death	21	3
Møller et al., 2003	799	34	Normal	Death	15	
			DR		24	
			RFP		50	
Hillis et al., 2004	250	13	E/e′ >15	Death	26	6

DR, delayed relaxation; DT, deceleration time; E/e′, ratio of mitral to anular E velocity; MR, mitral regurgitation; PN, pseudonormal inflow; RFP, restrictive filling pattern.

Pericardial Effusion

Transient pericardial effusion is not uncommon after acute myocardial infarction. It typically is seen in transmural or Q-wave myocardial infarction and only rarely in non–Q-wave myocardial infarction. Careful surveillance studies have demonstrated that 30% to 40% of patients with acute transmural infarction will have transient accumulation of small amounts of pericardial fluid (Fig. 15.35). Larger amounts of fluid, or fluid accumulation sufficient to result in hemodynamic compromise, is rare in uncomplicated myocardial infarction. The genesis of this effusion is assumed to be epicardial inflammation, and it may be seen in the absence of any symptoms specific for acute pericardial disease. Larger effusion or effusions with a hemorrhagic appearance should always prompt consideration of myocardial rupture.

A syndrome of delayed pericarditis has also been well described after myocardial infarction. The so-called Dressler syndrome appears to have become less frequent than originally described. This syndrome consists of development of recurrent pain with pericardial fluid, typically occurring 6 weeks to 3 months after myocardial infarction. The appearance and behavior of the effusion are similar to that due to any other cause, and as with the small effusions accumulating during the acute phase of myocardial infarction rarely leads to hemodynamic compromise.

The final scenario in which pericardial effusion is seen occurs with impeding or partial rupture of the free wall. This will be seen in the presence of infarct expansion and

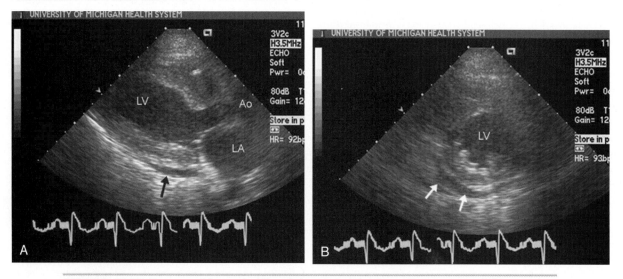

FIGURE 15.35. Parasternal long-axis (**A**) and short-axis (**B**) echocardiograms recorded in a patient with acute anteroapical myocardial infarction and a small pericardial effusion (*arrows*). AO, aorta; LA, left atrium; LV, left ventricle.

clinically in the presence of recurring chest pain and often with dynamic electrocardiographic changes but without additional enzyme level increases. Fluid accumulation in this instance represents inflammation of the thinned, expanded wall and/or direct extravasation of blood through a partial myocardial rupture. Figure 15.36 was recorded in a patient who developed recurrent pain and electrocardiographic changes 3 days after a transmural inferior wall myocardial infarction. In this setting, the presence of the pericardial effusion is an ominous warning that either partial rupture has occurred or rupture is impending. In most instances, there will be no distinguishing characteristics of the effusion seen in any of these three situations and the underlying pathology is assumed from either the timing or the clinical presentation. On occasion, the pericardial fluid may take on a cloudy appearance or contain vague homogeneous echo densities suggesting hemorrhage (Fig. 15.36).

Infarct Expansion

Even in the presence of acute infarction, myocardium with normal thickness has nearly normal tensile strength. Infarct expansion represents acute thinning of the ventricular wall with aneurysmal dilation, occurring 24 to 72 hours after transmural myocardial infarction. It represents an acute remodeling phenomenon and carries significant prognostic implications. This complication is not seen in nontransmural myocardial infarction. It is more common after anteroapical myocardial infarction than posterior distribution infarction. Echocardiographically, one detects a fairly typical aneurysmal bulge of the myocardium but without the appearance of dense scar. The wall in the area of infarct expansion consists of necrotic myocardial tissue, which, because it has expanded or been stretched over a larger endocardial surface area, may be only 4 to 6 mm in thickness rather than the normal 10 to 11 mm and have markedly reduced structural integrity. The thin necrotic wall has low tensile strength and is the precursor to most mechanical complications. Figure 15.37 schematizes this phenomenon. Figure 15.38 was recorded in a patient 1 day after acute anteroapical myocardial infarction and is an example of acute infarct expansion. This complication should be recognized because it is the precursor to mechanical complications such as free-wall rupture, ventricular septal rupture, and papillary muscle rupture. Early studies suggested a short-term, in-hospital mortality rate as high as 40% for patients with infarct expansion.

Free-Wall Rupture

Rupture of the free wall of the left ventricle is a nearly universally fatal event. In exceptional cases, rupture occurs with a timing such that immediate cardiovascular surgery and repair can be undertaken. In general, how-

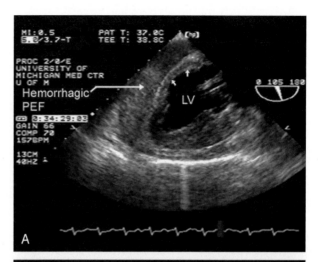

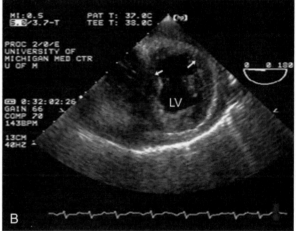

FIGURE 15.36. Transesophageal echocardiogram recorded in a patient with an inferior myocardial infarction. **A:** Recorded at 105 degrees; recorded at 0 degrees. Note the acute thinning of the inferior wall (*arrows*). **B:** Note the echo dense fluid filling pericardial space representing hemorrhage from a partial rupture of the infarcted inferior wall. LV, left ventricle.

ever, this is an instantaneously fatal event. As such, there are few recorded echocardiograms of patients with acute free-wall rupture. Figure 15.36 was recorded in a patient with free-wall rupture in which a large hemorrhagic pericardial effusion can be seen as well as acute aneurysm (infarct expansion) in the posterior wall. Free wall rupture most often results in instantaneous accumulation of massive compressive pericardial hemorrhage and death.

Ventricular Thrombus

Before the era of acute intervention for myocardial infarction. ventricular thrombus was reported in 25% to 40% of patients after anterior myocardial infarction. It is virtually always associated with anteroapical myocardial

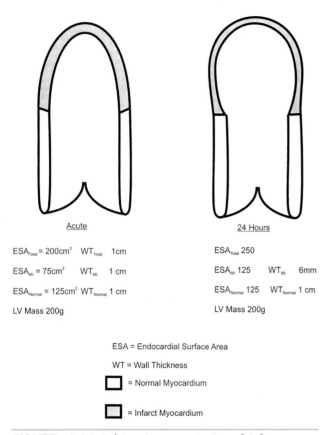

ESA$_{Total}$ = 200cm^2 WT$_{Total}$ 1cm

ESA$_{MI}$ = 75cm^2 WT$_{MI}$ 1 cm

ESA$_{Normal}$ = 125cm^2 WT$_{Normal}$ 1 cm

LV Mass 200g

ESA$_{Total}$ 250

ESA$_{MI}$ 125   WT$_{MI}$ 6mm

ESA$_{Normal}$ 125   WT$_{Normal}$ 1 cm

LV Mass 200g

ESA = Endocardial Surface Area

WT = Wall Thickness

☐ = Normal Myocardium

☐ = Infarct Myocardium

FIGURE 15.37. Schematic representation of infarct expansion. **Left:** Normal left ventricular geometry with acute transmural mitral infarction of the apical portions of the left ventricle is schematized. In the acute setting, there is similar thickness of both the infarct and noninfarct tissue. For this hypothetical example, an initial endocardial surface area of 200 cm^2 is assumed with uniform wall thickness of 1 cm, resulting in a left ventricular mass of 200 g. At the time of acute myocardial infarction, the total endocardial surface area is 200 cm^2, which is composed of 125 cm^2 of normal tissue and 75 cm^2 infarct tissue. Due to infarct expansion, apical dilation has occurred so that the total endocardial surface area is now 250 cm^2, which consists of 125 cm^2 normal tissue and 125 cm^2 infarct tissue. Because the total amount of myocardium has not increased, there is an obligatory thinning of the infarct tissue such that the wall thickness is now 6 mm in the infarct area versus 1.0 cm in the normal areas. The expanded area consists of necrotic myocardium with reduced tensile strength, which is the precursor for mechanical complications such as myocardial rupture.

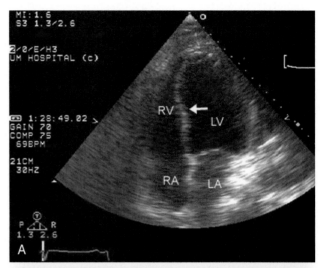

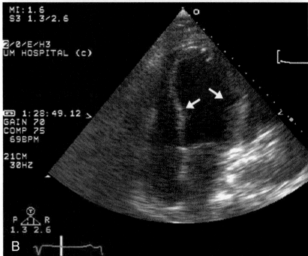

FIGURE 15.38. Apical four-chamber view recorded 36 hours after presentation with an extensive anteroapical ST-segment elevation myocardial infarction. **A:** Note in the image recorded in diastole that there is already abnormal left ventricular geometry with regional dilation of the distal septum (begins at *arrow*). This is more apparent in the image recorded in systole **(B)** where there is akinesis and dyskinesis of the distal septum and lateral walls (distal to the *arrows*). Because of the regional dilation, there is an obligatory thinning of the necrotic myocardium due to infarct expansion. LA, left atrium; LV, left ventricle; RA, right atrium; RV, right ventricle.

infarction with relatively extensive areas of abnormal wall motion. It is infrequently reported in inferior myocardial infarction. Figure 15.39 was recorded in a patient with acute myocardial infarction and thrombus formation. Several studies have examined the timing with which thrombi occur. The peak timing of early thrombus formation appears to be approximately 72 hours; however, in larger myocardial infarctions with large areas of apical akinesis and stagnant blood flow, they may form within hours of the acute event. A thrombus in acute myocardial infarction has the same characteristics as it does in chronic myocardial infarction and may be either laminar, pedunculated, or mobile. The likelihood of subsequent embolic events is greatest for thrombi that are either pedunculated or mobile and highest when a combination of features is seen. Two-dimensional echocardiography can be used to document resolution of a ventricular thrombus with anticoagulation therapy. Of note, several studies have demonstrated that patients are still at risk of formation of a ventricular thrombus even in the interventional and lytic era when thrombolytic therapy combined with heparin may have been administered.

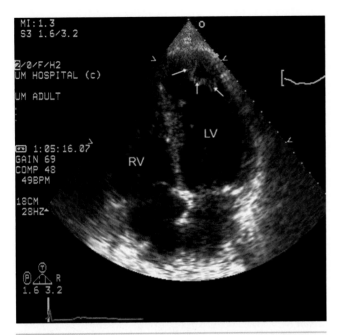

FIGURE 15.39. Apical four-chamber view recorded in a patient with an acute anterior apical myocardial infarction and early thrombus formation. Note the regional dilation of the left ventricle at the apex and the pedunculated, multilobulated mass protruding into the cavity of the left ventricle (*LV*) (*arrows*). RV, right ventricle.

Right Ventricular Infarction

Right ventricular infarction occurs most commonly (>90%) in conjunction with inferior myocardial infarction. On rare occasions, patients are noted with left anterior descending coronary artery distribution infarction and concurrent right ventricular involvement. This typically is due to a variation of coronary anatomy in which right ventricular branches arise from the left anterior descending coronary artery. The overwhelming majority of right ventricular infarctions, however, will be seen in the presence of inferior myocardial infarction due to occlusion of a proximal right coronary artery. In many instances, the wall motion abnormality of the inferior wall may be relatively small and overall left ventricular systolic function may appear preserved. Figures 15.40 and 15.41 were recorded in patients with inferior myocardial infarction and concurrent right ventricular infarction. With right ventricular infarction, dilation of the right ventricle and tricuspid anulus is common. Secondary tricuspid regurgitation is often seen. In many instances, more subtle degrees of right ventricular dysfunction will be present in which frank dilation and akinesis of the wall may not be noted. The elevation of right heart pressure may result in substantial amounts of right-to-left shunting through a patent foramen ovale. Figure 15.42 was recorded in a patient with an inferior myocardial infarction with right

ventricular involvement and marked desaturation. Note the substantial right-to-left shunt after intravenous arterial saline injection.

Evidence of right ventricular involvement may be transient because in many instances, the dysfunction is not due to true myocardial infarction but only transient ischemia. Concurrent mitral regurgitation or ventricular septal defect all increase the work of the right ventricle acutely and the combination of right ventricular involvement with either of these entities confers a substantially worse prognosis.

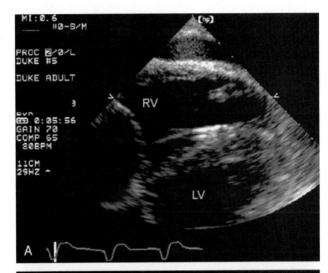

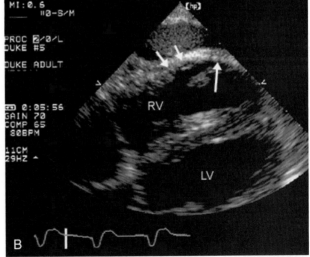

FIGURE 15.40. Subcostal view recorded in a patient with a limited inferior myocardial infarction and concurrent right ventricular infarction. **A:** Recorded in diastole. Note the dilated right ventricular cavity with relatively preserved right ventricular shape. **B:** Recorded in systole. Note the normal inward motion of the proximal right ventricular wall (*downward-pointing arrows*) and the dyskinesis of the apical portion of the right ventricular wall (*upward-pointing arrow*). LV, left ventricle; RV, right ventricle.

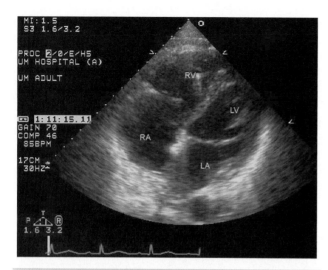

FIGURE 15.41. Off-axis four-chamber view recorded in a patient with an inferior myocardial infarction and right ventricular infarction. Note the dilation of the right ventricular cavity and the marked reduction in systolic function in the real-time image. LA, left atrium; LV, left ventricle; RA, right atrium; RV, right ventricle.

Acute Mitral Regurgitation

Mitral regurgitation occurs after acute myocardial infarction due to several different mechanisms. The first, closely related to infarct expansion, is rupture or partial rupture of the papillary muscle. This results in a portion of the mitral valve becoming flail and results in acute severe mitral regurgitation. In most patients, the anterolateral papillary muscle receives a dual blood supply from the left anterior descending and circumflex coronary arteries and is less likely to be involved by the ischemic process than is the posteromedial papillary muscle. Papillary muscle rupture should be suspected in a patient with acute myocardial infarction who subsequently develops a new holosystolic murmur and evidence of congestive heart failure. The differential diagnosis is obviously between papillary muscle rupture and acute ventricular septal defect. Although transthoracic echocardiography may suffice to establish the diagnosis, transesophageal echocardiography is often necessary to confirm the precise anatomic defect. Figures 15.43 and 15.44 were recorded in a patient with papillary muscle rupture in the setting of acute myocardial infarction. On occasion, one may image a patient with papillary muscle necrosis but without frank rupture. In these instances, one may note an abnormal shape of the papillary muscle.

Color flow imaging is crucial for evaluation of possible papillary muscle rupture. A partial flail leaflet most often results in an eccentric mitral jet, the direction of which is most often opposite to that of the involved leaflet. A posterior flail leaflet usually results in an anteriorly directed jet. The opposite is true for an anterior flail leaflet. Color

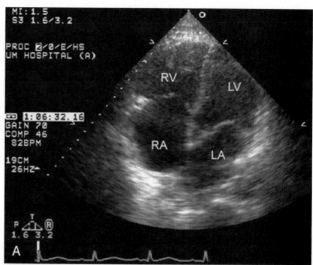

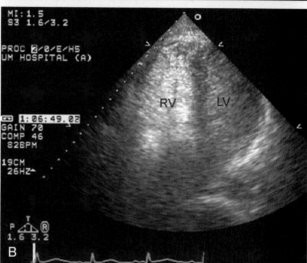

FIGURE 15.42. Apical four-chamber view recorded in the same patient depicted in Figure 15.41 with an inferior myocardial infarction complicated by right ventricular infarction. In this instance, marked arterial desaturation was noted. **A:** Note the marked dilation of the right ventricle (*RV*) and right atrium (*RA*). **B:** Image recorded after injection of intravenous saline shows marked opacification of the right ventricle with a substantial contrast effect in the left ventricle (*LV*) and left atrium (*LA*), indicative of a pathologic right to left shunt, subsequently documented to be due to a large patent foramen ovale.

flow Doppler allows clear separation of mitral regurgitation from ventricular septal defect in most instances. Often from a transthoracic window, the actual ruptured papillary muscle head cannot be directly visualized. However, detection of an eccentric mitral regurgitation jet with a relatively normal-sized left atrium is excellent indirect evidence that a mechanical disruption has occurred.

Transesophageal echocardiography provides incremental imaging in patients with suspected papillary muscle rupture. It is often necessary to fully exclude ventricular

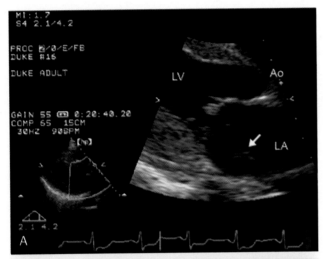

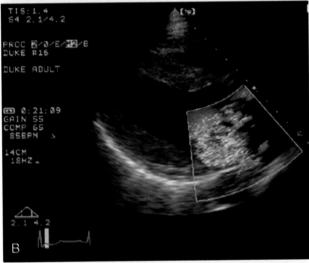

FIGURE 15.43. Parasternal long-axis view recorded in a patient with acute inferior myocardial infarction and rupture of the papillary muscle. **A:** Note the vague echo density in the left atrium (*LA*) (*arrow*), which represents the papillary muscle head. **B:** Note the severe mitral regurgitation seen with color flow Doppler imaging. Ao, aorta; LV, left ventricle.

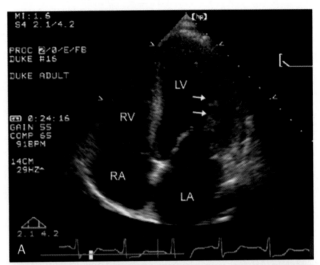

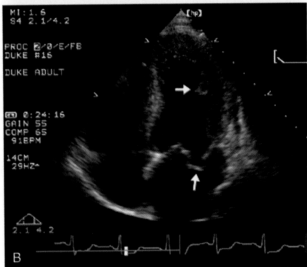

FIGURE 15.44. Apical four-chamber view recorded in the same patient depicted in Figure 15.43. **A:** Note the break in the continuity of the posterolateral papillary muscle with two portions of the papillary muscle head (*arrows*). **B:** Recorded in systole. Note the marked buckling of the mitral valve leaflet into the left atrium (*LA*) (*upward-pointing arrow*) and the ruptured papillary muscle base in the cavity of the left ventricle (*horizontal arrow*). LV, ventricle; RA, right atrium; RV, right ventricle.

septal defect, especially in patients who may have had preexisting mitral regurgitation. Figure 15.45 was recorded in a patient with papillary muscle rupture in whom transesophageal echocardiography allows visualization of the actual severed head of the papillary muscle, attached to the chordae tendineae and the flail leaflet.

In addition to anatomic disruption of the mitral valve apparatus, mitral regurgitation can be the result of functional disturbances in mitral valve coaptation. This is typically due to apical displacement of a papillary muscle, which tethers the leaflet tip and interferes with normal coaptation. Depending on the degree of displacement and which leaflet is involved, the mitral regurgitant jet may be central or eccentric and range from mild to severe (Fig. 15.46).

Ventricular Septal Rupture

Ventricular septal defect occurs in 3% to 5% of myocardial infarctions. As with other forms of mechanical disruption, it is virtually always associated with transmural rather than nontransmural myocardial necrosis, and acute infarct expansion is the precursor. It can occur at any point along the ventricular septum from the base to the apex. It can be seen in both left anterior descending and right coronary distribution myocardial infarction. It should be emphasized that the posterior septal perforator arteries at the base of the heart arise from the right coro-

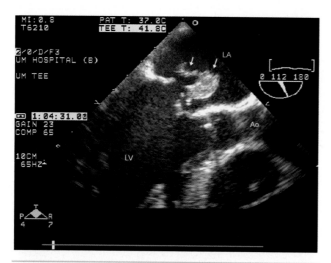

FIGURE 15.45. Transesophageal echocardiogram recorded in a longitudinal plane in a patient with inferior myocardial infarction and acute severe mitral regurgitation. This frame was recorded in systole, and a large portion of the papillary muscle head can be seen prolapsing into the left atrium (*LA*) (*arrows*). Ao, aorta; LV, left ventricle.

nary artery. Complete occlusion of a right coronary artery can result in infarction of the proximal inferior septum with infarct expansion and ventricular septal defect at the base of the heart. Figures 15.47 through 15.49 were recorded in patients with acute myocardial infarction and ventricular septal defect.

When evaluating patients for ventricular septal defect, it is often necessary to use nonconventional imaging planes. It is often most advantageous to first scan using color flow imaging in an effort to identify the pathologic left-to-right flow rather than scanning looking for the anatomic defect. Once the abnormal flow from the left ventricle to the right ventricle has been identified and its orientation maximized, color can then be turned off and anatomic gray scale imaging undertaken. As mentioned previously, the imaging plane in which the color flow jet has been best identified often does not correspond to traditional imaging planes. Ventricular septal defect after acute anterior myocardial infarction is unpredictable in location and can occur anywhere in the ventricular septum. These defects may take a serpiginous course through the ventricular myocardium, especially if only partial septal rupture has occurred.

Once the diagnosis of ventricular septal defect has been established, there are several other echocardiographic features that must be evaluated to determine prognosis. These include the status of overall left ventricular function, the presence of pulmonary hypertension, and the function of the right ventricle. When ventricular septal defect occurs as a consequence of a limited myocardial infarction and single-vessel disease, the remaining walls typically become hyperdynamic. Conversely, if a

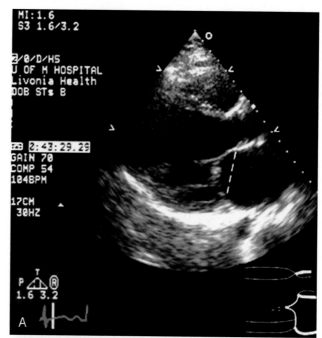

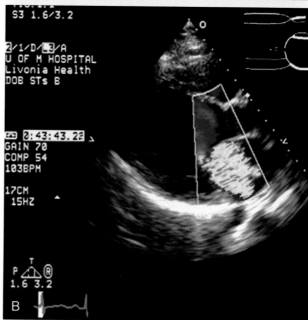

FIGURE 15.46. Parasternal long-axis view recorded in a patient with functional mitral regurgitation due to myocardial ischemia and subsequent malcoaptation of the mitral valve. **A:** Image recorded in end-systole demonstrates tethering of the mitral valve toward the apex. The *dashed line* denotes the plane of the mitral anulus. Note the "tenting" of the mitral leaflets into the cavity of the left ventricle. **B:** Image recorded in the same patient with color Doppler flow imaging reveals severe mitral regurgitation. In this instance, there is no anatomic disruption of the mitral valve apparatus and mitral regurgitation is due to functional abnormalities of mitral valve closure rather than an anatomic defect of the valve itself. The schematics denote normal (**A**) and abnormal (**B**) coaptation patterns for comparison.

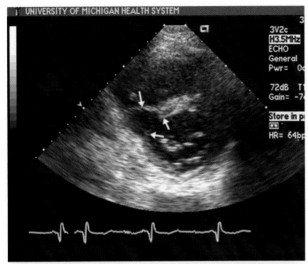

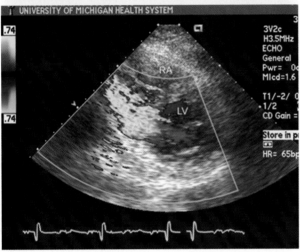

FIGURE 15.47. A. Parasternal short-axis view recorded in a patient with an extensive inferior and inferoseptal myocardial infarction with a partial rupture of the septum. Note the very thinwalled aneurysmal tissue extending from the inferior septum (*downward-pointing arrow*) and a relatively narrow entrance (*leftward-pointing arrows*). **B:** Note the color flow signal demonstrating marked turbulent flow from the cavity of the left ventricle (*LV*) into the pseudoaneurysm and subsequently into the right ventricular cavity. RA, right atrium.

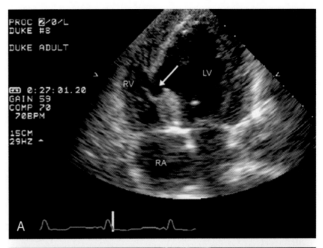

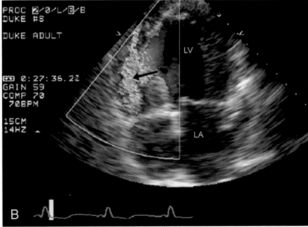

FIGURE 15.48. Apical four-chamber view recorded in a patient with acute inferoseptal and inferior myocardial infarction. Note the distinct break in the septal contour (*arrow*) **(A)** and the color flow signal traversing this ventricular septal defect (*arrow*) **(B)**. LA, left atrium; LV, left ventricle; RA, right atrium; RV, right ventricle.

previous infarction has occurred or if multivessel ischemia or infarction is present, the left ventricle may have global systolic dysfunction. The latter confers a substantially worse prognosis than does preserved left ventricular function. Additionally, small apical defects are substantially easier to approach from a surgical standpoint than are the large posterior ventricular septal defects and as such carry a more favorable surgical mortality. Concurrent ventricular septal defect and right ventricular infarction, which typically will be seen in inferior infarction, also carry a substantially worse prognosis.

CHRONIC CORONARY ARTERY DISEASE

Most chronic complications of coronary artery disease can be evaluated with echocardiography. These include sequelae of myocardial infarction such as aneurysm, pseudoaneurysm, chronic ventricular remodeling, chronic ischemic dysfunction ("ischemic cardiomyopathy"), and functional mitral regurgitation.

Left Ventricular Aneurysm

Before the era of urgent reperfusion strategies, with either thrombolytic or interventional therapy, left ventricular aneurysm was seen as the sequela of myocardial infarction in approximately 40% of anterior and 20% of posterior myocardial infarctions. Both pathologically and echocardiographically, an aneurysm is defined as a dis-

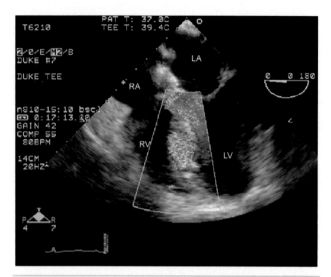

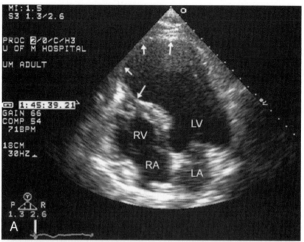

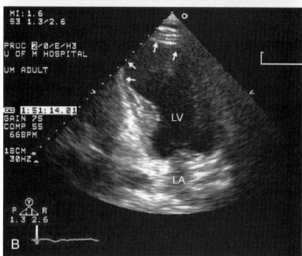

FIGURE 15.49. Transesophageal echocardiogram recorded in a transverse plane (0 degrees) in a patient with a ventricular septal defect after acute myocardial infarction. Note the turbulent color flow signal traversing the ventricular septum through the large ventricular septal defect. LA, left atrium; LV, left ventricle; RA, right atrium; RV, ventricle.

FIGURE 15.50. **A:** Apical four-chamber view recorded in a patient with a very large chronic anteroapical myocardial infarction and apical aneurysm. Note the normal thickness of the proximal 50% of the left ventricle (*LV*) with marked aneurysmal dilation, abnormal geometry, and wall thinning in the distal half of the ventricle. Note also in the two-chamber view (**B**) the involvement of the distal inferior wall with a distinct break in function and wall thickness (*arrows*). LA, left atrium; RA, right atrium; RV, right ventricle.

tinct break in the geometry of the left ventricular contour that is present in both diastole and systole with replacement of necrotic myocardium by fibrous scar tissue. By definition, it does not occur after nontransmural infarction. Approximately 6 weeks is required for scar formation. Acute infarct expansion may have a similar appearance but is seen within the 1 to 4 day timeframe. Figures 15.9 and 15.50 through 15.55 were recorded in patients with left ventricular aneurysms after myocardial infarction. Note the broad range of aneurysm size. Generally, a true aneurysm has a relatively wide mouth communicating with the aneurysmal cavity compared with a narrow neck that is seen in pseudoaneurysm. This results in a fairly broad gradual opening to the aneurysm as opposed to a distinct shelf-like opening.

There are several echocardiographic features that should be recorded if aneurysm resection is contemplated. The traditional indications for resection of a ventricular aneurysm are intractable heart failure and less commonly for control of arrhythmias. Mechanically, the aneurysm acts as a dead space reservoir with no ability to eject blood from its diastolic volume. The remaining myocardial walls may move normally; however, the aneurysmal cavity serves as a second output for ejection and thus compromises stroke volume. When contemplating aneurysm resection, it is essential to ensure that the basal portions of the cardiac walls have normal function. This can be accomplished by calculating an ejection fraction of the basal half of the left ventricle. A simplified method to evaluate basal function is to calculate basal fractional shortening or fractional area change using a two-dimen-

sional short-axis view at the base of the heart. Generally, if basal function is normal and the basal half ejection fraction or fractional shortening is greater than 35% or 18%, respectively, then aneurysm resection is more likely to be of clinical benefit. Figure 15.50 was recorded in a patient with well-preserved function at the base of the heart. In this patient, resection of the apical aneurysm results in removal of dead space and nonproductive diastolic volume, but the heart retains sufficient contractile myocardium to allow adequate overall cardiac performance postoperatively. Contrast this to Figure 15.9 in which there is more extensive proximal septal involvement and the basal half ejection fraction is pathologically de-

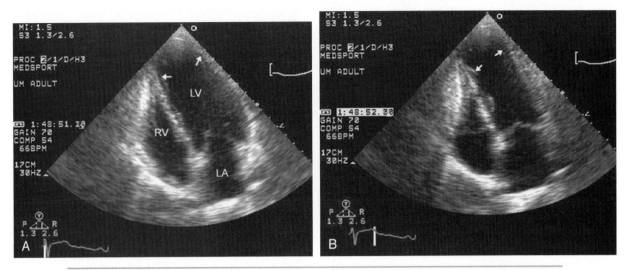

FIGURE 15.51. Apical four-chamber view recorded in a patient with a smaller apical aneurysm. **A:** Image recorded in diastole; note the loss of the normal tapering of the left ventricular apex. **B:** Image recorded in systole in which the abnormal geometry, and the distinct break between the normally functioning basal two-thirds of the ventricle and the aneurysm, is more apparent.

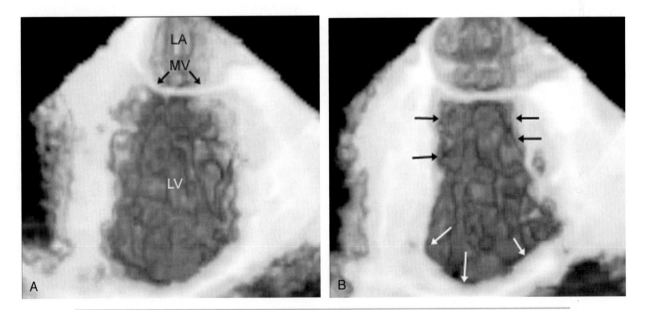

FIGURE 15.52. Three-dimensional reconstruction from a transesophageal echocardiogram recorded in a patient with a large anteroapical aneurysm. **A:** Image recorded in diastole reveals aneurysmal dilation of the distal 50% of the left ventricle. Note the loss of normal tapering toward the apex and the apical dilation. **B:** Image recorded in systole documents preserved function at the base of the heart (*black arrows*) with dyskinesis of the apical, aneurysmal segments (*white arrows*). LA, left atrium; LV, left ventricle; MV, mitral valve.

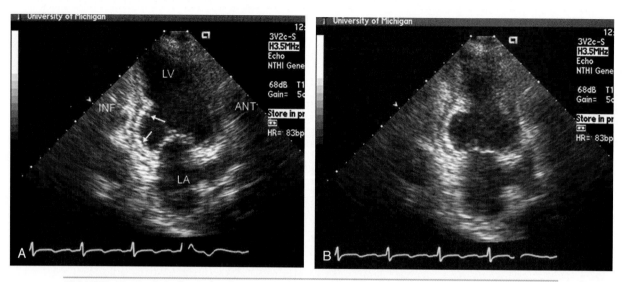

FIGURE 15.53. Apical two-chamber view recorded in diastole (**A**) and systole (**B**) in a patient with a remote inferior myocardial infarction and inferior aneurysm at the base of the heart. **A:** Recorded in diastole, note the abnormal geometry of the proximal inferior wall (*arrows*) (*INF*). This abnormality is even more prominent in the image recorded in systole (**B**) in which one can appreciate the preserved contractility of the distal inferior wall and anterior wall (*ANT*).

FIGURE 15.54. Apical two-chamber view recorded in a patient with a remote inferior myocardial infarction and a discrete basal aneurysm. In this instance, the outer wall of the aneurysm is noted by the *upward-pointing arrows*. Note the relatively narrow neck to the aneurysm and a laminar thrombus (*downward-pointing arrow*). In examples such as this, it may be difficult to separate a true aneurysm from a pseudoaneurysm. ANT, anterior wall; INF, inferior wall; LA, left atrium; LV, left ventricle.

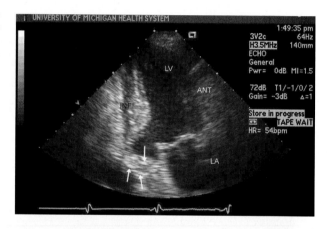

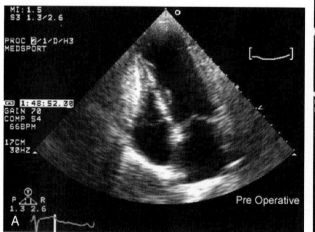

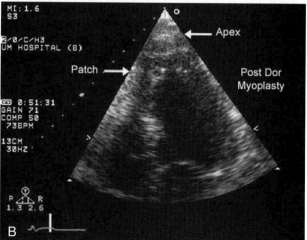

FIGURE 15.55. Apical four-chamber view recorded in a patient with an anteroapical aneurysm who subsequently underwent a Dor myoplasty for left ventricular remodeling. **A:** The preoperative image shows a large anteroapical aneurysm. **B:** Image recorded after the Dor myoplasty. Note the position of the patch and the obliterated apex of the left ventricle. The remaining left ventricular cavity has relatively normal geometry and systolic function.

creased. In this setting, traditional aneurysmectomy may not result in significant relief of congestive heart failure.

More recently, other approaches have been taken to control heart failure in patients with ventricular aneurysm. These have included reduction myoplasty and Dor myoplasty. In the reduction myoplasty, a large segment of the aneurysmal wall is resected, resulting in immediate remodeling of the left ventricle. In the Dor myoplasty, an intraventricular patch is placed that excludes a portion of the aneurysmal cavity without resecting the wall. The advantage of the Dor myoplasty is that the aneurysmal portion of the ventricular septum can also be excluded from the functional left ventricular cavity. Figure 15.55 was recorded in a patient after Dor myoplasty. In the postoperative echo (Fig. 15.55B), note the linear echo within the left ventricular cavity due to the intraventricular patch that separates a true functional left ventricle, composed of normally functioning myocardium as well as smaller portions of the aneurysmal wall, from the dead space aneurysm cavity. Echocardiography can play a valuable role in assessing feasibility of either of these approaches by determining the degree to which an aneurysm is located in the anterior septum and apex (which is more favorable for Dor myoplasty) and determining the function of the residual myocardium. After Dor myoplasty, it is not uncommon to see small degrees of residual blood flow into the apical dead space created by the intraventricular patch.

Pseudoaneurysm

Left ventricular pseudoaneurysm represents a contained rupture of the left ventricular free wall. In rare instances, a pseudoaneurysm can actually occur within the ventricular septum rather than along the free wall. It is important to recognize a pseudoaneurysm because the likelihood of spontaneous rupture is high. Unlike a true aneurysm in which the wall consists of dense fibrous tissue with excellent tensile strength, the wall of a pseudoaneurysm is composed of organizing thrombus and varying portions of the epicardium and parietal pericardium (Fig. 15.56). Pathologically, it is the sequela of myocardial rupture with hemorrhage into the pericardial space, which then becomes locally compressive. Local tamponade occurs, preventing further hemorrhage into the pericardium. Over time, the intrapericardial thrombus organizes, creating a wall to the pseudoaneurysm, however, with poor structural integrity. As such, it is at risk of spontaneous rupture, which is generally a fatal event.

Pseudoaneurysms can be separated from true aneurysms by several characteristics. Separation of true from pseudoaneurysms in the proximal posterior wall is often problematic, however. Figures 15.57 through 15.60 were recorded in patients with pseudoaneurysms. Note

the narrow opening to the pseudoaneurysm with an overhanging shelf-like edge. Traditionally, it is thought that if the size of the opening to the left ventricular cavity is less than the maximal dimension of the aneurysm, the defect is more likely to be a pseudoaneurysm. Because the pseudoaneurysm is composed of both a free aneurysmal

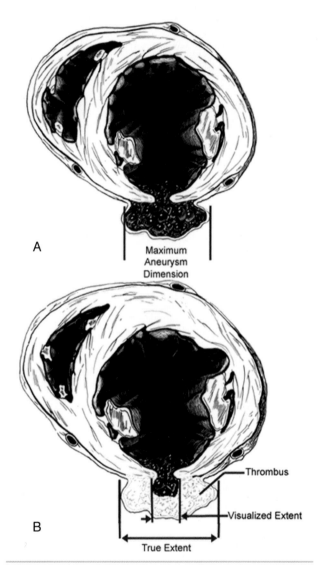

FIGURE 15.56. Schematic representation of a classic inferior pseudoaneurysm. **A:** Note the narrow opening to the relatively wide aneurysm that clearly extends beyond the border of the left ventricular epicardium. The pseudoaneurysm is contained by pericardial and epicardial tissue only and is predominantly filled by fresh thrombus or blood. **B:** A similar rendition of the pseudoaneurysm in which there has been substantial chronic thrombus formation within the pseudoaneurysm. In this instance, because the chronic thrombus has an echocardiographic signature similar to that of other tissue, only the smaller nonthrombosed portion of the pseudoaneurysm is directly visualized. This phenomenon may result in marked underestimation of the true size of the pseudoaneurysm because only its relatively narrow opening and the nonthrombosed portion may be visualized.

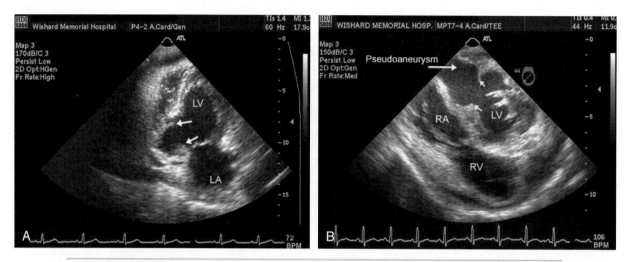

FIGURE 15.57. Off-axis transthoracic apical view **(A)** and transesophageal echocardiographic view **(B)** recorded in a patient with an inferior pseudoaneurysm. **A:** Note the proximal inferior wall aneurysm that appears to have a communication between the left ventricle (*LV*) and aneurysmal cavity that is relatively narrow (*arrows*). **B:** In the transesophageal echocardiogram, note the true extent of the pseudoaneurysm (*large arrow*) compared with the communication to the left ventricle (*small arrows*), which allows documentation that this is a pseudoaneurysm rather than a true aneurysm. LA, left atrium; LV, left ventricle; RA, right atrium; RV, right ventricle.

FIGURE 15.58. Transesophageal echocardiogram recorded in a patient with an inferior myocardial infarction and a very large pseudoaneurysm. In this example, the outer boundary of the pseudoaneurysm is as marked by the outer vertical lines (*O*) and the communication with the left ventricle (*LV*) by the inner vertical lines (*I*). In this example, the maximal dimension of the pseudoaneurysm actually exceeds the size of the left ventricle. The opening to the pseudoaneurysm is noted by the *smaller arrows*. LA, left atrium; MV, mitral valve.

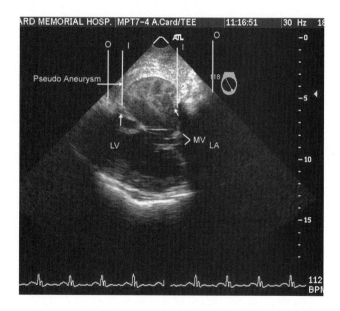

cavity and the organizing hematoma, its true size is often underrepresented on echocardiography because the organized hematoma has a soft-tissue density similar to that of many surrounding structures. It is therefore not uncommon to have the situation of a large pericardiac mass on chest radiograph or computed tomographic scan in the presence of what appears to be a modest size pseudoaneurysmal cavity detected with echocardiography. This phenomenon also makes it more difficult to assess the ratio of the size of the opening to the left ventricular cavity

to the actual aneurysm size because only the blood-filled aspect of the pseudoaneurysm may be easily visualized. This phenomenon is schematized in Figure 15.56B. Pseudoaneurysm at the base of the heart, most commonly after inferior myocardial infarction, may be difficult to separate from a true aneurysm. In this location, they may have a wider mouth than is traditionally taught and be difficult to distinguish from a true aneurysm. Their true nature is often only confirmed at the time of surgical inspection (or autopsy).

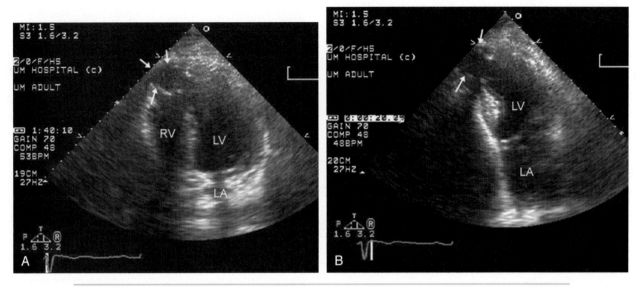

FIGURE 15.59. Apical view recorded in a patient with a chronic small apical pseudoaneurysm. **A:** An off-axis four-chamber view. **B:** A two-chamber view. In each instance, note the very discrete, nearly spherical pseudoaneurysm cavity bounded by a fairly echodense border, suggesting calcification in the rim. The pseudoaneurysm has a very narrow neck communicating with the cavity of the left ventricle near the apex. In this case, the pseudoaneurysm is the result of apical infarction noted to have occurred 5 years before recording this echocardiogram. LA, left atrium; LV, left ventricle; RV, right ventricle.

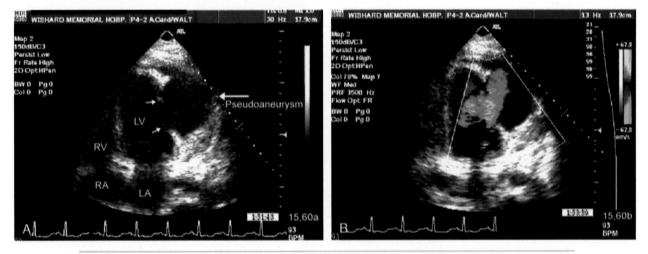

FIGURE 15.60. Apical four-chamber view recorded in a patient with a large pseudoaneurysm after lateral wall myocardial infarction. **A:** Note the very large pseudoaneurysm cavity communicating with the left ventricle by a relatively narrow neck (*arrows*). **B:** Image recorded with color flow Doppler imaging confirms the communication between the left ventricular cavity and the pseudoaneurysm. LA, left atrium; LV, left ventricle; RA, right atrium; RV, right ventricle.

Chronic Remodeling

After transmural myocardial infarction, a process of ventricular remodeling occurs. Remodeling refers to the tendency of the left ventricular chamber to gradually alter in size and geometry due to adverse effects of the myocardial infarction. Even a well-localized myocardial infarction will be surrounded by a dysfunctional border zone.

Within the border zone, myocardial dysfunction is due to a combination of factors including tethering, varying degrees of nontransmural necrosis, and abnormal regional wall stress in the regionally dilated segments. Over time, this results in progressive dilation of the ventricle at the margins of the myocardial infarction, even in the presence of a relatively healthy, normally perfused myocardium. Chronic remodeling is usually a complication of

Remodeling Schematic

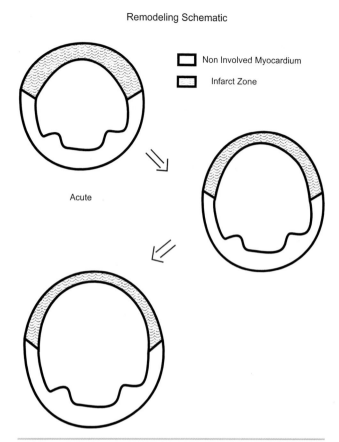

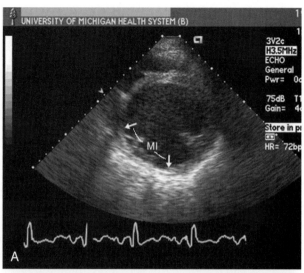

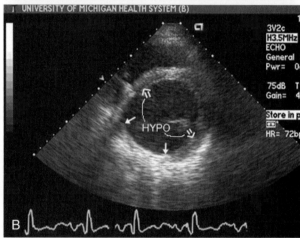

FIGURE 15.61. Schematic depiction of the remodeling phenomenon. The upper left schematic depicts a recent anterior and anteroseptal myocardial infarction (*shaded areas*) encompassing approximately 40% of the ventricular circumference. The remaining 60% is normal nonischemic, noninfarcted myocardium. The schematic in the middle depicts progressive thinning and dilation of the infarct segment so that it now represents approximately 50% of the ventricular circumference. The schematic at the bottom represents the long-term impact of the dilated infarct segment on the remaining normal, noninvolved myocardial segments. Over time, the dilation of the infarct segment results in progressive tethering of the adjacent normal border zone with subsequent secondary myocardial dysfunction and progressive dilation and malfunction of the previously noninvolved myocardium.

a larger anterior infarction and is rarely seen after posterior distribution infarction, and by definition will be seen after transmural rather than nontransmural necrosis. Figure 15.61 schematizes the remodeling process, and Figure 15.62 is an example of a patient with a relatively moderately sized inferior infarct who has had adverse remodeling over time. Ventricular remodeling is of clinical relevance because it results in dilation of the ventricular chamber and globally reduced contractile performance with reduction in left ventricular ejection fraction. Remodeling often also may result in malcoaptation of the mitral leaflets and secondary mitral regurgitation due to the apical and lateral displacement of the papillary mus-

FIGURE 15.62. Parasternal short-axis view recorded in a patient 2 years after extensive inferior myocardial infarction in whom there has been adverse remodeling. **A:** Recorded in diastole; note the extent of the inferior myocardial infarction (*MI*) (*arrows*) with wall thinning and scar formation. The remaining wall segments have normal myocardial texture and wall thickness. Note, however, that there is substantial dilation of the left ventricular cavity. **B:** Recorded in systole in which the adverse tethering effect can be noted. The infarct area is frankly dyskinetic, and there is a more extensive area of severe hypokinesis (*HYPO*) (*arrows*) encompassing approximately 50% of the left ventricular circumference. In this example, even the remote myocardial segments are hypokinetic due to adverse remodeling.

cles. Clinical studies have suggested that beta-blockers or angiotensin-converting enzyme blockade may prevent or retard adverse remodeling.

Mural Thrombus

Chronic thrombus formation is a not infrequent sequela of myocardial infarction. It is substantially more common after larger anterior myocardial infarctions, especially with involvement of the apex, than after inferior infarction. Before the lytic and urgent interventional era, left ventricular thrombus occurred in 25% to 40% of patients after the first anteroapical myocardial infarction. With the advent of lytic therapy, there has been a decline in this prevalence; however, thrombus formation is still seen after lytic therapy even with concurrent heparinization. The major risk of left ventricular thrombus is of subsequent embolization with stroke or major organ loss. The likelihood of embolic events is greatest in the first 2 weeks after the acute event and tapers off over the 6 weeks after myocardial infarction. After this time, there is presumed endothelialization of the thrombus with reduction in its embolic potential. There are several characteristics of ventricular thrombus that should be noted echocardiographically. These include not only size but also whether

it is a laminar thrombus forming a layer along the akinetic wall or whether it is pedunculated and protruding into the ventricle. Thrombi may be mobile. Mobility tends to be seen in fresher rather than chronic thrombi. Figures 15.63 through 15.65 were recorded in patients with myocardial infarction and illustrate the range of thrombi to be seen. Note in Figure 15.63 that there is an anteroapical wall motion abnormality with a purely laminar thrombus. This is a chronic thrombus, likely to be covered fully by an endothelial layer, and presumably has a relatively low embolic potential. Contrast this to the thrombi in Figures 15.64 and 15.65, which are pedunculated and mobile. Both a pedunculated character and mobility confer a greater likelihood of embolization with embolic rates reported as high as 40% when both mobility and protrusion into the cavity are noted. On occasion, fresh thrombi take on a cystic appearance. This is due to a combination of factors including varying degrees of maturity of the clot and results in acoustic boundaries between relatively fresh and more organized regions. This results in a relative echo lucency to the center of the thrombus. When seen in the presence of a wall motion abnormality in which thrombus would be expected, it is important to recognize this as such rather than make the diagnosis of presumed cyst or tumor.

In addition to frank thrombus formation, when using newer generation, high-frequency transducers, spontaneous contrast is occasionally noted in the left ventricular cavity. This typically will be seen immediately in the area of a regional wall motion abnormality. The etiology of the spontaneous contrast is presumably stagnant blood in the region of an aneurysmal dilation. Color flow imaging at low velocities can also demonstrate abnormal swirling patterns of blood.

On occasion, either the vague nature of a thrombus or technical limitations in the examination render it difficult

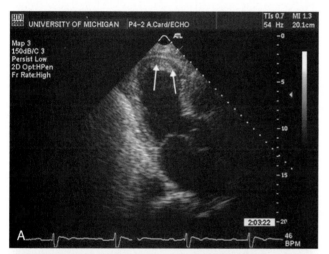

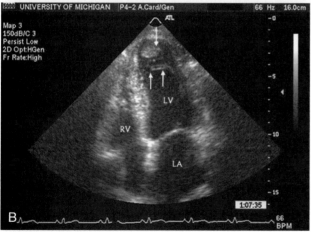

FIGURE 15.63. Apical long-axis **(A)** and four chamber **(B)** views recorded in a patient with an anteroapical myocardial infarction and a laminar apical thrombus. In each instance, note the laminar filling defect (*upward-pointing arrows*) in the apex of the left ventricle (*LV*), which is akinetic and dilated. **B:** Note the multiple laminar lines (*downward-pointing arrow*) with variable consistency of the thrombus suggesting chronicity. LA, left atrium; RV, right ventricle.

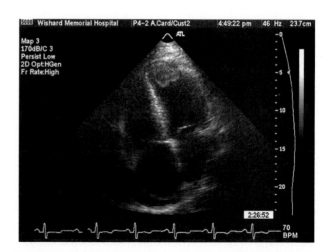

FIGURE 15.64. Apical four-chamber view recorded in a patient with an acute anteroapical myocardial infarction and a pedunculated, slightly mobile apical thrombus.

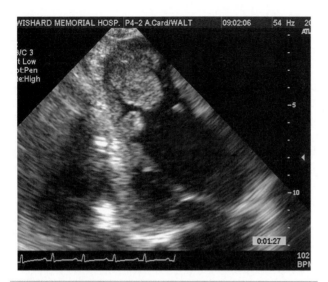

FIGURE 15.65. Apical two-chamber view recorded in a patient with an anteroapical myocardial infarction and multiple large pedunculated and mobile thrombi. Note the multiple masses protruding into the cavity of the left ventricular apex and the mobile nature of these thrombi in the real-time image.

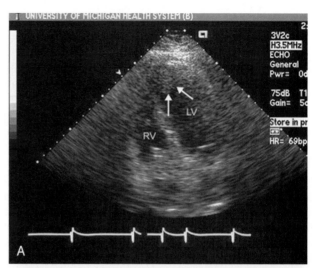

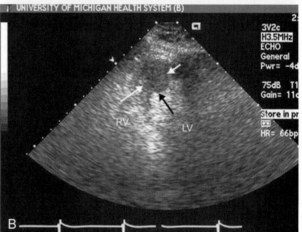

FIGURE 15.66. Apical four-chamber view recorded without **(A)** and with **(B)** intravenous contrast for left ventricular opacification. **A:** Note the vague suggestion of a filling defect in the apex of the left ventricle (*LV*) (*arrows*). **B:** After injection of intravenous contrast, the entire left ventricular cavity is opacified and the thrombus appears as a slightly mobile spherical filling defect in the left ventricular apex (*arrows*). RV, right ventricle.

to either exclude or confirm the presence of ventricular thrombus. The use of higher frequency, short-focus transducers can often result in higher quality imaging in the apex and resolve the dilemma. An additional echocardiographic tool to further evaluate the presence or absence of thrombus is the use of intravenous contrast. Using the newer generation perfluorocarbon-based agents, which pass into the left ventricular cavity, it is possible to fully opacify the left ventricular apex. In doing so, one may then detect a true fixed filling defect in the apex and thereby confirm the presence of ventricular thrombus. Figure 15.66 shows vague echoes in the left ventricular apex of uncertain etiology in a patient in whom contrast was used. Note that after contrast, there is a very distinct filling defect noted in the apex, diagnostic of a ventricular thrombus.

Mitral Regurgitation

As in acute myocardial infarction, mitral regurgitation occurs due to several mechanisms in chronic ischemic disease. The issue of papillary muscle rupture with acute severe mitral regurgitation was previously discussed. Chronic mitral regurgitation can occur through mechanisms other than frank papillary muscle rupture. Necrosis and subsequent scarring of a papillary muscle may result in retraction of either the anterior or posterior leaflet but is most common with the posterior leaflet. This results in a malcoaptation process, as shown in Figure 15.67. Figure 15.68 was recorded in a patient with previous myocardial infarction and papillary muscle dysfunc-

tion. It should be emphasized that papillary muscle dysfunction actually represents malfunction not only of the papillary muscle but also of the underlying ventricular wall. As a consequence of remodeling, the wall supporting the papillary muscle and the papillary muscle itself are apically and posteriorly displaced. This has the effect of functionally shortening the mitral valve apparatus for that leaflet, thus restricting its ability to close fully. This results in abnormal coaptation and mitral regurgitation. This is not infrequently accompanied by dilation of the mitral anulus to a variable degree. The degree of mitral regurgitation that results by this mechanism can range from trivial and inconsequential to severe and may be a cause of congestive heart failure. The severity of mitral regurgitation due to this mechanism is graded as for other

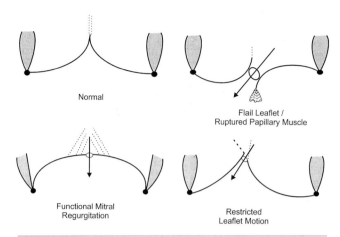

FIGURE 15.67. Schematic representation of normal and abnormal mitral valve closure patterns as they relate to ischemic heart disease. The normal closure pattern is noted in the upper left. Ischemia-related etiologies of mitral regurgitation due to abnormal coaptation are noted and include functional mitral regurgitation, a restricted posterior leaflet motion, and flail leaflet due to papillary muscle rupture. The regurgitant orifice is as noted by the *circle* and the direction of the regurgitant jet by the *arrow* in each instance.

forms of mitral regurgitation. Because the underlying pathophysiology may involve one leaflet more than the other, eccentric jets are not uncommon and caution regarding grading severity is advised, as discussed in Chapter 11.

Ischemic Cardiomyopathy

Ischemic cardiomyopathy is defined as chronic left ventricular dysfunction due to the sequelae of diffuse coronary artery disease. By definition, it excludes congestive heart failure due to discrete left ventricular aneurysm or acute complications of myocardial infarction. Several recent studies have demonstrated substantial areas of nontransmural infarction and fibrosis in most patients with diffuse left ventricular dysfunction and underlying coronary artery disease. This is often seen in the absence of clinical evidence of discrete myocardial infarction. In the typical ischemic cardiomyopathy, the left ventricle is composed of areas of normal myocardium, areas of transmural scar, and substantial areas of partial-thickness fibrosis. Echocardiographically, the left ventricle will be dilated and have diffuse wall motion abnormalities. On occasion, there may be one or more areas of discrete scar and frank akinesis, which allows the diagnosis of underlying coronary artery disease to be established. Figure 15.69 was recorded in a patient with chronic multivessel coronary artery disease and left ventricular systolic dysfunction. Because of the chronic nature of ischemic cardiomyopathy, varying degrees of mitral regurgitation are nearly ubiquitous and secondary pulmonary hypertension and tricuspid regurgitation are common. In many in-

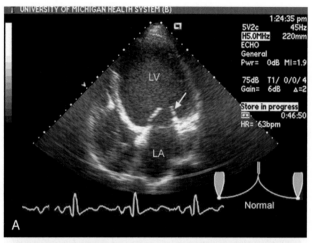

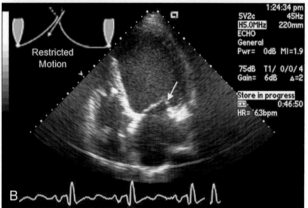

FIGURE 15.68. Apical four-chamber view recorded in a patient with an ischemic cardiomyopathy and restricted posterior leaflet motion. **A:** Recorded in diastole. Note the position of the posterior leaflet (*arrow*). In systole **(B)** there is normal motion of the anterior leaflet toward the tip of the posterior leaflet, which has remained tethered in position (*arrow*) due to the underlying wall motion abnormality. This abnormal coaptation results in functional mitral regurgitation. LA, left atrium; LV, left ventricle.

stances, there will be substantial areas of viable myocardium that may recover function if successfully reperfused. This issue is discussed further in Chapter 16.

It is often not possible to separate an ischemic from a nonischemic dilated cardiomyopathy. Clues to the former include patient age and cardiovascular risk factors as well as clinical information regarding previous ischemic events. In the absence of clinical evidence of previous infarction, detection of an area of frank scar frequently will establish the diagnosis of an ischemic etiology for chronic dysfunction. In many instances, it will not be possible to accurately separate the two entities and coronary arteriography will be necessary to establish or exclude the diagnosis. In some patients, there will be concurrent coronary disease and primary cardiomyopathy. Typically, these individuals will have significant left ventricular dys-

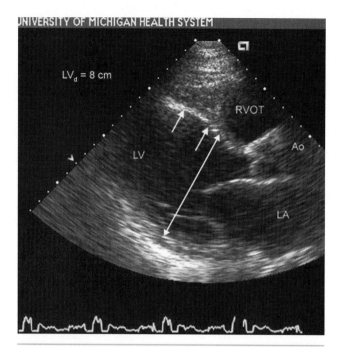

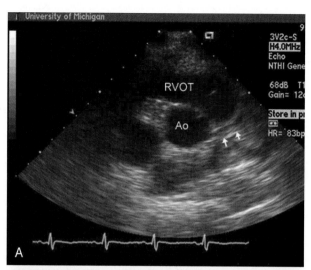

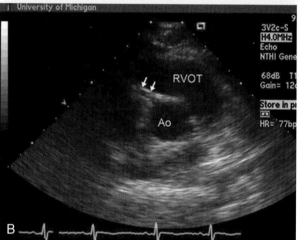

FIGURE 15.69. Parasternal long-axis echocardiogram recorded in a patient with an ischemic cardiomyopathy. Note the marked dilation of the left ventricular chamber that measures 8 cm at the mid ventricular level (*double-headed arrow*). Note also the areas of scar with akinesis in the anterior septum (*short arrows*) and the otherwise globally hypokinetic left ventricle. Ao, aorta; LA, left atrium; LV, left ventricle, RVOT, right ventricular outflow tract.

function and limited coronary artery disease, resulting in a situation in which the degree of left ventricular dysfunction is out of proportion to the severity of coronary disease. These individuals probably have the combination of nonischemic cardiomyopathy and incidental coronary disease.

DIRECT CORONARY VISUALIZATION

There are several clinical instances in which direct visualization of the epicardial coronary arteries can provide valuable clinical information. The ostia of the left main and right coronary arteries can be visualized in most adults and in virtually all children using transthoracic echocardiography. Additionally, a variable length of the left main and proximal left anterior descending coronary artery can likewise be visualized. Visualization is often feasible, even in patients for whom the remainder of the cardiac structures may be marginally visualized. The origin of both main coronary arteries can also be visualized using transesophageal echocardiography.

To visualize the origin of the left and right coronary arteries from a transthoracic echocardiogram, scanning is performed in a parasternal short-axis view at the base of the heart (Fig. 15.70). The proximal left main coronary artery is seen arising from the left coronary cusp at approx-

FIGURE 15.70. Parasternal short-axis echocardiogram recorded at the base of the heart demonstrates the origin of the left main coronary artery (*arrows*) **(A)** and the right coronary artery (*arrows*) **(B)**. Note that the takeoff of the two coronary arteries is not simultaneously visualized because the right coronary artery takeoff is slightly more cephalad than that of the left main coronary artery. Ao, aorta; RVOT, right ventricular outflow tract.

imately the 4-o'clock position. The ostium of the right coronary artery is closer to the sinotubular ridge and arises at approximately the 10-o'clock position. Typically, it is not possible to visualize the proximal portions of both coronary arteries simultaneously because the takeoff of the right coronary artery is more cephalad than that of the left. Additionally, a variable length of the left anterior descending coronary artery can be visualized using a modified parasternal long-axis view along the interventricular groove.

Using transesophageal echocardiography, both coronary ostia likewise can be visualized. Typically, the left main coronary artery is technically easier to visualize than the right. Figure 15.71 is a 30-degree scan of the proximal aorta showing a proximal portion of the left

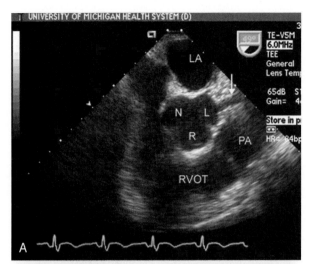

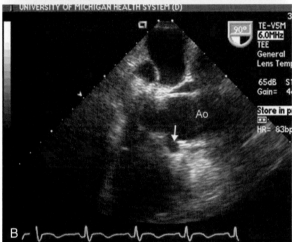

FIGURE 15.71. Transesophageal echocardiogram recorded in the short axis **(A)** and longitudinal axis **(B)** of the proximal aorta (*PA*). **A:** The takeoff of the left main coronary artery (*arrow*) is clearly visualized. **B:** The takeoff of the right coronary artery is clearly seen (*arrow*). Ao, aorta; L, left coronary cusp; LA, left atrium; N, non-coronary cusp; R, right coronary cusp; RVOT, right ventricular outflow tract.

in which the origin of a coronary artery from the pulmonary artery may lead to a cardiomyopathic process and in patients for whom echocardiographic screening as part of an athletic screen is indicated. If both coronary arteries are identified with normal origins, the likelihood of a coronary artery anomaly is low. If one or the other main coronary artery is not visualized, this is indirect evidence that there is a possible anomalous origin, from either the pulmonary artery or an anomalous location in the proximal aorta. Figures 15.73 and 15.74 were recorded in patients with anomalous coronary arteries.

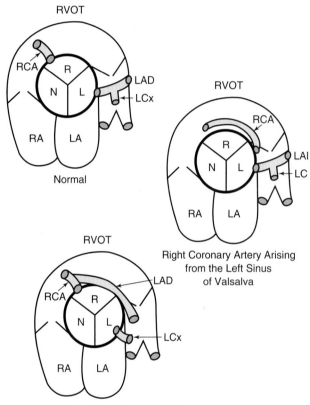

FIGURE 15.72. Schematic representation of normal and abnormal origins of the coronary arteries. The upper left schematic depicts the normal takeoff of the right coronary artery (*RCA*) and the left main coronary artery (LMCA) from the right and left Valsalva sinuses, respectively. The middle schematic depicts the anomalous origin of the right coronary artery from the left Valsalva sinus. The right coronary artery (RCA) courses between the aorta and right ventricular outflow tract (*RVOT*)/pulmonary artery. This course results in a marked angulation of the right coronary artery near its origin, which may result in coronary flow compromise. The lower left schematic depicts the origin of either the left coronary artery or circumflex from the right coronary artery or right Valsalva sinus. As with the anomalous origin of the right coronary artery from the left Valsalva sinus, the artery courses between the aorta and right ventricular outflow tract and may have an acute bend near its origin, which may result in compromise of flow. L, left coronary cusp; LA, left atrium; LAD, left anterior descending artery; N, non-coronary cusp; R, right coronary cusp; RA, right atrium.

main coronary artery. With minor withdrawal of the probe and rotation in a counterclockwise direction, it is possible to visualize the right coronary artery ostia as well. The takeoff of the left coronary artery is visualized in a longitudinal (120-degree) view as well.

There are several clinical instances in which visualization of the coronary arteries is of proven clinical benefit and others in which it may provide valuable clues to the presence of underlying disease. Clinical situations in which it is of proven benefit include identification of anomalous coronary artery takeoff and detection of aneurysms in Kawasaki disease.

There are several variations on anomalous coronary artery origin, some of which are schematized in Figure 15.72. Clinically, one should document the origin of both coronary arteries in childhood cases of cardiomyopathy

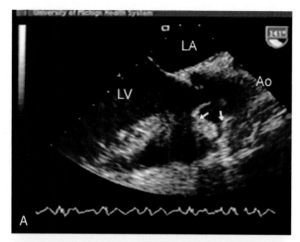

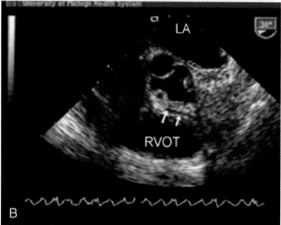

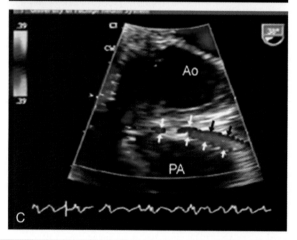

FIGURE 15.73. Transesophageal echocardiogram recorded in a patient with an anomalous origin of the left anterior descending coronary artery from the right Valsalva sinus. **A:** A longitudinal view of the aorta in which the normal origin of the right coronary artery can be seen (*downward-pointing arrow*). Additionally, a second smaller coronary artery arises closer to the aortic anulus (*leftward-pointing arrow*). **B:** Recorded in an orthogonal view, this artery can be seen to course between the aorta and right ventricular outflow tract (*arrows*). **C:** Expanded view of the anomalous left coronary artery with color flow Doppler imaging used to confirm coronary flow. Ao, aorta; LA, left atrium; LV, left ventricle; PA, pulmonary artery; RVOT, right ventricular outflow tract.

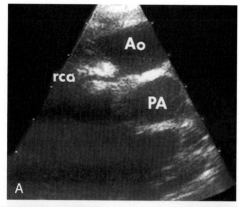

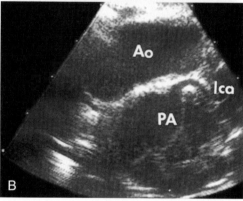

FIGURE 15.74. An anomalous left coronary artery (*lca*) is illustrated. **A:** The right coronary artery (*rca*) can be traced to the right coronary sinus of the aortic root (*Ao*). **B:** Angulation of the transducer permits recording of the left coronary artery arising from the main pulmonary artery (*PA*). (Courtesy of Gregory J. Ensing)

Variations on anomalous coronary artery origin include an anomalous origin of the right coronary artery from the left coronary sinus or the left or circumflex artery from the right coronary sinus. Less commonly, the left main coronary artery may arise in an anomalous location. A relatively common coronary anomaly is an anomalous origin of the right coronary artery from the left coronary cusp after which it then courses between the aorta and the pulmonary artery before assuming a relatively normal course. This anomaly has been associated with sudden cardiac death, presumably because of the acute angle that the coronary artery makes in arising from the left cusp before traversing posteriorly. The presumed mechanism of sudden death is acute kinking of the artery with reduction in flow at the time of or immediately after vigorous physical exercise. On occasion, the course of the anomalous coronary artery between the two great vessels can be directly visualized with either transthoracic echocardiography or transesophageal echocardiography.

An anomalous origin of a coronary artery from the pulmonary artery is an uncommon condition that leads to perfusion of the myocardium with desaturated blood. More often, a coronary steal phenomenon occurs in which there is retrograde flow in the anomalous artery. This results in effective bypassing of the myocardium into the low-pressure pulmonary circuit. This diversion of flow from the arterial origin into the low pressure pulmonary artery origin results in the myopathic process rather than perfusion of myocardium by low oxygen content blood. Because the anomalous coronary artery, arising from the pulmonary artery, represents a pathologic shunt, the vessel typically dilates in response to the high-volume flow. Additionally, because the entire myocardial blood flow volume is provided by the remaining normally connected arteries, they likewise dilate in response to the excess volume flow. Similar dilation of a coronary artery may be seen in cases of a coronary artery fistula in which the low resistance of flow into the atrium results in a pathologic increase in flow volume and subsequent coronary artery dilation (Fig. 15.75). On occasion, one may directly visualize the abnormal flow into a downstream chamber as a continuous turbulent flow signal (Fig. 15.76).

Kawasaki Disease

Kawasaki disease is an infectious/inflammatory disease, typically of childhood. Its major manifestations are arthralgia, rash, and fever, and it is associated with coronary arterial aneurysms. Detection of aneurysms by echocardiography is one of the clinical features for establishing the diagnosis of Kawasaki disease. Typically, the

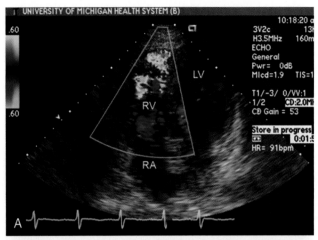
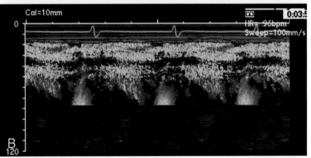

FIGURE 15.76. Apical view recorded in a patient status post-cardiac transplantation who has undergone multiple right ventricular endocardial biopsies. **A:** Note the continuous turbulent flow in the right ventricular apex, which is the result of an iatrogenic coronary artery fistula into the cavity of the right ventricle (*RV*). **B:** A color Doppler M-mode recording through that area demonstrates the continuous flow. LV, left ventricle; RA, right atrium.

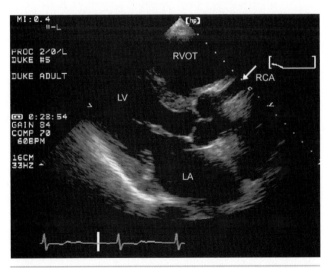

FIGURE 15.75. Parasternal long-axis view recorded in a patient with marked dilation of the proximal right coronary artery (*RCA*) due to a coronary artery fistula to the right atrium. A similar appearance may be noted in the anomalous takeoff of the left coronary artery from the pulmonary trunk due to compensatory high flow in the right coronary artery. LA, left atrium; LV, left ventricle; RVOT, right ventricular outflow tract.

aneurysms are present in the proximal portions of the coronary arteries and as such are visualized with transthoracic echocardiography. Because this is a childhood disease, in which coronary visualization is often less problematic, screening the coronary arteries with transthoracic echocardiography provides a reliable tool for establishing or excluding the diagnosis of the disease. The images in Figures 15.77 and 15.78 were recorded in patients with Kawasaki disease and demonstrate coronary artery aneurysms. Color flow imaging often demonstrates fairly limited color flow areas within the aneurysm. High-frequency scanning can frequently demonstrate thrombus lining the wall of an aneurysm. Two-dimensional echocardiography is used as a tool for follow-up of these aneurysms because their size and appearance may change over time.

Occasionally, one encounters an adult patient with a proximal coronary artery aneurysm of uncertain etiology. Many such aneurysms may represent the sequelae of previously unrecognized Kawasaki disease in childhood. Not infrequently the aneurysm is detected when echocardiog-

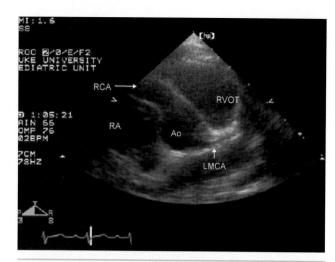

FIGURE 15.77. Parasternal short-axis view recorded at the base of the heart in a child with Kawasaki disease and aneurysmal dilation of the right coronary artery (*RCA*). Note the size and location of the aorta (*Ao*) and pulmonary artery and a markedly dilated right coronary artery that measures approximately 8 mm in diameter. LMCA, left main coronary artery; RA, right atrium; RVOT, right ventricular outflow tract.

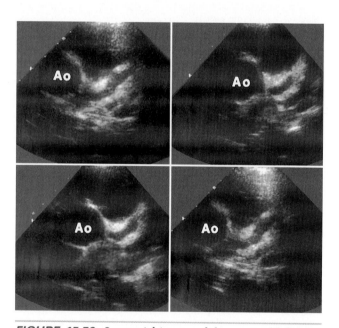

FIGURE 15.78. Sequential images of the proximal left coronary artery are recorded from the parasternal short-axis view. Multiple, fusiform dilated segments are apparent. Such coronary artery aneurysms are seen in patients with Kawasaki disease. Ao, aorta.

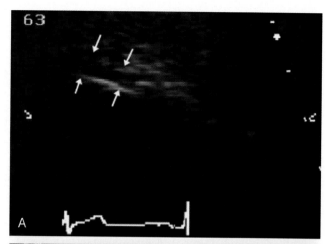

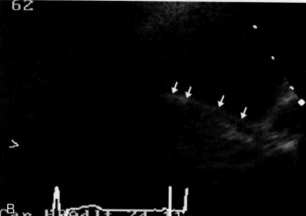

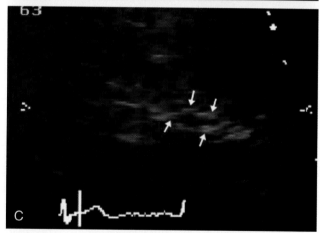

FIGURE 15.79. Transthoracic parasternal long-axis echocardiogram recorded along the axis of the interventricular groove imaging the mid portion of the left anterior descending coronary artery. **A:** A normal left anterior descending coronary artery. **B, C:** Varying degrees of diffuse and focal atherosclerotic disease are shown (*arrows*).

raphy is performed in a patient who is being evaluated for chest pain syndrome. On occasion, the aneurysms encountered in adult patients can reach substantial size, with aneurysms as large as 4 to 6 cm in diameter having been infrequently encountered.

Direct Visualization of Atherosclerosis

Coronary artery disease is typically a diffuse process. In most patients with significant obstructive disease, even if the major area of obstruction is more distal, there will be

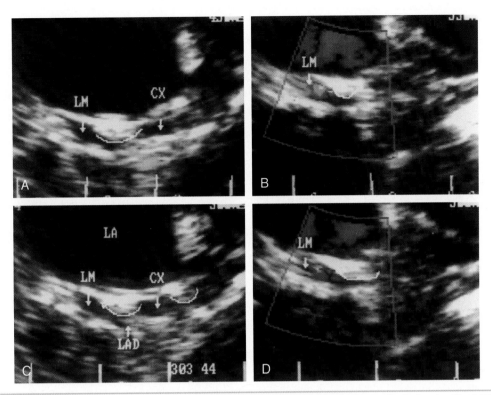

FIGURE 15.80. Transesophageal echocardiogram of a patient with an obstructive lesion (outline) **(A)** at the junction between the left main (*LM*) and the circumflex (*CX*) arteries. A second lesion (outline) **(C)** is visible in the circumflex artery. Doppler flow imaging **(B, D)** shows acceleration and aliasing in the left main artery proximal to the first stenotic lesion. LAD, left anterior descending artery.

involvement of the proximal coronary arteries. It has been well confirmed that patients with clinically significant coronary artery disease, irrespective of the location, frequently have thickening and/or calcification in the proximal left anterior descending coronary artery. This was demonstrated using transthoracic echocardiography in numerous studies and also forms the basis for screening for coronary artery disease using ultrafast computed tomography. As noted previously, it is possible to image the proximal portion of the left anterior descending coronary artery in most adult patients, even when routine anatomic imaging of the rest of the heart is suboptimal. Figures 15.79 and 15.80 were recorded in patients with varying degrees of thickening and/or calcification in the distal left main coronary artery or proximal left anterior descending coronary artery. Several clinical studies have demonstrated that the detection of calcification in the proximal coronary arteries is an accurate marker for the presence of clinically relevant coronary artery disease. Although an accurate means for identifying patients with obstructive coronary artery disease, this methodology has not had widespread acceptance for routine surveillance screening of patients, in large part due to the presumed difficulty of scanning and interpretation. Other ultrasound methodologies that can be used to detect the presence of obstructive coronary disease include trans-

esophageal echocardiographic scanning to evaluate the proximal coronary arteries for calcification and/or obstruction. In this instance, the data obtained are analogous to those described previously for transthoracic echocardiography.

Some investigators have reported success with using Doppler imaging of the lumen of the coronary artery from a transthoracic echocardiographic approach and thus measuring systolic and diastolic coronary flow waveforms (Fig. 15.81). Either nitroglycerin or dipyridamole has been given to alter coronary blood flow and the resulting changes in spectral Doppler flow profiles used as a marker for presence of coronary artery disease. Similarly, Doppler interrogation of coronary sinus flow, as a marker of antegrade coronary arterial flow, has been used to detect functional disturbances due to coronary artery disease. Similar measurements can be made of coronary sinus flow that provide an indirect assessment of coronary flow in the left coronary system.

See Chapter 18 for further discussion of the impact of anomalous coronary arteries in children, Chapter 22 for a discussion of neurogenic cardiac stunning, Chapters 3 and 19 for a discussion of intracoronary ultrasound, Chapter 17 for further discussion of ischemic cardiomyopathy, and Chapter 11 for further discussion of ischemic mitral regurgitation.

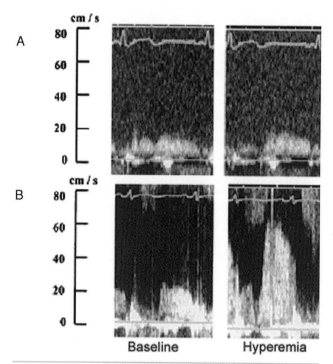

FIGURE 15.81. Transthoracic Doppler echocardiography recording flow in the mid portion of the left anterior descending coronary artery, at baseline (*left panels*) and during pharmacologically induced hyperemia (*right panels*). **B:** Recorded in a normal individual without coronary obstruction. Note the marked increase in coronary flow velocity during hyperemia. **A:** Image recorded in a patient with severe disease of the left anterior descending coronary artery reveals blunted flow at baseline and no augmentation during hyperemia. (From the American College of Cardiology Foundation, with permission.)

SUGGESTED READINGS

Angelini P, Velasco JA, Flamm S. Coronary anomalies: incidence, pathophysiology, and clinical relevance. Circulation 2002;105:2449–2454.

Baigrie RS, et al. The spectrum of right ventricular involvement in inferior wall myocardial infarction: a clinical, hemodynamic and noninvasive study. J Am Coll Cardiol 1983;1:1396–404.

Barzilai B, Davis VC, Stone PH, et al. Prognostic significance of mitral regurgitation in acute myocardial infarction. The MILIS Study Group. Am J Cardiol 1990;65:1169–1175.

Bourdillon PD, et al. Early recovery of regional left ventricular function after reperfusion in acute myocardial infarction assessed by serial two-dimensional echocardiography. Am J Cardiol 1989;63:641–646.

Bourdillon PD, et al. Regional wall motion index for infarct and noninfarct regions after reperfusion in acute myocardial infarction: comparison with global wall motion index. J Am Soc Echocardiogr 1989;2:398–407.

Burns RJ, et al. The relationships of left ventricular ejection fraction, end-systolic volume index and infarct size to six-month mortality after hospital discharge following myocardial infarction treated by thrombolysis. J Am Coll Cardiol 2002;39:30–36.

Cerisano G, et al. Doppler-derived mitral deceleration time: an early strong predictor of left ventricular remodeling after reperfused anterior acute myocardial infarction. Circulation 1999;99:230–236.

Cerisano G, et al. Prognostic implications of restrictive left ventricular filling in reperfused anterior acute myocardial infarction. J Am Coll Cardiol 2001;37:793–799.

Cerqueira MD, et al. Standardized myocardial segmentation and nomenclature for tomographic imaging of the heart. A statement for healthcare professionals from the Cardiac Imaging Committee of the Council on Clinical Cardiology of the American Heart Association. Circulation 2002;105:539–542.

Cheitlin MD, et al. ACC/AHA/ASE 2003 Guideline Update for the Clinical Application of Echocardiography: summary article. A report of the American College of Cardiology/American Heart Association Task Force on Practice Guidelines (ACC/AHA/ASE Committee to Update the 1997 Guidelines for the Clinical Application of Echocardiography). J Am Soc Echocardiogr 2003;16:1091–1110.

Daimon M, et al. Physiologic assessment of coronary artery stenosis by coronary flow reserve measurements with transthoracic Doppler echocardiography: comparison with exercise thallium-201 single piston emission computed tomography. J Am Coll Cardiol 2001;37:1310–1315.

Dawn B, et al. Two-dimensional and Doppler transesophageal echocardiographic delineation and flow characterization of anomalous coronary arteries in adults. J Am Soc Echocardiogr 2003;16:1274–1286.

Derumeaux G, et al. Tissue Doppler imaging differentiates transmural from nontransmural acute myocardial infarction after reperfusion therapy. Circulation 2001;103:589–596.

Eaton LW, et al. Regional cardiac dilatation after acute myocardial infarction: recognition by two-dimensional echocardiography. N Engl J Med 1979;300:57–62.

Edvardsen T, et al. Regional myocardial systolic function during acute myocardial ischemia assessed by strain Doppler echocardiography. J Am Coll Cardiol 2001;37:726–730.

Elhendy A, et al. Significance of resting wall motion abnormalities in 2-dimensional echocardiography in patients without previous myocardial infarction referred for pharmacologic stress testing. J Am Soc Echocardiogr 2000;13:1–8.

Feinberg MS, et al. Prognostic significance of mild mitral regurgitation by color Doppler echocardiography in acute myocardial infarction. Am J Cardiol 2000;86:903–907.

Figueras J, et al. Nature and progression of pericardial effusion in patients with a first myocardial infarction: relationship to age and free wall rupture. Am Heart J 2002;144:251–258.

Fleischmann KE, et al. Echocardiographic correlates of survival in patients with chest pain. J Am Coll Cardiol 1994;23:1390–1396.

Gibler WB, et al. A rapid diagnostic and treatment center for patients with chest pain in the emergency department. Ann Emerg Med 1995;25:1–8.

Gibson RS, et al. Value of early two dimensional echocardiography in patients with acute myocardial infarction. Am J Cardiol 1982;49:1110–1119.

Gillam LD, et al. A comparison of quantitative echocardiographic methods for delineating infarct-induced abnormal wall motion. Circulation 1984;70:113–122.

Godley RW, et al. Incomplete mitral leaflet closure in patients with papillary muscle dysfunction. Circulation 1981;63:565–571.

Gradus-Pizlo I, et al. Detection of subclinical coronary atherosclerosis using two-dimensional, high-resolution transthoracic echocardiography. J Am Coll Cardiol 2001;37:1422–1429.

Grigioni F, et al. Ischemic mitral regurgitation: long-term outcome and prognostic implications with quantitative Doppler assessment. Circulation 2001;103:1759–1764.

Hancock JE, et al. Determination of successful reperfusion after thrombolysis for acute myocardial infarction: a noninvasive method using ultrasonic tissue characterization that can be applied clinically. Circulation 2002;105:157–161.

Heger JJ, Weyman AE, Wann LS, et al. Cross-sectional echocardiographic analysis of the extent of left ventricular asynergy in acute myocardial infarction. [Journal Article] Circulation 1980;61(6):1113–8.

Hillis GS, et al. Noninvasive estimation of left ventricular filling pressure by E/e′ is a powerful predictor of survival after acute myocardial infarction. J Am Coll Cardiol 2004;43:360–367.

Homans DC, et al. Regional function and perfusion at the lateral border of ischemic myocardium. Circulation 1985;71:1038–1047.

Horowitz RS, et al. Immediate diagnosis of acute myocardial infarction by two-dimensional echocardiography. Circulation 1982;65:323–329.

Horowitz RS, Morganroth J. Immediate detection of early high-risk patients with acute myocardial infarction using two-dimensional echocardiographic evaluation of left ventricular regional wall motion abnormalities. Am Heart J 1982;103:814–822.

Jaarsma W, et al. Predictive value of two-dimensional echocardiographic and hemodynamic measurements on admission with acute myocardial infarction. J Am Soc Echocardiogr 1988;1:187–193.

Jiang L, et al. Quantitative three-dimensional reconstruction of aneurysmal left ventricles. *In vitro* and *in vivo* validation. Circulation 1995;91:222–230.

Jugdutt BI, et al. Evaluation of biventricular involvement in hypotensive patients with transmural inferior infarction by two-dimensional echocardiography. Am Heart J 1984;108:1417–1426.

Jugdutt BI, Sivaram CA. Prospective two-dimensional echocardiographic evaluation of left ventricular thrombus and embolism after acute myocardial infarction. J Am Coll Cardiol 1989;13:554–564.

Keren A, et al. Natural history of left ventricular thrombi: their appearance and resolution in the posthospitalization period of acute myocardial infarction. J Am Coll Cardiol 1990;15:790–800.

Kontos MC, et al. Comparison of 2-dimensional echocardiography and myocardial perfusion imaging for diagnosing myocardial infarction in emergency department patients. Am Heart J 2002;143:659–667.

Lee S, et al. Noninvasive evaluation of coronary reperfusion by transthoracic Doppler echocardiography in patients with anterior acute myocardial infarction before coronary intervention. Circulation 2003;108:2763–2768.

Lewis SJ, et al. Segmental wall motion abnormalities in the absence of clinically documented myocardial infarction: clinical significance and evidence of hibernating myocardium. Am Heart J 1991;121:1088–1094.

Lieberman AN, et al. Two-dimensional echocardiography and infarct size: relationship of regional wall motion and thickening to the extent of myocardial infarction in the dog. Circulation 1981;63:739–746.

Lima JA, et al. Impaired thickening of nonischemic myocardium during acute regional ischemia in the dog. Circulation 1985;71:1048–1059.

Lundgren C, et al. Comparison of contrast angiography and two-dimensional echocardiography for the evaluation of left ventricular regional wall motion abnormalities after acute myocardial infarction. Am J Cardiol 1990;65:1071–1077.

March KL, et al. Current concepts of left ventricular pseudoaneurysm: pathophysiology, therapy, and diagnostic imaging methods. Clin Cardiol 1989;12:531–540.

McGillem MJ, et al. Modification of the centerline method for assessment of echocardiographic wall thickening and motion: a comparison with areas of risk. J Am Coll Cardiol 1988;11:861–866.

Mehta SR, et al. Impact of right ventricular involvement on mortality and morbidity in patients with inferior myocardial infarction. J Am Coll Cardiol 2001;37:37–43.

Møller JE, et al. Pseudonormal and restrictive filling patterns predict left ventricular dilation and cardiac death after a first myocardial infarction: a serial color M-mode Doppler echocardiographic study. J Am Coll Cardiol 2000;36:1841–1846.

Møller JE, et al. Prognostic importance of systolic and diastolic function after acute myocardial infarction. Am Heart J 2003;145:147–153.

Moynihan PF, Parisi AF, Feldman CL. Quantitative detection of regional left ventricular contraction abnormalities by two-dimensional echocardiography. I. Analysis of methods. Circulation 1981;63:752–760.

Nidorf SM, et al. Benefit of late coronary reperfusion on ventricular morphology and function after myocardial infarction. J Am Coll Cardiol 1993;21:683–691.

Nishimura RA, et al. Role of two-dimensional echocardiography in the prediction of in-hospital complications after acute myocardial infarction. J Am Coll Cardiol 1984;4:1080–1087.

Parisi AF, et al. Quantitative detection of regional left ventricular contraction abnormalities by two-dimensional echocardiography. II. Accuracy in coronary artery disease. Circulation 1981;63:761–767.

Peels CH, et al. Usefulness of two-dimensional echocardiography for immediate detection of myocardial ischemia in the emergency room. Am J Cardiol 1990;65:687–691.

Picard MH, et al. Natural history of left ventricular size and function after acute myocardial infarction. Assessment and prediction by echocardiographic endocardial surface mapping. Circulation 1990;82:484–494.

Pierard LA, et al. Incidence and significance of pericardial effusion in acute myocardial infarction as determined by two-dimensional echocardiography. J Am Coll Cardiol 1986;8:517–520.

Roberts WC. Major anomalies of coronary arterial origin seen in adulthood. Am Heart J 1986;111:941–963.

Romano S, et al. Usefulness of echocardiography in the prognostic evaluation of non–Q-wave myocardial infarction. Am J Cardiol 2000;86:43G–45G.

Ryan T, et al. Quantitative two-dimensional echocardiographic assessment of patients undergoing left ventricular aneurysmectomy. Am Heart J 1986;111:714–720.

Sabia P, et al. Value of regional wall motion abnormality in the emergency room diagnosis of acute myocardial infarction. A prospective study using two-dimensional echocardiography. Circulation 1991;84(3 Suppl):I85–I92.

Sabia P, et al. Importance of two-dimensional echocardiographic assessment of left ventricular systolic function in patients presenting to the emergency room with cardiac-related symptoms. Circulation 1991;84:615–624.

Sasaki H, et al. Utility of echocardiography for the early assessment of patients with nondiagnostic chest pain. Am Heart J 1986;112:494–497.

Saeian K, Rhyne TL, Sagar KB. Ultrasonic tissue characterization for diagnosis of acute myocardial infarction in the coronary care unit. Am J Cardiol 1994;74:1211–1215.

St John Sutton M, et al. Left ventricular remodeling and ventricular arrhythmias after myocardial infarction. Circulation 2003;107:2577–2582.

Stamm RB, et al. Echocardiographic detection of infarct-localized asynergy and remote asynergy during acute myocardial infarction: correlation with the extent of angiographic coronary disease. Circulation 1983;67:233–244.

Visser CA, et al. Detection and quantification of acute, isolated myocardial infarction by two dimensional echocardiography. Am J Cardiol 1981;47:1020–1025.

Weinreich DJ, Burke JF, Pauletto FJ. Left ventricular mural thrombi complicating acute myocardial infarction. Long-term follow-up with serial echocardiography. Ann Intern Med 1984;100:789–794.

Weyman AE, et al. Importance of temporal heterogeneity in assessing the contraction abnormalities associated with acute myocardial ischemia. Circulation 1984;70:102–112.

Stress Echocardiography

Stress echocardiography is based on the fundamental causal relationship between induced myocardial ischemia and left ventricular regional wall motion abnormalities. The potential for using echocardiography for this purpose was first reported in 1979 when two groups of investigators demonstrated the proof of concept. Mason and colleagues used M-mode echocardiography to study 13 patients with coronary artery disease and 11 age-matched control subjects during supine bicycle exercise. Stress-induced wall motion changes were detected in 19 of 22 segments supplied by stenotic coronary arteries. Although this was the first demonstration of transient ischemia being detected with ultrasound, the inherent limitations of the M-mode technique were apparent. That same year, Wann and co-workers applied an early two-dimensional, 30-degree sector imaging system to demonstrate inducible wall motion abnormalities during supine bicycle exercise and subsequent improvement of the wall motion response after revascularization. These early studies were limited by image quality and a reliance on videotape analysis, factors that would slow the growth of the field in its early years.

In the 1980s, improvement in image quality and the development of digital acquisition technology, or *frame grabbers*, contributed to greater accuracy and increased the practicality of using stress echocardiography in clinical situations. Most important, the digitization of echocardiographic images reduced the problem of respiratory interference by permitting selection of cardiac cycles that were devoid of lung interference and the creation of cine loops that permitted side-by-side analysis of rest and stress images. This allowed more accurate interpretation of wall motion, largely by permitting relatively subtle changes in stress-induced wall motion to be detected. Digital technology also shortened the acquisition time for postexercise imaging and facilitated display, storage, and transmission of echocardiographic data. More than any other single factor, the application of digital imaging led to the rapid development of stress echocardiography as a clinical tool.

PHYSIOLOGIC BASIS

In the 1930s, Tennant and Wiggers observed the relationship between systolic contraction and myocardial blood supply to the left ventricle. With the induction of ischemia, these investigators demonstrated the rapid and predictable development of systolic bulging (or dyskinesis). This observation established the link between induced ischemia and transient regional myocardial dyssynergy, recorded echocardiographically as the development of wall motion abnormality after the application of a stressor (Fig. 16.1).

In the absence of a flow-limiting coronary stenosis, physiologic stress results in an increase in heart rate and contractility that is maintained via an increase in myocardial blood flow. Systolic wall thickening, endocardial excursion, and global contractility all increase, leading to a decrease in end-systolic volume (and an increase in the ejection fraction) compared with baseline. Although this response may be blunted in the setting of advanced age and/or hypertension or in the presence of beta-blocker therapy, absence of the hypercontractile state in response to stress should generally be considered an abnormal response.

In the presence of a coronary stenosis, the increase in myocardial oxygen demand that occurs in response to stress is not matched by an appropriate increase in supply. If the supply-demand mismatch persists, a complex sequence of events known as the ischemic cascade will develop (Fig. 16.2). Soon after the development of a regional perfusion defect, a wall motion abnormality will occur, characterized echocardiographically as a reduction in systolic thickening and endocardial excursion. The severity of the wall motion abnormality (hypokinesis versus dyskinesis) will depend on several factors, including the magnitude of the blood flow change, the spatial extent of the defect, the presence of collateral blood flow, left ventricular pressure and wall stress, and the duration of ischemia. Deterioration in regional wall motion, however, is a specific and predictable marker of regional ischemia

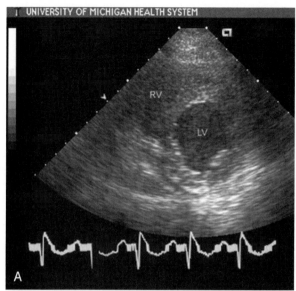

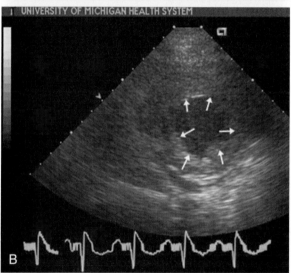

FIGURE 16.1. Short-axis views of a patient during an episode of acute ischemia in diastole **(A)** and systole **(B)**. With the onset of ischemia, anterior and lateral akinesis (*arrows*) develops almost immediately. LV, left ventricle; RV, right ventricle.

that generally precedes such traditional manifestations as angina or electrocardiographic abnormalities.

Once the stressor is eliminated, myocardial oxygen demand decreases and ischemia resolves. Normalization of wall motion may occur rapidly, although typically the complete recovery of normal function takes 1 to 2 minutes, largely depending on the severity and duration of ischemia. *Stunned myocardium* is the term applied when functional abnormalities persist after transient ischemia for a longer period. Although a reversible process, stunning may last days or even weeks if the ischemia is severe and prolonged.

The utility of echocardiography in conjunction with stress testing is contingent on the ability to record wall

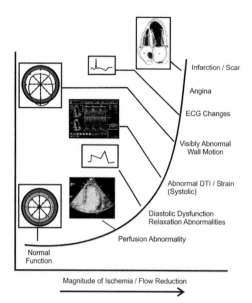

FIGURE 16.2. The ischemic cascade is the term used to describe the sequence of events that occur after the onset of ischemia. The temporal abnormalities develop in a predictable sequence, as demonstrated in this schematic. Wall motion abnormalities detectable by echocardiography generally develop after a perfusion defect but before electrocardiographic changes or angina. DTI, Doppler tissue imaging.

motion and left ventricular function at baseline and then to detect changes after the induction of stress, either exercise or pharmacologic (Table 16.1). At baseline, the presence of a regional wall motion abnormality generally implies the presence of previous myocardial damage, in most cases due to myocardial infarction. Less often, cardiomyopathy and stunned or hibernating myocardium cause resting wall motion abnormalities. Regional deterioration of left ventricular function during stress is a specific marker of ischemia. Although exercise-induced wall motion abnormalities may occasionally occur in normal individuals after prolonged, intense exercise, this type of response during stress testing is usually the result of significant coronary disease. A global decrease in left ventricular function in response to stress, however, may be due to other causes, such as hypertension or cardiomyopathy. Therefore, by comparing regional wall motion at baseline and during stress, the presence of inducible ischemia can be detected and localized.

Although most of the useful information gathered during stress echocardiography is dependent on two-dimensional imaging and the analysis of regional and global left ventricular function, several other useful parameters should also be considered. For example, Doppler techniques can be applied to measure changes in stroke volume that occur during stress. Analysis of mitral inflow velocity has been used to assess diastolic abnormalities in response to stress. As is discussed later, Doppler imaging has particular utility in the evaluation of

▶ TABLE 16.1 Causes of Wall Motion Abnormalities

Wall Motion Abnormalities at Rest	Wall Motion Abnormalities during Stress
Infarction	Ischemia
Cardiomyopathy	Translational cardiac motion
Myocarditis	Marked increase in blood pressure
Left bundle branch block	Cardiomyopathy
Hypertension/afterload mismatch	Rate-dependent left bundle branch block
Hibernating myocardium	
Stunned myocardium	
Toxins (e.g., alcohol)	
Postoperative state	
Paced rhythm	
Right ventricular volume/pressure overload	

patients with valvular heart disease, prosthetic valves, and hypertrophic cardiomyopathy. Stress testing in these patients can provide valuable information and has been used to assess the effectiveness of therapy and to make decisions regarding the timing of interventions.

More recently, the application of contrast echocardiography promises to revolutionize stress echocardiography by providing the simultaneous opportunity to assess regional myocardial perfusion in conjunction with wall motion analysis. Relative changes in myocardial perfusion in response to stressors form the basis of most nuclear stress techniques. Instead of relying on the development of wall motion abnormalities, perfusion methods depend on an ability to detect an abnormal blood flow (or perfusion) response. Because changes in myocardial perfusion precede regional systolic dysfunction, contrast echocardiography offers the potential for a more sensitive marker of myocardial ischemia.

METHODOLOGY

One of the advantages of stress echocardiography is its versatility with respect to the type of stress used (Table 16.2). Echocardiographic imaging can be applied to both exercise and pharmacologic stress for the detection of myocardial ischemia. Exercise echocardiography is

▶ TABLE 16.2 Types of Stressors Used in Stress
Echocardiography

Exercise	Nonexercise Stress
Treadmill	Dobutamine
Supine bicycle	Dipyridamole
Upright bicycle	Dipyridamole/dobutamine combination
Handgrip	Adenosine
Stair step	Pacing
	Ergonovine

most often performed using either treadmill or bicycle (upright or supine) exercise. The most common pharmacologic agent used in conjunction with echocardiography is dobutamine. Less commonly used stressors include isometric exercise such as handgrip, vasodilators such as dipyridamole or adenosine, and pacing, usually through a transesophageal approach. Modalities may even be combined. For example, handgrip may be used during dobutamine stress to increase workload and improve sensitivity.

Treadmill

Treadmill exercise is the most common form of stress testing in the United States. It provides a plethora of useful clinical information that has both diagnostic and prognostic value. These include exercise capacity, blood pressure response, and arrhythmias. It is safe and well tolerated and can be applied to a large percentage of the patients referred for stress testing. Because clinicians have become comfortable with this form of stress testing and because of the widespread availability of treadmill equipment, it is logical that stress echocardiography should be applied to this technique (Fig. 16.3).

Echocardiographic imaging in conjunction with treadmill exercise is intended not to alter the standard exercise protocol. Imaging is performed before and immediately after treadmill exercise, without affecting the exercise portion of the test. Thus, the advantages of treadmill exercise echocardiography include preserving the additional information already available from treadmill exercise, the widespread availability of this form of stress, and the relatively simple protocol created by the addition of echocardiographic imaging. The primary disadvantage of treadmill echocardiography stems from the difficulty in obtaining images while patients walk in an upright position. For this reason, imaging is limited to the immediate postexercise period. Because ischemia may resolve quickly after termination of exercise, it is incumbent on

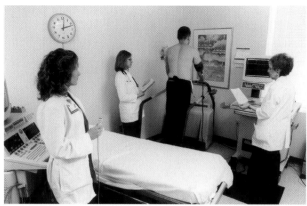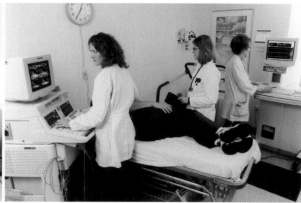

FIGURE 16.3. A treadmill exercise echocardiogram is being performed. The proximity of the echocardiography bed to the treadmill is critical so that postexercise images can be acquired immediately after termination of exercise.

the operator to complete postexercise imaging as soon as possible, certainly within 1 to 1.5 minutes after exercise. As soon as the exercise test ends, the patient must step off the treadmill and assume a recumbent position so that imaging can be completed quickly.

Although any available transthoracic view can be used in exercise echocardiographic protocols, the traditional approach has included the parasternal long- and short-axis and the apical four- and two-chamber views. The apical long-axis, the subcostal four-chamber, and short-axis views may also be included at the discretion of the operator. Image acquisition can be individualized, depending on available ultrasound windows but is always intended

to acquire images that provide more than one opportunity to examine each region of the left ventricle. In addition, some attention to right ventricular function and wall motion should also be a part of most stress echocardiographic protocols. Figure 16.4 is an example of a treadmill exercise echocardiogram showing the apical four- and two-chamber views. The resting or baseline images are on the left, and the postexercise images are on the right. Each quadrant contains annotated information about heart rate, stage, time of acquisition, etc. A typical treadmill exercise echocardiographic protocol is summarized in Table 16.3.

Resolution of induced wall motion abnormalities before postexercise imaging can be completed is a cause of false-negative results (Fig. 16.5). In this example, with treadmill exercise, anterior ischemia is evident in the long- and short-axis views, less obvious in the four-chamber view, and no longer present in the two-chamber view. This is because the wall motion abnormality resolved over the course of poststress image acquisition. As the heart rate decreases postexercise, wall motion recov-

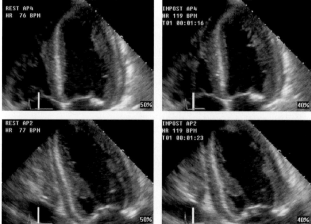

FIGURE 16.4. The standard format to display stress echocardiographic images is demonstrated. This example, from a treadmill exercise echocardiogram, demonstrates the four-chamber view at the top and the two-chamber images at the bottom. The resting study is displayed on the left, and the immediate postexercise images are on the right. Note that heart rate, exercise duration, and time of image acquisition are displayed for each quad.

▶ **TABLE 16.3 Protocol for Treadmill Exercise Echocardiography**

Patient is prepared for treadmill stress testing.
Instructions provided on transition from the treadmill to the examination table after exercise.
Rest echocardiographic images obtained, reviewed, and stored (both digitally and on videotape).
Standard treadmill exercise examination performed.
Patient moves as quickly as possible after exercise to the examination table.
Postexercise imaging acquired and recorded on videotape and digitally.
Digital images reviewed and representative loops selected.
Digital images stored on permanent medium.

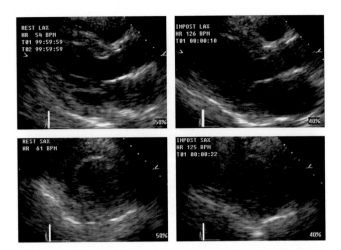

FIGURE 16.5. An example of rapid recovery of abnormal wall motion is demonstrated in a patient undergoing treadmill exercise. The resting study is normal. Postexercise, septal, and apical ischemia develops and is evident in the long- and short-axis views. The abnormality is less apparent in the four-chamber view and nearly resolved in the two-chamber view. Image acquisition was completed in approximately 75 seconds.

ers. If an adequate workload is achieved and postexercise images are acquired within 1 minute, the likelihood of a false-negative finding is minimized. Figure 16.6 is another example of rapid recovery, in this case during supine bicycle exercise. Note the obvious apical wall motion abnormality at peak exercise. Postexercise, there is near normalization of wall motion. Why some wall motion abnormalities normalize very quickly is not completely understood. Several investigators have compared peak and postexercise imaging during bicycle protocols and examined the frequency and possible causes of rapid recovery of wall motion abnormalities. Neither exercise duration, extent of disease, workload achieved, nor medical therapy is predictive of rapid recovery. Conversely, wall motion abnormalities that persist into late recovery generally indicate more severe epicardial coronary disease and/or multivessel disease.

Bicycle Ergometry

Stationary bicycle ergometry was the first form of exercise used in conjunction with echocardiography. Currently, both supine and upright bicycle ergometers are being used clinically. More recently, the availability of supine bicycle systems that permit a variety of patient positions have become popular. By providing an approximately 30-degree head-up tilt of the patient, a balance between comfort and image quality can be achieved (Fig. 16.7). To perform graded exercise, patients pedal at a constant cadence at increasing levels of resistance.

The primary advantage of bicycle stress echocardiography is the ability to image throughout exercise, particularly at peak stress. This not only avoids the potential problem of rapid recovery but also permits the onset of a wall motion abnormality to be documented. Exercise-induced wall motion abnormalities are more frequent, more extensive, and more easily visualized at peak compared with postexercise. Image acquisition at peak exercise is less rushed than postexercise imaging, so image quality is often better. The application of contrast to stress echocardiography is also easier using bicycle exercise compared with treadmill exercise. The major disadvan-

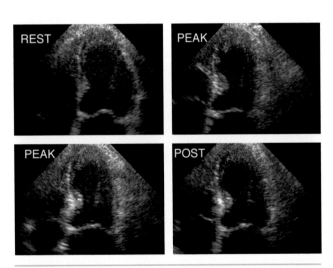

FIGURE 16.6. This study demonstrates rapid recovery during supine bicycle exercise. An obvious apical wall motion abnormality develops during exercise and is recorded at peak (right upper and left lower quads). Postexercise (right lower quad) wall motion is nearly normal. This is especially apparent in the two-chamber view.

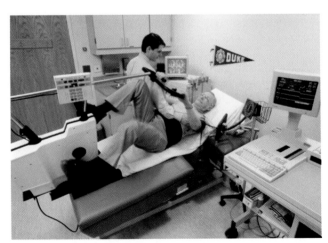

FIGURE 16.7. A supine bicycle exercise system is demonstrated. The patient is positioned to maximize comfort and to ensure optimal image acquisition. Imaging can be performed throughout the exercise protocol. See text for details.

▶ **TABLE 16.4 Protocol for Supine Bicycle Exercise Echocardigraphy**

Patient prepared for standard stress testing.
Patient instructed how to perform bicycle exercise.
Patient positioned on supine ergometer and secured in place.
Rest images obtained (table inclined to optimize images).
Exercise protocol begins at a workload of 25 W and a cadence of 60 rpm.
Workload increased by 25 W every 2 minutes.
Images monitored throughout exercise.
At peak exercise, a full series of images is obtained.
After cessation of exercise, wall motion is monitored to document resolution of induced ischemia.
Representative images are selected and rearranged for digital storage.

tage of bicycle exercise echocardiography is the problem of workload. Some patients find bicycling in the supine position very difficult, which may prevent an adequate level of stress to be achieved. However, supine posture appears to facilitate the induction of ischemia, perhaps by increasing venous return and preload or because it is associated with a greater blood pressure response. As a result, ischemia occurs at a lower heart rate during supine versus upright exercise. Again, the newer generation of bicycle ergometers increases the comfort and tolerability of supine exercise. Several protocols for bicycle echocardiography are in use today. One protocol using a supine bicycle ergometer is provided in Table 16.4.

Dobutamine Stress Echocardiography

Dobutamine is a synthetic catecholamine that causes both inotropic and chronotropic effects through its affinity for β_1, β_2, and α receptors in the myocardium and vasculature. Because of differences in affinity, the cardiovascular effects of dobutamine are dose dependent, with augmented contractility occurring at lower doses followed by a progressive chronotropic response at increasing doses. Peripheral effects may result in either predominant vasoconstriction or vasodilation, so changes in vascular resistance (i.e., blood pressure) are unpredictable. The net effect of these interactions is a combined increase in contractility and heart rate with an associated increase in myocardial oxygen demand. If coronary flow reserve is limited, myocardial oxygen demands will eventually exceed supply and ischemia will develop.

It should be noted that the mechanism of action of dobutamine is not identical to exercise. For example, the change in venous return that typically accompanies leg exercise is less pronounced with dobutamine. In addition, the autonomic nervous system–mediated changes in systemic and pulmonary vascular resistance are quite different with exercise compared with dobutamine. These dif-

ferences have implications for the determinants of the ischemic threshold during exercise and pharmacologic stress. For example, heart rate response is less important with dobutamine compared with exercise, and ischemia can often be induced even if target heart rate is not attained. The lower heart rate achieved during dobutamine infusion is offset by the greater augmentation in contractility. Thus, the two modalities are both capable of producing ischemia but do so by different mechanisms. As a result, the parameters that define an adequate level of stress are also different.

The primary application of dobutamine echocardiography is in patients unable or unwilling to exercise adequately. The ability of dobutamine to mimic the cardiac effects of exercise, coupled with the safety and versatility of the test, has contributed to the popularity of dobutamine echocardiography. A related application has been for the detection of viable myocardium in the setting of either stunned or hibernating myocardium. As with exercise, the goal is to produce a graded increase in cardiac workload that can be monitored for the development of ischemia. To do this, dobutamine is infused at increasing rates for 3- to 5-minute stages. Although this duration at each stage is insufficient to produce a steady-state effect, it generally yields a gradual and well-tolerated increase in both contractility and heart rate. Atropine is frequently used to augment the heart rate response. The use of atropine for this purpose has been shown to improve sensitivity, especially in patients taking beta-blockers. Although there is no universally agreed-on protocol for dobutamine administration, a commonly used approach is outlined in Table 16.5.

▶ **TABLE 16.5 Protocol for Dobutamine Stress Echocardiography**

Patient is prepared for standard stress testing.
Intravenous access is obtained.
Digital images are acquired at baseline (these loops are displayed and used as reference throughout the infusion).
Continuous electrocardiogram and blood pressure monitoring are established.
Dobutamine infusion is begun at a dose of 5 (or 10) μg/kg/min.
The infusion rate is increased every 3 minutes to doses of 10, 20, 30, and 40 μg/kg/min.
The echocardiogram, electrocardiogram, and blood pressure are monitored continuously.
Low-dose images are acquired at either 5 or 10 μg/kg/min (at the first sign of increased contractility).
Atropine in aliquots of 0.5 to 1.0 mg can be given during the mid- and high-dose stages to augment the heart rate response.
Mid-dose images are acquired at either 20 or 30 μg/kg/min.
Peak images are acquired before termination of the infusion.
Post-stress images are recorded after return to baseline.
The patient is monitored until he or she returns to baseline status.

▶ **TABLE 16.6 End Points and Reasons to Terminate the Dobutamine Infusion During Stress Testing**

Exceeding target heart rate of 85% age-predicted maximum
Development of significant angina[a]
Recognition of a new wall motion abnormality[b]
A decrease in systolic blood pressure >20 mm Hg from baseline[c]
Arrhythmias such as atrial fibrillation or nonsustained ventricular tachycardia
Limiting side effects or symptoms

[a]Decision may depend on clinical status of the patient and presence/extent of wall motion abnormality.
[b]Decision may depend on clinical status of the patient and extent/severity of the wall motion abnormality.
[c]Decision may depend on clinical status and left ventricular function and/or outflow tract gradient.

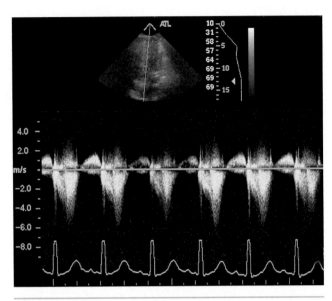

FIGURE 16.8. An example of an induced left ventricular outflow tract gradient during dobutamine stress testing is shown. This occurred in a patient with severe left ventricular hypertrophy who developed hyperdynamic wall motion at peak stress. Note the late peaking Doppler gradient.

The test may be terminated when one of several end points are reached (Table 16.6). Although such guidelines are essential, the decision to terminate the dobutamine infusion must be individualized. The ability to monitor wall motion is critically important to that decision. For example, atypical symptoms not associated with objective evidence of ischemia (i.e., a new wall motion abnormality) are not necessarily a reason to stop the test. A subtle or limited wall motion abnormality, particularly if well tolerated, also does not mandate termination. To assess the true extent of coronary disease, it is often prudent to continue the test under close monitoring. A decrease in blood pressure is sometimes an indication of extensive ischemia. During dobutamine infusion, however, hypotension may instead indicate the development of a left ventricular outflow tract gradient, and this can be easily recognized using Doppler imaging (Fig. 16.8). Finally, electrocardiographic evidence of ischemia is less reliable during dobutamine infusion than it is during exercise testing. Thus, neither ST-segment depression nor elevation occurring in the absence of a wall motion abnormality or typical symptoms is sufficient reason for terminating the dobutamine infusion.

The safety of dobutamine stress echocardiography has been examined in several series. Because of the short half-life of dobutamine, inducible ischemia can be readily reversed through termination of the infusion. In severe cases or when the ischemic manifestations persist, a short-acting intravenous beta-blocker (such as metoprolol or esmolol) is effective. In one series of 1,118 patients referred for dobutamine stress echocardiography, there were no incidents of death, myocardial infarction, or sustained ventricular tachycardia or fibrillation (Mertes et al., 1993). The most common side effects associated with dobutamine infusion were minor arrhythmias such as premature ventricular contractions, atrial arrhythmias, and minor symptoms such as palpitations or anxiety. Nonsustained ventricular tachycardia was seen in 3% of patients and was not a specific marker of coronary artery

disease. Rare isolated serious complications have been reported.

There are no absolute contraindications to dobutamine stress testing. Unstable patients, such as those with uncompensated heart failure for unstable angina, should rarely be subjected to stress testing of any kind. Dobutamine echocardiography has been safely performed in patients with recent myocardial infarction, extensive left ventricular dysfunction, abdominal aortic aneurysm, syncope, aortic stenosis, hypertrophic cardiomyopathy, history of ventricular tachycardia, and aborted sudden death. In each instance, the value of the expected diagnostic information must be balanced with the individualized risk to the patient. Unlike dipyridamole, dobutamine can be safely used in patients with bronchospastic lung disease.

Dipyridamole and Adenosine

Potent vasodilators such as dipyridamole and adenosine have been used in conjunction with echocardiography for the detection of coronary artery disease. Unlike dobutamine, these agents work by creating a maldistribution phenomenon by preventing the normal increase in flow in areas supplied by stenotic coronary arteries. In more extreme cases, flow may actually be diverted away from abnormal regions (so-called coronary steal), resulting in true ischemia. Adenosine is a potent and short-acting direct coronary vasodilator. Dipyridamole is slower acting and its effects result from inhibition of adenosine uptake. With both agents, the development of a wall motion abnormality is predicated on the ability to create sufficient maldistribution of regional blood flow to result in an ischemia-induced wall motion abnormality. Compared with dobutamine, these changes tend to be more subtle and short-lived.

The safety of dipyridamole and adenosine echocardiography is well established. However, both agents are substantially less popular compared with dobutamine as a pharmacologic stressor. The primary reason for this relates to the mechanism of action. It is conceivable that redistribution of regional blood flow can occur without an associated wall motion abnormality. Thus, vasodilator stress agents may be better suited to imaging techniques that rely on relative changes in perfusion rather than the development of a wall motion abnormality. This is the reason that dipyridamole and adenosine have been commonly used with nuclear imaging techniques. It also explains the renewed interest in these agents as contrast echocardiography gains support. As the application of contrast agents becomes more prevalent in stress echocardiography, the use of vasodilators has similarly experienced renewed popularity.

CHOOSING AMONG THE DIFFERENT STRESS MODALITIES

The wide range of choices in stress testing has the potential to create confusion for the clinician trying to select the optimal test for any given patient. Is the stress test necessary? Is any form of imaging required? Which stress modality is better: exercise or pharmacologic? What type of exercise works best with a given form of imaging? Although some of these decisions must be individualized, general guidelines can be provided. It is well established that all forms of imaging increase the accuracy of stress testing, particularly in those patients who have had or are likely to have a nondiagnostic stress electrocardiogram (ECG). Imaging also provides information on the location and extent of disease, contributing both to the diagnostic and prognostic value of the test. General guidelines for choosing among the various modalities are provided in Table 16.7.

For most patients, exercise is the preferred form of stress, provided the patient is capable of adequately performing either treadmill or bicycle exercise. The additional information available during an exercise stress test provides most of the advantage over pharmacologic testing. When compared in the same group of patients, exercise has generally been a more sensitive test for the detection of coronary disease compared with dobutamine. However, the superiority of exercise is modest and has not been a universal finding. In most clinical situations, exercise is preferred for the reasons listed previously. An exception to this general rule is when myocardial viability is an issue. In such cases, pharmacologic stress testing with dobutamine is preferred. Thus, dobutamine stress echocardiography is generally limited to patients who are unable to exercise adequately or to specifically address the question of viability.

When nonexercise stress is deemed necessary and echocardiography is the imaging modality, the weight of evidence and the general experience support the use of dobutamine as the stress agent. Because dobutamine is more likely to cause true ischemia rather than merely a flow mismatch, the induction of a wall motion abnormality, detectable with echocardiography, is more likely. However, as contrast techniques become more and more a routine part of stress echocardiography, the relative advantages of vasodilator stress testing will be reassessed.

Among the various forms of exercise echocardiography, both bicycle and treadmill techniques have been used successfully and are safe and well tolerated. Bicycle exercise has as its primary advantage the opportunity to image throughout exercise. The larger general experience with treadmill stress testing and the comfort that most clinicians have with the methodology and information available during a treadmill test must also be considered. Few studies have compared directly treadmill and bicycle exercise. In one series (Badruddin et al., 1999), in which treadmill exercise and supine bicycle exercise were performed in random order on 74 patients with suspected

▶ TABLE 16.7 **Comparison of the Different Stress Methodologies in Various Clinical Situations**

Clinical Question	Treadmill	Bicycle	Dobutamine
Chest pain evaluation	++	++	+
Post-myocardial infarction risk	++	++	++
Viability	−	−	++
Evaluation of dyspnea/fatigue	++	++	−
Preoperative risk assessment	+	+	++
Severity of valve disease	−	++	−
Pulmonary hypertension	−	++	−

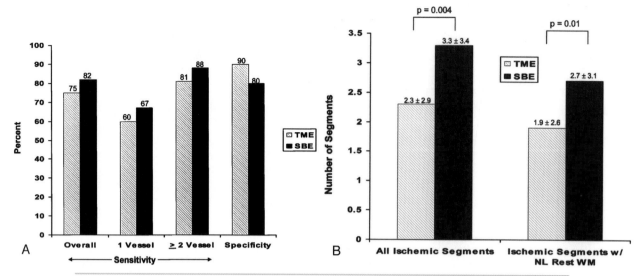

FIGURE 16.9. This graph is taken from a study that compared treadmill and bicycle exercise echocardiography in a series of 74 patients. Although not statistically significant, sensitivity was slightly higher for bicycle exercise, whereas specificity favored treadmill **(A)**. **B:** The extent of ischemia induced by each form of exercise is compared. Among patients who developed ischemia, the number of abnormal segments was significantly greater during bicycle exercise than during treadmill exercise. (From Badruddin SM, Ahmad A, Mickelson J, et al. Supine bicycle versus post-treadmill exercise echocardiography in the detection of myocardial ischemia: a randomized single-blind crossover trial. J Am Coll Cardiol 1999;33:1485–1490, with permission.)

coronary disease, the bicycle technique was found to be slightly more sensitive, whereas treadmill exercise was slightly more specific (Fig. 16.9A). Although mean exercise duration was considerably longer for bicycle exercise, overall workload, expressed as double product, was similar for the two tests. When an ischemic wall motion abnormality was induced, the extent of the defect was greater with bicycle exercise, most likely because imaging was performed during rather than after stress (Fig. 16.9B). Thus, both the treadmill and bicycle are acceptable forms of stress when echocardiographic imaging is used. Methods that permit imaging during exercise may allow both the presence and extent of disease to be more accurately determined. These advantages must be balanced by patient preference, exercise ability, and the availability of other types of diagnostic and prognostic data.

INTERPRETATION OF STRESS ECHOCARDIOGRAPHY

Most stress echocardiograms are analyzed based on a subjective assessment of regional wall motion, comparing wall thickening and endocardial excursion at baseline and during stress. The rest or baseline echocardiogram is first examined for the presence of global systolic dysfunction or regional wall motion abnormalities (Table 16.1). The presence of baseline wall motion abnormalities suggests

previous myocardial infarction. Other less likely possibilities include stunned or hibernating myocardium or a form of focal cardiomyopathy. Subtle abnormalities at baseline, such as hypokinesis of the inferior wall, may occur in the absence of coronary artery disease and represent a cause of false-positive results. Interventricular septal motion may be specifically altered in the presence of left bundle branch block, the postoperative state, ventricular pacing, or pressure or volume overload of the right ventricle.

Regardless of the form of stress, the normal response is the development of hyperdynamic wall motion (Table 16.8 and Fig. 16.10). Although this is generally true, some heterogeneity may be expected and not all left ventricular segments will necessarily display the same degree of hypercontractility. When examined quantitatively, this variability in the normal response is apparent and even mild hypokinesis may be present in normal subjects. Despite this caveat, a global increase in contractility should still be regarded as the normal response. Lack of hyperkinesis is abnormal and is most often caused by the development of regional myocardial ischemia. Other factors may also affect the ability to develop hyperkinesis. These include the presence of a nonischemic cardiomyopathy, treatment with beta-blocker therapy, left bundle branch block, and severe hypertension. In addition, submaximal exercise resulting in attainment of a low workload is often associated with the absence of a hyperkinetic response. If post-exercise imaging is performed after treadmill exercise, an

▶ **TABLE 16.8 Combination of Rest and Stress Wall Motion Responses**

Rest	Stress	Interpretation
Normal	Hyperkinetic	Normal
Normal	Hypokinetic/akinetic	Ischemic
Akinetic	Akinetic	Infarction
Hypokinetic	Akinetic/dyskinetic	Ischemic and/ or infarction
Hypokinetic/akinetic	Normal	Viable

excessive delay in image acquisition may miss the transient hyperkinesis and lead to a misinterpretation.

A limitation of this approach to interpretation is the subjective and nonquantitative nature of wall motion analysis. Several studies have examined the reproducibility of subjective wall motion scoring. In general, experienced interpreters agree in the majority of cases, and overall accuracy is reasonable. More quantitative and objective approaches, however, would have obvious advantages. Historically, such attempts have been limited by image quality and translational motion. In addition, the complexity and time-consuming nature of some methods greatly limited their acceptance. Calculation of the ejection fraction at rest and during stress, for example, is fraught with technical challenges and rarely performed in routine practice. A more practical approach involves the estimation of left ventricular volume changes during stress. The normal response to stress includes a decrease in both end-systolic and end-diastolic volume that can be visually appreciated using side-by-side inspection of images. Failure of the end-systolic size to decrease is an abnormal response. An increase in volume with stress often

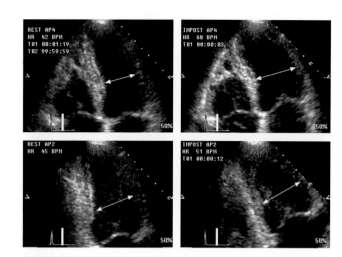

FIGURE 16.11. This treadmill exercise echocardiogram demonstrates an abnormal left ventricular volume response. These frames were taken at end-systole **(right)**. (Resting images on the **left.**) The postexercise images demonstrate a larger end-systolic volume compared with baseline, suggesting chamber enlargement in response to stress.

indicates severe and extensive (i.e., multivessel) disease. Supine bicycle exercise is an exception to this rule. With this form of stress, elevation of the legs increases venous return throughout exercise so left ventricular dilation at peak exercise may be a normal finding. Once exercise stops, the cavity usually will rapidly decrease in size. Figure 16.11 is an example of an abnormal volume response in a patient with extensive coronary disease. Note the increase in left ventricular systolic dimension, especially in the four-chamber view. The right ventricle also dilates, in this case, due to proximal right coronary artery ischemia.

More recently, strain rate imaging has been applied to stress echocardiography. This approach relies on tissue Doppler imaging to quantify myocardial deformation in response to applied stress. Strain is simply the change in length of a segment of tissue that occurs when force is applied. Strain rate is the first derivative of strain or how strain changes over time. When assessed using the Doppler technique, strain rate can be measured as the difference in velocity between two points normalized for the distance between them. Strain and strain rate have been examined as objective, quantifiable markers of ischemia during stress testing. One approach involves determining the myocardial velocity gradient, which is the difference between the systolic velocities of the endocardium versus the epicardium (normalized for wall thickness). Normally, the endocardium has a higher velocity than the epicardium, and this difference is frequently diminished with ischemia. Another approach relies on the delay in systolic shortening, sometimes called postsystolic shortening, that may occur with ischemia. This phenomenon is probably the equivalent of regional asynchrony or tardokinesis, both of which have been described as abnormal wall motion responses to

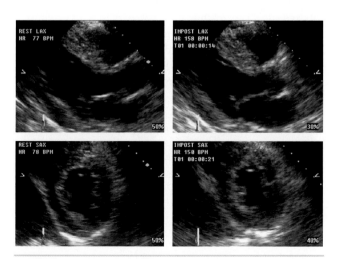

FIGURE 16.10. An example of a normal treadmill exercise echocardiogram, demonstrating a hyperdynamic response to stress, is provided. The resting study is on the left and postexercise images are on the right. Mild left ventricular hypertrophy is present.

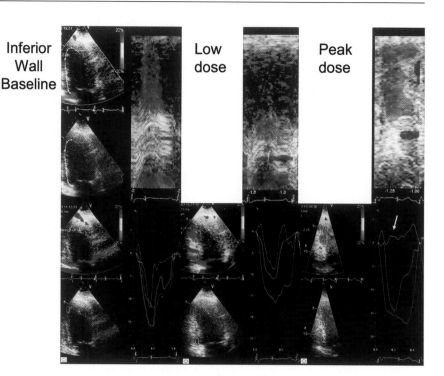

Inferior Wall Baseline — Low dose — Peak dose

FIGURE 16.12. An example of strain imaging of the inferior wall during dobutamine stress echocardiography is presented. Strain is normal in the apical, mid, and basal segments at rest (left). At peak dose, there is systolic lengthening of the basal segment (*arrow*). (Courtesy of T. Marwick, M.D.)

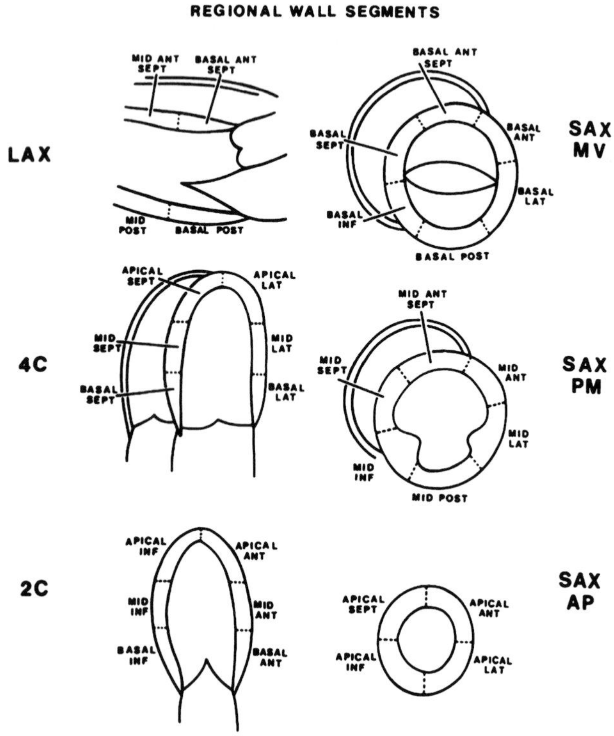

REGIONAL WALL SEGMENTS

FIGURE 16.13. The left ventricle can be divided into 16 segments that can be visualized from a series of long- and short-axis views. See text for details. LAX, long-axis; SAX, short-axis; MV, mitral valve; PM, papillary muscle; AP, apical; 2C, two-chamber; 4C, four-chamber.

stress. The potential to identify and even quantify such subtle manifestations of ischemia is an attractive feature of strain rate imaging. The theoretic advantages of strain rate imaging include a relative independence of translational motion and tethering, its inherently quantitative nature, the ability to distinguish active from passive motion, and the potential to examine wall motion throughout the cardiac cycle. Although more work is needed to validate the utility and accuracy of strain rate imaging during stress echocardiography, preliminary studies have been encouraging. Figure 16.12 is an example of strain imaging during dobutamine stress testing.

Several schemes for interpreting and reporting stress echocardiographic results are in clinical use. One approach (endorsed by the American Society of Echocardiography) divides the left ventricle into 16 segments (Fig. 16.13) and then grades each segment on a scale from 1 to 4 in which 1 is considered normal, 2 indicates hypokinesis, 3 indicates akinesis, and 4 corresponds to dyskinesis. Wall motion is analyzed at baseline, and a wall motion score index is generated according to the formula:

$$\text{Wall motion score index} = \frac{\sum_{1}^{16} \text{Segment scores}}{\text{No. of segments scored}}$$

[Eq. 16.1]

A similar approach is then taken for analysis of wall motion during stress. In this case, the development of hyperkinesis is assumed to be normal and assigned a score of 1. Thus, a normal study would be associated with a wall motion score index of 1.0 at both baseline and stress. Any score greater than 1.0 would indicate the presence of an abnormality. An increase in score would indicate either an increase in the extent and/or the severity of a wall motion abnormality. An example of wall motion scoring of a stress echocardiogram is provided in Figure 16.14. This approach has several advantages. It provides a systematic approach to wall motion analysis and encourages a thorough and standardized approach. Furthermore, it acknowledges the subjectivity of wall motion analysis but provides a quantitative reporting scheme that allows studies to be compared. The prognostic value of wall motion score index has been demonstrated in several studies.

Categorization of Wall Motion

Hypokinesis is the mildest form of abnormal wall motion. It is defined as the preservation of some degree of thickening and inward motion of the endocardium during systole but less than normal. It has been defined arbitrarily as less than 5 mm of endocardial excursion. The distinction between normal wall motion and hypokinesis is subtle, particularly in the setting of advanced age or beta-blocker therapy. Hypokinesis is most likely to be truly abnormal if it is limited to a region or territory that corresponds to the distribution of one coronary artery and is

associated with normal (or hyperdynamic) wall motion elsewhere. One particular form of hypokinesis is tardokinesis, which is used to describe delayed, sometimes postsystolic, inward motion or thickening. Analyzing wall motion frame by frame or trimming a cine loop to include only the first half of systole will help identify tardokinesis and distinguish it from other wall motion responses. Akinesis is defined as the absence of systolic myocardial thickening and endocardial excursion. Bear in mind that translational motion of the heart during systole can create the illusion of akinesis. However, wall thickening is less translation dependent and should be relied on in such cases. Dyskinesis is the most extreme form of a wall motion abnormality and is defined as systolic thinning and outward motion or bulging of the myocardium during systole. A left ventricular segment that is thin and/or highly echogenic indicates the presence of scar. Other less common wall motion responses have also been recognized. For example, early relaxation is used to describe a segment that appears to contract in early systole and then relaxes or dilates earlier than the other walls. It is a common cause of false-positive results because it is most likely a normal variant and not associated with ischemia. Again, trimming the cine loop to include only the first half of systole is a useful way to identify early relaxation and differentiate it from truly abnormal wall motion.

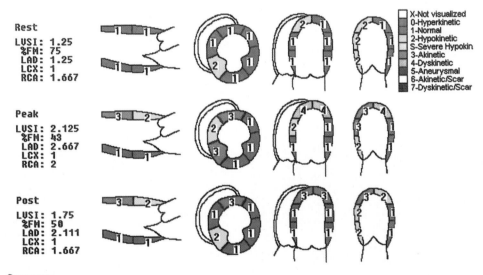

Summary:

Abnormal stress echo. Resting wall motion abnormalities, involving the apex and inferior walls. Worse with stress. New wall motion abnormalities involving the septum and apex.

CONCLUSIONS:

Evidence of prior MI with mild rest wall motion abnormalities, induced ischemia of the septum and apex.

FIGURE 16.14. An example of a stress echocardiographic report is provided, including a regional wall motion scoring summary. LVSI, left ventricle score index; %FM, percentage of normally functioning segments; MI, myocardial infarction. See text for details.

Wall Motion Response to Stress

By comparing wall motion at baseline and during stress, valuable diagnostic information is available (Table 16.8). Wall motion that increases or augments during stress is generally considered normal. The development of a wall motion abnormality during stress in an area normal at rest is most suggestive of ischemia. Segments that are abnormal at rest and remain unchanged with stress are generally best interpreted as showing evidence of infarction without additional ischemia. Hypokinetic areas that worsen during stress are usually labeled ischemic. These may represent a combination of previous nontransmural infarction and induced ischemia. Segments that are akinetic or dyskinetic at baseline, even if wall motion worsens during stress, are best interpreted as indicating infarction, and the ability to detect additional ischemia in such segments is limited. Occasionally, wall motion appears normal at rest and is unchanged with stress, i.e., neither hyper- nor hypokinetic. Some readers consider this abnormal and report it as an ischemic response. Although this may be the case, it is also the cause of many false-positive findings. Bear in mind that lack of hyperkinesis has multiple etiologies, including low workload, delayed postexercise imaging, beta-blockade, and cardiomyopathy. Elderly patients, especially women, may be unable to manifest a frankly hyperkinetic response. Therefore, to minimize false-positive results, consider these other possibilities before interpreting lack of hyperkinesis as an ischemic end point. A marked increase in blood pressure during exercise can also prevent the development of hyperkinesis or even result in global hypokinesis. An example of such a response is provided in Figure 16.15. Despite an adequate level of exercise and an ap-propriate heart rate response, the peak-exercise views are unchanged or, in some areas, mildly hypokinetic. This was due to a marked increase in blood pressure during exercise.

Finally, segments abnormal at baseline that improve with stress are uncommon and represent a special category. During exercise testing, these most likely indicate either a normal response or a localized abnormality in which the improvement is due to tethering from the surrounding normal myocardium. With dobutamine, however, improvement may indicate viability and the potential for recovery after revascularization. This topic is covered later in this chapter.

Localization of Coronary Artery Lesions

A practical application of stress echocardiography is to predict the presence of disease in specific coronary arteries or branches (Fig. 16.16). The relationship between left ventricular segments or territories and the corresponding artery distribution is covered in Chapters 6 and 15. A similar approach is applied to stress echocardiography. By recording the left ventricle in multiple views, an evaluation of the territories of each of the three main coronary arteries is possible. This allows a prediction of both the lo-

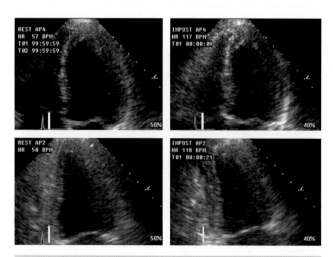

FIGURE 16.15. This exercise echocardiogram was performed in a patient who developed marked hypertension in response to exercise. The significant increase in blood pressure resulted in mild global hypokinesis. Failure to develop hyperdynamic wall motion is an abnormal response, but in this case was due to afterload mismatch.

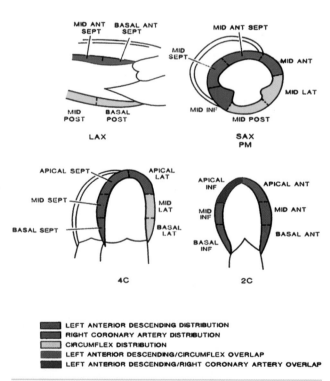

FIGURE 16.16. This schematic demonstrates the relationship between the coronary artery distribution and the corresponding left ventricular segments. With the four standard views, the territories of each of the main coronary arteries can be evaluated, as defined by the color scheme. Areas of overlap are indicated in green.

cation and the extent of disease to be made on the basis of wall motion. In general, stress echocardiography is more sensitive in patients with multivessel disease compared with single-vessel disease and more accurate for specifically identifying disease in the left anterior descending artery or right coronary artery compared with the left circumflex artery. Because of the variability in coronary artery distribution, accurate differentiation between lesions of the right coronary artery and left circumflex artery is not always possible. Figure 16.17 is an example of localized apical ischemia induced during dobutamine echocardiography. Wall motion is normal at the 20 μg/kg/min stage (heart rate, 72 bpm), but apical dyskinesis develops at the next stage, associated with a much higher heart rate. Figure 16.18 shows inferior

ischemia in a patient with a previous anterior myocardial infarction. At baseline, there is a small area of basal inferior akinesis. With stress, the entire inferior wall becomes dyskinetic at a low level of stress, whereas the anterior wall augments at higher dobutamine doses. In Figures 16.19 and 16.20, multivessel ischemia is demonstrated. In both, bicycle exercise echocardiography demonstrates multiple wall motion abnormalities induced in the setting of normal resting function.

Correlation with Symptoms and Electrocardiographic Changes

It should be apparent that the analysis of the stress echocardiogram is only one component of the compre-

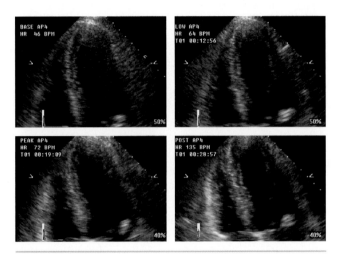

FIGURE 16.17. An example of an abnormal dobutamine stress echocardiogram is provided. The four-chamber view is shown and demonstrates apical and lateral ischemia. The abnormality is only apparent at peak stress (lower right quad).

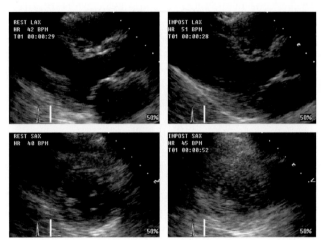

FIGURE 16.19. This exercise echocardiogram demonstrates multivessel ischemia involving the inferior, lateral, and apical segments. Extensive ischemia developed despite a modest heart rate response. In addition, note the akinesis of the right ventricular free wall, due to proximal right coronary artery disease.

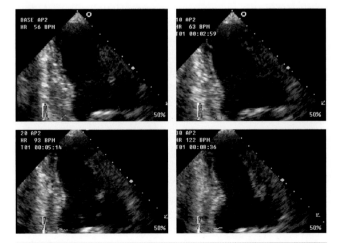

FIGURE 16.18. This dobutamine stress echocardiogram was performed in a patient with a previous anterior myocardial infarction. Inferior ischemia develops during the dobutamine infusion. See text for details.

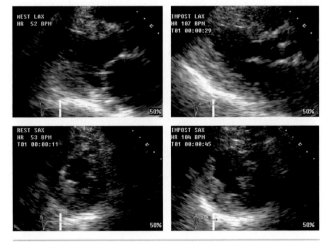

FIGURE 16.20. This bicycle exercise echocardiogram demonstrates multivessel ischemia involving the apex, septum, and inferior wall.

hensive stress test and that the other parameters, including the development of symptoms and/or ECG changes, cannot be ignored. In virtually every study that has examined the question, wall motion has been shown to be more sensitive and specific than either symptoms or ST-segment changes for the detection of coronary artery disease. In most instances, there is concordance among the various parameters that define ischemia. When a patient experiences typical chest pain in association with ECG and wall motion abnormalities, the diagnosis is straightforward. When results are discordant, however, certain assumptions must be made. Because wall motion is such a sensitive and specific marker of ischemia and because of the limitations in interpreting symptoms and ECG changes, the final report generally relies most heavily on the echocardiographic findings. In fact, one of the most common indications for stress echocardiography is to assess symptoms in patients who have had or would likely have an abnormal or nondiagnostic stress ECG. This would include patients with an abnormal ECG or left ventricular hypertrophy, and even women. In such cases, when the ECG is nondiagnostic, the added cost and inconvenience of imaging are most easily justified.

Wall motion changes in the absence of symptoms are usually an indication of painless ischemia, a common finding. There is some evidence that ischemia in the absence of chest pain and/or ST depression is less extensive and/or severe. More problematic is the situation of ischemic ECG changes in the absence of wall motion abnormalities. When this occurs in populations with a high likelihood of a false-positive stress ECG (e.g., women), a normal stress echocardiogram is strong evidence against coronary disease. However, in subsets of patients in whom the ECG is expected to be more reliable or when the changes are accompanied by typical symptoms, the possibility of a false-negative echocardiographic result must be entertained. In one study using bicycle exercise (Ryan et al., 1993), precise concordance between the ECG and echocardiogram occurred in approximately half of all cases, and the echocardiogram correctly classified patients in most instances of disagreement (Fig. 16.21). However, a positive ECG with a normal echocardiogram developed in 4% of cases. At catheterization, six of these patients had angiographic coronary artery disease, and the remaining seven did not. Thus, the two objective indicators of ischemia during stress testing provide concordant information most of time. When they disagree, echocardiography is more sensitive and specific and should be relied on in most instances. However, ignoring a markedly positive stress ECG, especially when accompanied by typical symptoms, is not advisable. A careful analysis of all echocardiographic images and all the available data should be undertaken.

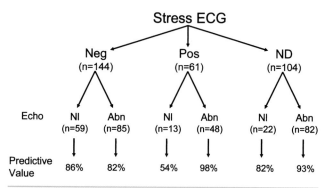

FIGURE 16.21. The relationship between the stress electrocardiogram (ECG) and the exercise echocardiogram is demonstrated in this schematic. This study compared the stress ECG with echocardiography in 309 patients undergoing upright bicycle exercise echocardiography. See text for details. Neg, negative; Pos, positive; ND, nondiagnostic; Nl, normal; Abn, abnormal. (From Ryan T, Segar DS, Sawada SG, et al. Detection of coronary artery disease with upright bicycle exercise echocardiography. *J Am Soc Echocardiogr* 1993;6:186–197, with permission.)

DETECTION OF CORONARY ARTERY DISEASE

The addition of imaging to routine stress testing has consistently led to an improvement in both sensitivity and specificity for the detection of coronary disease. Several studies have examined the accuracy of exercise echocardiography to detect coronary artery disease (Table 16.9). Using angiography as the standard for comparison, the overall sensitivity has ranged from 71% to 94%. Similar studies have been performed using dobutamine stress echocardiography, and a comparable range of sensitivity values has been reported (Table 16.10). The limitations of such comparisons are noteworthy. For example, differences in patient populations will explain much of this range. If a series includes a high percentage of patients with a condition, such as left ventricular hypertrophy, known to adversely affect accuracy, a lower sensitivity will be reported. Some of the variability of sensitivity values can be explained on the basis of the level of coronary artery stenosis considered significant in the different studies. The percentage of stenosis used to define a significant lesion varies from 50% to 75%, and quantitative angiographic techniques were used infrequently. It is likely that some 50% of lesions will not result in the development of ischemia during stress testing, thereby creating the potential for a false-negative result.

Another factor that affects the relevance of such studies is the inclusion of patients with resting wall motion abnormalities in many series. A resting wall motion abnormality is highly predictive of the presence of coronary disease, and in such patients, it is the extent rather than the presence of coronary artery disease that is important. Including patients with resting wall motion abnormalities

▶ TABLE 16.9 Accuracy of Exercise Echocardiography for the Detection of Angiographic Coronary Artery Disease

Ref.	Exercise	Significant CAD	No. of Total Patients	Sensitivity (%)	Sensitivity 1-VD (%)	Sensitivity MVD (%)	Specificity (%)	Accuracy (%)
Armstrong et al., 1987	TME	≥50%	123	88	81	93	86	88
Quinones et al., 1992	TME	≥50%	112	74	59	89	88	78
Hecht et al., 1993	SBE	≥50%	180	93	84	100	86	91
Ryan et al., 1993	UBE	≥50%	309	91	86	95	78	87
Mertes et al., 1993	SBE	≥50%	79	84	87	89	85	85
Beleslin et al., 1994	TME	≥50%	136	88	88	91	82	88
Roger et al., 1994	TME	≥50%	127	90			72	
Marwick et al., 1995[a]	TME	>50%	147	71	63	80	91	82
Marwick et al., 1995[b]	TME	>50%	161	80			81	81
Luotolahti et al., 1996	UBE	≥50%	118	94	94	93	70	92
Tian et al., 1996	TME	>50%	46	88	91	86	93	89
Marangelli et al., 1994	TME	>75%	80	89	76	97	91	90

[a]46% of patients had left ventricular hypertrophy.
[b]Women only.
CAD, coronary artery disease; LVH, left ventricular hypertrophy; MVD, multivessel disease; SBE, supine bicycle exercise; TME, treadmill exercise; UBE, upright bicycle exercise; 1-VD, single vessel disease.

▶ TABLE 16.10 Accuracy of Dobutamine Stress Echocardiography for the Detection of Angiographic Coronary Artery Disease

Ref.	Significant CAD	No. of Total Patients	Sensitivity (%)	Sensitivity 1-VD (%)	Sensitivity MVD (%)	Specificity (%)	Accuracy (%)
Sawada et al., 1991	≥50%	55	89	81	100	85	74
Marcovitz et al., 1992	≥50%	141	96	95	98	66	89
Marwick et al., 1993	≥50%	217	72	66	77	83	76
Takeuchi et al., 1993	≥50%	120	85	72	97	93	88
Ostojic et al., 1994	≥50%	150	75	74	81	79	75
Beleslin et al., 1994	≥50%	136	82	82	82	76	82
Pingitore et al., 1996	≥50%	110	84	78	88	89	85
Anthopoulos et al., 1996	≥50%	120	87	74	90	84	86
Dionisopoulos et al., 1997	≥50%	288	87	80	91	89	87
Elhendy et al., 1997	≥50%	306	74	59	83	85[a]	76
Hennessy et al., 1998	≥50%	218	89	81	97	50	83

[a]Specificity was 94% for men and 77% for women.
CAD, coronary artery disease; MVD, multivessel disease; 1-VD, single vessel disease.

will tend to increase the sensitivity of the stress test because patients will be correctly identified as having disease whether or not inducible ischemia occurs. In patients with normal wall motion at rest, the reported sensitivity of exercise echocardiography is somewhat lower. In one series (Ryan et al., 1988) of 64 patients with normal wall motion at rest, an inducible wall motion abnormality occurred in 78% of patients with angiographic disease. Finally, the subjective nature of wall motion interpretation, used in virtually all reported series, has important implications for understanding the practical limitations of sensitivity and specificity. If very subtle abnormalities (such as lack of hyperkinesis) are interpreted as abnormal, sensitivity will tend to be higher but at the expense of lower specificity. If only the most obvious wall motion abnormalities are interpreted as positive, mild disease will be missed, and sensitivity will decrease and specificity will increase. It is not surprising then that studies that report the highest sensitivity will likewise demonstrate very modest specificity and vice versa.

In addition to the degree of coronary artery narrowing, other factors that affect the sensitivity of the test include the presence of multivessel disease, the level of stress achieved, and image quality. Sensitivity is consistently higher among patients with multivessel coronary disease compared with those with single-vessel disease. The location of disease may also affect accuracy. Stenoses in the left anterior descending and right coronary artery are detected more reliably than lesions in the left circumflex artery. Another potential cause of false-negative results during dobutamine stress echocardiography is the presence of left ventricular hypertrophy. Studies have shown that patients with increased wall thickness, in the setting of normal left ventricular mass (i.e., small left ventricular chamber size), have a disproportionately high frequency of false-negative results. This combination of thick walls and small left ventricular cavity size, termed *concentric remodeling*, is a common finding in elderly patients with hypertension. In one large series (Smart et al., 2000), this group of patients accounted for a majority of the false-negative results. The authors postulated that a blunted increase in end-systolic wall stress at peak dobutamine infusion may account for the reduced sensitivity in this subgroup (Fig. 16.22). From a practical standpoint, physicians who interpret dobutamine stress echocardiographic studies should be aware of this phenomenon. Patients with concentric remodeling, especially those with hyperdynamic wall motion and/or a reduced blood pressure response during dobutamine infusion, may not manifest wall motion abnormalities in the presence of angiographic coronary artery disease. Figure 16.23 is an example of a false-negative dobutamine stress echocardiogram in a patient with moderate left ventricular hypertrophy and a small cavity, that is, concentric remodeling. Note the hyperdynamic response to stress.

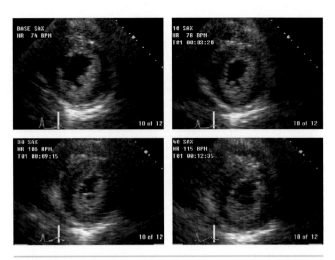

FIGURE 16.23. An example of a false-negative dobutamine stress echo is presented from a patient with significant left ventricular hypertrophy. Despite the presence of coronary artery disease, a wall motion abnormality did not develop.

Addressing the issue of specificity in studies comparing stress echocardiography with angiography is limited by referral bias. When angiography is used as the gold standard, the reported specificity of exercise echocardiography ranges from 64% to 100%, although in most series, values of 80% to 90% are found. Because of referral bias, the number of patients with "normal" stress echocardiograms in such series is often quite low. An alternative approach uses the concept of normalcy rate. This approach examines the likelihood that the stress echocardiogram will be interpreted as normal in a group of patients with a very low pretest likelihood of disease. Applied to stress echocardiography, normalcy rates of 92% to 100% have been reported. As is discussed later, a normal wall motion response during stress echocardiography, even in the presence of known coronary artery disease, confers a favorable prognosis in most cases. Among the most common causes of false-positive results is left bundle branch block. Figure 16.24 is an example of left bundle branch block in a patient undergoing treadmill stress echocardiography. One rest view and three postexercise views are displayed. Note the abnormal septal motion, both at rest and with stress. However, there is preservation of myocardial thickening. This is evidence against ischemia as the cause of abnormal endocardial excursion. This confusing picture can sometimes be clarified by trimming the loops to avoid the first few frames of systole.

Another form of bias in published studies that likely affects both sensitivity and specificity is test verification bias. This phenomenon results in a distortion of true accuracy because published series include selected patients with a high percentage of angiographic referrals, that is, the decision to perform angiography depends on the results of the test being studied. This leads to a misleading increase in sensitivity and decrease in specificity com-

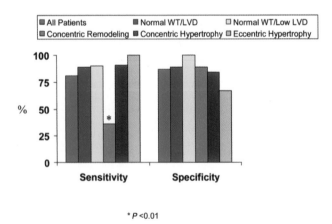

*P <0.01

FIGURE 16.22. The effect of concentric remodeling on the sensitivity and specificity of dobutamine stress echocardiography is demonstrated in this graph. In this series, the majority of the false-negative results occurred in patients with evidence of concentric remodeling. In this small subgroup, sensitivity was significantly reduced compared with all other subgroups. See text for details. WT, wall thickness; LVD, left ventricular minor-axis dimension. (From Smart SC, Knickelbine T, Malik F, et al. Dobutamine-atropine stress echocardiography for the detection of coronary artery disease in patients with left ventricular hypertrophy. Importance of chamber size and systolic wall stress. Circulation 2000;101:258–263, with permission.)

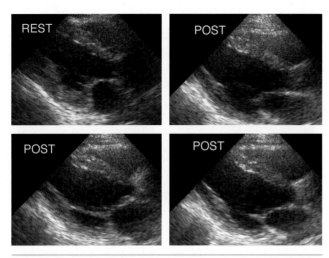

FIGURE 16.24. This treadmill exercise echocardiogram was performed in a patient with left bundle branch block. Abnormal wall motion is present at rest and postexercise. Left bundle branch block is a common cause of false-positive results. See text for details.

pared with how the test would likely perform in an unselected population. Test verification bias has been demonstrated in exercise echocardiography (Roger et al., 1997). When adjusted for, true sensitivity is lower than reported, whereas specificity is higher. Because of differences in the prevalence of coronary disease, the decrease in sensitivity is greater in women than in men. This phenomenon has been shown to plague virtually all forms of stress testing. Recognizing that it occurs and understanding its impact are key to the optimal use of stress echocardiography in clinical practice.

Localization of coronary artery disease is an additional goal of stress echocardiography. The ability to examine the entire left ventricle and to correlate coronary anatomy with wall motion territories is now well established (Fig. 16.16). Through the use of multiple views, the entire left ventricle can be evaluated and the regions supplied by each coronary artery can be independently assessed. In most series, detection (and localization) of ischemia is highest for the territory supplied by the left anterior descending artery and somewhat lower for the right coronary artery. A limitation of stress echocardiography is the ability to specifically identify left circumflex coronary artery ischemia and to distinguish between lesions in the right coronary and left circumflex artery. Acknowledging this problem, investigators who have grouped lesions into anterior or posterior (right or left circumflex coronary artery) distribution have demonstrated a high level of accuracy for localizing disease.

Comparison with Nuclear Techniques

An alternative approach to assessing accuracy involves the comparison of stress echocardiography and nuclear perfusion techniques. Several studies have addressed this important issue and have generally demonstrated a high degree of correlation between the different modalities (Table 16.11). In one series (Quinones et al., 1992) in which 289 patients were subjected to simultaneous treadmill exercise echocardiography and tomographic thallium scintigraphy, the concordance between the tests was 87%. Overall accuracy is generally similar, although nuclear techniques may be more sensitive, whereas echocardiography is generally more specific when compared with angiography. Echocardiographic and nuclear imaging have also been compared using dobutamine stress, and similar levels of accuracy have been found.

▶ **TABLE 16.11** Comparing the Accuracy of Stress Echocardiography and Stress Nuclear Imaging Techniques

			Echocardiography		Nuclear	
Ref.	*Stress*	*No. of Patients*	*Sensitivity (%)*	*Specificity (%)*	*Sensitivity (%)*	*Specificity (%)*
Marwick et al., 1993	Dob-echo Aden-MIBI	97	85	82	86	71
Forster et al., 1993	Dob-echo Dob-MIBI	105	75	89	83	89
Marwick et al., 1993	Dob-echo Dob-MIBI	217	72	83	76	67
Quinones et al., 1992	Exer-echo Exer-thal	292	74	88	75	81
Hecht et al., 1993	Exer-echo Exer-thal	71	88	87	80	84
Fragasso et al., 1999	Dob-echo Exer-MIBI	101	88	80	98	36
San Roman et al., 1995	Dob-echo Dob-MIBI	102	78	88	87	70

Dob, dobutamine; Aden, adenosine; Exer, exercise; MIBI, sestamibi; thal, thallium.

A meta-analysis (Fleischmann et al., 1998) of the clinical reports that have compared echocardiographic and nuclear imaging during exercise has been reported. Analysis of the pooled data revealed almost identical sensitivity values but higher specificity for exercise echocardiography. Thus, summary receiver operator curves revealed that echocardiography better discriminated between patients with and without disease (Fig. 16.25). The relative cost-effectiveness of the different strategies to test for coronary disease has also been examined and compared (Kuntz et al., 1999 and Garber et al., 1999). Because of the inherently lower costs and similar overall accuracy, stress echocardiography performs well in such analyses. The results of these models underscore the importance of relative accuracy and operator dependency. For most types of patients and levels of disease severity, exercise echocardiography is an attractive cost-effective alternative to both nonimaging treadmill testing and nuclear techniques.

It should be recognized that both tests are operator dependent and often rely on subjective interpretation of results. Thus, the relative superiority of one technique versus the other is largely a matter of expertise. The advantages of stress echocardiography include the versatility of the technique with respect to the availability of additional diagnostic information, the lower cost of the test, and the opportunity to avoid radiation exposure. In addition, stress echocardiography is more convenient for the patient because the need to return for late imaging is avoided.

APPLICATIONS OF STRESS ECHOCARDIOGRAPHY

The accuracy and versatility of stress echocardiography support its use in a variety of settings. It has both diagnostic and prognostic utility. Echocardiographic imaging should be seen as a supplement to routine stress testing that increases both the sensitivity and specificity of the test for diagnosing ischemia. In addition, the opportunity to assess left ventricular function and wall motion at rest provides further value. Some of the accepted indications for stress echocardiography are provided in Table 16.12.

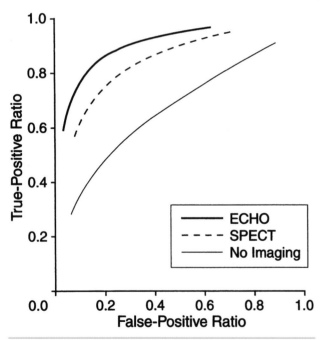

FIGURE 16.25. Comparative summary receiver operator characteristic curves are shown for exercise echocardiography (ECHO), exercise single photon emission computed tomography, and nonimaging exercise testing. The horizontal axis represents the false-positive ratio (1-specificity), and the vertical axis represents the true-positive ratio (sensitivity). (From Fleischmann KE, Hunink MG, Kuntz KM, et al. Exercise echocardiography or exercise SPECT imaging? A meta-analysis of diagnostic test performance. JAMA 1998;280:913–920, with permission.)

▶ **TABLE 16.12 Indications for Echocardiography in Diagnosis and Prognosis of Chronic Ischemic Heart Disease**

Indication	*Class*
1. Diagnosis of myocardial ischemia in symptomatic individuals[a]	I
2. Assessment of global ventricular function at rest	I
3. Assessment of myocardial viability (hibernating myocardium) for planning revascularization[b]	I
4. Assessment of functional significance of coronary lesions (if not already known) in planning percutaneous transluminal coronary angioplasty[a]	I
5. Diagnosis of myocardial ischemia in selected patients with an intermediate or high pretest likelihood of coronary artery disease[a]	IIb
6. Assessment of an asymptomatic patient with positive results from a screening treadmill test	IIb
7. Assessment of global ventricular function with exercise[a]	IIb
8. Screening of asymptomatic persons with a low likelihood of coronary artery disease	III
9. Routine periodic reassessment of stable patients for whom no change in therapy is contemplated	III
10. Routine substitution for treadmill exercise testing in patients for whom electrocardiographic analysis is expected to suffice	III

[a]Exercise or pharmacologic stress echocardiogram
[b]Dobutamine stress echocardiogram
Cheitlin MD, Alpert JS, Armstrong WF, et al. ACC/AHA Guidelines for the Clinical Application of Echocardiography. A report of the American College of Cardiology/American Heart Association Task Force on Practice Guidelines (Committee on Clinical Application of Echocardiography). Developed in collaboration with the American Society of Echocardiography. Circulation. 1997;95(6):1686–1744.

In the following section, some of these specific indications are discussed in detail.

Prognostic Value of Stress Echocardiography

Several features of the resting echocardiogram are known to provide prognostic information. Among these, wall motion, left ventricular function, and mass are well established determinants of the risk of future cardiovascular events. The treadmill test alone (without imaging) also offers powerful prognostic information. It is not surprising then that the combination of exercise parameters and echocardiographic data should provide incremental information on risk status. Specifically, the development of a wall motion abnormality as a marker of inducible ischemia has been shown in several studies to be a powerful predictor of high-risk status. Although most studies have focused on inducible ischemia as the primary predictor, exercise duration, workload achieved, blood pressure response, and ECG changes are simultaneously available and should be incorporated into the overall determination of prognosis. The echocardiogram itself offers a range of information, including resting left ventricular function and mass. Although the presence or absence of a new wall motion abnormality is important, additional data from the stress echocardiogram should also be evaluated. These include the extent and severity of the wall motion abnormality, the volume response of the left ventricle (assessed at end-systole), the number of coronary arteries that are involved, and changes in right ventricular function. Only after all these available parameters have been evaluated is a complete determination of risk possible.

The prognostic value of stress echocardiography has been evaluated in several settings (Table 16.13). Among patients with normal wall motion before and immediately after exercise, the likelihood of a coronary event over the ensuing 1 to 3 years is very low. McCully and colleagues (1998) examined 1,325 patients, of whom 35% had an intermediate (26%–69%) and 10% had a high (≥70%) pretest probability of disease. All patients were characterized as having a normal exercise echocardiogram. Event-free survival at 1, 2, and 3 years was 99%, 98%, and 97%, respectively. Predictors of events, by multivariate analysis, were age, low exercise workload, angina, and left ventricular hypertrophy.

In contrast, an abnormal exercise echocardiogram generally identifies patients at increased risk of cardiac events. The echocardiographic findings that have been correlated with risk include a new wall motion abnormality, rest and exercise wall motion score index, and end-systolic volume response. In most series, echocardiographic evidence of ischemia was the most potent marker of high-risk status and has consistently been a better discriminator than other variables, such as

exercise-induced ST-segment depression (Fig. 16.26). It is also apparent that stress echocardiography provides more than simply a binary result, i.e., normal or abnormal. In one large series, the postexercise wall motion score index was linearly related to event rate, suggesting that both the extent and severity of disease determine risk (Fig. 16.27). The prognostic value of stress echocardiography has also been compared with nuclear techniques. In most such series, echocardiography has provided similar or superior discriminatory power (Fig. 16.28). Thus, high-risk status correlates best with the presence of inducible ischemia. Other echocardiographic findings, including left ventricular ejection fraction, also contribute prognostic information, as does treadmill variables such as workload, blood pressure, ECG, and symptoms. In multivariate models, however, nonechocardiographic parameters such as age, symptoms, and diabetes frequently contribute independent prognostic data. Figures 16.29 through 16.31 are examples of abnormal exercise echocardiograms demonstrating the range of positivity that the test can provide.

There is an extensive body of literature demonstrating the value of dobutamine echocardiography for risk assessment. Bear in mind that patients who are referred for dobutamine echocardiography are inherently different from patients undergoing exercise testing. The very fact that pharmacologic stress is being performed instead of exercise suggests that the patient is incapable of exercising, itself an ominous prognostic sign. It is no surprise, therefore, that event rates after dobutamine echocardiography are generally higher compared with exercise. Still, risk stratification is possible, but a normal dobutamine echocardiogram has a more modest event-free survival compared with a normal exercise echocardiogram. In addition to the presence or absence of ischemia, myocardial viability can also be assessed, and this finding conveys significant information on risk. The prognostic implications of viability are covered later in this chapter.

Stress Echocardiography After Myocardial Infarction

Stress testing after myocardial infarction is used both to identify high- and low-risk subsets and to predict the location and extent of coronary disease. When applied to this population, it must be recognized that most patients will have a resting wall motion abnormality. The goal of the test is to identify ischemia at a distance and, in doing so, to predict both the likelihood of multivessel disease and the presence of inducible ischemia. In this setting, a normal response would be the development of hyperdynamic wall motion in all regions remote from the infarct. Therefore, the most important positive finding is the detection of a new wall motion abnormality remote from the site of previous infarction.

▶ **TABLE 16.13 Studies Examining the Prognostic Value of Stress Echocardiography**

Ref.	Type of Stress	Inclusion/ Exclusion	No. of Patients	Duration of F/U	Event-free Survival Negative Echo	Event-free Survival Positive Echo	Event Rate Negative Echo	Event Rate Positive Echo	Best Predictor of Events
Heupler et al., 1997	TME	Women only	508	41 ± 10 mo	96%	55%	4%	31%	Ischemia by echo
Krivokapich et al., 1999	Dob		558	1 y			3% MI/death 10% all events	9% MI/death 34% all events	Rest WMA
Yao et al., 2003	TME, Dob		1,500	2.7 ± 1.0 y			0.9%	4.2% overall (1.4% TME, 4.7% Dob)	Peak WMSI
Krivokapich et al., 1993	TME		360	1 y			3% hard events 9% all events	11% hard events 34% all events	≤6 min on Bruce Ischemia by echo
Chuah et al., 1998	Dob		860	3 y	98% 1y 97% 2y 96% 3y	93% 1y 88% 2y 86% 3y	4%	14%	Hx of CHF No. of abnormal segments
Sawada et al., 1990	TME	Normal stress echoes only	148	28 ± 5 mo			0.9%		
McCully et al., 1998	TME	Normal stress echoes only	1,325	Median 23 mo	99% 1y 98% 2y 97% 3y				Low workload Hypotension Angina on TME
McCully et al., 2002	TME	Abnormal stress echo, but with good exercise capacity	1,874	3.1 ± 1.6 y			1.6% w/ normal LVESV response	2.9% w/ abnormal LVESV response	Hx of MI Abnormal LVESV response
Smart et al., 1999	Dob	Rest EF < 40%	350	>18 mo			Hard events: 66% w/ ischemia treated medically, 10% revascularized	Hard events: 66% w/ ischemia treated medically, 10% w/ ischemia	Ischemia by echo
Poldermans et al., 1999	Dob		1,734	1 y			1.2% annual, over 5-y period	5.4% w/ induced WMA 6.8% w/ rest + induced WMA	Ischemia by echo
Cortigiani et al., 1998	Dip, Dob	Women with chest pain	456	32 ± 19 mo	99.2% (hard events, 3 y)	69.5% (hard events, 3 y)			New/worsening WMA
Sicari et al., 2003	Dip, Dob	Multicenter	7,333	2.6 y	92%	71%			Peak WMSI
Bholasigh et al., 2003	Dob	CPU pts, negative troponin T	377	6 mo			0.3% MI/death, 4% all events	12% MI/death, 31% all events	Ischemia by echo
Steinberg et al., 1997	Dob	Long-term (>5 y) F/U	120	5 y			5% (hard events, 5 y)	13% (hard events, 5 y)	Ischemia by echo
Marwick et al., 1997	TME		463	44 ± 11 mo	90% (all events, 4.5 y)	61% ischemia only 29% ischemia + scar			Ischemia by echo

Dip, dipyridamole; Dob, dobutamine; CPU, chest pain unit; CHF, congestive heart failure; echo, echocardiography; F/U, follow-up; Hx, history; LVESV, left ventricular end-systolic volume; MI, myocardial infarction; Pts, patients; TME, treadmill exercise; WMA, wall motion abnormality; WMSI, wall motion score index; EF, ejection fraction; y, years; m, months.

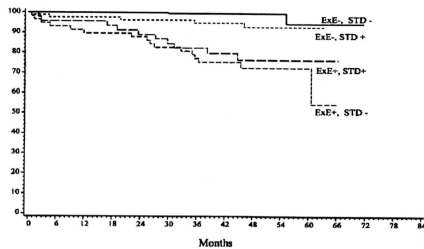

Months

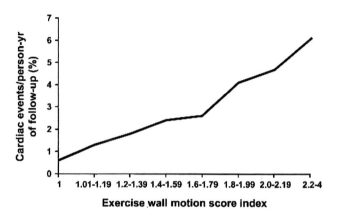

Exercise wall motion score index

FIGURE 16.26. The prognostic value of exercise echocardiography and the stress electrocardiogram (ECG) are compared in this series of 500 patients. Event-free survival over 5 years is compared among four groups. These four groups are defined by the presence or absence of abnormal echocardiographic results (ExE+ and ExE−, respectively) and those with a positive or negative stress ECG (STD+ and STD−, respectively). The lowest event rate occurred in those patients with a negative exercise echocardiogram. See text for details. (From Marwick TH, Mehta R, Arheart K, et al. Use of exercise echocardiography for prognostic evaluation of patients with known or suspected coronary artery disease. J Am Coll Cardiol 1997;30:83–90, with permission.)

FIGURE 16.27. The annual cardiac event rate is plotted against the postexercise wall motion score index from a series of 5,798 consecutive patients referred for evaluation of chest pain syndromes. (From Arruda-Olson AM, Juracan EM, Mahoney DW, et al. Prognostic value of exercise echocardiography in 5,798 patients: is there a gender difference? J Am Coll Cardiol 2002;39:625–631, with permission.)

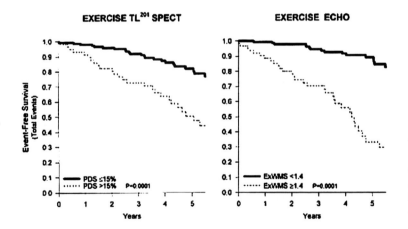

FIGURE 16.28. The prognostic value of exercise single photon emission computed tomography (SPECT) **(left)** and exercise echocardiography **(right)** are compared in a series of 248 patients followed for a mean of 3.7 years. The top panels include total cardiac events, and the bottom panels compare only ischemic events and cardiac death. For each graph, two groups were defined to provide the greatest difference in event-free survival. The prognostic value of the two tests was similar. (From Olmos LI, Dakik H, Gordon R, et al. Long-term prognostic value of exercise echocardiography compared with exercise 201Tl, ECG, and clinical variables in patients evaluated for coronary artery disease. Circulation 1998;98:2679–2686, with permission.)

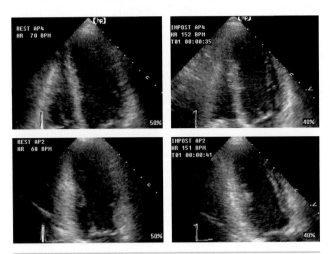

FIGURE 16.29. An example of a mildly positive treadmill exercise echocardiogram is provided. The resting study is normal. Postexercise, inferoapical ischemia is recorded. The abnormality developed at a high workload.

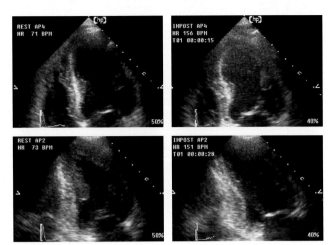

FIGURE 16.31. A markedly positive treadmill exercise echocardiogram is demonstrated. Inferior, septal, and anteroapical ischemia is evident, consistent with three-vessel coronary disease.

Exercise echocardiography has been used to detect multivessel disease and to identify high-risk cohorts (Figs. 16.32 and 16.33). This ability, combined with a functional assessment of exercise capacity in a patient recovering from myocardial infarction, accounts for the prognostic value of the test. In these two examples, high-risk status is suggested both by the presence of a resting wall motion abnormality and, more important, by the extent of induced ischemia. In contrast, Figure 16.34 is an example of limited ischemia in a patient studied after an apical infarct. The apex is hypokinetic at baseline and becomes dyskinetic at peak exercise, whereas the remainder of the left ventricle demonstrates a normal hyperdynamic response. Dobutamine echocardiography can also be used for this purpose (Fig. 16.35). In this example, a patient

with a remote history of inferior myocardial infarction undergoes stress testing. A shallow inferobasal aneurysm is present, but the remaining areas become hyperdynamic with dobutamine, conferring low-risk status.

Evidence of ischemia not only predicts high-risk status but also correlates with the likelihood of multivessel coronary disease. In one series (Carlos et al., 1997), dobutamine echocardiographic evidence of multivessel involvement was a better predictor of future events than angiographic evidence of multivessel disease. Thus, absence of evidence of inducible ischemia by stress echocardiography identifies patients recovering from infarction with a favorable prognosis in whom further testing may

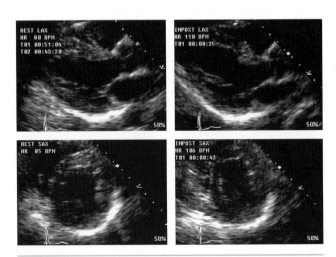

FIGURE 16.30. An abnormal exercise echocardiogram is provided. The resting study is normal. Post-exercise, the distal septum and apex become ischemic.

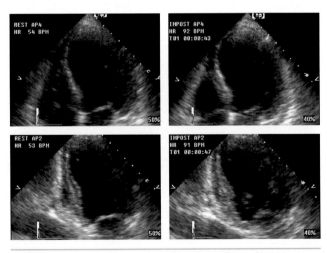

FIGURE 16.32. This supine bicycle echocardiogram was recorded in a patient after anterior myocardial infarction. The study demonstrates worsening of the anteroapical wall motion abnormality, the development of inferior ischemia, and dilation of the left ventricle. These abnormalities developed within 2 minutes of exercise and at a very low heart rate.

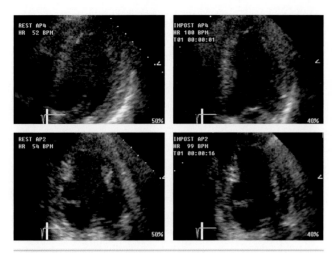

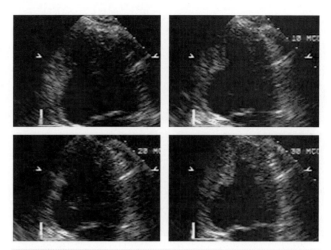

FIGURE 16.33. This bicycle exercise echocardiogram was performed in a patient with a history of inferior myocardial infarction. The study demonstrates the development of anterior ischemia that is extensive and severe. A shallow inferobasal aneurysm is also present.

FIGURE 16.35. This dobutamine stress echocardiogram was performed in a patient with a previous inferior myocardial infarction. An inferobasal aneurysm is demonstrated in the two-chamber view. With dobutamine, there is a normal hyperdynamic response in all other areas. No evidence of ischemia was detected.

be unnecessary. Inducible ischemia, on the other hand, is a powerful indicator of high risk and suggests the need for further testing, specifically angiography.

Stress Echocardiography After Revascularization

Stress testing after revascularization is used to evaluate the initial success of the procedure, to look for recurrence of disease, and to assess symptoms in patients with known coronary disease. Some of the accepted in-

dications for stress echocardiography after revascularization are provided in Table 16.14. The limitations of symptoms and the stress ECG in this setting underscore the importance of imaging. Exercise echocardiography has been used before and after angioplasty to localize disease and to document objective improvement after the procedure. Mertes and colleagues (1993) used bicycle stress echocardiography to evaluate patients 6 months after a percutaneous coronary intervention. They reported a sensitivity of 83% and a specificity of 85% for the detection of significant coronary stenoses.

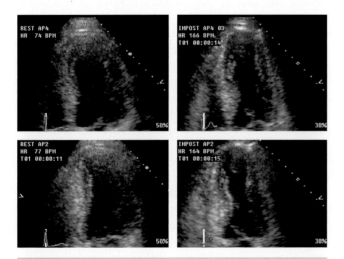

FIGURE 16.34. This exercise echocardiogram was performed in a patient with a history of anterior myocardial infarction. At rest, a limited apical wall motion abnormality is present. At peak exercise, the apex becomes dyskinetic, but there is a hyperdynamic response in all other areas.

▶ **TABLE 16.14 Indications for Echocardiography in Assessment of Interventions in Chronic Ischemic Heart Disease**

Indication	Class
1. Assessment of left ventricular function when needed to guide institution and modification of drug therapy in patients with known or suspected left ventricular dysfunction	I
2. Assessment for restenosis after revascularization in patients with atypical recurrent symptoms[a]	I
3. Assessment for restenosis after revascularization in patients with typical recurrent symptoms[a]	IIa
4. Routine assessment of asymptomatic patients after revascularization	III

[a]Exercise or pharmacologic stress echocardiography.

Cheitlin MD, Alpert JS, Armstrong WF, et al. ACC/AHA Guidelines for the Clinical Application of Echocardiography. A report of the American College of Cardiology/American Heart Association Task Force on Practice Guidelines (Committee on Clinical Application of Echocardiography). Developed in collaboration with the American Society of Echocardiography. Circulation. 1997;95(6):1686–1744.

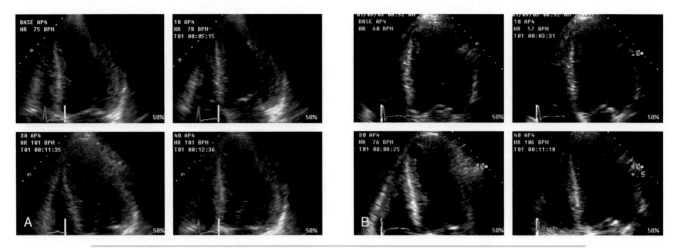

FIGURE 16.36. Two dobutamine stress echocardiograms are provided from a patient with diabetes and peripheral vascular disease. **A:** Extensive wall motion abnormalities are induced during dobutamine infusion, consistent with multivessel ischemia. The patient then underwent surgical revascularization. **B:** A dobutamine stress echocardiogram performed 4 months after surgery is provided. Note the striking improvement in the left ventricular response to stress. A higher heart rate is achieved, and only a moderate-sized apical wall motion abnormality is apparent.

Similar results have been reported using stress echocardiography after coronary artery bypass surgery. In this setting, stress echocardiography has been successfully used to detect the presence of stenotic grafts, nonrevascularized coronary arteries, and diseased native vessels distal to the surgical anastomosis. A practical application in this setting is to provide objective evidence of ischemia in a subset of patients with a high likelihood of atypical symptoms. Figure 16.36 is an example of stress echocardiography before and after revascularization. In this example, a patient undergoes dobutamine stress echocardiography and multivessel ischemia is detected at a low heart rate. Four months later, after surgical revascularization, another dobutamine study is performed. A much higher heart rate and improved wall motion response are demonstrated.

Preoperative Risk Assessment

To assess preoperative risk prior to noncardiac surgery, a resting echocardiogram alone does not appear to provide sufficient prognostic data. Stress echocardiography, however, has been well studied for this purpose (Table 16.15). Most series applying stress echocardiography to the patient before noncardiac surgery have used dobutamine stress. The majority of patients in the published literature were evaluated before major peripheral vascular surgery and therefore included patients who frequently are unable to exercise. In this high-risk subset, dobutamine stress echocardiography has consistently demonstrated value and the presence or absence of an inducible wall motion abnormality has been the most potent determinant of relative risk. The absence of an inducible wall motion abnormality confers a very favorable prognosis, with

a negative predictive value of 93% to 100%. In this setting, predictive value refers to the test's ability to identify patients who subsequently experience perioperative events. In part, this very high negative predictive value is confounded by the inclusion of patients with a low pretest likelihood of coronary disease in whom the added value of stress testing is questionable. When examined critically, the discriminatory ability of the test is greatest when it is confined to patients with intermediate or high-risk of disease.

The presence of an induced wall motion abnormality substantially increases the relative risk to the individual patient. The positive predictive value of an inducible wall motion abnormality has ranged from 7% to 33% when *hard* events are used as the end point. An intermediate-risk subgroup includes those patients with a resting wall motion abnormality but no evidence of ischemia. A resting wall motion abnormality, most likely indicating previous myocardial infarction, has also been associated with a much lower risk compared with those with induced ischemia. Most of these patients can safely undergo elective surgery, with an overall perioperative risk similar to that of the "normal" group.

The ability to assess risk is not confined to the immediate perioperative period. In long-term follow-up after vascular surgery (Poldermans et al., 1997), the results of the dobutamine echocardiogram were similarly predictive of late cardiac events, occurring as long as 2.5 years after the index procedure. In a meta-analysis examining the value of dipyridamole thallium and dobutamine echocardiography before vascular surgery (Shaw et al., 1996), the presence of an inducible wall motion abnormality on echocardiography provided the greatest ability to discriminate between high- and low-risk status.

▶ **TABLE 16.15** **Stress Echocardiography for Preoperative Risk Assessment Before Noncardiac Surgery**

			Positive Predictive Value		
Ref.	No. of Patients	Patients with Ischemia (%)	All Events (%)	Hard Events (%)	Negative Predictive Value (%)
Lalka et al., 1992	60	50	29	23	93
Eichelberger et al., 1993	75	36	19	7	100
Langan et al., 1993	74	24	20	17	100
Poldermans et al., 1993	131	27	43	14	100
Davila Roman et al., 1993	88	23	20	10	100
Poldermans et al., 1995	302	24	38	24	100
Plotkin et al., 1998	80	8		33	100
Bossone et al., 1999	46	9		25	100
Das et al., 2000	530	40		15	100
Pellikka et al., 1996	80	24	29		98

Stress Echocardiography in Women

There is some evidence that stress testing is applied less frequently in women than in men. The relatively lower prevalence of disease and the higher rates of a false-positive ECG response complicate stress testing in women. The limitations of the stress ECG in this population have led some investigators to recommend an imaging stress test in most if not all circumstances. Several series have examined the role of both exercise and dobutamine stress echocardiography in this large patient subset. The majority of these studies have demonstrated that wall motion analysis increases both the sensitivity and the specificity of the test. Most series report a sensitivity of 80% to 90% and a specificity of 85% to 90%. In addition to its accuracy, studies have shown stress echocardiography to be a cost-effective method to evaluate chest pain in women. Other investigators have explored the possibility that stress echocardiography is less accurate in women than in men. It now appears clear that no significant gender difference exists, with respect to both the diagnostic and the prognostic value of the test. It is often used in the setting of an asymptomatic positive stress ECG, when a false-positive finding is suspected.

Assessment of Myocardial Viability

The capacity of dysfunctional myocardium to recover spontaneously or improve after revascularization has been recognized for many years. The term viable is commonly used to refer to myocardium that has the potential for functional recovery, that is, is either stunned or hibernating. Distinguishing viable from nonviable myocardium in patients with resting left ventricular dysfunction has been extensively examined using a variety of imaging techniques including echocardiography. To begin the analysis, the resting echocardiogram has some utility for predicting viability; the more severe the wall motion abnormality is at rest, the less likely it is to be viable. Dyskinetic regions,

for example, are less likely than hypokinetic segments to recover. Thin, scarred segments are also likely to be nonviable. However, the resting echocardiogram is neither sensitive nor specific for this purpose. The use of dobutamine echocardiography is based on the observation that viable myocardium will augment in response to β-adrenergic stimulation, whereas nonviable myocardium will not. In practice, dobutamine is infused at incremental rates while wall motion and endocardial thickening are carefully monitored. The biphasic response, augmentation at low dose followed by deterioration at higher doses, is most predictive of the capacity for functional recovery after revascularization. Sustained improvement and "no change" are patterns that correlate with nonviability, that is, lack of improvement after revascularization. Figures 16.37 through 16.39 are examples of viability in patients

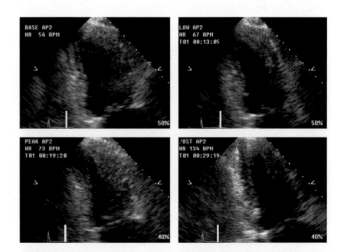

FIGURE 16.37. Myocardial viability is demonstrated during dobutamine echocardiography in a patient with a previous inferior myocardial infarction. The inferior wall is hypokinetic at baseline. Augmentation of wall motion and wall thickening develops at low-dose dobutamine. At peak dose, inferior akinesis is evident. This is an example of a biphasic response.

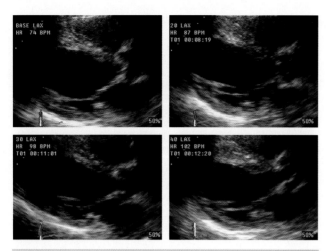

FIGURE 16.38. A dobutamine echocardiogram is performed in a patient with ischemic cardiomyopathy. Extensive wall motion abnormalities at baseline are evident. With dobutamine infusion, anterior and lateral viability is demonstrated.

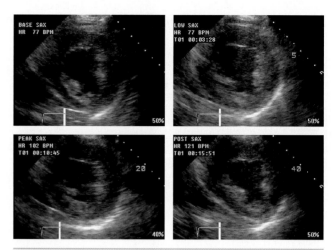

FIGURE 16.40. Dobutamine echocardiography was performed in this patient with ischemic cardiomyopathy. Multiple resting wall motion abnormalities are present. No improvement occurs with the dobutamine infusion, suggesting absence of viable myocardium.

with multivessel coronary disease. An example of absence of viability is provided in Figure 16.40.

With an improvement in resting left ventricular function after revascularization as the end point, dobutamine echocardiography has been tested in two clinical scenarios. Early studies focused on patients soon after myocardial infarction, in whom stunning may have been the predominant pathologic process. Later, the test was extended to include patients with chronic coronary disease and ischemic cardiomyopathy (Table 16.16). In most series, sensitivity (for predicting functional recovery) has ranged from 80% to 85% with slightly higher specificity (85%–90%). The amount of myocardium identified as viable

correlates fairly well with the degree of improvement in global function after revascularization and with long-term outcome. When compared with nuclear techniques, dobutamine echocardiography provides generally concordant results. However, nuclear techniques will identify significantly more segments (and patients) as viable. In most series, sensitivity favors nuclear methods, whereas dobutamine echocardiography is consistently more specific. Thus, all the methods appear to provide a similar positive predictive value. That is, evidence of viability by any of the techniques is predictive of the potential for functional recovery after revascularization. However, the negative predictive value varies widely among the different modalities, and in many series, dobutamine echocardiography is favored.

The prognostic value of this application has also been examined. Although these studies are observational and randomized trials are not yet available, they demonstrate the important link between evidence of viability and management. The presence of viability identifies patients in whom revascularization is associated with a significant survival advantage compared with medical management (Fig. 16.41). Absence of viability is associated with no significant outcome advantage, whether medical or surgical therapy is implemented. These results were confirmed in a meta-analysis that included more than 3,000 patients studied with either echocardiographic or nuclear methods (Allman et al., 2002). Among patients with viability, surgical revascularization improved prognosis compared with medical therapy. In patients without viability, outcome was similar regardless of treatment strategy (Fig. 16.42). This is in contrast to the results of a multicenter registry in which medically treated patients with viability had a better prognosis than patients without viability

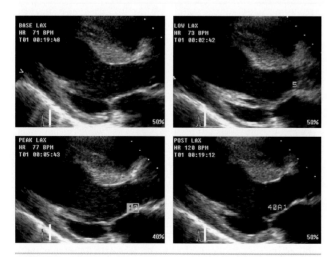

FIGURE 16.39. This example is taken from a patient with ischemic cardiomyopathy and severe left ventricular dysfunction. With dobutamine infusion, there is sustained improvement in the septum, apex, and lateral walls. The inferior and posterior walls remain akinetic.

▶ TABLE 16.16 **Assessment of Myocardial Viability Using Dobutamine Echocardiography**

Ref.	*Patient Population*	*Total Patients*	*Sensitivity (%)*	*Specificity (%)*	*Comments*
Pierard et al., 1990	Recent MI	17	83	73	Recent anterior MI, Rx with thrombolysis
Smart et al., 1993	Recent MI	51	86	90	Recent MI, Rx with thrombolysis
Cigarroa et al., 1993	Chronic CAD	25	82	86	DSE results compared with post-CABG echocardiography
La Canna et al., 1994	Chronic CAD	33	87	82	Analyzed by individual segments
Arnese et al., 1995	Chronic CAD	38	74	95	Before CABG, compared with thallium
Senior et al., 1995	Chronic CAD	45	87	82	
Bax et al., 1996	Chronic CAD	17	85	63	Compared with PET and thallium
Vanoverschelde et al., 1996	Chronic CAD	73	88	77	Defined as WMSI improved by >3.5
Perrone-Filardi et al., 1996	Chronic CAD	40	79	83	Concordance with thallium better in hypokinetic than akinetic segments

CAD, coronary artery disease; CABG, coronary artery bypass surgery; DSE, dobutamine stress echocardiography; MI, myocardial infarction; PET, positron emisson tomography; Rx, treatment; WMSI, wall motion score index.

(Picano et al., 1998). However, this study focused on patients early after acute myocardial infarction, with moderate to severe left ventricular dysfunction, all of whom were treated medically. In this subset, sustained improvement conferred a survival advantage, whereas ischemia identified a high-risk cohort.

USE OF MYOCARDIAL CONTRAST TECHNIQUES IN STRESS ECHOCARDIOGRAPHY

The application of contrast echocardiographic techniques to stress testing falls into two distinct categories: left ventricular opacification for border enhancement and myo-

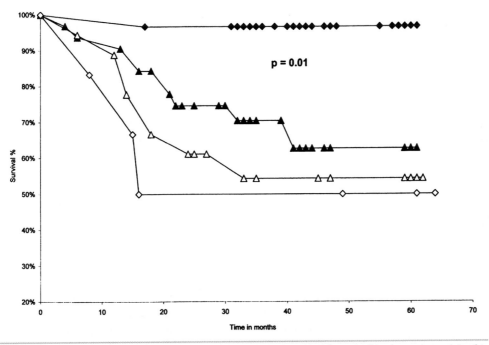

FIGURE 16.41. The relationship among viability, management, and survival is demonstrated in this study. All patients underwent dobutamine stress echocardiography and were classified on the basis of the presence or absence of viable myocardium. Patients were subsequently managed either medically or with revascularization. Event-free survival curves according to viability status and management are shown. Only those patients with evidence of viability who underwent revascularization had a survival benefit compared with the other three groups. **Solid diamond,** revascularization with myocardial viability; **solid triangle,** medical therapy with myocardial viability; **open triangle,** medical therapy without myocardial viability; **open diamond,** revascularization without myocardial viability. (From Senior R, Kaul S, Lahiri A. Myocardial viability on echocardiography predicts long-term survival after revascularization in patients with ischemic congestive heart failure. J Am Coll Cardiol 1999;33:1848–1854, with permission.)

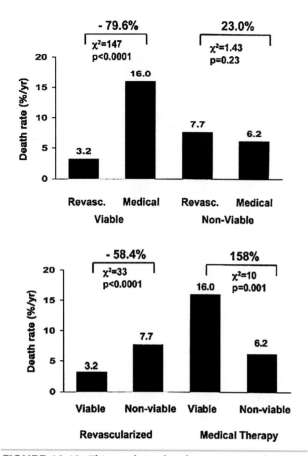

FIGURE 16.42. This graph is taken from a meta-analysis that included both echocardiographic and nuclear approaches to detecting myocardial viability. Pooled data from 24 clinical studies involving more than 3,000 patients were analyzed. The relationship between viability and management is examined in this bar graph. **A:** The death rate among patients with viable myocardium was significantly higher among those treated medically compared with those who underwent revascularization. Among patients with no evidence of viability, the death rate was similar regardless of management. **B:** Among patients treated medically, those with evidence of myocardial viability had a significantly higher death rate compared with those patients without viability. (From Allman KC, Shaw LJ, Hachamovitch R, et al. Myocardial viability testing and impact of revascularization on prognosis in patients with coronary artery disease and left ventricular dysfunction: a meta-analysis. *J Am Coll Cardiol* 2002;39:1151–1158, with permission.)

cardial perfusion imaging. The concept of using an intravenous contrast agent to improve left ventricular border detection is predicated on its ability to cross the pulmonary circuit and provide sufficient left-sided chamber opacification. As such, this application is not limited to stress echocardiography but has utility whenever image quality adversely affects wall motion assessment. By improving endocardial border detection, the accuracy with which systolic function and wall motion analysis can be ascertained is increased. Studies have confirmed, in properly selected patients, that the use of contrast for left ventricular opacification improves the reproducibility and ac-

curacy of wall motion analysis. This topic is covered in greater detail in Chapter 4.

The application of contrast agents to detect stress-induced myocardial perfusion abnormalities is an area of intense clinical investigation. In theory, a perfusion defect must precede the development of a wall motion abnormality so a method to assess myocardial perfusion should increase the sensitivity of the test to detect ischemia. After intravenous injection, the distribution of the contrast agent parallels blood flow and can be visualized (the contrast effect) as it traverses the microvasculature of the tissue, generating a time-intensity curve. Thus, perfusion can be assessed as a relative change (rest versus stress), a regional difference (e.g., lateral wall versus septum), or more quantitatively based on changes in the rate of flow or blood volume. An echocardiographic test that combines wall motion assessment with the simultaneous ability to evaluate perfusion changes in response to stress would have considerable utility. There is now ample evidence that contrast echocardiography, using second- and third-generation agents and novel acquisition algorithms, can detect and localize perfusion abnormalities during stress echocardiography.

In practice, various protocols and acquisition algorithms have been proposed. To date, no one approach has proven consistently superior. These protocols differ with respect to contrast administration and image acquisition. The options include bolus versus continuous infusion of the agent and continuous versus intermittent triggered imaging. Regardless of the protocol, the intensity and time course of the contrast effect within the myocardium are evaluated and are assumed to correlate with tissue blood volume. More detailed information regarding these and other contrast echocardiographic techniques are provided in Chapter 4. As it applies to stress echocardiography, in most cases, the perfusion information serves as a supplement to wall motion for the diagnosis of coronary artery disease. Both exercise and pharmacologic stress modalities can be used for this purpose. Most studies have relied on vasodilator stress (dipyridamole or adenosine) to induce regional changes in blood flow as a marker of coronary artery disease. After perfusion is evaluated in the resting study, the stress test is performed and perfusion imaging is repeated, usually during peak stress.

An example of a perfusion stress echocardiogram is provided in Figure 16.43. This study used vasodilator stress and intermittent triggered imaging during continuous infusion of an experimental agent. Images were acquired during diastole using the power Doppler mode. At rest, the displayed image was recorded from the fourth cycle after bubble destruction, long enough for the contrast to adequately replenish within the tissue. At peak stress, because of vasodilation, filling in of the bubbles should occur more quickly and in a normal case should

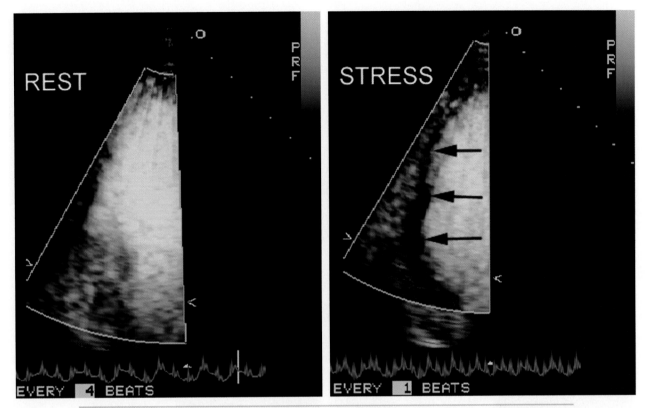

FIGURE 16.43. An example of an abnormal myocardial contrast perfusion stress echocardiogram is provided. Using vasodilator stress, apical long-axis imaging is performed at rest **(left)** and at peak stress **(right)**. Posterior perfusion is normal at baseline, but there is abnormal perfusion in the mid and basal posterior wall with stress (*arrows*). See text for details. (Courtesy of J. Jollis, M.D.)

be completed within one or two cycles. The stress image (Fig. 16.43B) demonstrates perfusion after a one-cycle delay. By demonstrating a delay in the rate of replenishment of the microbubbles, a perfusion defect is detected. The case illustrates posterior hypoperfusion (compared with a normally perfused anterior wall) in a patient with left circumflex coronary artery disease. In Figure 16.44, another investigational agent is used, again during vasodilator stress. After bubble destruction, real-time power Doppler imaging is performed. The study illustrates delayed refilling of the apical and lateral myocardium (compared with other areas) at peak stress in a patient with three-vessel coronary artery disease.

The use of these newer contrast agents for the specific purpose of perfusion imaging has not yet been approved by the U.S. Food and Drug Administration. However, both experimental and clinical studies have demonstrated the feasibility of myocardial contrast echocardiography to detect hypoperfused regions during stress. Studies comparing this technique with nuclear imaging or coronary angiography have been promising. Larger, well-designed validation studies are under way, and continued refinement of the techniques and protocols can be expected.

STRESS ECHOCARDIOGRAPHY IN VALVULAR HEART DISEASE

Stress echocardiography has a limited role in the evaluation of patients with other forms of heart disease. During routine stress testing, in patients with known or suspected coronary disease, important valvular abnormalities are occasionally identified with Doppler. In one series involving 1,272 consecutive patients (Gaur et al., 2003), significant mitral regurgitation was detected in 5% of patients, aortic regurgitation in 13%, and aortic or mitral stenosis in approximately 1% each. Even in patients who had a previous Doppler study as part of a routine echocardiogram, an important new Doppler finding was recorded in 9%. This suggests that a limited Doppler study should be a part of most stress echocardiographic examinations.

Stress echocardiography can also be used specifically for the assessment of valvular heart disease. For example, in patients with mitral stenosis of "borderline" severity, the response to exercise can be helpful, particularly to correlate symptoms with objective evidence of disease. Some patients with relatively mild disease will have a significant increase in mean gradient during exercise. This may be accompanied by an inappropriate increase in pul-

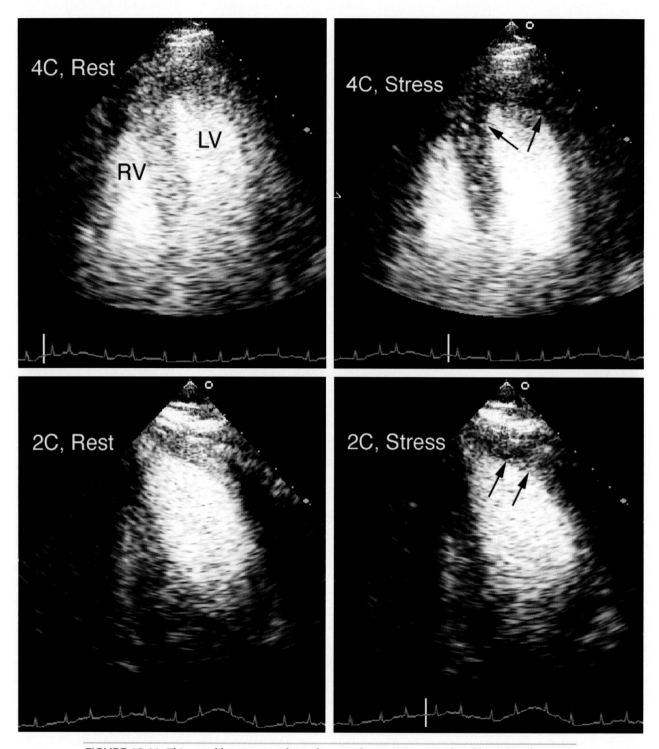

FIGURE 16.44. This vasodilator stress echocardiogram demonstrates apical and lateral perfusion abnormalities. Apical four-chamber (*4C*) **(top)** and two-chamber (*2C*) **(bottom)** views are shown at rest (at left) and peak stress (at right). Using intermittent triggered imaging, myocardial perfusion at baseline is uniformly normal. With stress, there is hypoperfusion of the apical and distal anterior and lateral walls (*arrows*). LV, left ventricle; RV, right ventricle. (Courtesy of J. Jollis, M.D.)

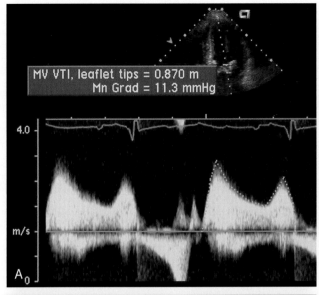

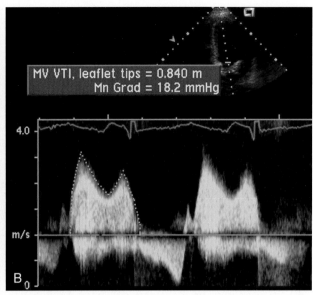

FIGURE 16.45. Supine bicycle exercise echocardiogram from a patient with mitral stenosis is provided. **A:** Doppler interrogation of mitral inflow demonstrates an 11 mm Hg mean gradient. **B:** At low exercise workload, the mean mitral valve gradient has increased to 18 mm Hg. **C:** At peak exercise, a significant increase in mean gradient (26 mm Hg) is demonstrated.

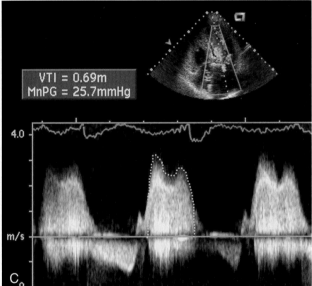

monary artery pressure that also can be documented with the Doppler technique. Stress echocardiography has also been used in patients with mitral stenosis to select candidates for balloon mitral valvuloplasty and to document the improved hemodynamics after the procedure (Fig. 16.45).

Detecting dynamic mitral regurgitation using exercise Doppler techniques is also possible. Unexpected worsening of mitral regurgitation severity can be recorded during stress with color Doppler imaging. Exercise-induced worsening of mitral regurgitation has been reported in the absence of ischemia or left ventricular dilation. In patients with valvular aortic stenosis, Doppler can be used to quantify the change in gradient during exercise in asymptomatic patients. Again, the test may be useful in clinical decision making in patients with exertional symp-

toms whose stenosis appears borderline on the resting study. Stress echocardiography has particular value in patients with left ventricular dysfunction and a moderate aortic valve gradient. In such cases, the resting study often fails to differentiate between moderate and severe aortic stenosis based on gradient alone. Dobutamine, by increasing transvalvular flow, can be used to distinguish moderate stenosis in the setting of poor left ventricular function from critical aortic stenosis. This topic is covered more fully in Chapter 10.

Exercise echocardiography has also been used to study prosthetic valve function. Pressure gradients across normally functioning prostheses often increase substantially during exercise. Stress echocardiographic techniques have proven valuable in understanding and quantifying the hemodynamic differences among the various types of prosthetic valves. Exercise hemodynamics may also provide evidence of patient-prosthesis mismatch. Other applications of stress echocardiography include the detection of exercise-induced changes in pulmonary artery pressure in patients with chronic lung disease, the evaluation of the dynamic outflow tract gradient in patients with hypertrophic obstructive cardiomyopathy, and the assessment of doxorubicin cardiomyopathy.

SUGGESTED READINGS

Afridi I, Grayburn PA, Panza JA, et al. Myocardial viability during dobutamine echocardiography predicts survival in patients with coronary artery disease and severe left ventricular systolic dysfunction. J Am Coll Cardiol 1998;32:921–926.

Allman KC, Shaw LJ, Hachamovitch R, et al. Myocardial viability testing and impact of revascularization on prognosis in patients with coronary artery disease and left ventricular dysfunction: a meta-analysis. J Am Coll Cardiol 2002;39:1151–1158.

Anthopoulos LP, Bonou MS, Kardaras FG, et al. Stress echocardiography in elderly patients with coronary artery disease: applicability, safety and prognostic value of dobutamine and adenosine echocardiography in elderly patients. J Am Coll Cardiol 1996;28:52–59.

Armstrong WF, O'Donnell J, Dillon JC, et al. Complementary value of two-dimensional exercise echocardiography to routine treadmill exercise testing. Ann Intern Med 1986;105:829–835.

Armstrong WF, O'Donnell J, Ryan T, et al. Effect of prior myocardial infarction and extent and location of coronary disease on accuracy of exercise echocardiography. J Am Coll Cardiol 1987;10:531–538.

Arnese M, Fioretti PM, Cornel JH, et al. Akinesis becoming dyskinesis during high-dose dobutamine stress echocardiography: a marker of myocardial ischemia or a mechanical phenomenon? Am J Cardiol 1994;73:896–899.

Arruda-Olson AM, Juracan EM, Mahoney DW, et al. Prognostic value of exercise echocardiography in 5,798 patients: is there a gender difference? J Am Coll Cardiol 2002;39:625–631.

Bach DS, Hepner A, Marcovitz PA, et al. Dobutamine stress echocardiography: prevalence of a nonischemic response in a low-risk population. Am Heart J 1993;125:1257–1261.

Badruddin SM, Ahmad A, Mickelson J, et al. Supine bicycle versus post-treadmill exercise echocardiography in the detection of myocardial ischemia: a randomized single-blind crossover trial. J Am Coll Cardiol 1999;33:1485–1490.

Bax JJ, Cornel JH, Visser FC, et al. Prediction of recovery of myocardial dysfunction after revascularization: comparison of fluorine-18 fluorodeoxyglucose/thallium-201 SPECT, thallium-201 stress-reinjection SPECT and dobutamine echocardiography. J Am Coll Cardiol 1996;28:558–564.

Beleslin BD, Ostojic M, Stepanovic J, et al. Stress echocardiography in the detection of myocardial ischemia. Head-to-head comparison of exercise, dobutamine, and dipyridamole tests. Circulation 1994;90:1168–1176.

Bholasingh R, Cornel JH, Camp O, et al. Prognostic value of predischarge dobutamine stress echocardiography in chest pain patients with a negative cardiac troponin T. J Am Coll Cardiol 2003;41:596–602.

Bossone E, Martinez FJ, Whyte RI, et al. Dobutamine stress echocardiography for the preoperative evaluation of patients undergoing lung volume reduction surgery. J Thorac Cardiovasc Surg 1999;118:542–546.

Carlos ME, Smart SC, Wynsen JC, et al. Dobutamine stress echocardiography for risk stratification after myocardial infarction. Circulation 1997;95:1402–1410.

Cheitlin MD, Alpert JS, Armstrong WF, et al. ACC/AHA Guidelines for the Clinical Application of Echocardiography. A report of the American College of Cardiology/American Heart Association Task Force on Practice Guidelines (Committee on Clinical Appliaction of Echocardiography). Developed in collaboration with the American Society of Echocardiography. Circulation. 1997;95(6):1686–1744.

Chuah SC, Pellikka PA, Roger VL, et al. Role of dobutamine stress echocardiography in predicting outcome in 860 patients with known or suspected coronary artery disease. Circulation 1998;97:1474–1480.

Cigarroa CG, deFilippi CR, Brickner ME, et al. Dobutamine stress echocardiography identifies hibernating myocardium and predicts recovery of left ventricular function after coronary revascularization. Circulation 1993;88:430–436.

Cortigiani L, Dodi C, Paolini EA, et al. Prognostic value of pharmacological stress echocardiography in women with chest pain and unknown coronary artery disease. J Am Coll Cardiol 1998;32:1975–1981.

Das MK, Pellikka PA, Mahoney DW, et al. Assessment of cardiac risk before nonvascular surgery: dobutamine stress echocardiography in 530 patients. J Am Coll Cardiol 2000;35:1647–1653.

Davila-Roman VG, Waggoner AD, Sicard GA, et al. Dobutamine stress echocardiography predicts surgical outcome in patients with an aortic aneurysm and peripheral vascular disease. J Am Coll Cardiol 1993;1:957–963.

Dionisopoulos PN, Collins JD, Smart SC, et al. The value of dobutamine stress echocardiography for the detection of coronary artery disease in women. J Am Soc Echocardiogr 1997;10:811–817.

Eichelberger JP, Schwarz KQ, Black ER, et al. Predictive value of dobutamine echocardiography just before noncardiac vascular surgery. Am J Cardiol 1993;72:602–607.

Elhendy A, Geleijnse ML, van Domburg RT, et al. Gender differences in the accuracy of dobutamine stress echocardiography for the diagnosis of coronary artery disease. Am J Cardiol 1997;80:1414–1418.

Fleischmann KE, Hunink MG, Kuntz KM, et al. Exercise echocardiography or exercise SPECT imaging? A meta-analysis of diagnostic test performance. JAMA 1998;280:913–920.

Forster T, McNeill AJ, Salustri A, et al. Simultaneous dobutamine stress echocardiography and technetium-99m isonitrile single-photon emission computed tomography in patients with suspected coronary artery disease. J Am Coll Cardiol 1993;21:1591–1596.

Fragasso G, Lu C, Dabrowski P, et al. Comparison of stress/rest myocardial perfusion tomography, dipyridamole and dobutamine stress echocardiography for the detection of coronary disease in hypertensive patients with chest pain and positive exercise test. J Am Coll Cardiol 1999;34:441–447.

Garber AM, Solomon NA. Cost-effectiveness of alternative test strategies for the diagnosis of coronary artery disease. Ann Intern Med 1999;130:719–728.

Gaur A, Yeon SB, Lewis CW, et al. Valvular flow abnormalities are often identified by a resting focused Doppler examination performed at the time of stress echocardiography. Am J Med 2003;114:20–24.

Hecht HS, DeBord L, Shaw R, et al. Supine bicycle stress echocardiography versus tomographic thallium-201 exercise imaging for the detection of coronary artery disease. J Am Soc Echocardiogr 1993;6:177–185.

Hecht HS, DeBord L, Shaw R, et al. Digital supine bicycle stress echocardiography: a new technique for evaluating coronary artery disease. J Am Coll Cardiol 1993;21:950–956.

Hecht HS, DeBord L, Sotomayor N, et al. Supine bicycle stress echocardiography: peak exercise imaging is superior to postexercise imaging. J Am Soc Echocardiogr 1993;6:265–271.

Heinle SK, Noblin J, Goree-Best P, et al. Assessment of myocardial perfusion by harmonic power Doppler imaging at rest and during adenosine stress: comparison with 99m Tc-sestamibi SPECT imaging. Circulation 2000;102:55–60.

Hennessy T, Sioban Hennessy M, Codd MB, et al. Detection of coronary artery disease using dobutamine stress echocardiography in patients with an abnormal resting ECG. Int J Cardiol 1998;64:293–298.

Heupler S, Mehta R, Lobo A, et al. Prognostic implications of exercise echocardiography in women with known or suspected coronary artery disease. J Am Coll Cardiol 1997;30:414–420.

Kaul S, Senior R, Dittrich H, et al. Detection of coronary artery disease with myocardial contrast echocardiography: comparison with 99mTc-sestamibi single-photon emission computed tomography. Circulation 1997;96:785–792.

Krivokapich J, Child JS, Gerber RS, et al. Prognostic usefulness of positive or negative exercise stress echocardiography for predicting coronary events in ensuing twelve months. Am J Cardiol 1993;71:646–651.

Krivokapich J, Child JS, Walter DO, et al. Prognostic value of dobutamine stress echocardiography in predicting cardiac events in patients with known or suspected coronary artery disease. J Am Coll Cardiol 1999;33:708–716.

Kuntz KM, Fleischmann KE, Hunink MG, et al. Cost-effectiveness of diagnostic strategies for patients with chest pain. Ann Intern Med 1999;130:709–718.

La Canna G, Alfieri O, Giubbini R, et al. Echocardiography during infusion of dobutamine for identification of reversibly dysfunction in patients with chronic coronary artery disease. J Am Coll Cardiol 1994;23:617–626.

Lalka SG, Sawada SG, Dalsing MC, et al. Dobutamine stress echocardiography as a predictor of cardiac events associated with aortic surgery. J Vasc Surg 1992;15:831–840.

Langan EM III, Youkey JR, Franklin DP, et al. Dobutamine stress echocardiography for cardiac risk assessment before aortic surgery. J Vasc Surg 1993;18:905–911.

Ling LH, Pellikka PA, Mahoney DW, et al. Atropine augmentation in dobutamine stress echocardiography: role and incremental value in a clinical practice setting. J Am Coll Cardiol 1996;28:551–557.

Luotolahti M, Saraste M, Hartiala J. Exercise echocardiography in the diagnosis of coronary artery disease. Ann Med 1996;28:73–77.

Marangelli V, Iliceto S, Piccinni G, et al. Detection of coronary artery disease by digital stress echocardiography: comparison of exercise, transesophageal atrial pacing and dipyridamole echocardiography. J Am Coll Cardiol 1994;24:117–124.

Marcovitz PA, Armstrong WF. Accuracy of dobutamine stress echocardiography in detecting coronary artery disease. Am J Cardiol 1992;69:1269–1273.

Marcovitz PA, Shayna V, Horn RA, et al. Value of dobutamine stress echocardiography in determining the prognosis of patients with known or suspected coronary artery disease. Am J Cardiol 1996;78:404–408.

Martin TW, Seaworth JF, Johns JP, et al. Comparison of adenosine, dipyridamole, and dobutamine in stress echocardiography. Ann Intern Med 1992;116:190–196.

Marwick T, D'Hondt AM, Baudhuin T, et al. Optimal use of dobutamine stress for the detection and evaluation of coronary artery disease: combination with echocardiography or scintigraphy, or both? J Am Coll Cardiol 1993;22:159–167.

Marwick T, Willemart B, D'Hondt AM, et al. Selection of the optimal nonexercise stress for the evaluation of ischemic regional myocardial dysfunction and malperfusion. Comparison of dobutamine and adenosine using echocardiography and 99mTc-MIBI single photon emission computed tomography. Circulation 1993;87:345–354.

Marwick TH, Anderson T, Williams MJ, et al. Exercise echocardiography is an accurate and cost-efficient technique for detection of coronary artery disease in women. J Am Coll Cardiol 1995;26:335–341.

Marwick TH, D'Hondt AM, Mairesse GH, et al. Comparative ability of dobutamine and exercise stress in inducing myocardial ischaemia in active patients. Br Heart J 1994;72:31–38.

Marwick TH, Mehta R, Arheart K, et al. Use of exercise echocardiography for prognostic evaluation of patients with known or suspected coronary artery disease. J Am Coll Cardiol 1997;30:83–90.

Marwick TH, Torelli J, Harjai K, et al. Influence of left ventricular hypertrophy on detection of coronary artery disease using exercise echocardiography. J Am Coll Cardiol 1995;26:1180–1186.

Mason SJ, Weiss JL, Weisfeldt ML, et al. Exercise echocardiography: detection of wall motion abnormalities during ischemia. Circulation 1979;59:50–59.

McCully RB, Roger VL, Mahoney DW, et al. Outcome after abnormal exercise echocardiography for patients with good exercise capacity: prognostic importance of the extent and severity of exercise-related left ventricular dysfunction. J Am Coll Cardiol 2002;39:1345–1352.

McCully RB, Roger VL, Mahoney DW, et al. Outcome after normal exercise echocardiography and predictors of subsequent cardiac events: follow-up of 1,325 patients. J Am Coll Cardiol 1998;31:144–149.

Mertes H, Erbel R, Nixdorff U, et al. Exercise echocardiography for the evaluation of patients after nonsurgical coronary artery revascularization. J Am Coll Cardiol 1993;21:1087–1093.

Mertes H, Sawada SG, Ryan T, et al. Symptoms, adverse effects, and complications associated with dobutamine stress echocardiography. Experience in 1118 patients. Circulation 1993;88:15–19.

Nihoyannopoulos P, Marsonis A, Joshi J, et al. Magnitude of myocardial dysfunction is greater in painful than in painless myocardial ischemia: an exercise echocardiographic study. J Am Coll Cardiol 1995;25:1507–1512.

Olmos LI, Dakik H, Gordon R, et al. Long-term prognostic value of exercise echocardiography compared with exercise 201Tl, ECG, and clinical variables in patients evaluated for coronary artery disease. Circulation 1998;98:2679–2686.

Ostojic M, Picano E, Beleslin B, et al. Dipyridamole-dobutamine echocardiography: a novel test for the detection of milder forms of coronary artery disease. J Am Coll Cardiol 1994;23:1115–1122.

Pellikka PA, Roger VL, Oh JK, et al. Safety of performing dobutamine stress echocardiography in patients with abdominal aortic aneurysm ≤4 cm in diameter. Am J Cardiol 1996;77:413–416.

Perrone-Filardi P, Pace L, Prastaro M, et al. Assessment of myocardial viability in patients with chronic coronary artery disease. Rest-4-hour-24-hour 201Tl tomography versus dobutamine echocardiography. Circulation 1996;94:2712–2719.

Picano E, Lattanzi F, Masini M, et al. High dose dipyridamole echocardiography test in effort angina pectoris. J Am Coll Cardiol 1986;8:848–854.

Picano E, Sicari R, Landi P, et al. Prognostic value of myocardial viability in medically treated patients with global left ventricular dysfunction early after an acute uncomplicated myocardial infarction: a dobutamine stress echocardiographic study. Circulation 1998;98:1078–1084.

Pierard LA, De Landsheere CM, Berthe C, et al. Identification of viable myocardium by echocardiography during dobutamine infusion in patients with myocardial infarction after thrombolytic therapy: comparison with positron emission tomography. J Am Coll Cardiol 1990;15:1021–1031.

Pingitore A, Picano E, Colosso MQ, et al. The atropine factor in pharmacologic stress echocardiography. Echo Persantine (EPIC) and Echo Dobutamine International Cooperative (EDIC) Study Groups. J Am Coll Cardiol 1996;27:1164–1170.

Plotkin JS, Benitez RM, Kuo PC, et al. Dobutamine stress echocardiography for preoperative cardiac risk stratification in patients undergoing orthotopic liver transplantation. Liver Transpl Surg 1998;4:253–257.

Poldermans D, Arnese M, Fioretti PM, et al. Improved cardiac risk stratification in major vascular surgery with dobutamine–atropine stress echocardiography. J Am Coll Cardiol 1995;26:648–653.

Poldermans D, Arnese M, Fioretti PM, et al. Sustained prognostic value of dobutamine stress echocardiography for late cardiac events after major noncardiac vascular surgery. Circulation 1997;95:53–58.

Poldermans D, Fioretti PM, Boersma E, et al. Long-term prognostic value of dobutamine-atropine stress echocardiography in 1737 patients with known or suspected coronary artery disease: a single-center experience. Circulation 1999;99:757–762.

Poldermans D, Fioretti PM, Forster T, et al. Dobutamine stress echocardiography for assessment of perioperative cardiac risk in patients undergoing major vascular surgery. Circulation 1993;87:1506–1512.

Porter TR, Xie F, Silver M, et al. Real-time perfusion imaging with low mechanical index pulse inversion Doppler imaging. J Am Coll Cardiol 2001;37:748–753.

Quinones MA, Verani MS, Haichin RM, et al. Exercise echocardiography versus 201Tl single-photon emission computed tomography in evaluation of coronary artery disease. Analysis of 292 patients. Circulation 1992;85:1026–1031.

Rallidis L, Cokkinos P, Tousoulis D, et al. Comparison of dobutamine and treadmill exercise echocardiography in inducing ischemia in patients with coronary artery disease. J Am Coll Cardiol 1997;30:1660–1668.

Robertson WS, Feigenbaum H, Armstrong WF, et al. Exercise echocardiography: a clinically practical addition in the evaluation of coronary artery disease. J Am Coll Cardiol 1983;2:1085–1091.

Roger VL, Jacobsen SJ, Pellikka PA, et al. Gender differences in use of stress testing and coronary heart disease mortality: a population-based study in Olmsted County, Minnesota. J Am Coll Cardiol 1998;32:345–352.

Roger VL, Pellikka PA, Bell MR, et al. Sex and test verification bias. Impact on the diagnostic value of exercise echocardiography. Circulation 1997;95:405–410.

Roger VL, Pellikka PA, Oh JK, et al. Identification of multivessel coronary artery disease by exercise echocardiography. J Am Coll Cardiol 1994;24:109–114.

Ryan T, Segar DS, Sawada SG, et al. Detection of coronary artery disease with upright bicycle exercise echocardiography. J Am Soc Echocardiogr 1993;6:186–197.

Ryan T, Vasey CG, Presti CF, et al. Exercise echocardiography: detection of coronary artery disease in patients with normal left ventricular wall motion at rest. J Am Coll Cardiol 1988;11:993–999.

Salustri A, Ciavatti M, Seccareccia F, et al. Prediction of cardiac events after uncomplicated acute myocardial infarction by clinical variables and dobutamine stress test. J Am Coll Cardiol 1999;34:435–440.

San Roman JA, Rollan MJ, Vilacosta I. Echocardiography and MIB-SPECT scintigraphy during dobutamine infusion in the diagnosis of coronary disease. Rev Esp Cardiol 1995;48:606–614.

Sawada SG, Ryan T, Fineberg NS, et al. Exercise echocardiographic detection of coronary artery disease in women. J Am Coll Cardiol 1989;14:1440–1447.

Schiller NB, Shah PM, Crawford M, et al. Recommendations for quantitation of the left ventricle by two-dimensional echocardiography. American Society of Echocardiography Committee on Standards, Subcommittee on Quantitation of Two-Dimensional Echocardiograms. J Am Soc Echocardiogr 1989;2:358–367.

Senior R, Kaul S, Lahiri A. Myocardial viability on echocardiography predicts long-term survival after revascularization in patients with ischemic congestive heart failure. J Am Coll Cardiol 1999;33:1848–1854.

Shaw LJ, Eagle KA, Gersh BJ, et al. Meta-analysis of intravenous dipyridamole-thallium-201 imaging (1985 to 1994) and dobutamine echocardiography (1991 to 1994) for risk stratification before vascular surgery. J Am Coll Cardiol 1996;27:787–798.

Shimoni S, Zoghbi WA, Iskander S, et al. Real-time assessment of myocardial perfusion and wall motion during bicycle and treadmill exercise echocardiography: comparison with single photon emission computed tomography. J Am Coll Cardiol 2001;37:741–747.

Sicari R, Pasanisi E, Venneri L, et al. Stress echo results predict mortality: a large-scale multicenter prospective international study. J Am Coll Cardiol 2003;41:589–595.

Smart SC, Dionisopoulos PN, Knickelbine TA, et al. Dobutamine-atropine stress echocardiography for risk stratification in patients with chronic left ventricular dysfunction. J Am Coll Cardiol 1999;33:512–521.

Smart SC, Knickelbine T, Malik F, et al. Dobutamine-atropine stress echocardiography for the detection of coronary artery disease in patients with left ventricular hypertrophy. Importance of chamber size and systolic wall stress. Circulation 2000;101:258–263.

Smart SC, Sawada S, Ryan T, et al. Low-dose dobutamine echocardiography detects reversible dysfunction after thrombolytic therapy of acute myocardial infarction. Circulation 1993;88:405–415.

Smart S, Wynsen J, Sagar K. Dobutamine-atropine stress echocardiography for reversible dysfunction during the first week after acute myocardial infarction: limitations and determinants of accuracy. J Am Coll Cardiol 1997;30:1669–1678.

Steinberg EH, Madmon L, Patel CP, et al. Long-term prognostic significance of dobutamine echocardiography in patients with suspected coronary artery disease: results of a 5-year follow-up study. J Am Coll Cardiol 1997;29:969–973.

Takeuchi M, Araki M, Nakashima Y, et al. Comparison of dobutamine stress echocardiography and stress thallium-201 single-photon emission computed tomography for detecting coronary artery disease. J Am Soc Echocardiogr 1993;6:593–602.

Tian J, Zhang G, Wang X, et al. Exercise echocardiography: feasibility and value for detection of coronary artery disease. Chin Med J 1996;109:381–384.

Tischler MD, Niggel J. Exercise echocardiography in combined mild mitral valve stenosis and regurgitation. Echocardiography 1993;10:453–457.

Tischler MD, Plehn JF. Applications of stress echocardiography: beyond coronary disease. J Am Soc Echocardiogr 1995;8:185–197.

Tsoukas A, Ikonomidis I, Cokkinos P, et al. Significance of persistent left ventricular dysfunction during recovery after dobutamine stress echocardiography. J Am Coll Cardiol 1996;30:621–626.

Vanoverschelde JL, D'Hondt AM, Marwick T, et al. Head-to-head comparison of exercise-redistribution-reinjection thallium single-photon emission computed tomography and low dose dobutamine echocardiography for prediction of reversibility of chronic left ventricular ischemic dysfunction. J Am Coll Cardiol 1996;28:432–442.

Voigt JU, Exner B, Schmiedehausen K, et al. Strain-rate imaging during dobutamine stress echocardiography provides objective evidence of inducible ischemia. Circulation 2003;107:2120–2126.

Wann LS, Faris JV, Childress RH, et al. Exercise cross-sectional echocardiography in ischemic heart disease. Circulation 1979;60:1300–1308.

Yao SS, Qureshi E, Sherrid MV, et al. Practical applications in stress echocardiography: risk stratification and prognosis in patients with known or suspected ischemic heart disease. J Am Coll Cardiol 2003;42:1084–1090.

Yuda S, Khoury V, Marwick TH. Influence of wall stress and left ventricular geometry on the accuracy of dobutamine stress echocardiography. J Am Coll Cardiol 2002;40:1311–1319.

Chapter 17

Cardiomyopathies

CLINICAL AND ECHOCARDIOGRAPHIC OVERVIEW

Cardiomyopathy represents a diverse group of diseases intrinsic to the myocardium. By strict definition, they are a primary myocardial disorder and not related to the effects of conditions such as preexisting valve disease, hypertension, and coronary artery disease. From a practical standpoint, severe dysfunction due to diffuse coronary disease and the effects of chronic ischemia is often considered a form of cardiomyopathy (ischemic cardiomyopathy). Traditionally, cardiomyopathies are divided into dilated or congestive and nondilated or restrictive forms. Some forms of cardiomyopathy may present either as a dilated cardiomyopathy or restrictive cardiomyopathy. An additional subset includes true hypertrophic cardiomyopathy, which can either be nonobstructive or obstructive.

DILATED CARDIOMYOPATHY

There are multiple etiologies for dilated cardiomyopathy that fall into the general categories of ischemic and nonischemic (Table 17.1). Clinically, cardiomyopathies share a constellation of symptoms that can be present to varying degrees, including congestive heart failure, low-output state, fatigue, dyspnea, arrhythmias, and sudden cardiac death. Echocardiography serves as a definitive tool for establishing the presence and type of cardiomyopathy, may provide information regarding the specific etiology, and can be used to accurately track the physiologic abnormalities associated with the cardiomyopathy. The American College of Cardiology/American Heart Association guidelines for management of congestive heart failure consider echocardiography a Class I diagnostic test, implying that it is generally indicated and useful in all patients with congestive heart failure and suspected cardiomyopathy. Additionally, echocardiography and Doppler imaging can provide valuable prognostic information and serve as a guide to success of therapy.

▶ **TABLE 17.1 Classification of Cardiomyopathy and Diseases Resulting in Acute or Chronic Left Ventricular Dysfunction**

Dilated cardiomyopathy
  Idiopathic cardiomyopathy
  Familial cardiomyopathy
  Noncompacted myocardium
  Postpartum cardiomyopathy
  Hemachromatosis
  Infectious
    Postviral myocarditis
    Human immunodeficiency virus related
    Legionella infection
    Sepsis (gram negative)
  Toxic cardiomyopathy
    Adriamycin
    Alcohol
    Carbon monoxide poisoning
    Other chemotherapy
High-output cardiomyopathy
  Tachycardia-mediated cardiomyopathy
  Thyrotoxicosis
  Nutritional (beriberi, thiamine deficiency)
  Peripheral left-to-right shunt lesions
  Anemia
Hypertrophic cardiomyopathy
  Asymmetric septal hypertrophy (idiopathic hypertrophic cardiomyopathy)
    Obstructive vs. nonobstructive
  Concentric hypertrophic cardiomyopathy
  Isolated apical hypertrophic cardiomyopathy
  Atypical hypertrophic cardiomyopathy
Restrictive cardiomyopathy
  Idiopathic
  Infiltrative
    Amyloidosis
    Glycogen storage diseases
    Hemachromatosis
  Post-radiation therapy
  Endocardial fibroelastosis
Other
  Friedreich ataxia
  Muscular dystrophies

Although the primary diagnostic features of dilated cardiomyopathy are left ventricular dilation and systolic dysfunction, other secondary features are nearly ubiquitous and substantially contribute to the development of symptoms. These include diastolic dysfunction with chronic elevation of left atrial pressure, secondary mitral regurgitation, and secondary pulmonary hypertension. The primary and secondary abnormalities seen in dilated cardiomyopathy are listed in Table 17.2. The most common clinical presentation of dilated cardiomyopathy is congestive heart failure symptoms with shortness of breath and exercise intolerance. Depending on severity and duration, patients with dilated cardiomyopathy can present with New York Heart Association Class I to IV symptoms.

The echocardiographic features of dilated cardiomyopathy parallel the primary and secondary findings noted in Table 17.2. Left ventricular dilation is ubiquitous and a requisite component for establishing the diagnosis. The degree of dilation can be mild or substantial with left ventricular internal dimensions of as large as 8.0 cm occasionally being encountered. The distribution of systolic dysfunction within the left ventricular walls is dependent on whether the cardiomyopathy has an ischemic etiology. Classically, if an ischemic etiology is present, there will be greater regional variation in systolic dysfunction than if the process is nonischemic. It should be emphasized, however, that in documented nonischemic cardiomyopathy, there will be regional variation in the degree of systolic dysfunction, typically with the proximal portions of the inferoposterior and posterior lateral walls having preserved function when compared with other left ventricular segments. As a consequence of dilation and systolic dysfunction, the left ventricle takes on a more spherical geometry that further contributes to the deterioration of left ventricular systolic function because the spherical geometry interferes with the contractile efficiency of the myocardial fibers. Normally, the long axis dimension of the left ventricle exceeds the minor axis dimension (diameter) with a ratio of 1.6:1 or greater. With progressive dilation, the minor axis increases disproportionally, and the ratio of long to minor axis decreases. Typically, a ratio (sphericity index) of less than 1.5:1 implies marked pathologic remodeling. The increasing spherical geometry results in apical and lateral displacement of the papillary muscles. This has the result of effectively reducing the length of the mitral apparatus as compared with the anulus and results in secondary functional mitral regurgitation.

Figures 17.1 through 17.7 depict several features of dilated cardiomyopathy. Notice in Figure 17.1 the relatively mild left ventricular dilation and relative preservation of normal ventricular geometry. When comparing diastolic and systolic frames, ventricular systolic dysfunction is clearly present, but the ejection fraction is reduced to only

▶ TABLE 17.2 Echocardiographic Abnormalities in Cardiomyopathy

Left ventricular dilation
  Increasing sphericity of left ventricular geometry
  Apical and lateral displacement of papillary muscles
    Functional mitral regurgitation
  Left ventricular thrombus
Left atrial dilation
  Atrial fibrillation
  Left atrial thrombosis/stasis of blood
Pulmonary hypertension
Tricuspid regurgitation
Right ventricular dilation

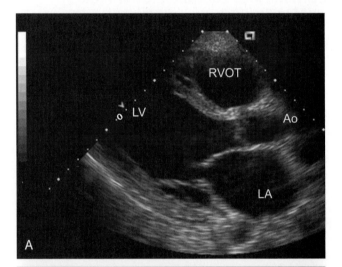
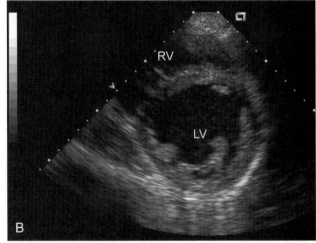

FIGURE 17.1. Parasternal views recorded in a patient with a dilated cardiomyopathy. **A:** Parasternal long-axis view recorded in end-diastole. Note the dilation of the left ventricle (65 mm) and left atrium (50 mm). **B:** End-diastolic short-axis view. Note the normal circular geometry of the left ventricle and the uniform wall thickness. In real time, all walls are uniformly hypokinetic. Ao, aorta; LA, left atrium; LV, left ventricular; RV, right ventricle; RVOT, right ventricular outflow tract.

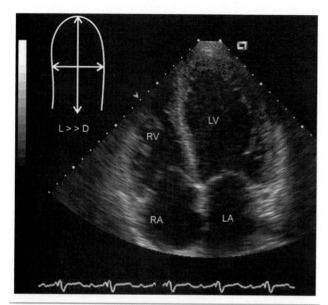

FIGURE 17.2. Apical four-chamber view recorded in the same patient as in Figure 17.1. Note the relatively normal bullet-shape geometry of the left ventricle (*LV*) and the modest four-chamber enlargement. In this example, normal left ventricular geometry has been preserved, with a long-axis dimension (*L*) significantly greater than the short-axis (*D*) dimension, as noted in the schematic in the upper left. LA, left atrium; RA, right atrium; RV, right ventricle.

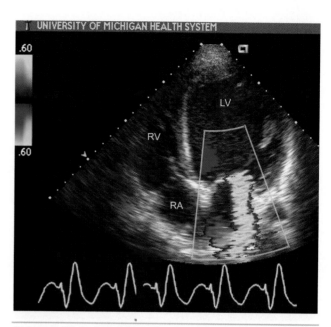

FIGURE 17.4. Apical four-chamber view recorded in a patient with a dilated cardiomyopathy and functional mitral regurgitation that is the result of lateral displacement of the papillary muscles. Note the mitral regurgitation jet, with the color flow Doppler signal filling approximately 40% of the left atrial area. LV, left ventricle; RA, right atrium; RV, right ventricle.

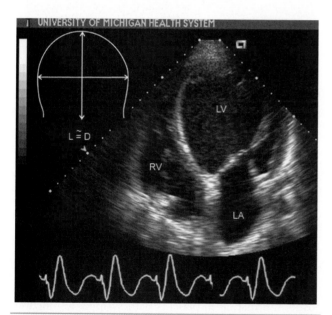

FIGURE 17.3. Apical four-chamber view recorded in a patient with a dilated cardiomyopathy and abnormal ventricular geometry. Note the relatively spherical shape of the left ventricle in which the long-axis dimension (*L*) and short-axis dimension (*D*) are essentially equal. This has resulted in lateral displacement of the papillary muscles and retraction of the mitral apparatus toward the apex. LA, left atrium; LV, left ventricle; RV, right ventricle.

35%. Figure 17.3 is a more extreme example of long-standing dilated cardiomyopathy in which the left ventricle has taken on a more spherical geometry. Note the relationship of the maximal lateral dimension to the length, which is increased compared with the geometry seen in normal individuals and increased compared with the milder dilated cardiomyopathy presented in Figure 17.1. Figure 17.4 depicts secondary mitral regurgitation due to the apical and posterior displacement of the papillary muscles, resulting in abnormal coaptation of the mitral valve leaflets.

Figure 17.5 depicts a classic ischemic cardiomyopathy. Note the thin, scarred inferior and inferoposterior walls and generalized hypokinesis of the remaining walls. This image would be consistent with an established extensive inferior myocardial infarction with milder degrees of secondary left ventricular dysfunction in the remaining segments, resulting in the appearance of global systolic dysfunction and reduced ventricular performance.

Once the diagnosis has been established, it is clinically useful to quantify the degree of systolic dysfunction. Parameters that have diagnostic and prognostic importance include any of the linear- or area-based measurements of left ventricular size from which the derived parameters of fractional shortening and fractional area change can be calculated. Additionally, the left ventricular cavity volume can be determined from several methods (the Simpson

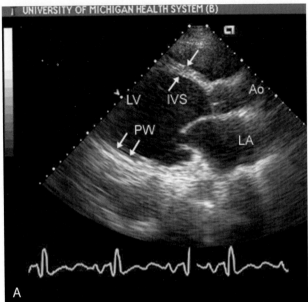

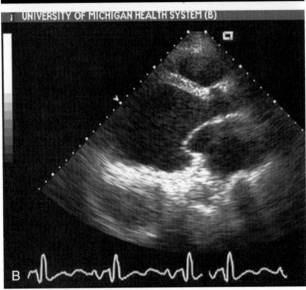

FIGURE 17.5. Parasternal long-axis view recorded in a patient with a classic ischemic cardiomyopathy. **A:** Recorded in end-diastole. Note the dilated left ventricle (*LV*) and the relative preservation of ventricular septal thickness (*upper arrows*) as compared with the thinned posterior wall (*lower arrows*) (*PW*). **B:** End-systolic frame. Note the hypokinesis of the anterior septum and akinesis of the posterior wall. Ao, aorta; IVS, interventricular septum; LA, left atrium.

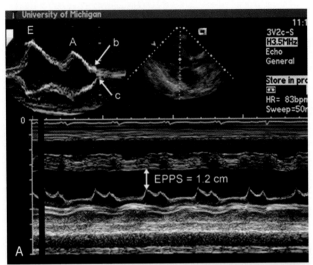

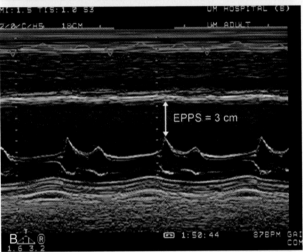

FIGURE 17.6. M-mode echocardiograms recorded in patients with cardiomyopathy and systolic dysfunction. In each case, note the increased E-point to septal separation (*EPSS*) indicative of a reduced ejection fraction. **A:** The E-point to septal separation is 1.2 cm as compared with 3.0 cm (**B**). This suggests that the ejection fraction for the patient represented in **B** is substantially worse than that in **A**. The inset in **A** demonstrates a classic B-bump in mitral valve closure. Note that the smooth continuation between the A point and the closure point (*c*) is interrupted by transient reopening of the mitral valve denoted by the B-bump.

rule is the most often used) from which the stroke volume and ejection fraction can be calculated. Other parameters of systolic function can be derived from Doppler echocardiography. All the different modalities described in Chapter 6 can be used to characterize and quantify left ventricular systolic dysfunction in dilated cardiomyopathy. Those that have the most diagnostic and prognostic relevance include end-diastolic and systolic volumes and ejection fraction.

There are several M-mode findings that provide diagnostic information in patients with systolic dysfunction. The first of these is the E-point to septal separation (EPSS) defined as the distance (in millimeters) from the anterior septal endocardium to the maximal early opening point (E-point) of the mitral valve (Fig. 17.6). Because the internal dimension of the left ventricle is proportional to diastolic left ventricular volume and the maximal excursion of the mitral valve in diastole is proportional to the mitral stroke volume, the ratio of the two dimensions

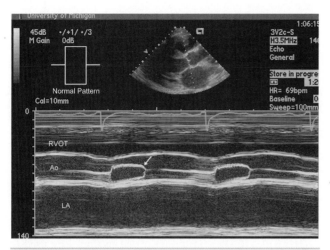

FIGURE 17.7. M-mode echocardiogram recorded through the aortic valve in a patient with a dilated cardiomyopathy and reduced stroke volume. Note the gradual curved closure of the aortic valve at end-systole (*arrow*). This is due to the progressively diminishing forward flow as a consequence of severe systolic dysfunction. The small inset in the upper left schematizes the normal opening and closing pattern of the aortic valve. Ao, aorta; LA, left atrium; RVOT, right ventricular outflow tract.

▶ **TABLE 17.3 Role of Doppler Echocardiography in Cardiomyopathy**

Assessment of forward flow
  Doppler-based left ventricular outflow tract time velocity integral (TVI)
  Volume-based left ventricular stroke volume
  Cardiac output
Assessment of diastolic properties of the left ventricle
  Mitral inflow pattern
    E_m/A_m ratio
      Response to Valsalva maneuver
    Deceleration time
    Dispersion of E-wave velocity
    Isovolumic relaxation time
    Color Doppler M-mode velocity of propagation (V_p)
  Pulmonary vein flow
    Systolic/diastolic flow ratio
    Pulmonary vein A-wave duration
  Anular Doppler tissue imaging
    E_a/A_a ratio
    E_m/E_a ratio
Assessment of diastolic properties of the right ventricle
  Doppler flow in the hepatic veins
  Superior vena caval Doppler flow

will be proportional to the ejection fraction. As such, limited mitral valve opening (manifested by a greater distance between the E-point and the septum) is an indirect indicator of a reduced ejection fraction. The normal EPSS is 6 mm, with progressively larger EPPS representing a lower ejection fraction.

Evaluation of aortic valve motion also provides clues to left ventricular performance. Normally, the aortic valve has crisp opening and closing points and as such opens as a "box" when viewed with M-mode echocardiography. Reduced forward flow results in a more gradual closure during systole so that there is rounding of the aortic valve closing due to reduced forward flow (Fig. 17.7).

DOPPLER EVALUATION OF SYSTOLIC AND DIASTOLIC FUNCTION

The use of Doppler techniques to determine systolic and diastolic dysfunction is described in Chapters 6 and 8. Doppler parameters, which can be employed to evaluate systolic and diastolic dysfunction in cardiomyopathy are listed in Table 17.3. Stroke volume can be determined by recording the time velocity integral (TVI) in the left ventricular outflow tract. This represents the integral of flow velocity over time and, when multiplied by the cross-sectional area of the left ventricular outflow tract, provides actual volume of flow. Figure 17.8 schematizes this concept, and Figure 17.9 shows examples of left ventricular outflow tract TVI in patients with dilated cardiomyopathy and varying degrees of systolic dysfunction. Once

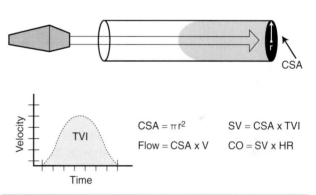

$$CSA = \pi r^2 \qquad SV = CSA \times TVI$$
$$Flow = CSA \times V \qquad CO = SV \times HR$$

FIGURE 17.8. Schematic illustration outlining determination of stroke volume in the left ventricular outflow tract from which cardiac output can also be obtained. Pulsed wave Doppler imaging is used to interrogate flow in a defined area such as the left ventricular outflow tract. The cross-sectional area (*CSA*) can be calculated from the radius. Pulsed Doppler imaging is used to determine the time velocity integral (*TVI*) of flow. Stroke volume (*SV*) is calculated as the product of CSA and TVI. Cardiac output (*CO*) can be calculated as stroke volume times heart rate (*HR*). This calculation can be performed for any laminar flow through a relatively tubular structure such as the left ventricular outflow tract.

this per-beat stroke volume has been determined, the cardiac output can be calculated as the product of the heart rate and forward stroke volume. This calculation assumes that aortic insufficiency is not present. As previously noted, the major source of error in this calculation is the measurement of left ventricular outflow tract area, which relies on the square of the radius. For any individual pa-

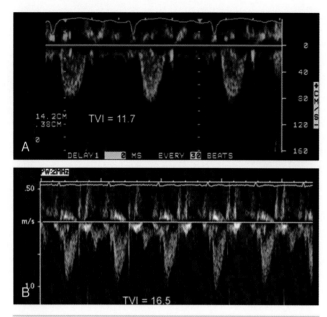

FIGURE 17.9. Examples of the time velocity integral (*TVI*) in patients with cardiomyopathy and reduced forward stroke volume. **A:** Note the time velocity integral of 11.7 cm compared with the time velocity integral of 16.5 cm **(B)**, which implies substantially greater forward flow in the lower panel.

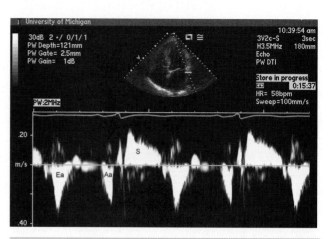

FIGURE 17.10. Demonstration of the methodology used to determine anular velocities using Doppler tissue imaging (DTI). The upper image is a four chamber apical view in which a pulsed sample volume has been placed in the lateral anulus. The lower panel is the DTI spectral Doppler recorded from this position. There are three components to this recording. The first is the upward moving systolic (S) velocity of the anulus. The second and third are the biphasic downward motion occurring in diastole (Ea and Aa, respectively). With normal systolic and diastolic function of the left ventricle, Ea typically exceeds the Aa velocity.

tient, one can assume the outflow tract area remains a constant, and, therefore, comparison of the TVI alone provides a reliable means for comparing the left ventricular stroke volume at different time points or when evaluating the impact of acute therapy.

An indirect and nonvolumetric measure of left ventricular systolic function that can be employed in dilated cardiomyopathy is measurement of the descent of the base of the heart. With ventricular contraction, there is motion of the anulus of the heart toward the apex. The magnitude of this motion can be determined with M-mode echocardiography but more recently has been evaluated using Doppler tissue imaging. In this technique, a sample volume is placed either in the lateral anulus or the proximal ventricular septum (Fig. 17.10). A spectral display of the Doppler tissue profile then allows determination of the velocity with which the anulus moves toward the base in systole. There is a direct relationship between the anular velocity and the left ventricular ejection fraction, such that the lower the systolic velocity is, the lower the ejection fraction. Doppler tissue imaging of anular motion can also be used to determine diastolic motion, which parallels the information provided from mitral valve inflow parameters.

A final means for assessing left ventricular systolic function is calculation of the left ventricular dP/dt (see Chapter 6 for detailed methodology). This can be done from inspection of the continuous wave Doppler profile

of mitral regurgitation. To perform this calculation, the sweep speed should be set at 100 mm/sec and a high-quality Doppler signal acquired with the continuous wave beam aligned parallel to the direction of flow. Figure 17.11 is an example of the range of left ventricular dP/dt encountered in patients with dilated cardiomyopathy. This noninvasively determined dP/dt correlates well with values determined by cardiac catheterization and has been shown to have prognostic significance in patients with dilated cardiomyopathy. A dP/dt less than 600 mm Hg/sec has been associated with a worsened prognosis.

Assessment of Diastolic Function

Assessment of diastolic function in dilated cardiomyopathy provides valuable clues to the pathology underlying the development of symptoms. Currently, this is most commonly evaluated with Doppler interrogation of diastolic inflow patterns. One M-mode finding has retained clinical relevance, which is the b bump of mitral valve closure (Fig. 17.6A). The b bump has been associated with elevated left atrial pressure, which in turn reflects ventricular end-diastolic pressure, typically exceeding 20 mm Hg. When combined with a suspected pseudonormal pattern of mitral valve inflow, it may provide essential information regarding elevated diastolic pressures.

A hierarchy of diastolic flow profiles can be seen when interrogating the mitral valve in patients with dilated car-

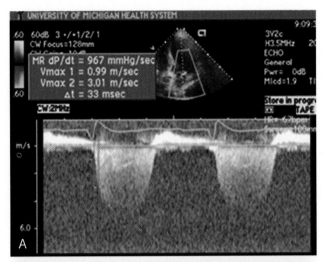

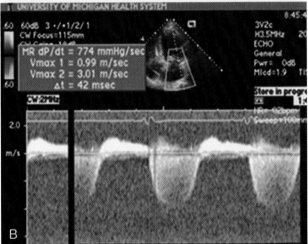

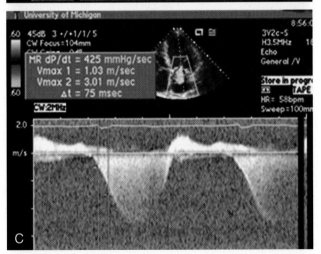

FIGURE 17.11. Examples of left ventricular dP/dt calculated from the continuous wave Doppler spectral display of mitral regurgitation in three patients with dilated cardiomyopathy and varying degrees of left ventricular systolic dysfunction. **A:** Left ventricular dP/dt is relatively preserved at 967 mm Hg/sec. **B, C:** Moderate and marked reduction in left ventricular dP/dt is noted.

diomyopathy. These are schematized in Figure 17.12. As discussed in Chapter 6, it is important to integrate multiple observations of diastolic function to reliably determine the status of left atrial filling pressures and overall diastolic function. The echocardiographic and Doppler parameters that can be used to evaluate diastolic dysfunction in dilated cardiomyopathy are listed in Table 17.3. This includes a number of essential observations that should be obtained in individuals with cardiomyopathy and include mitral valve inflow patterns and Doppler tissue imaging for anular velocity.

Pulmonary vein flow Doppler recordings can be obtained from an apical view in most patients. Normal pulmonary vein flow occurs in both ventricular systole and diastole, and there is a brief retrograde flow that corresponds to atrial contraction (A-wave reversal). Figure 17.12 schematizes the progressive decrease in systolic flow and the increasingly prominent A-wave reversal with progressively more severe diastolic dysfunction. Because of its ease of acquisition and quantitative nature, Doppler tissue imaging of the mitral anulus has largely supplanted pulmonary vein flow analysis in most laboratories.

As noted in Figure 17.12, there is a hierarchy of abnormalities of diastolic function beginning with delayed relaxation and progressing to end-stage "restrictive" and irreversible physiology that implies markedly elevated left ventricular diastolic pressure. Many patients with intermediate levels of diastolic dysfunction will have a pseudonormal pattern in which the mitral valve E/A ratio is nor-

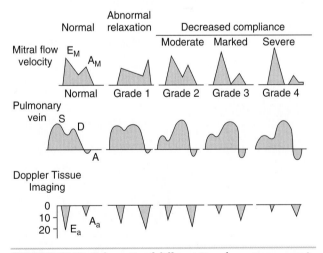

FIGURE 17.12. Schematic of different Doppler patterns seen in healthy subjects and patients with varying stages of diastolic dysfunction. **Top:** The mitral inflow pattern recorded from the apex of the left ventricle. **Middle:** Pulmonary vein flow. **Bottom:** Doppler tissue imaging recorded from the mitral valve anulus. In general, the appearance of grade 4 dysfunction is similar to that of grade 3. Clinically, grade 4 is considered irreversible, whereas the grade 3 pattern will revert to grade 2 with maneuvers that reduce LV filling acutely or after successful therapy. See text for further details. A, A-wave reversal; D, diastole; S, systole.

mal in the presence of diastolic dysfunction. This pattern can be seen either as the patient progresses from mild diastolic dysfunction to more severe stages (grade 1 to 3 in Fig. 17.12) or as a patient is treated and has reduced left ventricular diastolic pressures and improves from grade 3 to 1. There are several ancillary measures that can help identify the pseudonormal pattern including evaluating pulmonary vein flow (Fig. 17.13), Doppler tissue imaging of the mitral anulus (Fig. 17.14), or reevaluating the mitral inflow pattern during the Valsalva maneuver. During the Valsalva maneuver, flow into the left heart is reduced

and left atrial and ventricular diastolic pressure is decreased, resulting in a reduction in the E-wave velocity and reversal of the pseudonormal E/A ratio to reveal a pattern of abnormal relaxation (Fig. 17.15).

By combining the mitral valve inflow pattern with information from Doppler tissue imaging of the anulus, an index of mitral valve (E_m) to anular E velocity (E_a) can be obtained. This index E_m/E_a is linearly related to left atrial filling pressure, as can be seen in Figures 17.14 and 17.16. The majority of individuals with E_m/E_a of 20 or more have markedly elevated pulmonary papillary wedge pressures of 25 mm Hg or more, and individuals with E_m/E_a of less than 10 generally have low left atrial filling pressures. E_m/E_a values between 10 and 20 have been associated with a broad range of filling pressures. This measure appears independent of heart rate and, because it relies only on early filling velocities, is also valid in patients in atrial fibrillation.

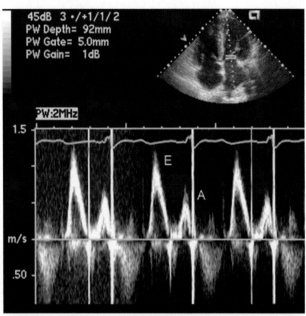

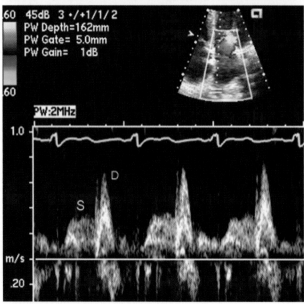

FIGURE 17.13. Example of a patient with a pseudonormal mitral inflow pattern (grade 2 diastolic dysfunction). Note the E/A ratio of approximately 1.8 but the reduced systolic velocity in the pulmonary veins. D, diastole, S, systole.

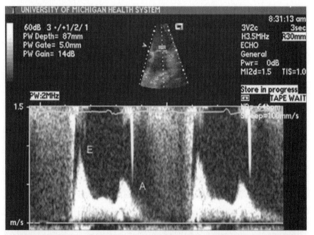

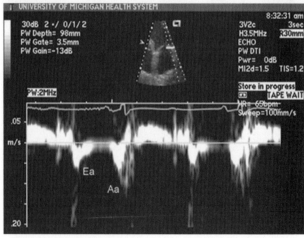

FIGURE 17.14. Mitral inflow pattern **(A)** and anular Doppler tissue imaging velocities **(B)** recorded in a patient with diastolic dysfunction. Note the normal mitral valve E/A ratio but the reduced E_a/A_a ratio, implying diastolic dysfunction. In this example, the mitral E velocity is 100 cm/sec and the anular E_a velocity is approximately 5 cm/sec. The ratio E_m/E_a is 20, implying markedly elevated left atrial pressure (Fig. 17.16).

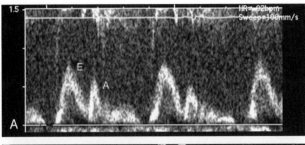

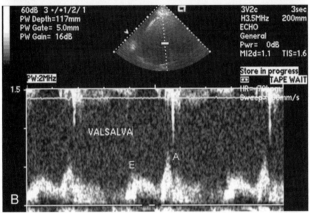

FIGURE 17.15. Effect of the Valsalva maneuver on the mitral inflow pattern in a patient with diastolic dysfunction. **A:** Note the normal E/A ratio. During the Valsalva maneuver **(B)**, left atrial and left ventricular volume is diminished and a reversed E/A ratio is uncovered.

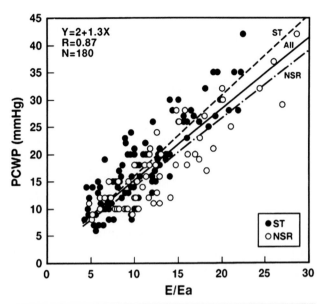

FIGURE 17.16. Graphic representation of pulmonary capillary wedge pressure (*PCWP*) and mitral E/anular E_a ratio. Note the direct relationship between pulmonary capillary wedge pressure and the ratio E_m/E_a in which the majority of patients with an E_m/E_a ratio less than 10 have a pulmonary capillary wedge pressure less than 15 mm Hg, whereas those with a ratio more than 20 typically have a pulmonary capillary wedge pressure more than 20 mm Hg. (From Nagueh SF, Mikati I, Kopelen HA, et al. Doppler estimation of left ventricular filling pressure in sinus tachycardia. A new application of tissue Doppler imaging. Circulation 1998;98:1644–1650, with permission.)

Other echocardiographic modalities that can be used to evaluate diastolic dysfunction include color M-mode echocardiography of mitral valve inflow. From this, a velocity of propagation (V_p) of inflow can be calculated from the slope of the leading edge of the M-mode color flow signal. In normal hearts, V_p exceeds 50 mm/sec with progressively lower V_p implying greater degrees of diastolic dysfunction. Measurement of V_p appears to be a relatively preload independent marker of diastolic dysfunction. Figure 17.17 is a color Doppler M-mode image recorded in a patient with marked systolic and diastolic dysfunction. In Figure 17.17A, a normal mitral valve inflow pattern is noted for comparison. With marked diastolic dysfunction, there is a reduction in the velocity of inflow that is seen as a flattened slope of the mitral valve color flow profile and a decrease in depth toward the apex to which the flow propagates in an organized manner.

Myocardial Performance Index

The myocardial performance index is a unitless number reflecting global left ventricular performance. It is defined as the ratio of the total isovolumic times (isovolumetric contraction and relaxation) to ejection time (Figs. 17.18 and 17.19). It is calculated from Doppler spectral tracings of the left ventricular outflow tract and mitral valve inflow. Normally, this value is 0.40 or less, with increasing values representing progressively worse left ventricular performance. It has been shown to provide independent prognostic information in patients with heart failure due to dilated cardiomyopathy.

Secondary Findings in Dilated Cardiomyopathy

The anatomic and pathologic secondary features of dilated cardiomyopathy that can be detected with echocardiography are listed in Table 17.2. Some of these secondary findings such as left atrial dilation and right heart involvement are nearly ubiquitous and an essential part of establishing the diagnosis. Others such as secondary mitral regurgitation, thrombus formation, and secondary pulmonary hypertension occur to a variable degree and are dependent on both the severity and duration of cardiomyopathy.

As noted previously, some degree of left atrial dilation is ubiquitous and dependent on the duration of cardiomyopathy. The left atrium can dilate to substantial dimensions, and left atrial dimensions of 8 and 9 cm are occasionally encountered. More recently, left atrial area or volume has been measured from the apical view. Recent

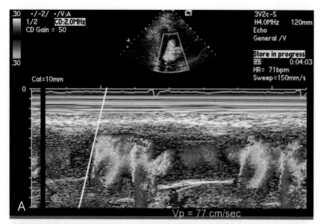

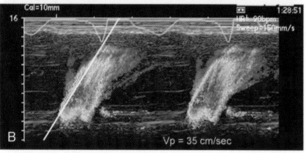

FIGURE 17.17. Color Doppler M-mode imaging of mitral inflow in a patient with normal systolic and diastolic function **(A)** and abnormal systolic and diastolic function **(B)**. **A:** Note the relatively steep slope of the color Doppler M-mode signal with a velocity of propagation (V_p) of 77 cm/sec compared with the relatively flat slope in **B** (V_p = 35 cm/sec), which was recorded in a patient with combined systolic and diastolic dysfunction.

data have suggested a strong relationship between the left atrial area and prognosis. In the setting of left ventricular dysfunction, left atrial dilation, whether quantified as a linear dimension or area, is a marker of more severe and more long-standing ventricular dysfunction. Left atrial dilation is largely due to elevated diastolic pressures in the left ventricle and often concurrent mitral regurgitation. It may also be due to a myopathic process in the atrial wall. All this results in a heightened likelihood of developing atrial fibrillation or flutter. As a consequence of left atrial dilation, especially if seen in the presence of poor atrial mechanical function or atrial fibrillation, left atrial spontaneous contrast is not uncommonly encountered, most often with transesophageal imaging. Occasionally, spontaneous contrast may be seen in the body of the left ventricle as well (Fig. 17.20).

Formation of mural thrombus in patients with dilated cardiomyopathy is less frequent than in patients with myocardial infarction. Thrombus is diagnosed when an echo-dense filling defect is noted in the ventricular cavity (Figs. 17.21 and 17.22), which may be laminar, pedunculated, or mobile.

Because of the increasing spherical geometry of the left ventricle, normal coaptation of the mitral valve leaflets becomes interrupted as the papillary muscles are dis-

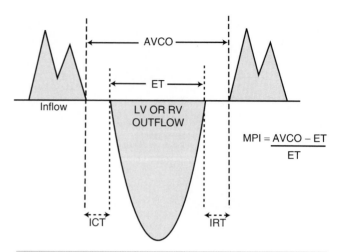

FIGURE 17.18. Schematic outlining the calculation of the myocardial performance index (_MPI_). In this schematic, the atrioventricular valve (formula can be used for either the mitral or tricuspid valve) inflow and ventricular outflow velocities are simultaneously displayed. In actual practice, the velocities may be recorded from slightly different angles and measurements made separately. The myocardial performance index is calculated as noted on the schematic. Normal MPI, ≤0.40, with progressively larger MPI implying worsened myocardial performance. AVCO, atrioventricular valve closure to opening interval; ICT, isovolumic contraction time; IRT, isovolumic relaxation time; LV, left ventricle; RV, right ventricle.

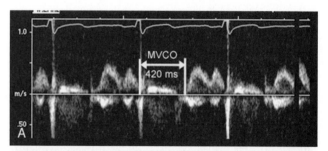

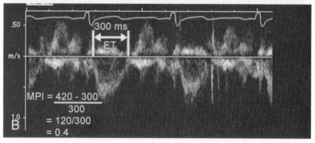

FIGURE 17.19. Demonstration of the Doppler spectral recordings required to calculate the myocardial performance index. **A:** Recording of mitral inflow from which the atrioventricular valve closure to opening interval is calculated. **B:** Recorded from the left ventricular outflow tract, from which the ejection time (_ET_) can be determined. In this instance, the value for myocardial performance index (_MPI_) was 0.4, as noted in the calculations superimposed on the figure. MVCO, mitral valve closure to opening time.

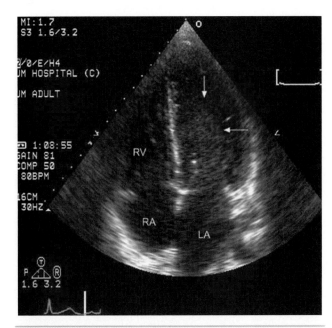

FIGURE 17.20. Apical four-chamber view recorded in a patient with a dilated cardiomyopathy and spontaneous echo contrast (*arrows*) in the cavity of the left ventricle. In the real-time image, there is a vague cloud-like echo density with a swirling motion in the left ventricular cavity. LA, left atrium; RA, right atrium; RV, right ventricle.

placed apically and laterally. This results in a shortened length of coaptation of the mitral valve leaflets which ordinarily coapt along a several-millimeter length of their edge (the *zona coapta*). With displacement of the papillary muscles, functional mitral regurgitation occurs as the leaflets coapt only at their tips or occasionally fail to make contact at all during systole. Figures 17.23 through 17.26 depict varying degrees of papillary muscle dysfunction in patients with dilated cardiomyopathy and functional mitral regurgitation. The quantitation of mitral regurgitation is undertaken in a manner identical to that described in Chapter 11 for other etiologies of mitral regurgitation.

Because of either concurrent involvement of the right ventricle or secondary pulmonary hypertension and subsequent tricuspid anular dilation, tricuspid regurgitation is frequently noted in advanced cardiomyopathy (Fig. 17.27). The tricuspid regurgitation jet can be used to determine right ventricular systolic pressure as for any other cause of pulmonary hypertension.

ETIOLOGY OF DILATED CARDIOMYOPATHY

It is often not possible to determine the etiology of a dilated cardiomyopathy with echocardiography. Table 17.1 lists a number of the dilated cardiomyopathies, some of which can be specifically identified using echocardiographic techniques. Generally, the most common distinction to be made is between an ischemic and nonischemic cardiomyopathy. Distinguishing features of an ischemic

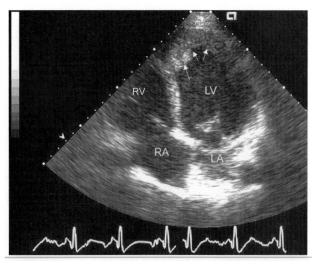

FIGURE 17.21. Apical four-chamber view recorded in a patient with a dilated cardiomyopathy and a pedunculated thrombus in the left ventricular apex (*arrows*). LA, left atrium; LV, left ventricle; RA, right atrium; RV, right ventricle.

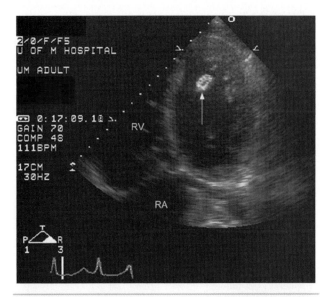

FIGURE 17.22. Apical four-chamber view recorded in a patient with a dilated cardiomyopathy, severe systolic dysfunction, and a mobile thrombus in the left ventricle (*arrow*). In the real-time image, the bright echo density can be seen to be highly mobile and to arise from a more laminar component of the apical thrombus. RA, right atrium; RV, right ventricle.

cardiomyopathy include a relatively greater degree of regional heterogeneity of systolic function often with areas of frank scar or aneurysm formation. When either a substantial area of scar, conforming to a well-defined coronary territory or left ventricular aneurysm is noted, the likelihood of an ischemic etiology is high. Figure 17.5 was recorded in a patient with a classic ischemic cardiomyopathy. There was global left ventricular dysfunction with frank akinesis with a shallow aneurysm in the posterior wall, allowing an echocardiographic diagnosis of ischemic cardiac disease to be made. Often patients will

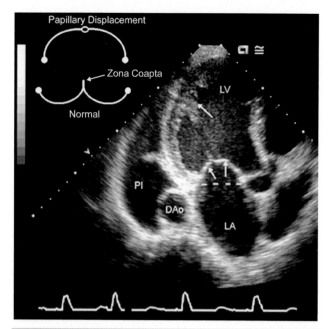

FIGURE 17.23. Apical long-axis view recorded in a patient with a dilated cardiomyopathy and posterior and lateral displacement of the papillary muscles (*arrow*). The *dotted line* indicates the plane of the mitral anulus. Note that the closed mitral valve leaflets bow into the cavity of the left ventricle (*arrows*). The functional shortening of the mitral apparatus compared with the dimension of the ventricle results in tip-to-tip coaptation of the mitral leaflets and secondary mitral regurgitation. The normal coaptation pattern and abnormal pattern are schematized in the upper left. DAo, descending thoracic aorta; LA, left atrium; LV, left ventricle; Pl, pleural effusion.

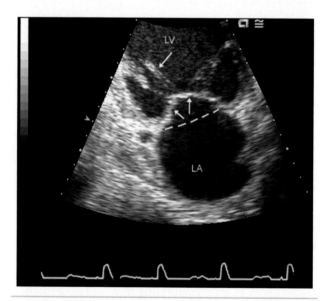

FIGURE 17.24. Expanded view recorded in the same patient is noted in Figure 17.23. The *dotted line* represents the plane of the mitral anulus. Note that the entire length of both mitral leaflets is displaced apically from the anulus (*arrows*) with abnormal tip to tip coaptation. Both papillary muscles have been displaced apically (*downward-pointing arrow*). LA, left atrium; LV, left ventricle.

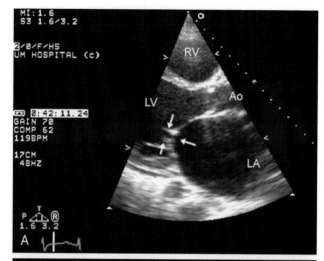

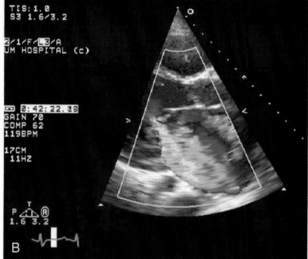

FIGURE 17.25. Parasternal long-axis echocardiogram recorded in a patient with a dilated cardiomyopathy and functional mitral regurgitation. **A:** Recorded in mid-systole. Note the leaflet tips are coapting tip to tip (*vertical arrows*). In this instance, there is failure of coaptation and the actual regurgitant orifice can be directly visualized (*horizontal arrow*). **B:** Recorded with color flow Doppler imaging, moderate to severe mitral regurgitation is revealed that can be seen to arise from the area of the non-coapted leaflets. Ao, aorta; LA, left atrium; LV, left ventricle; RV, right ventricle.

present with a dilated and globally hypokinetic ventricle but no obvious evidence of myocardial infarction. In these instances, there may be no echocardiographic features that allow an ischemic versus nonischemic etiology to be firmly established. Even in the presence of a nonischemic cardiomyopathy, there will be regional variation in left ventricular systolic dysfunction, typically with the proximal inferoposterior and posterior lateral walls having preserved function when compared with the other regions. Because of heterogeneity in regional wall stress, the degree of dysfunction can also vary when apical and basal segments are compared.

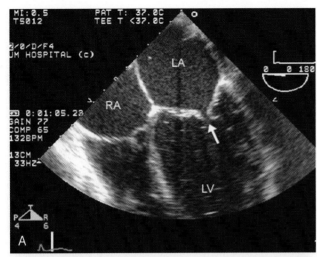

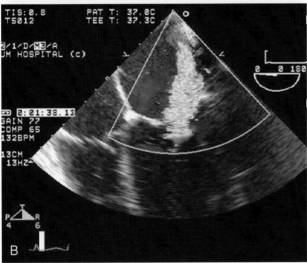

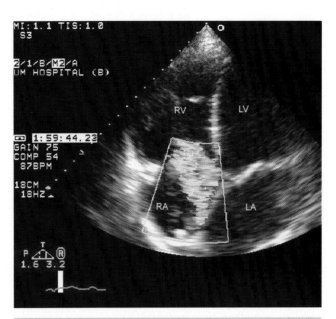

FIGURE 17.27. Apical four-chamber view recorded in a patient with a dilated cardiomyopathy and secondary right ventricular dysfunction. Due to the combination of right ventricular dysfunction and pulmonary hypertension, the tricuspid anulus is dilated, and there is evidence of moderate secondary tricuspid regurgitation and elevated right ventricular systolic pressure. In this example, the right ventricular systolic pressure and, by inference, the pulmonary artery systolic pressure can be calculated as 70 mm Hg from the continuous wave Doppler image, which revealed a right ventricular-right atrial gradient of 55 mm Hg. LA, left atrium; LV left ventricle; RA, right atrium; RV, right ventricle.

FIGURE 17.26. Transesophageal echocardiogram recorded in the same patient depicted in Figure 17.25. **A:** Recorded in midsystole. There is failure of coaptation due to lateral displacement of the papillary muscles and tethering of the mitral valve toward the apex. The actual gap between the leaflet tips can be visualized (*arrow*). **B:** Color flow Doppler was used to demonstrate the mitral regurgitation jet that arises centrally from the area denoted by the *arrow* in **A**. LA, left atrium; LV, left ventricle; RA, right atrium.

One form of dilated cardiomyopathy that can be diagnosed with near certainty using echocardiographic techniques is noncompaction of the myocardium. Developmentally, the ventricular myocardium begins as a series of sinusoids that then compress or compact into the organized myocardial fibers. Occasionally during development, compaction fails to occur and the ventricular myocardium persists in the embryonic noncompacted state, which does not provide the requisite level of contractile efficiency to protect ventricular geometry. Typically, these individuals will present in either childhood or the second or third decade of life, often with arrhythmias, left ven-

tricular dilation, and global systolic dysfunction. Figure 17.28 was recorded in a patient with noncompacted myocardium. Note the honeycombed appearance of the myocardium, most prominent at the apex. This type of appearance initially could be confused with multiple ventricular thrombi, but its generalized diffuse nature including at the base of the heart is a distinguishing characteristic that allows the diagnosis of noncompaction to be made.

Many dilated cardiomyopathies are the sequelae of acute myocarditis that may not have been clinically recognized. If echocardiographic imaging is performed early in the course of this disease, one classically will note relatively preserved wall thickness and chamber size with global systolic dysfunction. If there is no spontaneous recovery of the myocarditis, progressive dilation and wall thinning with increasing left ventricular dysfunction will typically occur. More often, however, patients present after the chambers have dilated and thinned and therefore are indistinguishable from cardiomyopathy from other etiologies.

Poorly controlled hypertension results in hypertensive cardiovascular disease and, when long-standing, the appearance of a dilated cardiomyopathy. In this instance,

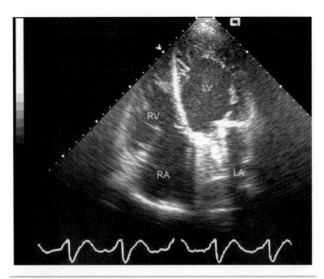

FIGURE 17.28. Apical four-chamber view recorded in a patient with a dilated cardiomyopathy due to noncompaction of the ventricular myocardium. Note the fairly thick network of sinusoidal spaces in the apex. On occasion, this appearance could be confused with thrombus; however, its generalized nature throughout the majority of the ventricular myocardium is classic for noncompacted myocardium. LA, left atrium; LV, left ventricle; RA, right atrium; RV, right ventricle.

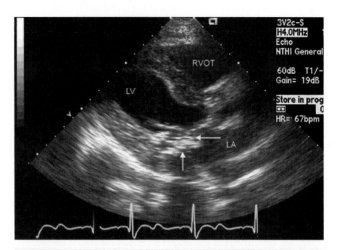

FIGURE 17.29. Parasternal long-axis view recorded in a patient with end-stage renal disease. Note the uniform left ventricular hypertrophy and the extensive mitral anular calcification (*arrows*). In this instance, there was significant systolic dysfunction as well. LA, left atrium; LV, left ventricle; RVOT, right ventricular outflow tract.

left ventricular hypertrophy typically persists in the presence of chamber dilation and global dysfunction. This combination of hypertrophy with moderate degrees of dilation and global dysfunction is fairly typical of hypertensive cardiovascular disease with subsequent left ventricular dysfunction but also could be mimicked by a variety of infiltrative diseases.

Long-standing renal disease typically in a patient on dialysis can also result in a fairly characteristic cardiomyopathy. Figure 17.29 was recorded in a patient with insulin-dependent diabetes and long-standing end-stage renal disease on dialysis. The concurrent metabolic abnormalities and hypertension resulted in anular calcification with marked left ventricular hypertrophy. Left ventricular systolic dysfunction and congestive heart failure are present due to a combination of metabolic effects and the effects of long-standing hypertrophy. On occasion, such individuals have shown improvement in ventricular function after either renal transplantation or more aggressive dialysis regimens.

DETERMINATION OF PROGNOSIS IN DILATED CARDIOMYOPATHY

Several echocardiographic and Doppler findings can be related to prognosis in dilated cardiomyopathy. These are listed in Table 17.4. As with all other imaging techniques, including radionuclide ventriculography and contrast ventriculography, any of the systolic indices such as ejec-

tion fraction can be accurately calculated and are related to prognosis.

Doppler ultrasound techniques also can be used to derive prognostic indices. The most commonly employed technique is interrogation of mitral valve inflow patterns. The Doppler finding carrying the most important prognostic information is that of the so-called restrictive pattern (Fig. 17.30). This is characterized as a high E/A ratio, typically greater than 2.5, in association with a short deceleration time (typically <130–150 milliseconds). This pattern indicates a near end-stage degree of diastolic dysfunction in which the left ventricle has dilated to the point of reaching mechanical and pericardial constraint. This pattern also implies marked elevation of end-diastolic and left atrial pressures and as such is often seen in individuals with the more marked degrees of left atrial dilation and secondary pulmonary hypertension. The adverse

▶ **TABLE 17.4 Echocardiographic and Doppler Predictors of Adverse Prognosis in Cardiomyopathy**

Left ventricular size and function
    Left ventricular internal dimension
    Left ventricular end-diastolic volume >75 mL/m²
    Left ventricular end-systolic volume >55 mL/m²
    Left ventricular ejection fraction <0.4
    Sphericity index <1.5
    Left ventricular dP/dt <600 mm Hg/sec
    Myocardial performance index >0.4
Diastolic properties of the left ventricle
    Restrictive mitral inflow pattern
    Pseudonormal mitral inflow pattern

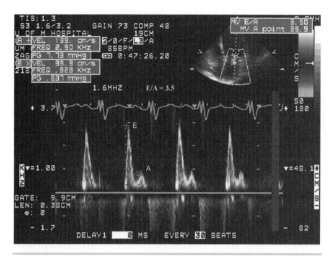

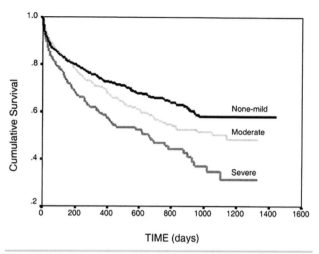

FIGURE 17.30. Pulsed Doppler mitral inflow pattern recorded in a patient with a dilated cardiomyopathy and severe diastolic dysfunction. Note the E/A ratio of approximately 3.0 with a short deceleration time. This is the pattern seen in grade 3 or 4 diastolic dysfunction.

FIGURE 17.32. Relationship of survival to the severity of mitral regurgitation in patients with cardiomyopathy and reduced systolic function. Note the progressively worse outcome comparing patients with none to mild, moderate, and severe mitral regurgitation. (From Koelling TM, Aaronson KD, Cody RJ, et al. Prognostic significance of mitral regurgitation and tricuspid regurgitation in patients with left ventricular systolic dysfunction. Am Heart J 2002;144:524–529, with permission.)

prognosis associated with a restrictive filling pattern has been demonstrated in numerous studies. Figure 17.31 outlines the outcome in a series of patients with dilated cardiomyopathy, stratified by the ejection fraction and the presence or absence of restrictive filling. Note the relatively benign outcome in individuals with relatively preserved left ventricular function versus those with reduced left ventricular function and the incrementally worse prognosis when a restrictive filling pattern is present.

Additionally, the left ventricular dP/dt, calculated from mitral regurgitation spectral velocity, also has been shown to carry prognostic information with the likelihood of events being inversely proportional to positive and negative dP/dt.

The presence of mitral and tricuspid regurgitation also affects prognosis. As a general rule, more severe mitral regurgitation is the sequela of greater left ventricular dilation and changes in geometry, and, as such, the impact of mitral regurgitation independent of the underlying process is difficult to establish. Several studies have demonstrated, however, that increasing degrees of mitral and tricuspid regurgitation correlate with a worsening prognosis. Figure 17.32 represents the mortality rates in a large series of individuals with congestive heart failure, systolic dysfunction, and varying degrees of mitral regurgitation. Severe mitral regurgitation in the presence of systolic dysfunction in patients with congestive heart failure carries a prognosis substantially worse than that of individuals with lesser degrees of mitral regurgitation.

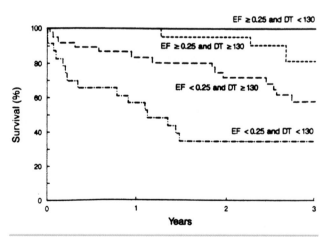

FIGURE 17.31. Graphic representation of survival in patients with dilated cardiomyopathy stratified by ejection fraction (*EF*) and mitral valve deceleration time (*DT*). Note the relatively benign prognosis with an EF of 0.25 or more. For the subsets of patients with an EF of less than 0.25, there was a substantially worse outcome for the subset with a DT of less than 130 milliseconds compared with those with a DT of 130 milliseconds or more. (From Rihal CS, Nishimura RA, Hatle LK, et al. Systolic and diastolic dysfunction in patients with clinical diagnosis of dilated cardiomyopathy. Relation to symptoms and prognosis. Circulation 1994;90:2772–2779, with permission.)

THERAPEUTIC DECISIONS

Although decisions regarding specific forms of medical and nonmedical therapy should be made on clinical grounds and incorporating all available data, the echocardiogram can play a valuable role in stratifying patients into different therapeutic subtypes. Obviously, detection of a dilated cardiomyopathy with systolic dysfunction identifies a patient for whom afterload reduction therapy, typically with an angiotensin-converting enzyme inhibitor, is clinically warranted and has been shown to provide symptomatic and prognostic benefit. Similarly, avoidance of this type of therapy in individuals with other types of cardiomyopathy (e.g., hypertrophic) allows appropriate decision making regarding therapy. Identification of individuals with restrictive physiology identifies an end-stage subpopulation for whom very aggressive management is indicated, and when combined with other parameters such as the E_m/E_a ratio may identify a subset of patients likely to be volume overloaded for whom aggressive diuretic therapy may be beneficial. It should be emphasized, however, that individual decisions regarding appropriate specific therapies should be made using a combination of clinical, echocardiographic, and other information and not solely echocardiographic observations.

Biventricular Pacing for Congestive Heart Failure

A recent approach to treatment of congestive heart failure symptoms in patients with dilated cardiomyopathy has been biventricular pacing. A subset of patients with dilated cardiomyopathy and left bundle branch block have marked mechanical dyssynchrony, which results in inefficient left ventricular contraction and reduced stroke volume. Early attempts at identifying patients most likely to benefit from biventricular pacing involved measurement of the QRS duration. Recently, studies using echocardiography or radionuclide ventriculography for wall motion analysis have suggested that identifying patients on the basis of mechanical dyssynchrony may be a more appropriate and accurate means for identifying patients likely to benefit. The hypothesis underlying biventricular pacing is that simultaneously pacing the ventricular septum and lateral wall of the left ventricle will result in simultaneous contraction of both left ventricular walls as opposed to the dyssynchronous contraction seen in the native left bundle branch block. Clinical studies have demonstrated that successful biventricular pacing results in an improved left ventricular ejection fraction, reduction in left ventricular volumes, often reduction in the magnitude of secondary mitral regurgitation, and improvement in symptomatic and functional status.

By identifying patients with more marked degrees of mechanical dyssynchrony, echocardiography can play a valuable role in appropriately selecting patients for this expensive new technology. The hypothesis is that only those patients with more marked degrees of mechanical dyssynchrony will benefit from biventricular pacing. The simplest method for determining the magnitude of mechanical dyssynchrony is to determine the delay between contraction of the septum and posterior wall using either M-mode echocardiography or more recently Doppler tissue imaging. A second role that echocardiography can play is in optimizing the atrioventricular delay for atrioventricular pacing. A complete titration of atrioventricular delay can be done while monitoring a variety of parameters of left ventricular performance, including severity of mitral regurgitation, left ventricular ejection fraction, and the TVI of the left ventricular outflow tract (Fig. 17.33). In general, a relatively short atrioventricular delay results in maximal improvement in left ventricular performance during atrioventricular pacing.

Other parameters of left ventricular performance that can be followed include the dP/dt of left ventricular pressure generation, which can be derived from the spectral display of mitral regurgitation. Because there is dyssynchronous contraction of the left ventricular walls, pressure generation within the cavity of the left ventricle is not efficient, as contraction of the lateral wall may not begin until well after that of the septal wall. This results in a relatively narrow time window in which all walls are contracting simultaneously and a more gradual generation of pressure development within the left ventricular cavity. Resynchronization with biventricular pacing results in a greater time of mutual contraction of all left ventricular walls and hence the steeper increase in pressure generation within the left ventricle, which is manifested as an increased dP/dt during biventricular pacing. Newer generations of biventricular pacemakers will allow programming of the delay between left ventricular and right ventricular activation and will probably increase the need for detailed echocardiographic/Doppler monitoring for optimizing these devices. Figure 17.34 is an example of a patient with a dilated cardiomyopathy and marked left ventricular dyssynchrony who has undergone biventricular pacing. Over a 6-month period, there was a progressive increase in the left ventricular ejection fraction from 15% to 40%, with improvement of all other parameters including the left ventricular dP/dt and severity of mitral regurgitation.

Cardiac Transplantation

Cardiac transplantation remains a therapeutic option for patients with congestive heart failure or other end-stage cardiovascular disease. Although the operative approach to transplantation is relatively straightforward, the evaluation and management of patients after cardiac transplant remain challenging. Current practice mandates that repeat endomyocardial biopsy be performed to screen for cardiac rejection. Several echocardiographic and noninvasive procedures have been evaluated as markers of transplant rejection in an effort to find a less invasive means of monitoring rejection. To date, accuracy is not

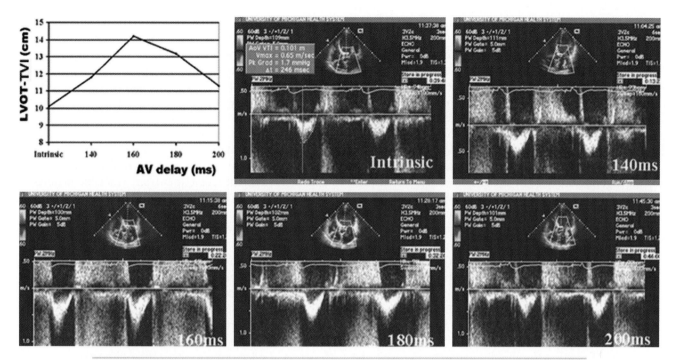

FIGURE 17.33. Impact of varying atrioventricular (*AV*) delay during biventricular pacing on left ventricular outflow tract time velocity integral (*TVI*). Five examples of the left ventricular outflow tract (*LVOT*) spectral Doppler imaging are presented during intrinsic rhythm and during biventricular pacing at AV delay ranging from 140 to 200 milliseconds. A graphic demonstration of the AV delay versus Doppler tissue imaging is shown in the upper left. Note the maximal forward flow occurs during biventricular pacing with AV delay of 160 milliseconds in this patient.

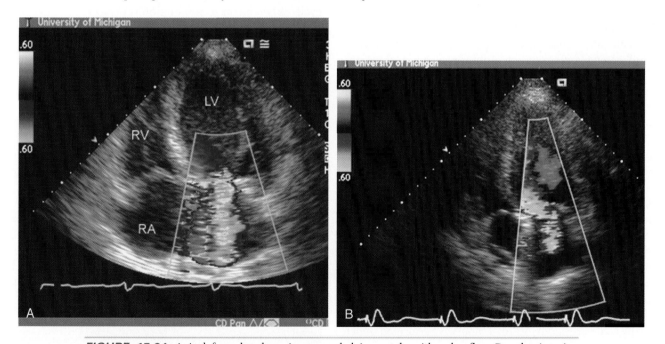

FIGURE 17.34. Apical four-chamber view recorded in systole with color flow Doppler imaging recorded in a patient before (**A**) and 6 months after (**B**) institution of biventricular pacing. **A:** Note the markedly dilated left ventricle with relatively spherical geometry and the presence of moderate mitral regurgitation. **B:** Note the substantial decrease in left ventricular internal dimension, the more bullet-shaped geometry, the smaller cavity area at an equivalent time in the cardiac cycle, and the marked decrease in severity of mitral regurgitation. LV, left ventricle; RA, right atrium; RV, right ventricle.

sufficient to warrant their widespread application, and none has had widespread acceptance.

One of the earliest echocardiographic findings in acute rejection was pericardial effusion and increased left ventricular wall thickness, presumably due to inflammation and myocardial edema. Although occasionally noted at the time of acute fulminant rejection, this sign has not been a reliable indicator in all patients with rejection and is not present in milder and moderate forms of rejection.

Other echocardiographic features that have been evaluated have included serial evaluation of left ventricular systolic function, which may decrease with acute severe rejection or after long-standing rejection of lesser severity. Unfortunately, reduction in left ventricular systolic function is an end-stage phenomenon and therefore cannot be relied on for early monitoring of rejection. Patients who have undergone cardiac transplantation have an accelerated rate of coronary atherosclerosis, even if both the donor and recipient are relatively young. This has been referred to as transplant vasculopathy. In these individuals, premature coronary artery disease develops, the sequela of which is acute myocardial infarction. Because the transplanted heart is denervated, these infarcts, although sometimes of substantial magnitude, are often clinically "silent." As such, development of congestive heart failure in a patient after cardiac transplantation should result in an echocardiographic search for occult myocardial infarction.

Doppler echocardiography has been used in various formats for detection of cardiac rejection. The earlier studies relied on evaluation of mitral valve E/A ratios under the assumption that early rejection would result in worsening diastolic function. Diastolic function of the transplanted heart, even in the absence of rejection, is often abnormal, and, as such, no given Doppler parameter showed significant discriminatory ability for separation of rejection from nonrejection in patients. More recently, Doppler tissue imaging has been used to evaluate mitral anular or direct myocardial motion in transplant recipients. Early results have been encouraging, and this technique may provide an earlier marker of rejection than previously described echocardiographic or Doppler parameters. At this time, however, no single or combination of echocardiographic or Doppler parameters should be considered as a reliable indicator of the presence or absence of milder forms of cardiac rejection. As such, endomyocardial biopsy will continue to be necessary. In many centers, endomyocardial biopsy is performed under direct echocardiographic surveillance.

Ventricular Assist Devices

Modern therapy of end-stage cardiovascular disease involves a wide range of medical and mechanical options. As noted previously, echocardiography plays a major role in the diagnosis of dilated cardiomyopathy, determination of appropriate therapy, assessment of prognosis, and effectiveness of therapy. One of the newer and more aggressive forms of therapy is a temporary left ventricular assist device, some of which can be implanted and function using portable power sources. Echocardiography plays an instrumental role in determining the success of this type of therapy and in evaluating patients for possible management outside the hospital. The mechanism by which the more common devices work is to place an inlet cannula in the left ventricular apex from which blood flows to a pulsatile pump (Fig. 17.35). Blood is then pumped into the ascending aorta. Hydrodynamically, there are several underlying cardiac factors that must be determined before placement of such a device. If aortic insufficiency is present or develops, then injection of blood, via the outlet cannula, into the ascending aorta, can result in worsening aortic regurgitation, left ventricular dysfunction, and a low-output state. Second, most patients who are candidates for long-term outpatient therapy should be identified on the basis of having some residual left ventricular function. Under ordinary operating circumstances with the left ventricular assist device operating at normal capacity, the aortic valve remains consistently closed (Fig. 17.36). By reducing the rate of the left ventricular assist device, one allows the native left ventricle an opportunity to contract and eject blood during an intrinsic systolic cycle. When intrinsic contraction is preserved to a degree sufficient to result in a forward-going stroke volume, aortic valve opening can be noted. Echocardiographic screening of patients with a left ventricular assist device

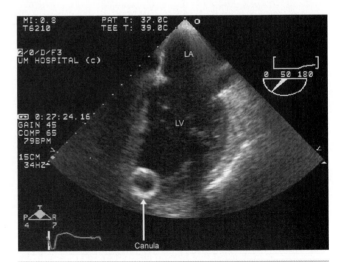

FIGURE 17.35. Transesophageal echocardiogram recorded in a patient with a left ventricular assist device. The dense circular echo in the apex of the left ventricle (*LV*) represents the tip of the inlet cannula (*arrow*), which draws blood from the left ventricular cavity to be pumped by the device into the ascending aorta. LA, left atrium.

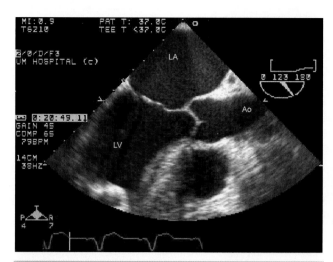

FIGURE 17.36. Transesophageal echocardiogram recorded in a longitudinal view of the left ventricular outflow tract in a patient with an implantable left ventricular assist device. Note the aortic valve is closed during systole (see electrocardiogram). In a real-time image, one can appreciate the opening and closing of the mitral valve but the persistently closed aortic valve. Ao, aorta; LA, left atrium; LV, left ventricle.

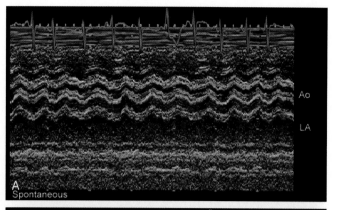

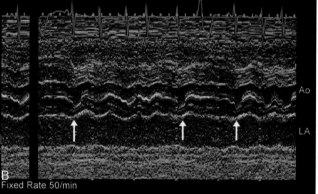

FIGURE 17.37. M-mode echocardiograms recorded in a patient with a left ventricular assist device during spontaneous device function (**A**) and with the device set at a fixed rate of 50 per minute (**B**). **A:** Note that the aortic valve remains closed continuously through the entire recording. **B:** There is intermittent opening of the aortic valve (*arrows*), indicative of sufficient residual ventricular function to overcome aortic diastolic pressure, which provides some degree of forward flow. Ao, aorta; LA, left atrium.

before discharge should be performed to ensure that there is an underlying level of left ventricular contraction sufficient to provide stroke volume and cardiac output sufficient to avoid instantaneous patient demise in the event of a catastrophic failure of the device. This can be done by observation of aortic valve motion either with two-dimensional or M-mode echocardiography or by Doppler interrogation of the left ventricular outflow tract (Fig. 17.37). An additional feature that should be evaluated is the absence of insufficiency of the valve in the inlet cannula placed in the left ventricular apex. Insufficiency of this valve results in ineffective mechanical support and represents a device failure that should be corrected.

This is a rapidly evolving field for which several different competing devices are available. The specific role to be played by echocardiography will vary with the nature of the device and the nature of the information required, whether determining suitability for the device or suitability for discharge.

INFILTRATIVE AND RESTRICTIVE CARDIOMYOPATHY

True isolated restrictive cardiomyopathy represents a relatively infrequent cause of congestive heart failure. In the pure forms, systolic function is preserved and heart failure symptoms are due to diastolic dysfunction. Several etiologies of restrictive cardiomyopathy are outlined in Table 17.1. The classic restrictive cardiomyopathy is infiltrative in nature as typified by cardiac amyloidosis. Although cardiac amyloid may be the prototypical disease causing restrictive cardiomyopathy, it is by no means the most common situation in which to identify heart failure with restrictive-type filling patterns. A number of diseases including end-stage hypertensive cardiovascular disease, hypertrophic cardiomyopathy, idiopathic restrictive cardiomyopathy, and restrictive heart disease of the elderly all present with similar pathophysiologic derangement and symptoms of congestive heart failure.

The underlying abnormality in restrictive cardiomyopathy is primary stiffening of the left ventricular myocardium and subsequent congestive heart failure due purely to diastolic dysfunction. In many of the restrictive cardiomyopathies, however, especially later in their course, a component of systolic dysfunction may be present. The pathologic stiffening of the left ventricle shifts the left ventricular compliance curve dramatically to the left and upward, such that for any given intraventricular volume, left ventricular diastolic pressures are elevated. The elevated diastolic pressure is transmitted in turn to the left atrium and pulmonary veins where it results in symptoms due to pulmonary congestion. The left and right ventricular chamber sizes typically are normal or near normal, and there is secondary and often marked dilation of both atria. This secondary atrial dilation is commonly associated with atrial fibrillation and stasis of blood flow in the atria. Secondary pulmonary hypertension may often be seen as well.

Echocardiographic Evaluation of Restrictive Cardiomyopathy

The echocardiographic hallmark of restrictive cardiomyopathy is normal ventricular size and systolic function with evidence of pathologic diastolic stiffening. Diastolic dysfunction may be often accompanied by varying degrees of increased wall thickness, whether due to left ventricular hypertrophy, as in end-stage hypertensive cardiovascular disease, or infiltration, as typified by amyloid. Biatrial enlargement is nearly ubiquitous. Varying degrees of concurrent systolic dysfunction may be noted in end-stage cases. Figures 17.38 and 17.39 were recorded in patients

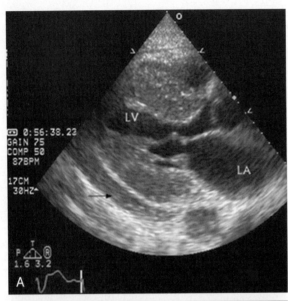

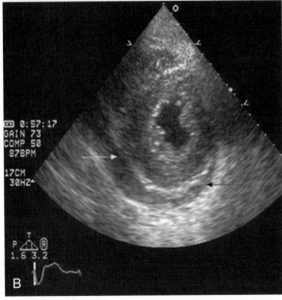

FIGURE 17.38. Parasternal long-axis **(A)** and short-axis **(B)** views recorded in a patient with cardiac amyloidosis. There is evidence of pericardial effusion (*arrow*). Note the uniform thickening of the ventricular myocardium with abnormal myocardial texture. LA, left atrium; LV, left ventricle.

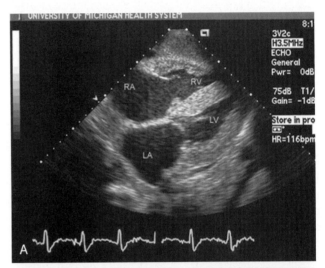

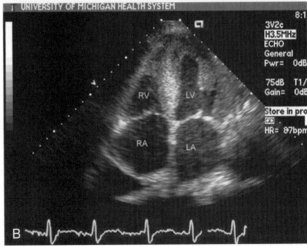

FIGURE 17.39. Subcostal **(A)** and apical four-chamber **(B)** views recorded in a patient with classic cardiac amyloidosis. In each view, note the uniform hypertrophy of the walls with abnormal myocardial texture. The myocardium is substantially brighter than normal and in real-time may take on a speckled appearance. There is secondary biatrial enlargement noted in this example. LA, left atrium; LV, left ventricle; RA, right atrium; RV, right ventricle.

with classic cardiac amyloid. Note the marked increase in ventricular wall thickness associated with abnormal myocardial texture and the involvement of the cardiac valves by the amyloid process. It should be emphasized that the findings in cardiac amyloid vary with its severity and duration. In early phases, abnormal texture may be a subtle finding and Doppler inflow patterns may suggest delayed relaxation rather than a restrictive pattern.

Figure 17.40 was recorded in a patient with the idiopathic restrictive cardiomyopathy most commonly seen in the elderly. In this instance, mild left ventricular hypertrophy without abnormal texture is present and there is marked dilation of both atria. In some instances in which an idiopathic restrictive cardiomyopathy has been detected in a relatively young patient, the underlying substrate may have been a previously unrecognized hypertrophic cardiomyopathy. Figure 17.41 depicts the Doppler examination of mitral inflow and anular velocities in the same patient presented in Figure 17.40. Note the exaggerated E/A ratio of 4.0 and the markedly reduced anular E_a velocity of 4 cm/sec.

Doppler evaluation is essential to confirm the diagnosis of restrictive cardiomyopathy. Early in the course of an infiltrative process such as amyloid, mitral inflow shows a pattern of delayed relaxation (Fig. 17.42). In advanced restrictive myopathy, one classically encounters a pathologically elevated E/A ratio of mitral valve inflow (typically ≥2.0) with a shortened deceleration time (typically <160 milliseconds) (Fig. 17.41). In distinction to constrictive pericarditis, there is less respiratory variation in E-wave velocity. Concurrent with abnormalities in mitral valve inflow, there are distinctive abnormalities in pulmonary vein flow as typified in Figure 17.13B. Color M-mode imaging of mitral valve inflow can also be used to document the abnormal filling pattern in restrictive cardiomyopathy (Fig. 17.17). Doppler tissue imaging of the mitral anulus or proximal septum reveals abnormally low diastolic Doppler velocities of the anulus in patients with restrictive cardiomyopathy (Figs. 17.41 and 17.42). The pattern of diastolic abnormality is distinct from that seen in constriction, and this can be a valuable tool for separation of a constrictive process, in which anular E_a velocities are normal.

The majority of symptoms in restrictive cardiomyopathy are due to left ventricular involvement and subsequent pulmonary congestion. It should be emphasized, however, that restrictive cardiomyopathy is often a global process, and similar pathology can be noted in the right ventricle, including varying degrees of hypertrophy and infiltration and abnormalities of tricuspid inflow and he-

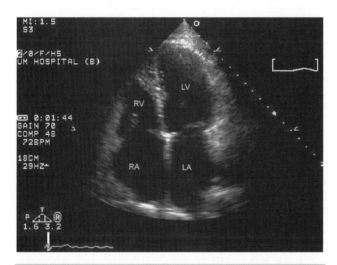

FIGURE 17.40. Apical four-chamber view recorded in a patient with an idiopathic restrictive cardiomyopathy. This was a 70-year-old patient with refractory congestive heart failure and atrial fibrillation. Note the marked biatrial enlargement and normal right and left ventricular sizes. Left ventricular systolic function was normal. LA, left atrium; LV, left ventricle; RA, right atrium; RV, right ventricle.

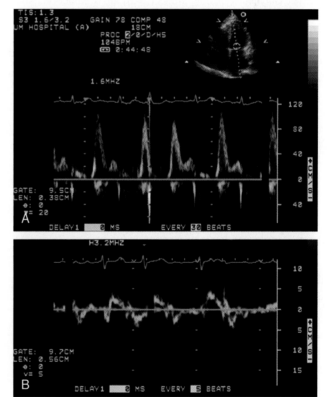

FIGURE 17.41. Pulsed Doppler imaging of mitral inflow **(A)** and anular Doppler tissue imaging **(B)** recorded in a patient with restrictive cardiomyopathy and evidence of significant diastolic dysfunction. **A:** Note the mitral E_m/A_m ratio of approximately 3.5 and the short deceleration time, typical of a restrictive process. **B:** Note the marked reduction in anular E_a velocity. In this example, the ratio of E_m/E_a is more than 25, indicative of a marked elevation in left atrial pressure.

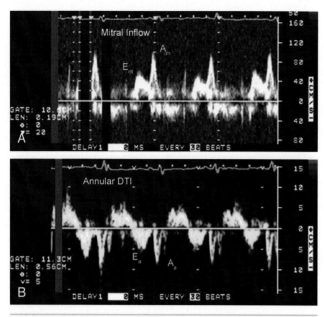

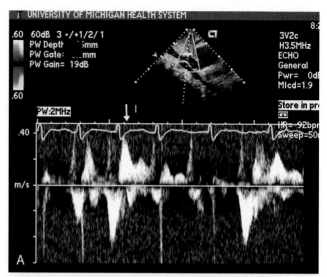

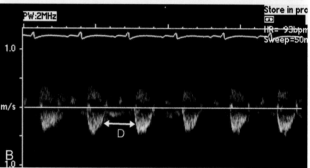

FIGURE 17.42. Pulsed Doppler of mitral inflow **(A)** and anular Doppler tissue imaging (*DTI*) **(B)** recorded in a patient with cardiac amyloid, revealing grade 1 diastolic dysfunction. Note the reduced mitral E/A ratio, which is paralleled by the Doppler tissue imaging of anular motion in diastole.

patic vein flow, which are similar to those seen on the left side. Figure 17.43 was recorded from the hepatic veins of patients with restrictive cardiomyopathy.

Other diseases can be associated with restrictive cardiomyopathy including hemachromatosis and glycogen storage diseases such as Fabry disease. Both of these are far less commonly encountered in general practice than are amyloid heart disease and the idiopathic forms seen in the elderly patients. Figure 17.44 was recorded in a patient with glycogen storage disease in which pathologic hypertrophy of the posterior wall is noted in association with Doppler evidence of restrictive filling.

Constrictive Versus Restrictive Heart Disease

Clinically, it is often difficult to differentiate between constrictive pericarditis and restrictive cardiomyopathy. Both entities can present with evidence of low-output and congestive heart failure symptoms with preserved ventricular function. Table 17.5 outlines some of the distinguishing echocardiographic and Doppler parameters that can assist in separation of these two entities. It should be emphasized that most of these observations were made in patients with either classic calcific pericarditis or classic restriction due to cardiac amyloid. In routine practice, both pericardial constriction and restrictive cardiomyopathy may be present in incomplete forms with variable involvement of cardiac chambers, and no single distinguishing feature is fully accurate for separation of the two entities.

FIGURE 17.43. Hepatic vein pulsed Doppler recordings from two patients with documented, restrictive cardiomyopathy showing the variability in inflow patterns that can be seen. **A:** Note the loss of smooth multiphasic flow out of the hepatic vein and the distinct inspiratory reversal of flow (*downward-pointing arrow*). **B:** Recorded in a patient with cardiac amyloid and abnormal hepatic vein flow. Note the lack of any respiratory variation and the forward flow out of the hepatic vein, which is confined exclusively to the systolic portion of the cardiac cycle. Note that there is little or no flow during diastole (*D*) (*double-headed arrow*). In this example, there also is no respiratory reversal of flow.

In many instances, there will be little confusion differentiating between constrictive pericarditis and restrictive cardiomyopathy if classic anatomic findings are present. As such, when a patient presents with symmetrically hypertrophied walls with abnormal myocardial texture, diffuse valve thickening, biatrial enlargement, and a restrictive mitral inflow pattern, the diagnosis of cardiac amyloid is reasonably assured and constrictive pericarditis is less of a clinical consideration. For other, less classic forms of restrictive cardiomyopathy, the underlying left ventricular anatomy may not provide a definitive answer and further evaluation of cardiac physiology with Doppler interrogation may be necessary. One of the more reliable discriminators between constrictive pericarditis and restrictive car-

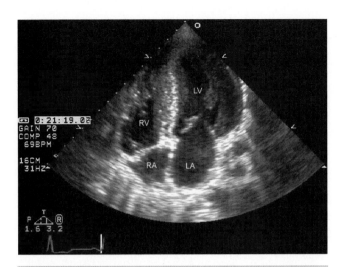

FIGURE 17.44. Apical four-chamber view recorded in a patient with glycogen storage disease. Note the increased wall thickness with mildly abnormal myocardial texture. In real-time, the ventricle was globally hypokinetic.

HYPERTROPHIC CARDIOMYOPATHY

Hypertrophic cardiomyopathy occurs either in sporadic or familial forms. The genetics of the disease are highly variable with respect to the specific gene mutation and degree of penetrance. As of this writing, more than 20 different distinct genetic mutations, each resulting in a specific alteration in troponin or myoglobin structure, have been identified. All forms of hypertrophic cardiomyopathy have in common inappropriate left ventricular hypertrophy often with abnormal myofibril orientation. The classic form, idiopathic hypertrophic cardiomyopathy, results in dynamic left ventricular outflow tract obstruction, mitral regurgitation, a high prevalence of arrhythmias, and sudden cardiac death in susceptible individuals. Hypertrophic cardiomyopathy represents a diverse spectrum of disease with varying degrees of hypertrophic expression even among a given family. Table 17.1 outlines the varying anatomic types of hypertrophic cardiomyopathy.

Echocardiographic Evaluation of Hypertrophic Cardiomyopathy

Earlier echocardiographic studies of hypertrophic cardiomyopathy used M-mode echocardiography. With this technique, a septal to posterior wall thickness ratio of 1.3:1 was considered evidence of inappropriate septal hypertrophy. It should be emphasized that there are a number of other disease states such as pulmonary hypertension with right ventricular hypertrophy and inferior wall infarction in the presence of left ventricular hypertrophy that will also result in a similar septal to posterior wall thickness ratio.

Two-dimensional echocardiography is currently the primary tool for screening and evaluation of known or

diomyopathy is the respiratory variation in E-wave amplitude of the mitral valve inflow. With constrictive pericarditis, there is typically exaggerated (>25%) respiratory variation of mitral inflow E-wave velocity compared with normal respiratory variation in restrictive cardiomyopathy. Other findings such as behavior of pulmonary and hepatic vein flow can be more problematic to accurately record, and the distinguishing observations are far more subtle. Anular E-wave velocity using Doppler tissue imaging also appears to be a relatively simple and highly discriminatory tool for distinguishing these two entities. Most reports have suggested that E-wave velocities are substantially greater, typically more than 20 cm/sec, in constrictive pericarditis compared with restrictive cardiomyopathy in which the E_a velocity is often less than 10 cm/sec.

▶ **TABLE 17.5 Separation of Constrictive Pericarditis from Restrictive Cardiomyopathy**

	Constriction	*Restriction*
Atrial size	Normal	Dilated
Pericardial appearance	Thick/bright	Normal
Septal motion	Abnormal	Normal
Septal position	Varies with respiration	Normal
Mitral E/A	Increased (≥2.0)	Increased (≥2.0)
Deceleration time	Short (≤160 ms)	Short (≤160 ms)
Anular E_m	Normal	Reduced (≤10 cm/sec)
Pulmonary hypertension	Rare	Frequent
Left ventricular size/function	Normal	Normal
Mitral/tricuspid regurgitation	Infrequent	Frequent (TR > MR)
Isovolumic relaxation time	Varies with respiration	Stable with respiration
Respiratory variation of mitral E velocity	Exaggerated (≥25%)	Normal

MR, mitral regurgitation; TR, tricuspid regurgitation.

suspected hypertrophic cardiomyopathy. The presence, magnitude, and distribution of left ventricular hypertrophy can be accurately determined, and, when combined with M-mode echocardiography, color flow and spectral Doppler imaging can fully delineate the entire spectrum of hemodynamic abnormalities seen in hypertrophic cardiomyopathy. For evaluation of hypertrophic cardiomyopathy, a detailed complete hemodynamic assessment using all Doppler modalities is essential in all patients. Figures 17.45 through 17.59 were recorded in patients with hypertrophic obstructive cardiomyopathy (previously referred to as idiopathic hypertrophic cardiomyopathy). Note the marked thickening of the proximal anterior septum and relative sparing of the other walls in Figure 17.45. M-mode echocardiography (Fig. 17.46B) recorded in the same patient presented in Figure 17.45 reveals what appears to be isolated septal hypertrophy with normal wall thickness. Inspection of the short-axis view in Figure 17.45, however, reveals that the hypertrophy is far more generalized than what would have been appreciated from only the parasternal long-axis view or M-mode echocardiography. Commonly, there is a spectrum of hypertrophy in the left ventricle with maximal involvement in the anterior septum and little or no involvement in the true posterior wall. There is an intermediate level of involvement in the lateral wall and inferior septum. This pattern is substantially more common than true isolated septal hypertrophy.

Figure 17.47 was recorded in a patient with milder hypertrophic cardiomyopathy. Note the proximal septal hypertrophy but relatively preserved area of the left ventricular outflow tract. Doppler imaging through the outflow tract revealed no evidence of obstruction at rest (Fig. 17.48). After exercise, a gradient of 34 mm Hg was provoked. Other maneuvers that can be used to provoke a gradient in hypertrophic cardiomyopathy include inhalation of amyl nitrate, rapid standing from a squatting position, and infusion of an isotope such as dobutamine.

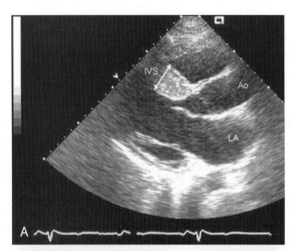

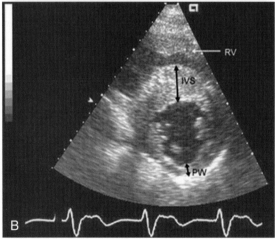

FIGURE 17.45. Parasternal long-axis **(A)** and short-axis **(B)** views recorded in a patient with classic hypertrophic cardiomyopathy. In both the long-axis and short-axis views, note the marked thickening of the interventricular septum (*arrows*) and the normal thickness of the posterior wall (*PW*) (*arrows*). In the short axis view, note that there is a spectrum of hypertrophy of the left ventricle, with maximum hypertrophy in the septum, no hypertrophy of the true posterior wall, and intermediate hypertrophy of the lateral and true inferior wall. Ao, aorta; IVS, interventricular septum; LA, left atrium; RV, right ventricle.

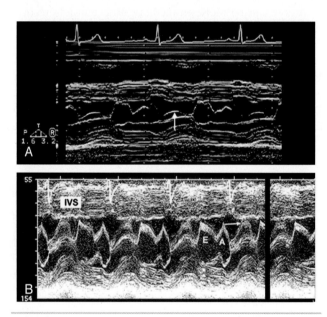

FIGURE 17.46. M-mode echocardiograms recorded in patients with hypertrophic cardiomyopathy demonstrating systolic anterior motion of the mitral valve (*arrow*). **A:** There is only mild systolic anterior motion present, which does not contact the ventricular septum. Obstruction of left ventricular outflow would not be expected with this pattern. **B:** Recorded in the same patient depicted in Figure 17.45. Note the thickness of the interventricular septum (*IVS*) and the dramatic systolic anterior motion (*arrow*), indicative of significant outflow tract obstruction.

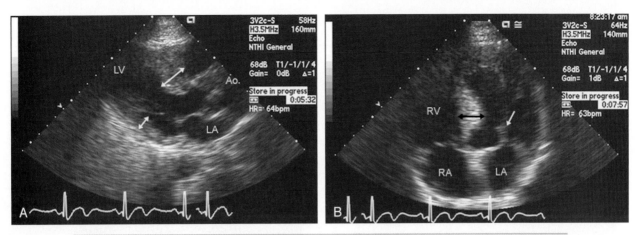

FIGURE 17.47. Parasternal long-axis (**A**) and apical four chamber (**B**) views recorded in a 50-year-old patient with a mild, asymptomatic hypertrophic cardiomyopathy. Both views reveal the relative hypertrophy of the proximal ventricular septum (*double-headed arrows*). **B:** There is relatively mild systolic anterior motion of the mitral valve (*white arrow*) without contact with the ventricular septum. Ao, aorta; LA, left atrium; LV, left ventricle; RA, right atrium; RV, right ventricle.

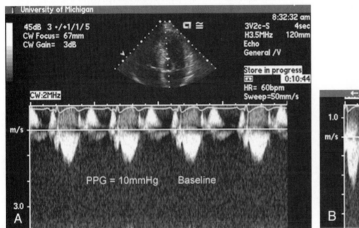
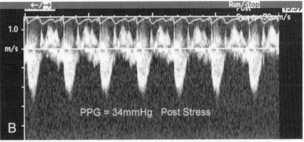

FIGURE 14.48. Continuous wave Doppler recordings through the left ventricular outflow tract of the patient recorded in Figure 17.47. **A:** Recorded under resting basal conditions revealing a peak gradient of 10 mm Hg. Close scrutiny reveals presystolic flow acceleration in the left ventricular outflow tract. **B:** Recorded immediately after exercise reveals a provokable gradient of 34 mm Hg. PPG, peak pressure gradient.

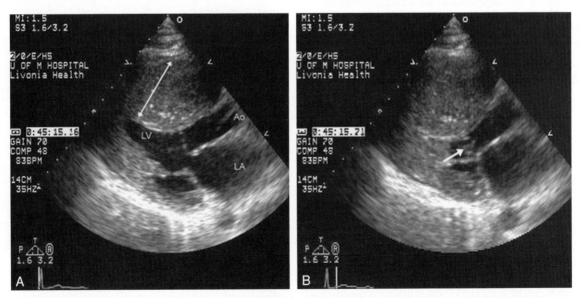

FIGURE 17.49. Parasternal long-axis view recorded in diastole (**A**) and systole (**B**) in a patient with hypertrophic cardiomyopathy and massive hypertrophy of the ventricular septum (*arrow*). In this instance, the anterior septum measures approximately 4 cm in thickness. **B:** Note the systolic anterior motion of the mitral valve (*arrow*), which appears as a mass of echoes in the left ventricular outflow tract. Ao, aorta; LA, left atrium; LV, left ventricle.

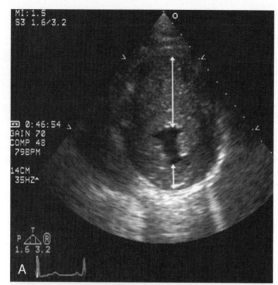

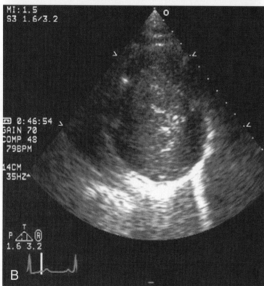

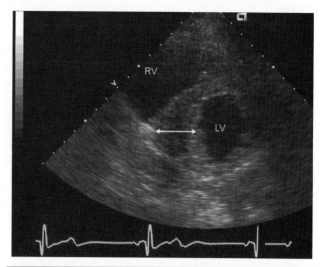

FIGURE 17.51. Parasternal short-axis image recorded in a patient with hypertrophic cardiomyopathy in which the hypertrophy was confined to the proximal inferior wall and inferior septum (*arrow*). There was no evidence of dynamic outflow tract obstruction in this patient. LV, left ventricle; RV, right ventricle.

FIGURE 17.50. Parasternal short-axis view recorded in the same patient depicted in Figure 17.47. Note the massive hypertrophy of the ventricular septum (*long arrow*) with lesser degrees of hypertrophy present throughout the entire circumference of the left ventricle (*short arrow*). **B:** Recorded at mid-systole. Note the almost complete cavity obliteration due to the marked hypertrophy.

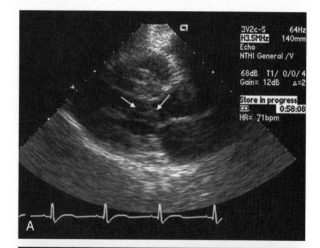

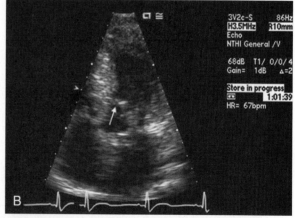

FIGURE 17.52. Parasternal long-axis (**A**) and apical four-chamber (**B**) views recorded a patient with a hypertrophic cardiomyopathy with systolic anterior motion of the mitral valve seen in both views (*arrows*).

Figures 17.49 and 17.50 were recorded in a patient with a more concentric form of hypertrophic cardiomyopathy. In the short-axis view, note the almost complete cavity obliteration in systole due to the marked hypertrophy. Often the concentric forms of hypertrophic cardiomyopathy are not obstructive. Symptoms develop in patients with the nonobstructive form due to pathologic stiffness of the left ventricular myocardium and elevated diastolic pressures as well as the small stroke volume due to small diastolic vol-

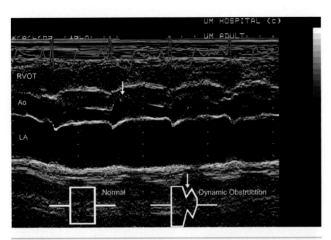

FIGURE 17.53. M-mode echocardiogram recorded in a patient with a hypertrophic cardiomyopathy demonstrates systolic notching of the aortic valve (*arrow*). Normal closure is schematized in the inset. Ao, aorta; LA, left atrium; RVOT, right ventricular outflow tract.

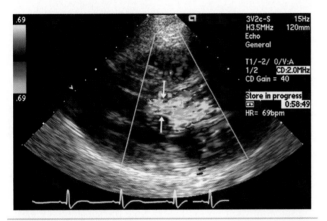

FIGURE 17.54. Parasternal long-axis view (systolic frame) recorded with color flow Doppler imaging in a patient with hypertrophic cardiomyopathy and systolic anterior motion of the mitral valve demonstrates marked turbulence in the left ventricular outflow tract. Note the relatively narrow width of the turbulent jet at the level of the mitral valve (*arrows*).

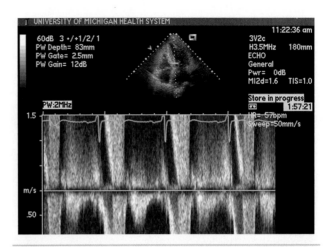

FIGURE 17.55. Pulsed wave Doppler imaging recorded in the left ventricular outflow tract of a patient with hypertrophic cardiomyopathy and dynamic outflow tract obstruction. As the sample volume is moved from the apex toward the aortic valve along the septum, the outflow tract velocity exceeds the Nyquist limit and aliasing occurs.

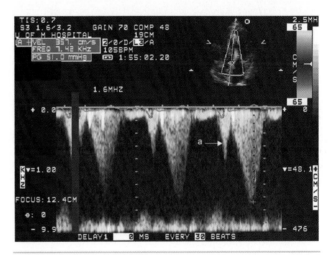

FIGURE 17.56. Continuous wave Doppler image recorded through the left ventricular outflow tract in a patient with hypertrophic cardiomyopathy. Note the relatively late peaking systolic gradient with peak pressure gradient of 51.0 mm Hg. Also note the prominent presystolic flow in the outflow tract (*a*) due to atrial contraction against a highly noncompliant and hypertrophied left ventricle.

umes. Occasionally, hypertrophic cardiomyopathy is encountered in which the pathologic hypertrophy is confined to the posterior or lateral wall of the left ventricle (Fig. 17.51) or to the right ventricular wall.

Assessment of the Left Ventricular Outflow Tract in Obstructive Cardiomyopathy

A major sequela of hypertrophic cardiomyopathy is dynamic left ventricular outflow obstruction. M-mode echocardiography was initially used to document the presence of outflow tract obstruction. The M-mode abnormalities associated with dynamic outflow tract obstruction were systolic anterior motion of the mitral valve and abnormal aortic valve motion in systole. It is now recognized that systolic anterior motion of the mitral valve occurs because of an abnormal geometric relationship of papillary muscles and the mitral supporting apparatus combined with hyperdynamic left ventricular ejection. This results in anterior displacement of varying portions of the mitral valve apparatus in systole. Systolic anterior motion can be identified on M-mode (Fig. 17.46) or two-dimensional scanning (Figs. 17.49 and 17.52) and should be characterized by the area of the mitral valve having abnormal motion (chordal or leaflet),

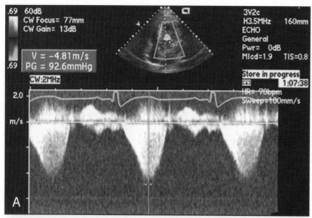

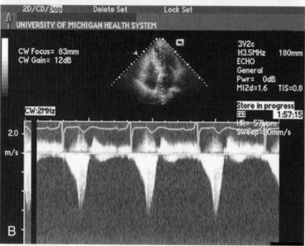

FIGURE 17.57. A, B: Continuous wave Doppler recordings from two patients with hypertrophic cardiomyopathy and dynamic outflow tract obstruction. In each instance, note the late peaking systolic gradient resulting in a dagger-shaped contour to the spectral display. This is more dramatically illustrated in **B**.

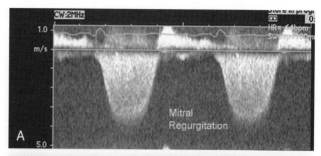

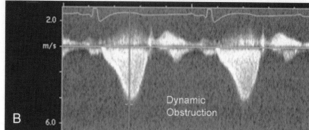

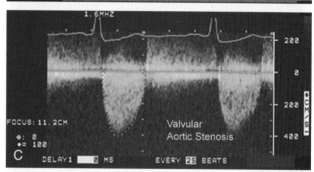

FIGURE 17.58. Comparison of the spectral display of mitral regurgitation **(A)**, dynamic outflow tract obstruction **(B)**, and valvular aortic stenosis **(C)**. **A–C:** The images have been aligned so that for each image the first QRS complex the is at roughly the same location on the figure. Note the substantially earlier onset of flow in the mitral regurgitation signal **(A)** compared with dynamic obstruction **(B)** or valvular aortic stenosis **(C)**. The dynamic outflow tract obstruction profile shows a classically late-peaking dagger profile compared with the symmetric flow profile in valvular aortic stenosis and mitral regurgitation.

the degree to which the systolic anterior motion results in contact of the valvular apparatus with the ventricular septum, and the duration of contact with the ventricular septum. Obstruction is more likely to be present when systolic anterior motion persists for 40% of the systolic cycle and directly makes contact with the ventricular septum. Detection of systolic anterior motion of the mitral valve is indirect evidence of left ventricular outflow tract obstruction. Figure 17.53 is an M-mode echocardiogram of aortic valve motion in a patient with an obstructive hypertrophic cardiomyopathy.

The ejection dynamics of obstructive hypertrophic cardiomyopathy allow for relatively normal early left ventricular ejection during which the aortic valve opens normally. Obstruction occurs in mid- to late-systole concurrent with late-phase left ventricular contraction at which point ejection transiently diminishes. The reduction in flow volume out the left ventricular outflow tract results in partial closure of the aortic valve, often with a

secondary opening as final ejection occurs. This results in a single notch or occasionally several discrete high-amplitude notches of aortic valve motion. Of note, the degree to which there is preclosure and notching of the aortic valve is not uniform among the three aortic valve cusps.

Doppler interrogation of the left ventricular outflow tract provides direct documentation and quantitation of outflow tract obstruction. Dynamic outflow tract obstruction results in marked turbulence in the outflow tract, which can be detected with color flow Doppler (Fig. 17.54). Pulsed Doppler imaging can be used to track the ejection velocities along the left ventricular outflow tract at which point, when significant dynamic outflow tract obstruction is present, the velocity will exceed the Nyquist

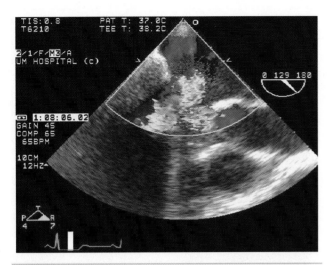

FIGURE 17.59. Two-dimensional echocardiogram with color flow Doppler imaging depicts mitral regurgitation in hypertrophic cardiomyopathy. Systolic anterior motion of the mitral valve results in abnormal coaptation of the leaflets and secondary mitral regurgitation.

limit and aliasing will occur (Fig. 17.55). Continuous wave Doppler imaging provides a higher fidelity analysis of left ventricular outflow tract ejection dynamics and gradients but as a stand-alone technique does not identify the location of obstruction. In a hypertrophic cardiomyopathy with evidence of systolic anterior motion of the mitral valve, the level of anatomic obstruction is rarely in question, and hence the use of continuous wave Doppler imaging for high-resolution quantitation combined with anatomic assessment frequently provides a full assessment of the location and degree of outflow tract obstruction. Figures 17.56 and 17.57 are continuous wave Doppler recordings from which the true peak velocities can be recorded without aliasing. There are several characteristics of continuous wave Doppler imaging that relate to the dynamic nature of outflow tract obstruction. In Figure 17.57, note the relatively late peak of the maximal gradient. This has been described as a dagger-shaped profile in distinction to the spectral profile of mitral regurgitation or aortic stenosis (Fig. 17.58). The late peaking of the outflow tract gradient is evidence of the dynamic nature of the gradient that develops toward mid- and end-systole rather than being related to a fixed obstruction in which the gradient occurs early in systole at the time of maximal volumetric flow. It should be recognized that as this maximal gradient is occurring in late-systole, after the majority of left ventricular ejection has occurred, it is not truly obstructive with respect to volume of flow because the majority of the left ventricular stroke volume has been ejected at the time that the "obstruction" develops. Often there is evidence of presystolic forward flow in the left ventricular outflow tract (Fig. 17.56). This occurs when atrial contraction results

in acceleration of flow as the A-wave related flow volume is transmitted to the outflow tract because of a highly noncompliant left ventricle.

Occasionally, one encounters an individual in whom the two-dimensional echocardiographic anatomy would be consistent with hypertrophic cardiomyopathy but in whom no direct or indirect evidence of obstruction can be found. It should be emphasized that many of the signs, symptoms, and adverse clinical sequelae of hypertrophic cardiomyopathy are independent of outflow tract obstruction and that the absence of obstruction should not preclude establishing this diagnosis and instituting appropriate therapy. On occasion, it is clinically useful to attempt to provoke an outflow tract gradient (Fig. 17.48). Physiologically, any maneuver that either increases contractility, reduces left ventricular volume, or decreases resistance to left ventricular outflow may unmask an occult gradient. Repeating Doppler and M-mode echocardiography at the time of such maneuvers as changes in body position (squatting to standing) or pharmacologic provocation (amyl nitrate inhalation) can be used to document the presence of a provokable gradient.

Mitral Regurgitation in Hypertrophic Cardiomyopathy

Mitral regurgitation is a common finding in obstructive hypertrophic cardiomyopathy. The etiology of the mitral regurgitation is the malcoaptation of the leaflets due to tethering that occurs during systolic anterior motion (Fig. 17.59). The severity of mitral regurgitation can range from mild to severe, and mitral regurgitation often is an independent contributor to development of symptoms. The jet typically arises centrally but may take an eccentric course in the left atrium and often is present in mid- to late-systole during the time of maximal systolic anterior motion rather than being truly holosystolic. Because dynamic outflow tract obstruction occurs in these individuals, intracavitary left ventricular pressure increases in mid- and late-systole. This results in an atypical mitral regurgitation contour in which the maximal mitral regurgitation velocity is late rather than early as in structural mitral regurgitation (Figs. 17.58 and 17.60). Occasionally confusion arises when looking for an outflow tract gradient if one mistakenly interrogates mitral regurgitation with a late peak and confuses it with the dynamic outflow tract obstruction. Often the mitral regurgitation signal will have a later onset than the outflow tract flow profile, and frequently the peak velocities are in a supraphysiologic range (Fig. 17.60). When one encounters a hypertrophic cardiomyopathy with mitral regurgitation and a late peaking velocity of 6 m/sec, confusion with the mitral regurgitation jet should be considered.

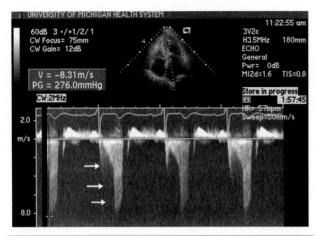

FIGURE 17.60. Continuous wave Doppler recording through the area of the left ventricular outflow tract in a patient with hypertrophic cardiomyopathy and mitral regurgitation. On the basis of the direction of the interrogation line alone, it is difficult to determine the etiology of this signal. Note, however, the relatively faint early systolic boundary (*arrows*), typical of mitral regurgitation and a peak gradient of 276 mm Hg, which is far more likely to represent the gradient from the left ventricle to the left atrium due to mitral regurgitation than through the left ventricular outflow tract.

Other Variants of Hypertrophic Cardiomyopathy

A relatively infrequent form of hypertrophic cardiomyopathy is the isolated apical variant. This form is more common in Asian populations and is associated with deep symmetric T-wave inversion in the anterior precordial leads on the electrocardiogram in many instances. Figure 17.61 was recorded in a patient with an apical hypertrophic cardiomyopathy. Note the normal wall thickness at the base of the heart and the pathologic thickness toward the apex. The degree of thickening increases from base to apex, resulting in a markedly diminished apical cavity and a spade-shaped left ventricular cavity. Apical hypertrophic cardiomyopathy can occasionally be overlooked on echocardiography, especially when scanning with low-frequency transducers. In this instance, the low frequency transducer penetrates through the relatively less echogenic myocardium and only the epicardium is visualized.

Several additional maneuvers can be used to identify an apical or mid-ventricular hypertrophic cardiomyopathy when it is not apparent on routine clinical scan. The first is to use relatively shallow focal depths and high-frequency transducers. Additionally, by employing color flow Doppler imaging in the apex, at a relatively low Nyquist limit, one can appreciate the blood pool tissue boundary and often identify a convergence zone near the apex that represents an area of left ventricular narrowing at the apical or mid-ventricular level (Fig. 17.62).

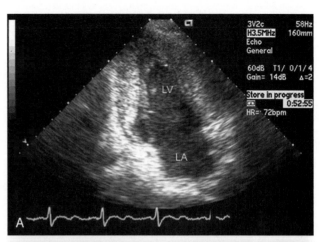

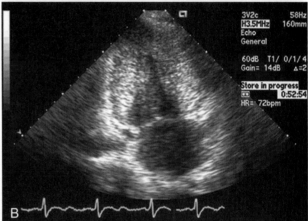

FIGURE 17.61. Apical two-chamber view recorded in a patient with classic apical hypertrophy variant of hypertrophic cardiomyopathy. **A:** Note the progressively greater wall thickness when comparing the base to the apical portions. **B:** Recorded at end-systole, revealing a classic spade-shaped ventricular cavity. LA, left atrium; LV, left ventricle.

Contrast echocardiography using transpulmonary agents to opacify the left ventricle can also be used to confirm the presence of apical hypertrophic cardiomyopathy. After opacification of a left ventricular cavity with contrast, the true extent of hypertrophy can be appreciated, and the abnormal contour of the left ventricular cavity can be clearly documented.

Mid-Cavitary Obstruction

An additional form of hypertrophic cardiomyopathy involves selective hypertrophy and obstruction at the mid-left ventricular level. This finding may represent the effects of long-standing hypertension with relatively small left ventricular cavities in some individuals. It is quite likely that there is a distinct anatomic subtype of hypertrophic cardiomyopathy resulting in this pattern as well. In this instance, color flow Doppler imaging will often

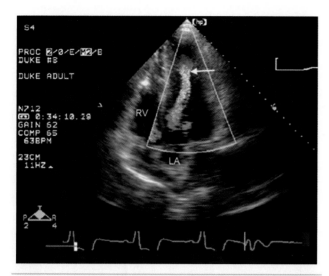

FIGURE 17.62. Apical four-chamber view with color flow Doppler imaging recorded in a patient with an apical hypertrophic cardiomyopathy and apical aneurysm. This image was recorded in systole. Note the apically located convergence zone and relatively narrow flow profile at the apex of the left ventricle consistent with obstruction at that level. In this example, there is a discrete apical aneurysm due to localized infarction. LA, left atrium; RV, right ventricle.

identify a narrow constricted area of the left ventricular cavity in systole, and continuous wave Doppler imaging will identify a high velocity consistent with the hemodynamic gradient, typically at the level of the mid-papillary muscle levels. This type of hypertrophic cardiomyopathy may be more difficult to identify because there typically will not be evidence of systolic anterior motion of the mitral valve. Because image detail is dependent on lateral resolution, when imaging from the apex, the actual degree of narrowing at the mid left ventricular level may be underappreciated. Evaluation of the color flow signal in systole may often be the first evidence of mid-cavitary obstruction (Fig. 17.63). Similarly, intravenous contrast for left ventricular opacification can be used to identify the true boundary of the left ventricular cavity and the degree to which there is narrowing at the mid left ventricular level (Fig. 17.64).

Conditions Mimicking Hypertrophic Cardiomyopathy

Several clinical situations mimic true obstructive hypertrophic cardiomyopathy. The first is the so-called acquired hypertrophic cardiomyopathy of the hypertensive elderly (Fig. 17.65). This is a variation of hypertensive cardiovascular disease in which there has been a relatively greater degree of hypertrophy of the ventricular septum, which when combined with the normal increase in septal angulation seen in the elderly results in a variable degree of outflow tract obstruction. The obstruction occasionally

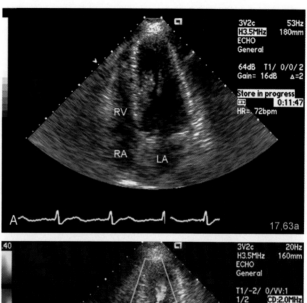

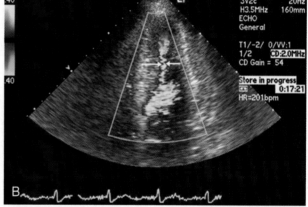

FIGURE 17.63. Apical four-chamber views recorded in systole in a patient with mid-cavity obstruction. **A:** Note the suggestion of near cavity obliteration at the level of the papillary muscles, which is confirmed using color flow Doppler imaging (**B**), where one can see the very narrow residual cavity of the left ventricle (*arrows*). LA, left atrium; RA, right atrium; RV, right ventricle.

reaches levels similar to those seen in a true genetically based hypertrophic cardiomyopathy. Systolic anterior motion of the mitral valve can result in secondary mitral regurgitation. The diagnosis is established clinically when one encounters the anatomic appearance of an obstructive hypertrophic cardiomyopathy in an elderly patient with long-standing hypertension.

A second clinical situation in which echocardiographic and Doppler abnormalities mimicking hypertrophic cardiomyopathy are encountered is in patients with intravascular volume depletion, especially if concurrently on inotropic agents. This syndrome is not infrequently encountered in intensive care units where a hypotensive patient with relatively low intravascular volume is placed on inotropic support. Often there has been an underlying history of hypertension, and the relatively low intravascular volumes with augmented contractility due to these agents result in hyperdynamic motion of the ventricle with an ac-

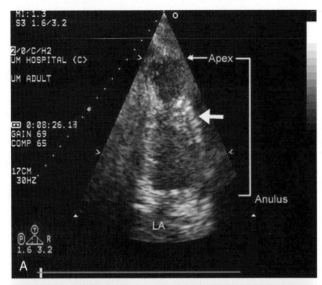

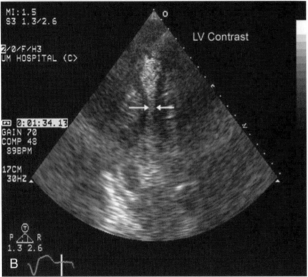

FIGURE 17.64. Apical two-chamber view recorded in a patient with midcavity obstruction. **A:** Note the location of the apex and the anulus. At the level of the left ventricle (*arrow*), there is nearly complete cavity obstruction. **B:** Recorded after injection of intravenous contrast for left ventricular opacification. Note the very narrow left ventricular cavity in its mid-portion (*arrows*) representing mid-cavity obstruction. LA, left atrium; LV, left ventricle.

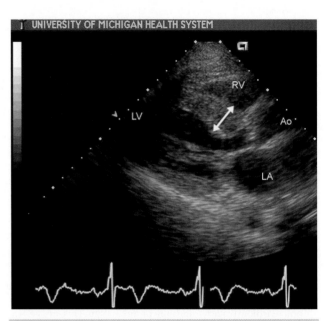

FIGURE 17.65. Parasternal long-axis view recorded in an elderly hypertensive patient with hypertensive hypertrophic cardiomyopathy of the elderly. The combination of septal angulation and disproportionate proximal septal hypertrophy results in an anatomic pattern, mimicking classic hypertrophic cardiomyopathy. Systolic anterior motion and varying degrees of outflow tract obstruction may also be encountered. Ao, aorta; LA, left atrium; LV, left ventricle; RV, right ventricle.

quired form of dynamic outflow tract obstruction. The acquired dynamic outflow tract obstruction and systolic anterior motion of the mitral valve can occasionally result in significant degrees of mitral regurgitation and detection of clinically significant murmurs. The combination of mitral regurgitation, a small ventricular cavity, and outflow tract obstruction leads to progressive hypotension for which an inappropriate increase in inotropic agents is occasionally employed. Detection of a small hyperdynamic ventricle with outflow tract obstruction in this setting is an indication for volume resuscitation and discontinua-

tion or decrease in inotropic support, which often result in relief of the entire syndrome. This issue is discussed further in Chapter 19.

Several anatomic variants or other primary diseases may mimic the echocardiographic appearance of the hypertrophic cardiomyopathy. One of the more commonly encountered is prominent right ventricular muscle bundle or trabeculation, lying along the right ventricular side of the anterior ventricular septum. With either M-mode echocardiography or isolated parasternal long-axis imaging the overlying trabeculation may be confused with an intrinsic portion of the ventricular septum. This results in erroneous measurement of septal thickness, mimicking true septal hypertrophy, which when compared with the normal thickness of the posterior wall leads to the erroneous diagnosis of hypertrophic cardiomyopathy. Similarly, any entity resulting in right ventricular hypertrophy will also result in isolated septal hypertrophy (Fig. 17.66). In this instance, the septal hypertrophy represents the contribution of right ventricular hypertrophy rather than intrinsic disease of the left ventricular septum. The septal thickness is increased; this may also mimic hypertrophic cardiomyopathy. Full evaluation of the right ventricle will often reveal evidence of right ventricular hypertrophy and more Doppler evidence of right ventricular hypertension. Additionally, there will not be evidence of dynamic left

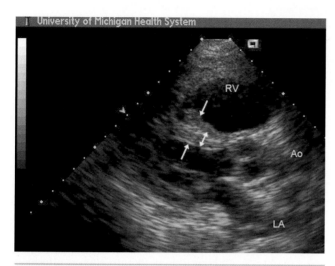

FIGURE 17.66. Patient with pulmonary hypertension and right ventricular hypertrophy in which the right ventricular hypertrophy has resulted in the appearance of septal hypertrophy, mimicking a hypertrophic cardiomyopathy. Careful scrutiny of the septal echoes, however, reveals that the hypertrophy is constituted almost entirely by hypertrophied right ventricular trabeculation and does not represent hypertrophy of the left ventricular portion of the septum. The true septal dimension is noted by the *double-headed arrow*, whereas the apparent (septal and trabeculation) dimension is noted by the two *inward-pointing arrows*. Ao, aorta; LA, left atrium; RV, right ventricle.

ventricular outflow tract obstruction. It is quite common to see disproportionate septal hypertrophy meeting the classic criteria of the septal to posterior wall thickness of 1:3:1 in patients with pulmonary hypertension. Recognition of the underlying disease as pulmonary hypertension with right ventricular hypertrophy should avoid confusion with true hypertrophic cardiomyopathy.

End-Stage Hypertrophic Cardiomyopathy

One occasionally encounters a patient who presents with inappropriate ventricular hypertrophy (i.e., in the absence of hypertension) and significant left ventricular systolic dysfunction. This pattern can represent the end-stage of a hypertrophic cardiomyopathy in which the hyperdynamic left ventricular contraction has "burned out" and the patient is left with global ventricular hypokinesis. Because of the decrease in contractility, systolic anterior motion and dynamic outflow tract obstruction are no longer present and the patient presents as having a mildly dilated but hypertrophied cardiomyopathy. The diagnosis of end-stage hypertrophic cardiomyopathy can be made only when previous clinical and echocardiographic evidence has documented a typical hypertrophic cardiomyopathy but is occasionally suspected when patients present who have no other etiology for the combination of hypertrophy and systolic dysfunction. Additionally, one

occasionally encounters patients with long-standing hypertrophic cardiomyopathy and myocardial infarction but without obstructive coronary artery disease. The etiology of the full-thickness infarct may be compression of the intramyocardial coronary arteries. This phenomenon can also be seen in the apical variant of hypertrophic cardiomyopathy.

Therapeutic Decision Making and Monitoring in Hypertrophic Cardiomyopathy

Obstructive hypertrophic cardiomyopathy often represents a frustrating and difficult management challenge. Medical therapy directed at decreasing contractility with beta-blockers or calcium channel blockers has provided only limited benefit. Reduction in outflow tract gradients by surgical myotomy-myectomy, or by alcohol ablation of a septal perforator, has had substantial success with respect to alleviating hemodynamic abnormalities including mitral regurgitation and outflow tract obstruction. Echocardiographic monitoring of these procedures is discussed in Chapter 19. After successful septal reduction therapy (either operative or interventional), one notes acute and dramatic thinning of the proximal septum (Fig. 17.67) and the absence of further Doppler evidence of outflow tract obstruction or of mitral regurgitation.

Atrioventricular pacing represents another therapeutic option in hypertrophic cardiomyopathy for which echocardiographic screening can play a role in patient selection. The patient most likely to benefit from dual-chamber pacing is one in whom the native atrioventricular relationship has resulted in an abnormally short diastolic filling period. Echocardiographic and Doppler monitoring can be performed during trials of various pacing intervals to document the atrioventricular pacing interval that results in a decrease in outflow tract obstruction and a concurrent increase in forward stroke volume. The ventricular dyssynchrony that results from pacing at the right ventricular apex may also reduce the degree of dynamic outflow tract obstruction. In addition to acute monitoring of therapy such as dual-chamber pacing, echocardiography and Doppler imaging can be used to track the long-term success of these procedures as well.

MYOCARDITIS

Acute myocarditis is typically a viral or postviral process. It results in the acute onset of left ventricular systolic dysfunction of varying degrees, which can range from mild and clinically undetectable to fulminant and fatal over a short course. Although myocarditis often is the sequela of viral infection, not all patients will have evidence of an antecedent acute febrile and presumably viral illness.

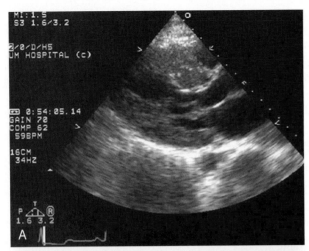

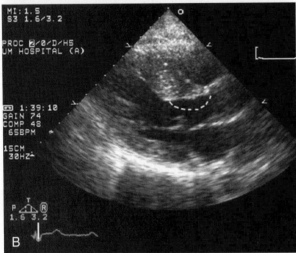

FIGURE 17.67. Parasternal long-axis view recorded in a patient before **(A)** and after **(B)** alcohol septal ablation of the proximal septum for hypertrophic cardiomyopathy. Both images are recorded in early systole. **A:** Note the marked hypertrophy of the proximal septum that narrows the left ventricular outflow tract. **B:** Note the relative thinning of the proximal septum and a substantial widening of the left ventricular outflow tract. **B:** *Dotted lines* denote the original boundary of the hypertrophied proximal septum. LA, left atrium; LV, left ventricle; RVOT, right ventricular outflow tract.

Clinically, patients with acute viral myocarditis present with tachycardia, hypotension, and shortness of breath. Atrial fibrillation is not uncommon. The clinical course of myocarditis is highly variable with complete or nearly complete resolution occurring in a matter of weeks in some patients. A minority of patients will have an acute fulminant and rapidly fatal course. The majority will have a less fulminant course and experience some degree of recovery of function but often are left with a degree of left ventricular dysfunction.

Two-dimensional echocardiography should be an early and universally used tool in suspected myocarditis. The echocardiographic findings of myocarditis are near-

normal ventricular dimensions with a global decrease in systolic function. As with cardiomyopathy, there may be some regional variation in the degree to which function is diminished. Subsequent to the initial insult, ventricular dilation may result in varying degrees of mitral or tricuspid regurgitation. Additionally, inflammation of the visceral pericardium may result in pericardial effusion, which is typically small in the majority of patients. Figure 17.68 was recorded in a patient with acute viral myocarditis. Note the normal chamber sizes and global systolic dysfunction. Once the diagnosis has been clinically established, echocardiography should be used for serial follow-up because there will be varying degrees of improvement in left ventricular function. The degree to which recovery of function occurs plays a role in decision making with respect to the type and duration of therapy such as afterload reduction, diuretics, and other modalities.

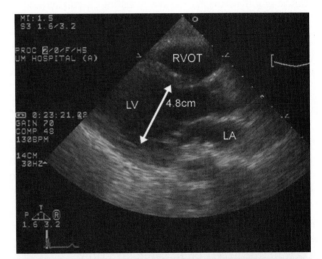

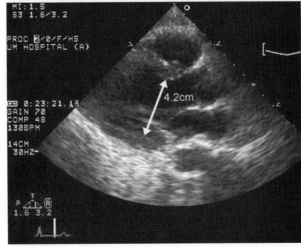

FIGURE 17.68. Parasternal long-axis view recorded in a patient with acute myocarditis. Note the normal left ventricular internal dimension of 4.8 cm. The ventricle is globally hypokinetic with an ejection fraction of approximately 25%. LA, left atrium; LV, left ventricle; RA, right atrium; RV, right ventricle.

On occasion, the pattern of involvement in acute myocarditis suggests a specific etiology. Lymphocytic and giant cell myocarditis may present with predominantly anterior wall and right ventricular involvement. Either of these two diagnoses should be considered when myocarditis is associated with a focal distribution of wall motion abnormalities.

POSTPARTUM CARDIOMYOPATHY

Postpartum cardiomyopathy remains a poorly defined entity in which features of cardiomyopathy with ventricular dilation, systolic dysfunction, and secondary mitral regurgitation occur in the peripartum period. Most women present shortly after childbirth, although a subset will have the initial clinical and echocardiographic presentation late in the third trimester of pregnancy. The etiology of this entity remains in dispute. It has been linked to preeclampsia and has been occasionally ascribed to a viral etiology. At this point, a firm etiology for the entity has not been established. The severity of left ventricular dysfunction ranges from mild to fulminant, and the time course of recovery is variable.

Echocardiography and Doppler imaging employed in peripartum cardiomyopathy reveal findings identical to those for any other dilated cardiomyopathy. The degree of chamber dilation is dependent on the timing of the examination with respect to onset. Near-normal chamber sizes may be encountered early in the course of the disease. As with other forms of cardiomyopathy, mitral regurgitation may be encountered as a secondary finding. The diagnosis of peripartum cardiomyopathy is made in the context of a cardiomyopathy first noted in the peripartum period.

CHAGAS MYOCARDITIS

Chagas disease is the sequela of an infection with *Trypanosoma cruzi*. This type of myocarditis typically results in focal involvement that is often apical in location, resulting in a narrow-neck aneurysm (Fig. 17.69). The disease is endemic to South America and rarely if ever is encountered in individuals without travel to endemic areas.

ENDOCARDIAL FIBROELASTOSIS AND HYPEREOSINOPHILIC SYNDROME

Endocardial fibroelastosis occurs in several forms, including congenital and tropical and nontropical acquired forms. Endocardial fibroelastosis is also associated with the hypereosinophilic syndrome. Endocardial fibroelastosis results in inflammation of the endocardium with subsequent creation of a thick endocardial layer. Due to the inflammatory process, there is overlying thrombus and the appearance of an obliterative apical process (Fig. 17.70). The process involves both ventricles and may be more prominent at the apex. Both global systolic dysfunction and variable degrees of diastolic dysfunction occur. In late stages, it has the appearance of a dilated cardiomyopathy

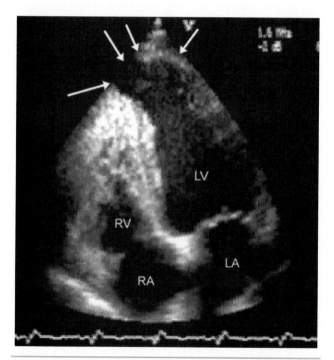

FIGURE 17.69. Apical four-chamber view recorded in a patient with Chagas myocarditis. Note the discrete apical aneurysm (*arrows*) typically seen in this disease. LA, left atrium; LV, left ventricle; RA, right atrium; RV, right ventricle. (Courtesy of Wilson Mathias, M.D.)

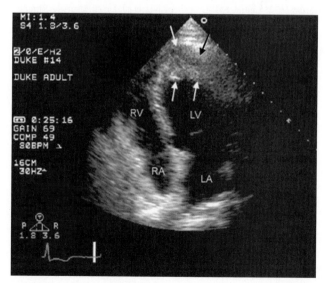

FIGURE 17.70. Apical four-chamber view recorded in a patient with hypereosinophilic syndrome and endocardial fibrosis. The boundary of the true apex is noted by the downward pointing arrows. Note the homogeneous mass obliterating the left ventricular apex, which represents a combination of inflammatory material and superimposed thrombus.

with restrictive physiology. Also common in hypereosinophilia syndrome is selective involvement of the posterior mitral valve leaflet, resulting in mitral regurgitation.

SUGGESTED READINGS

Agmon Y, Connolly HM, Olson U, et al. Noncompaction of the ventricular myocardium. J Am Soc Echocardiogr 1999;12:859–863.

Alizad A, Seward JB. Echocardiographic features of genetic diseases: part 1. Cardiomyopathy. J Am Soc Echocardiogr 2000;13:73–86.

Ammash NM, Seward JB, Bailey KR, et al. Clinical profile and outcome of idiopathic restrictive cardiomyopathy. Circulation 2000;101: 2490–2496.

Aurigemma GP, Gottdiener JS, Shemanski L, et al. Predictive value of systolic and diastolic function for incident congestive heart failure in the elderly: the cardiovascular health study. J Am Coll Cardiol 2001;37:1042–1048.

Bargiggia GS, Bertucci C, Recusani F, et al. A new method for estimating left ventricular dP/dt by continuous wave Doppler-echocardiography. Validation studies at cardiac catheterization. Circulation 1989;80:1287–1292.

Beithardt OA, Sinha AM, Schwammenthal E, et al. Acute effects of cardiac resynchronization therapy on functional mitral regurgitation in advanced systolic heart failure. J Am Coll Cardiol 2003;41:765–770.

Chen C, Rodriguez L, Lethor JP, et al. Continuous wave Doppler echocardiography for noninvasive assessment of left ventricular dP/dt and relaxation time constant from mitral regurgitant spectra in patients. J Am Coll Cardiol 1994;23:970–976.

Dujardin KS, Tei C, Yeo TC, et al. Prognostic value of a Doppler index combining systolic and diastolic performance in idiopathic-dilated cardiomyopathy. Am J Cardiol 1998;82:1071–1076.

Fans R, Coats AJ, Henein MY. Echocardiography-derived variables predict outcome in patients with nonischemic dilated cardiomyopathy with or without a restrictive filling pattern. Am Heart J 2002;144: 343–350.

Felker GM, Boehmer JP, Hruban RH, et al. Echocardiographic findings in fulminant and acute myocarditis. J Am Coll Cardiol 2000;36: 227–232.

Garcia MJ, Palac RT, Malenka DJ, et al. Color M-mode Doppler flow propagation velocity is a relatively preload-independent index of left ventricular filling. J Am Soc Echocardiogr 1999;12:129–137.

Garcia MJ, Smedira NG, Greenberg NL, et al. Color M-mode Doppler flow propagation velocity is a preload insensitive index of left ventricular relaxation: animal and human validation. J Am Coll Cardiol 2000;35:201–208.

Garcia MJ, Thomas JD, Klein AL. New Doppler echocardiographic applications for the study of diastolic function. J Am Coll Cardiol 1998;32:865–875.

Klein AL, Hatle UK, Taliercio CP, et al. Prognostic significance of Doppler measures of diastolic function in cardiac amyloidosis. A Doppler echocardiography study. Circulation 1991;83:808–816.

Koelling TM, Aaronson KD, Cody RJ, et al. Prognostic significance of mitral regurgitation and tricuspid regurgitation in patients with left ventricular systolic dysfunction. Am Heart J 2002;144:524–529.

Lakkis NM, Nagueh SF, Kleiman NS, et al. Echocardiography-guided ethanol septal reduction for hypertrophic obstructive cardiomyopathy. Circulation 1998;98:1750–1755.

Morales FJ, Asencio MC, Oneto J, et al. Deceleration time of early filling in patients with left ventricular systolic dysfunction: functional and prognostic independent value. Am Heart J 2002;143:1101–1106.

Nagueh SF, Kopelen HA, Quinones MA. Assessment of left ventricular filling pressures by Doppler in the presence of atrial fibrillation. Circulation 1996;94:2138–2145.

Nagueh SF, Mikati I, Kopelen HA, et al. Doppler estimation of left ventricular filling pressure in sinus tachycardia. A new application of tissue Doppler imaging. Circulation 1998;98:1644–1650.

Nishimura RA, Abel MD, Hatie LK, et al. Relation of pulmonary vein to mitral flow velocities by transesophageal Doppler echocardiography. Effect of different loading conditions. Circulation 1990;81: 1488–1497.

Nishimura RA, Hayes DL, Ilstrup DM, et al. Effect of dual-chamber pacing on systolic and diastolic function in patients with hypertrophic cardiomyopathy. Acute Doppler echocardiographic and catheterization hemodynamic study. J Am Coll Cardiol 199627:421–430.

Oechslin EN, Attenhofer Jost CH, Rojas JR, et al. Long term follow-up of 34 adults with isolated left ventricular noncompaction: a distinct cardiomyopathy with poor prognosis. J Am Coll Cardiol 2000;36: 493–500.

Ommen SR, Nishimura RA, Appleton CP, et al. Clinical utility of Doppler echocardiography and tissue Doppler imaging in the estimation of left ventricular filling pressures: a comparative simultaneous Doppler-catheterization study. Circulation 2000;102:1788–1794.

Rihal CS, Nishimura RA, Hatle LK, et al. Systolic and diastolic dysfunction in patients with clinical diagnosis of dilated cardiomyopathy. Relation to symptoms and prognosis. Circulation 1994;90: 2772–2779.

Rossvoll O, Hatle LK. Pulmonary venous flow velocities recorded by transthoracic Doppler ultrasound: relation to left ventricular diastolic pressures. J Am Coll Cardiol 1993;21:1687–1696.

Saxon LA, De Marco T, Schafer J, et al. Effects of long-term biventricular stimulation for resynchronization on echocardiographic measures of remodeling. Circulation 2002;105:1304–1310.

Senni M, Rodeheffer RJ, Tribouilloy CM, et al. Use of echocardiography in the management of congestive heart failure in the community. J Am Coll Cardiol 1999;33:164–170.

Shapiro LM, McKenna WJ. Distribution of left ventricular hypertrophy in hypertrophic cardiomyopathy: a two-dimensional echocardiographic study. J Am Coll Cardiol 1983;2:437–444.

Tabata T, Thomas JD, Klein AL. Pulmonary venous flow by Doppler echocardiography: revisited 12 years later. J Am Coll Cardiol 2003;41:1243–1250.

Temporelli PL, Corra U, Imparato A, et al. Reversible restrictive left ventricular diastolic filling with optimized oral therapy predicts a more favorable prognosis in patients with chronic heart failure. J Am Coll Cardiol 1998;31:1591–1597.

Ward RP, Weinert L, Spencer KT, et al. Quantitative diagnosis of apical cardiomyopathy using contrast echocardiography. J Am Soc Echocardiogr 2002;15:316–322.

Webb JG, Sasson Z, Rakowski H, et al. Apical hypertrophic cardiomyopathy: clinical follow-up and diagnostic correlates. J Am Coll Cardiol 1990;15:83–90.

Chapter 18

Congenital Heart Diseases

Congenital heart diseases are broadly defined as those cardiac anomalies that are present at birth. By their very nature, such defects have their origin in embryonic development. Most congenital cardiac lesions constitute gross structural abnormalities with a spectrum of associated hemodynamic derangements. It is not surprising that the various echocardiographic techniques are ideally suited to the study of patients with congenital heart disease. Perhaps nowhere in cardiology have these methods played a more vital role in diagnosis and management. Historically, the emergence of two-dimensional echocardiography must be viewed as a milestone in the diagnostic approach to congenital heart disease. The tomographic nature of the technique and the unlimited number of imaging planes permit the anatomy and relationships of the cardiac structures to be defined, even in the presence of complex congenital malformations. For the noninvasive assessment of cardiac structure and function, echocardiography plays a preeminent role as the most accurate and widely applied method.

The echocardiographic approach to patients with congenital heart lesions differs substantially from that used to evaluate other forms of cardiac disease. Imaging in children has both advantages and disadvantages compared with adults. The smaller patient size permits the use of higher frequency transducers, thereby enhancing image quality. The presence of less heavily calcified bone and the absence of hyperinflated lungs in most children increase the available acoustic windows and generally contribute to improved image quality. Unfortunately, the smaller patient size also creates practical problems for image acquisition. Children are more likely to be uncooperative and may have other malformations (such as a chest deformity) that complicate imaging.

Adults with congenital heart disease present an entirely different array of challenges to the echocardiographer. The decision to intervene in these patients frequently hinges on the adequacy of previous interventions and the presence and severity of pulmonary vascular disease. In patients who have undergone surgery, an accurate assessment may be difficult. When details of the clinical history are unavailable, the echocardiographer is often called on to determine which surgical procedures have been performed. The options for further intervention often depend on the echocardiographic results. As the patient with congenital heart disease ages, the superimposition of other medical conditions (such as hypertension or coronary disease) further complicates his or her evaluation and management. Both image acquisition and interpretation can be challenging and time-consuming. The diversity and complexity of congenital cardiac malformations obviate even the most basic assumptions regarding chamber orientation and great vessel relationships. These problems are magnified in the patient who has undergone a surgical procedure previously. Therefore, the initial evaluation of the patient with suspected congenital heart disease mandates a thorough and systematic echocardiographic approach, often using additional views beyond those obtained during the standard examination.

This chapter focuses on the role of echocardiography in the adolescent and adult with congenital heart disease. Guidelines for the use of echocardiographic techniques in this growing patient population are provided in Table 18.1. The chapter is not intended as an exhaustive description of all forms of congenital heart disease. Lesions that are seen more commonly in adult patients are emphasized, whereas those considered less relevant are covered only superficially. Finally, the evaluation of the postoperative patient is covered in some detail.

THE ECHOCARDIOGRAPHIC EXAMINATION: A SEGMENTAL APPROACH TO ANATOMY

The initial echocardiographic examination of the patient with suspected congenital heart disease requires a sequential and systematic approach to cardiac anatomy. Such a method is necessary to detect cardiac malpositions and to diagnose complex congenital heart disease. The first step in this sequential approach is to determine

▶ **TABLE 18.1 Indications for Echocardiography in the Adult Patient with Congenital Heart Disease**

	Class
1. Patients with clinically suspected congenital heart disease, as evidenced by signs and symptoms such as a murmur, cyanosis, or unexplained arterial desaturation, and an abnormal electrocardiogram or radiograph suggesting congenital heart disease	I
2. Patients with known congenital heart disease on follow-up when there is a change in clinical findings	I
3. Patients with known congenital heart disease for whom there is uncertainty as to the original diagnosis or when the precise nature of the structural abnormalities or hemodynamics is unclear	I
4. Periodic echocardiograms in patients with known congenital heart lesions and for whom ventricular function and atrioventricular valve regurgitation must be followed (e.g., patients with a functionally single ventricle after a Fontan procedure, transposition of the great vessels after a Mustard procedure, L-transposition and ventricular inversion, and palliative shunts)	I
5. Patients with known congenital heart disease for whom following pulmonary artery pressure is important (e.g., patients with moderate or large ventricular septal defects, atrial septal defects, single ventricle, or any of the above with an additional risk factor of pulmonary hypertension)	I
6. Periodic echocardiography in patients with surgically repaired (or palliated) congenital heart disease with the following: change in clinical condition or clinical suspicion of residual defects, left or right ventricular function that must be followed, or the possibility of hemodynamic progression or a history of pulmonary hypertension	I
7. To direct interventional catheter valvotomy, radiofrequency ablation valvotomy interventions in the presence of complex cardiac anatomy	I
8. A follow-up Doppler echocardiographic study, annually or once every 2 years, in patients with known hemodynamically significant congenital heart disease without evident change in clinical condition	IIb
9. Multiple repeat Doppler echocardiography in patients with a repaired patent ductus arteriosus, atrial septal defect, ventricular septal defect, coarctation of the aorta, or bicuspid aortic valve without change in clinical condition	III
10. Repeat Doppler echocardiography in patients with known hemodynamically insignificant congenital heart lesions (e.g., small atrial septal defect, small ventricular septal defect) without a change in clinical condition	III

Adapted from Cheitlin MD, Alpert JS, Armstrong WF, et al. ACC/AHA Guidelines for the Clinical Application of Echocardiography: a report of the American College of Cardiology/American Heart Association Task Force on Practice Guidelines (Committee on Clinical Application of Echocardiography) developed in collaboration with the American Society of Echocardiography. Circulation 1997;95:1686–1744, with permission.

atrial situs and to assess the venous inflow patterns to the atria. Then, atrioventricular connections are defined and ventricular morphology and position are determined. Finally, ventriculoarterial relationships are evaluated. In most cases, this approach permits the identification of even the most complex forms of congenital heart disease (Table 18.2).

Cardiac Situs

Determination of atrial situs is best accomplished by using the subcostal views. In atrial *situs solitus*, the normal situation, the morphologic right atrium is to the right and the morphologic left atrium is to the left. *In situs inversus*, the opposite occurs, creating a mirror image effect. Atrial and visceral situs are almost always concordant. Thus, a right-sided liver and left-sided stomach are usually associated with atrial *situs solitus*. In the rare cases when atrial and abdominal situs are discordant, however, the

likelihood of complex congenital lesions is high. By using two-dimensional echocardiography, the location and morphology of the atria can be determined. The morphologic right atrium always contains the eustachian valve, and its appendage is shorter and broader than that of the left atrium. The left atrium lacks the eustachian valve and has a more rounded shape than the right atrium. The left atrial appendage is long and thin and has a narrower atrial junction compared with that of the right.

Although venous inflow does not define atrial morphology, the patterns of systemic and pulmonary venous return are helpful in determining situs. This spatial relationship is best evaluated using a transverse imaging plane through the upper abdomen. Normally, the abdominal aorta lies to the left and the inferior vena cava lies to the right of the spine. Compared with the vena cava, the aorta appears larger, more rounded, and more pulsatile. When in doubt, color flow imaging can be used to differentiate between the two vessels by demonstrating higher

▶ TABLE 18.2 **A Segmental Approach to Cardiac Situs and Malpositions**

Atrial situs
  Visceral situs (and visceroatrial concordance)
  Atrial morphology (*situs solitus* or *inversus*)
  Venous inflow patterns
Ventricular localization
  Ventricular morphology (D-loop or L-loop)
  Atrioventricular concordance (atrioventricular valve
    morphology)
  Base-to-apex axis (levocardia or dextrocardia)
Great artery connections
Identification of the great arteries
Ventriculoarterial concordance or transposition
**Spatial relationship between the great arteries and ventricular
  septum**

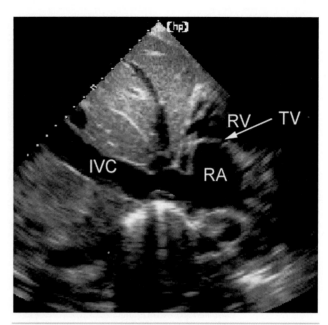

FIGURE 18.2 Subcostal long-axis view of a normal subject is provided. The inferior vena cava (*IVC*) can be seen entering the right atrium (*RA*). RV, right ventricle; TV, tricuspid valve.

velocity and primarily systolic flow in the aorta (Fig. 18.1). The opposite spatial relationship is characteristic of *situs inversus*. By tracing the course of the inferior vena cava and hepatic veins in the subcostal long-axis view, the right atrium generally can be identified in its usual position anterior and to the right of the left atrium (Fig. 18.2).

The pulmonary venous connections to the left atrium may be visualized using the apical and suprasternal window (Fig. 18.3). Color Doppler imaging is particularly helpful in identifying the pulmonary veins as they enter the left atrium. In adults, it is usually impossible to record the insertion of all four pulmonary veins using transthoracic echocardiography. With transesophageal echocardiography, however, the pulmonary venous drainage pat-

tern can be defined more precisely. Because of the possibility of anomalous pulmonary venous drainage, the relationship between the pulmonary veins and the left atrium is not constant, and their connections should not be used to define atrial morphology.

Ventricular Morphology

Once visceroatrial situs and venous connections are established, the orientation and morphology of the ventricles should be determined. During normal embryogenesis, the straight heart tube folds to the right (a D-loop) and then pivots to occupy a position within the left side of the chest. This positioning results in the right ventricle developing anteriorly and to the right of the left ventricle. The base-to-apex axis points leftward and most of the cardiac mass lies within the left side of the chest. If the initial fold in the heart tube is leftward, an L-loop develops, with the morphologic right ventricle to the left of the morphologic left ventricle. Thus, atrioventricular discordance occurs in the presence of *situs solitus* and an L-loop or *situs inversus* and a D-loop.

Ventricular morphology is readily assessed with two-dimensional echocardiography. Features that are useful in distinguishing the right and left ventricles are listed in Table 18.3. The presence of muscle bundles, particularly the moderator band, gives the right ventricle a trabeculated endocardial surface (Fig. 18.4). In contrast, the left ventricle is characterized by a smooth endocardial surface. This distinction is apparent using echocardiography and serves as one of the more reliable characteristics

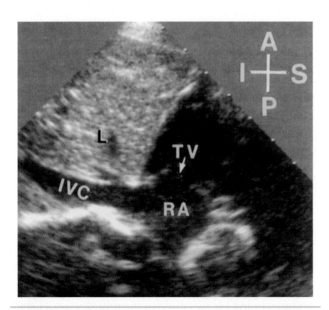

FIGURE 18.1. Subcostal short-axis view of the subject with situs solitus. The liver (*L*) and inferior vena cava (*IVC*) are on the patient's right, and the aorta (*Ao*) is to the patient's left. With the use of color flow imaging, flow within the aorta is detected. S, spine; A, anterior; P, posterior; R, right: L, left.

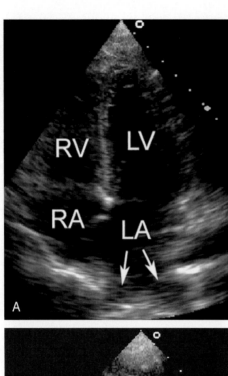

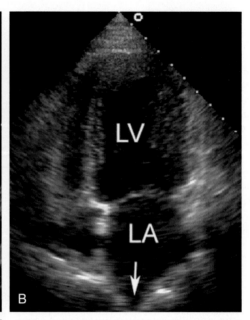

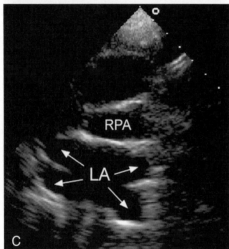

FIGURE 18.3 Apical four- **(A)** and two-chamber **(B)** views from a patient demonstrate the entrance of the pulmonary veins (*arrows*) into the left atrium (*LA*). **C:** A suprasternal short-axis view shows the posterior region of the left atrium, below the right pulmonary artery (*RPA*), where the pulmonary veins enter (*arrows*). LV, left ventricle; RA, right atrium; RV, right ventricle.

▶ **TABLE 18.3 Echocardiographic Characteristics of Right and Left Ventricles**

Right Ventricle	*Left Ventricle*
Trabeculated endocardial surface	Smooth endocardial surface
Three papillary muscles	Two papillary muscles
Chordae insert into ventricular septum	Ellipsoidal geometry
Infundibular muscle band	Mitral atrioventricular valve with two leaflets with relatively basal insertion
Moderator band	
Triangular cavity shape	
Tricuspid atrioventricular valve with relatively apical insertion	

when determining ventricular morphology. The structure and position of the atrioventricular valves are additional echocardiographic clues that are useful in distinguishing the right and left ventricles. If two ventricles are present, the atrioventricular valves associate with the correspond-ing ventricle and identification of the mitral and tricuspid valves defines the respective chambers. The tricuspid valve is more apically displaced, has three leaflets (and three papillary muscles) and chordal insertions into the septum. The mitral valve has a more basal septal attach-

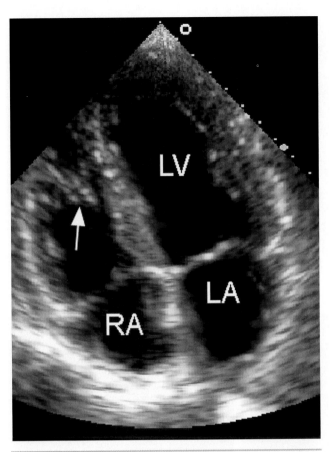

FIGURE 18.4 Apical four-chamber view from a healthy subject with a prominent moderator band (*arrow*), which represents a normal structure that is occasionally confused with thrombus or tumor. LA, left atrium; LV, left ventricle; RA, right atrium;

ment and has two leaflets, which insert into two papillary muscles but not the septum. All these features can be assessed with echocardiography. The four-chamber view allows the echocardiographer to determine ventricular morphology and the relative positions of the atrioventricular valves. The short-axis views permit definition of the papillary muscles and chordal insertions. The relative positions of the atrioventricular valves and the presence or absence of chordal insertions into the septum are the most helpful echocardiographic features when attempting to determine ventricular identity.

Great Artery Connections

The final step in the segmental approach to cardiac anatomy involves identification of the great arteries and their respective connections. In the normal heart with concordant connections, the morphologic left ventricle gives rise to the aorta and the pulmonary artery serves as the outlet of the right ventricle. In the presence of normal ventricular orientation, this arrangement results in an anterior and leftward pulmonary artery and a posterior and

rightward aorta with a left-sided aortic arch and descending aorta. The great arteries originate in orthogonal planes creating a "sausage and circle" appearance on short-axis imaging, which results from the rotation during development of the right ventricular outflow tract and pulmonary artery (the "sausage") around the ascending aorta (the "circle"). Discordant ventriculoarterial connections, or transposition, occur when the great arteries arise from the opposite ventricle. Two forms of transposition exist. In D-transposition, ventricular relationship is normal, with the morphologic right ventricle located to the right of the morphologic left ventricle. In L-transposition, atrioventricular discordance is present (because of formation of an L-loop during embryogenesis) so that the morphologic right ventricle lies to the left of the morphologic left ventricle.

Two-dimensional echocardiography permits accurate identification of the great arteries and their origins and relationship. The short-axis view at the base of the heart is most helpful when assessing these features. In the normal heart, the pulmonary valve lies slightly anterior and to the left of the aortic valve (Fig. 18.5). The pulmonary artery then courses posteriorly and bifurcates, with the right pulmonary artery passing immediately below the aortic arch. These findings are best appreciated in the parasternal long- and short-axis and subcostal views. The proximal aorta is optimally recorded from the parasternal window and the suprasternal notch (Fig. 18.6). To identify the great arteries, the course of the vessel and the presence or absence of a bifurcation are the most reliable echocardiographic signs. The presence of a right aortic arch can also be detected by assessing from the suprasternal short-axis view the course of the brachiocephalic vessels as they leave the arch.

ABNORMALITIES OF RIGHT VENTRICULAR INFLOW

The right ventricular inflow tract and tricuspid valve are visualized using the apical and subcostal four-chamber views, the short-axis view at the base, and the medially angulated parasternal long-axis view. The most important congenital pathologic entities involving the tricuspid valve are Ebstein anomaly and tricuspid atresia (discussed subsequently). Ebstein anomaly consists of apical displacement of the septal and posterior (and sometimes the anterior) leaflets of the tricuspid valve into the right ventricle. Typically, the leaflets are elongated and redundant with abnormal chordal attachments. This results in "atrialization" of the basal portion of the right ventricle as the functional orifice is displaced apically relative to the anatomic anulus. Ebstein anomaly is a spectrum of abnormalities, depending on the extent of apical displacement of the valve, the distal attachments of the leaflets,

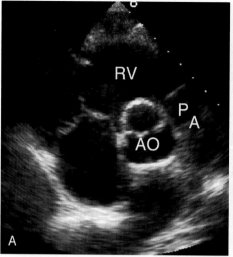 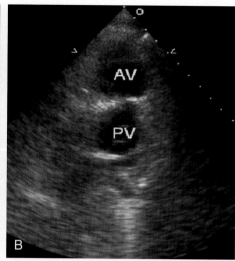

FIGURE 18.5 Parasternal short-axis echocardiograms from a healthy subject **(A)** and a patient with D-transposition of the great arteries **(B)**. In the healthy subject, the aortic valve (*AV*) is posterior and the right ventricular (*RV*) outflow tract and pulmonary artery (*PA*) appear to wrap around the aorta. With transposition, the aorta is anterior and the two great vessels arise in parallel. PV, pulmonary valve.

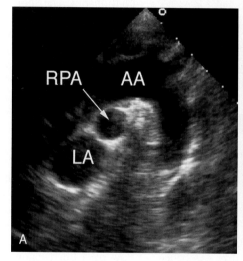 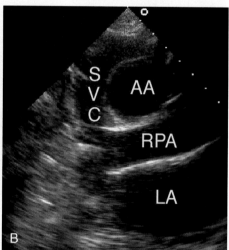

FIGURE 18.6 Suprasternal long- **(A)** and short-axis **(B)** views from a healthy subject. The right pulmonary artery (*RPA*) passes below the aortic arch (*AA*) and above the left atrium (LA). The superior vena cava (*SVC*) can be seen to the right of the aortic arch.

the size and function of the remaining right ventricle, the degree of tricuspid regurgitation, and the presence of right ventricular outflow tract obstruction (usually from the redundant anterior tricuspid valve leaflet).

The best echocardiographic view for the evaluation of Ebstein anomaly is the four-chamber view. The characteristic features identified in this plane are shown schematically in Figure 18.7. Of principal importance is the accurate recording of the level of insertion of the septal leaflet of the tricuspid valve relative to the anulus. Apical displacement of this insertion site is optimally assessed in this view and is the key to diagnosis (Fig. 18.8). Because the tricuspid valve is normally positioned more apically than the mitral valve, abnormal apical displacement is relative, and some investigators have suggested measuring the distance between insertion sites of the two atrioventricular valves. When normalized for body surface area, a distance of greater than 8 mm/M^2 is indicative

of Ebstein anomaly. Other investigators have advocated a maximal displacement of more than 20 mm as the diagnostic criterion in adults.

The four-chamber and medially angulated parasternal views may be used to assess the severity of Ebstein anomaly and to determine surgical options. The degree of atrialization of the ventricle, the extent of leaflet tethering, and the magnitude of deformity or dysplasia of the valve leaflets are important features with implications for surgical repair (Fig. 18.9). The extent of chordal attachments between the anterior leaflet and the anterior free wall should be assessed in multiple views. If tethering is significant, valve replacement rather than repair may be required. The greater the degree of atrialization is, the worse the prognosis. If the area of the functional right ventricle is less than one-third of the total right ventricular area, overall prognosis is poor. Because of the complexity of right ventricular geometry, an accurate measure

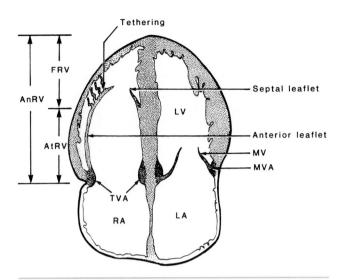

FIGURE 18.7 Schematic of anatomic abnormalities in Ebstein anomaly. RA, right atrium; LA, left atrium; LV, left ventricle; MV, mitral valve; MVA, mitral valve anulus; TVA, tricuspid valve anulus; AnRV, anatomic right ventricle; FRV, functional right ventricle; AtRV, atrialized right ventricle.

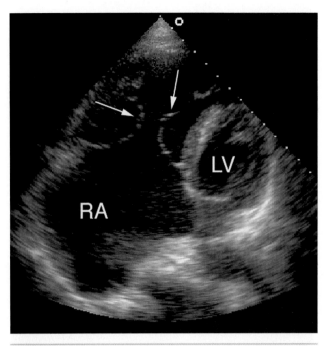

FIGURE 18.9 A more extreme form of Ebstein anomaly is demonstrated. The tricuspid valve (*arrows*) is markedly abnormal, and there is tethering of the leaflets, which prevented normal coaptation and resulted in significant tricuspid regurgitation. The right atrium (*RA*) is severely dilated. LV, left ventricle.

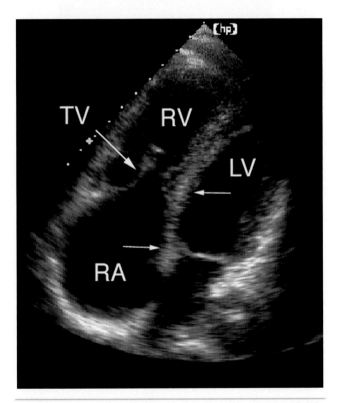

FIGURE 18.8 A four-chamber view from a patient with Ebstein anomaly is shown. The *arrows* indicate the degree of apical displacement of the tricuspid valve (*TV*), which had restricted motion. Note that the functional portion of the right ventricle (*RV*) is fairly well preserved. LV, left ventricle; RA, right atrium.

of the size of the functional right ventricle is difficult, and all available views should be used (Fig. 18.10). Doppler echocardiography should be used to detect tricuspid regurgitation, which is commonly seen in patients with Ebstein anomaly (Fig. 18.11). A redundant anterior tricuspid valve leaflet may cause functional right ventricular outflow tract obstruction, which can also be detected with Doppler imaging. In severe cases, pulmonary atresia may be present, although it is rarely seen in adults.

Ebstein anomaly may be associated with a variety of other abnormalities that can be detected with echocardiography, namely, atrial septal defect, mitral valve prolapse, and left ventricular dysfunction. The etiology of the left ventricular dysfunction is not known, but its presence is associated with a poor prognosis. Surgical options in patients with Ebstein anomaly include tricuspid valve repair or replacement. After surgical repair, echocardiography plays a role in assessing the success of the procedure and the function of the tricuspid valve.

ABNORMALITIES OF LEFT VENTRICULAR INFLOW

Pulmonary Veins

Obstruction of left ventricular inflow can occur at several levels (Table 18.4). Pulmonary vein stenosis may be seen

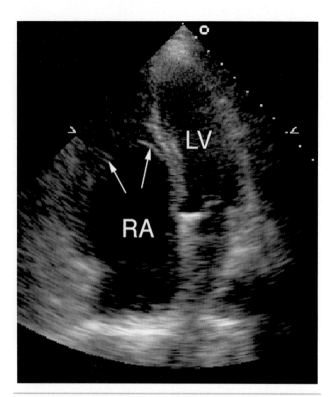

FIGURE 18.10 In this patient with Ebstein anomaly, apical displacement of the tricuspid valve (*arrows*) resulted in significant atrialization of the right ventricle, resulting in a small functional right ventricle. Note how the interventricular septum bows toward the left ventricle (*LV*). RA, right atrium.

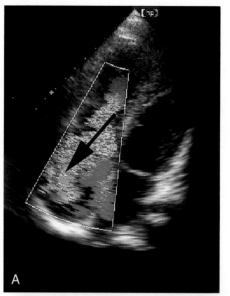

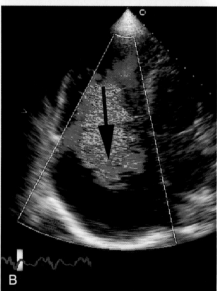

FIGURE 18.11 A, B: In patients with Ebstein anomaly, tethering and restricted motion of the tricuspid valve often lead to significant tricuspid regurgitation. These color Doppler images are from the same patients illustrated in Figures 18.9 and 18.10. In both cases, severe tricuspid regurgitation is documented.

as an isolated entity or in association with other congenital lesions. In one form, discrete areas of stenosis involving one or more pulmonary veins occur at or near the junction with the left atrium. Alternatively, hypoplasia of the pulmonary veins may be present. The echocardiographic diagnosis of the discrete form of pulmonary vein stenosis is contingent on the ability to visualize the entrance of the veins into the left atrium, which is optimally recorded using the apical and subcostal four-chamber views. In younger patients, a posteriorly angulated suprasternal short-axis view (sometimes referred to as the "crab view") can also be obtained (Fig. 18.3C). Usually, only the right or left upper pulmonary veins are imaged. Because of the proximity of the transducer to the left atrium, transesophageal echocardiography is superior for recording the insertion of the pulmonary veins (Fig. 18.12A). An approach to pulmonary vein visualization using this technique is covered in detail in Chapter 7. In most patients, all four veins can be visualized. Echocardiography has also been used for the diagnosis of pulmonary vein obstruction from compression by an extrinsic mass or secondary to stricture after an atrial fibrillation ablation procedure.

Visualizing pulmonary vein stenosis with two-dimensional echocardiography is rarely possible, and Doppler imaging is the primary means of securing a noninvasive diagnosis. Color Doppler imaging is useful when attempting to identify venous inflow and to detect the turbulent flow associated with stenosis. Because of the increase in velocity distal to the stenosis, color Doppler imaging may record a jet of blood entering the left atrium near the posterior wall. Turbulent flow in the posterior left atrium may be the initial echocardiographic abnormality and should suggest the possibility of a stenotic pulmonary vein. Then, pulsed Doppler imaging can be used to assess the inflow pattern and determine flow velocity. Normally,

▶ **TABLE 18.4 Levels of Obstruction of Left Ventricular Inflow**

Pulmonary veins
  Pulmonary vein stenosis (discrete)
  Hypoplastic pulmonary veins
  Extrinsic compression
Left atrium
  Cor triatriatum
  Supravalvular stenosing ring
Mitral valve
  Hypoplastic mitral valve
  Congenital mitral stenosis
    Parachute mitral valve
    Anomalous mitral arcade
    Double-orifice mitral valve

biphasic antegrade pulmonary venous flow (during ventricular systole and early diastole) is recorded (Fig. 18.12B). With stenosis, the flow velocity increases and becomes turbulent and more continuous. An example of mild pulmonary vein stenosis in an adult is presented in Figure 18.13.

Left Atrium

Obstruction of left ventricular filling also occurs at the atrial level, usually because of a fibrous membrane that impedes the flow of blood through the chamber. These membranes may be located in the middle of the atrium, effectively partitioning the left atrium into two chambers (a condition known as cor triatriatum), or they may occur

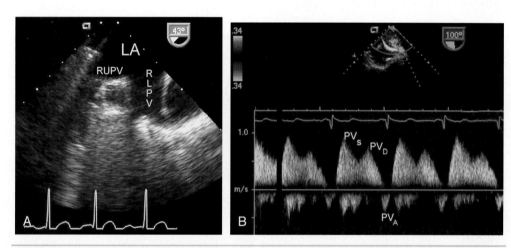

FIGURE 18.12 A: A transesophageal echocardiogram shows the entrance of the right lower (*RLPV*) and right upper (*RUPV*) pulmonary veins into the left atrium (*LA*). **B:** Flow in the left upper pulmonary vein is recorded from transesophageal echocardiography. In this example, moderately increased flow velocity is the result of left-to-right shunting through an atrial septal defect. PV_S, PV_D, and PV_A refer to pulmonary vein flow during systole, diastole, and atrial systole, respectively.

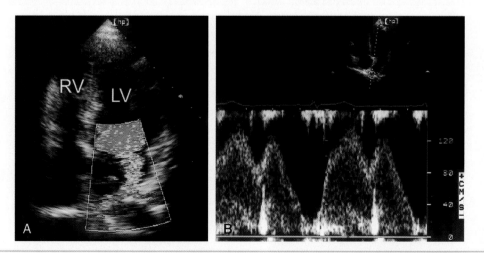

FIGURE 18.13 A patient with pulmonary vein stenosis is shown. **A:** Color Doppler imaging demonstrates a turbulent jet that appears to originate from the right upper pulmonary vein as it enters the left atrium. **B:** Pulsed Doppler imaging reveals nearly continuous antegrade flow and increased velocity. LV, left ventricle; RV, right ventricle.

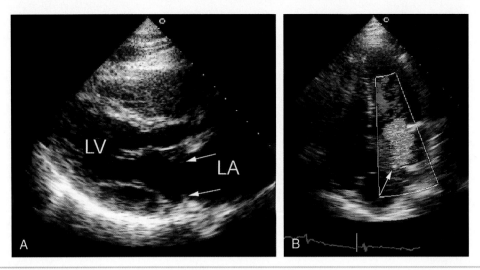

FIGURE 18.14 Cor triatriatum is demonstrated from the parasternal long-axis **(A)** and four-chamber **(B)** views. The membrane (*arrows*) within the left atrium (*LA*) is much better seen from the apical window. In such cases, color Doppler imaging is useful to demonstrate turbulent flow through the defect in the membrane (*arrow*). LV, left ventricle.

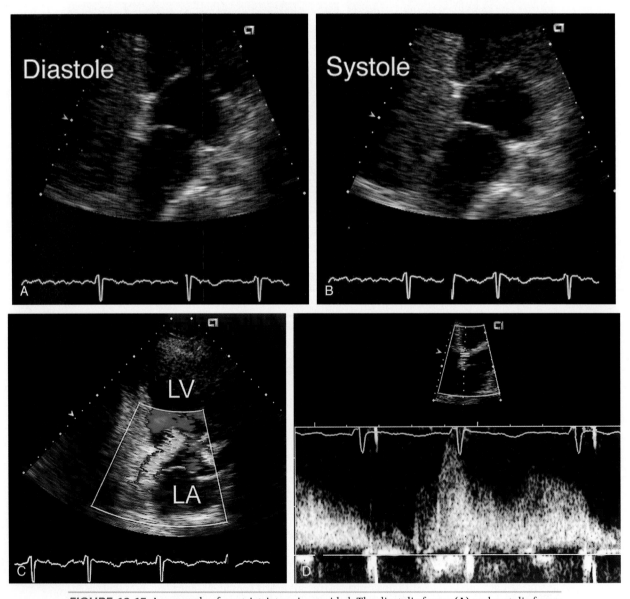

FIGURE 18.15 An example of cor triatriatum is provided. The diastolic frame **(A)** and systolic frame **(B)** demonstrate the relationship of the membrane to the mitral valve. **C:** Color Doppler imaging reveals the perforation within the membrane and the turbulent flow into the lower portion of the left atrium (*LA*). **D:** Pulsed Doppler imaging is used to assess flow velocity across the membrane, which has an appearance similar to that of mitral stenosis. LV, left ventricle.

at or near the level of the mitral anulus (a supravalvular stenosing ring). Such membranes are readily detected and localized with two-dimensional echocardiography. The membrane is visualized as a linear, echogenic structure extending from the anterosuperior to the posterolateral wall. In most cases, the superior "chamber" receives the pulmonary veins and the inferior "chamber" is associated with the atrial appendage and mitral valve (which is usually normal). Because of the orientation of the membrane, the four-chamber view is often optimal because it places the membrane perpendicular to the beam. Note in Figure 18.14 the improved visualization of the membrane from an apical window compared with the parasternal view. The obligatory perforation connecting the two is most often posterior and may be multiple. This communication

may be difficult to record with echocardiography. Color Doppler imaging usually permits localization of the opening in the membrane so that the pressure gradient can be assessed with pulsed Doppler imaging (Fig. 18.15). When the transthoracic study is suboptimal, transesophageal echocardiography should be used for evaluating this entity. Figure 18.16 is an example of cor triatriatum assessed from the transesophageal approach.

Distinguishing among the different levels of left ventricular inflow obstruction requires a combination of two-dimensional imaging and Doppler imaging and is best accomplished using the parasternal long-axis and apical four-chamber views. An example of a supravalvular stenosing ring is presented in Figure 18.17. In contrast to cor triatriatum, these membranes are closer to the mitral

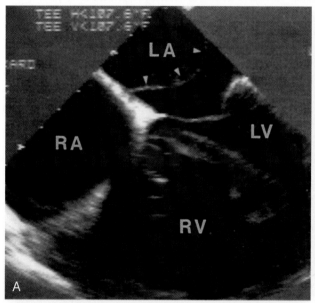

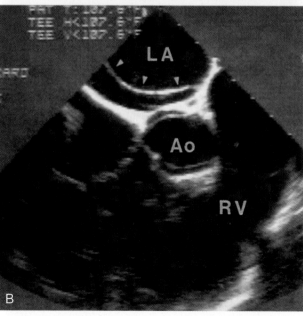

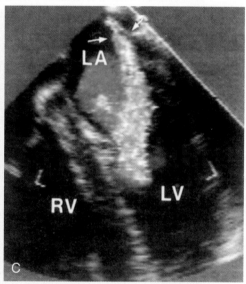

FIGURE 18.16 A transesophageal four-chamber echocardiogram from a patient with cor triatriatum (**A**). The membrane within the left atrium (*LA*) is indicated by *arrowheads*. Note the dilated right atrium (*RA*) and right ventricle (*RV*). In the transverse plane (**B**), the membrane is clearly visualized. **C:** Color flow imaging during diastole reveals turbulent flow through the defect in the membrane (*arrows*). LV, left ventricle; Ao, aorta.

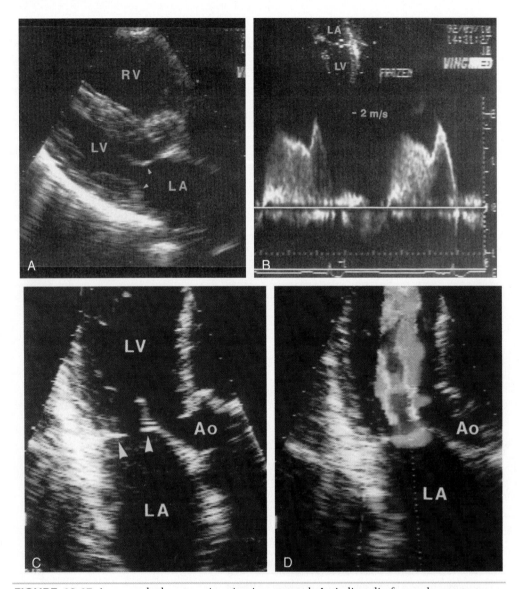

FIGURE 18.17 A supravalvular stenosing ring is presented. **A:** A diastolic frame demonstrates restricted opening of the mitral valve (*arrowheads*). The left atrium (*LA*) and right ventricle (*RV*) are dilated; however, the stenosing ring is not well visualized. **B:** A Doppler recording through the mitral valve indicates significant obstruction with increased flow velocity and a prolonged pressure half-time. **C:** An apical long-axis view demonstrates the stenosing ring (*arrowheads*). **D:** Color flow imaging in diastole reveals turbulent flow through the mitral orifice. Mitral regurgitation was also present. LV, left ventricle; Ao, aorta.

valve and may actually adhere to the valve leaflets. In the example presented, the membrane was not well visualized in the long-axis view, although restricted mobility of the mitral leaflets was apparent. Absence of anterior leaflet doming excludes the possibility of rheumatic mitral stenosis, and the presence of the supravalvular membrane was detected from the apical window. By using color Doppler imaging, identification of flow acceleration and turbulence at the level of the anulus rather than the leaflet tips is an additional clue to distinguish a supravalvular ring from mitral valve stenosis. Continuous wave Doppler imaging can then be used to assess the severity of the obstruction. The proximity of the membrane to the valve can

lead to leaflet damage, the result of high-velocity turbulent flow. Leaflet thickening and mitral regurgitation may develop as a consequence. Caution must be used when diagnosing a supravalvular stenosing ring with echocardiography. Differentiating between a thickened and calcified mitral anulus and a stenosing ring may be difficult, leading to both false-positive and false-negative results. Associated anomalies are seen frequently with both cor triatriatum and supravalvular stenosis. Atrial septal defect and persistent left superior vena cava are especially common and are readily detected with echocardiography. These entities may also occur in association with aortic coarctation and subaortic stenosis (Shone complex).

Mitral Valve

Congenital mitral stenosis is far less common than rheumatic mitral valve disease. Several anatomic variations exist (Table 18.4), and all can be diagnosed accurately with echocardiography. Because rheumatic mitral stenosis is so much more common in adults, however, the diagnosis of congenital mitral stenosis is often missed. Figure 18.18 is an example of a parachute mitral valve. In this condition, all the chordae insert into a single, large papillary muscle (hence the term "parachute"). The parasternal short-axis view is most helpful in determining the number, size, and location of the papillary muscles. The long-axis view reveals deformity and thickening of the mitral valve, restricted leaflet excursion, and chordal thickening and fusion. Because many of these features are common to rheumatic mitral valve disease, proper diagnosis is sometimes difficult and relies on detecting the presence of a single papillary muscle. The degree of stenosis is variable and is best assessed with Doppler imaging (Fig. 18.19). Because the inflow jet is often eccentric, color flow mapping is helpful for proper orientation of the Doppler beam. A supravalvular stenosing ring may coexist, thereby complicating the Doppler assessment.

Other congenital forms of mitral stenosis include anomalous mitral arcade and double-orifice mitral valve. In arcade-type mitral stenosis, the chordae insert into multiple small papillary muscles. Both stenosis and regurgitation are possible. Double-orifice mitral valve occurs because of duplication of the mitral orifice with or without fusion of subvalvular chordal structures. Usually, all the chordae associated with each orifice insert into the same papillary muscle, a situation similar to parachute mitral valve. The diagnosis is made by visualization of two separate orifices in the short-axis view (Fig. 18.20). The presence and severity of stenosis are variable in this condition. Other forms of congenital mitral valve pathology, including mitral valve prolapse and cleft mitral valve, are discussed elsewhere.

ABNORMALITIES OF RIGHT VENTRICULAR OUTFLOW

Right Ventricle

Narrowing of the right ventricular outflow tract can occur on several levels, and obstruction may be present at multiple sites within an individual patient. Subvalvular pul-

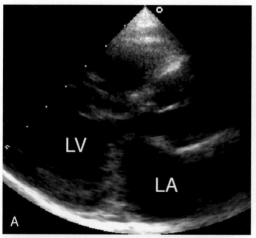

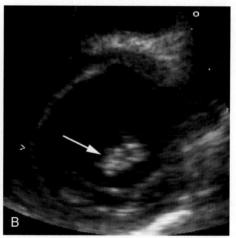

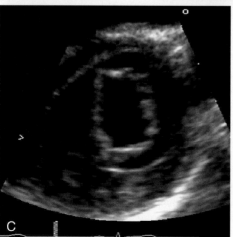

FIGURE 18.18 An example of parachute mitral valve is demonstrated. **A:** The long-axis view reveals thickened mitral leaflets that dome in diastole. **B:** A short-axis view at the mid-ventricular level demonstrates the chordae converging on a single papillary muscle (*arrow*). **C:** The orifice of the abnormal mitral valve is shown from the short-axis view. Although the orifice is large, a mild degree of subvalvular gradient was present. LA, left atrium; LV, left ventricle.

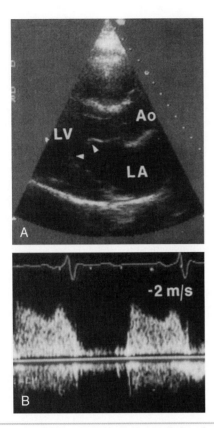

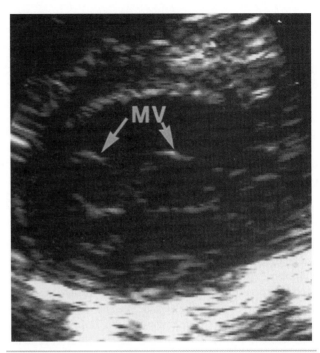

FIGURE 18.20 Parasternal short-axis view from a patient with double-orifice mitral valve (*MV*). In this case, the degree of functional mitral stenosis was insignificant.

FIGURE 18.19 Parasternal long-axis view **(A)** and continuous wave Doppler recording of mitral inflow **(B)** from a child with a parachute mitral valve. The echocardiogram reveals a thickened mitral valve with restricted leaflet mobility and chordal fusion (*arrowheads*). The left atrium (*LA*) is dilated. Color flow imaging revealed a turbulent and anteriorly directed jet. Continuous wave Doppler imaging demonstrates significantly increased inflow velocity and a prolonged pressure half-time consistent with mitral stenosis. Ao, aorta; LV, left ventricle.

monary stenosis usually involves the infundibulum and is less common than valvular stenosis. Infundibular pulmonary stenosis may be the result of discrete fibromuscular narrowing or hypertrophied subvalvular muscle bundles (also called double-chambered right ventricle) (Fig. 18.21). In many cases, a ventricular septal defect is also present. Right ventricular outflow tract narrowing is occasionally secondary to stenosis at a more distal level. For example, valvular pulmonary stenosis may lead to right ventricular hypertrophy, the development of subvalvular muscle bundles, and subsequent outflow tract narrowing.

Two-dimensional echocardiography is well suited to the evaluation of the right ventricular outflow tract. The parasternal short-axis and the subcostal four-chamber views are ideal for assessing the complex geometry of this region and for determining the level and severity of stenosis. The use of Doppler imaging to measure the pressure gradient may be challenging, however. Orienting the ultrasound beam parallel to the outflow tract jet requires considerable effort and the use of all available windows. Furthermore, localization of the site of stenosis may be difficult if narrowing occurs at more than one level (Fig. 18.22). Typically, subvalvular stenosis is a dynamic form of obstruction with maximal velocity occurring in late systole, a pattern that is analogous to the outflow jet seen in hypertrophic cardiomyopathy. The magnitude of reduction in pulmonary artery flow can affect development of the pulmonary arteries, which can be an important factor in surgical planning. Therefore, an evaluation of children with any form of right ventricular outflow tract obstruction should include an assessment of the pulmonary arteries. This includes patients with tetralogy of Fallot, in whom the type and timing of surgical repair are determined in part by the size of the pulmonary arteries.

A rare congenital abnormality of the right ventricle is arrhythmogenic right ventricular dysplasia (Fig. 18.23). This condition is characterized by dysplasia of the right ventricular myocardium, the extent of which varies considerably. Functionally, the dysplastic myocardium results in a form of right ventricular cardiomyopathy with decreased contractility and a propensity for ventricular arrhythmias. A spectrum of echocardiographic findings exists, depending on the extent of involvement. Thinning and hypokinesis of the free wall are characteristic. The systolic dysfunction may appear regional or, in cases of extensive dysplasia, global. Associated valvular pathology is not a feature of this condition.

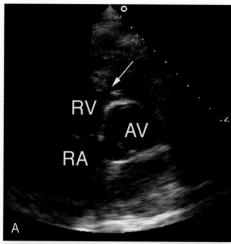

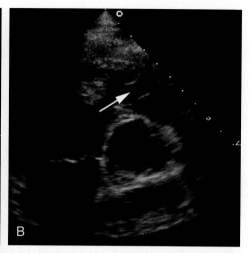

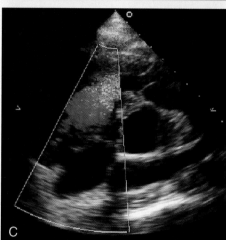

FIGURE 18.21 A series of short-axis images demonstrate infundibular right ventricular (*RV*) narrowing. **A:** Note the presence of muscle bundles in the area of the right ventricular outflow tract (*arrow*). **B:** The relationship of the subvalvular narrowing to the pulmonary valve (*arrow*) is demonstrated. **C:** Color Doppler imaging demonstrates turbulence in this area. Dynamic subvalvular stenosis is present with a late-peaking gradient. RA, right atrium; AV, aortic valve; RA, right atrium.

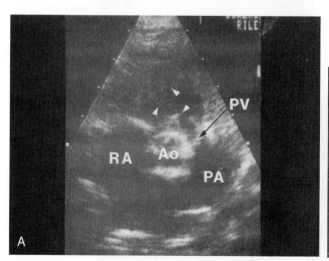

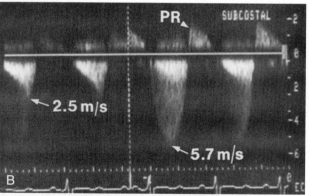

FIGURE 18.22 Two-dimensional echocardiogram **(A)** and Doppler recording **(B)** from a patient with combined subvalvular and valvular pulmonary stenosis. From the parasternal short-axis view **(A)**, right ventricular hypertrophy and infundibular narrowing are apparent (*arrowheads*). The pulmonary valve is not well visualized in this view, but thickening and immobility of the valve were apparent on real-time imaging. **B:** From the subcostal window, Doppler imaging demonstrates both subvalvular and valvular obstruction. On the left side is a dynamic subvalvular gradient. The maximal velocity occurs in late systole and suggests a peak gradient of approximately 25 mm Hg. On the right side, the maximal gradient at the level of the valve is 130 mm Hg. Pulmonary regurgitation (*PR*) is also present. Ao, aorta; PA, pulmonary artery; PV, pulmonary valve; RA, right atrium.

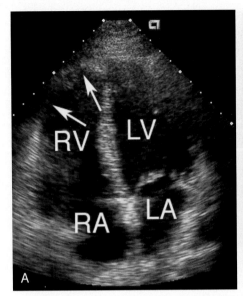
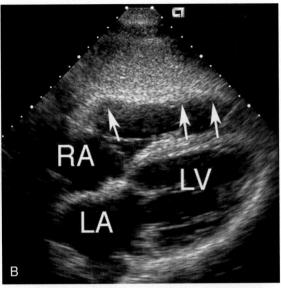

FIGURE 18.23 Extensive right ventricular involvement in a patient with arrhythmogenic right ventricular dysplasia is shown. **A:** The apical four-chamber view demonstrates dilation of the right ventricle (*RV*) and hypokinesis of the right ventricular free wall (*arrows*). **B:** A subcostal view reveals segmental right ventricular dysfunction in some aneurysmal dilation near the apex (*arrows*). LA, left atrium; LV, left ventricle; RA, right atrium.

Pulmonary Valve

Stenosis of the pulmonary valve is a fairly common congenital lesion that may occur in isolation or in association with other cardiac defects. The most frequently encountered form is characterized by fusion of the cusps and incompletely formed raphae, resulting in a dome-like structure with a narrowed orifice. Typically, the valve anulus is normal in size. With severe stenosis, right ventricular hypertrophy may lead to variable degrees of subvalvular narrowing.

In adults, the morphology of the stenotic pulmonary valve is best visualized in the parasternal short-axis plane through the base of the heart. With two-dimensional echocardiography, the cusps appear thickened, have decreased excursion, and dome in systole (Fig. 18.24). Poststenotic pulmonary artery dilation is frequently evident, but its presence does not correlate with severity. In most cases, right ventricular size and function are normal, and trabeculation of the right ventricular walls is increased. Calcification of the valve is characteristic in adults, but not children, with this disorder. Less common, dysplasia of the pulmonary valve will cause valvular stenosis at birth, due to myxomatous thickening of the leaflets (Fig. 18.25). When pulmonary stenosis is severe, evidence of right ven-

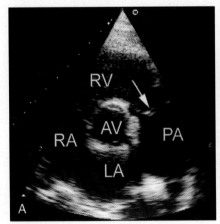
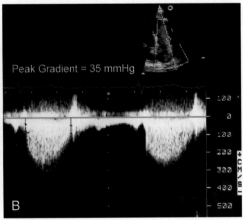

FIGURE 18.24 An example of valvular pulmonary stenosis is presented. **A:** A basal short-axis view demonstrates a thickened pulmonary valve (*arrow*). **B:** Doppler imaging demonstrates a peak gradient of 35 mm Hg. AV, aortic valve; LA, left atrium; PA, pulmonary artery; RV, right ventricle.

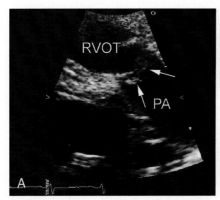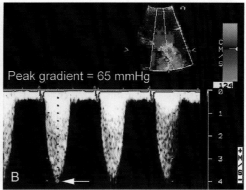

FIGURE 18.25 An example of dysplastic pulmonary valve stenosis is provided. **A:** The pulmonary valve (*arrow*) is markedly thickened and immobile. Doming during systole is present. **B:** A maximal pressure gradient of approximately 65 mm Hg is demonstrated. PA, pulmonary artery; RVOT, right ventricular outflow tract.

tricular pressure overload will be present. The degree of septal flattening and right ventricular enlargement correlate roughly with the severity of stenosis. Figure 18.26 is an example of extreme right ventricular pressure overload secondary to severe valvular pulmonary stenosis.

Although two-dimensional echocardiography is essential for the morphologic diagnosis of pulmonary stenosis, the technique is limited for assessing the severity of obstruction. Neither the degree of cusp thickening nor the presence of right ventricular hypertrophy provides a quantitative measure of severity. Doppler imaging is the technique of choice to measure the severity of pulmonary stenosis. Using the modified Bernoulli equation, the peak instantaneous pressure gradient can be calculated (Figs. 18.25 and 18.26). Several clinical studies have demonstrated an excellent correlation between Doppler imaging and catheterization-derived pressure gradients in patients

with pulmonary stenosis. In most patients, optimal alignment of the Doppler beam with the stenotic jet uses the parasternal short-axis view. In some individuals, use of a lower interspace is necessary to better align with a superiorly directed jet. In patients with pulmonary artery dilation, anterior displacement of the valve precludes proper beam alignment from the parasternal window. In this situation, the subcostal or suprasternal approach is usually adequate. In children, particularly, the subcostal approach provides optimal beam alignment and permits detection of the maximal jet velocity.

In children with pulmonary stenosis, surgical valvotomy or balloon valvuloplasty is often performed to relieve the obstruction. After such interventions, Doppler echocardiography may be used for serial evaluation and to detect residual stenosis (Fig. 18.27). The magnitude of associated pulmonary insufficiency and abnormalities of

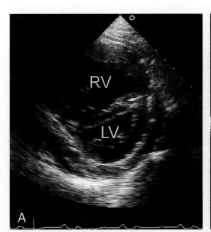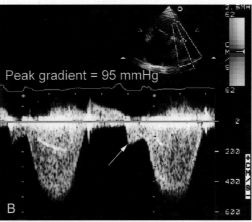

FIGURE 18.26 **A:** A patient with severe pulmonary stenosis demonstrates septal flattening with a dilated and hypertrophied right ventricle (*RV*). These findings are consistent with right ventricular pressure overload. **B:** Severe pulmonary stenosis is confirmed with a maximal pressure gradient of approximately 95 mm Hg. Note the presence of presystolic flow through the pulmonary valve at the time of right atrial systole (*arrow*). LV, left ventricle.

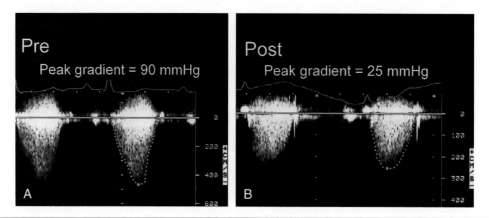

FIGURE 18.27 A case of pulmonary stenosis is shown before (*Pre*) **(A)** and after (*Post*) **(B)** valvuloplasty. The procedure resulted in a decrease in pulmonary valve gradient from 90 to 25 mm Hg.

right ventricular diastolic filling can also be assessed. In patients with combined valvular and infundibular stenosis, the presence of serial obstructions may result in overestimation by continuous wave Doppler imaging of the catheterization-derived pressure gradient.

Pulmonary Artery

Pulmonary artery stenosis (also referred to as peripheral or supravalvular pulmonary stenosis) can occur at any level and often involves multiple sites. Several morphologic forms exist, including discrete membrane-like lesions, long tubular stenoses, and tubular hypoplasia. These anomalies frequently are associated with other congenital cardiac and extracardiac lesions (e.g., Williams syndrome). The ability to detect pulmonary artery stenoses with echocardiography depends on the location of the lesions. Proximal lesions can be visualized from the parasternal short-axis window. Figure 18.28 is an example of peripheral pulmonary stenosis involving the right branch. In most such cases, the diagnosis is apparent from two-dimensional echocardio-

graphic imaging. Color Doppler imaging should be used to demonstrate turbulence and acceleration of flow within the stenotic segment. The echocardiographer must bear in mind, however, that a more common cause of turbulent flow within the main pulmonary artery is patent ductus arteriosus. More peripheral stenoses may be impossible to visualize, especially in older patients. In children, the subcostal four-chamber and the suprasternal views may permit detection of distal lesions. The diagnosis should be considered in a patient with unexplained right ventricular hypertrophy, particularly in the presence of a pulsatile proximal pulmonary artery.

ABNORMALITIES OF LEFT VENTRICULAR OUTFLOW

Congenital abnormalities of left ventricular outflow usually involve obstruction of flow, and several important forms exist. These lesions may be categorized as subvalvular, valvular, or supravalvular (which includes coarctation of

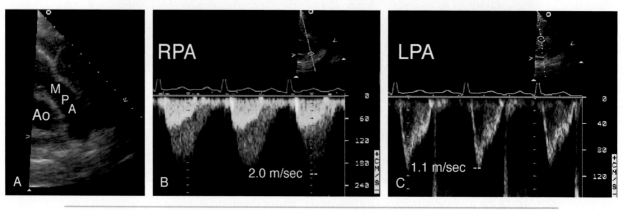

FIGURE 18.28 An example of pulmonary artery stenosis is demonstrated. **A:** The main pulmonary artery (*MPA*) appears normal. **B:** Flow through the right pulmonary artery (*RPA*) demonstrates increased velocity and acceleration. **C:** Normal flow velocity through the left pulmonary artery (*LPA*). Ao, aorta.

▶ **TABLE 18.5** **Classification of the Various Congenital Forms of Left Ventricular Outflow Tract Obstruction**

Subvalvular
   Discrete membranous stenosis
   Fibromuscular tunnel
   Hypertrophic obstructive cardiomyopathy
Valvular
   Unicuspid
   Bicuspid
   Dysplastic
Supravalvular
   Discrete (membranous or "hourglass")
   Aortic hypoplasia or atresia
   Interrupted aortic arch
   Coarctation of the aorta

the aorta) (Table 18.5). The subvalvular forms are heterogeneous and include hypertrophic cardiomyopathy, which is discussed in Chapter 17. The most important forms are the valvular lesions, which are common causes of stenosis in children (the unicuspid or congenitally stenotic aortic valve) and in adults (the bicuspid valve). The form of supravalvular obstruction encountered most frequently in the adult patient is coarctation of the aorta. This section includes a discussion of the lesions that occur at each of these different levels in order, but the focus is on those anomalies that are most common in adults.

Subvalvular Obstruction

Two types of subvalvular aortic stenosis are discussed here: the discrete form and the fibromuscular type of subaortic obstruction. Together, these lesions account for less than 20% of all cases of left ventricular outflow ob-

struction in children and both are uncommon in adult patients. Discrete subaortic stenosis results from a thin, fibrous membrane or ridge that forms a crescentic barrier within the outflow tract just below the aortic valve. The membrane usually extends from the anterior septum to the anterior mitral leaflet. The degree of obstruction to flow is variable, and aortic regurgitation develops in approximately 50% of patients. With two-dimensional echocardiography, these membranes are seen as a discrete linear echo in the left ventricular outflow tract perpendicular to the interventricular septum. Because the membranes are parallel to the beam, recording these structures from the parasternal long-axis window may require the use of multiple transducer positions (Fig. 18.29). In many cases, the membranes are detected more easily from the apical views (where the ultrasound beam is oriented perpendicular to the structure) (Fig. 18.30). Transesophageal echocardiography has also been used in the assessment of patients with subvalvular obstruction. Doppler imaging plays an essential role in the evaluation of these patients. After the location and orientation of the jet are visualized with color flow imaging, continuous wave Doppler imaging can be used to estimate the peak pressure gradient across the membrane (Fig. 18.31). In the absence of aortic valve stenosis, this value correlates well with the catheterization-derived measure of obstruction. In the presence of multiple serial stenoses, however, Doppler imaging may overestimate the catheterization-measured gradient. The presence and severity of aortic regurgitation can also be assessed with Doppler techniques (Fig. 18.29). M-mode echocardiography can also be helpful in assessing subvalvular obstruction. Midsystolic partial closure with reopening of the leaflets in late systole is indicative of a subvalvular pressure gradient.

Membranous subaortic stenosis is distinguished from a subaortic fibromuscular ridge or tunnel with two-

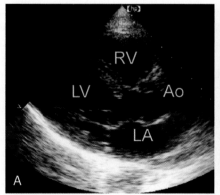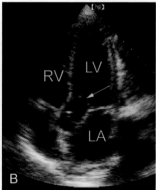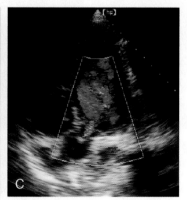

FIGURE 18.29 An example of a subaortic membrane is provided. **A:** Long-axis view reveals narrowing below the aortic valve, which appears structurally normal. The presence of the membrane (*arrow*) and its relationship to the aortic valve is better appreciated from the apical four-chamber view (**B**). **C:** Mild aortic regurgitation is demonstrated by Doppler imaging. Ao, aorta; LA, left atrium; LV, left ventricle; RV, right ventricle.

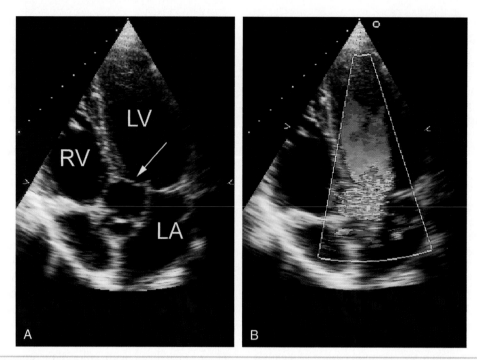

FIGURE 18.30 A: A subaortic membrane is readily apparent in this apical four-chamber view. **B:** The presence of the membrane results in turbulence in the left ventricular outflow tract, proximal to the aortic valve. This high-velocity, turbulent flow can result in damage to the aortic cusps. LA, left atrium; LV, left ventricle; RV, right ventricle.

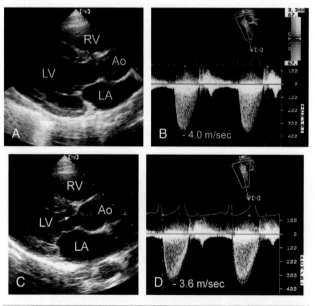

FIGURE 18.31 These two cases demonstrate the continuum between a discrete subaortic membrane and a fibromuscular ridge. **A:** A discrete membrane is demonstrated. Note how the membrane attaches to and deforms the base of the anterior mitral leaflet. A 60 mm Hg peak systolic gradient is confirmed **(B)**. **C:** A fibromuscular ridge (*arrow*) in association with a membrane is located just below the aortic valve. In this patient, the peak gradient across the subvalvular obstruction is approximately 52 mm Hg **(D)**. Ao, aorta; LA, left atrium; LV, left ventricle; RV, right ventricle.

dimensional echocardiography. Tunnel-type subaortic obstruction, rarely seen in adults, is characterized by diffuse thickening and narrowing of the left ventricular outflow tract with associated concentric left ventricular hypertrophy. A fibromuscular ridge may also obstruct the outflow tract (Fig. 18.31). This entity is similar to discrete membranous subaortic stenosis, but the obstruction is thicker and less discrete and appears more muscular (Fig. 18.32). These different forms of subaortic obstruction probably exist as a continuum, with a thin discrete membrane at one extreme and a diffuse tunnel at the other. Differentiating among individual cases may, therefore, be difficult and somewhat arbitrary. All these forms of subaortic obstruction are frequently associated with ventricular septal defects. Occasionally, other congenital cardiac anomalies are associated with subvalvular left ventricular outflow tract obstruction, including accessory mitral valve chordae, anomalous papillary muscle insertion, and abnormal insertion of the anterior mitral leaflet.

Valvular Aortic Stenosis

Aortic stenosis may be present at birth (a congenitally stenotic aortic valve) or may develop over time in a congenitally abnormal, but not stenotic, valve. In the former, the valve may be acommissural (resembling a volcano and more typical of pulmonary stenosis) or unicuspid unicommissural (with a slit-like orifice, resembling an ex-

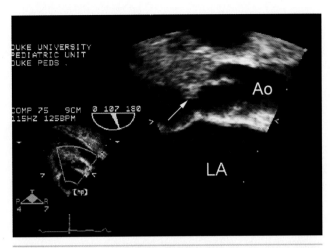

FIGURE 18.32 An example of a fibromuscular ridge below the aortic valve is demonstrated on transesophageal echocardiography. A ring of fibrous tissue results in moderate subvalvular narrowing and involves the base of the anterior mitral leaflet (*arrow*). Ao, aorta; LA, left atrium.

clamation point). A bicuspid or tricuspid valve can also be stenotic at birth because of commissural fusion or dysplasia. Most often, such valves will be functionally normal at birth but gradually become stenotic over time because of progressive fibrosis and calcification. In other cases, degeneration of the valve leads to predominant aortic regurgitation. Quadricuspid valves are rare and have a similar natural history.

Bicuspid aortic valve is estimated to occur in 1% to 2% of the general population, making it the single most common congenital cardiac anomaly. As just noted, these valves often are functionally normal at birth (Fig. 18.33). Two-dimensional echocardiography plays a major role in detection of this entity. Direct visualization of the aortic cusps is possible from the parasternal short-axis view through the base of the heart. During diastole, the cusps of a normal tricuspid valve are closed within the plane of the scan and the commissures form a "Y" (sometimes referred to as an inverted Mercedes-Benz sign). A *true* bicuspid valve has two cusps of nearly equal size, two associated sinuses, and a single linear commissure. A raphe may be present and, if present, creates the illusion of three separate cusps. By observing valve opening in systole, however, the number of distinct cusps is apparent. Fusion of two of the cusps may create the appearance of a bicuspid valve, but the presence of three distinct sinuses will establish this difference. Confirming the presence of a bicuspid aortic valve with echocardiography requires high-resolution images from the short-axis view for adequate visualization of valve morphology. A unicuspid valve has a single slit-like commissure, and the opening is eccentric and restricted. The stenotic tricuspid valve has three cusps with variable degrees of commissural fusion. Thus, an accurate assessment of functional anatomy requires an analysis of the number of apparent cusps, the

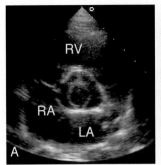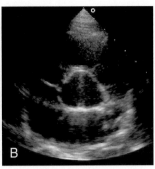

FIGURE 18.33 A bicuspid aortic valve is demonstrated from the short-axis view. The systolic frame (**A**) demonstrates a circular orifice. **B:** During diastole, a vertical commissure is seen between the two cusps. LA, left atrium; RA, right atrium; RV, right ventricle.

degree of cusp separation, and a recording of their mobility and excursion during systole.

Whereas the short-axis view is useful for determining the number of commissures and the degree, if any, of commissural fusion, movement of the cusps out of the imaging plane during systole precludes accurate determination of the presence and severity of stenosis. In fact, normal systolic excursion of the bodies of the cusps recorded from the short-axis view may lead to underestimation of the severity of congenital aortic stenosis. Thus, the short-axis view is useful when evaluating aortic valve anatomy but should never be used to exclude the possibility of congenital aortic stenosis. The long-axis views have several advantages for this purpose. The thickness and excursion of the cusps can be assessed. Normally, they appear as thin, delicate structures that appear to open completely in systole and are aligned parallel to and against the aortic walls. With congenital aortic stenosis, the cusps are thickened and appear to dome during systole, the result of restricted motion of the tips relative to the more mobile bodies of the cusps (Fig. 18.34). A qualitative estimate of severity is pos-

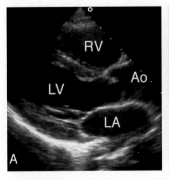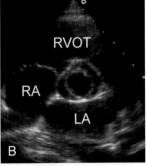

FIGURE 18.34 A functionally normal bicuspid aortic valve from a young patient is shown. **A:** Long-axis view demonstrates doming of the valve in systole. **B:** Basal short-axis view confirms that the valve is bicuspid but with no evidence of stenosis. Ao, aorta; LA, left atrium; LV, left ventricle; RA, right atrium; RV, right ventricle; RVOT, right ventricular outflow tract.

sible, based on the thickness and immobility of the cusps, the extent of leaflet tip separation in systole, the degree of left ventricular hypertrophy, and the presence of post-stenotic aortic root dilation.

Doppler imaging should be used to complete the non-invasive assessment of aortic stenosis and to provide a quantitative evaluation of severity. The apical, right parasternal, and suprasternal windows should be used to ensure that the maximal velocity is obtained. Then, through the use of the modified Bernoulli equation, the peak pressure gradient can be calculated. Both peak instantaneous and mean pressure gradients can be derived, and in children, the mean gradient is often used for clinical decision making. The values obtained with this approach correlate well with catheterization-derived gradients. Inherent differences exist between the two methods, and discrepancies should not necessarily be viewed as an error on the part of one or the other technique. In children especially, anxiety and increased activity during the examination will lead to an increase in flow velocity (both proximal and distal to the valve) and will thereby increase the measured pressure gradient. To calculate aortic valve area, the continuity equation can be used. It should be emphasized that the application of Doppler imaging to quantify aortic stenosis is similar in children and adults. The basic principles underlying these applications are covered in detail in Chapters 8 and 10.

In adults with congenital aortic stenosis, an important application of the Doppler technique is to assess patients after valvotomy, primarily to detect restenosis. Because these valves have been instrumented, assessing restenosis using morphologic criteria from two-dimensional echocardiography may be difficult. Doppler imaging is an ideal technique for the serial follow-up of these patients to assess both stenosis and regurgitation (Fig. 18.35), although the orientation of the jet may be eccentric after valvotomy and proper alignment of the Doppler beam may be difficult.

Supravalvular Aortic Stenosis

The least common site for congenital aortic stenosis is in the supravalvular area. Three morphologic types of supravalvular aortic stenosis have been described: (1) fibromuscular thickening producing an hourglass-shaped narrowing above the sinuses (the most common form), (2) a discrete fibrous membrane in a normal-sized aorta, usually located near the sinotubular junction, and (3) diffuse hypoplasia of the ascending aorta, often involving the origins of the brachiocephalic arteries. Because of the presence of stenosis above the aortic valve and coronary ostia, two additional features often accompany these anomalies: (1) dilation of the coronary arteries, sometimes with ostial obstruction and (2) thickening and fibrosis of the aortic cusps, usually with an element of aortic regurgitation. Williams syndrome includes supravalvular aortic stenosis, elfin facies, mental retardation, and, occasionally, peripheral pulmonary stenosis. Isolated supravalvular aortic stenosis with or without peripheral pulmonary stenosis may be inherited as an autosomal dominant trait.

The parasternal long-axis view or a high right parasternal view is most helpful for diagnosing supra-

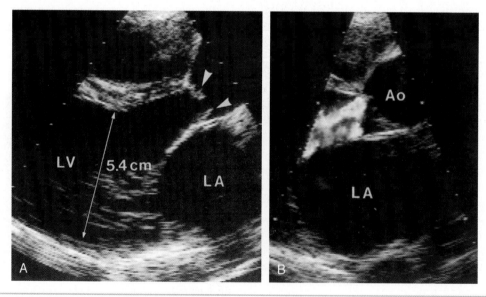

FIGURE 18.35 Parasternal long-axis views from a patient with congenital aortic stenosis after valvotomy. **A:** The aortic cusps are thickened and moderately immobile. Systolic doming is present. The left ventricle (*LV*) is dilated at 5.4 cm. The left atrium (*LA*) and aorta (*Ao*) are also dilated. **B:** Color flow imaging reveals moderate aortic regurgitation.

valvular aortic stenosis. In the normal aorta, the vessel diameter is greatest at the level of the sinuses. At the sinotubular junction, the diameter decreases slightly and approximates the size of the aortic anulus. With supravalvular aortic stenosis, an hourglass deformity occurs that is characterized by a segment of gradual tapering and then widening of the lumen (Fig. 18.36). The aortic walls usually appear thickened and echogenic. Aortic cusp fibrosis is often present, but poststenotic dilation of the ascending aorta is not a feature of this anomaly. A hypoplastic aorta is characterized by more diffuse and extensive narrowing with variable involvement of the branch vessels.

Assessing the severity of supravalvular aortic stenosis relies on two-dimensional echocardiography for accurate visualization of the magnitude and linear extent of the narrowing. Careful assessment of the aortic valve and the coronary arteries is an essential part of the evaluation of these patients. Proximal coronary artery dilation or ostial stenosis may be detected from the parasternal short-axis view at the base of the heart. Doppler imaging can be used to estimate the peak pressure drop across the site of aortic narrowing. In the presence of a discrete, isolated stenosis, the pressure gradient derived from Doppler imaging is an accurate reflector of severity. As noted previously, however, if the stenoses are multiple or tubular, the correlation between Doppler imaging and catheterization-derived gradients may be poor.

COARCTATION OF THE AORTA

This relatively common condition is the result of localized narrowing of the descending aorta near the origin of the ductus arteriosus. The lesion consists of a ridge-like indentation of the posterolateral wall of the aorta resulting from thickening and infolding of the aortic media. It is typically located just distal to the origin of the left subclavian artery and the specific location may be "preductal" or "postductal" depending on the position of the ridge of tissue relative to the ductus (or ligamentum) arteriosus. It is often associated with other forms of congenital heart disease, especially bicuspid aortic valve and mitral valve malformations.

Echocardiographic detection of coarctation requires both an index of suspicion and careful recording of the descending aorta from the suprasternal window. In children, the evaluation of this portion of the aorta is relatively straightforward. In adults, however, the assessment can be technically demanding and both false-negative and false-positive results occur. The goal is to record the arch and descending aorta in the long axis from the suprasternal notch. False-negative results usually result from an inability to image the most distal portion of the arch (where the narrowing occurs). False-positive findings are the result of a tangential imaging plane through the vessel, creating the illusion of narrowing. The origins of the carotid and subclavian arteries serve as landmarks when localizing the juxtaductal area. The location of the left subclavian artery relative to the coarctation is an important factor in surgical management. If an area of stenosis is suspected, care should be taken to ensure proper beam alignment. If the aortic lumen can be seen beyond the narrowing, the likelihood of a false-positive result is reduced (Fig. 18.37). Dilation and exaggerated pulsation of the proximal aortic arch are further evidence of significant coarctation.

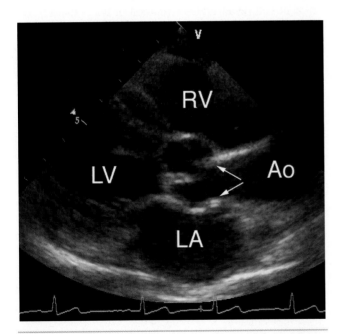

FIGURE 18.36 A child with supravalvular aortic stenosis is presented. The narrowing begins at the sinotubular junction (*arrows*) and is associated with increased echogenicity of the vessel walls. Ao, aorta; LA, left atrium; LV, left ventricle; RV, right ventricle. (Courtesy of T. R. Kimball, M.D., and S.A. Witt, R.D.C.S.)

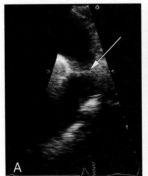
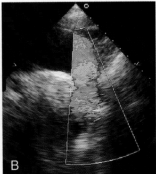

FIGURE 18.37 Aortic coarctation is demonstrated from the suprasternal notch. **A:** The descending aorta can be seen with a shelf-like narrowing in the mid-portion (*arrow*). **B:** Color Doppler imaging demonstrates acceleration of flow and turbulence at the level of the coarctation.

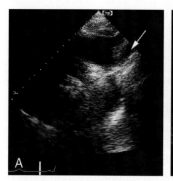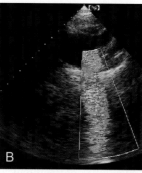

FIGURE 18.38 A: The location of the coarctation relative to the branch arteries is demonstrated. The left subclavian artery (*arrow*) is seen proximal to the site of obstruction. **B:** Color Doppler imaging demonstrates turbulence at the site of the coarctation.

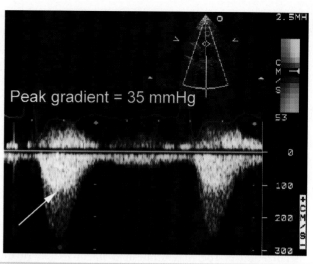

Peak gradient = 35 mmHg

FIGURE 18.39 Continuous wave Doppler imaging demonstrates a peak systolic pressure gradient of 35 mm Hg across the coarctation. Superimposed within the systolic flow signal is a darker jet (*arrow*) that corresponds to flow proximal to the stenosis. Note the absence of flow during diastole.

An example of coarctation of the aorta in an adult patient is shown in Figure 18.38. Note the location of a shelf-like constriction just beyond the origin of the left subclavian artery. Dilation of the ascending aorta is also apparent. When two-dimensional echocardiographic imaging is diagnostic of (or suspicious for) coarctation, Doppler imaging should be performed to aid in the diagnosis and to provide an estimation of the pressure gradient. As a first step, color Doppler imaging can be used to detect acceleration and turbulence within the region of narrowing. The absence of Doppler evidence of acceleration and turbulence of flow should alert the examiner to the possibility of a false-positive two-dimensional echocardiographic result. Color Doppler imaging also permits more accurate alignment of the continuous wave Doppler beam. Figure 18.39 is an example of a Doppler recording of flow across an aortic coarctation. To estimate the peak pressure gradient, the Bernoulli equation can be used. When this equation is applied to aortic coarctation, however, it may be inappropriate to ignore the proximal aortic flow velocity. As a general rule, if this proximal velocity is less than 1.5 m/sec, it can be ignored and the simplified equation can be used. If it is greater than 1.5 m/sec, the expanded Bernoulli equation is necessary. In this way, a more accurate pressure gradient is obtained. The persistence of a high-velocity flow signal into diastole is another useful clue to the severity of the stenosis. A pressure gradient throughout the cardiac cycle indicates a more severe form of obstruction compared with a pressure gradient that is confined to systole (Fig. 18.40). In this example, color Doppler imaging reveals persistence of turbulent antegrade flow across the coarct. Then, the presence of a diastolic gradient is confirmed with continuous wave Doppler imaging. Because coarctation gradients are flow dependent, low-level exercise, usually in the form of leg lifts, can be performed to assess the response to stress. In many cases, exercise will not cause a significant increase in the peak gradient, but will result in the development or increase in the diastolic gradient. In borderline cases, this response can be helpful in clinical decision making.

Although Doppler imaging is sensitive for the detection of coarctation, false-negative results can occur in the presence of a patent ductus arteriosus. Left-to-right runoff of blood flow through the ductus reduces the jet velocity through the coarctation and leads to an underestimation of the pressure gradient. This can also occur in the presence of well-developed collaterals. In such cases, the Doppler gradient will be an underestimation of the actual severity of obstruction. False-positive results are even less common. Occasionally, a mild increase (1.5–2 m/sec) in descending aortic flow velocity will be misinterpreted as evidence of coarctation. In the absence of turbulence or echocardiographic evidence of vessel narrowing, this should generally be attributed to normal acceleration around the arch. Long-term follow-up after repair of aortic coarctation relies heavily on echocardiographic methods for the detection of restenosis. Estimation of the restenosis gradient by Doppler imaging is possible and correlates well with catheterization-derived values (Fig. 18.41).

Aortic atresia and interrupted aortic arch are severe and uncommon forms of left ventricular outflow obstruction. They may be diagnosed *in utero* or shortly after birth by using echocardiographic techniques. Interruption of the aortic arch may be thought of as an extreme form of coarctation. The length of the "missing" segment varies, as does the relative insertion sites of the arch vessels. With echocardiography, the diagnosis rests on visualization of the aortic arch as it abruptly terminates, and it is usually best seen from the suprasternal window. A patent ductus arteriosus (usually large) will also be present. When aortic arch interruption is suspected, a careful search for a right aortic arch should be undertaken to avoid confusion between these two entities.

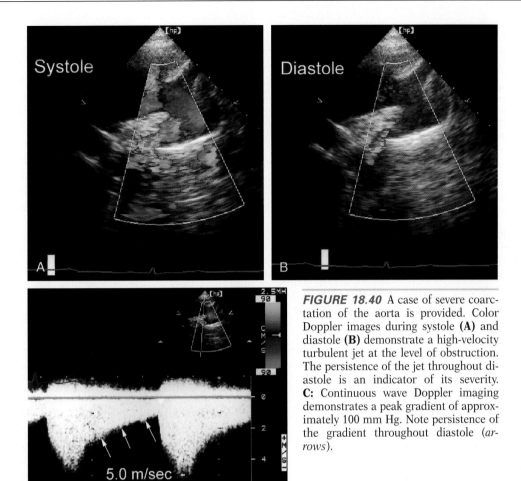

FIGURE 18.40 A case of severe coarctation of the aorta is provided. Color Doppler images during systole **(A)** and diastole **(B)** demonstrate a high-velocity turbulent jet at the level of obstruction. The persistence of the jet throughout diastole is an indicator of its severity. **C:** Continuous wave Doppler imaging demonstrates a peak gradient of approximately 100 mm Hg. Note persistence of the gradient throughout diastole (*arrows*).

ABNORMALITIES OF CARDIAC SEPTATION

Defects in septation between the cardiac chambers constitute the largest single group of congenital cardiac malformations. These developmental anomalies may involve the atrial septum, the ventricular septum, or the conotruncus (the infundibulum or outlet portion of the ventricles). Within each category, specific lesions are designated on the basis of their embryologic origin and anatomic site. These anomalies often occur in association with other complex lesions; the focus of this section is on those conditions in which septation defects are the primary cardiac anomaly.

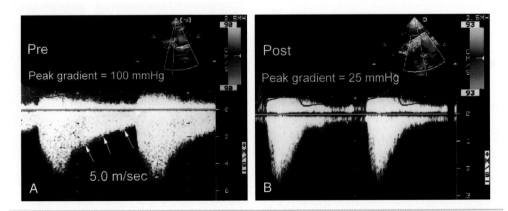

FIGURE 18.41 Balloon angioplasty can be used to treat coarctation of the aorta. These Doppler recordings were obtained before (*Pre*) **(A)** and after (*Post*) **(B)** balloon dilation of a coarct. The procedure resulted in a decrease in the peak gradient from approximately 100 to 25 mm Hg.

Atrial Septal Defect

There are four types of atrial septal defect, which correspond to abnormal development at specific stages of embryogenesis and to specific locations within the atrial septum (Fig. 18.42A). The most common type is the ostium secundum defect, located in the area of the fossa ovalis or middle of the atrial septum. In the adult population, this type comprises approximately two-thirds of all cases. The ostium primum defect involves the lower (or primum) portion of the atrial septum and accounts for approximately 15% of atrial septal defects seen in adults. This type may occur alone or in association with defects in the inlet portion of the ventricular septum and atrioventricular valves (i.e., as a component of an endocardial cushion defect). The sinus venosus defect is slightly less common (approximately 10% of cases) and occurs in the superior and posterior septum, near the junction of the superior vena cava. Defects in the area of the coronary sinus are rare and are not discussed.

Atrial septal defects usually are single and vary considerably in size. Direct visualization of the atrial septum with two-dimensional echocardiography is the most accurate means by which to diagnose these lesions. The presence of an atrial septal defect is often first suspected, however, on the basis of indirect echocardiographic findings. Right ventricular dilation in an otherwise healthy young patient should always suggest this possibility. Abnormal motion of the interventricular septum is another clue to its presence. Typically, septal motion in the presence of an atrial septal defect is characterized by brisk anterior movement in early systole or flattened motion throughout systole.

Two-dimensional echocardiography permits a more direct assessment of an atrial septal defect (Fig. 18.42B). As with M-mode echocardiography, right ventricular dilation and paradoxic septal motion can be detected. In the parasternal short-axis view, the abnormal ventricular septal geometry indicative of a right ventricular volume overload can be confirmed. This abnormal geometry is characterized by leftward displacement (or flattening) of the septum in diastole, the result of a right ventricular diastolic volume overload. During systole, the normal transseptal pressure gradient is restored and the septum regains its normal circular geometry. Rounding of the septum in early systole causes it to be displaced anteriorly (from its abnormal posterior position in late diastole). Figure 18.43 is from a patient with right ventricular volume overload due to an atrial septal defect. Septal flattening in diastole is present but reverses in systole, with restoration of normal circular geometry.

More directly, two-dimensional echocardiography allows visualization of atrial septal defects. To assess the presence, location, and size of an atrial septal defect, multiple echocardiographic views are required, and an appreciation of the advantages and limitations of each is essential. In the apical four-chamber view, the atrial septum is

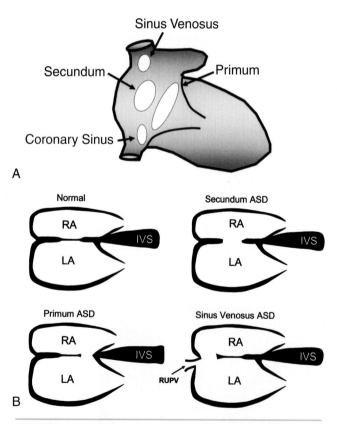

FIGURE 18.42 These schematics illustrate the different types of atrial septal defect. **A:** The relationship of the different types of atrial septal defects viewed from the perspective of the right heart is shown. **B:** The differences among the types of atrial septal defect (*ASD*) from a subcostal four-chamber perspective. See text for details. IVS, interventricular septum; LAA, left atrial appendage; LA, left atrium; RA, right atrium; RUPV, right upper pulmonary vein.

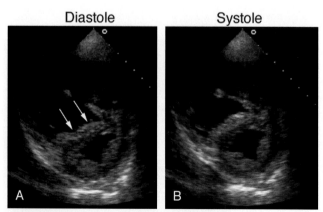

FIGURE 18.43 Right ventricular volume overload results in septal flattening during diastole (*arrows*) **(A)** with restoration of normal septal curvature during systole (*arrows*) **(B)**.

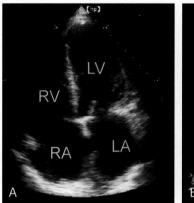
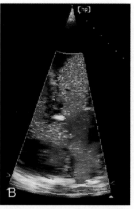

FIGURE 18.44 A secundum atrial septal defect is demonstrated from the apical four-chamber view. In this case, the defect is readily apparent on two-dimensional imaging **(A)**. Left-to-right shunting through the defect is confirmed **(B)** with color Doppler imaging. LA, left atrium; LV, left ventricle; RA, right atrium; RV, right ventricle.

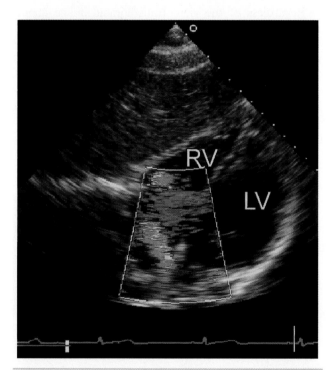

FIGURE 18.45 From the subcostal view, a secundum atrial septal defect is detected with color Doppler imaging. This view places the atrial septum more perpendicular to the ultrasound beam. Color Doppler imaging demonstrates a left-to-right shunt. LV, left ventricle; RV, right ventricle.

located in the far field, relatively parallel to the ultrasound beam. Although the diagnosis of an ostium primum defect can often be made with confidence from this view, detection of a secundum defect is considerably more difficult. Shadowing and echo dropout (particularly in the area of the fossa ovalis) create the potential for false-positive results. To aid in diagnosis, contrast and/or color

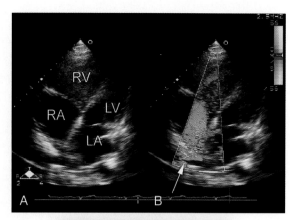
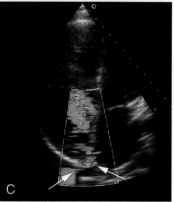

FIGURE 18.46 A sinus venosus defect is shown. **A:** This four-chamber view demonstrates a dilated right heart, but suggests that the atrial septum is intact. **B:** Color Doppler imaging reveals a defect in the most superior portion of the atrial septum, near the entrance of the superior vena cava (*arrow*). **C:** Flow through anomalous pulmonary vein as it enters the left atrium at the site of the defect (*arrows*) is shown. LA, left atrium; LV, left ventricle; RA, right atrium; RV, right ventricle.

flow imaging can be performed. These techniques will usually allow distinction between echo dropout and a true septal defect (Fig. 18.44).

The subcostal four-chamber view places the atrial septum perpendicular to the ultrasound beam and thereby obviates many of the limitations of the apical approach (Fig. 18.45). From this window, the fossa ovalis is seen as a thin central region within the atrial septum. The presence and approximate size of secundum defects can be assessed accurately in more than 90% of cases. This view is also ideal when distinguishing among defects of the primum, secundum, and sinus venosus type. In fact, this is the only transthoracic view in which sinus venosus defects are consistently visualized. Careful interrogation of the most superior and posterior portions of the atria is necessary to detect smaller sinus venosus defects (Figs. 18.46–18.48). By rotating the imaging plane into a subcostal sagittal view, the dimensions of the atrial septal defect can be assessed. In a minority of adult patients, the entrance of the superior vena cava and pulmonary veins

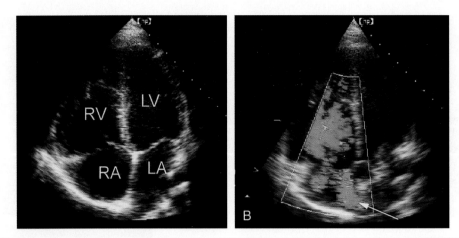

FIGURE 18.47 From the apical four-chamber view **(A)**, marked dilation of the right atrium (*RA*) and right ventricle (*RV*) is evident, but the atrial septum appears intact. **B:** By superior angulation of the scan plane, color Doppler imaging (*arrow*) was able to demonstrate a sinus venosus defect. LA, left atrium; LV, left ventricle.

frequently can be identified, thereby permitting diagnosis of anomalous pulmonary venous drainage (although this diagnosis usually requires transesophageal imaging). Finally, the subcostal views are helpful for the detection of an atrial septal aneurysm. These aneurysms consist of thin, billowing tissue in the area of the fossa ovalis that moves with the cardiac and respiratory cycles and usually protrudes into the right atrial cavity.

Regardless of the view, transthoracic image quality may preclude an acute diagnosis in some adult patients. To overcome this problem, the first step should involve color Doppler imaging and, in some cases, contrast echocardiography. By aligning the Doppler sample volume perpendicular to the atrial septum in the subcostal view, flow across the defect can be recorded (Fig. 18.49). In the usual case, pulsed Doppler imaging will demon-

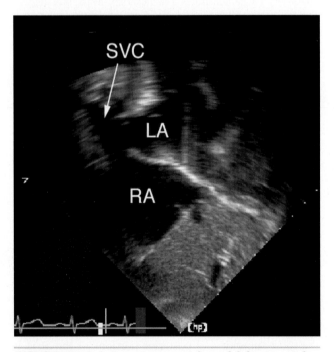

FIGURE 18.48 A sinus venosus atrial septal defect in an infant is detected from the subcostal view. By adjusting the scan plane to record the superior and posterior portion of the atrial septum, the defect can be seen. Note the relationship between the septal defect and the entrance of the superior vena cava (*SVC*) (*arrow*). LA, left atrium; RA, right atrium.

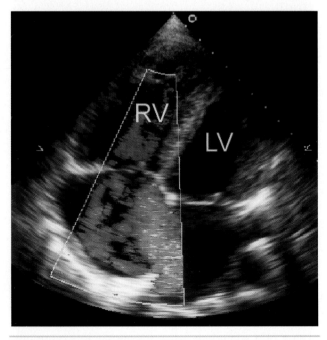

FIGURE 18.49 A large secundum atrial septal defect is present. The right heart is dilated and color Doppler imaging confirms left-to-right shunting through the atrial septum. LV, left ventricle, RV, right ventricle.

strate low-velocity, left-to-right flow extending from mid-systole to mid-diastole, with a second phase of flow coincident with atrial systole. A brief period of right-to-left shunting may also be recorded in early systole. Because the pressure difference between the atria is relatively small, a high-velocity jet will not be present. The respiratory phase will also affect the flow pattern. Care must be taken to avoid confusing the low-velocity shunt flow with normal venous and atrioventricular valve flow. Although color flow imaging can confirm the presence of an atrial septal defect, false-positive results can occur due to improper gain settings. In addition, caval flow streaming along the right side of the atrial septum can sometimes be mistaken for flow through an atrial septal defect.

As a next step, quantitation of shunt size can be determined with Doppler techniques. This assessment requires determination of left and right ventricular stroke volume, which can be derived from aortic and pulmonary flow velocity profiles (Fig. 18.50). In children, this method has been used to estimate the direction and magnitude of the shunt (i.e., the net shunt ratio or Qp/Qs). Correlation between Doppler imaging and catheterization techniques for this measurement is good. In adults, however, technical problems limit the accuracy and utility of this approach.

Contrast echocardiography is another technique for detecting intracardiac shunting. The apical four-chamber view usually is optimal because it allows simultaneous visualization of all four chambers. After intravenous injection of agitated saline, the right side of the heart is rapidly and completely opacified. The demonstration of contrast echoes in the left atrium suggests right-to-left shunting at the atrial level (Fig. 18.51). This phenomenon occurs both in the presence and absence of elevated pressure in the right side of the heart, even when the predominant shunt is left to right. The magnitude of this shunt, however, is often small and transient and may easily be missed. Contrast-containing blood within the left atrium also occurs in the presence of a pulmonary arteriovenous malformation. Direct evidence of a left-to-right shunt relies on the appearance of noncontrast-containing blood within the right atrium (a so-called negative contrast effect). Unfortunately, noncontrast-enhanced blood may enter the right atrium across an atrial septal defect, via the coronary sinus, through a left ventricle-to-right atrium communication, or from the inferior vena cava. Slow motion and frame-by-frame analysis of the echocardiogram is necessary to distinguish among these possibilities. It should be recognized that contrast echocardiography has certain limitations for detecting atrial septal defects. First, the method is not quantitative. Shunting is a transient phenomenon reflecting the instantaneous pressure gradient across the atrial septum. The appearance of right-to-left

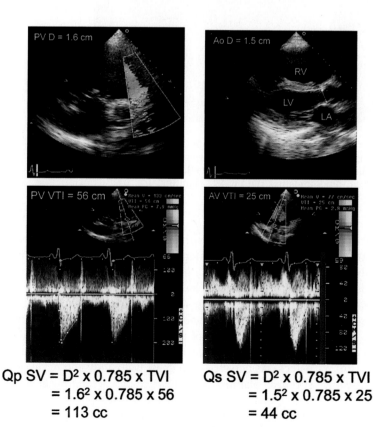

FIGURE 18.50 In the presence of an intracardiac shunt, Qp/Qs provides a means to quantify the magnitude of shunting. In this example from a patient with a large secundum atrial septal defect, stroke volume (*SV*) through the pulmonary **(left)** and aortic **(right)** valves are measured and the Qp/Qs is determined.

$$Qp\ SV = D^2 \times 0.785 \times TVI$$
$$= 1.6^2 \times 0.785 \times 56$$
$$= 113\ cc$$

$$Qs\ SV = D^2 \times 0.785 \times TVI$$
$$= 1.5^2 \times 0.785 \times 25$$
$$= 44\ cc$$

$$Qp/Qs = 113/44 = 2.5$$

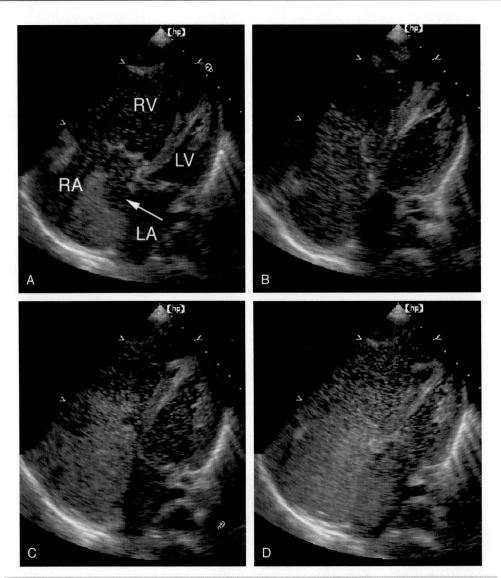

FIGURE 18.51 Contrast echocardiography can be used to demonstrate intracardiac shunting through an atrial septal defect. In this example, sequential images after intravenous contrast injection demonstrate the appearance of bubbles in the right heart. A negative contrast effect is indicated by the *arrow* **(A)**. Subsequent images reveal predominantly right-to-left shunting. LA, left atrium; LV, left ventricle; RA, right atrium; RV, right ventricle.

shunting should not be misconstrued as evidence of pulmonary hypertension. Conversely, an apparent "negative" contrast effect within the right atrium must be analyzed carefully to avoid false-positive results. Finally, evidence of shunting at the atrial level may occur with a patent foramen ovale and does not by itself confirm the presence of an atrial septal defect. These concepts are also discussed in Chapter 4.

The most accurate technique for evaluating the integrity of the interatrial septum is transesophageal echocardiography. The proximity and orientation of the septum relative to the esophagus permit the entire structure to be adequately visualized in virtually every patient (Fig. 18.52). The presence, location, and size of the defect can be determined with confidence. When percutaneous device closure is contemplated, the test is often required to accurately size the defect and to determine the feasibility of successful closure. Atrial septal defects are not necessarily round, so their dimensions should be measured in multiple planes to ensure proper sizing. Figure 18.53 is an example of incremental information provided by the transesophageal study. In this patient, a secundum defect was detected on a chest wall study and device closure was planned. The presence of a *second* atrial septal defect was confirmed with the transesophageal echocardiogram, and the plan was altered accordingly. In addition, transesophageal echocardiography is often used when contrast echocardiography demonstrates shunting,

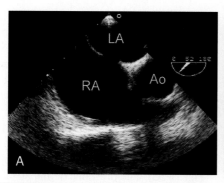
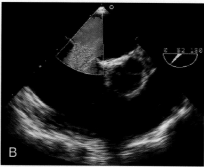

FIGURE 18.52 A secundum atrial septal defect is detected during transesophageal echocardiography. **A:** The location and size of the defect are evident. **B:** Color Doppler imaging reveals flow predominantly from the left atrium (*LA*) to the right atrium (*RA*). Ao, aorta.

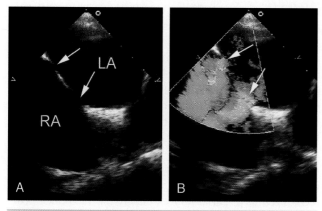

FIGURE 18.53 A: This transesophageal echocardiogram demonstrates two separate small secundum atrial septal defects (*arrows*). **B:** Left-to-right shunting is confirmed with color flow imaging (*arrows*). LA, left atrium; RA, right atrium.

but a defect cannot be visualized on transthoracic imaging. In this situation, the transesophageal approach is necessary to differentiate between a patent foramen ovale and a true atrial septal defect. Thus, for the diagnosis of

an atrial septal defect, the sensitivity of transesophageal echocardiography approaches 100%.

In adult patients, transesophageal echocardiography is particularly advantageous in the assessment of sinus venosus defects. This is primarily because these defects are the ones most likely to be missed on a transthoracic study. In addition, the possibility of partial anomalous pulmonary venous drainage is best evaluated using this technique. Typically, the right upper pulmonary vein will drain into the confluence created by the septal defect and the entrance of the superior vena cava. Although this can usually be seen in children from a chest wall study, in adults, this determination is rarely possible without resorting to transesophageal imaging. Figure 18.54 provides an example of sinus venosus atrial septal defect detected using transesophageal echocardiography. Note the relationships among the defect, the superior vena cava, and the superior rim of the atrial septum.

Diagnosis of an ostium primum atrial septal defect is easily accomplished with two-dimensional echocardiography. Such defects result from failure of partitioning of the atrioventricular canal and frequently involve the ven-

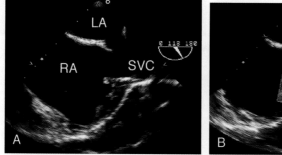
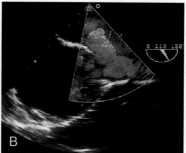

FIGURE 18.54 Transesophageal echocardiography is often required to detect and characterize a sinus venosus defect in adult patients. **A:** The defect is visualized at the junction of the superior vena cava (*SVC*). Flow through the defect is confirmed with color Doppler imaging (**B**). LA, left atrium; RA, right atrium.

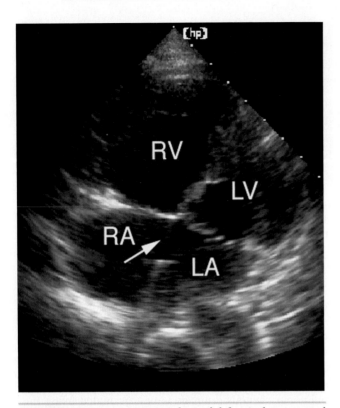

FIGURE 18.55 A primum atrial septal defect is demonstrated on transthoracic echocardiography. Note the location of the defect (*arrow*) relative to the septal leaflets of the mitral and tricuspid valves. LA, left atrium; LV, left ventricle; RA, right atrium; RV, right ventricle.

tricular septum as well. Thus, an ostium primum defect may occur alone (partial atrioventricular canal) or in association with defects in the inlet ventricular septum (complete atrioventricular canal or endocardial cushion defect). Absence of tissue in the most inferior portion of the atrial septum (at the level of insertion of the septal leaflets of the atrioventricular valves) is diagnostic and serves to distinguish ostium primum from secundum defects. This determination can be made from any of several views, although the apical four-chamber view is often best (Fig. 18.55). The presence of any atrial septal tissue above the base of the atrioventricular valves excludes the diagnosis of a primum defect. Atrioventricular canal defects are also associated with a lack of separate fibrous atrioventricular valve rings. As a consequence, both atrioventricular valves lie in the same plane (rather than more apical displacement of the tricuspid valve). This finding is also readily apparent from the four-chamber view.

Once an ostium primum atrial septal defect is detected, it is essential to assess for the presence of associated abnormalities, including (1) an inlet ventricular septal defect, (2) a cleft mitral valve, (3) the presence and severity of atrioventricular valve regurgitation, and (4) partial attachment of the septal leaflet of the mitral valve to the interventricular septum. Cleft mitral valve, often seen in the presence of an ostium primum defect, is detected more easily from the parasternal short-axis view by careful scanning at the tips of the mitral leaflets (Fig. 18.56). The cleft will generally be recognized as a gap at approximately the 12 o'clock posi-

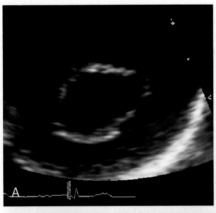
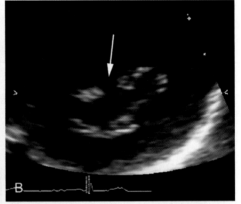
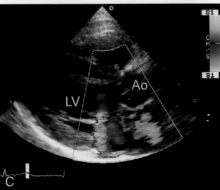

FIGURE 18.56 Primum atrial septal defect is often associated with a cleft mitral valve. **A:** The mitral orifice is demonstrated from the short-axis view. **B:** By scanning slightly more apically, the cleft in the anterior leaflet is demonstrated (*arrow*). **C:** Such patients often have a posteriorly directed jet of mitral regurgitation. Ao, aorta; LV, left ventricle.

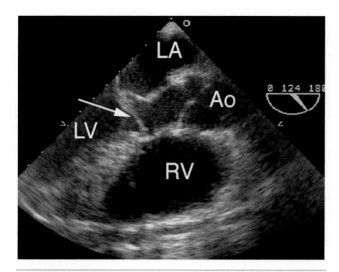

FIGURE 18.57 Abnormal insertion of a portion of the anterior mitral leaflet is sometimes present in patients with primum atrial septal defect. In this transesophageal echocardiogram, a portion of the anterior leaflet is displaced anteriorly into the left ventricular outflow tract (*arrow*). Ao, aorta; LA, left atrium; LV, left ventricle; RV, right ventricle.

tion. Mitral regurgitation is invariably present and often oriented in an eccentric direction. Abnormal insertion of the anterior mitral valve leaflet is best appreciated from the parasternal long-axis view (Fig. 18.57). By varying the angulation of the transducer, the displaced attachment site can be visualized.

The management of patients with an atrial septal defect continues to evolve. A key factor in clinical decision making is the presence and severity of pulmonary hypertension. Figure 18.58 is an example of a large secundum defect in a middle-aged woman. The study demonstrates significant enlargement of the right heart and evidence of severe pulmonary hypertension. Surgical repair remains the mainstay of therapy, and many patients are able to undergo surgery without the need for cardiac catheterization, based on a thorough echocardiographic assessment. Echocardiography also plays a vital role in the percutaneous approach to atrial septal defect closure (Fig. 18.59). In these patients, transesophageal echocardiography is critical for selecting candidates for repair based on the size and location of the defect as well as the presence of

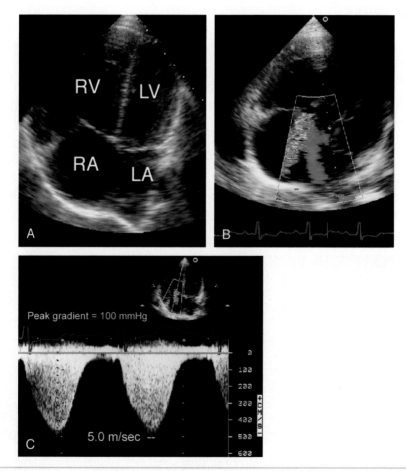

FIGURE 18.58 Severe pulmonary hypertension developed in this patient with a large secundum atrial septal defect. **A:** Absence of tissue in the region of the atrial septal is evident and the right heart is dilated. **B:** Color Doppler imaging demonstrates both tricuspid regurgitation (mosaic pattern) and low-velocity systolic flow (in red) through the defect. **C:** High-velocity tricuspid regurgitation is demonstrated, indicating a right ventricular systolic pressure of greater than 100 mm Hg. LA, left atrium; LV, left ventricle; RA, right atrium; RV, right ventricle.

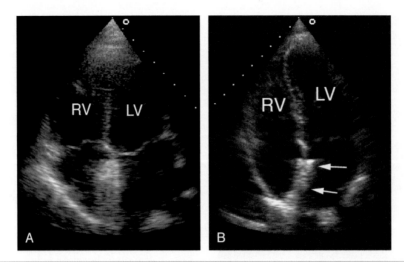

FIGURE 18.59 Percutaneous closure of an atrial septal defect using an Amplatzer® device is demonstrated in two patients. Such devices appear on echocardiography as echogenic structures within the area of the atrial septum. **A:** Two devices (*arrows*) were needed to occlude two separate defects. Color Doppler imaging can be used to detect residual shunting across the defects. LA, left atrium; LV, left ventricle.

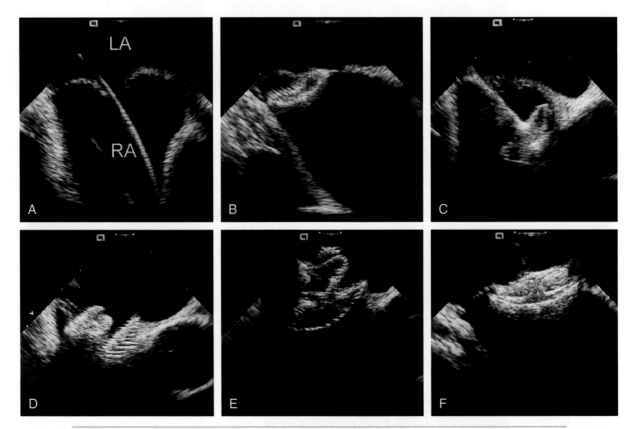

FIGURE 18.60 **A–F:** During device closure of an atrial septal defect, intracardiac echocardiography is often use to guide deployment of the device. This series of echocardiograms demonstrates placement of an Amplatzer closure device across a secundum atrial septal defect. After the left atrial (*LA*) device is positioned, the structure is secured against the atrial septum before the right atrial component is engaged. Then, the deployment catheter is released, allowing the device to straddle the septum and obscure the defect. See text for details. LA, left atrium; RA, right atrium.

an adequate rim of septal tissue to allow stabilization of the device. Then, during the procedure, either transesophageal or intracardiac echocardiography is necessary to guide device deployment and to determine the success of the procedure (Fig. 18.60). As three-dimensional echocardiography continues to develop, it is likely that this technique's ability to provide an *en face* view will permit the size, shape, and location of the defect to be more accurately characterized.

Ventricular Septal Defect

This lesion is one of the most common cardiac anomalies encountered in the pediatric population. The interventricular septum is composed of a membranous portion and a muscular portion (Fig. 18.61). The membranous septum is small and located directly below the aortic valve. Its right ventricular surface is adjacent to the septal leaflet of the tricuspid valve. On the left, the membranous septum forms the superior border of the left ventricular outflow tract. The remainder of the interventricular septum is composed of muscular tissue that extends out from the membranous septum in an inferior, apical, and anterior direction. Three regions are identified: the inlet septum (lying posterior to the membranous septum and between the two atrioventricular valves), the trabecular septum (extending from the membranous septum toward the cardiac apex), and the outlet or infundibular septum (extending anteriorly from the membranous septum and lying above

the trabecular septum and below the great arteries). The outlet septum straddles the crista supraventricularis.

Ventricular septal defects are rarely limited to the membranous septum but more often extend into one of the three muscular regions. To describe such defects, the designation "perimembranous" is preferred to "membranous." Perimembranous defects are by far the most common variety of ventricular septal defect, accounting for approximately 80% of all cases. Next most common are the trabecular ventricular septal defects, which may be multiple and vary considerably in size and location. Defects of the inlet and outlet septa are less common. Inlet ventricular septal defects occur infrequently in isolation but may be a component of endocardial cushion defects. Outlet ventricular septal defects, when they abut both semilunar valves, are referred to as supracristal or doubly committed subarterial defects. These anatomic distinctions have important clinical implications with regard to the chance of spontaneous closure, the surgical approach, risk of conducting system involvement, and likelihood of associated valvular dysfunction (e.g., aortic regurgitation).

The accuracy of echocardiography for detecting a ventricular septal defect depends on its size and location. The ventricular septum is curved and therefore does not lie in a single plane. Multiple views are required to examine the entire septal region, and a single imaging plane will neither interrogate the complete structure nor detect every defect (Fig. 18.62). Visualization of a ventricular septal defect in more than one imaging plane is the most direct

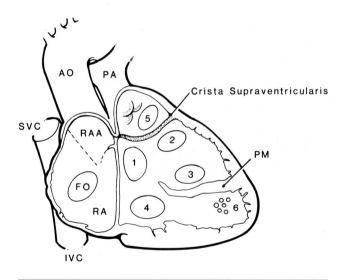

FIGURE 18.61 Schematic of the right ventricular surface of the interventricular septum diagramming common locations of ventricular septal defects. Ao, aorta; FO, foramen ovale; IVC, inferior vena cava; PA, pulmonary artery; PM, papillary muscle; RA, right atrium; SVC, superior vena cava; RAA, right atrial appendage; region 1, membranous interventricular septum; region 2, outflow interventricular septum; region 3, trabecular septum; region 4, inflow septum; region 5, subarterial region; region 6, distal multiple "Swiss cheese" septal defects.

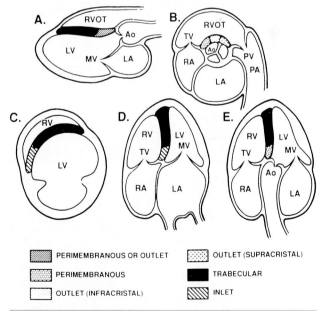

FIGURE 18.62 Schematic diagram of the location of the various types of ventricular septal defect when viewed using two-dimensional echocardiography. See text for details. Ao, aorta; LA, left atrium; LV, left ventricle; MV, mitral valve; PV, pulmonary valve; RA, right atrium; RV, right ventricle; RVOT, right ventricular outflow tract; TV, tricuspid valve.

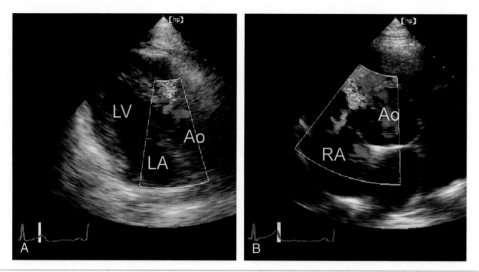

FIGURE 18.63 A perimembranous ventricular septal defect is demonstrated. **A:** The apical long-axis view demonstrates a turbulent jet crossing the septum just below the aortic valve. **B:** A basal short-axis view confirms the location of the defect to the perimembranous area. Ao, aorta; LA, left atrium; LV, left ventricle; RA, right atrium.

means of diagnosis. In general, false-negative findings are more common than false-positive results. The sensitivity of two-dimensional echocardiography for diagnosis of a ventricular septal defect depends on location. Sensitivity is highest for inlet and outlet defects (approaching 100%),

slightly less for perimembranous defects (80%–90%), and least for trabecular defects (as low as 50% in some earlier studies but considerably higher with modern equipment and techniques). The reasons for this low detection rate are that trabecular defects can occur anywhere within a

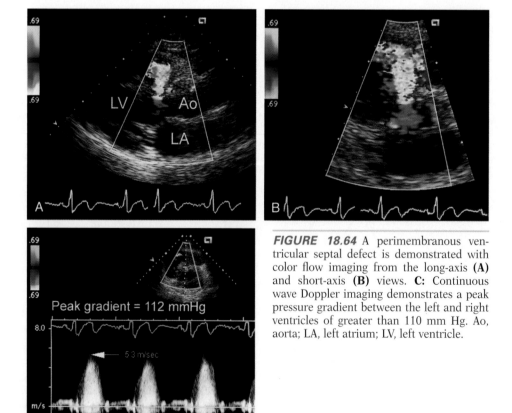

FIGURE 18.64 A perimembranous ventricular septal defect is demonstrated with color flow imaging from the long-axis **(A)** and short-axis **(B)** views. **C:** Continuous wave Doppler imaging demonstrates a peak pressure gradient between the left and right ventricles of greater than 110 mm Hg. Ao, aorta; LA, left atrium; LV, left ventricle.

fairly large area, are sometimes small, and may be multiple. Furthermore, the shape of the defect is often complex, and the orifice may be obscured in systole because of myocardial contraction.

Perimembranous defects are visible in the parasternal long- and short-axis views but generally are not seen from the four-chamber view. Slight medial angulation of the long-axis plane is required to record this area. When this adjustment is done, the membranous septum is located superior to and just below the aortic valve. From this perspective, however, distinguishing between perimembranous and outlet defects (both above and below the crista supraventricularis) may not be possible. For this purpose, the short-axis view is superior. When the scan plane is oriented just below the aortic anulus, both the membranous and outlet septa are visualized. Perimembranous defects are located medially, usually near the septal leaflet of the tricuspid valve (Figs. 18.63 and 18.64).

Outlet defects are more anterior and leftward, relative to the aortic anulus (Fig. 18.65). The short-axis view further permits classification of outlet defects as being either above or below the crista supraventricularis. Defects below the crista are to the right of midline, whereas supracristal ventricular septal defects are far leftward and adjacent to the pulmonary valve (Fig. 18.66). Supracristal defects are optimally detected from a high parasternal long-axis or parasternal short-axis view. In the long-axis plane, lateral angulation and rotation permit visualization of both the aortic and pulmonary valves, with the defect adjacent to both. Supracristal defects are often relatively small and may be missed, particularly if color flow imaging is not used. Once detected, a careful interrogation of the aortic valve is mandatory to exclude cusp prolapse and associated aortic regurgitation. This finding may be accompanied by Valsalva sinus enlargement, usually involving the right sinus.

The apical four-chamber view permits visualization of both the inlet and trabecular ventricular septum. By tilting the scanning plane inferiorly, the inlet portion of the septum is imaged in the area between the atrioventricular valves. In infants and young children, scanning anteriorly also allows recording of the outlet portion. Although the septum is parallel to the beam in this projection, the four-chamber view is ideal for detecting inlet ventricular septal defects (Fig. 18.67). This view should also be used to assess the relative position of the two atrioventricular valves. In the presence of an uncomplicated inlet ventricular septal defect, the normal apical displacement of the tricuspid valve is preserved. If both valves are in the same plane, an atrioventricular canal defect is present. Because most inlet defects are large, care must be taken to avoid confusing this lesion with a double-inlet left ventricle.

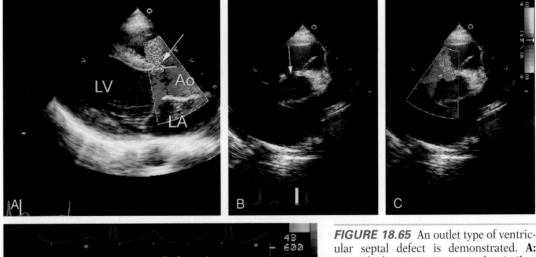

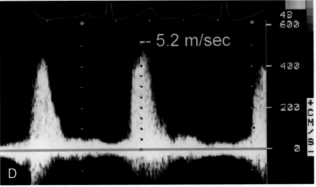

FIGURE 18.65 An outlet type of ventricular septal defect is demonstrated. **A:** From the long-axis view, note the similarity between this type of defect and a perimembranous defect. The distinction is apparent from the short-axis views **(B, C)**. The defect is more anterior and leftward (*arrow*) relative to the tricuspid valve. **D:** A high-velocity jet confirms that the defect is small and restrictive with normal right heart pressure. Ao, aorta; LA, left atrium; LV, left ventricle.

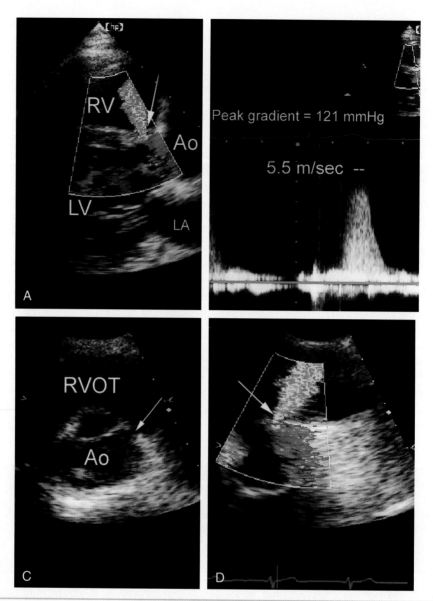

FIGURE 18.66 A restrictive supracristal ventricular septal defect is demonstrated. **A:** Medial angulation of the long-axis view allows the defect to be seen using color Doppler imaging. This view also permits optimal alignment for determining the peak pressure gradient, using continuous wave Doppler imaging **(B)**. **C:** Short-axis view demonstrates the relationship of the defect (*arrow*) to the two semilunar valves. This is confirmed, using color Doppler imaging **(D)**. RV, right ventricle; LV, left ventricle; LA, left atrium; RVOT, right ventricular outflow tract.

Malalignment between the septa can also be detected from the four-chamber view. When the atrial and ventricular septa are not aligned, it is essential that the chordal attachments of the atrioventricular valves are carefully assessed. It is crucial to differentiate between a straddling atrioventricular valve (in which some chordae traverse the defect to insert into the opposite ventricle) and an overriding valve (which overlies the defect but has no chordae extending through to the opposite ventricle). In the former case, the presence of chordae crossing the defect greatly complicates surgical repair (Fig. 18.68).

Chordal attachments crossing an inlet ventricular septal defect may obscure the defect, leading to a false-negative interpretation.

Defects in the trabecular, or muscular, portion of the muscular septum may be difficult to record with two-dimensional echocardiography. All available imaging planes should be used to exclude the possibility of small defects in this region (Fig. 18.69). Trabecular defects may appear as narrow, irregular channels through the muscular septum. Thus, the orifice on one side of the septum may be displaced from the orifice on the other side, pre-

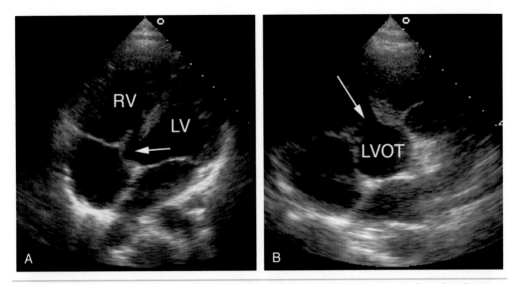

FIGURE 18.67 An example of an inlet ventricular septal defect is provided. In the four-chamber view, the inlet portion of the septum is absent and the relationship between the defect and the septal leaflets of the mitral and tricuspid valve is apparent (*arrow*) **(A)**. **B:** From the basal short-axis view, the proximity of the septal defect to the tricuspid valve is shown (*arrow*). LV, left ventricle; LVOT, left ventricular outflow tract; RV, right ventricle.

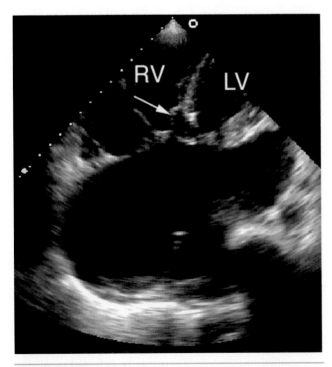

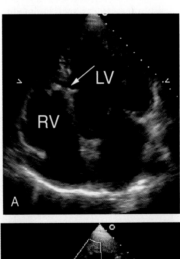

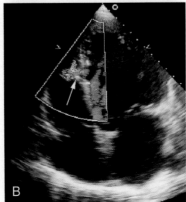

FIGURE 18.68 An inlet ventricular septal defect in association with atrioventricular canal is shown. Note the presence of chordae crossing the defect (*arrow*). A large primum atrial septal defect is also noted. LV, left ventricle; RV, right ventricle.

FIGURE 18.69 A trabecular ventricular septal defect is shown. The presence of the defect (*arrow*) is suggested on two-dimensional imaging **(A)** and confirmed with color Doppler imaging (*arrow*) **(B)**. LV, left ventricle; RV, right ventricle.

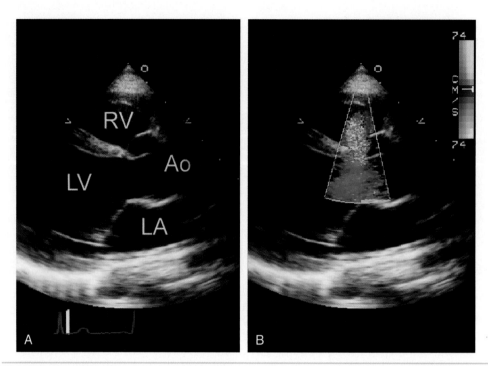

FIGURE 18.70 Small ventricular septal defects may not be apparent on two-dimensional imaging **(A)**, but their presence can be confirmed using color Doppler imaging **(B)**. In this example, the septum appears intact, but medial angulation and the use of color Doppler imaging confirm the presence of a small defect. Ao, aorta; LA, left atrium; LV, left ventricle; RV, right ventricle.

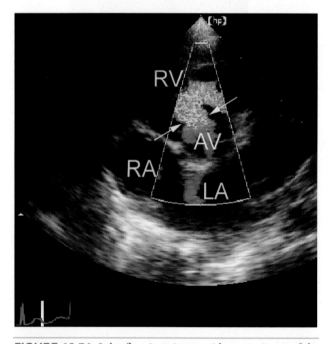

FIGURE 18.71 Color flow imaging provides an estimate of the size of a ventricular septal defect. The dimensions of the color flow jet through the defect correlate fairly well with defect size (*arrows*). AV, aortic valve; LA, left atrium; RA, right atrium; RV, right ventricle.

cluding visualization of the entire course in one plane. Once a trabecular defect is identified, it is essential to recognize the possibility of multiple defects and a careful search should be undertaken. Defects located in the apical portion of the septum are especially likely to be multiple (so-called Swiss cheese defects). In such cases, detection is greatly facilitated by the simultaneous use of color Doppler imaging.

Whenever a ventricular septal defect is suspected, Doppler imaging is crucial as an aid in diagnosis and to characterize the flow direction and velocity. Flow through a small restrictive ventricular septal defect is recorded with Doppler imaging as a turbulent, high-velocity systolic jet crossing the septum from left to right. To detect such jets, the right ventricular septal surface is carefully and systematically scanned with color Doppler imaging. Small defects appear as thin jets of turbulent flow within (and on the right ventricular side of) the septum (Fig. 18.70). Larger defects are characterized by a wider jet when imaged with color Doppler imaging (Fig. 18.71). When the location of the defect is unknown, the left parasternal, apical, and subcostal windows should be used for screening. Once the jet is identified, the Doppler beam can be oriented parallel to flow to permit recording of the peak jet velocity. With restrictive defects, the jet velocity is high, reflecting the high pressure gradient between the ventricles during systole (Fig. 18.72). With larger defects, the pressure gradient is

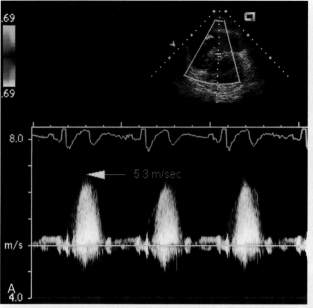

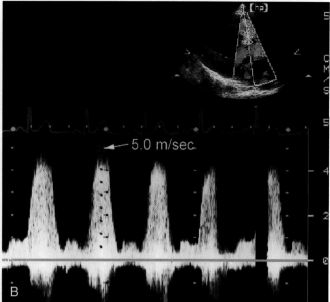

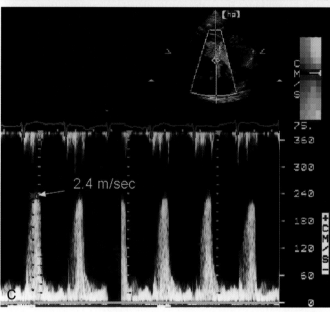

FIGURE 18.72 With proper beam alignment, the pressure gradient across a ventricular septal defect can be measured. These examples demonstrate both high **(A, B)** and low **(C)** jet velocities, suggesting either normal or elevated right ventricular pressure, respectively. **C:** Low-velocity flow through the defect is consistent with only a 25 mm Hg systolic pressure difference between the left and right ventricles. This was recorded from a patient with Eisenmenger syndrome. See text for details.

less, and, hence, the jet velocity is lower. In the presence of a large ventricular septal defect and elevated right ventricular pressure, there may be relatively little flow across the defect. The flow can be assessed by using pulsed Doppler and color flow imaging and indicates the presence of Eisenmenger physiology.

The pressure gradient (PG) between the ventricles can be estimated using the modified Bernoulli equation:

$$PG \text{ (mm Hg)} = 4 \times (\text{peak velocity})^2 \qquad \text{[Eq. 18.1]}$$

If the systolic blood pressure is determined by cuff recording of the upper extremity and no left ventricular outflow tract obstruction is present, the left ventricular (LV)

systolic pressure can be determined. Then, right ventricular (RV) systolic pressure is calculated from the equation(s):

$$PG = LV \text{ (systolic) pressure} - RV \text{ (systolic) pressure, or} \qquad \text{[Eq. 18.2]}$$

$$RV \text{ pressure} = LV \text{ pressure} - PG, \text{ or by substitution} \qquad \text{[Eq. 18.3]}$$

$$RV \text{ pressure} = \text{cuff systolic blood pressure} - [4 \times (\text{peak velocity})^2] \qquad \text{[Eq. 18.4]}$$

In the absence of right ventricular outflow tract obstruction, this value is equal to the pulmonary artery systolic pressure. Thus, a noninvasive estimate of the pres-

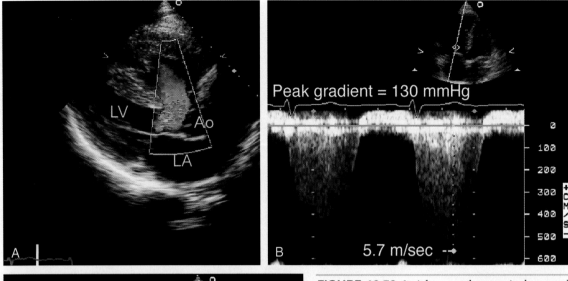

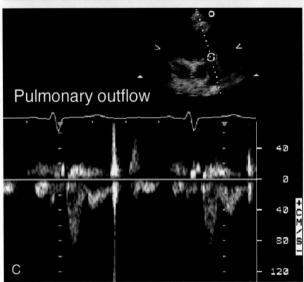

FIGURE 18.73 A: A large outlet ventricular septal defect is demonstrated, resulting in Eisenmenger syndrome. **B:** High-velocity tricuspid regurgitation confirms markedly elevated right ventricular systolic pressure. **C:** Pulsed Doppler recording of pulmonary valve flow is consistent with pulmonary hypertension. Ao, aorta; LA, left atrium; LV, left ventricle.

ence and severity of pulmonary hypertension can be made. Alternatively, right ventricular systolic pressure can be calculated from the peak velocity of the tricuspid regurgitation (TR) jet using a similar equation (Fig. 18.73):

$$\text{RV systolic pressure} = \text{RA pressure} + [4 \times (\text{TR velocity})^2]$$
$$[\text{Eq. 18.5}]$$

By using one or both of these approaches, an accurate measure of right ventricular pressure can be obtained in most patients.

A variety of associated lesions or complications occur in the setting of a ventricular septal defect, most of which are readily detected using echocardiography. Among the most common is the ventricular septal aneurysm, a thin membrane of tissue that usually arises from the margin of the defect, sometimes by incorporation of a portion of tricuspid septal leaflet tissue. Such aneurysms are commonly associated with perimembranous ventricular sep-

tal defects. Although aneurysms are usually patent, they represent one mechanism for spontaneous closure of a ventricular septal defect. The parasternal long- and short-axis views are most useful in detecting a ventricular septal aneurysm (Fig. 18.74). They are seen as thin, membranous pouches that bulge through the defect often with a windsock appearance. They may be highly mobile, often protruding through the defect into the right ventricle during systole. Once detected, they should be interrogated with color flow imaging (Fig. 18.75) to determine the patency of the aneurysm. If the tricuspid valve is involved, the presence and severity of associated tricuspid regurgitation should be determined.

An unusual type of ventricular defect involves a direct communication between the left ventricle and right atrium, sometimes called a Gerbode defect. This can occur because the more apically positioned septal leaflet of the tricuspid valve creates a small region of septum between the left ventricle and right atrium (Fig. 18.76). In

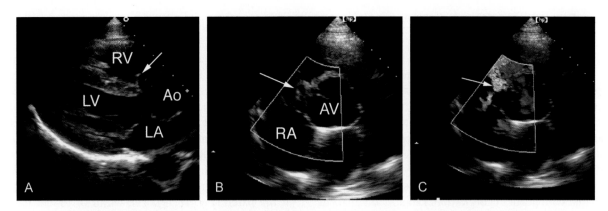

FIGURE 18.74 Spontaneous closure of ventricular septal defect occurs, usually resulting in aneurysm formation (*arrow*) that may be complete or partial. This can be recorded from either the long-axis (**A**) or short-axis (**B**) view. **C:** Color Doppler imaging demonstrates residual shunting through the aneurysm. Ao, aorta; LA, left atrium; LV, left ventricle; RV, right ventricle.

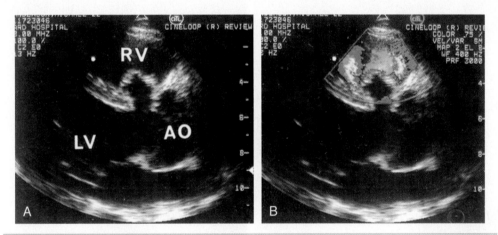

FIGURE 18.75 A:. Two-dimensional echocardiogram from a patient with a perimembranous ventricular septal defect and a large ventricular septal aneurysm. **B:** Color flow imaging in the parasternal long-axis view discloses left-to-right shunting at multiple sites, indicated by the turbulent mosaic flow at the edges of the aneurysm. AO, aorta; LV, left ventricle; RV, right ventricle.

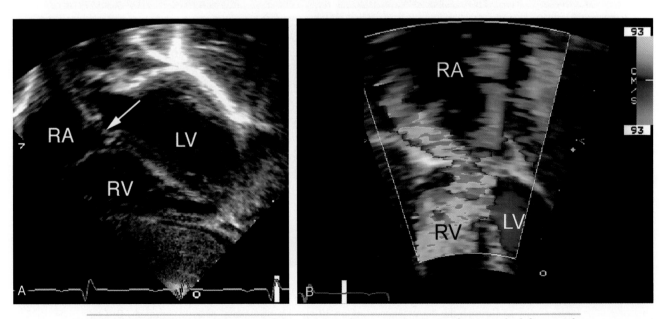

FIGURE 18.76 An unusual type of defect involves direct communication between the left ventricle (*LV*) and right atrium (*RA*). **A:** The presence of a defect is suggested from this subcostal view (*arrow*). **B:** Color Doppler imaging confirms left-to-right shunting from the left ventricle into both the right atrium and right ventricle (*RV*). The images are inverted, as is customary in many pediatric echocardiography laboratories.

the illustration provided, the septal defect can be seen below the aortic valve, but above the tricuspid valve. Color Doppler imaging demonstrates a degree of left-to-right shunting that enters both the right atrium and ventricle.

Another complication associated with ventricular septal defects is aortic regurgitation, which occurs most commonly with outlet defects in which the support of the valve is undermined by an absence of myocardium below the anulus (Fig. 18.77). Perimembranous defects are also associated with aortic regurgitation. Prolapse of an aortic cusp through the defect occasionally is recorded. The finding of aortic regurgitation in a patient with a ventric-

ular septal defect has important implications. Surgical closure is often recommended, even in the absence of a large shunt, to reduce the risk of progressive aortic valve dysfunction.

After surgical repair, echocardiography can be used to determine the integrity of the ventricular septal defect patch (Fig. 18.78). Color flow imaging is the most sensitive technique for detection of a residual shunt, which is recorded as a turbulent, high-velocity jet at the periphery of the patch (Fig. 18.79). The width of the jet has been correlated with the magnitude of the shunt and the likelihood of the need for reoperation. Percutaneous closure of

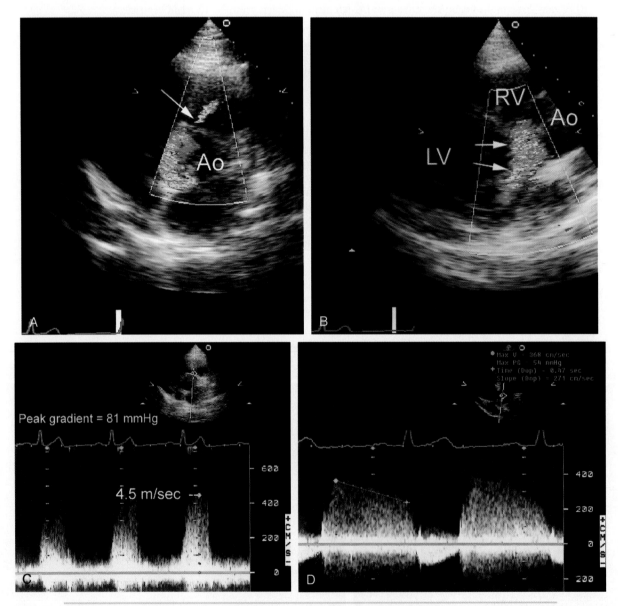

FIGURE 18.77 **A:** A supracristal ventricular septal defect (*arrow*) is detected using color Doppler imaging. **B:** Associated aortic regurgitation is demonstrated (*arrows*). **C:** Doppler imaging confirms a high-velocity jet through the defect, suggesting an 80 mm Hg transseptal pressure gradient. **D:** Continuous wave Doppler imaging of the aortic regurgitation jet. Ao, aorta; LA, left atrium; LV, left ventricle; RV, right ventricle.

Before   After

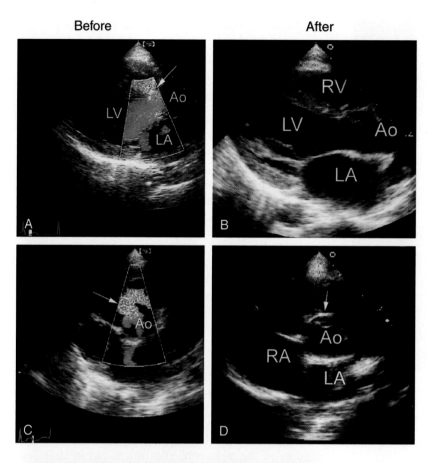

FIGURE 18.78 A moderate-sized outlet ventricular septal defect is shown before **(A, C)** and after **(B, D)** surgical repair. **A, C:** Color Doppler imaging demonstrates flow through the septal defect (*arrows*). **B, D:** Recorded after surgery. The patch used to close the septal defect is visualized on two-dimensional imaging (*arrow*). Ao, aorta; LA, left atrium; LV, left ventricle; RA, right atrium; RV, right ventricle.

FIGURE 18.79 Doppler imaging from a basal short-axis view demonstrates residual shunting (*arrow*) after surgical closure of a perimembranous ventricular septal defect. Ao, aorta.

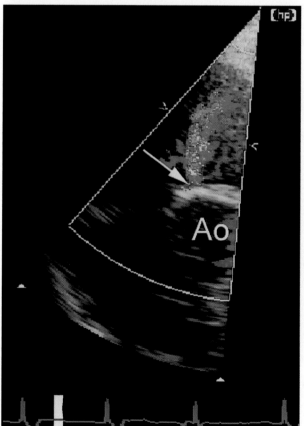

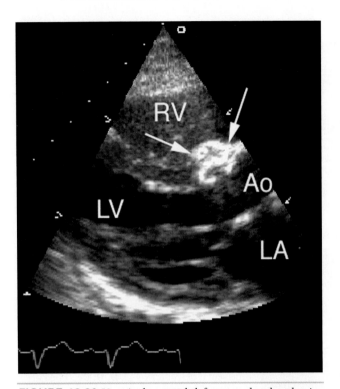

FIGURE 18.80 Ventricular septal defects can be closed using percutaneous techniques. This illustration demonstrates closure of a perimembranous defect using an Amplatzer® device. Ao, aorta; LA, left atrium; LV, left ventricle; RV, right ventricle.

ventricular septal defects is now possible. Figure 18.80 is an example of closure of a perimembranous defect using an Amplatzer device.

Endocardial Cushion Defect

Division of the common atrioventricular canal into left and right sides occurs by fusion of the superior and inferior endocardial cushions. Failure to do so results in an atrioventricular septal defect with various combinations of ostium primum atrial septal defect, inlet ventricular septal defect, and structural abnormalities of the atrioventricular valves. Thus, an endocardial cushion defect is a spectrum of lesions including partial atrioventricular canal (implying separate atrioventricular orifices), complete atrioventricular canal (a common atrioventricular orifice), and isolated inlet ventricular septal defect.

Two-dimensional echocardiography permits detailed assessment of virtually every morphologic feature of endocardial cushion defect. The primum portion of the atrial septum, the inlet ventricular septum, atrioventricular valve morphology, ventriculoatrial septal malalignment, and ventricular outflow tract obstruction can be accurately assessed. The four-chamber view generally yields the most diagnostic information on this entity (Fig. 18.81). Importantly, the presence and size of the atrial and ventricular septal defects can be determined and the anatomy of the atrioventricular valves can be assessed. Because the valve leaflets move freely within the defect, accurate assessment of these features requires real-time imaging. During systole, the atrioventricular valve as-

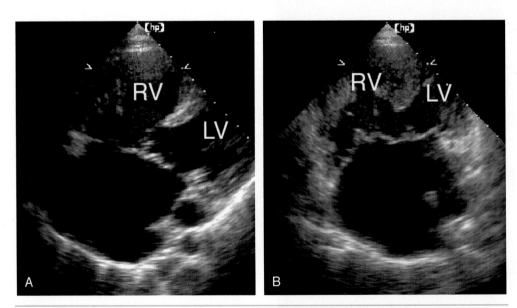

FIGURE 18.81 A complete atrioventricular canal is demonstrated in a child. The four-chamber view **(A)** reveals no evidence of atrial septal tissue. A large inlet ventricular septal defect is also present and the common atrioventricular valve appears to float within the defect. **B:** A modified four-chamber view better demonstrates the ventricular septal defect. LV, left ventricle; RV, right ventricle.

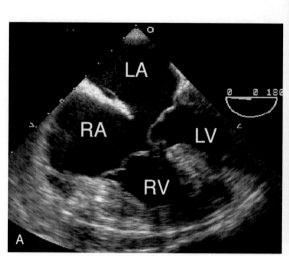 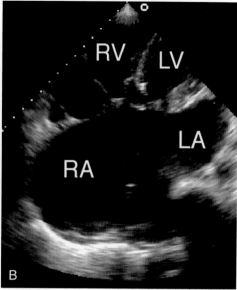

FIGURE 18.82 Complete atrioventricular canal may be associated with a straddling atrioventricular valve. **A:** Recorded during transesophageal imaging. **B:** A transthoracic four-chamber view. In both studies, chordae can be seen crossing the inlet defect. LA, left atrium; LV, left ventricle; RA, right atrium; RV, right ventricle.

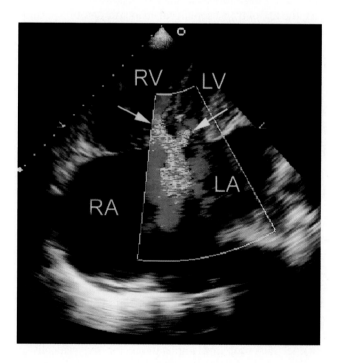

FIGURE 18.83 Atrioventricular valve regurgitation is demonstrated using color flow imaging in this patient with complete atrioventricular canal. Note how the regurgitant jets (*arrows*) appear to originate from both sides of the atrioventricular valve in a criss-cross fashion. LA, left atrium; LV, left ventricle; RA, right atrium; RV, right ventricle.

sumes a basal position, obscuring the primum atrial septal defect but permitting assessment of the size of the inlet ventricular septal defect and the presence of atrioventricular valve regurgitation. As the valve opens in diastole, the atrial portion of the defect can be examined. Chordal attachments and the presence of straddling (Fig. 18.82) can also be determined. Although atrioventricular valve regurgitation can be detected from the four-chamber view (Fig. 18.83), the presence of a cleft anterior mitral valve

leaflet is better recorded from the parasternal short-axis view (Fig. 18.84). The short-axis view also permits visualization of both the atrial and ventricular septal defects (Fig. 18.85). In the four-chamber view, the presence of left ventricle-to-right atrial shunting can be detected by using color flow imaging (Fig. 18.83).

Because of the broad spectrum of anomalies that may occur in the setting of an endocardial cushion defect, echocardiography plays a major role in determining the

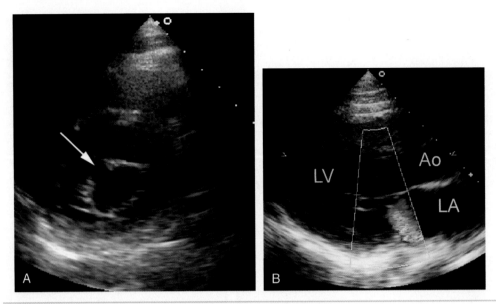

FIGURE 18.84 An example of a cleft mitral valve (*arrow*) is demonstrated (**A**) in association with eccentric and posteriorly directed mitral regurgitation (**B**). Ao, aorta; LA, left atrium; LV, left ventricle.

feasibility of surgical repair. Specifically, the relative size of the ventricles, the presence of septal malalignment, and the extent of the atrial and ventricular communications should be established. The morphology of the atrioventricular valves is also critical in planning reparative surgery. Echocardiography allows the anatomy of the valves and their chordal insertions to be determined. The presence of a straddling or overriding valve and the degree of valvular regurgitation can also be assessed. During surgery, the use of transesophageal echocardiography permits assessment of the adequacy of repair. Most importantly, the presence and severity of residual atrioventricular valve regurgitation can be determined.

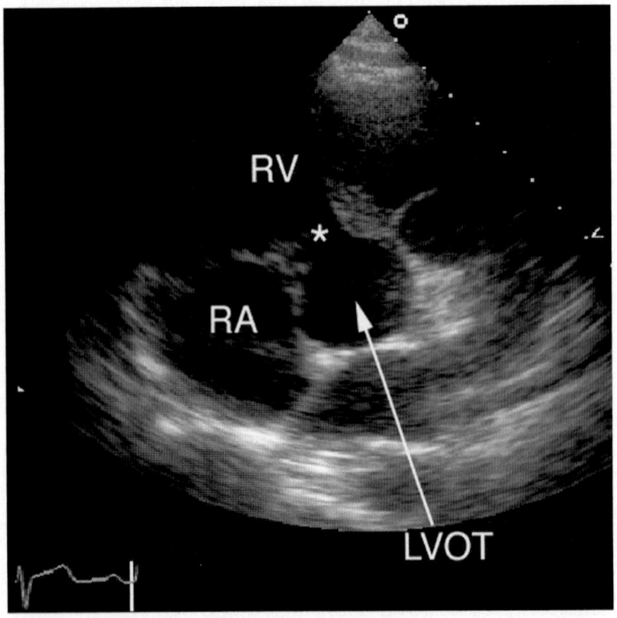

ABNORMAL VASCULAR CONNECTIONS AND STRUCTURES

Patent Ductus Arteriosus

The ductus arteriosus is the normal fetal vascular channel that connects the descending aorta and the main pulmonary artery, providing a conduit for blood from the right ventricle to the thoracic aorta. Failure of the ductus to close shortly after birth is abnormal, giving rise to the term patent ductus arteriosus. This persistent patency of the ductus may be desirable or undesirable, depending on the presence of other associated anomalies. For example, in the presence of pulmonary atresia, the persistent patency of the ductus may be the only source of pulmonary blood flow. Expedient and accurate detection of this vascular channel has profound implications for the critically ill newborn. Later in life, patent ductus arteriosus is one of the important causes of a left-to-right shunting and volume overload of the left ventricle. The functional significance of a patent ductus arteriosus depends on the size of the channel, the pulmonary vascular resistance, and the presence and degree of left ventricular dysfunction.

Both echocardiography and Doppler imaging are crucial in the assessment of patients with patent ductus arteriosus. The first step in imaging a ductus is knowing where to look for it. The pulmonary arterial end of the

FIGURE 18.85 The short-axis view below the aortic valve is useful to assess the inlet ventricular septal defect (*asterisk*) associated with atrioventricular canal. LVOT, left ventricular outflow tract; RA, right atrium; RV, right ventricle.

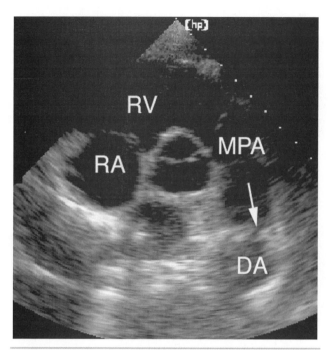

FIGURE 18.86 A patent ductus arteriosus is barely visualized (*arrow*) entering the distal main pulmonary artery (*MPA*) from the descending aorta (*DA*) in this short-axis view. RA, right atrium; RV, right ventricle.

short-axis view, angling the imaging plane in a leftward and superior direction allows visualization of the bifurcation of the pulmonary artery (Fig. 18.86). Clockwise rotation permits recording of a greater length of the descending aorta so that the entire ductus may be visualized. From the suprasternal window, the ductus is seen as a narrow channel extending from the inferior border of the aorta to the pulmonary trunk. Unfortunately, this view has significant limitations, particularly in adults. The ductus can be recorded directly in only a few patients and care must be taken to avoid mistaking the left pulmonary artery for a large ductal channel. In addition, the ductus is often aligned such that it is parallel to the ultrasound beam and is therefore subject to the limitations of lateral resolution.

Doppler imaging improves the diagnostic sensitivity by directly visualizing left-to-right flow through the channel. In ducti too small to be detected with two-dimensional echocardiographic imaging, a narrow jet of turbulent flow on color Doppler imaging may be the first indication of a patent ductus arteriosus. This flow is usually best seen from the high parasternal short-axis view as a retrograde mosaic jet entering the distal pulmonary artery from the posterolateral direction (Figs. 18.87 and 18.88). The orientation of the jet within the pulmonary artery varies, and distinguishing it from normal pulmonary flow or pulmonary regurgitation may require slow-motion and freeze-frame analysis.

In addition to its role in diagnosis, echocardiography is also used to estimate the magnitude of the shunt and the degree of pulmonary artery hypertension. The left-to-right shunt associated with a patent ductus results in volume overload of the left ventricle. The degree of left atrial

ductus is located to the left of the pulmonary trunk and adjacent to the left pulmonary artery. The aortic insertion is opposite to and just beyond the origin of the left subclavian artery. The aortic orifice of the channel is usually larger than the pulmonary end, giving the ductus a funnel shape. For direct visualization, the suprasternal and high parasternal short-axis views are used. In the parasternal

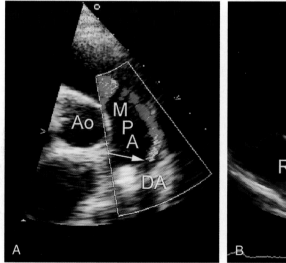
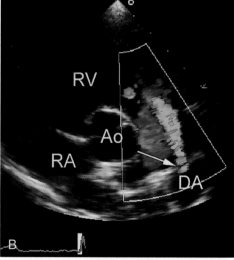

FIGURE 18.87 Two examples of patent ductus arteriosus visualized with color flow imaging are demonstrated from the basal short-axis view. **A:** Note how the jet hugs the lateral wall of the main pulmonary artery (*MPA*). Ao, aorta; DA, descending aorta; RV, right ventricle.

Before

After

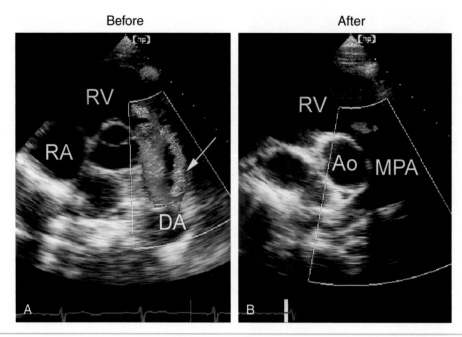

FIGURE 18.88 A patient with a patent ductus arteriosus before **(A)** and after **(B)** coil occlusion is shown. After closure of the defect, the shunt is no longer present and only trivial pulmonary regurgitation is apparent. Ao, aorta; DA, descending aorta; MPA, main pulmonary artery; RA, right atrium; RV, right ventricle.

and left ventricular dilation is a useful marker of the magnitude of shunting. A dilated and hyperdynamic left side of the heart is an indication of volume overload and, in the absence of other causes, suggests the presence of a significant left-to-right shunt. Doppler imaging also plays a role in this area. In most cases, high-velocity turbulent flow occurs continuously in a left-to-right direction, reaching a peak in late systole (Fig. 18.89). With Doppler

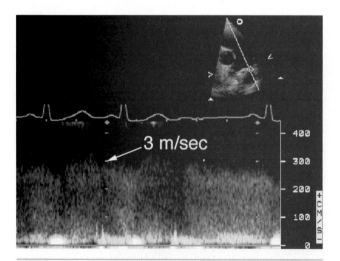

FIGURE 18.89 Continuous wave Doppler imaging can be used to measure the velocity of flow through a patent ductus arteriosus. Continuous flow is typically present, and the maximal velocity can be used to estimate the pressure gradient across the ductus. In this example, a peak gradient of only 36 mm Hg is present, suggesting elevated pulmonary artery pressure.

imaging, the peak pressure gradient can be calculated by using the modified Bernoulli equation. This method permits a quantitative estimate of pulmonary artery pressure. If the ductus is relatively long (>7 mm), however, the simplified Bernoulli equation may be inaccurate. Bidirectional shunting always implies elevated pulmonary vascular resistance. In this situation, flow occurs from right to left in early systole and from left to right in late systole and diastole. As pulmonary pressure increases, the duration and extent of right-to-left shunt flow in diastole increase.

Abnormal Systemic Venous Connections

A persistent left superior vena cava is the most common congenital anomaly involving the systemic veins. It occurs in approximately 0.5% of the general population and 3% to 10% of patients with congenital heart disease. In most cases, the left superior vena cava drains into the right atrium via the coronary sinus. As such, it has no physiologic consequences (aside from a predisposition to arrhythmias and heart block) and venous return is essentially normal. Less often, it drains into the left atrium or a pulmonary vein, resulting in a right-to-left shunt. Associated lesions, especially defects of the atrial septum, are common. Diagnosis of a persistent left superior vena cava frequently occurs after a dilated coronary sinus is detected with echocardiography. Coronary sinus dilation is usually the result of anomalous drainage to the sinus, either from a persistent left superior vena cava or an anom-

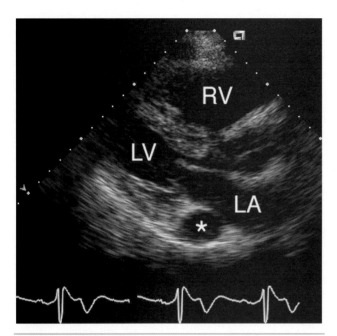

FIGURE 18.90 A dilated coronary sinus (*asterisk*) is shown in this parasternal long-axis view. LA, left atrium; LV, left ventricle; RV, right ventricle.

alous pulmonary vein. Occasionally, the degree of coronary sinus enlargement is so great that the structure is mistaken for something else, such as a pericardial effusion, pulmonary vein, or descending aorta.

The coronary sinus is best visualized in the parasternal long-axis view as a circular structure in the posterior atrioventricular groove (Fig. 18.90). Its location anterior to the pericardium distinguishes it from other venous and arterial structures, especially the descending aorta. In the

parasternal short-axis view, the coronary sinus can be recorded as a tubular, crescent-shaped structure lying within the atrioventricular groove and communicating with the right atrium. From the four-chamber view, posterior angulation of the beam will demonstrate the coronary sinus in long axis, coursing behind the left atrium and emptying into the right atrium (Fig. 18.91). Occasionally, a Chiari network is seen where the coronary sinus empties into the posterior right atrium.

Direct visualization of a left superior vena cava is easier in children than in adults. The vessel can be seen from the suprasternal window as a vertical structure to the left of the aortic arch (Fig. 18.92). This view is particularly helpful in determining whether both vena cavae are present, to assess their relative size, and to detect an innominate vein. The connections between the cavae and the atria should also be examined using a combination of two-dimensional and color Doppler imaging. In this example (Fig. 18.92), the drainage of the left superior vena cava into the left atrium is clearly visualized using color flow imaging. Color Doppler imaging may be used to distinguish higher velocity arterial flow (which, at usual gain settings, appears as red or blue laminar flow in systole) from venous flow (which is often not detected with color flow imaging). Pulsed Doppler imaging can be used to confirm venous flow, by recording low-velocity, phasic flow in a superior-to-inferior direction.

Contrast-enhanced echocardiography is of great value in the differential diagnosis of a dilated coronary sinus and to assess abnormal vena caval connections (Fig. 18.93). If injection into the left arm results in opacification of the coronary sinus *before* the right atrium and ventricle, the diagnosis of a persistent left superior vena cava

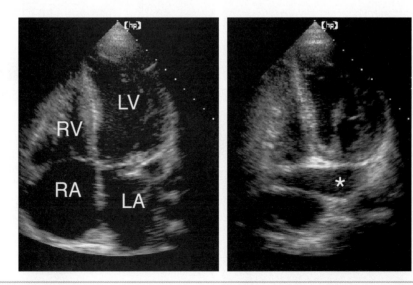

FIGURE 18.91 A dilated coronary sinus is recorded from the apical view. **A:** The four-chamber view reveals only mild dilation of the right-sided chambers. By directing the ultrasound beam steeper relative to the chest wall **(B)**, the coronary sinus is recorded (*asterisk*). LA, left atrium; LV, left ventricle; RA, right atrium; RV, right ventricle.

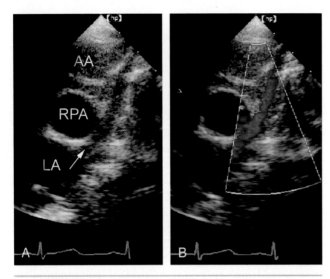

FIGURE 18.92 A persistent left superior vena cava is demonstrated from the suprasternal view. **A:** The vessel is seen just to the left of the aortic arch (*AA*) and appears connected to the left atrium (*LA*) (*arrow*). **B:** Color Doppler imaging demonstrates low-velocity flow directed inferiorly into the left atrium. RPA, right pulmonary artery.

is likely. If the same injection leads to left atrial opacification, abnormal drainage of the vena cava (either left or common) is present. This pattern of drainage is unusual and typically is associated with other cardiac lesions. Injection into the right arm should then be performed. In the presence of a left superior vena cava (draining into either the left or right atrium), this injection should lead to the normal sequence of opacification (i.e., no opacification of the coronary sinus).

Abnormal Pulmonary Venous Connections

Anomalous pulmonary venous return may be total or partial. Total anomalous pulmonary venous return is characterized by drainage of all four pulmonary veins into a systemic venous tributary of the right atrium or into the right atrium itself. The connections may be above or below the diaphragm and may involve an element of obstruction. Some degree of interatrial admixing is mandatory and provides the only access for pulmonary venous blood to the left heart. The degree and direction of the shunt depend on the size of the interatrial communica-

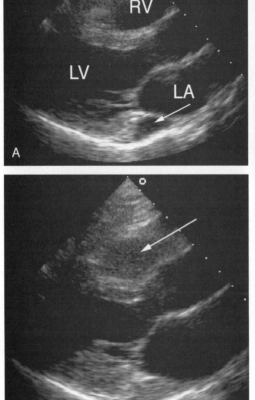

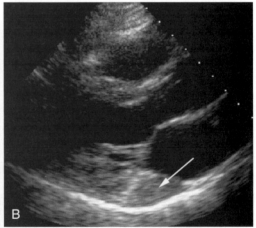

FIGURE 18.93 After contrast injection into a left arm vein, this sequence demonstrates evidence of a persistent left superior vena cava draining into the coronary sinus. **A:** A dilated coronary sinus is evident (*arrow*). **B:** Contrast is seen within the coronary sinus (*arrow*) before opacification of the right ventricle. **C:** Bubbles are visualized within the right ventricle (*arrow*) a few beats later. See text for details. LA, left atrium; LV, left ventricle; RV, right ventricle.

tion and the relative compliance of the two ventricles. Associated cardiac anomalies are present in more than one-third of patients. Survival beyond infancy without surgical palliation or repair is unlikely, so this entity is not encountered in the adult population.

Partial anomalous pulmonary venous return is present when some but not all (usually one or two) of the pulmonary veins connect to the right rather than the left atrium. The situation occurs in 10% of patients with an ostium secundum atrial septal defect and in more than 80% of patients with a sinus venosus defect (Fig. 18.46). The most common anomalous connections (in decreasing order of frequency) are (1) right upper pulmonary vein connecting to the right atrium or superior vena cava (accounting for more than 90% of cases and often in association with a sinus venosus atrial septal defect), (2) left pulmonary veins connecting to an innominate vein, and (3) right pulmonary veins connecting to the inferior vena cava. The physiologic consequences of partial anomalous pulmonary venous drainage may be minor, especially if only one pulmonary vein is involved. If more of the pulmonary venous drainage is diverted to the right side of the heart, evidence of right atrial and right ventricular volume overload will be present.

The echocardiographic diagnosis of total anomalous pulmonary venous return relies on visualization of the termination of the four pulmonary veins and detection of a venous confluence with connection to the right atrium, coronary sinus, or vena cava. In total anomalous pulmonary venous return, the venous confluence may be located posterior, inferior, or superior to the left atrium

(Fig. 18.94). The parasternal, apical, suprasternal, and subcostal views all play a role in diagnosis because the confluence may be small and difficult to image. Imaging the pulmonary veins behind or near the left atrium does not prove that they connect to the left atrium. A careful search for the pulmonary veins entering the left atrium should be undertaken. If normal connections are not seen, a pulmonary venous confluence and abnormal connection to the right atrium should be sought. As discussed previously, a dilated coronary sinus is sometimes the initial echocardiographic abnormality detected, and this finding should always prompt a search for anomalous pulmonary venous drainage. Doppler imaging is often useful in this setting to determine the direction of flow within venous channels. The direction of venous flow may allow differentiation between a normal systemic vein and an anomalous pulmonary vein (Fig. 18.95).

Partial anomalous pulmonary venous return may be difficult to diagnose because of the technical problems in identifying all four pulmonary venous connections to the left atrium. Unless all four vessels are identified, it is impossible to completely exclude the possibility of an anomalous vein. In most cases, this diagnosis is considered when an atrial septal defect and/or dilation of the right side of the heart is detected. Most often, the anomaly involves the right pulmonary veins and the abnormal connection is usually near the right side of the atrial septum or the base of the superior vena cava. The suprasternal, apical four-chamber, and subcostal views should be used. By using the subcostal window, the superior portion of the interatrial septum is consistently seen so this is the

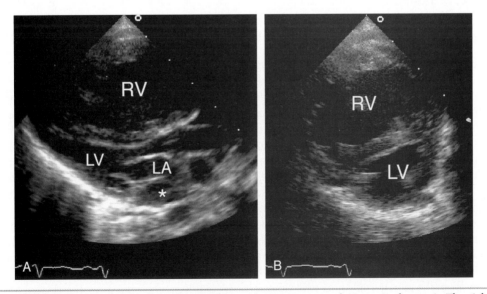

FIGURE 18.94 An infant with total anomalous pulmonary venous drainage is shown. **A:** The right ventricle (*RV*) is markedly dilated and the septum encroaches on the left ventricle (*LV*). Note the dilated coronary sinus (*asterisk*). **B:** Right ventricular enlargement and septal flattening are again demonstrated. In this patient, all four pulmonary veins drained into the coronary sinus and then to the right atrium. LA, left atrium.

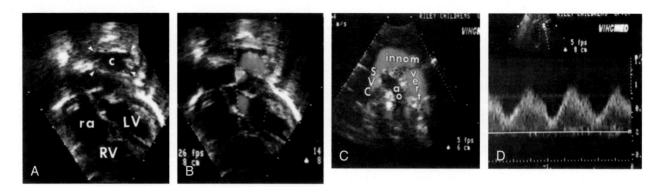

FIGURE 18.95 A: The apical four-chamber view in an infant with total anomalous pulmonary venous return reveals a structure posterior and superior to the left atrium representing the pulmonary venous confluence (*c*). The *arrowheads* indicate the entrance of the pulmonary veins. **B:** Low-velocity flow within the confluence is demonstrated using color flow imaging. **C:** A suprasternal short-axis view reveals the presence of a vertical vein (*vert*), the innominate vein (*innom*), and the superior vena cava (*SVC*). Color flow imaging demonstrates red flow within the vertical vein (directed toward the transducer) and blue flow in the innominate vein and superior vena cava (directed away from the transducer). **D:** Superiorly oriented flow in the vertical vein was confirmed by using pulsed Doppler imaging. A normal venous structure in this region would be expected to drain toward the heart, i.e., away from the transducer. ao, aorta; ra, right atrium; LV, left ventricle; RV, right ventricle. (Courtesy of Gregory J. Ensing.)

view most likely to yield a diagnosis. By clockwise rotation of the transducer, the entry of the right upper pulmonary vein and superior vena cava can be recorded. Color Doppler imaging is often helpful for identifying the pulmonary veins and their continuity (or lack thereof) with the left atrium. Transesophageal echocardiography can also be diagnostic of this condition. The proximity of the transducer to the left atrium makes this an ideal technique to assess pulmonary venous connections and the presence or absence of a pulmonary venous confluence.

Abnormalities of the Coronary Circulation

The most important congenital abnormalities involving the coronary circulation include anomalous origin of the coronary arteries and coronary artery fistulae. Coronary artery aneurysms, which may be congenital but more commonly are the result of Kawasaki disease, are also discussed in this section. Anomalous origin of a coronary artery is present in approximately 1% of patients undergoing cardiac catheterization. Origin of the left circumflex artery from the right coronary sinus and origin of the right coronary artery from the left sinus are the most frequently encountered variants. These anomalies are of particular relevance when the course of the aberrant artery passes between the aorta and the pulmonary trunk. The ostia and proximal coronary arteries can be imaged with echocardiography from the parasternal short-axis view at the base. This view permits determination of the size and initial course of the arteries. In adults, transesophageal echocardiography generally provides higher quality images of the proximal coronary arteries, and anomalous

vessels can be identified with a high degree of accuracy. An inability to record the origin of the coronary artery from this view raises the possibility of an aberrant vessel.

Coronary artery anatomy may be especially important in certain forms of complex congenital heart disease, such as tetralogy of Fallot and transposition of the great arteries. Here, assessment of coronary artery anomalies and vessel diameter has implications for prognosis and surgical repair. Anomalous origin of the left coronary artery from the pulmonary trunk is one of the causes of heart failure in the neonate. In such patients, the right coronary artery is dilated and the left coronary ostium is absent from the aortic root. The left coronary artery may be visualized but does not connect with the aorta. By using a high parasternal view of the pulmonary trunk (similar to that used to evaluate a patent ductus arteriosus), the vessel can be seen arising from the posterior wall of the pulmonary trunk (Fig. 18.96). Searching for coronary arteries is often easiest using color Doppler imaging.

A coronary artery fistula is a rare anomaly that results from the abnormal connection between a coronary artery and another vessel or chamber (either a coronary vein, pulmonary artery, or the right ventricle). This connection results in a left-to-right shunt and a continuous murmur, which is often confused with a patent ductus arteriosus. Two-dimensional echocardiography reveals dilation of the involved coronary artery that is uniform and often severe. In children, the course of the dilated vessel can be followed by the use of multiple imaging planes and simultaneous color flow imaging. The fistula itself may be difficult to image. Color Doppler imaging and/or contrast-enhanced echocardiography are useful when attempting

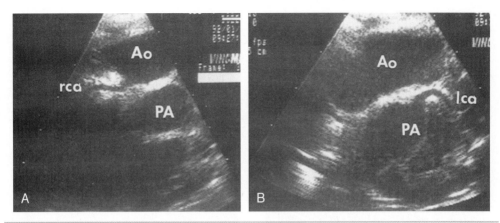

FIGURE 18.96 An anomalous left coronary artery (*lca*) is illustrated. **A:** The right coronary artery (*rca*) can be traced to the right coronary sinus of the aortic root (*Ao*). **B:** Angulation of the transducer permits recording of the left coronary artery arising from the main pulmonary artery (*PA*). (Courtesy of Gregory J. Ensing, MD.)

to follow the path of the vessel (Fig. 18.97). Detection of turbulent flow within the right ventricle or pulmonary artery may identify the site of the fistulous connection (Fig. 18.98). If the left-to-right shunt is large, chamber dilation may also be apparent.

Coronary artery aneurysms usually occur in association with Kawasaki disease. These aneurysms appear as localized dilated segments, usually with a fusiform shape. They often are multiple, may occur anywhere along the vessel, and sometimes are lined with thrombus. Detection requires the use of multiple imaging planes to record as much as possible of the distal arteries (Fig. 18.99). In young patients, the entire left main coronary artery and the

proximal segments of the right, left circumflex, and left anterior descending arteries can be seen from the parasternal short-axis view. The parasternal long-axis view of the right ventricular outflow tract may permit recording of the more distal left anterior descending artery, whereas the apical four-chamber view can be used to assess the left circumflex and right coronary arteries. As noted previously, transesophageal echocardiography can also be used effectively to examine the coronary arteries. The diameter of the coronary artery aneurysms should be measured because the size has prognostic implications. The presence of a pericardial effusion should also be sought. Its presence increases the likelihood of coronary artery aneurysms.

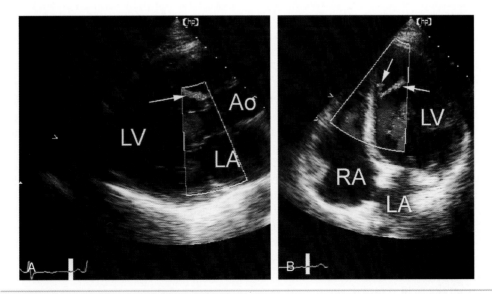

FIGURE 18.97 An echocardiogram recorded from a patient with multiple coronary artery fistulae, detected using color Doppler imaging. **A:** Parasternal long-axis view demonstrates a fistulous connection between the right coronary artery and right ventricle (*arrow*). **B:** From the apical four-chamber view, multiple fistulae (*arrows*) can be seen entering the left ventricle (*LV*) along the interventricular septum. Ao, aorta; RA, right atrium.

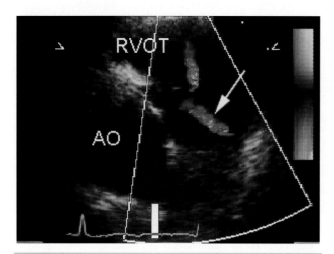

FIGURE 18.98 An example of a coronary artery fistula, with connection between the right coronary artery and the proximal pulmonary artery is shown. Color Doppler imaging demonstrates the jet from the right coronary artery entering the proximal pulmonary artery (*arrow*). Mild pulmonary regurgitation is also demonstrated in this diastolic frame. AO, aorta; RVOT, right ventricular outflow tract.

CONOTRUNCAL ABNORMALITIES

Tetralogy of Fallot

Tetralogy of Fallot is the most common form of cyanotic congenital heart disease and is one of the few such lesions that may escape diagnosis until later in life. This anomaly has four anatomic features: (1) anterior and rightward displacement of the aortic root, (2) ventricular septal defect, (3) right ventricular outflow tract obstruction, and (4) right ventricular hypertrophy. The echocardiographic evaluation includes *de novo* diagnosis of the lesion, a determination of the options for surgical intervention, and postoperative assessment of the adequacy of repair.

The critical developmental defect in tetralogy of Fallot is malalignment of the infundibular septum, resulting in a nonrestrictive infundibular (and sometimes perimembranous) septal defect and overriding of the aorta. Both of these fundamental anatomic features are optimally assessed using the parasternal long-axis view, which permits the viewer to determine the presence of the ventricular septal defect and the degree of aortic overriding (Fig. 18.100). Discontinuity between the infundibular septum and the anterior aortic root is readily apparent. Proper transducer position and angulation are necessary to ensure accurate assessment of the degree of aortic overriding. This feature is variable, ranging from minimal to extreme. In the latter case, the aortic valve may appear to arise exclusively from the right ventricle and resembles a double-outlet right ventricle. Most investigators follow the "50% rule" to make this distinction. If more than 50% of the aorta overlies the left ventricle, the proper designation should be tetralogy of Fallot. If more than 50% of the

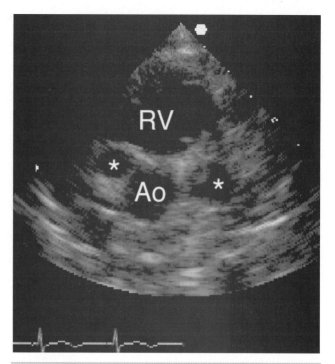

FIGURE 18.99 An example of coronary artery aneurysms from a patient with Kawasaki disease is provided. This basal short-axis view shows multiple, large, saccular aneurysms (*asterisks*) in the proximal left and right coronary arteries. Ao, aorta; RV, right ventricle.

aorta overlies the right ventricle, double-outlet right ventricle is present.

The short-axis view allows the echocardiographer to determine the extent and size of the septal defect. More important, the right ventricular outflow tract can be assessed. Narrowing can occur on multiple levels. In most cases, it is the displacement of the infundibular septum that produces the subvalvular narrowing that is characteristic of tetralogy of Fallot. In general, the greater the aortic overriding is, the more severe the subpulmonary stenosis. Various combinations of infundibular hypoplasia and muscular hypertrophy may be present. Stenosis may also involve the pulmonary anulus and/or valve. Less often, the proximal pulmonary arteries are hypoplastic, resulting in supravalvular stenosis. In the most extreme situation, pulmonary atresia is present and perfusion of the lungs depends on systemic to pulmonary artery collaterals and a patent ductus arteriosus.

By using the parasternal short-axis and subcostal coronal views, each of these potential levels of obstruction must be carefully evaluated (Fig. 18.101). Color Doppler imaging is often helpful in assessing the location of the narrowed, turbulent flow. Continuous wave Doppler imaging is then used to determine the pressure gradient across the various levels of obstruction. Determining the size of the pulmonary arteries is important in planning any surgical intervention, and it is best accomplished

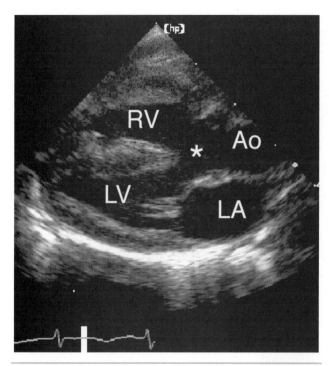

FIGURE 18.100 Long-axis image from a patient with tetralogy of Fallot demonstrates the overriding aorta (*Ao*) and a large subaortic ventricular septal defect (*asterisk*). Right ventricular hypertrophy is also present. LA, left atrium; LV, left ventricle; RV, right ventricle.

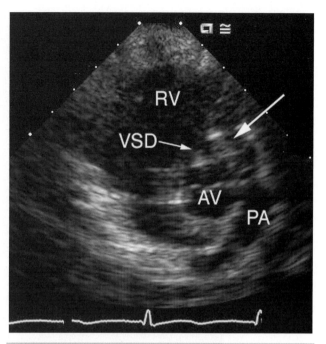

FIGURE 18.101 A child with tetralogy of Fallot is illustrated. Subvalvular (infundibular) pulmonary stenosis due to anterior deviation of the conal septum is indicated by the *large arrow*. The ventricular septal defect (*VSD*) (*large arrow*) is also shown. AV, aortic valve; PA, pulmonary artery; RV, right ventricle; VSD, ventricular septal defect. (Courtesy of T.R. Kimball, M.D., and S.A. Witt, R.D.C.S.)

from the short-axis and suprasternal views. The relative sizes of the right and left pulmonary arteries can be compared. In infants, care must be taken to avoid confusing the left pulmonary artery with a patent ductus arteriosus. The diameter of the right pulmonary artery is best assessed as it passes below the aortic arch (as recorded from the suprasternal long-axis view). Coronary artery anatomy must also be examined preoperatively, and this assessment generally can be accomplished by using two-dimensional echocardiographic techniques. A coronary artery branch crossing the right ventricular outflow tract (either an aberrant left anterior descending or conus branch) has important implications for surgical repair.

After repair of tetralogy of Fallot, echocardiography plays a key role in assessing the surgical results. From the parasternal long-axis view, the ventricular septal defect patch is seen as a linear structure passing obliquely from the septum to the anterior aortic root (Fig. 18.102). The oblique course is a consequence of the aortic overriding. Residual shunting may be detected with Doppler imaging, usually at the margins of the patch. Next, right ventricular size and contractility should be assessed. These parameters have important long-term prognostic implications. Finally, the right ventricular outflow tract is interrogated. Evidence of residual stenosis may be recorded with Doppler imaging (Fig. 18.103). The location and severity of any residual obstruction should be as-

certained. In most cases, pulmonary regurgitation also is present. The magnitude varies considerably but is sometimes severe. The clinical implications of chronic, severe pulmonary regurgitation after repair of tetralogy of Fallot are not firmly established, although close follow-up and serial assessment with echocardiography is recommended.

Transposition of the Great Arteries

The term transposition is used to describe a discordant ventriculoarterial connection in which the aorta arises from the morphologic right ventricle and the pulmonary artery arises from the left ventricle. Transposition can exist with either *situs solitus* or *situs inversus*. For simplicity, this section is a discussion of transposition in the presence of *situs solitus* only. The distinction between D-transposition and L-transposition is important and often is a source of confusion. In D-transposition, there is atrioventricular concordance and the morphologic right ventricle lies to the right of the morphologic left ventricle. In L-transposition, there is ventricular inversion and atrioventricular discordance. Thus, the morphologic right ventricle is to the left of the morphologic left ventricle. In both cases, the great arteries arise from the "incorrect" ventricle. With normal conotruncal development, the pulmonary artery arises anterior and to the left of the aorta.

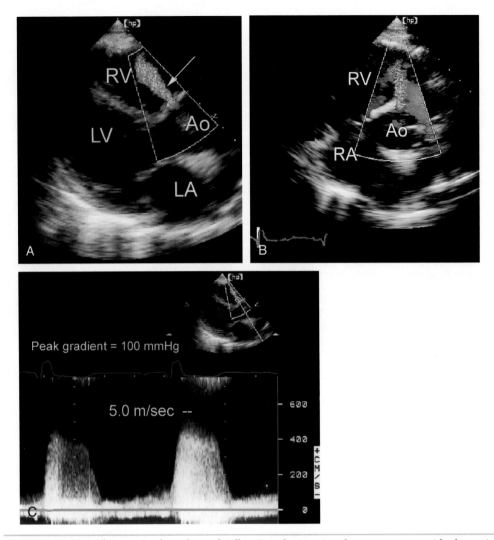

FIGURE 18.102 After repair of tetralogy of Fallot, Doppler imaging demonstrates a residual ventricular septal defect at the margin of the surgically placed patch. The left-to-right jet is demonstrated in the long-axis **(A)** and short-axis **(B)** views. **C:** The velocity of the jet is recorded with continuous wave Doppler imaging. Ao, aorta; LA, left atrium; LV, left ventricle; RA, right atrium; RV, right ventricle.

FIGURE 18.103 Doppler recording of right ventricular outflow tract velocity from the same patient illustrated in Figure 18.102. There is mild residual stenosis with a peak gradient across the pulmonary valve of 30 mm Hg. No evidence of significant pulmonary regurgitation is present.

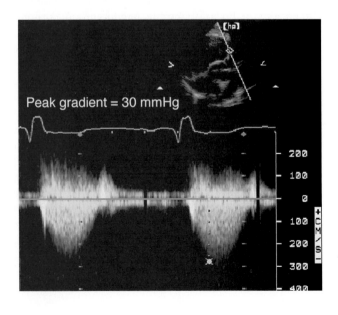

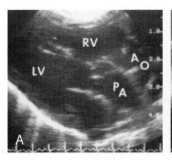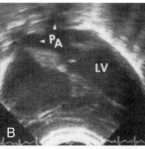

FIGURE 18.104 Example of D-transposition of the great arteries. **A:** Parasternal long-axis view demonstrates a normal ventricular relationship with the right ventricle (*RV*) anterior to the left ventricle (*LV*). Ventriculoarterial discordance is present with the aorta (*Ao*) arising from the right ventricle after the pulmonary artery (*PA*) arising from the left ventricle. In this view alone, the identity of the great arteries is not clear. **B:** A modified subcostal four-chamber view demonstrates a bifurcating great artery arising from the left ventricle. This image confirms that this vessel is the pulmonary artery and secures the diagnosis of transposition. (Courtesy of Gregory J. Ensing, MD.)

Its initial course is posterior and then it bifurcates into right and left branches. The aortic valve is more posterior and rightward, and the course of the aorta is oblique with reference to the pulmonary artery. The aorta does not bifurcate but forms an arch as it passes posteriorly and inferiorly. Thus, the outflow tracts and great arteries of the right and left sides of the heart appear to wrap around one another in a spiral fashion. Transposition results in a more parallel alignment of the great arteries. With two-dimensional echocardiography, this positioning has been described as a "double-barrel" appearance rather than the normal "circle and sausage" orientation (Fig. 18.5).

D-Transposition

The echocardiographic diagnosis of D-transposition requires demonstration of a right-sided right ventricle giving rise to an aorta and a left-sided left ventricle giving rise to a pulmonary artery. In children, this anatomic structure is best evaluated from the subcostal four-chamber view, which allows all these features of D-transposition to be displayed (Figs. 18.104 and 18.105). In adults, however, this assessment is technically challenging. More often, the parasternal short-axis and apical four-chamber views provide most of the diagnostic information (Fig. 18.106). In the short-axis view, the aortic valve is usually anterior and to the right of the pulmonary valve, and the great arteries arise in parallel. It should be emphasized that this spatial relationship between the great arteries is not essential for the diagnosis, and the aorta occasionally lies directly anterior or slightly to the left of the pulmonary valve. These arrangements are easily discerned from the short-axis view at the base (Figs. 18.105 and 18.106). Because the semilu-

nar valves occupy different levels (the aortic valve being slightly more cranial), they usually are not seen in the same short-axis plane. In the long-axis view, this parallel relationship of the great arteries can often be recorded in the longitudinal plane. By demonstrating that the anterior vessel arches posteriorly and the posterior vessel bifurcates, the diagnosis of D-transposition is established. Transesophageal echocardiography can be used to identify the great vessels (Fig. 18.107) but is usually not required. Visualization of the ostia of the coronary arteries and the brachiocephalic branch vessels also serves to identify the aorta.

The presence of ventriculoarterial discordance alone will necessarily result in the creation of two parallel circuits and is incompatible with life. Therefore, admixture of arterial and venous blood is a prerequisite for survival and can occur at any level. An atrial septal defect, usually the secundum variety, is present in most patients. The size and direction of the interatrial shunt can be assessed with Doppler techniques. When venous admixing is inadequate, an atrial septostomy is often performed as a palliative measure. This intervention can be performed under echocardiographic guidance. Echocardiography also plays a vital role in selecting candidates for this procedure and in determining its success (as judged by the size of the resulting defect).

Approximately one-third of patients with D-transposition have a ventricular septal defect. The location of these defects is variable. In most, the defect involves the outlet septum and may be associated with pulmonary artery overriding. Care must be taken to avoid confusing this condition with tetralogy of Fallot or a double-outlet right ventricle. In D-transposition, more than 50% of the pulmonary artery is committed to the left ventricle and there is pulmonary-mitral continuity. These features are optimally assessed from the parasternal long-axis view.

Additional associated lesions include subaortic (i.e., right ventricular outflow tract) stenosis and tricuspid (i.e., systemic atrioventricular) valve abnormalities. Subpulmonary (left ventricular outflow tract) obstruction may also be present, and several anatomic forms have been described. In most cases, this form of obstruction is dynamic because of systolic bowing of the septum into the left ventricle. Doppler techniques can be used to assess the pressure gradient across such stenoses. Ventricular function and size are important parameters that should be assessed with echocardiography. The right ventricle, because it must pump against the systemic vascular resistance, becomes dilated and hypertrophied. Conversely, the left ventricle is often small and relatively thin walled. The normal septal curvature is reversed with the right ventricle assuming a rounded configuration and the left ventricle becoming more crescent-shaped. Coronary artery anomalies are present in more than one-third of patients. Detection requires careful recording of the ostia

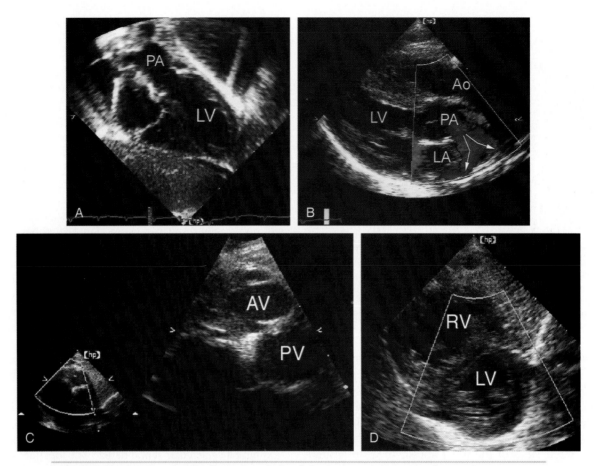

FIGURE 18.105 An example of D-transposition of the great arteries in an infant is shown. **A:** From the subcostal view, the pulmonary artery (*PA*) can again be seen to arise from the anatomic left ventricle (*LV*). **B:** By demonstrating bifurcation of the great artery that arises from the posterior left ventricle, ventriculoarterial discordance is confirmed. **C:** A short-axis view at the base of the heart demonstrates the parallel course of the great arteries with an anterior aortic valve (*AV*). **D:** The right ventricle (*RV*) is seen anterior and rightward of the left ventricle. It is dilated and hypertrophied. Ao, aorta; LA, left atrium.

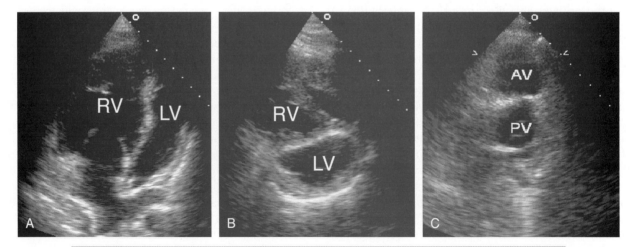

FIGURE 18.106 In patients with D-transposition of the great arteries, the anatomic right ventricle acts as the systemic ventricle. **A:** From the four-chamber view, note that the right ventricle (*RV*) is dilated and hypokinetic. Similar findings are apparent in the short-axis view **(B)**. **C:** The transposed great artery relationship is demonstrated. AV, aortic valve; LV, left ventricle; PV, pulmonary valve.

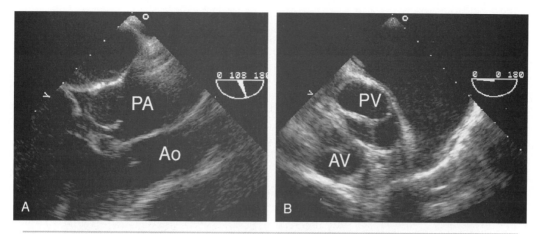

FIGURE 18.107 In D-transposition of the great arteries, the relationship between the vessels is readily demonstrated using transesophageal echocardiography. **A:** The parallel course of the great arteries is shown. **B:** From a short-axis plane, the side-by-side relationship of the semilunar valves is illustrated, with the aortic valve (*AV*) in a more anterior position. Ao, aorta; PA, pulmonary artery; PV, pulmonary valve.

and initial course of the vessels as they arise from the aortic root. An approach similar to that described in the section on tetralogy of Fallot should be used.

The evaluation of patients after surgical correction of D-transposition relies heavily on echocardiographic techniques. Two distinct surgical procedures have been performed for treatment of this condition. In the past, the most common form of palliation for D-transposition was an intraatrial baffle (also known as a Mustard, Senning, or atrial switch) procedure. A baffle connects the vena cava to the mitral valve (and hence the pulmonary circuit) by diverting blood flow across the atrial septum while simultaneously allowing pulmonary venous blood to be

routed over the baffle to the tricuspid valve (and on to the systemic circuit). Echocardiographic evaluation relies on direct visualization of the newly created systemic and pulmonary venous atria and careful assessment of right (i.e., systemic) ventricular function (Fig. 18.106). The presence and severity of tricuspid regurgitation should also be determined with Doppler imaging.

In the parasternal long-axis view, the baffle is seen as an oblique, linear echo within the anatomic left atrium (Fig. 18.108). The pulmonary venous atrium is superior and posterior while the systemic venous atrium is in communication with the mitral valve. Medial or rightward angulation may permit visualization of the junction of the

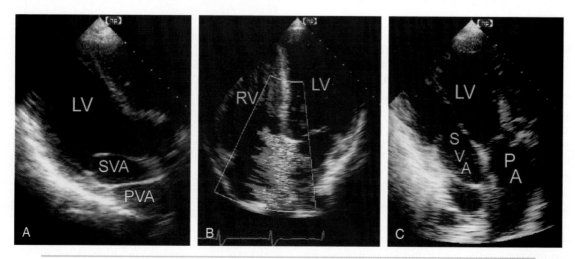

FIGURE 18.108 A Mustard repair is shown in a patient with D-transposition of the great arteries. The intraatrial baffle is well visualized. **A:** From the long-axis view, the relationship of the systemic venous atrium (*SVA*) and pulmonary venous atrium (*PVA*) is shown. **B:** Systemic atrioventricular valve regurgitation is seen with color Doppler imaging. **C:** An apical view demonstrates the pulmonary artery (*PA*) arising from the posterior left ventricle (*LV*). RV, right ventricle.

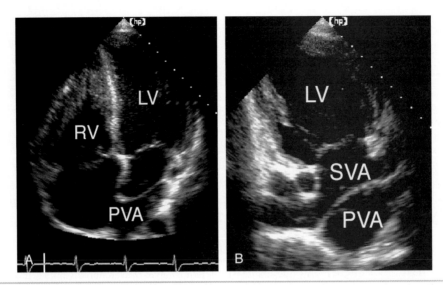

FIGURE 18.109 A Mustard repair of transposition of the great arteries is provided. From the apical window, by tilting the transducer at different angles, the various limbs of the baffle can be visualized. **A:** The pulmonary venous atrium (*PVA*) can be seen in association with the anatomic right atrium. **B:** The systemic venous atrium (*SVA*) diverts blood through the mitral valve. LV, left ventricle; RV, right ventricle.

pulmonary venous atrium with the right ventricle. From the apical and subcostal four-chamber views, most regions of the baffle can be assessed. Shallow angulation of the transducer allows most of the pulmonary venous atrium to be recorded and is useful in detecting obstruction within this region (Fig. 18.109). By tilting the transducer more posteriorly, the junction between the inferior vena cava and the systemic venous atrium (an uncommon site of obstruction) is visible. Obstruction within the superior vena caval limb of the baffle is more common, but it may be difficult to visualize, particularly in adults. The subcostal and suprasternal short-axis views can be used for this purpose.

Leaks within the baffle can be detected by using contrast echocardiography from the four-chamber view (Fig. 18.110). With this technique, right-to-left baffle leaks can be diagnosed with high sensitivity. Color Doppler imaging also permits these leaks to be identified and localized. Obstruction within the baffle can also be detected with contrast echocardiography or color Doppler imaging (Fig. 18.111). Obstruction within the superior vena cava is assessed from the suprasternal notch. With a normally functioning baffle, color Doppler imaging can be used to follow the undisturbed, low-velocity flow from the vena cava to the systemic venous atrium. Pulsed Doppler imaging can identify obstruction as a continuous, turbulent flow in excess of 1 m/sec. Obstruction within the pulmonary venous atrium requires the use of Doppler techniques for detection. First, color Doppler imaging is used to search for turbulence within the conduit. Then, pulsed Doppler imaging can be applied to measure the increased velocity within the structure. A diastolic flow velocity that is

greater than 2 m/sec suggests significant obstruction. Lower velocity turbulent flow does not exclude the possibility of obstruction, however. Transesophageal echocardiography has been used to more accurately assess intraatrial baffles. Use of this technique may be particularly important in adults in whom transthoracic image quality is sometimes a limitation.

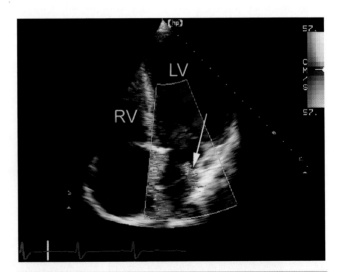

FIGURE 18.110 From a patient with Mustard repair of transposition of the great arteries, a baffle leak is demonstrated with color Doppler imaging (*arrow*). The shunt, which is physiologically similar to an atrial septal defect, allows blood to flow from the pulmonary venous atrium (below) to the systemic venous atrium (above). LV, left ventricle; RV, right ventricle.

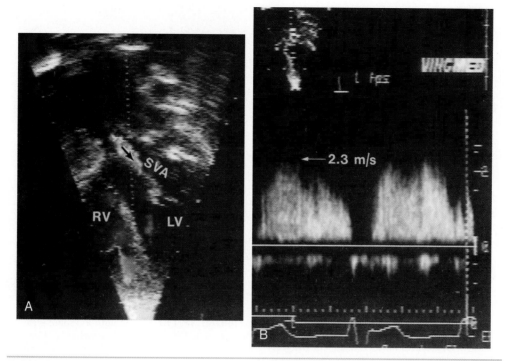

FIGURE 18.111 A: Color flow imaging in a 9-year-old patient with an intraatrial baffle demonstrates turbulence within the systemic venous atrium (*SVA*) (*arrow*). **B:** Pulsed Doppler imaging reveals significantly elevated velocity in this region, consistent with obstruction within the systemic venous atrium as it connects with the superior vena cava. LV, left ventricle; RV, right ventricle.

The arterial switch procedure is currently the standard approach for anatomic correction of D-transposition. This method has several practical and theoretic advantages over the intraatrial baffle procedure and has now become the operation of choice in most situations. The procedure involves transection of both great arteries and reanastomosis of the pulmonary artery to the right ventricle and the aorta to the left ventricle. Thus, the normal structure-function relationships of the ventricles are restored. Selecting infants for this procedure depends in part on coronary artery anatomy, and echocardiography can be used for this determination. Echocardiographic evaluation after the arterial switch procedure should focus on assessment of left and right ventricular function and the detection of any newly created structural problems, either involving the ventricles, the great artery anastomoses, or the origin of the coronary arteries. Both supravalvular aortic and pulmonary narrowing have been reported. Some degree of structural distortion of the origins of the great arteries does occur commonly without significant stenosis. Therefore, Doppler imaging must be used to determine the severity of any apparent narrowing seen with two-dimensional echocardiography. The ostia of the coronary arteries should also be visualized. This study is best performed in the parasternal short-axis view. The ability to demonstrate the proximal coronary arteries with echocardiography suggests that this technique may be helpful in detecting narrowing or kinking of the reimplanted vessels.

L-Transposition

In simplest terms, L-transposition can be thought of as isolated ventricular inversion in which the morphologic right ventricle is to the left of the morphologic left ventricle. The echocardiographic diagnosis rests on demonstrating abnormal atrioventricular and ventriculoarterial connections. Determining ventricular morphology and establishing the spatial relationships of the two chambers are accomplished as described previously. The discordant connections are detected by using multiple echocardiographic windows. From the four-chamber view, the presence of ventricular inversion usually can be established (Fig. 18.112A). Apical displacement of the left-sided tricuspid valve can also be demonstrated. In the long-axis view, direct continuity between the pulmonary valve and anterior mitral leaflet is apparent. In most cases, the ventricles are oriented in a side-by-side fashion, which creates some unusual and confusing echocardiographic views. For example, the parasternal long-axis plane may be vertical. In the short-axis view, the septum also appears more vertical (i.e., perpendicular to the frontal plane). The great arteries arise in parallel, with the aorta usually positioned leftward, anterior, and superior to the pulmonary valve. This is best appreciated from the basal short-axis view (Fig. 18.112B). This relationship contrasts with D-transposition, in which the aortic valve is anterior and usually rightward of the pulmonary valve.

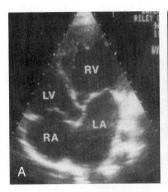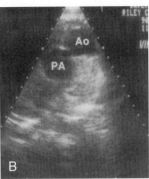

FIGURE 18.112 Apical four-chamber (**A**) and high parasternal short-axis (**B**) views from a patient with L-transposition of the great arteries. **A:** Ventricular inversion is demonstrated. The dilated and trabeculated right ventricle (*RV*) receives blood from the morphologic left atrium (*LA*). The displaced tricuspid valve is apical to the right-sided mitral valve. **B:** The two great arteries arise in parallel and the aorta (*Ao*) is anterior and to the left of the pulmonary artery (*PA*). LV, left ventricle; RA, right atrium.

Associated anomalies are a common and important feature of L-transposition. Structural abnormalities of the left-sided tricuspid valve occur in most patients. Apical displacement of the leaflet insertions (an Ebstein-like deformity) and tricuspid regurgitation may occur. A perimembranous ventricular septal defect is present in approximately 70% of cases. Less often, left ventricular outflow tract obstruction (valvular or subvalvular pulmonary stenosis) is present and can be assessed with Doppler imaging. Finally, right (i.e., systemic) ventricular function is frequently abnormal and should be examined carefully. Gradual deterioration in function of the right side of the heart may occur over time. Echocardiography plays an important role in the detection of this problem and in the assessment of any associated tricuspid regurgitation.

Double-Outlet Right Ventricle

In a double-outlet right ventricle, both great arteries arise predominantly from the right ventricle. A ventricular septal defect is present and is the sole outlet for the left ventricle. Partial septal overriding of the posterior great vessel may occur, but the posterior artery is primarily (>50%) committed to the right ventricle. In most cases, a muscular infundibulum or conus supports both great vessels, resulting in a separation (or lack of fibrous continuity) between the posterior semilunar valve and the anterior mitral leaflet. The echocardiographic evaluation of patients with a double-outlet right ventricle includes an assessment of the great artery relations, determination of the size and type of ventricular septal defect, and detection of the presence of any associated lesions (especially pulmonary stenosis and atrial septal defect). The echocardiographic diagnosis of a double-outlet right ventricle is based on the demonstration that both great arteries arise

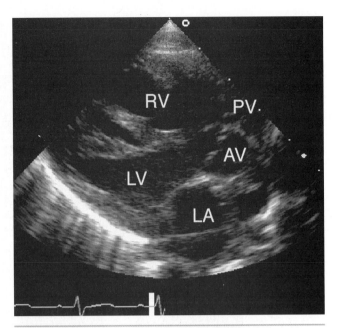

FIGURE 18.113 A child with a double-outlet right ventricle is illustrated. A large subaortic ventricular septal defect is present. There is minimal anterior deviation of the conal septum, and the great arteries are normally related. AV, aortic valve; LA, left atrium; LV, left ventricle; PV, pulmonary valve; RV, right ventricle.

to the right of the ventricular septum (i.e., are primarily committed to the right ventricle). The origin of the great arteries in relation to the septum is best visualized from the parasternal long-axis and subcostal coronal views (Fig. 18.113). These views also help to determine the lack of fibrous continuity between the posterior semilunar valve and the anterior mitral valve leaflet. This finding is not mandatory for diagnosis, however, because complete absorption of the conus below the posterior semilunar valve will allow fibrous continuity with the atrioventricular valve to be established.

Once the diagnosis is made, the great vessel relationships should be determined. Four spatial arrangements are possible: (1) normal (pulmonary artery anterior and to the left of the aorta), (2) side-by-side (aorta to the right but in the same transverse plane), (3) dextromalposition (aorta anterior and to the right), and (4) levomalposition (aorta anterior and to the left). This determination is made by using the parasternal long- and short-axis and subcostal four-chamber views (Fig. 18.114). The approach is similar to that used in the assessment of transposition. A normal great vessel relationship is rare and may be confused with tetralogy of Fallot. When the two vessels appear side by side in the short-axis view, determining their respective identity requires superior angulation to detect bifurcation of the pulmonary artery.

The ventricular septal defect is usually large and may be either subaortic (the most common), subpulmonary

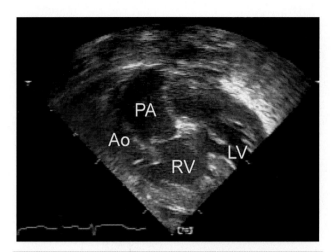

FIGURE 18.114 An example of a double-outlet right ventricle is provided, viewed from the parasternal long-axis. A large subpulmonary ventricular septal defect is present, and both great vessels arise from the right ventricle (*RV*). The aorta (*Ao*) is anterior and slightly rightward of the pulmonary artery (*PA*), a relationship properly referred to as dextromal-position. LV, left ventricle. (Courtesy of T.R. Kimball, M.D., and S.A. Witt, R.D.C.S.)

(the Taussig-Bing form), doubly committed, or noncommitted. The defect is easily appreciated from multiple echocardiographic views. Next, the possibility of pulmonary stenosis (valvular and/or subvalvular) must be assessed. This condition is present in approximately 50% of patients and usually is most easily detected from the parasternal long-axis view. Doppler techniques should be used to assess the pressure gradient and any associated regurgitation. Other anomalies that may be detected with echocardiography include atrial septal defect, subaortic stenosis, patent ductus arteriosus, and mitral valve abnormalities. Surgical repair of a double-outlet right ventricle is complex and depends in part on the great artery relationships. Echocardiographic assessment after repair should focus on the evaluation of the ventricular septal defect patch, the presence of outflow obstruction, and the possibility of semilunar valve regurgitation.

Persistent Truncus Arteriosus and Aortopulmonary Window

Persistent truncus arteriosus is characterized by the presence of a single great vessel arising from the base of the heart and dividing into systemic and pulmonary arteries. An outlet ventricular septal defect and a single semilunar valve are other essential features. This lesion is the result of a failure of partitioning involving the conus, truncus arteriosus, and aortic sac. The truncal valve is often large and structurally abnormal, sometimes with significant regurgitation. It is positioned directly over the ventricular septal defect and usually originates equally from the two ventricles. The origin of the pulmonary arteries from the

truncus is variable and used to classify the various types of truncus arteriosus. By far, the most common is type I, in which a short main pulmonary artery arises from the truncus before dividing into left and right branches. In type II, no main pulmonary artery is present and the left and right branches arise separately from the posterior wall of the truncus. These two forms account for more than 90% of all cases.

The echocardiographic diagnosis relies on the demonstration of a single large great artery arising from the base of the heart and overriding an outlet ventricular septal defect. In the parasternal long-axis view, the size of the great vessel and septal defect, as well as the degree of overriding, can be assessed (Fig. 18.115). The posterior truncal wall is seen in fibrous continuity with the anterior mitral leaflet. Because these features are shared by other conotruncal lesions (tetralogy of Fallot and pulmonary atresia with ventricular septal defect), the diagnosis cannot be made from the parasternal long-axis alone. The echocardiographer must evaluate the pulmonary arteries as they branch from the truncus, which is best accomplished from the parasternal short-axis view at the base. Here, the absence of the pulmonary valve and the origin of the pulmonary arteries from the posterior truncal wall are diagnostic of this entity. Both pulmonary arteries must be assessed to exclude the possibility of unilateral absence of one artery. Classification of the anatomic type is usually possible, and the number of truncal valve leaflets can often be determined. As many as six cusps may be present. The magnitude of truncal valve regurgitation and the relative sizes of the two ventricles are determined from the apical four-chamber view. From the suprasternal view, the presence of a right-sided aortic arch can be identified. Branch pulmonary artery stenosis, sometimes associated with truncus, can also be detected (Fig. 18.116). Other possible anomalies in patients with truncus arteriosus include atresia of the ductus arteriosus and anomalous origin of the coronary arteries.

An aortopulmonary window is a related anomaly involving the conotruncus in which the ventricular septum is intact, two semilunar valves are present, and two great arteries arise from the base of the heart. Incomplete partitioning of the truncus results in a communication between the proximal aorta and the main pulmonary artery, usually just above the semilunar valves. The anatomic defect bears many similarities to a ductus arteriosus and the two are sometimes confused. With echocardiography, the subcostal four-chamber view may be useful in establishing this diagnosis. The presence or absence of the proximal truncal septum distinguishes an aortopulmonary window (in which it is present) from truncus arteriosus (in which it is absent). The identification of two semilunar valves clearly differentiates these entities. Finally, Doppler imaging has proven useful in detecting an aortopul-

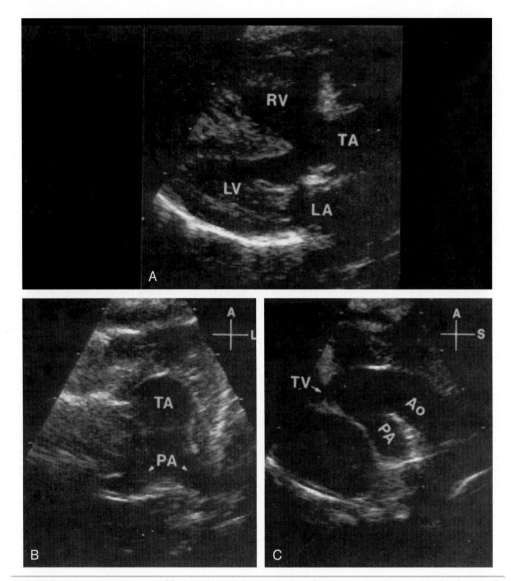

FIGURE 18.115 **A:** Parasternal long-axis view in a patient with truncus arteriosus reveals a large subarterial ventricular septal defect and an overriding great artery, the truncus arteriosus (*TA*). **B:** High parasternal short-axis view demonstrates the origin of the pulmonary artery (*PA*) from the posterior wall of the truncus arteriosus which bifurcates into a right and left branch. **C:** Long-axis view at the same level again reveals the origin of the pulmonary artery from the posterior wall of the truncus arteriosus. The position of the truncal valve (*TV*) is indicated (*arrow*). This is an example of type I truncus arteriosus. Ao, aorta; LA, left atrium; LV, left ventricle; RV, right ventricle.

monary window and in assessing the size of the communication.

ABNORMALITIES OF VENTRICULAR DEVELOPMENT

Abnormalities of ventricular development may occur as a primary disorder, such as hypoplastic left heart syndrome, or may be secondary to other conditions, such as right ventricular hypoplasia resulting from tricuspid atre-

sia. In either situation, hypoplasia of one or both ventricles is the primary functional anomaly.

Hypoplastic Left Heart Syndrome

Hypoplasia of the left ventricle is usually associated with atresia of the aortic and mitral valves, endocardial thickening, and a small left atrium and is properly referred to as hypoplastic left heart syndrome. The aortic diameter is reduced but increases in size beyond the ductus arteriosus, which is dilated. The echocardio-

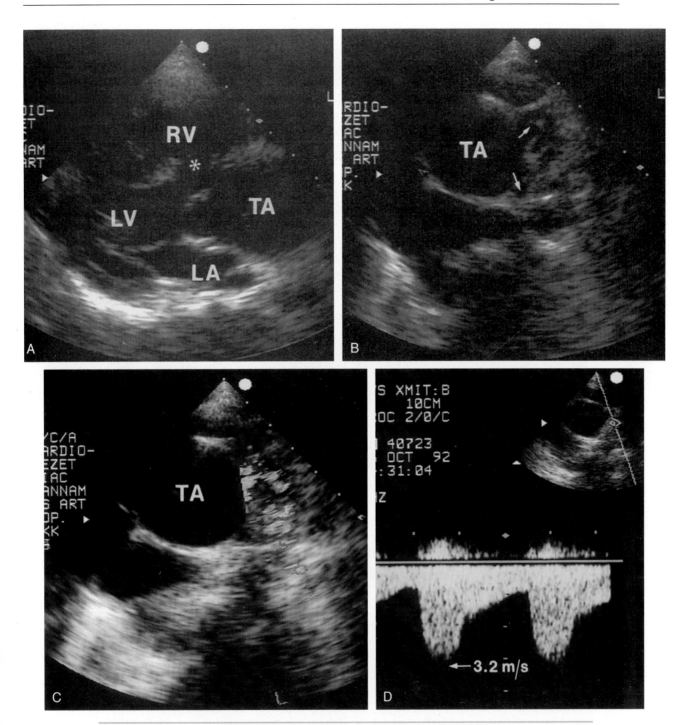

FIGURE 18.116 An example of truncus arteriosus, type II, in a young child. **A:** Parasternal long-axis view demonstrates the truncus arteriosus (*TA*) and a large ventricular septal defect (*asterisk*). **B:** Short-axis view again demonstrates the truncus arteriosus. The small pulmonary arteries are barely visualized arising separately from the posterior truncal wall (*arrows*). **C:** Color flow imaging from the same view demonstrates turbulent flow within the proximal pulmonary arteries. **D:** Continuous wave Doppler imaging reveals stenosis near their origin. The maximal velocity within the proximal pulmonary artery was 3.2 m/sec, consistent with a peak systolic gradient of approximately 40 mm Hg. LA, left atrium; LV, left ventricle; RV, right ventricle. (Courtesy of K. Kádár, Hungarian Institute of Cardiology.)

graphic diagnosis is based on the presence of an abnormally small and underdeveloped left ventricle, usually in association with a dilated right ventricle (Fig. 18.117). The ventricular septum should be carefully evaluated for the presence of a septal defect. The mitral valve, aortic valve, and aortic arch should also be assessed. In the short-axis view, the relative sizes of the two ventricles can be determined. The diameter of the aortic root can be measured and is usually less than 5 mm. A dilated pulmonary artery can be seen connecting to an enlarged ductus arteriosus. The entire aortic arch must be carefully evaluated from the parasternal and suprasternal views. The dimensions of the vessel and the severity of coarctation should be determined. These features have important implications for surgical repair. The ductus should be identified and carefully dif-

ferentiated from the main pulmonary artery. In planning surgical intervention, several other anatomic features should be analyzed, right ventricular systolic function most importantly. The presence and severity of tricuspid regurgitation must also be determined. Finally, the atrial septum should be assessed for the presence of a defect.

A rare form of ventricular dysplasia, noncompaction of left ventricular myocardium, occurs because of arrested endomyocardial morphogenesis resulting in failure of trabecular "compaction" of the developing myocardium. This condition leads to a "spongy" appearance of the myocardium, characterized by prominent ventricular trabeculations and deep intertrabecular recesses. These structural abnormalities are readily detected using two-dimensional echocardiography (Fig. 18.118).

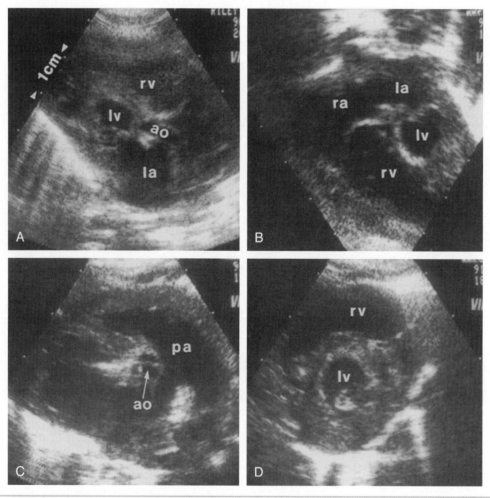

FIGURE 18.117 Serial images from an infant with hypoplastic left heart syndrome. **A:** Parasternal long-axis view demonstrates hypoplasia of the left ventricle (*lv*) and ascending aorta (*ao*). **B:** Apical four-chamber view again reveals a small left ventricle with a normally developed right ventricle (*rv*). An atrial septal defect is also present. **C:** Parasternal short-axis view at the base illustrates the hypoplastic aorta relative to a normal pulmonary artery (*pa*). **D:** A more apical parasternal short-axis view again demonstrates left ventricular hypoplasia. ra, right atrium; la, left atrium.

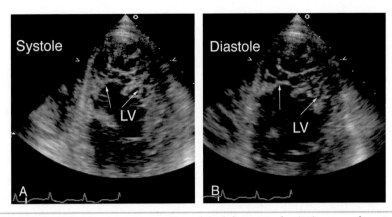

FIGURE 18.118 An example of noncompaction of the left ventricular (*LV*) myocardium is illustrated. Systolic **(A)** and diastolic **(B)** images are provided. The left ventricular apex has a thickened, spongiform appearance (*arrows*).

Single Ventricle

In the simplest definition, single ventricle refers to a condition in which a single pumping chamber receives inflow from both atria (i.e., has two inlet regions and is connected to two atrioventricular valves). A second or rudimentary chamber may be present, but it has no inlet portion (hence, is not a ventricle). The rudimentary chamber is sometimes referred to as an outlet chamber or rudimentary pouch. Based on the morphology, location, and trabecular pattern of the pumping and rudimentary chambers, the heart is referred to as a univentricular heart of either right, left, or indeterminate ventricular type. The most common form of single ventricle is the left ventricular type, also referred to as double-inlet left ventricle. Ventriculoarterial connections are also variable. Unfortunately, the diagnosis and classification of the univentricular heart are complex and considerable controversy exists regarding nomenclature and definitions.

With echocardiography, the type of single ventricle can be determined. In the left ventricular type, the rudimentary chamber is anterior and superior to the pumping chamber. In the right ventricular type, it is located more posteriorly. Because the location of the rudimentary chamber varies, the echocardiographic views used to assess this structure must also vary. For the left ventricular type, the parasternal long- and short-axis views usually provide the best opportunities to visualize the rudimentary chamber and intervening trabecular septum. For the right ventricular type, the four-chamber view is often best. In either case, the short-axis and four-chamber views are critical to demonstrate two side-by-side inlets without an intervening inlet septum (Fig. 18.119). This finding establishes the diagnosis and distinguishes single ventricle from other conditions in which two distinct pumping chambers are not readily apparent, including hypoplastic left or right heart (which has associated atrioventricular and semilunar valve hypoplasia), tricuspid atresia (char-

acterized by a blind-ending right atrium), and a large ventricular septal defect (in which an inlet septum separates the inflow of the two atrioventricular valves). Once the rudimentary chamber is identified, the interventricular communication, or bulboventricular foramen, should be sought. Evidence of flow restriction through the foramen can be assessed with Doppler techniques.

Once the diagnosis of single ventricle is made, the echocardiographic evaluation should focus on two related issues that have important implications for repair. First,

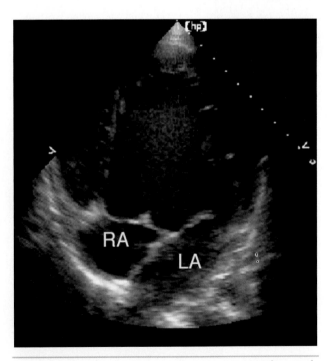

FIGURE 18.119 An apical view from a patient with a single ventricle (left-ventricular type) is shown. No evidence of interventricular septal tissue is recorded. Two atrioventricular valves are present, and the atrial septum is well visualized. LA, left atrium; RA, right atrium.

the specific type of atrioventricular connections should be established. In most cases, two separate inlet connections through two distinct atrioventricular valves are present (i.e., a double-inlet ventricle). Alternatively, in the setting of an indeterminate type of single ventricle, a single, large, common atrioventricular valve may be present. One of the atrioventricular connections may be absent, a condition that may be difficult to distinguish from tricuspid atresia or hypoplastic left heart. Finally, the two valves themselves must be assessed carefully for the presence of straddling or overriding. As discussed previously, the insertion of the chordae relative to the trabecular septum has implications for proper classification as well as surgical repair.

Next, the ventriculoarterial connections should be determined. Although any form of connection may occur, some are more likely than others. For example, with left ventricular type single ventricle, discordant ventriculo-arterial connections are common, usually with the aorta arising from the rudimentary (anterior) chamber and the pulmonary artery from the (posterior) ventricle. Although this relationship is not properly referred to as "transposition," it bears many of the typical echocardiographic features. With the right ventricular type single ventricle, the most common connections are double outlet from the ventricle or single outlet with pulmonary atresia.

Tricuspid Atresia

This condition is discussed here because the presence of an atretic tricuspid valve invariably leads to some degree of right ventricular hypoplasia. As a consequence, this lesion may be confused with some of the other disorders included in this section. Tricuspid atresia is characterized by an imperforate tricuspid valve, hypoplasia of the morphologic right ventricle, an interatrial communication, and a normally developed left ventricle and mitral valve. In contrast to single ventricle, the hypoplastic chamber has an inlet portion (although it is atretic), and therefore it is properly called a ventricle. The interatrial communication is most often a patent foramen ovale and is therefore restrictive. A larger secundum defect is present in approximately 25% of patients. The clinically important variable features of tricuspid atresia include the ventriculoarterial communication (concordant or transposed), the presence and size of a ventricular septal defect, and the presence and magnitude of obstruction to pulmonary blood flow.

The echocardiographic diagnosis of tricuspid atresia is made from the four-chamber view from which the imperforate tricuspid valve can be visualized directly (Fig. 18.120). The presence of severe valvular hypoplasia (rather than atresia) is established by detecting remnants of the tricuspid valve apparatus. In either case, the inlet is imperforate. When the atresia is caused by a membrane, considerable motion in the area of the anulus may be present. Doppler imaging is useful for confirming the absence of flow through the inlet. The size and function of the hypoplastic right ventricle can be determined, and the presence of mitral regurgitation can also be assessed. The parasternal long-axis view is used to examine the septum for defects and to help determine the great artery relationships. Because any form of great artery connections is possible, the exact position of the posterior great vessel relative to the septum must also be noted. By scanning superiorly, the presence or absence of transposition can usu-

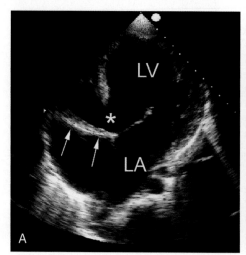
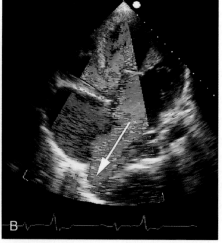

FIGURE 18.120 An example of tricuspid atresia is shown. **A:** The atretic tricuspid valve is indicated by the *arrows* and the *asterisk* denotes the ventricular septal defect. A hypoplastic right ventricle is present but not well seen in this view. A large atrial septal defect is evident. **B:** Significant mitral regurgitation is documented using color Doppler imaging. LA, left atrium; LV, left ventricle.

ally be determined. In the short-axis view, the right ventricular outflow tract and pulmonary valve can be evaluated for the presence of outflow obstruction. Confirming the diagnosis of pulmonary artery atresia, however, requires the use of multiple imaging planes. The subcostal views may be helpful in assessing the size of the interatrial communication. Dilation of the right atrium and bowing of the septum into the left atrium suggests a small, restrictive communication. From the suprasternal notch, the size and continuity of the pulmonary arteries can be assessed.

ECHOCARDIOGRAPHIC EVALUATION DURING AND AFTER SURGERY

Echocardiography is extremely useful for clinical decision making in patients undergoing palliative or reparative surgical procedures. Intraoperative echocardiography, both epicardial and transesophageal, permits additional diagnoses to be made and allows the adequacy of repair to be determined before completion of the operation. Subsequently, echocardiography compares favorably with cardiac catheterization for the detection of postoperative residua. Valvular lesions, conduit dysfunction, residual shunting, and pulmonary pressure can be accurately assessed in postoperative patients without the need for invasive procedures.

Systemic Artery to Pulmonary Artery Shunts

Over the years, various shunts have been devised to increase pulmonary artery flow by a systemic artery to pulmonary artery anastomosis. Today, they are used less often in favor of primary repair. Their extensive use in the past, however, accounts for the fact that they are still encountered frequently in adult postoperative patients. Fortunately, the most common shunt seen today, the modified Blalock-Taussig shunt, is also the one that is easiest to image. This shunt is a vascular connection between the subclavian or innominate artery and a branch pulmonary artery. Thus, it may be relatively long and can be created on either the right or left side. A direct anastomosis is commonly performed (a native shunt) or a prosthetic conduit (either Dacron or Gore-Tex®) may be used. In several situations, one might wish to evaluate a Blalock-Taussig shunt. Demonstrating the presence of such a shunt and its patency is of obvious clinical importance. Dysfunction because of stenosis can also be assessed. Finally, by determining the gradient across the conduit, the pulmonary artery pressure can be estimated.

Blalock-Taussig shunts are best viewed from the suprasternal notch or a high parasternal window (Fig. 18.121). A right-sided shunt may be seen in the suprasternal short-axis view. As the right pulmonary artery passes below the aortic arch, the insertion of the conduit can often be recorded. A left-sided shunt may be more difficult to record. From the suprasternal notch, the scan plane is tilted far to the left to include the left pulmonary artery. When the shunt cannot be observed directly, Doppler imaging and color flow imaging are often helpful for identification. The patency of a shunt and the presence of kinking or stenosis (usually at the distal insertion site) can also be determined with Doppler imaging. If a nonimaging probe is used, however, care must be taken to avoid mistaking the Blalock-Taussig shunt for a patent ductus arteriosus. The pressure gradient across the shunt can be measured by using the modified Bernoulli equation, and this value can be used to estimate the pulmonary pressure, both in systole and diastole (Fig. 18.121B). The pe-

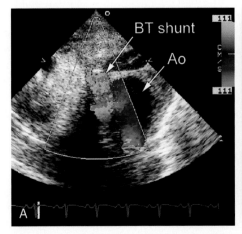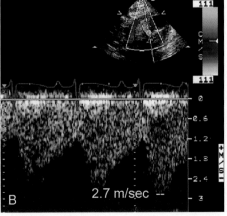

FIGURE 18.121 **A:** An example of a right Blalock-Taussig shunt (*BT shunt*) is demonstrated. Color Doppler imaging is useful to follow to the course of the conduit as it passes alongside the aorta (*Ao*) and enters the pulmonary artery. **B:** Continuous wave Doppler imaging is used to evaluate the velocity of flow through the shunt.

ripheral systolic and diastolic pressures are determined
from the sphygmomanometer and the pressure gradient
is subtracted from these values to derive the pulmonary
pressures. The amount of shunt flow can also be estimated from the Doppler tracing. Low-velocity retrograde
diastolic flow in the descending aorta indicates antegrade
flow through the shunt. Another type of shunt designed to
increase pulmonary blood flow is the Glenn shunt (Fig.
18.122). This involves anastomosis of the superior vena
cava into the right pulmonary artery. This can be in the
form of an end-to-end connection (the classic Glenn
shunt, in which caval flow is diverted solely into the right
pulmonary circuit) or as an end-to-side connection (bidirectional Glenn, in which caval flow is directed to both
lungs).

Pulmonary Artery Bands

A pulmonary artery band can be recorded as a linear
echogenic structure positioned transversely across the
main pulmonary artery (usually in its middle portion).
They are best evaluated from the parasternal short-axis
and subcostal views (Fig. 18.123A). A band can become
displaced and its abnormal position can often be detected
with two-dimensional echocardiography. The degree of
stenosis created by these structures cannot be judged reliably with echocardiography alone, although poststenotic dilation is suggestive of significant narrowing.
Doppler imaging should be used to estimate the pressure
gradient across a band (Fig. 18.123B). The correlation between the Doppler estimate and the catheterization-
measured gradient is high. Furthermore, in the presence

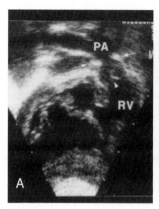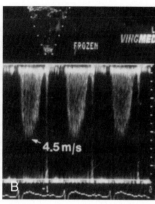

FIGURE 18.123 A pulmonary artery band is shown. **A:** Subcostal view demonstrates the right ventricle (*RV*), outflow tract,
and pulmonary artery (*PA*). The *arrows* indicate the location of
the pulmonary artery band immediately distal to the valve (*arrowhead*). **B:** Continuous wave Doppler recording through the
band reveals a maximal velocity of 4.5 m/sec consistent with a
peak systolic gradient of approximately 80 mm Hg.

of a nonrestrictive ventricular septal defect, when right
and left ventricular systolic pressures are approximately
equal, the pulmonary artery systolic pressure can be estimated as the brachial systolic pressure minus the gradient across the band (provided there is no left ventricular
outflow tract obstruction). In patients who have had a
pulmonary artery band removed, the echocardiographic
findings may be confusing. Residual narrowing and scar
tissue at the site of the banding make it difficult to determine whether the band is still in place. No echocardiographic signs alone can reliably make this distinction.

The Fontan Procedure

For lesions such as single ventricle and tricuspid atresia,
in which abnormal right ventricular structure or function
prevents adequate pulmonary blood flow, the Fontan procedure is frequently used for effective palliation. The
Fontan anastomosis is a connection between the systemic
atrium and the pulmonary circuit that is designed to increase pulmonary blood flow. The Fontan circuit can be
created in a variety of ways. In many cases, a direct anastomosis using pericardial tissue is placed between the
right atrial appendage and the pulmonary artery. In other
situations, a valved or nonvalved conduit is used. Intraatrial conduits, connecting the inferior vena cava to the
pulmonary artery, are also placed.

Visualization of the Fontan anastomosis is often challenging. Optimal evaluation is facilitated by knowledge of
the specific type of connection that was created surgically.
The course of most of these connections is retrosternal,
further complicating their echocardiographic detection.
High parasternal and subcostal views are usually most effective (Fig. 18.124). There have been a variety of modifi-

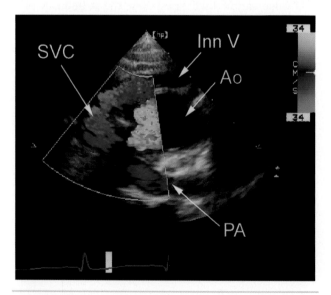

FIGURE 18.122. A Glenn shunt augments pulmonary blood
flow by connecting the superior vena cava (*SVC*) to the
right pulmonary artery (*PA*). Ao, aorta; Inn V, innominate vein.

cations and improvements in the original Fontan concept. For example, the Fontan connection may instead involve an internal conduit, sometimes called a lateral tunnel Fontan (Fig. 18.125). These conduits are more easily visualized and appear as a circular insert within the right atrium. Once the connection is visualized, Doppler imaging plays an important role in assessing the flow pattern and in determining the presence of dysfunction. Normal pulmonary artery flow after a Fontan procedure is biphasic, with one peak in late systole and a larger peak in late

diastole during atrial contraction. Augmentation of flow velocity is normally seen during inspiration. Abnormal systemic ventricular function is suggested by reduced or absent late diastolic flow and diminished respiratory variation in the flow pattern. Transesophageal echocardiography can also be used to assess the Fontan connection.

Fontan connections may also be fenestrated, purposely allowing right-to-left shunting. This is usually done in the setting of increased pulmonary vascular resistance to "decompress" the right atrium when pulmonary vascular re-

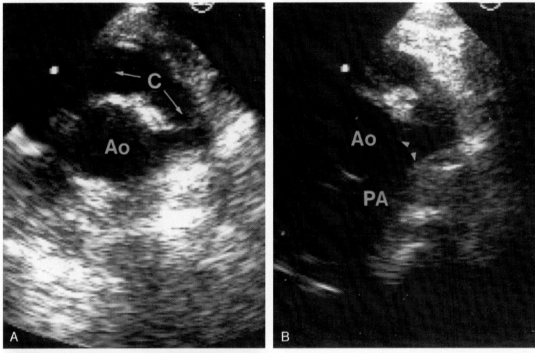

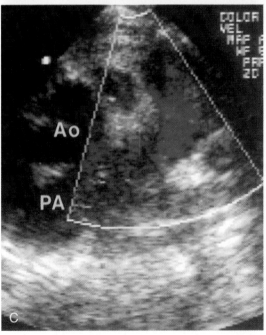

FIGURE 18.124 A: Short-axis view at the base of the heart in a patient with tricuspid atresia demonstrates a Fontan conduit (*C*) (*arrows*) passing anterior and left of the aorta (*Ao*). **B:** Angulation of the scan plane permits demonstration of the distal anastomosis of the conduit into the pulmonary artery (*PA*) (*arrowheads*). **C:** Color flow imaging in the same plane demonstrates flow within the conduit without significant turbulence, which suggests the absence of significant obstruction within the conduit.

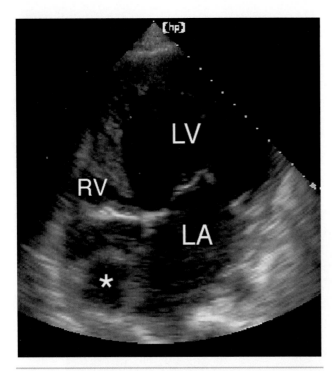

FIGURE 18.125 This type of Fontan employs an internal conduit and is sometimes called a lateral tunnel Fontan. The conduit can be seen in cross section (*asterisk*) within the right atrium in this patient with tricuspid atresia. LA, left atrium; LV, left ventricle; RV, right ventricle.

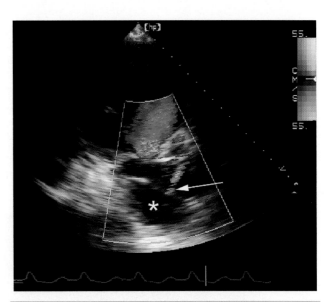

FIGURE 18.126 One modification of the Fontan procedure involves creating a fenestration to allow shunting between the Fontan connection (*asterisk*) and pulmonary venous (i.e., left) atrium, a type of right-to-left shunt. This can be assessed using color Doppler imaging (*arrow*). Continuous wave Doppler imaging can also be performed to estimate the gradient across the pulmonary circuit.

sistance is high. Such fenestrations usually are created at the time of surgery in high-risk patients and closed at a later time. The shunt flow can be easily visualized using color Doppler imaging (Fig. 18.126). The velocity of the shunt flow, assessed with continuous wave Doppler imaging, reflects the pressure gradient between the Fontan and the left atrium and is therefore a useful indicator of the total pressure gradient across the pulmonary circuit.

Right Ventricle to Pulmonary Artery Conduits

Both valved and nonvalved conduits have been used to shunt blood from the right ventricle to the pulmonary artery (e.g., in cases of pulmonary atresia or severe tetralogy of Fallot). One specific type of repair, called a Rastelli procedure, is performed in the setting of transposition of the great arteries with associated ventricular septal defect and pulmonary stenosis or atresia. A part of this complex repair includes a conduit from the right ventricle to the pulmonary artery. The echocardiographic evaluation of these structures requires an approach similar to that just described for left ventricle to aorta conduits. The conduits are best recorded from the high parasternal or subcostal windows (Fig. 18.127). Conduit obstruction can occur at the proximal or distal insertion site (usually because of problems in surgical positioning), at the valve (from primary tissue degeneration), or diffusely (the result of development of a

neointimal peel). Turbulence on color flow imaging may provide the initial evidence of conduit stenosis (Figs. 18.128 and 18.129). Regurgitation, diagnosed with Doppler imaging, is present in many of these valved conduits.

FETAL ECHOCARDIOGRAPHY

Fetal echocardiography provides a valuable new means to better understand intrauterine growth and development of the heart and great vessels. The prenatal diagnosis of structural heart disease and the physiologic evaluation of fetal arrhythmias are perhaps the most important insights provided by this technique. The long-term effects of ultrasound energy on the developing fetus, however, are unknown. This fact may be particularly important when the higher energy levels associated with Doppler techniques are used. To date, no detrimental effects in humans have been demonstrated. Still, it is advisable to avoid excess exposure of the fetus by keeping the examination time as short as possible and using the lowest possible power setting. There are several potential indications for performing fetal echocardiography. Evaluation of the heart in the setting of retarded fetal growth or fetal distress is often recommended. Whenever extracardiac anomalies are detected during fetal ultrasound examination, cardiac assessment may be beneficial. The presence of chromosomal abnormalities detected with amniocentesis is strongly correlated with congenital heart disease and is another accepted indication for fetal echocardiography.

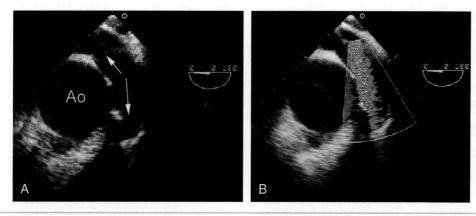

FIGURE 18.127 A right ventricle-to-pulmonary artery conduit (*arrows*) is shown from a patient with pulmonary atresia. The prosthetic material of the conduit is highly echogenic **(A)**. **B:** Using color Doppler imaging, flow through the conduit is demonstrated. Ao, aorta.

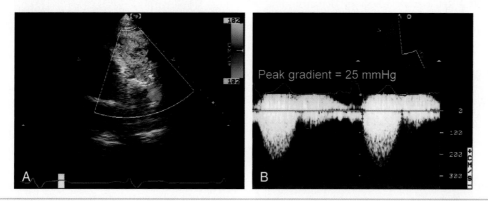

FIGURE 18.128 Mild obstruction is demonstrated in this patient who underwent a Rastelli repair. **A:** Color Doppler imaging demonstrates turbulent flow through the right ventricle-to-pulmonary artery conduit. **B:** Continuous wave Doppler imaging reveals a 25 mm Hg peak gradient through the conduit.

The test should also be performed as part of the assessment of fetal arrhythmias. Finally, whenever congenital heart disease is suspected for other reasons, such as maternal exposure to teratogenic substances or a parental history of previous children with congenital lesions, the examination should be considered.

The performance of a fetal echocardiogram requires experience and a systematic approach. Guidelines for training have been formulated, and only qualified individuals should perform this highly specialized examination. A brief description of the examination is presented here for interest only. The first step is to determine the position and orientation of the fetus within the uterus. Within the thorax, the heart, because of its motion, is usually the easiest and most recognizable structure to examine. The four-chamber view is most important and should be recorded first (Fig. 18.130). For orientation, the left atrium is identified by the presence of the septum primum and the pulmonary veins. Cardiac situs can be determined by identifying the systemic veins and the position of the atria relative to the liver and spleen. Next, the atrioventricular valves are identified, with the tricuspid valve slightly more

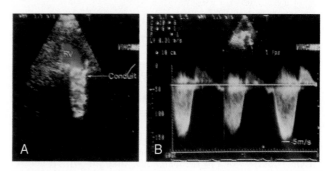

FIGURE 18.129 An example of a right ventricle-to-pulmonary artery conduit is provided. **A:** Color flow imaging demonstrates acceleration and turbulence within the conduit as indicated by the mosaic blood flow pattern. **B:** Continuous wave Doppler imaging demonstrates severe obstruction. The maximal flow velocity was 5.0 m/sec, suggesting a peak pressure gradient within the conduit of approximately 100 mm Hg. RV, right ventricle.

apical than the mitral valve. The outlet portions of the heart are then evaluated. Cardiac measurements can be made and compared with normal values that have been defined for all gestational ages. Doppler techniques can be

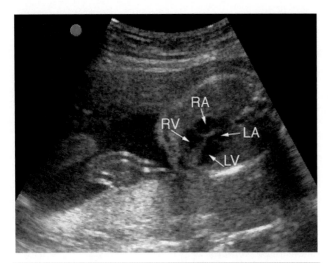

FIGURE 18.130 A fetal echocardiogram demonstrating a structurally normal heart from the four-chamber view is provided. LA, left atrium; LV, left ventricle; RA, right atrium; RV, right ventricle.

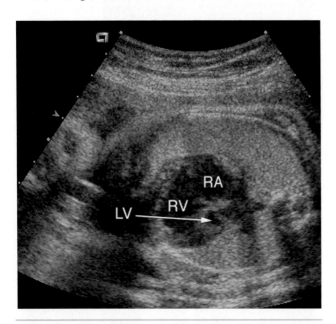

FIGURE 18.131 An example of hypoplastic left heart syndrome is shown. Note the size of the left ventricle (*LV*) compared with the right heart structures. RA, right atrium; RV, right ventricle. (Courtesy of T.R. Kimball, M.D., and S.A. Witt, R.D.C.S.)

used to visualize blood flow through the heart, great vessels, and umbilical vessels. Assessment of fetal arrhythmias is best accomplished by using a combination of M-mode and Doppler recordings. When these arrhythmias are present, a careful search for structural heart disease is mandatory. With this approach, a wealth of diagnostic information is available. Figure 18.131 is an example of hypoplastic left heart syndrome diagnosed in a fetus. Knowledge of complex congenital heart disease before delivery allows therapeutic interventions to begin immediately af-

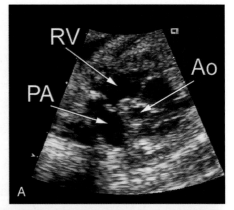

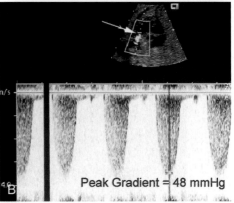

FIGURE 18.132 An echocardiogram recorded from a fetus with pulmonary stenosis. **A:** A basal short-axis view reveals a thickened pulmonary valve that domes in systole. **B:** Continuous wave Doppler imaging demonstrates a peak valvular gradient of 48 mm Hg. Ao, aorta; PA, pulmonary artery; RV, right ventricle.

ter birth and can be life saving for such patients. In Figure 18.132, valvular pulmonary stenosis is diagnosed *in utero*. In both of these examples, knowledge about the presence and severity of congenital cardiac defects facilitated management of labor and delivery and allowed perinatal care to be optimized.

The critical role of echocardiography in prenatal diagnosis is evident, and both the accuracy and safety of the test are now well established. The structures in these images are small, however, and random movements of the fetus make for a challenging and time-consuming examination. Despite these factors, fetal echocardiography has provided clinicians with earlier diagnosis of heart disease and a better understanding of fetal hemodynamics.

SUGGESTED READINGS

Barron JV, Sahn DJ, Valdes-Cruz LM, et al. Clinical utility of two-dimensional Doppler echocardiographic techniques for estimating pulmonary to systemic blood flow ratios in children with left-to-right shunting atrial septal defect, ventricular septal defect of patent ductus arteriosus. J Am Coll Cardiol 1984;3:169.

Barron JV, Sanches-Ugarte T, Keirns C, et al. Calcification of patent ductus arteriosus detected by two-dimensional echocardiography. Am Heart J 1987;114:446.

Bevilacqua M, Sanders SP, VanPraagh S, et al. Double-inlet single left ventricle: Echocardiographic anatomy with emphasis on the morphology of the atrioventricular valves and ventricular septal defect. J Am Coll Cardiol 1991;18:559.

Brandenburg J, Tajik AJ, Edwards WD, et al. Accuracy of 2-dimensional echocardiographic diagnosis of congenitally bicuspid aortic valve: Echocardiographic-anatomic correlation in 115 patients. Am J Cardiol 1983;51:1469.

Carvalho JS, Rigby ML, Shinebourne EA, et al. Cross sectional echocardiography for recognition of ventricular topology in atrioventricular septal defect. Br Heart J 1989;61:285.

Cheitlin MD, Alpert JS, Armstrong WF, et al. ACC/AHA Guidelines for the Clinical Application of Echocardiography: a report of the American College of Cardiology/American Heart Association Task Force on Practice Guidelines (Committee on Clinical Application of Echocardiography) developed in collaboration with the American Society of Echocardiography. Circulation 1997;95:1686–1744.

Chin TK, Perloff JK, Williams RG, et al. Isolated noncompaction of left ventricular myocardium: a study of eight cases. Circulation 1990;82:507.

Cohen M, Fuster V, Steele PM, et al. Coarctation of the aorta: long-term follow-up and prediction of outcome after surgical correction. Circulation 1989;80:840.

Dittman H, Jacksch R, Voelker W, et al. Accuracy of Doppler echocardiography in quantification of left to right shunts in adult patients with atrial septal defect. J Am Coll Cardiol 1988;11:338.

Frommelt PC, Snider AR, Meliones JN, et al. Doppler assessment of pulmonary artery flow patterns and ventricular function after the Fontan operation. Am J Cardiol 1991;68:1211.

Garg A, Shrivastava S, Radhakrishnan S, et al. Doppler assessment of interventricular pressure gradient across isolated ventricular septal defect. Clin Cardiol 1990;13:717.

George L, Waldman JD, Mathewson JW, et al. Two dimensional echocardiographic discrimination of normal from abnormal great artery relationships. Clin Cardiol 1983;6:327.

Gill HK, Splitt M, Sharland GK, et al. Patterns of recurrence of congenital heart disease: an analysis of 6,640 consecutive pregnancies evaluated by detailed fetal echocardiography. J Am Coll Cardiol 2003;42:923.

Gleason MM, Chin AJ, Andrews BA, et al. Two dimensional and Doppler echocardiographic assessment of neonatal arterial repair for transposition of the great arteries. J Am Coll Cardiol 1989;13:1320.

Gutgesell HP, Huhta JC. Cardiac septation in atrioventricular canal defect. J Am Coll Cardiol 1986;8:1421.

Gutgesell NP, Cheatham J, Latson LA, et al. Atrioventricular valve abnormalities in infancy: Two-dimensional echocardiographic and angiocardiographic comparison. J Am Coll Cardiol 1983;2:531.

Hausmann D, Daniel WG, Mugge A, et al. Value of transesophageal color Doppler echocardiography for detection of different types of atrial septal defects in adults. J Am Soc Echocardiogr 1992;5:481.

Henry WL, Maron BJ, Griffith JM. Cross sectional echocardiography in the diagnosis of congenital heart disease: identification of the relation of the ventricles and great arteries. Circulation 1977;56:267.

Hiraishi S, Horiguchi Y, Misawa H, et al. Noninvasive Doppler echocardiographic evaluation of shunt flow dynamics of the ductus arteriosus. Circulation 1987;75:1146.

Horneffer PJ, Zahka KG, Rowe SA, et al. Long term results of total repair of tetralogy of Fallot in childhood. Ann Thorac Surg 1990;50:179.

Hsu YH, Santulli T, Wong AL, et al. Impact of intraoperative echocardiography on surgical management of congenital heart disease. Am J Cardiol 1991;67:1279.

Huhta JC, Carpenter RJ, Moise KJ, et al. Prenatal diagnosis and postnatal management of critical aortic stenosis. Circulation 1987;75:573.

Huhta JC, Glasow P, Murphy DJ, et al. Surgery without catheterization for congential heart defects: management of 100 patients. J Am Coll Cardiol 1987;9:823.

Huhta JC, Seward JB, Tajik AJ, et al. Two-dimensional echocardiographic spectrum of univentricular atrioventricular connection. J Am Coll Cardiol 1985;5:149.

Jureidini SB, Appleton RS, Nouri S, et al. Detection of coronary artery abnormalities in tetralogy of Fallot by two-dimensional echocardiography. J Am Coll Cardiol 1998;14:960.

Kaulitz R, Stumper OFW, Geuskens R, et al. Comparative values of the precordial and transesophageal approaches in the echocardiographic evaluation of atrial baffle function after an atrial correction procedure. J Am Coll Cardiol 1990;16:686.

Klewer SE, Samson RA, Donnerstein RL, et al. Comparison of accuracy of diagnosis of congenital heart disease by history and physical examination versus echocardiography. Am J Cardiol 2002;89:1329.

Kronzon I, Tunick PA, Freedberg RS, et al. Transesophageal echocardiography is superior to transthoracic echocardiography in the diagnosis of sinus venosus atrial septal defect. J Am Coll Cardiol 1991;17:537.

Lang D, Oberhoffer R, Cook A, et al. Pathologic spectrum of malformations of the tricuspid valve in prenatal and neonatal life. J Am Coll Cardiol 1991;17:1161.

Lipshultz SE, Sanders SP, Mayer JE, et al. Are routine preoperative cardiac catheterization and angiography necessary before repair of ostium primum atrial septal defect? J Am Coll Cardiol 1988;11:373.

Ludomirsky A, Tani L, Murphy DJ, et al. Usefulness of color-flow Doppler in diagnosing and in differentiating supracristal ventricular septal defect from right ventricular outflow tract obstruction. Am J Cardiol 1991;67:194.

Mair DD, Hagler DJ, Julsrud PR, et al. Early and late results of the modified Fontan procedure for double-inlet left ventricle: the Mayo Clinic experience. J Am Coll Cardiol 1991;18:1727.

Martin RP, Qureshi SA, Ettedgui JA, et al. An evaluation of right and left ventricular function after anatomical correction and intra-atrial repair operations for complete transposition of the great arteries. Circulation 1990;82:808.

Marx GR, Allen HD. Accuracy and pitfalls of Doppler evaluation of the pressure gradient in aortic coarctation. J Am Coll Cardiol 1986;7:1379.

Mehta RH, Helmcke F, Nanda NC, et al. Transesophageal Doppler color flow mapping assessment of atrial septal defect. J Am Coll Cardiol 1990;16:1010.

Meissner MD, Panidis LP, Eshaghpour E, et al. Corrected transposition of the great arteries: evaluation by two-dimensional and Doppler echocardiography. Am Heart J 1986;111:599.

Moises VA, Maciel BC, Hornberger LK, et al. A new method for noninvasive estimation of ventricular septal defect shunt flow by Doppler color flow mapping: imaging of the laminar flow convergence region on the left septal surface. J Am Coll Cardiol 1991;18:824.

Mullen MJ, Dias BF, Walker F, et al. Intracardiac echocardiography guided device closure of atrial septal defects. J Am Coll Cardiol 2003;41:285.

Musewe NN, Smallhorn JF, Benson LN, et al. Validation of Doppler-derived pulmonary arterial pressure in patients with ductus arteriosus under different hemodynamic states. Circulation 1987;76:1081.

Nihoyannopoulos P, Karas S, Sapsford RN, et al. Accuracy of two-dimensional echocardiography in the diagnosis of aortic arch obstruction. J Am Coll Cardiol 1987;10:1072.

Nishimura RA, Pieroni DR, Bierman FZ, et al. Second natural history study of congenital heart defects. Aortic stenosis: echocardiography. Circulation 1993;87(Suppl 11):1–66.

Pieroni DR, Nishimura RA, Bierman FZ, et al. Second natural history study of congenital heart defects. Ventricular septal defect: echocardiography. Circulation 1993;87(Suppl 1):1–80.

Quaegebeur JM, Sreeram N, Fraser AG, et al. Surgery for Ebstein's anomaly: the clinical and echocardiographic evaluation of a new technique. J Am Coll Cardiol 1991;17:722.

Qureshi SA, Richheimer R, McKay R, et al. Doppler echocardiographic evaluation of pulmonary artery flow after modified Fontan operation: Importance of atrial contraction. Br Heart J 1990;64:272.

Ramaciotti C, Keren A, Silverman NH. Importance of (perimembranous) ventricular septal aneurysm in the natural history of isolated perimembranous ventricular septal defect. Am J Cardiol 1986;57:268.

Reeder GS, Currie PJ, Hagler DJ, et al. Use of Doppler techniques (continuous-wave, pulsed-wave, and color flow imaging) in the noninvasive hemodynamic assessment of congenital heart disease. Mayo Clin Proc 1986;61:725.

Rhodes JF, Qureshi AM, Preminger TJ, e al. Intracardiac echocardiography during transcatheter interventions for congenital heart disease. Am J Cardiol 2003;92:1482.

Roberson DA, Muhiudeen IA, Silverman NH, et al. Intraoperative transesophageal echocardiography of atrioventricular septal defect. J Am Coll Cardiol 1991;18:537.

Rychik J, Norwood WI, Chin AJ. Doppler color flow mapping assessment of residual shunt after closure of large ventricular septal defects. Circulation 1991;84(Suppl 3):111.

Sanders SP, Parness IA, Colan SD. Recognition of abnormal connections of coronary arteries with the use of Doppler color flow mapping. J Am Coll Cardiol 1989;13:922.

Schmidt KG, Cassidy SC, Silverman NH, et al. Doubly committed subarterial ventricular septal defects: Echocardiographic features and surgical implications. J Am Coll Cardiol 1988;12:1538.

Sharif DS, Huhta JC, Marantz P, et al. Two-dimensional echocardiographic determination of ventricular septal defect size: correlation with autopsy. Am Heart J 1989;117:1333.

Shiina A, Seward JB, Tajik AJ, et al. Two-dimensional echocardiographic surgical correlation in Ebstein's anomaly: preoperative determination of patients requiring tricuspid valve plication vs. replacement. Circulation 1983;68:534.

Shub C, Dimopoulos IN, Seward JB, et al. Sensitivity of two-dimensional echocardiography in the direct visualization of atrial septal defects utilizing the subcostal approach: experience with 154 patients. J Am Coll Cardiol 1983;2:127.

Silverman NH. An ultrasonic approach to the diagnosis of cardiac situs, connections, and malpositions. Cardiol Clin 1983;1:473.

Silverman NH, Golbus MS. Echocardiographic techniques for assessing normal and abnormal fetal cardiac anatomy. J Am Coll Cardiol 1985;5:20.

Simpson IA, Sahn DJ, Valdes-Cruz LM, et al. Color Doppler flow mapping in patients with coarctation of the aorta: new observations and improved evaluation with color flow diameter and proximal acceleration as predictors of severity. Circulation 1988;77:736.

Simpson IA, Valdes-Cruz LM, Yoganathan AP, et al. Spatial velocity distribution and acceleration in serial subvalve tunnel and valvular obstructions: an *in vitro* study using Doppler color flow mapping. J Am Coll Cardiol 1989;13:241.

Smallhorn J, Grow R, Freedom R, et al. Pulsed Doppler echocardiographic assessment of the pulmonary venous pathway after the Mustard or Senning procedure for transposition of the great arteries. Circulation 1986;73:765.

Smallhorn JF. Intraoperative transesophageal echocardiography in congenital heart disease. Echocardiography 2002;8:799.

Smallhorn JF, Burrows P, Wilson G, et al. Two-dimensional and pulsed Doppler echocardiography in the postoperative evaluation of total anomalous pulmonary venous connection. Circulation 1987;76:298.

Sreeram N, Kaulitz R, Stumper OFW, et al. Comparative roles of intraoperative epicardial and early postoperative transthoracic echocardiography in the assessment of surgical repair of congenital heart defects. J Am Coll Cardiol 1990;16:913.

Sreeram N, Walsh K. Diagnosis of total anomalous pulmonary venous drainage by Doppler color flow imaging. J Am Coll Cardiol 1992;19:1577.

Stamper O, Sutherland GR, Geuskens R, et al. Transesophageal echocardiography in evaluation and management after a Fontan procedure. J Am Coll Cardiol 1991;17:1152.

Valdes-Cruz LM, Horowitz S, Mesel E, et al. A pulsed Doppler echocardiographic method for calculating pulmonary and systemic blood flow in atrial level shunts: validation studies in animals and initial human experience. Circulation 1984;69:80.

Van der Velde ME, Parness LA, Colan SD, et al. Two-dimensional echocardiography in the pre- and postoperative management of totally anomalous pulmonary venous connection. J Am Coll Cardiol 1991;18:1746.

Van Praagh R. Diagnosis of complex congenital heart disease: morphologic-anatomic method and terminology. Cardiovasc Intervent Radiol 1984;7:115.

Van Praagh S, Vangi V, Hee Sul J, et al. Tricuspid atresia or severe stenosis with partial common atrioventricular canal: anatomic data, clinical profile and surgical considerations. J Am Coll Cardiol 1991;17:932.

Van Hare GG, Silverman NH. Contrast two-dimensional echocardiography in congenital heart disease: techniques, indications and clinical utility. J Am Coll Cardiol 1989;13:673.

Vick III GW, Murphy DJ, Ludomirsky A, et al. Pulmonary venous and systemic ventricular inflow obstruction in patients with congenital heart disease: detection by combined two-dimensional and Doppler echocardiography. J Am Coll Cardiol 1987;9:580.

Weintraub R, Shiota T, Elkadi T, et al. Transesophageal echocardiography in infants and children with congenital heart disease. Circulation 1992;86:711.

Wolf WJ, Casta A, Sapire DW. Atrial septal aneurysms in infants and children. Am Heart J 1987;113:1149.

Wren C, Oslizlok P, Bull C. Natural history of supravalvular aortic stenosis and pulmonary artery stenosis. J Am Coll Cardiol 1991;15:1625.

Chapter 19

ICU and Operative/Perioperative Applications

In addition to its widespread use in ambulatory and hospitalized patients with cardiac disease, echocardiography plays a valuable role in the management of patients in medical and surgical intensive care units with shock, hypoxia, and other critical illnesses. The use of transesophageal echocardiography in the operating room and perioperative period has greatly enhanced our understanding of intraoperative hemodynamics. Additionally, echocardiography can be used as a primary or secondary imaging tool during a variety of catheterization-based procedures such as balloon valvotomy, atrial septostomy, percutaneous atrial septal defect closure, and pericardiocentesis. This chapter explores different uses of echocardiographic techniques in the intensive care and operating room arenas.

EVALUATION OF PATIENTS IN AN INTENSIVE CARE UNIT

The use of echocardiography in the coronary care unit is well established and is discussed in Chapter 15. Echocardiography can play a valuable role in management of patients in medical intensive care units with a broad range of problems such as hypoxia, acute febrile illnesses, hypotension, and shock. Surveillance studies have suggested that as many as one-fourth of patients hospitalized in a medical intensive care unit without overt evidence of cardiovascular disease have an underlying cardiovascular abnormality that may mimic a noncardiac condition and/or complicate therapy. Its use is similar in patients in a postsurgical intensive care unit. Table 19.1 outlines a number of the clinical disorders often encountered in an intensive care unit in which echocardiography plays a substantial role in patient management. It should be emphasized that in many instances the role of echocardiography will be to exclude cardiovascular disease as a cause of hemodynamic or other instability and hence allow the clinician to appropriately direct attention to noncardiovascular conditions.

▶ **TABLE 19.1 Use of Echocardiography in the Intensive Care Unit**

Surveillance
  Confirm/exclude occult cardiac disease
  Source of murmur
Hemodynamics
  Hypotension
  Assess volume status
  Left ventricular function
    Regional wall motion abnormality
    Global dysfunction
    Transient dysfunction (sepsis, stunning)
  Right ventricular function
  Outflow tract obstruction
  Valvular stenosis/insufficiency
Hypoxia
  Right ventricular function
  Right ventricular pressure
  Intracardiac shunt
  Pulmonary embolus
Infections
  Bacterial endocarditis

Hypotension and Shock

In dealing with patients with hypotension and shock, one must distinguish among a cardiac etiology resulting in primary reduction in cardiac output, a purely noncardiac entity such as hemorrhage with hypovolemia, and other cardiac entities resulting in hemodynamic instability such as acute valvular insufficiency and identify concurrent cardiac abnormalities that may either complicate diagnosis or therapy. Figures 19.1 through 19.5 were all recorded in patients with hypotension and/or shock in a medical or surgical intensive care unit. Figure 19.1 was recorded in a patient hospitalized with sepsis, hypotension, and malperfusion. The echocardiogram documented severe left ventricular systolic dysfunction that, in this case, was transient and improved after treatment of the gram-

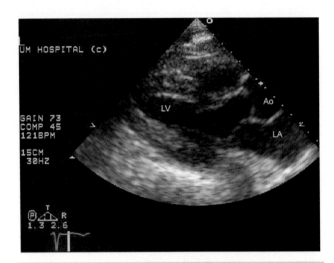

FIGURE 19.1. Parasternal long-axis echocardiogram recorded in a 30-year-old patient with gram-negative sepsis. Note the normal size of the left ventricle (*LV*). This image was recorded at end-systole and depicts significant global hypokinesis, which is more apparent in the real-time image. Left ventricular function normalized after successful treatment of the bacterial infection. Ao, aorta; LA, left atrium; LV, left ventricle.

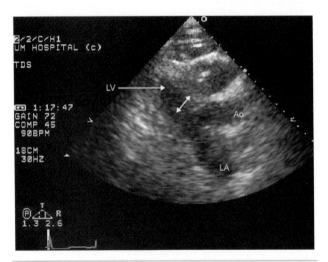

FIGURE 19.2. Parasternal long-axis view recorded in an elderly patient with hypotension and shock who initially presented with pneumonia. Note the very small left ventricular cavity (*double-headed arrow*) with normal systolic function suggesting that hypovolemia is the etiology for hypotension. Ao, aorta; LA, left atrium; LV, left ventricle.

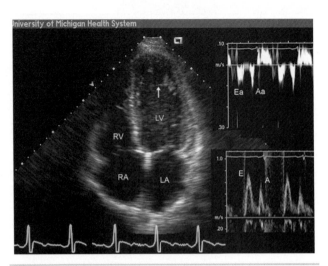

FIGURE 19.3. Apical four-chamber view recorded in a patient with hypotension and shock after an acute febrile illness. Note the global hypokinesis of the left ventricle (*LV*) consistent with an underlying cardiomyopathy. The Doppler pattern (*insets*) is consistent with a pseudonormal pattern (grade 2 diastolic dysfunction). In this instance, there was no recovery of function with treatment of the underlying illness. Incidental note is made of a pseudochord in the left ventricular apex (*arrow*). LA, left atrium; RA, right atrium; RV, right ventricle.

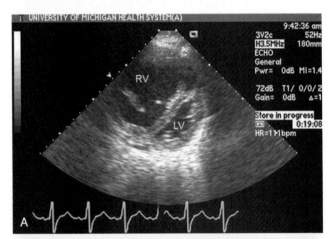

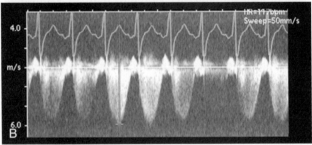

FIGURE 19.4. Parasternal short-axis view recorded in a 37-year-old woman presenting with a febrile illness and hypotension. **A:** Note the massively dilated and hypertrophied right ventricle (*RV*) and the small slit-like left ventricle (*LV*) consistent with a severe right ventricular pressure overload. **B:** The spectral Doppler of tricuspid regurgitation demonstrates a tricuspid regurgitation gradient suggesting systemic right ventricular systolic pressure, which in this case was due to previously unrecognized primary arterial pulmonary hypertension.

negative sepsis. In the other examples, note the broad range of underlying cardiovascular abnormalities that have resulted in similar degrees of hypotension and organ malperfusion.

Because of the critically ill nature of these patients and the fact that many are often on ventilatory support, routine transthoracic echocardiography often results in suboptimal image quality. It is often feasible, however, to evaluate the status of left ventricular function and exclude left ventricular systolic dysfunction as a cause of hy-

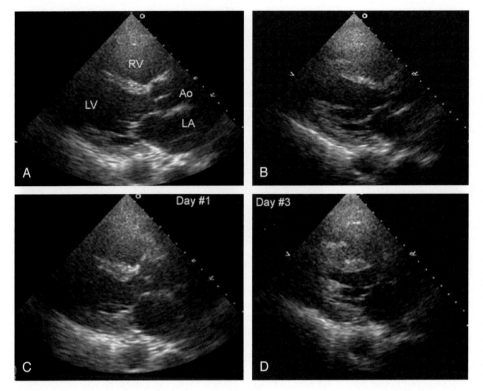

FIGURE 19.5. Serial parasternal long-axis echocardiograms recorded in a 23-year-old patient 4 hours after renal transplantation who developed hypotension and was unable to be weaned from the ventilator. For each pair of images diastole is on that top and systole is on the bottom. **A, C:** Images recorded at the time of clinical deterioration reveal septal akinesis with otherwise global hypokinesis. **B, D:** Images recorded 2 days later demonstrate complete recovery of function. In this instance, the left ventricular dysfunction was due to myocardial stunning of uncertain provocation and was not related to obstructive coronary disease. Ao, aorta; LA, left atrium; LV, left ventricle; RV, right ventricle.

potension even in poor-quality images. Figure 19.2 was recorded in a patient with hypotension and shock. The transthoracic echocardiogram, although of suboptimal quality, clearly reveals a small, underfilled left ventricle with preserved systolic function consistent with hypovolemia with preserved left ventricular systolic function.

The routine use of second harmonic imaging and intravenous contrast for left ventricular opacification is beneficial to enhance visualization of left ventricular function in ventilated patients in an intensive care unit (Fig. 19.6). Although it may be possible to determine the status of left and right ventricular function from transthoracic echocardiography using contrast echocardiography, in many patients to further evaluate valvular anatomy and hemodynamics may require transesophageal echocardiography. Several studies have demonstrated the incremental value of transesophageal echocardiography for elucidating the underlying mechanism of hypotension or hypoxia in pa-

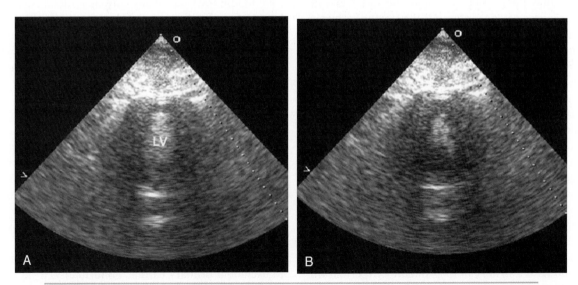

FIGURE 19.6. Parasternal short-axis view recorded in an obese patient in a medical intensive care unit undergoing mechanical ventilation. Note in the diastolic image **(A)** the normal chamber size and left ventricular hypertrophy, and the normal systolic function **(B)**. LV, left ventricle.

tients hospitalized in an intensive care unit with a broad range of underlying disorders.

A not uncommon source of hypotension in critically ill patients, especially in a surgical or trauma intensive care unit, is hemorrhage and hypovolemia. This can be documented on an echocardiogram when a small left ventricular volume and hyperdynamic motion are noted (Fig. 19.2). This is reliable evidence of intravascular volume depletion and has obvious therapeutic implications. On occasion, one encounters a patient with progressive hypotension in whom intravenous pressors have been employed without benefit and with even further deterioration. There is a subset of patients, many of whom have a history of hypertension, who with volume depletion develop a syndrome of acquired dynamic left ventricular outflow tract obstruction. Physiologically, this mimics a true obstructive hypertrophic cardiomyopathy. Dynamic left ventricular outflow tract obstruction and systolic anterior motion of the mitral valve with secondary mitral regurgitation may be seen. The overall hemodynamic result of this syndrome is progressive hypotension with the development of a prominent systolic murmur (due either to outflow tract obstruction, mitral regurgitation, or both). The etiology of the hypotension in this situation is the relatively low stroke volume of the left ventricle due to hypovolemia complicated by outflow tract obstruction. Gradients exceeding 100 mm Hg in the left ventricular outflow tract have been noted due to this phenomenon. In many instances, hemodynamics as assessed with right heart catheterization may be misleading and result in inappropriate decision making. In this instance, right heart catheterization will reveal an elevated pulmonary capillary wedge pressure that is then assumed to reflect left ventricular filling volume. When the syndrome of significant mitral regurgitation with outflow tract obstruction is identified, one then recognizes that the elevated pulmonary capillary wedge pressure is the result of a hyperdynamic but noncompliant left ventricle and mitral regurgitation. Failure to appreciate this phenomenon results in the inappropriate course of increasing pressor support and diuretics, which obviously has the effect of worsening rather than improving the clinical situation. Figure 19.7 was recorded in a patient with this syndrome. Recognition of hypovolemia with dynamic outflow tract obstruction should lead to the appropriate management decision to resuscitate the patient with fluids and withdraw agents aimed at increasing contractility and/or reducing vascular resistance.

More commonly, previously unrecognized diastolic dysfunction results in pulmonary congestion and heart failure in patients hospitalized with medical illnesses or in the postoperative period. These patients typically are elderly and have a history of long-standing hypertension. In the operative or postoperative period, overly aggressive fluid resuscitation may result in congestive heart failure.

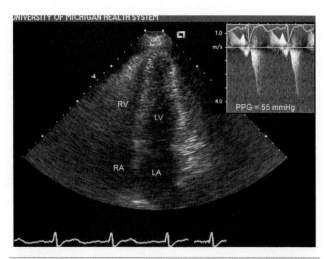

FIGURE 19.7. Apical four-chamber view (end-systolic) recorded in a 60-year-old patient with hypotension and a gastrointestinal bleed. At end-systole, note the small left ventricular cavity with hyperdynamic motion and cavity obliteration at the mid left ventricle. Continuous wave Doppler imaging revealed a mid-cavity gradient of 55 mm Hg. In this instance, the obstruction is related to hypovolemia and a heightened adrenergic state on the background of hypertension and left ventricular hypertrophy rather than to a true hypertrophic cardiomyopathy. LA, left atrium; LV, left ventricle; RA, right atrium; RV, right ventricle.

The echocardiogram will typically reveal normal systolic function and left ventricular hypertrophy (Fig. 19.8). Mitral inflow patterns may be highly variable and show either delayed relaxation or a restrictive filling pattern. Because an intravascular volume overload is present, a pseudonormal pattern is not uncommon.

Occasionally after an intrathoracic procedure or major chest trauma, transthoracic echocardiography results in total failure to visualize any cardiac structures. This may be associated with strong and occasionally dynamic reverberation signals (Fig. 19.9). When this scenario is encountered, one should suspect either substantial amounts of subcutaneous air or a pneumothorax or pneumomediastinum.

Evaluation of Hypoxia

An additional common use of echocardiography in an intensive care unit is evaluation of unexplained hypoxia or inability to wean from ventilatory support. Etiologies of hypoxia that can be documented by echocardiography are also listed in Table 19.1. An acute pulmonary embolus is an obvious cause of hypoxia. This issue is discussed in Chapter 22. A comprehensive echocardiographic examination is useful in patients with hypotension and shock to exclude a primary cardiac abnormality; if no primary cardiac abnormality is identified, including right-to-left shunting, then the etiology of hypoxia can reliably be as-

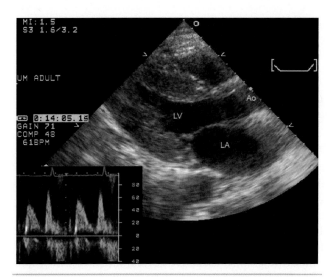

FIGURE 19.8. Parasternal long-axis echocardiogram recorded in a 50-year-old patient with long-standing hypertension admitted to an intensive care unit with ketoacidosis. Note the left ventricular hypertrophy and normal systolic function in this end-systolic image. The accompanying Doppler profile confirms the presence of diastolic dysfunction, which may make this patient susceptible to pulmonary congestion during aggressive volume resuscitation. Ao, aorta; LA, left atrium; LV, left ventricle.

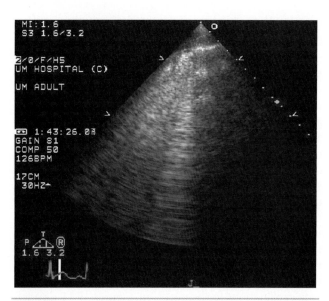

FIGURE 19.9. Attempt to obtain a parasternal long-axis echocardiogram in a patient after a motor vehicle accident. Identical images were obtained from multiple transthoracic transducer positions and reveal only ultrasound "noise." In the real-time image, notice the oscillating nature of the echoes in the near field. These images are consistent with subcutaneous air secondary to chest trauma.

sumed to be noncardiac and appropriate diagnostic and therapeutic efforts are then directed to pulmonary or other causes. A cause of hypoxia in the intensive care unit that is uniquely evaluated by echocardiography is the opening of a patent foramen ovale with subsequent right-to-left shunting and arterial desaturation (Fig. 19.10). This generally requires not only the presence of a patent foramen ovale but also a concurrent process that elevates right heart pressure such as pulmonary hypertension, acute pulmonary embolus, or right ventricular dysfunction. Additionally, reactive pulmonary hypertension of any etiology, including that provoked by bronchospasm, can result in elevation of right heart pressure to a point that a patent foramen becomes a source for significant right-to-left shunting.

An additional source of right-to-left shunting is a pulmonary arteriovenous malformation (AVM). AVMs are seen in chronic liver disease as well as in Osler-Weber-Rendu syndrome. Most AVMs result in clinically inconsequential degrees of shunting and rarely result in clinically relevant, or even detectable, hypoxia. On occasion, large or multiple AVMs may result in substantial right-to-left shunting with clinically relevant hypoxia. Separation of an AVM from atrial level communication is discussed in Chapter 4 and relies on timing of contrast appearance in the left heart, which is delayed when an AVM is present. The basis for this echocardiographic finding is that before its appearance in the left heart, contrast must pass through the entire pulmonary vascular circuit. This typi-

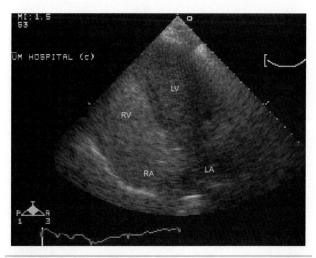

FIGURE 19.10. Apical four-chamber view recorded in a patient with obstructive lung disease and significant hypoxia. Note on this contrast echocardiogram the significant opacification of the left ventricular cavity after an intravenous injection of agitated saline. This is indicative of a significant right-to-left shunt due to opening of a patent foramen ovale. LA, left atrium; LV, left ventricle; RA, right atrium; RV, right ventricle.

cally takes three to six cardiac cycles depending on cardiac output. The pulmonary circuit then acts as a reservoir of contrast that continues to flow into the left side of the heart even after the initial intravenous bolus has begun clearing from the right heart.

Echocardiography in the Emergency Department

For patients presenting to the emergency department with hypotension, shock, or major trauma (especially thoracic), many of the same considerations noted above regarding use of echocardiography in the intensive care unit apply. Obviously for patients with major trauma, hemorrhagic shock is a consideration. Echocardiography can quickly document a small, underfilled ventricle in that syndrome. Additionally, in patients with major blunt chest trauma, such as after a high-speed motor vehicle accident, echocardiography can be instrumental in documenting cardiac involvement including myocardial contusion or pericardial effusion. Additionally, by confirming the absence of significant cardiac involvement, echocardiography allows the clinician to redirect efforts to alternate explanations for hypotension. Figures 19.11 through 19.13 were recorded in patients presenting to an emer-

gency department after various forms of trauma in which echocardiography played a crucial role in rapidly establishing the diagnosis.

PRE-, INTRA-, AND PERIOPERATIVE ECHOCARDIOGRAPHY

The use of echocardiography in conjunction with cardiac and noncardiac surgical procedures can be divided into use before surgery, in the operating room, which typically is confined to transesophageal or epicardial echocardiography, and in the perioperative period (Table 19.2). Although the most common echocardiographic modality to use in the operating room is transesophageal echocardiography, there are several situations in which transthoracic or other probes designed for epicardial

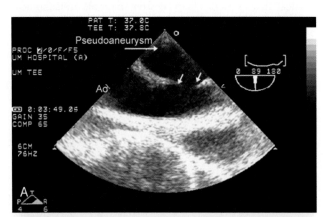

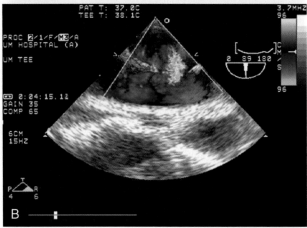

FIGURE 19.11. Transesophageal echocardiogram performed on an emergent basis in a young patient with hypotension, shock, and a left plural effusion after a high-speed motor vehicle accident. **A:** The transesophageal echocardiogram identifies a break in the contour of the aorta (*arrows*) with color flow **B:** demonstrating communication between the lumen of the aorta and the extraaortic space consistent with aortic rupture and pseudoaneurysm. Ao, aorta.

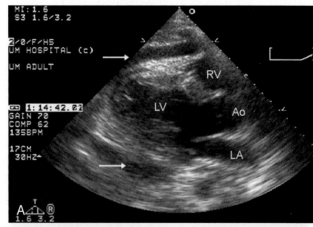

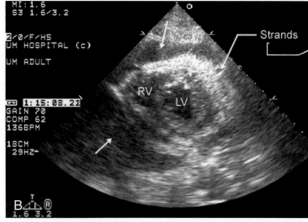

FIGURE 19.12. Parasternal long-axis echocardiogram recorded in a young patient after a gunshot wound to the chest with hypotension and shock. Note in both the parasternal long-axis **(A)** and short-axis **(B)** views that there is a "cloudy" pericardial effusion (*arrows*) consistent with acute hemorrhage into the pericardium. In the real-time image, also note the area of apical akinesis consistent with direct myocardial or coronary arterial injury. Ao, aorta; LA, left atrium; LV, left ventricle; RV, right ventricle.

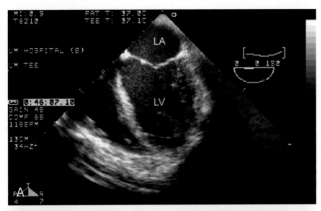

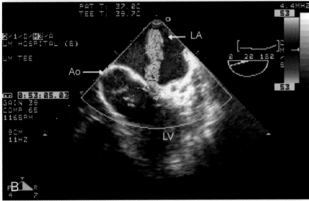

FIGURE 19.13. Transesophageal echocardiogram recorded in a young patient with a stab wound to the chest with hypotension, shock, and a loud murmur. **A:** In the longitudinal view, note the severe global hypokinesis of both the left and right ventricles, the etiology of which is presumed to be coronary injury. **B:** Note the abnormal communication between the left ventricular cavity and left atrium (*LA*) consistent with a direct penetrating injury in that area. Ao, aorta; LV, left ventricle.

scanning in the open chest, typically covered with a sterile sheath, are used for direct application to the heart or vascular structures.

The most common intraoperative application of transesophageal echocardiography is in the monitoring of valvular, congenital, or other complex cardiovascular surgical procedures. This includes mitral valve repair and aortic valve repair and implantation of newer bioprostheses as well as some aortic aneurysm repair. Intraoperative transesophageal echocardiography has become the standard of care for confirming the success of mitral valve repair and is also used to assess the success of valve replacement with respect to residual gradients and paravalvular regurgitation. Preoperative echocardiography can be instrumental in assessing the feasibility and likelihood of success of virtually all forms of valve surgery. There are several entities noted on echocardiography that have a direct bearing on the nature of the surgery to be undertaken. When considering a patient for aortic valve

▶ **TABLE 19.2 Echocardiography in the Operating Room**

Preoperative
Assess need for valvular surgery
Left ventricular function
Pulmonary artery pressure
Predict complications
Aortic atheroma
Aortic valve procedures
Anular size
Left ventricular outflow tract size
Aortic dilation/aneurysm
Mitral valve procedures
Anular calcification
Mechanism of regurgitation
Feasibility of repair
Intraoperative
Monitor LV and RV function for noncardiac procedures
Placement of cannulas, occlusive devices
Postoperative
Success of valve repair/replacement
Detect complications (see Table 19.3)

LV, left ventricle; RV, right ventricle.

replacement, the size of the left ventricular outflow tract and the degree, if any, of subvalvular septal hypertrophy have a direct bearing on the surgical technique with respect to the need for an outflow tract widening procedure or concurrent myectomy, each of which will increase the complexity and risk of aortic valve replacement. As part of the assessment of a patient for aortic valve replacement, it is essential to evaluate the proximal ascending aorta for significant dilation and the need for an aortic root procedure as well as an aortic valve replacement. There are several features of mitral valve disease that also have a direct bearing on the likelihood of success and risk of surgical mitral valve replacement. Patients who have a heavily calcified mitral anulus have an increased surgical risk due to the possibility of separation of the left ventricular myocardium from the anulus at the time of manipulating the heart and may also require debulking of the heavy calcific deposits. Finally, implanting a sewing ring into a calcified anulus results in a greater than unusual likelihood of paravalvular mitral regurgitation, which may have long-term consequences with respect to the overall success of the surgical procedure.

Transesophageal echocardiography plays several roles with respect to valve surgery. The first is its preoperative role in assessing the feasibility and nature of the repair or replacement to be performed. Selection of patients for surgical repair of a mitral valve is also discussed in Chapter 11. Determination of the feasibility of mitral valve repair relies heavily on the preoperative transesophageal echocardiogram. In general, posterior leaflet pathology is more easily repaired than anterior, and in general any disease process that scars or foreshortens the mitral valve apparatus results in anatomy less likely to be successfully repaired than diseases associated with excess or redundant tissue.

Role of Echocardiography in Mitral Valve Surgery

When performing transesophageal echocardiography for the purpose of assessing mitral valve anatomy before intended mitral valve repair, it is important that a thorough and detailed evaluation of the mitral valve be undertaken in a systematic fashion. The primary purpose of the examination is to determine the underlying anatomic abnormality responsible for the regurgitation or stenosis. It is important to recognize that there are three different viewing perspectives on mitral valve anatomy (Fig. 19.14). The surgeon will be viewing the mitral valve from within the left atrium so that the anterolateral commissures will be to the left of the field of view and the medial commissures to the right. When viewed with either transesophageal or transthoracic echocardiography, this orientation will be reversed (assuming traditional recom-

mended viewing formats on a video screen). Also, depending on whether the reference is a transthoracic or transesophageal echocardiogram, the anterior and posterior leaflets of the mitral valve will vary in position compared with the surgical perspective. Figure 19.14 depicts all three perspectives of the mitral valve in relation to the aorta and left atrial appendage.

There are multiple imaging planes available from transesophageal echocardiography, each of which will interrogate a different aspect of mitral valve anatomy. Figure 19.15 depicts the location of each of the scallops of the anterior and posterior mitral valve leaflets as they relate to different transesophageal imaging planes. Even with substantial experience, it is occasionally difficult to identify the precise site of pathology and much experience

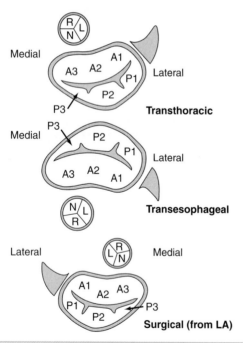

FIGURE 19.14. Schematic representation of the mitral valve from multiple perspectives. **Bottom:** The mitral valve from the surgical perspective, from inside the left atrium. **Top:** The mitral valve as viewed from a traditional transthoracic parasternal short-axis view. **Middle:** The mitral valve is seen from a transesophageal approach at the mid-gastric level. In each instance, the proximal aorta is as noted in the schematic, as is the left atrial appendage. The three distinct scallops of the anterior (A1, A2, A3) and posterior (P1, P2, P3) leaflets are also schematized. L, left coronary sinuses; N, non-coronary sinuses; R, right coronary sinuses.

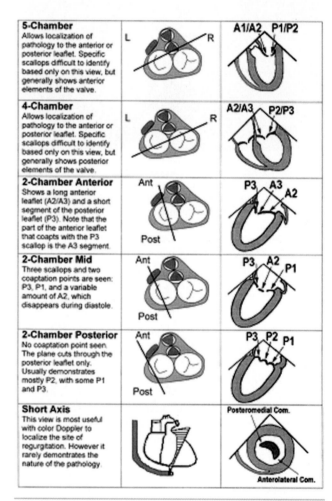

FIGURE 19.15. Summary figure of multiple transesophageal echocardiographic views for visualizing the mitral valve in relation to preoperative planning. A1, A2, A3, anterior scallops; Ant, anterior; P1, Com., commissure; P2, P3, posterior scallops; Post, posterior. (From Lambert AS, Miller JP, Merrick SH, et al. Improved evaluation of the location and mechanism of mitral valve regurgitation with a systematic transesophageal echocardiography examination. Anesth Analg 1999;88:1205–1212, with permission.)

is necessary before being able to render consistently accurate interpretations of mitral valve pathology with respect to the precise anatomy responsible for a regurgitant lesion.

Figures 19.16 through 19.28 were recorded in patients with moderate and severe mitral regurgitation in whom mitral valve repair was undertaken. Figures 19.16 through 19.18A were recorded in a patient with dilated cardiomyopathy and mitral regurgitation. The mitral valve is anatomically normal; however, there is failure of coaptation, resulting in severe mitral regurgitation. In this instance, the mechanism of regurgitation can be seen to be apical displacement of the papillary muscles in the dilated and spherical left ventricle. Note the central location of the mitral regurgitation jet that arises at the area of noncoaptation of the mitral leaflets (Fig. 19.17). This type of mitral regurgitation can be addressed by placement of an anular ring, which corrects the abnormal coaptation of the mitral valve. In a similar fashion, Figure 19.19 was recorded in a patient with a previous inferior myocardial infarction and significant mitral regurgitation due to malcoaptation, predominantly due to restricted motion of the posterior mitral valve leaflet. In this instance, there has been scarring of the posterior papillary muscle that functionally foreshortens the anatomically normal posterior leaflet and re-

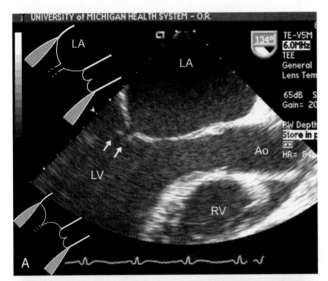

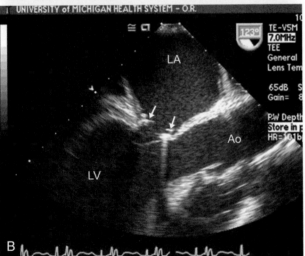

FIGURE 19.16. Pre- and postoperative transesophageal echocardiograms recorded in a patient with left ventricular dysfunction and mitral regurgitation due to failure of mitral valve coaptation. Longitudinal views recorded at end-systole are presented. **A:** Pre-repair, note the apical displacement of the mitral valve tips and the failure to coapt (*arrows*) in this systolic frame. The schematic in the upper left of **A** depicts the effect of apical and lateral tethering of the papillary muscles with incomplete valve coaptation. Normal coaptation is depicted in the lower schematic. **B:** Recorded after successful repair by placement of an anular ring (*arrows*). Ao, aorta; LA, left atrium; LV, left ventricle; RV, right ventricle.

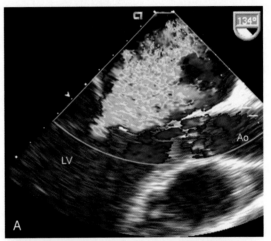

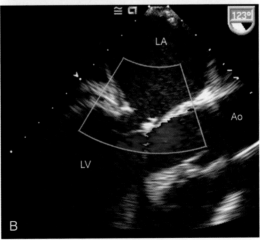

FIGURE 19.17. Color Doppler flow images corresponding to the images presented in Figure 19.16 are shown. **A:** Note the severe mitral regurgitation arising centrally with the *vena contracta* location identified by the area of noncoaptation in Figure 19.16A. **B:** A systolic frame recorded after placement of a mitral ring. Note the absence of mitral regurgitation after ring placement. Ao, aorta; LA, left atrium; LV, left ventricle.

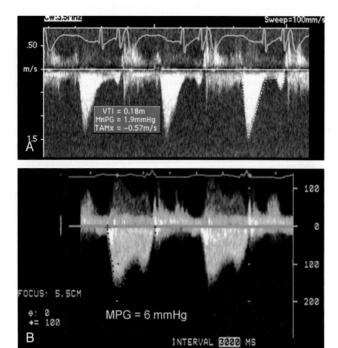

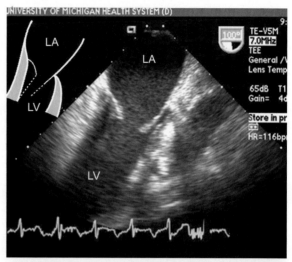

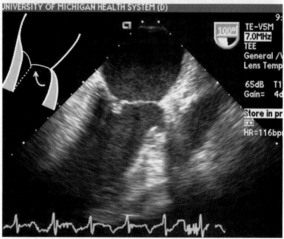

FIGURE 19.18. A: Continuous wave Doppler recording through the mitral orifice after placement of a mitral ring demonstrates a mean pressure gradient of 1.9 mm Hg after repair (same patient presented in Figure 19.16). **B:** Recorded in a patient with a less ideal repair and a residual gradient of 6 mm Hg.

FIGURE 19.19. Transesophageal echocardiogram recorded in diastole **(top)** and systole **(bottom)** a patient with an inferior myocardial infarction and tethered motion of the posterior mitral valve leaflet, leading to significant mitral regurgitation. The leaflet motion is schematized for each image as well. In this instance, surgical remodeling of the mitral anulus will result in normal coaptation of the mitral valve and resolution of mitral regurgitation. Note in the real-time image the absence of motion of the posterior leaflet. LA, left atrium; LV, left ventricle.

sults in malcoaptation. This type of mitral regurgitation is likewise correctable with a mitral anular ring. Contrast this to the patients illustrated in Figures 19.20–19.22 where there is a flail leaflet of the mitral valve. In this instance, regurgitation is due to anatomic disruption of the mitral valve and the repair will necessitate resection of the flail scallop with reapposition of the intact margins.

In addition to evaluating the feasibility of repair in native valve disease, transesophageal echocardiography can also assist in determining the feasibility of a re-repair in patients who have previously undergone a mitral valve procedure. If failure of the repair is due to problems with structural integrity of the mitral valve tissue, it is unlikely a repeat repair will provide a durable benefit. Conversely, if it is due to a technical problem with a mitral valve ring, a repeat surgical procedure may be beneficial. Figures 19.23 and 19.24 were recorded in a patient who had previously undergone a successful mitral valve repair for a flail posterior leaflet and had an excellent symptomatic response. Three months postoperatively, he developed recurrent symptoms and was noted to have mitral regurgitation on physical examination. Note from the baseline images (Figs. 19.23A and 19.24A) that the anular ring is no longer attached to the mitral anulus. This allowed apical and lateral displacement of the papillary muscles to interfere with normal mitral coaptation and resulted in significant functional mitral regurgitation, as can be seen

in Figure 19.24A. In this instance, the mitral anular ring was resuspended, recreating normal coaptation of the mitral valve (Fig. 19.23B) and completely eliminating mitral regurgitation.

Typically, transesophageal echocardiography suffices for complete evaluation of mitral valve anatomy including determination of the portion of the mitral leaflet that is flail. Additionally, three-dimensional reconstruction can be used to enhance the assessment of mitral anatomy and the precise determination of the location of a flail leaflet. Figure 19.25 is a three-dimensional reconstruction from a transesophageal echocardiogram of a patient with a flail posterior leaflet, in which the precise

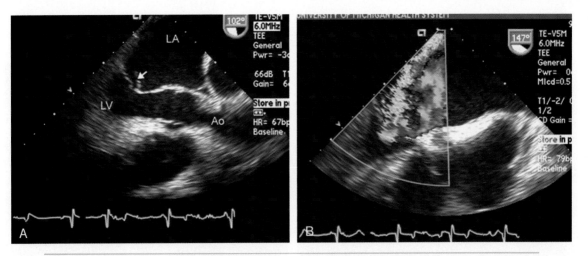

FIGURE 19.20. Transesophageal echocardiogram recorded in a longitudinal view of a flail anterior mitral valve leaflet. **A:** Note the chordal attachments in the left atrium (*LA*) (*arrow*) in systole. **B:** Note the more posteriorly directed eccentric mitral regurgitation jet consistent with a partial flail of the anterior mitral valve leaflet. Ao, aorta; LV, left ventricle.

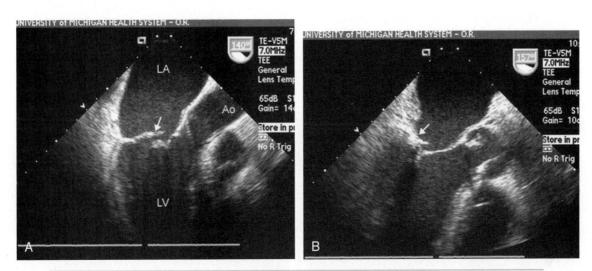

FIGURE 19.21. Intraoperative transesophageal echocardiogram recorded in a patient with a flail posterior leaflet (P2). Recorded before **(A)** and after **(B)** surgical repair. **A:** Note the portion of the posterior leaflet behind the anterior leaflet in systole (*arrow*). **B:** A mitral ring has been placed (*arrow*), and the flail portion of the posterior leaflet has been resected. LA, left atrium; LV, left ventricle.

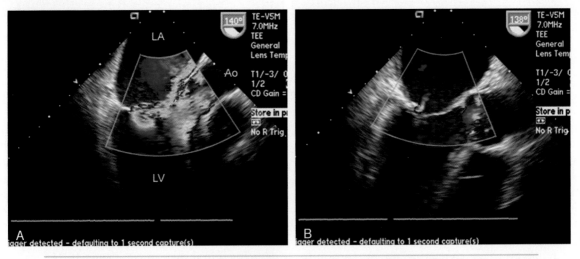

FIGURE 19.22. Intraoperative transesophageal echocardiogram with color flow Doppler imaging recorded in the same patient presented in Figure 19.21. **A:** Recorded before repair and demonstrates a highly eccentric anteriorly directed mitral regurgitation jet. **B:** Recorded after repair and reveals only trivial residual mitral regurgitation. LA, left atrium; LV, left ventricle.

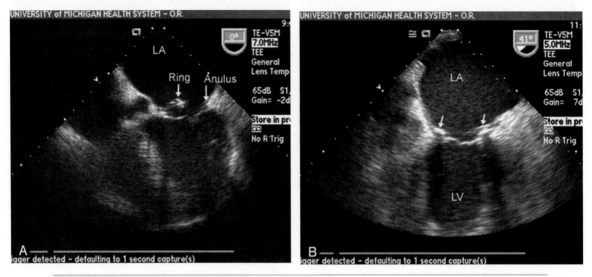

FIGURE 19.23. Transesophageal echocardiogram recorded in the horizontal plane in a patient who had previously undergone mitral repair with an anular ring. **A:** Note the separation between the anulus and the ring consistent with ring dehiscence. This has resulted in severe functional mitral regurgitation as can be seen in Figure 19.24. **B:** Recorded after re-repair and demonstrates that the ring is now reattached to the anulus with improved leaflet coaptation. LA, left atrium; LV, left ventricle.

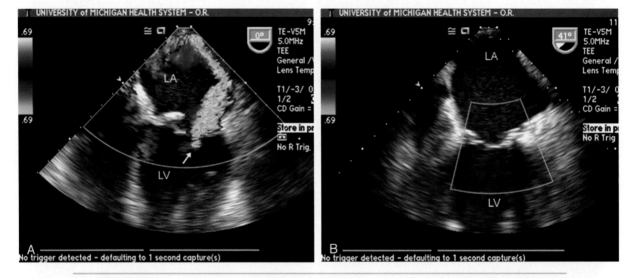

FIGURE 19.24. Intraoperative transesophageal echocardiogram recorded in the same patient depicted in Figure 19.23. **A:** Recorded before repeat repair and demonstrates severe mitral regurgitation due to apical displacement of the mitral valve. Note the location of the convergence zone well into the left ventricular cavity (*arrow*). **B:** Recorded after repair and confirms the absence of residual mitral regurgitation. LA, left atrium; LV, left ventricle.

location and overall extent of disrupted tissue are far better appreciated than on two-dimensional echocardiography.

It should be emphasized that the intracardiac hemodynamics in an anesthetized and ventilated open chest patient are radically different than hemodynamics in the awake or mildly sedated patient. For this reason, there can be marked differences in the apparent severity of mitral regurgitation when comparing an intraoperative transesophageal echocardiogram with one performed on an ambulatory patient. In general, diseases resulting in functional mitral regurgitation will tend to have a reduction in the severity of mitral regurgitation when comparing the intraoperative with the preoperative studies. There is far less reduction in the apparent severity of mitral regurgitation for patients with anatomic disruption of a valve leaflet. Figure 19.26 was recorded in a patient undergoing mitral valve repair. Figure 19.26A was recorded

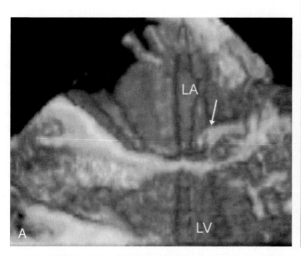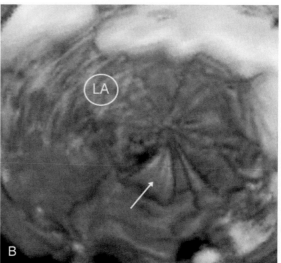

FIGURE 19.25. Three-dimensional reconstruction from a transesophageal echocardiogram in a patient with a flail posterior mitral valve leaflet. **A:** A horizontal view demonstrates the flail portion of the posterior leaflet. **B:** A surgical perspective from within the left atrium (*LA*) is shown and demonstrates the flail leaflet prolapsing into the cavity of the left atrium (*arrow*). LV left ventricle.

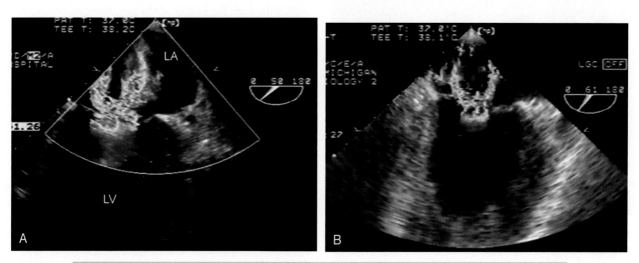

FIGURE 19.26. Transesophageal echocardiogram recorded under conscious sedation in an outpatient (**A**) and in the operating room with general anesthesia and mechanical ventilation (**B**). Blood pressure and heart rate were virtually identical during both echocardiograms. Note the substantially greater size of the mitral regurgitation jet in the outpatient ambulatory transesophageal echocardiogram compared with that seen in the operating room. LA, left atrium; LV, left ventricle.

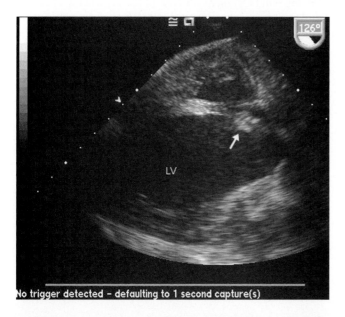

FIGURE 19.27. Intraoperative transesophageal echocardiogram recorded in a patient after complex mitral valve repair including an anular ring and chordal transposition. In this longitudinal view from a low esophageal position, note the prominent chordae and the area of thickening (*arrow*) on the anterior mitral valve leaflet, which is the site of surgical transplantation of chordae. LV, left ventricle.

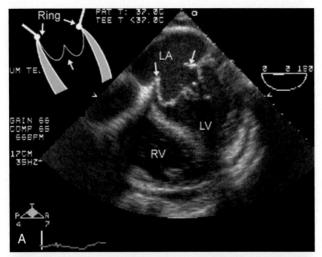

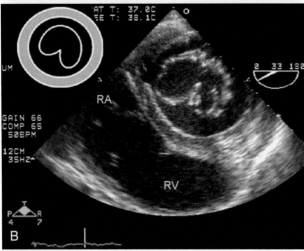

FIGURE 19.28. **A:** Horizontal plane. Intraoperative transesophageal echocardiogram recorded in a patient after a mitral valve repair that included an anular ring (*arrows*) **(A)** and an Alfieri stitch. This image was recorded in end-diastole. Note the unusual opening appearance of the mitral valve in which the motion of the tips is limited by the stitch, resulting in the belly of the leaflet protruding further into the left ventricular cavity than the tips in this instance (see schematic). **B:** Lower esophageal short-axis view of the open mitral valve demonstrates the restricted motion at the midportion due to the presence of the stitch, resulting in a nearly figure 8 appearance to the opening. LA, left atrium; LV, left ventricle; RA, right atrium; RV, right ventricle.

provide intact chordae to the previously flail leaflet (Fig. 19.27). Finally, prosthetic chords can be attached to a flail mitral leaflet and subsequently to a papillary muscle to replace chordal structures that are damaged beyond repair. The goal of mitral valve repair is to reduce the severity of mitral regurgitation to no more than mild without creating iatrogenic mitral stenosis. In the examples presented, note the smaller anular dimensions due to an anular ring as well as the areas of thickening on the mitral valve that represent areas of resection. The most common repair is resection of the redundant portion of a flail posterior leaflet with reapproximation of the intact edges. A mitral anular ring is then placed. This has the effect of converting the mitral valve from a two-leaflet structure to essentially a unileaflet valve with an anterior leaflet providing the mobile valvular structure.

An additional method for repair of mitral valve regurgitation is to place an anular ring in conjunction with a stitch through the center of the anterior and posterior mitral valve leaflets to further restrict mobility (Alfieri stitch). This results in limitation of motion of the mitral valve in diastole and more of a figure 8 opening pattern in the short-axis view (Fig. 19.28).

After surgical repair, it is important to determine the severity of any residual mitral regurgitation or iatrogenic stenosis. Although many investigators stress the importance of making this determination at normal systolic blood pressures, it should be emphasized that systolic blood pressure is not the only hemodynamic factor that alters the apparent severity of mitral regurgitation. Although restitution of normal blood pressure does not guarantee accuracy of the assessment of regurgitation that may be present subsequently, it should be emphasized that the assessment of regurgitation should not be undertaken in patients who are overtly hypotensive or incompletely volume resuscitated at the time of evaluation.

Assessment of iatrogenic mitral stenosis is undertaken using pulsed and continuous wave Doppler tracings. Typically after mitral valve repair, a mean gradient of 2 to 4 mm Hg will be present because of the narrowing effects of anular ring and the essential reduction in the total length and volume of mitral valve tissue (Fig. 19.18). Transmitral gradients exceeding 5 or 6 mm Hg should be viewed as a possible indicator of iatrogenic stenosis (Fig. 19.18B). It should be emphasized that intraoperative hemodynamics may be misleading, especially if the patient is on inotropic support or significantly tachycardiac.

There are several complications of mitral valve repair. In patients with redundant mitral valve tissue and a normally contracting or hyperdynamic left ventricle, placement of the mitral ring along with reduction in left ventricular volume allows systolic anterior motion of the residual mitral valve tissue into the left ventricular outflow tract (Fig. 19.29). Mild degrees of systolic anterior motion are not uncommon, especially in patients receiv-

in a lightly sedated patient preoperatively and reveals severe mitral regurgitation. The lower panel was recorded in the same patient during an intraoperative study and reveals substantially less mitral regurgitation. Of note, blood pressure and heart rate were equivalent at the time of the two examinations.

Mitral valve repair typically involves placement of an anular ring (Figs. 19.16, 19.21, and 19.23) with or without concurrent repair of mitral leaflet tissue itself. More complex repairs may include transposition of a portion of a leaflet and its attached chordae to the opposite leaflet to

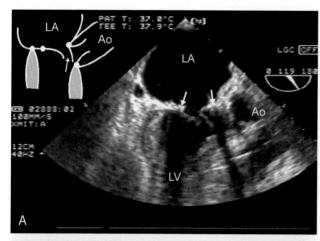

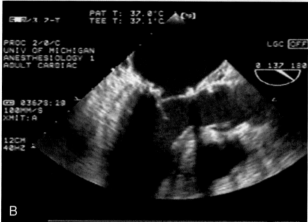

FIGURE 19.29. Intraoperative transesophageal echocardiogram recorded in a patient after mitral valve repair who developed systolic anterior motion of the anterior mitral valve associated with dynamic left ventricular outflow tract obstruction and mitral regurgitation (Fig. 19.30). **A:** Note at the time of maximal systolic motion of the leaflet into the outflow tract that there is separation of the mitral leaflets (*arrows*), creating a regurgitant orifice (see schematic). **B:** Image recorded after volume resuscitation and withdrawal of inotropic agents shows a larger left ventricular cavity and a marked reduction in the systolic anterior motion of the mitral valve. Ao, aorta; LA, left atrium; LV, left ventricle.

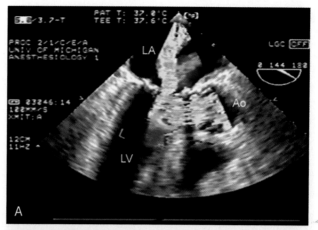

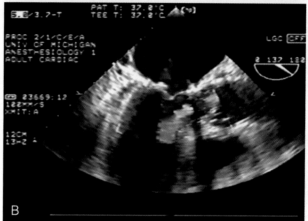

FIGURE 19.30. Transesophageal echocardiogram with color flow Doppler imaging recorded in the same patient presented in Figure 19.29. **A:** Color flow Doppler image corresponding to that in Figure 19.29A. Note the marked turbulence in the left ventricular outflow tract and the mitral regurgitation that arises through the regurgitant channel noted in the schematic in Figure 19.29. **B:** Image corresponds to that in Figure 19.29B and reveals substantially less turbulence in the left ventricular outflow tract and almost complete resolution of mitral regurgitation after volume replenishment and withdrawal of inotropic agents. Ao, aorta; LA, left atrium; LV, left ventricle.

ing inotropic therapy. If there is evidence of significant mitral regurgitation or outflow tract obstruction, further evaluation is usually necessary. This syndrome can result in significant dynamic outflow obstruction, mimicking hypertrophic cardiomyopathy. Mitral regurgitation may be induced as part of this syndrome as well (Fig. 19.30). If outflow obstruction is significant and does not respond to volume resuscitation and reduction in inotropic therapy, modification of the surgical repair or placement of a prosthetic valve may be necessary.

Although intraoperative transesophageal echocardiography is employed in most patients undergoing mitral valve repair, it is less often used in patients undergoing replacement with a prosthetic valve. For patients who are undergoing repeat mitral valve replacement, for those in whom the initial indication for valve replacement is paravalvular regurgitation or endocarditis, or in patients with a heavily calcified mitral anulus, intraoperative transesophageal echocardiography is often used to confirm the successful "seating" of the valve ring within the anulus and to confirm that there is no paravalvular mitral regurgitation (Fig. 19.31).

Aortic Valve Procedures

Transesophageal echocardiography plays less of a role in aortic valve procedures than it does in mitral valve procedures. There are several instances in which it provides in-

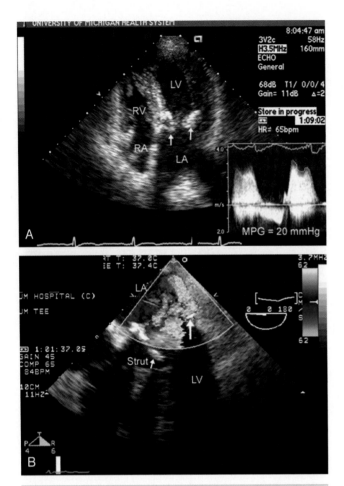

FIGURE 19.31. Pre- and postoperative echocardiograms recorded in a patient with left ventricular hypertrophy and heavy anular calcification resulting in severe functional mitral stenosis. **A:** Preoperative apical four-chamber view reveals left ventricular hypertrophy and marked calcification of the mitral anulus (*arrows*). Note the significant transmitral gradient with a mean pressure gradient of 20 mm Hg (*inset*). **B:** A transesophageal echocardiogram revealing moderate to severe paravalvular mitral regurgitation (*arrow*) due to lack of complete "seating" of the prosthetic valve ring in the calcified mitral anulus. LA, left atrium; LV, left ventricle; RA, right atrium; RV, right ventricle.

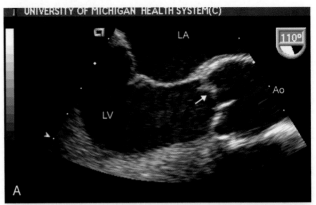

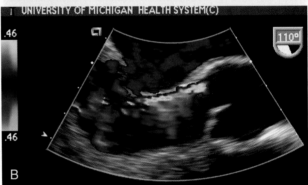

FIGURE 19.32. Transesophageal echocardiogram recorded in a longitudinal view in a patient with a small aortic valve perforation due to endocarditis (healed at the time of this echocardiogram). Note the area of focal thickening on the noncoronary cusp **(A)** and the aortic regurgitation jet arising from a perforation in the area of the healed vegetation **(B)**. Limited cusp disruption such as that depicted here constitutes favorable anatomy for aortic valve repair. Ao, aorta; LA, left atrium; LV, left ventricle.

cremental clinical information, including determination of the feasibility and evaluation of the success of aortic valve repair and in sizing the aortic anulus and proximal aorta for placement of some of the newer bioprostheses.

The aortic valve is less amenable to repair than is the mitral valve. Aortic valve repair has been attempted for at least three decades and has met with variable success. Typically, a repairable aortic valve will have regurgitation due to a limited perforation or prolapse of one cusp edge. If a perforation is present, a small pericardial or other biologic patch can be placed successfully in many instances. If there is malcoaptation due to prolapse of an edge, this can often be surgically approached by resecting a small wedge of tissue and then placing buttressing sutures in the proximal commissures to effectively shorten the coaptation line. Patients with other forms of regurgitation such as that due to marked valve destruction secondary to endocarditis, aortic insufficiency coexisting with aortic stenosis, or advanced fibrosis of a bicuspid leaflet typically are not candidates for repair. Figures 19.32 and 19.33 were recorded in patients with aortic insufficiency for whom aortic root or aortic valve repair was performed. Notice in Figure 19.32 that there is an isolated perforation that is amenable to repair, and in Figure 19.33, an unremarkable three-leaflet valve is present with a central aortic insufficiency jet due to malcoaptation. In this setting, replacement of the aortic root with restitution of normal sinotubular geometry allowed normal aortic cusp coaptation and resolution of aortic regurgitation.

An additional area in which feasibility of repair can be determined with transesophageal echocardiography is aortic insufficiency associated with type I aortic dissection. In the presence of aortic dissection, there are multiple etiologies for aortic insufficiency (Fig. 19.34). Aortic

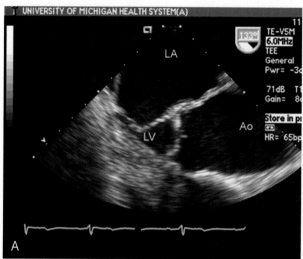

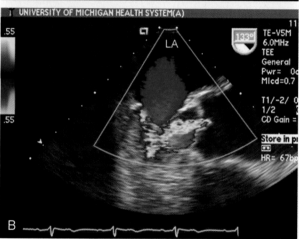

FIGURE 19.33. Transthoracic echocardiogram recorded in a patient with dilation of the ascending aorta and aortic regurgitation secondary to effacement of the sinotubular junction. Note the progressive dilation of the aorta from the anulus to the ascending aorta **(A)** and the area of central aortic regurgitation **(B)**. This type of aortic regurgitation is correctable by graft replacement of the ascending aorta, which narrows the sinotubular junction and results in competence of the aortic valve. Ao, aorta; LA, left atrium; LV, left ventricle.

insufficiency due to dilation of the sinotubular junction often can be corrected with a valve-sparing procedure as can aortic insufficiency due to disruption of the base of the aortic cusp secondary to dissection propagating toward the anulus. Figures 19.35 through 19.37 were recorded in patients in whom a valve-sparing procedure could be performed at the time of aortic dissection repair.

A final area in which transesophageal echocardiography is used for intraoperative decision making is in the evaluation of patients for placement of newer bioprostheses, including cryopreserved homografts and new stentless porcine prostheses. The human homograft includes the donor anulus, aortic cusps, and ascending aorta and must be sized to the recipient heart. Because homograft

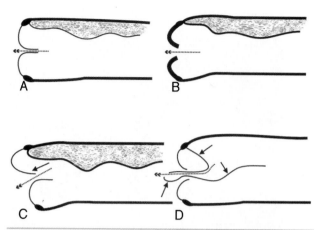

FIGURE 19.34. Multiple mechanisms can be responsible for aortic insufficiency in aortic dissection including effacement or dilation of the sinotubular junction resulting in malcoaptation of the aortic valve **(A)**, aortic dissection in the presence of intrinsic aortic valve disease **(B)**, disruption of the insertion of an aortic cusp **(C)**, and prolapse of the intimal dissection flap through the aortic valve, which serves as a conduit for aortic regurgitation **(D)**.

valves are in short supply and once thawed cannot be refrozen, it is imperative to ensure a good match between the available homograft valve and the patient under consideration. This is typically done with the preoperative transesophageal echocardiogram.

After implantation, it is imperative that the echocardiographer appreciates the full range of appearance of these valves. Depending on the implantation technique, the valve may be nearly indistinguishable from a normal native valve or there may be substantial areas of excess fluid and tissue accumulation when the valve is implanted with an inclusion technique. In this technique, the bioprosthesis is implanted within the donor aorta, resulting in a double-density wall to the aorta either circumferentially or more commonly localized to the noncoronary cusp area. Figure 19.38 was recorded in a patient after implantation of a stentless porcine prosthesis using an inclusion technique. Notice the double density of the aortic wall in the noncoronary cusp area and the soft tissue and fluid collection between the donor and recipient aortic walls, mimicking an aortic abscess. There is a broad range of appearance immediately after surgery. Typically, 3 to 6 weeks after this type of implantation, the free space between the bioprosthesis and the recipient aorta has been obliterated and the appearance of the wall is markedly changed (Fig. 19.38B). In the long term, these valves may be nearly indistinguishable from a native aortic valve.

A rare complication after aortic valve replacement for severe aortic stenosis is the development of dynamic outflow tract obstruction. This complication is easily detected with intraoperative transesophageal echocardiography. There is a subset of patients, typically female and

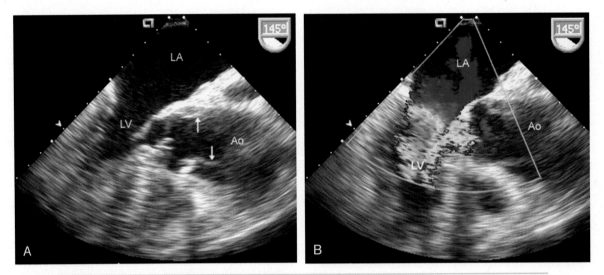

FIGURE 19.35. Transesophageal echocardiogram recorded in a patient with an acute type A dissection. Note the dissection flap in the proximal aorta (*arrows*), the mobility of which is apparent in the real-time image. **B:** Note the severe aortic regurgitation, which is secondary to disruption of normal aortic anatomy rather than disruption of the aortic valve cusps. Ao, aorta; LA, left atrium; LV, left ventricle.

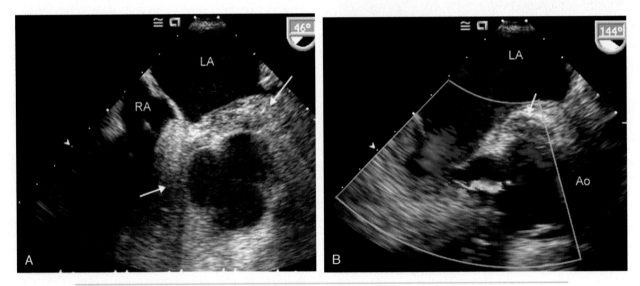

FIGURE 19.36. Postoperative transesophageal echocardiogram recorded in the same patient presented in Figure 19.35. The ascending aorta has been replaced from the sinotubular junction distally and surgical remodeling has been performed on the left and noncoronary sinuses. **A:** Note the homogeneous echo densities (*arrows* in A and B) surrounding the aorta, which is a result of the surgical repair. **B:** Color flow Doppler image recorded in an orthogonal view reveals only mild residual aortic regurgitation (*arrow*). Ao, aorta; LA, left atrium; RA, right atrium.

elderly, who have severe aortic stenosis, marked left ventricular hypertrophy, and a small left ventricular cavity. These patients have developed severe left ventricular hypertrophy over a long period of time, typically measured in decades. After relief of the afterload obstruction due to critical aortic stenosis, the ventricle becomes hyperdynamic and a pattern mimicking acquired hypertrophic cardiomyopathy of the elderly is unmasked. This can result in hemodynamic instability and hypotension in the perioperative period. Transesophageal echocardiography can identify this syndrome when there is evidence of a small hyperdynamic left ventricle with dynamic outflow tract obstruction, with or without secondary mitral regurgitation, after aortic valve replacement. Some investigators have suggested that the combination of a small preoperative cavity with marked left ventricular hypertrophy accurately predicts development of this syndrome and that the surgical procedure should include not only

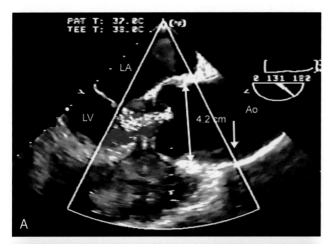

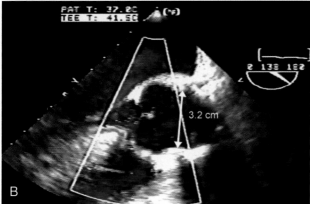

FIGURE 19.37. Pre- **(A)** and postoperative **(B)** transesophageal echocardiograms recorded in a longitudinal view in a patient with a type A dissection and aortic insufficiency due to efface-ment of the sinotubular junction. **A:** Note the dilation of the sino-tubular junction, which measures 4.2 cm compared with an an-ular dimension of approximately 2.8 cm. The false lumen of the dissection is partially thrombosed at this level (*arrow*). Note the central aortic regurgitation jet, which is due to incomplete coap-tation of the aortic valve cusps. **B:** Recorded after graft replace-ment of the ascending aorta from the sinotubular junction into the arch. Note that the sinotubular junction now mea-sures 3.2 cm and the absence of residual aortic insuffi-ciency. LA, left atrium; LV, left ventricle.

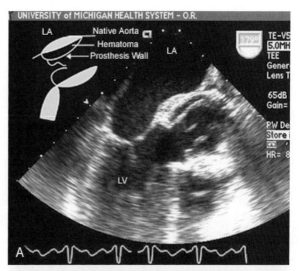

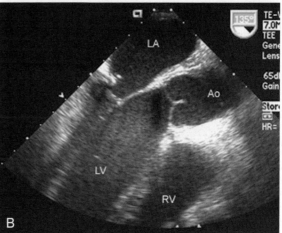

FIGURE 19.38. Intraoperative transesophageal echocardio-gram recorded in a patient after aortic valve replacement using a new stentless aortic valve prosthesis and an "inclusion" tech-nique. **A:** Note the free space between the prosthesis wall and the native aorta in this intraoperative echocardiogram. **B:** Over time, this free space disappears and there will be smooth conti-nuity between the included prosthesis and the native aortic wall. Ao, aorta; LA, left atrium; LV, left ventricle; RV, right ventricle.

aortic valve replacement but also proximal myotomy-myectomy.

One complication of aortic valve replacement, espe-cially if a concurrent myectomy or anular enlarging pro-cedure has been performed, is creation of a ventricular septal defect. Because the defect may be quite small and located underneath the sewing ring, it may be difficult for a surgeon to directly visualize the defect. Postopera-tive transesophageal echocardiography typically will easily identify these defects and allow the surgeon to make a decision regarding the necessity of returning the patient to cardiopulmonary bypass for further repair (Fig. 19.39).

A complication unique to surgical myectomy is the cre-ation of a coronary fistula in the area of the myectomy (Fig.

19.40). As a consequence of surgical excision of septal muscle, an intramural coronary artery may be sheared off and result in a fistula in the left ventricular outflow tract. These are not noted at the time of the actual procedure be-cause the patient is on cardiopulmonary bypass and the heart is arrested. They are rarely of clinical concern.

In many institutions, mitral valve replacement with a prosthetic valve is accomplished by leaving the posterior mitral valve leaflet and the associated papillary muscle and chordae intact. This protects against adverse remod-eling of the left ventricle, which can be seen if the entire apparatus is severed. A potential complication of leaving residual mitral valve tissue is that the retained chordae can interrupt function of a disk prosthesis. This is a com-plication that can be screened for intraoperatively but un-

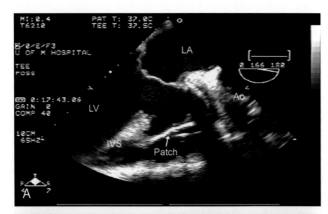

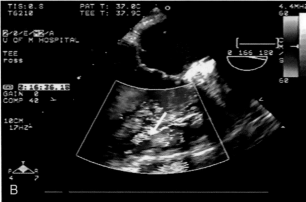

FIGURE 19.39. A: Intraoperative transesophageal echocardiogram recorded in a patient after complex aortic valve replacement necessitated by a narrow left ventricular outflow tract and small aortic anulus. The surgical procedure consisted of a myectomy and patch graft (Kono procedure) for widening the left ventricular outflow tract. **B:** In this immediate postoperative echocardiogram, note the high-velocity jet just below the aortic prosthesis consistent with a ventricular septal defect at the margin of the patch (*arrow*). Ao, aorta; IVS, interventricular septum; LA, left atrium; LV, left ventricle.

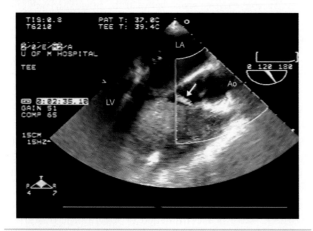

FIGURE 19.40. Transesophageal echocardiogram recorded in a longitudinal view in a patient after a myectomy for hypertrophic cardiomyopathy. Immediately below the aortic valve, note the diastolic Doppler flow signal arising from within the myocardium and projecting into the left ventricular outflow tract (*arrow*). This represents a small coronary fistula that is the result of severing an intramyocardial blood vessel at the time of myectomy. Ao, aorta; LA, left atrium; LV, left ventricle.

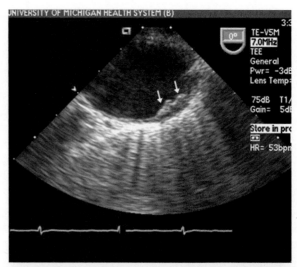

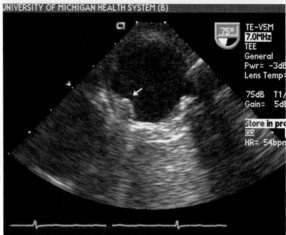

FIGURE 19.41. A, B: Intraoperative transesophageal echocardiogram recorded in a patient undergoing elective cardiac surgery. These images are recorded of the arch and demonstrate focal atheroma in the arch (*arrows*). Placement of a cannula at this site would be likely to result in embolization of atheroma.

fortunately may be a delayed development rather than an immediate postoperative complication.

Miscellaneous Applications

There are several miscellaneous applications of echocardiography in the operating room, including assessment of aortic atherosclerosis and assisting with placement of cannulae or other devices. When operating on patients with atherosclerotic heart or vascular disease, it is not uncommon to encounter significant amounts of aortic atherosclerosis. These areas are preferably avoided when placing aortic cannulae or cross clamps. Most surgeons rely on palpation of the aorta to assess for underlying atheroma at the site of intended cannulation or device placement. In many centers, transesophageal or, less often, direct epicardial imaging is used to evaluate the location and extent of underlying atheroma before instrumenting the aorta at that location (Fig. 19.41).

On rare occasions, transesophageal echo guidance is necessary to assist in placement of catheters, such as a retrograde cardioplegia catheter. Because radiographic landmarks usually suffice, it is rare to require ultrasound guidance for placement of an intraaortic balloon pump, although it may be occasionally useful to avoid areas of marked atheroma. There are several other procedures for which transesophageal echo guidance is used. One is in percutaneous placement of an occlusive balloon or perfusion device in the aorta. In some centers, a minimally invasive approach to cardiopulmonary bypass is used in select patients. This requires placement of an occlusive balloon device and perfusion cannulae in the proximal descending aorta. Transesophageal echocardiography is occasionally used to ensure appropriate placement and function of these occlusive devices.

Intraoperative Complications of Cardiac Surgery

The echocardiographer involved in intraoperative evaluation should be aware of the full range of cardiac compli-

cations that can occur at the time of cardiovascular surgery. Many of these complications are listed in Table 19.3. It is imperative to recognize the characteristics of ventricular performance and aortic flow for a patient on cardiopulmonary bypass. While on complete bypass, the left ventricle will be unloaded and its diastolic volume is reduced. In this situation, even in the beating heart, the ventricle will appear globally hypokinetic (Fig. 19.42). Once fully removed from bypass and after appropriate volume resuscitation, ventricular size and function should return to baseline or possibly be improved compared with base-

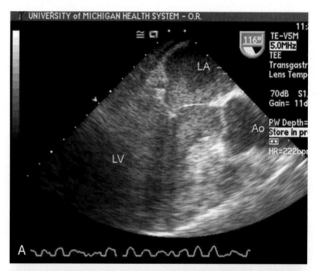

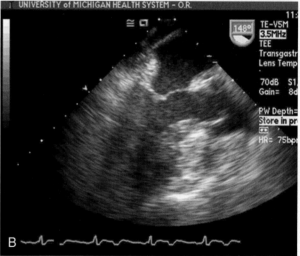

FIGURE 19.42. Transesophageal echocardiograms recorded in a patient on complete (**A**) and partial (**B**) cardiopulmonary bypass. **A:** Note that while on complete bypass, the left atrium (*LA*) and left ventricle (*LV*) are filled with homogeneous echoes consistent with marked stasis of blood flow. Note the fibrillating left ventricle (*LV*). Also note the relative absence of stasis in the aorta (*Ao*), which receives flow from a cardiopulmonary bypass cannula. **B:** Recorded after restoration of sinus rhythm and while on partial (1.5 L/min) cardiopulmonary bypass. Again, note the underfilled left ventricle with the poor ventricular function due to reduced filling and the substantial clearing of the spontaneous contrast within the chambers.

TABLE 19.3 Complications Detected with Intraoperative Transesophageal Echocardiography

"Intracardiac" air
    Intracavitary
    Intercavitary
    Myocardial
    Individual targets
Right ventricular dysfunction
Left ventricular dysfunction
    Regional
    Global
Following myectomy
    Ventricular septal defect
    Residual obstruction
    Coronary fistula
Following aortic valve replacement
    Paravaluar regurgitation
    Patient-prosthesis mismatch
    Outflow tract obstruction
Following mitral valve repair
    Residual mitral regurgitation
    Iatrogenic mitral stenosis
    Systolic anterior motion–dynamic outflow obstruction
Following mitral valve replacement
    Paravalvular regurgitation
    Chordal interference with disc function
Following repair of congenital heart lesions
    Residual shunt
    Baffle integrity
    Right ventricular function

line, depending on the nature of the surgery and its success and the use of inotropic agents. Partial bypass, or incomplete volume restoration, results in intermediate levels of ventricular performance. While on complete bypass, continuous nonphasic flow will be seen in the aorta (Fig. 19.43).

One of the major considerations after cardiac surgery is the presence and location of any residual intracardiac air. Individual small contrast targets indicative of small microbubbles (similar in size and character to those seen during saline contrast injection) are not uncommon after any cardiac procedure. Intracardiac air typically can take on one of three appearances. It should be recalled that air is an intense echo reflector, and a significant pocket of air will result in both acoustic shadowing and reverberation. As such, the appearance of air may be that of a single bright linear line with shadowing behind it. It should also be emphasized that air will float to the surface of the blood pool, and, as such, a free air collection would be expected to be seen in the more anterior locations (assuming supine patient position). The most common sites

to find significant pockets of residual air are the left atrial appendage, the pulmonary veins, and along the atrial septum. Figures 19.44 and 19.45 were recorded in patients with intracardiac air after mitral valve procedures. Note the appearance is that of a single bright linear echo with reverberation and shadowing. This echo often has an oscillatory appearance to it as the air rises to the surface of the blood pool. This type of echo represents a variable but typically clinically relevant amount of intracardiac air that should be identified and addressed before the patient is removed from cardiopulmonary bypass. Often the visualized air pocket may be trapped between two cardiac structures (intercardiac), such as the aorta and left atrial wall, as opposed to being contained within a cardiac chamber (intracardiac). It may not be possible to distinguish extracardiac air from true intracavity air. If it is not in an anterior location and does not migrate with physical motion, it is more likely to be noncavitary.

A second appearance of intracardiac air is that of an air embolus to the level of the myocardium. This typically will present as a bright white area in the ventricular myocardium, much as would be expected during purposeful myocardial perfusion echocardiography (Fig. 19.46). Typically, this results in reduced myocardial blood flow in that area, and the myocardial region not only has pathologic echo intensity but frequently systolic dysfunction as well. A related phenomenon is an air embolus to a major coronary artery that has interrupted flow, resulting in a wall motion abnormality but that has not resulted in dif-

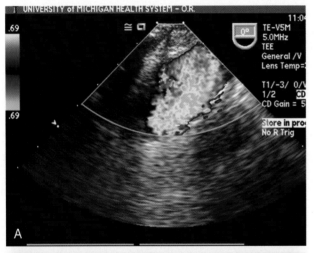

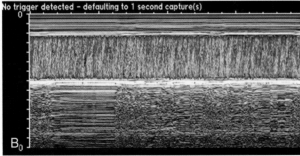

FIGURE 19.43. Intraoperative transesophageal echocardiogram of the aortic arch during cardiopulmonary bypass. **A:** Note the continuous high-velocity flow in the aortic arch on the color flow image, which is also appreciated in the color Doppler M-mode image **(B)**. This is the result of continuous flow into the aorta from the cardiopulmonary bypass apparatus and does not represent pathology.

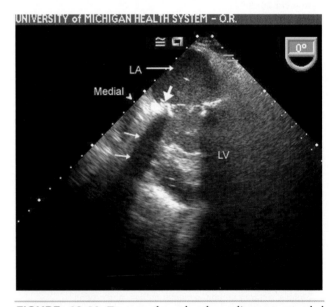

FIGURE 19.44. Transesophageal echocardiogram recorded immediately after mitral valve replacement. Note the individual small air targets within the left atrium (*LA*) and the larger more discrete air "pocket" (*large arrow*) resulting in a distinct shadow distally (*smaller arrows*). In this view, the air pocket is medially located and may not represent true intracavitary air. LV, left ventricle.

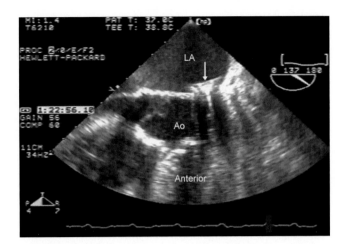

FIGURE 19.45. Intraoperative transesophageal echocardiogram recorded after mitral valve surgery. In this longitudinal view, note the discrete air "pocket" (*arrow*) in the left atrium (*LA*) resulting in distal shadowing. Also note the side lobe artifact arising from the main target. In the real-time image, note the oscillatory nature of this signal, confirming that it as an air pocket. In this instance, the air pocket is located anteriorly, which would be the anticipated area of free intracavitary air versus the more medial location noted in Figure 19.44. Ao, aorta.

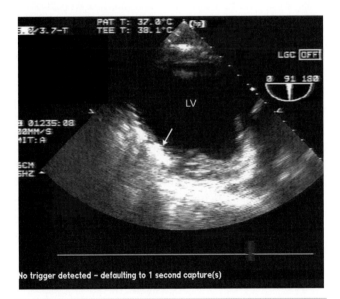

FIGURE 19.46. Intraoperative transesophageal echocardiogram recorded in a longitudinal view at the mid-esophagus. This patient had undergone bypass surgery and placement of a mitral anular ring. Note the bright oscillating echoes that appear in the wall of the myocardium (*arrow*). It may be difficult to determine that this air is truly myocardial or whether it is trapped in apical trabeculae. LV, left ventricle.

fuse air accumulation within the myocardium. This is typically identified as a regional wall motion abnormality, corresponding to a coronary distribution but without evidence of air in the myocardium. Obviously, this type of appearance could be due to any other factor resulting in interruption of coronary blood flow.

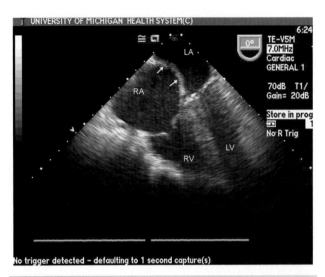

FIGURE 19.47. Intraoperative transesophageal echocardiogram recorded in a patient after aortic valve replacement and bypass surgery in whom there was difficulty weaning from cardiopulmonary bypass. Note the small, underfilled left ventricle (*LV*) and the markedly dilated right ventricle (*RV*) and right atrium (*RA*) due to severe right ventricular dysfunction. Note also the persistent bulging of the atrial septum into the left atrium (*LA*) (*arrows*), indicative of markedly elevated right atrial pressures.

An additional appearance of intracardiac air is that of small pockets of air trapped within trabeculae at the left ventricular or right ventricular apex. This will be seen almost exclusively after valvular procedures in which the cavity of the left ventricle has been emptied and exposed to air. Typically, if air is in this location, physical motion of the heart in that area by the surgeon may dislodge at least a portion of it and confirm its nature as being trapped in trabeculae rather than being truly intramyocardial.

Additional cardiac complications that can be screened for with intraoperative transesophageal echocardiography include the development of new or worsening systolic function of either the left or right ventricle. Because the right ventricle is typically more exposed and less well preserved by the cardioplegia solution, some degree of right ventricular dysfunction is common after cardiac procedures. The severity and likelihood of right ventricular dysfunction are directly related to the complexity and duration of the procedure. On occasion, clinically relevant degrees of right ventricular dysfunction that may interfere with overall cardiac output are encountered. Right ventricular dysfunction of the transplanted heart is a worrisome complication because these patients frequently have a degree of pulmonary hypertension that exacerbates the right ventricular dysfunction occurring as a result of the transplantation procedure. Intraoperative transesophageal echocardiography is extremely useful for detecting and following the progress of this complication. Figure 19.47 was recorded in a patient in whom preoperative right ventricular function was normal, but, after a lengthy operative course, the right ventricle was noted to be dilated and hypokinetic. Although resulting in significant degrees of right ventricular dysfunction initially, recovery of right ventricular function may occur over the ensuing several days. A secondary complication that can be seen in patients who develop right ventricular dysfunction is opening of a patent foramen ovale resulting in right-to-left shunting and systemic hypoxia. This syndrome can lead to difficulty in weaning from ventilatory support and on occasion has required surgical closure of a patent foramen ovale. This complication can be screened for both in the operating room and in the perioperative period in the intensive care unit.

Left ventricular function should be reassessed immediately after cardiac procedures. Systolic dysfunction can occur either regionally, where it is assumed to be the result of interruption of flow to a discrete coronary artery territory, or globally, which can have several etiologies. Figure 19.48 was recorded in a patient after a cardiac surgical procedure in whom global right and left ventricular dysfunction was noted immediately postoperatively. When a regional abnormality is noted, corresponding to a well-defined coronary circulation, direct visual inspection for the integrity of bypass grafts to ensure that there is no kink or other anatomic disruption is clearly in order (Fig. 19.49).

A final intraoperative complication that should be considered is that of iatrogenic aortic dissection. This typi-

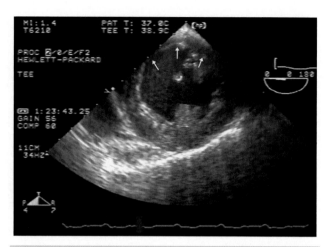

FIGURE 19.49. Intraoperative transesophageal echocardiogram recorded in a patient after multivessel coronary artery bypass surgery. Preoperatively, the patient had normal left ventricular systolic function. In this image, recorded immediately after discontinuation of cardiopulmonary bypass, note the significant area of inferior wall akinesis (*arrows*) suggesting graft failure.

cally occurs at the site of aortic cannulation. As part of the postoperative evaluation, the ascending aorta, arch, and descending thoracic aorta should be screened for integrity of the wall and to ensure that there is no evidence of iatrogenic dissection. Iatrogenic dissection may be limited and clinically silent but on occasion may result in major organ malperfusion with inadequate urine output or bowel or limb ischemia. Figure 19.50 was recorded in a patient after otherwise uncomplicated mitral valve repair and coronary artery bypass surgery. During the course of the surgical procedure, the patient became progressively oliguric, and postoperative transesophageal echocardiography demonstrated a new aortic dissection extending from the arch to beyond the gastroesophageal junction.

Operative Monitoring for Noncardiac Procedures

Transesophageal echocardiography is occasionally used to monitor cardiac function during noncardiac procedures. Typically, this has been confined to either high-risk patients or to patients undergoing high-risk procedures such as liver transplantation or major vascular procedures. Echocardiographic monitoring is most often used for determination of left ventricular systolic function and volume status. It should be emphasized that in patients with significant hypertension and coexistent organic heart disease, right heart catheterization may not provide an accurate assessment of true ventricular preload. Because of the marked left ventricular hypertrophy and diastolic dysfunction, left ventricular filling pressures as

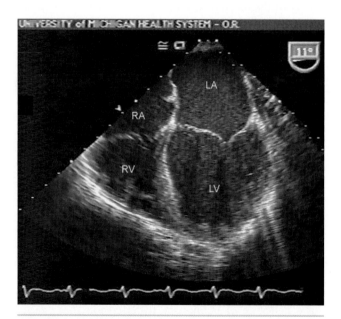

FIGURE 19.48. Intraoperative transesophageal echocardiogram recorded immediately after removing a patient from cardiopulmonary bypass after an otherwise an uncomplicated procedure. Note the marked dilation of the left ventricle (*LV*) and the severe global hypokinesis representing severe diffuse myocardial stunning. LA, left atrium; RA, right atrium; RV, right ventricle.

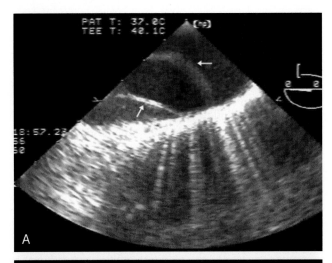

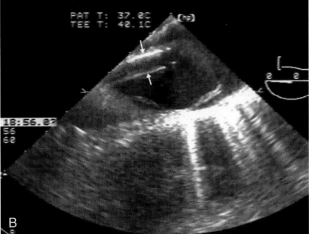

FIGURE 19.50. Intraoperative transesophageal echocardiogram recorded in a patient immediately after cardiac surgery. Note the dissection in the arch (*arrows*) **(A)** and the position of the cannula at the origin of the dissection flap (*arrows*) **(B)**.

measured by right heart catheterization are high; however, the ventricle itself is small and underfilled, resulting in reduced stroke volume, hypotension, and poor perfusion. Recognition of this pattern of a small, underfilled ventricle in the presence of hypotension with elevated filling pressure by right catheterization allows the appropriate therapy of volume resuscitation to be undertaken rather than the inappropriate maneuver of combined diuretics and pressors.

Transesophageal echocardiography can also be used for online monitoring of regional ventricular function. Development of a new regional wall motion abnormality is assumed to represent myocardial ischemia or infarction in progress. Although accurate for detection of infarction or ischemia in progress, there are unfortunately few options available for acutely changing the course of this complication, and, as such, the ability of online monitoring of regional function to alter clinical management

is rather limited. Detection of new regional wall motion abnormalities during the course of surgery may, however, identify a subset of patients for whom more intensive postoperative monitoring and care will be in order.

Delayed Cardiac Surgery Complications

Occasionally after bypass surgery, there may be an immediate deterioration in a patient's clinical status after being removed from cardiopulmonary bypass and transferred to the intensive care unit. The differential of this is extensive and includes pericardial fluid and hemorrhage. Additionally, attention should be paid to the possibility of early graft closure. In this instance, one anticipates seeing a regional wall motion abnormality conforming to the distribution of either a native vessel or one of the implanted grafts. Figure 19.51 was recorded in a patient 24 hours after otherwise uncomplicated bypass surgery who subsequently developed hypotension and new electrocardiographic changes. The transthoracic echocardiogram revealed evidence of myocardial ischemia in the left anterior descending distribution, prompting reevaluation for the integrity of the previously placed bypass graft. Occasionally after mitral valve repair, a delayed syndrome of dynamic outflow tract obstruction may result in the development of a new systolic murmur and hypotension. Measurement of hemodynamics with right heart catheterization may be misleading in this situation. Figure 19.52 was recorded in a patient 48 hours after mitral valve repair who developed this syndrome.

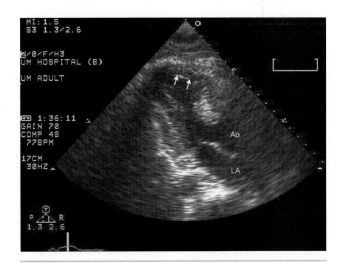

FIGURE 19.51. Transthoracic echocardiogram recorded 24 hours after an otherwise uncomplicated coronary bypass surgery in a patient who subsequently developed new electrocardiographic changes. Note the dyskinesis of the apical septum (*arrows*) in a distribution typical for left anterior descending coronary artery ischemia or infarction. Ao, aorta; LA, left atrium.

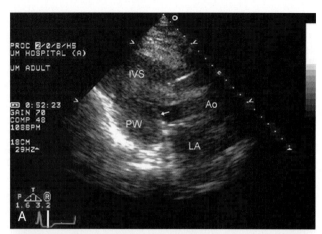

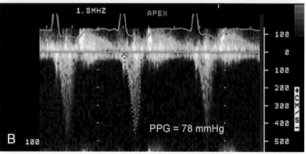

FIGURE 19.52. Parasternal long-axis echocardiogram recorded 24 hours after placement of a mitral ring for mitral regurgitation after the patient developed significant hypotension and a new systolic murmur. **A:** Note the systolic anterior motion of the mitral valve (*arrow*) and the small hyperdynamic left ventricle. **B:** Continuous wave Doppler image recorded from the apex reveals a late-peaking gradient in the left ventricular outflow tract of 78 mm Hg. Ao, aorta; IVS, interventricular septum; LA, left atrium; PW, posterior wall.

There are several additional complications that can occur after cardiac surgery. These include localized intrapericardial or mediastinal hematoma and obstruction of venous inflow. Typically, intrapericardial hematoma is suspected in a patient 1 to 5 days after cardiac surgery in whom hypotension and hemodynamic compromise occur. Because the hematoma may not be circumferential, typical signs of tamponade may be absent. Because of the critically ill nature of these patients and the interference created by recent surgical wounds, transesophageal echocardiography may be necessary to identify this complication. Figures 19.53 through 19.55 were recorded in patients after cardiac surgery in whom hemodynamic instability was the indication for study. There is a tremendous range of hematoma noted that may or may not be associated with free pericardial fluid. Variants of intrapericardial hematoma are noted in which only one cardiac chamber may be compressed. Additionally, intrapericardial hematoma may selectively compress either vena caval blood flow or pulmonary vein flow. As some degree of pericardial effusion and even hematoma is not uncommon after cardiac surgery and often causes no hemodynamic em-

barrassment, it is important to integrate a full range of observations when determining the clinical relevance of pericardial hematoma. Clinically relevant pericardial hematomas usually result in distortion of chamber geometry and/or evidence of reduced cardiac filling. Figure 19.53 was recorded in a patient in whom pericardial hematoma had impeded venous inflow to the heart and thus resulted in the appearance of hypovolemia but in the absence of obvious blood loss. Because of the difficulty in separating organized hematoma from consolidated lung tissue and other intrathoracic structures, correlative imaging with computed tomography is often employed to confirm the findings noted on echocardiography. Hemodynamic compromise in the early postoperative period, if accompanied by echocardiographic evidence of pericardial fluid or hematoma, may appropriately lead to reexploration of the chest without the need for additional testing.

A final short-term complication of intrathoracic procedures that can be identified with transesophageal echocardiography is pulmonary vein stenosis after lung transplantation or pulmonary vein isolation done for atrial fibrillation ablation. This results in obstruction of flow from the transplanted lung and may result in unilateral pulmonary edema of the recently transplanted lung. After lung transplantation, complete transesophageal echocardiographic evaluation should include visualization of all four pulmonary veins for diameter, flow turbulence, and determination of gradients. This is often a difficult examination to perform. Figure 19.56 was recorded in a patient after lung transplantation with poor oxygenation and unilateral pulmonary edema. Notice the anatomic stenosis of the pulmonary vein associated with a marked reduction in pulmonary vein flow compared with the nonobstructed contralateral pulmonary veins.

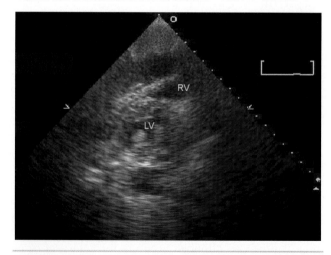

FIGURE 19.53. Transthoracic echocardiogram recorded in a patient 36 hours after cardiac surgery who subsequently developed progressive hypotension. Note the significant circumferential pericardial effusion and the small compressed right (*RV*) and left (*LV*) ventricles.

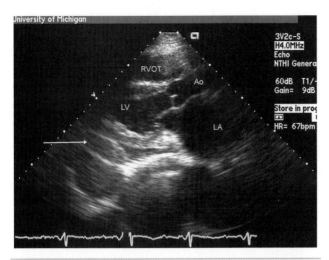

FIGURE 19.54. Parasternal long-axis echocardiogram recorded in a patient 48 hours after cardiac surgery who developed hypotension. Note the small pericardial effusion with organized components consistent with thrombus (*arrow*) and the normal size and contour of all visualized chambers. The preserved chamber size is indirect evidence that this pericardial effusion may not be hemodynamically significant and that another etiology for hypotension should be considered Ao, aorta; LA, left atrium; LV, left ventricle; RVOT, right ventricular outflow tract.

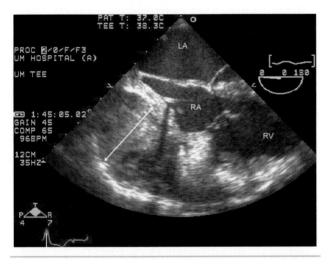

FIGURE 19.55. Transesophageal echocardiogram recorded in a patient with hemodynamic compromise 36 hours after cardiac surgery. Note the large (*double-headed arrow*) consolidated hematoma predominantly adjacent to and compressing the right atrium (*RA*). LA, left atrium; RV, right ventricle.

MONITORING OF NONOPERATIVE AND OTHER INTERVENTIONAL PROCEDURES

There are several cardiovascular procedures, typically performed in an intensive care unit or cardiac catheterization laboratory, for which online echocardiographic monitoring may be advantageous. Some authorities have recommended online monitoring of pericardiocen-

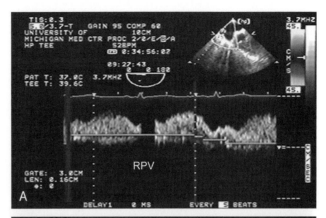

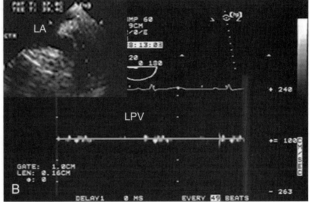

FIGURE 19.56. Transesophageal echocardiogram recorded in a patient 24 hours after single lung transplantation. **A:** Doppler recording of pulmonary vein flow from a right pulmonary vein (*RPV*) reveals normal flow velocity and contour. **B:** Recorded in a left pulmonary vein (*LPV*) revealing absent pulmonary venous inflow suggesting pulmonary vein obstruction. LA, left atrium.

tesis as a means of reducing complication rates, specifically cardiac perforation. Thorough preprocedure echocardiography probably suffices to determine the amount and distribution of fluid from which the likelihood of cardiac injury can be anticipated. When a large circumferential effusion is detected, careful attention to procedural detail is usually all that is necessary to avoid cardiac injury. Conversely, for smaller fluid collections or for loculated or otherwise atypically distributed fluid, online monitoring of the pericardiocentesis needle may help increase the likelihood of successful drainage and reduce the likelihood of cardiac perforation. Localization of a pericardiocentesis needle is not always as successful as one might anticipate. The needle tip can be difficult to identify. An additional maneuver to ensure that the needle tip is within the pericardial space is to inject a small amount of agitated saline contrast. If the contrast appears in the pericardial space, this is excellent evidence that the pericardial needle is in the space and that guidewire placement can then appropriately be undertaken (Fig. 19.57).

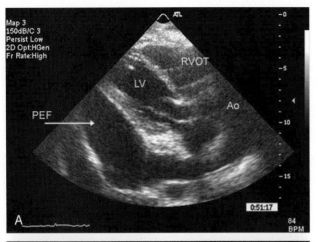

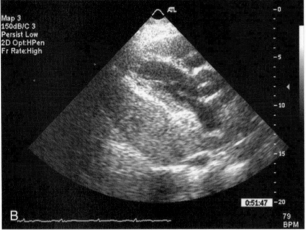

FIGURE 19.57. Transthoracic echocardiogram recorded in a patient with a large pericardial effusion undergoing pericardiocentesis. **A:** Note the clear posterior pericardial effusion (*PEF*) (*arrow*). **B:** Recorded after injection of agitated saline through a pericardiocentesis needle, which confirms the location of the needle in the pericardial space. Ao, aorta; LV, left ventricle; RVOT, right ventricular outflow tract.

Cardiac Interventional Procedures

There are several procedures requiring transatrial catheter placement that can be monitored with transesophageal echocardiography. More recently, success has been demonstrated in monitoring these procedures with high-frequency intracardiac probes (Figs. 19.58 and 19.59). Procedures that require crossing the atrial septum include mitral valvuloplasty, percutaneous atrial septal defect closure, and atrial septostomy for severe pulmonary hypertension in adults. Information to be gained from transesophageal echocardiography includes a thorough preprocedure assessment of atrial septal anatomy. An atrial septum that is in neutral position with a well-defined foramen ovale represents less of a technical challenge to atrial septal puncture than does an atrial septum whose geometry is markedly distorted by pressure over-

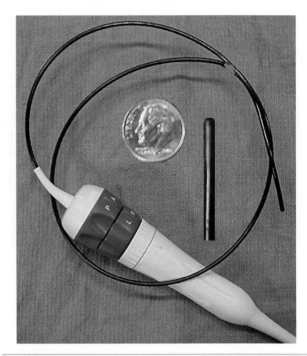

FIGURE 19.58. Dedicated single-plane two-dimensional probe developed for intracardiac ultrasound. The two blue rings on the white handle allow flexion of approximately 60 degrees in two different planes. The middle is an expanded view of the tip of catheter. The probe is approximately 10-French in size.

load on either the right or left side. Figure 19.60 illustrates examples of different atrial septal geometry posing varying degrees of technical challenge for atrial septal puncture and subsequent transatrial procedures.

Percutaneous balloon mitral valvuloplasty is occasionally monitored using transesophageal echocardiography (Fig. 19.61). The transesophageal echocardiogram can be used to identify left atrial or left atrial appendage thrombus, which may represent a contraindication to the procedure, to characterize the anticipated technical difficulty of the procedure and to monitor appropriate placement of the transseptal needle and guidewire. The transesophageal echocardiogram can confirm the presence of the guidewire in the left atrium. Additionally, transesophageal echo with color flow imaging can confirm the presence and size of the atrial septal defect created for balloon passage, and, subsequently, can confirm the course of the dilation balloon from the right atrium into the left atrium and across the mitral valve. After the procedure, transesophageal echocardiography can be used to determine the presence and severity of mitral regurgitation that may have occurred as a complication of the procedure and to confirm transmitral gradients. Similar monitoring can also be done using an intracardiac imaging catheter.

An increasingly employed strategy for both adult and pediatric patients with atrial septal defect is percutaneous

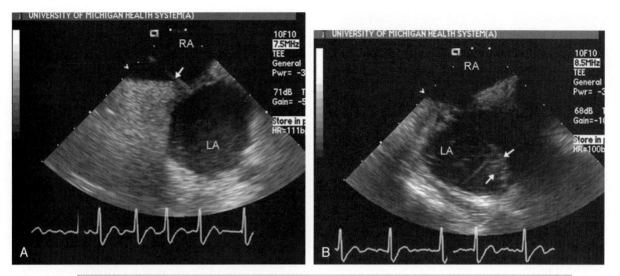

FIGURE 19.59. Intracardiac echocardiogram recorded in a patient undergoing atrial septal puncture for performance of an electrophysiologic procedure. **A:** Note the position of the needle (*arrow*) in the thickened atrial septum. **B:** Note the cloud of ultrasound contrast (*arrows*) created after injection of agitated saline through the transseptal catheter, confirming its location in the left atrium (*LA*). RA, right atrium.

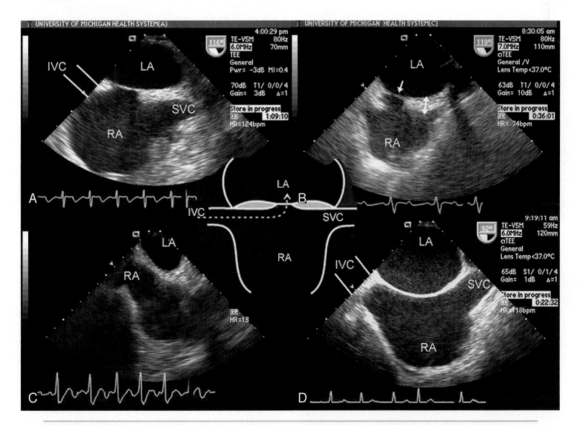

FIGURE 19.60. Transesophageal echocardiograms recorded in patients being considered for interventional procedures that require crossing the atrial septum. Atrial septal puncture is technically easiest in individuals in whom the atrial septum is thin and located in a "neutral" position **(upper left)**. **Upper right:** An atrial septum in "neutral" position but with significant lipomatous atrial hypertrophy. Obviously puncture will be difficult if not impossible at the areas of lipomatous infiltration (*double-headed arrows*), and the catheter position is ideal in the foramen (*single arrow*). **Lower left:** A diffusely and uniformly thickened atrial septum that may present technical difficulties for successful puncture in crossing the atrial septum. **Lower right:** An atrial septum that is distorted due to marked left-to-right bowing as a consequence of mitral stenosis, which may also complicate transseptal puncture. In the schematic, the *dotted line* represents the path of a transseptal catheter passed from the inferior vena cava (*IVC*) across the area of the foramen ovale. LA, left atrium; RA, right atrium; SVC, superior vena cava.

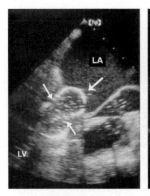 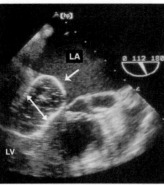

FIGURE 19.61. Transesophageal echocardiogram recorded at the time of percutaneous mitral balloon valvotomy. **Left:** Note the partially inflated balloon within the mitral orifice. Note the narrowing (*arrows*) of the mid-portion of the balloon due to constraint by the stenotic orifice. **Right:** Recorded after complete balloon dilation (*double-headed arrow*). LA, left atrium; LV, left ventricle. (Courtesy of Steven A. Goldstein, M.D.)

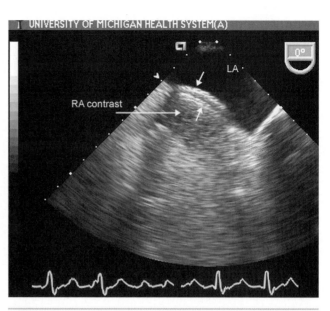

FIGURE 19.63. Transesophageal echocardiogram recorded after placement of an atrial septal closure device (*small arrows*). Intravenous contrast has been injected to confirm the lack of persistent shunting. The right and left sides of the device are noted by the *arrows*. LA, left atrium; RA, right atrium.

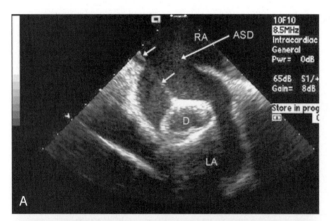

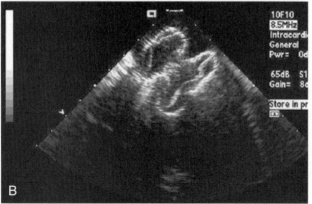

FIGURE 19.62. Intracardiac echocardiogram recorded in a patient at the time of placement of an occluder device for closure of a secundum atrial septal defect. **A:** Recorded after passing the left atrial portion of the device (*D*). **B:** Recorded after both the left and right sides had been placed. ASD, atrial septal defect; D, device; LA, left atrium; RA, right atrium.

closure. There are several clinically available devices, each of which typically consists of an umbrella-like structure that is passed in a folded position across the atrial septal defect. The device is then expanded and pulled back against the left side of the atrial septum. Once this occluder portion is in place, a second device is passed along the guidewire and attached to the right side of the atrial septum. Transesophageal echocardiography is usually employed to monitor placement of the device to ensure its appropriate location and that it has successfully reduced the degree of intracardiac shunting. Figures 19.62 through 19.64 were recorded in patients undergoing percutaneous atrial septal defect closure using one of these devices. Notice in Figure 19.64 that the device has resulted in a more rigid-appearing atrial septum. Typically, color Doppler flow imaging and contrast echocardiography, using agitated saline, are employed at the end of the procedure to ensure that there is no significant residual right-to-left shunting.

Transesophageal echocardiography is typically employed before percutaneous closure of an atrial septal defect to precisely determine the size of the defect and its location and the adequacy of a rim of tissue surrounding the defect that is large enough and has enough structural integrity to allow placement of a mechanical occluder device. Figure 19.65 was recorded in patients with atrial septal defects being considered for percutaneous closure. Notice in Figure 19.65A the size of the atrial septal defect, which is well below the occluder size, and the presence of an adequate tissue rim surrounding this secundum atrial

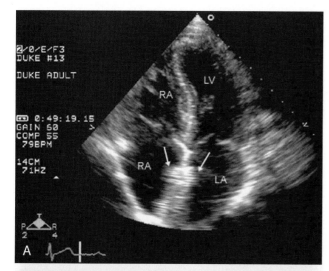

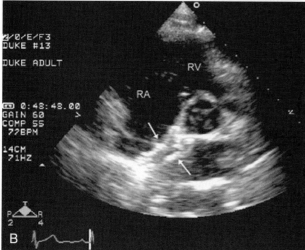

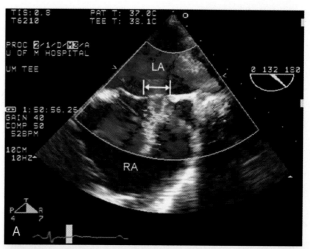

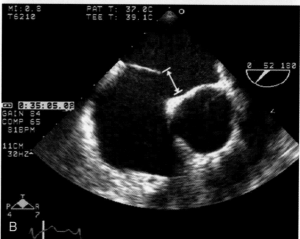

FIGURE 19.64. Transthoracic echocardiogram recorded in apical four-chamber **(A)** and parasternal short-axis **(B)** views in a patient after placement of an atrial closure device. Note the thickened appearance to the atrial septum. With close inspection, both the right atrial and left atrial sides of the closure device can be clearly identified. LA, left atrium; LV, left ventricle; RA, right atrium; RV, right ventricle.

FIGURE 19.65. Transesophageal echocardiograms recorded in two patients being considered for closure of atrial septal defect. **A:** Recorded in a patient with a classic secundum atrial septal defect measuring approximately 1 cm (*arrows*). Note the structural integrity of the atrial septum on either side of the defect and the excellent rim of tissue for placing a closure device. **B:** Recorded in a patient with a slightly larger atrial septal defect (*arrows*) with less structural integrity to the residual atrial septum and lack of a rim at the more superior portion of the defect, which may render percutaneous closure problematic. LA, left atrium; RA, right atrium.

septal defect. This echocardiogram would be consistent with an atrial septal defect with the location, size, and tissue integrity to allow percutaneous closure. Compare this with the atrial septal defect depicted in Figure 19.65B in which there is less adequate tissue rim for attachment of a device. Three-dimensional echocardiography and intracardiac echocardiography have both been used to enhance the assessment of feasibility of arterial septal defect closure. Figure 19.66 is a three-dimensional echocardiogram recorded in a patient with an atrial septal defect. The spatial resolution of three-dimensional echocardiography allows a more refined assessment of the exact location and size of the atrial septal defect as well as the degree to which an appropriate rim for device attachment is present.

A final interventional procedure, often monitored with transesophageal or intracardiac echocardiography is the creation of an atrial septostomy. This procedure involves balloon perforation of the atrial septum in an effort to create a small atrial septal defect and allow communication of blood between the atria. Atrial septostomy was frequently employed in cyanotic infants with tricuspid atresia. In adult patients, it may be used as part of the management for patients with end-stage pulmonary hypertension for whom the limiting factor for systemic cardiac output is the pathologically elevated pulmonary vascular resistance and reduced right ventricular output. By creating an atrial septal defect, shunting of nonoxy-

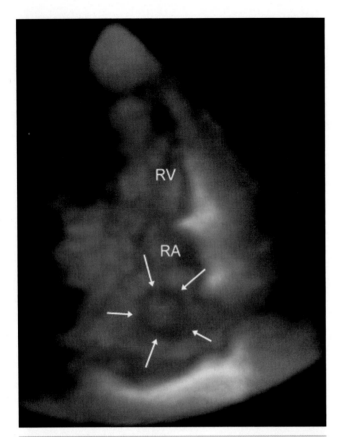

FIGURE 19.66. Three-dimensional echocardiogram recorded in a patient with an atrial septal defect demonstrates the excellent spatial resolution of this technique for defining atrial septal anatomy and suitability for percutaneous closure. Note the complete rim of tissue surrounding the defect (*arrows*). RA, right atrium; RV, right ventricle.

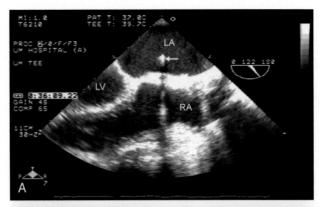

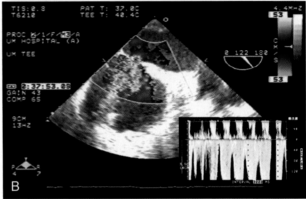

FIGURE 19.67. Transesophageal echocardiograms recorded at the time of creating an atrial septostomy in a patient with an intraaortic balloon pump and severe left ventricular dysfunction and dilation. **A:** Recorded in a longitudinal view confirming the location of a guiding catheter across the atrial septum with the tip of the catheter in the left atrium (*LA*) (*arrow*). **B:** Recorded with color flow Doppler imaging after creation of a septostomy with a dilating balloon confirming the presence of an iatrogenically created atrial septal defect measuring approximately 6 mm. Continuous wave Doppler image recorded through the defect demonstrates continuous flow from left to right (*small inset*). LV, left ventricle; RA, right atrium.

genated blood from right to left is allowed, which typically has little impact on atrial oxygen saturation but which may allow substantially greater degrees of left ventricular filling and enhanced left ventricular cardiac output. It is also occasionally used in patients with severe left ventricular dysfunction to decompress the left heart while on an assist device (Fig. 19.67).

Other Applications in the Catheterization Laboratory

On occasion, the echocardiographer may be called to the catheterization or interventional laboratory to assist in evaluating a patient who has acutely deteriorated during a procedure. Echocardiography plays an instrumental role in diagnosing perforation with iatrogenic pericardial effusion and for reassessing left ventricular global and regional wall motion quickly and accurately as it does in the postoperative intensive care unit. Evidence of regional left ventricle dysfunction supports a diagnosis of interruption of blood flow of any etiology including the iatrogenic

coronary dissection, acute closure after a percutaneous intervention, or a spontaneous event. Occasionally, transesophageal echocardiography (Fig. 19.68) may be necessary for a complete evaluation.

EVALUATION OF PATIENTS AFTER CARDIAC TRANSPLANTATION

After cardiac transplantation, echocardiography plays a number of roles. It is important for the echocardiographer to recognize the anticipated appearance of a heart after cardiac transplantation. The majority of cardiac transplantation is accomplished with an atrial wall to atrial wall anastomosis. This results in the eventual postoperative atrium being composed of the donor atrial wall as well as the recipient atrial wall and pulmonary veins.

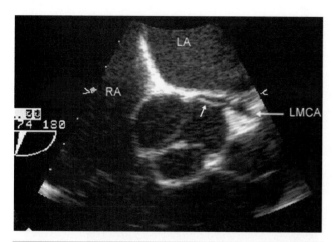

FIGURE 19.68. Transesophageal echocardiogram performed on an emergent basis in the cardiac catheterization laboratory in a patient who developed chest pain and electrocardiographic changes after diagnostic catheterization. Note the limited dissection (*arrow*) in the left Valsalva sinus, which extends into the left main coronary artery (*LMCA*) (*arrow*). RA, right atrium; LA, left atrium.

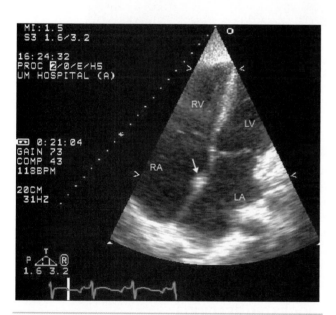

FIGURE 19.69. Apical four-chamber view recorded in a patient several years after orthotopic cardiac transplantation. Note the biatrial enlargement and the echo density along the atrial septum, which represents a prominent atrial suture line (*arrow*). Residual right ventricular and right atrial dilation are also present. LA, left atrium; LV, left ventricle; RA, right atrium; RV, right ventricle.

This anastomotic approach avoids the potential problem of pulmonary vein stenosis. It results in the appearance of prominent suture lines along the atrial wall, which should not be confused with thrombus or other pathologic mass (Fig. 19.69). This also results in the appearance of a dilated left atrium in the vast majority of patients. The left atrial enlargement is often most pronounced when viewed

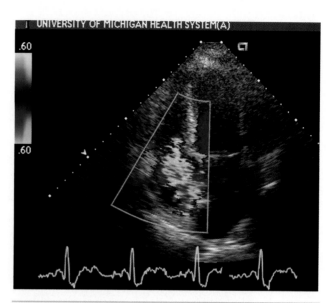

FIGURE 19.70. Apical four-chamber view recorded in a patient several years after cardiac transplantation demonstrates moderate to severe tricuspid regurgitation, the etiology of which typically is a combination of residual right ventricular dysfunction and potential injury from multiple transvenous myocardial biopsies.

from apical four-chamber view. Other common sequelae of cardiac transplantation are variable degrees of right ventricular dysfunction. Right ventricular dysfunction after cardiac transplantation is multifactorial and often relates to relatively poor preservation of right ventricular myocardium during the harvesting and transplantation process as well as the impact on the recipient's preexisting pulmonary hypertension, which is often seen in end-stage heart disease. Due to right ventricular dilation, variable degrees of tricuspid regurgitation are nearly ubiquitous (Fig 19.70).

After cardiac transplantation patients are followed for the development of cardiac rejection. Numerous attempts have been made to use echocardiographic parameters to monitor patients for cardiac rejection. Unfortunately, no echocardiographic parameter has been demonstrated to provide sufficient sensitivity and specificity when compared with the standard of cardiac biopsy. Patients with acute severe rejection frequently will have the appearance of left ventricular wall thickening (pseudohypertrophy) and systolic dysfunction. Unfortunately, this appearance is seen only in patients with advanced cardiac rejection or when the diagnosis is otherwise not in doubt (Fig. 19.71). Other echocardiographic techniques such as tissue characterization, Doppler tissue imaging, and evaluation of diastolic properties of the left ventricle have all been evaluated as markers of cardiac rejection; however, none have been demonstrated to have an adequate sensitivity to replace myocardial biopsy.

In many centers, percutaneous myocardial biopsy may be performed with ultrasound rather than fluoro-

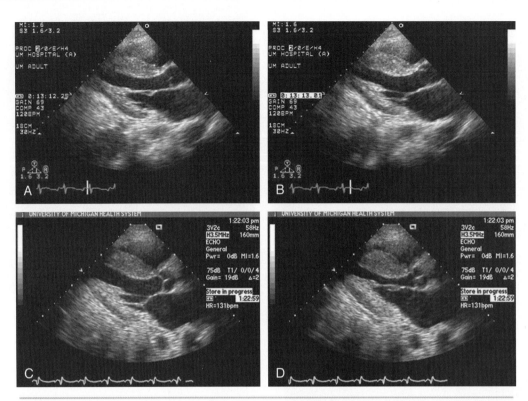

FIGURE 19.71. Parasternal long-axis echocardiograms recorded in a patient with acute severe rejection. Diastolic frames are on the left, systolic on the right. **A, B:** Recorded at the time of presentation with acute severe rejection and reveals apparent left ventricular hypertrophy and severe global hypokinesis. The follow-up echocardiogram **(C, D)** was recorded approximately 3 weeks later after aggressive immunosuppressive therapy and reveals significant recovery of function.

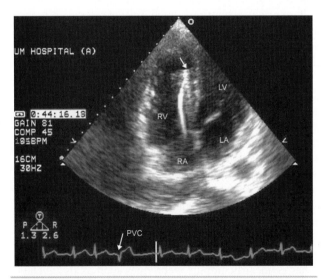

FIGURE 19.72. Apical four-chamber view recorded at the time of transvenous right ventricular biopsy performed for monitoring of cardiac rejection. Note the position of the bioptome along the apical portion of the right side of the ventricular septum (*arrow*). Also note the premature ventricular contraction (*PVC*), which has been provoked by the procedure. LA, left atrium; LV, left ventricle; RA, right atrium; RV, right ventricle.

scopic guidance. This is typically done by imaging from an apical four-chamber view at which time the bioptome can be seen to enter the right atrium and right ventricle (Fig. 19.72). Echocardiography is used to identify the appropriate site for biopsy (apical septum rather than free wall) and to screen for complications such as the iatrogenic right ventricular perforation and pericardial effusion.

SUGGESTED READINGS

Abraham TP, Kon ND, Nomeir AM, et al. Accuracy of transesophageal echocardiography in preoperative determination of aortic anulus size during valve replacement. J Am Soc Echocardiogr 1997;10: 149–154.

Bach DS, LeMire MS, Eberhart D, et al. Impact of intraoperative postpump aortic regurgitation with stentless aortic bioprostheses. Semin Thorac Cardiovasc Surg 1999;11(Suppl 1):88–92.

Bach DS, Deeb GM, Bolling SF. Accuracy of intraoperative transesophageal echocardiography for estimating the severity of functional mitral regurgitation. Am J Cardiol 1995;76:508–512.

Bossone E, DiGiovine B, Watts S, et al. Range and prevalence of cardiac abnormalities in patients hospitalized in a medical ICU. Chest 2002;122(4):1370–6.

Chaliki HP, Click RL, Abel MD. Comparison of intraoperative transesophageal echocardiographic examinations with the operative findings: prospective review of 1918 cases. J Am Soc Echocardiogr 1999;12:237–240.

Chenzbraun A, Pinto FJ, Schnittger I. Transesophageal echocardiography in the intensive care unit: impact on diagnosis and decision-making. Clin Cardiol 1994;17:438–444.

Chu E, Fitzpatrick AP, Chin MC, et al. Radiofrequency catheter ablation guided by intracardiac echocardiography. Circulation 1994;89:1301–1305.

Chu E, Kalman JM, Kwasman MA, et al. Intracardiac echocardiography during radiofrequency catheter ablation of cardiac arrhythmias in humans. J Am Coll Cardiol 1994;24:1351–1357.

Click RL, Abel MD, Schaff HV. Intraoperative transesophageal echocardiography: 5-year prospective review of impact on surgical management. Mayo Clin Proc 2000;75:241–247.

Cooke JC, Gelman JS, Harper RW. Echocardiologists' role in the deployment of the Amplatzer atrial septal occluder device in adults. J Am Soc Echocardiogr 2001;14:588–594.

Currie PJ, Stewart WJ. Intraoperative echocardiography in mitral valve repair for mitral regurgitation. Am J Cardiac Imaging 1990;4:192–206.

Dabaghi SF, Rokey R, Rivera JM, et al. Comparison of echocardiographic assessment of cardiac hemodynamics in the intensive care unit with right-sided cardiac catheterization. Am J Cardiol 1995;76:392–395.

Grewal KS, Malkowski MJ, Piracha AR, et al. Effect of general anesthesia on the severity of mitral regurgitation by transesophageal echocardiography. Am J Cardiol 2000;85:199–203.

Heidenreich PA, Stainback RF, Redberg RF, et al. Transesophageal echocardiography predicts mortality in critically ill patients with unexplained hypotension. J Am Coll Cardiol 1995;26:152–158.

Hurrell DG, Nishimura RA, Symanski JD, et al. Echocardiography in the invasive laboratory: utility of two-dimensional echocardiography in performing transseptal catheterization. Mayo Clin Proc 1998;73:126–131.

Ionescu AA, West RR, Proudman C, et al. Prospective study of routine perioperative transesophageal echocardiography for elective valve replacement: clinical impact and cost-saving implications. J Am Soc Echocardiogr 2001;14:659–667.

Kaul S, Stratienko AA, Pollock SG, et al. Value of two-dimensional echocardiography for determining the basis of hemodynamic compromise in critically ill patients: a prospective study. J Am Soc Echocardiogr 1994;7:598–606.

Kodavatiganti R. Intraoperative assessment of the mitral valve by transesophageal echocardiography: an overview. Ann Cardiac Anaesth 2002;5:127–134.

Krishnamoorthy KM, Tharakan JA, Titus T, et al. Usefulness of transthoracic echocardiography for identification of left atrial thrombus before balloon mitral valvuloplasty. Am J Cardiol 2003;92:1132–1134.

Lambert AS, Miller JP, Merrick SH, et al. Improved evaluation of the location and mechanism of mitral valve regurgitation with a systematic transesophageal echocardiography examination. Anesth Analg 1999;88:1205–1212

Martin F, Sanchez PL, Doherty E, et al. Percutaneous transcatheter closure of patent foramen ovale in patients with paradoxical embolism. Circulation 2002;106:1121–1126.

Mazic U, Gavora P, Masura J. The role of transesophageal echocardiography in transcatheter closure of secundum atrial septal defects by the Amplatzer septal occluder. Am Heart J 2001;142:482–438.

Michel-Cherqui M, Ceddaha A, Liu N, et al. Assessment of systematic use of intraoperative transesophageal echocardiography during cardiac surgery in adults: a prospective study of 203 patients. J Cardiothorac Vasc Anesth 2000;14:45–50.

Mullen MJ, Dias BF, Walker F, et al. Intracardiac echocardiography guided device closure of atrial septal defects. J Am Coll Cardiol 2003;41:285–292.

Nowrangi SK, et al. Impact of intraoperative transesophageal echocardiography among patients undergoing aortic valve replacement for aortic stenosis. J Am Soc Echocardiogr 2001;14:863–866.

Oh CC, Click RL, Orszulak TA, et al. Role of intraoperative transesophageal echocardiography in determining aortic anulus diameter in homograft insertion. J Am Soc Echocardiogr 1998;11:638–642.

Poelaert JI, Trouerbach J, De Buyzere M, et al. Evaluation of transesophageal echocardiography as a diagnostic and therapeutic aid in a critical care setting. Chest 1995;107:774–779.

Poelaert J, Schmidt C, Colardyn F. Transoesophageal echocardiography in the critically ill. Anaesthesia 1998;53:55–68.

Reichert CL, Visser CA, Koolen JJ, et al. Transesophageal echocardiography in hypotensive patients after cardiac operations. Comparison with hemodynamic parameters. J Thorac Cardiovasc Surg 1992;104:321–326.

Schmidlin D, Schuepbach R, Bernard E, et al. Indications and impact of postoperative transesophageal echocardiography in cardiac surgical patients. Crit Care Med 2001;29:2143–2148.

Shanewise JS, Cheung AT, Aronson S, et al. ASE/SCA guidelines for performing a comprehensive intraoperative multiplane transesophageal echocardiography examination: recommendations of the American Society of Echocardiography Council for Intraoperative Echocardiography and the Society of Cardiovascular Anesthesiologists Task Force for Certification in Perioperative Transesophageal Echocardiography. Anesth Analg 1999;89:870–884.

Sohn DW, Shin GJ, Oh JK, et al. Role of transesophageal echocardiography in hemodynamically unstable patients. Mayo Clin Proc 1995;70:925–931.

Stevenson JG, Sorensen GK, Gartman DM, et al. Transesophageal echocardiography during repair of congenital cardiac defects: identification of residual problems necessitating reoperation. J Am Soc Echocardiogr 1993;6:356–365.

Stewart WJ, Currie PJ, Salcedo EE, et al. Intraoperative Doppler color flow mapping for decision-making in valve repair for mitral regurgitation. Technique and results in 100 patients. Circulation 1990;81:556–566.

Diseases of the Aorta

Evaluation of the intrathoracic portion of the aorta and of aortic disease has become a major use of transesophageal echocardiography. Although transthoracic echocardiography provides only a limited view of the proximal ascending aorta and a small portion of the descending aorta behind the left atrium, transesophageal echocardiography provides a high-resolution view of the entire length of the aorta from the aortic valve to approximately the diaphragm. Both normal anatomy and pathologic states can be identified with an accuracy equivalent to that of the competing techniques of computed tomography and magnetic resonance imaging. The speed with which this can be accomplished, often in a portable or intensive care unit setting, confers obvious advantages with respect to the emergency evaluation of aortic dissection, suspected aortic trauma, or in the otherwise critically ill. Transthoracic echocardiography retains a valuable role for screening and serial follow-up of diseases such as Marfan syndrome, which predominantly affects the proximal ascending aorta. Multiple diseases affect different portions of the aorta. These are outlined in Table 20.1 and include dilation (anuloaortic ectasia) and aneurysm formation, atherosclerosis, acute and chronic dissection, coarctation, and various forms of arteritis.

NORMAL AORTIC ANATOMY

The normal aorta can be considered to consist of six discrete segments. These are schematized in Figures 20.1 and 20.2 and consist of the anulus, Valsalva sinuses, sinotubular junction, ascending tubular aorta, the arch, and the descending thoracic aorta. The proximal portion, from the anulus to the proximal ascending aorta, is commonly referred to as the aortic root. The aortic anulus represents the junction of the proximal ascending aorta with the left ventricular outflow tract. It is part of the fibrous skeleton of the heart and is contiguous with the anterior mitral valve leaflet and perimembranous septum. Because the anulus is a fibrous structure, it is relatively

resistant to dilation and represents a relatively stable dimension to which the remaining aortic sizes can be indexed. Typically, the aortic anulus measures 13 ± 1.0 mm/M^2. The normal aorta dilates at the level of the sinuses by approximately 6 mm/M^2 and then tapers to within 2 to 3 mm of anular size at the sinotubular junction (Fig. 20.1). Normally there are three Valsalva sinuses of roughly equal size. The right and left sinuses contain the ostia of the right and left coronary arteries, respectively. The takeoff of the left coronary artery can be visualized from both transthoracic and transesophageal echocardiography in the left Valsalva sinus where its position is relatively closer to the anulus than is the takeoff

▶ **TABLE 20.1 Diseases Affecting the Aorta**

Atherosclerotic
  Aneurysm
  Atheroembolic disease
  Rupture
  Pseudoaneurysm
  Penetrating ulcer
  Dissection
  Intramural hematoma
Non-atherosclerotic
  Cystic medial necrosis
  Aneurysm
  Aortic dissection
  Intramural hematoma
  Anuloaortic ectasia
Inflammatory/infectious
  Takayasu arteritis
  Giant cell arteritis
  Endocarditis
Miscellaneous
  Trauma
  Intraluminal thrombus
  Poststenotic dilation
  Hypertension
  Aortic insufficiency/Stenosis
  Iatrogenic injury

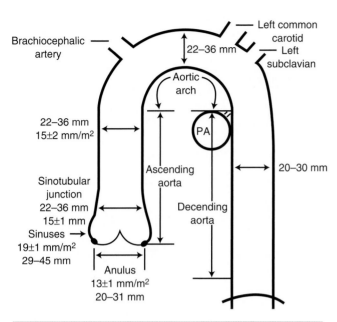

FIGURE 20.1. Schematic of normal aortic anatomy. The thoracic aortic can be characterized as having three distinct segments. The ascending aorta consists of that portion that extends from the anulus to the innominate artery and includes the three Valsalva sinuses, the three cusps of the aortic valve, the sinotubular junction, the ostia of the coronary arteries, and the proximal ascending aorta. The arch is defined as that portion that extends from a left innominate to the *ligamentum arteriosum* and includes the great vessels arising off of the arch. The descending thoracic aorta extends from the *ligamentum arteriosum* to the level of the diaphragm. The normal dimensions of the aorta are noted on the schematic and vary with location. Dimensions are given both indexed to body surface area (*BSA*) and as the range anticipated in routine adult echocardiography. PA, right pulmonary artery.

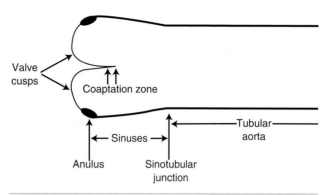

FIGURE 20.2. Detailed schematic of the proximal aorta. The relative dimensions of the anulus, Valsalva sinuses, sinotubular junction, and proximal ascending aorta can be appreciated. In the normal disease-free state, the sinuses dilate symmetrically so that their greatest dimension exceeds that of the anulus by approximately 6 mm/m^2 of body surface area. At the level of the sinotubular junction, the aorta narrows to within 2 to 3 mm of its anular dimension and then gradually tapers throughout its course. Note that the aortic cusps coapt along a 2 to 3 mm coaptation zone and do not meet tip to tip.

ECHOCARDIOGRAPHIC EVALUATION

As noted previously, only the proximal 4 to 5 cm of the ascending aorta and arch can be evaluated with transthoracic echocardiography. Typically, the proximal aorta can be seen in its long and short axis from the parasternal view. Figure 20.3 is a parasternal long-axis view of the heart with superior angulation that emphasizes visualization of the normal ascending aorta. Note the relative dimensions of the anulus, sinuses, sinotubular junction, and ascending aorta, which can be accurately determined from this transthoracic image. The suprasternal notch provides an additional window for visualization of the arch and great vessels of the aorta. Figure 20.4 was recorded in a normal individual in whom the majority of the arch and great vessels can be easily visualized. Imaging from the suprasternal view often is more feasible in children and adolescents than in adult patients. It should be emphasized that placement of the ultrasound probe in the suprasternal notch not infrequently results in mild patient discomfort, of which the examiner should be aware. Finally, transthoracic echocardiography can visualize a limited portion of the descending thoracic aorta in both its long- and short-axis view as it courses behind the left atrium. Figure 20.5 is a depiction of the normal descending thoracic aorta as visualized behind the left atrium. In the parasternal long-axis view, the descending thoracic aorta appears as a circular structure behind the left atrium. On occasion, it can be confused with a dilated coronary sinus; however, the proximity of the coronary sinus to the atrioventricular groove as well as the more

of the right coronary artery, which tends to be more superior and closer to the sinotubular junction.

The geometry of the sinotubular junction is a crucial feature of normal aortic valve coaptation. Insertion of aortic valve cusps is continuous from the level of the anulus up through the sinuses to the level of the sinotubular junction. Dilation of the sinotubular junction can result in splaying of the coaptation line of the aortic cusps resulting in secondary aortic insufficiency. The dimension of the normal ascending aorta is similar to that of the sinotubular junction. The ascending aorta terminates at the left innominate artery (brachiocephalic artery) where the aortic arch begins and continues to the left subclavian and ligamentum arteriosum. The three major branch vessels of the arch, the right innominate artery, and the left carotid and subclavian arteries can be visualized in the majority of patients from a suprasternal transthoracic as well as a transesophageal approach. The dimension of the ascending aorta, arch, and descending thoracic aorta are all similar with slight tapering in the descending thoracic aorta.

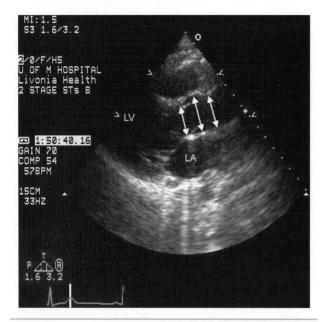

FIGURE 20.3. Transthoracic parasternal long-axis view of the normal aorta. This view includes the normal attachment of the anterior mitral valve leaflet to the posterior wall of the aorta and also visualization of the left atrium. Note the similar relationship in size of the anatomically viewed aorta compared with the schematic in Figure 20.2. *Arrows,* internal limits of the aorta.

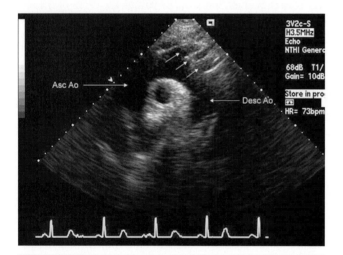

FIGURE 20.4. Transthoracic view of the arch of the aorta from a suprasternal view. Note the normal caliber of the arch of the aorta, which is similar to that of the proximal ascending aorta, and the orientation of the innominate artery and left carotid and subclavian arteries (*arrows*). AscAo, ascending aorta; DescAo, descending aorta.

rigid shape of the aorta should be accurate discriminating features.

Transesophageal echocardiography provides a substantially broader window to aortic anatomy and pathology than does transthoracic echocardiography. The aorta

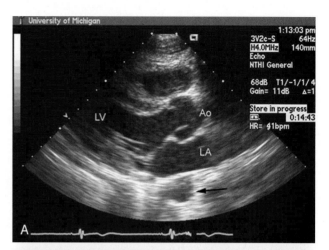

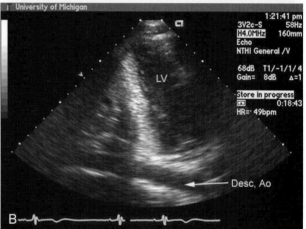

FIGURE 20.5. Transthoracic echocardiograms depict the appearance of a normal descending thoracic aorta. **A:** Parasternal long-axis view of the heart in which the normal circular descending thoracic aorta can be seen behind the left atrium (*arrow*). **B:** Longitudinal view of the descending thoracic aorta coursing behind the heart.

can be visualized from the anulus through the ascending and arch portions and the descending thoracic aorta to the level of the gastroesophageal junction. Figures 20.6 through 20.9 are transesophageal echocardiographic images recorded in a patient with a normal thoracic aorta. The relative sizes of the anulus, sinuses, sinotubular junction, and proximal ascending aorta can be appreciated in Figure 20.6. By imaging at a 30-degree image plane, the three sinuses and aortic cusps can be visualized simultaneously (Fig. 20.7). The arch and descending portions of the aorta can be easily appreciated as well (Figs. 20.8 and 20.9).

Typically, transesophageal echocardiographic imaging of the aorta begins with imaging of the ascending aorta with the probe behind the left atrium. Generally, the proximal 5 to 10 cm of the ascending aorta can be vi-

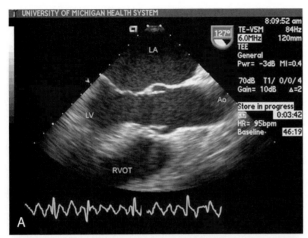

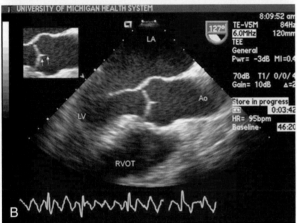

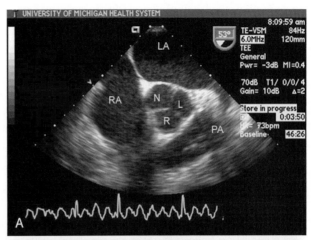

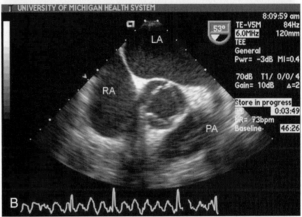

FIGURE 20.6. Transesophageal longitudinal view of the heart including visualization of the ascending aorta. Transesophageal echocardiogram of the ascending aorta recorded in a normal disease-free individual. **A:** Longitudinal (127-degree) view that provides imaging analogous to that of the transthoracic long-axis view seen in Figure 20.3. Again note the symmetric dilation at the level of the sinuses and the narrowing at the level of the sinotubular junction. **B:** Image recorded in systole demonstrates closure of the aortic cusps along a 2 to 3 mm length (*arrows in the small inset*).

FIGURE 20.7. Transesophageal echocardiogram recorded at 53-degree probe rotation at the base of the heart. These images were acquired at the same transducer position as those in Figure 20.6. With this probe orientation, a short-axis view of the aorta is obtained at the level of the sinuses, revealing the left (*L*), right (*R*), and non (*N*) coronary sinuses. The left atrium (*LA*), right atrium (*RA*), and proximal pulmonary artery (*PA*) are well visualized. **A:** Image recorded in diastole, and three symmetric sinuses are noted as well as three coaptation lines of the cusps. **B:** Image recorded in systole and shows the relatively triangular and symmetric opening of all three cusps.

sualized by scanning at a 120-degree imaging plane with the transesophageal probe in this position. By rotating the imaging plane to a 30-60 degree view, a series of short-axis views of the proximal ascending aorta can be obtained including a short-axis view of aortic valve closure (Fig. 20.7). The descending thoracic aorta is imaged next by inserting the probe deeper toward the gastroesophageal junction, rotating it 180 degrees to face posteriorly and scanning at a 0-degree imaging plane. The probe can then be slowly withdrawn along the length of the aorta and a continuous series of short-axis views of the thoracic aorta obtained (Fig. 20.8). At any point along the course of the aorta, the probe can be rotated to a 90-degree plane for a longitudinal view of the aorta. In

elderly patients, the aorta tends to become more tortuous, and slight rotation of the probe is frequently necessary to maintain the short axis of the aorta in the center of the imaging plane. When visualizing the arch, it should be emphasized that the probe will be at a relatively shallow depth (20 to 30 cm from the incisors), which results in a more dramatic curvature of the probe in the oropharynx. This probe position is less well tolerated by many patients than are deeper probe positions. The arch is best visualized by slowly withdrawing the probe to the level of the left subclavian artery, and as the probe is further withdrawn, it is rotated clockwise to obtain an elongated view of the arch (Fig. 20.9). At the point that the arch is seen at the apex of the scanning

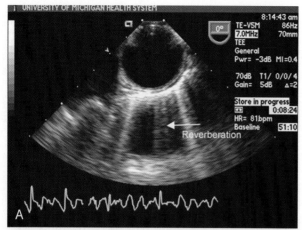

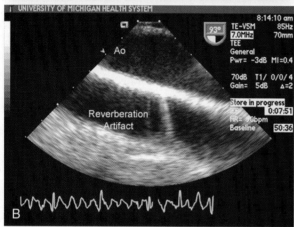

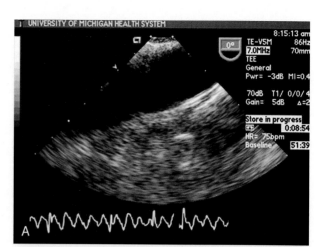

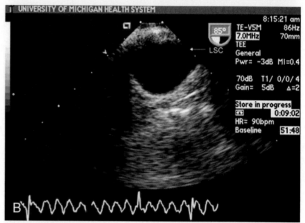

FIGURE 20.8. Transesophageal echocardiogram of the descending thoracic aorta. **A:** Recorded at 0 degrees and provides a short-axis view of a circular and symmetric normal aorta with little or no atherosclerotic disease. Because of the highly reflective nature of the aortic wall, a reverberation artifact mimicking a second aorta behind the real image is frequently encountered. **B:** Recorded with the imaging plane at 90 degrees providing a longitudinal view of the descending thoracic aorta.

FIGURE 20.9. Transesophageal echocardiographic view of the arch of the aorta. **A:** Recorded with the imaging plane at 0 degrees with marked clockwise rotation of the probe. In occasional patients, even more marked probe angulation can allow visualization of the ascending aorta to a level near to the sinotubular junction. **B:** Recorded from the same transducer position with the probe at a 85-degree angle providing a short-axis view of the apex of the arch. The takeoff of the left subclavian (*LSC*) can often be visualized from this view.

plane, the multiplane probe can be rotated to a 90-degree angle and a short-axis view of the apex of the arch can be recorded. By rotating clockwise and counterclockwise, the takeoff of the great vessels can often be visualized from this view.

A final ultrasound modality that has been used in evaluation of the aorta is intravascular ultrasound (Fig. 20.10). This can be performed with high-frequency (20–30 MHz) transducers or more recently with an intracardiac probe operating at 5.5 to 10 MHz. These higher frequency probes provide a highly detailed, high-resolution view of intraaortic anatomy including visualization of intimal and medial layers when using the higher frequency probes. Intravascular ultrasound has been used in the di-

agnosis and management of aortic dissection and as a primary imaging tool to monitor therapeutic fenestration performed for acute aortic dissection. Intravascular ultrasound has the advantage of being able to image the entire aorta, from the root to the iliac artery. It clearly demonstrates the true and false lumens, the dissection flap, and thrombosed false lumen. It can also demonstrate the origin of each of the abdominal aortic branches (iliac artery, mesenteric branches, renal arteries), detecting whether they arise from true or false lumen. Intimal tear sites can also be imaged. Determination of aortic segment dimensions by this technique correlate precisely with computed tomographic and transesophageal echocardiographic measurements.

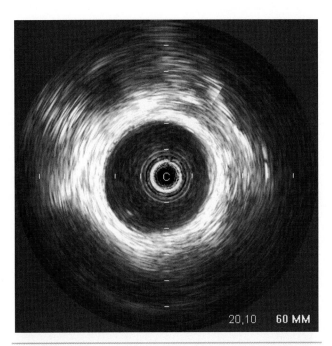

FIGURE 20.10. Intravascular ultrasound (*IVUS*) of the thoracic aorta. The intravascular ultrasound probe is in the lumen of the descending thoracic aorta. Note the circular smooth lumen of the aorta. From approximately 2 o'clock to 4 o'clock there is minimal intimal thickening, consistent with early atheroma formation.

AORTIC DILATION AND ANEURYSM

Dilation of the aorta can occur at any point along its course. It is important to recognize that identification of disease in one portion of the aorta should be an indication for evaluation of the full extent of the aorta because many diseases affecting one portion of the aorta can also have manifestations in other areas. Dilation of the aorta can either be primary or secondary. Idiopathic dilation and tortuosity have often been referred to as anuloaortic ectasia. It is unclear whether this is a distinct disease entity or related to the effects of aging, hypertension, or unrecognized primary disease of the aorta. Primary aortic dilation occurs with cystic medial necrosis, as typified by Marfan syndrome, but is also seen in other connective tissue diseases. Cystic medial necrosis is also seen as a secondary feature of many other forms of chronic aortic pathology. This process results in weakening of the medial layers with subsequent dilation and aneurysm formation of the aorta. When associated with Marfan syndrome, it characteristically involves the ascending aorta and sinuses. Secondary dilation of the aorta can occur in volume or pressure overload states such as aortic insufficiency or hypertension. Poststenotic aortic dilation occurs in patients with valvular aortic stenosis.

Dilation of the proximal ascending aorta can often be appreciated from the transthoracic parasternal long-axis view. Figures 20.11 through 20.14 were recorded in patients with varying degrees of ascending aortic dilation. As noted previously, the aortic anulus is a relatively stable structure that does not dilate. Proximal aortic dilation is far more common and predominates in the sinuses, sinotubular junction, and ascending aortic areas. In Figure 20.12, note the gradual dilation of the aorta as it extends from the anulus to the ascending aorta. There has been effacement or loss of tapering at the sinotubular junction in this instance. The ascending aorta then progressively dilates. Frank aneurysms can occur in the ascending aorta but typically do so past the sinotubular junction and are better visualized with transesophageal echocardiography. Figures 20.13 through 20.15 were recorded in patients with ascending aortic aneurysms. Note the fairly broad range of both dilation and asymmetry that can be seen in ascending aortic aneurysms.

For patients with dilation or aneurysm of the ascending aorta, the likelihood of rupture or spontaneous dissection is directly related to the degree of dilation. Typically, a threshold of 55 mm is considered an indication for prophylactic aortic surgery in an effort to reduce the likelihood of a catastrophic event such as rupture or dissec-

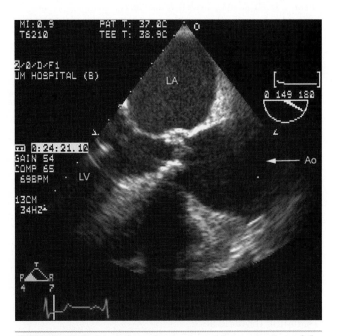

FIGURE 20.11. Transthoracic parasternal long-axis view of the ascending aorta recorded in a patient with significant valvular aortic stenosis and proximal aortic dilation. Note the dilation of the aorta at the level of the sinuses, sinotubular junction, and proximal ascending aorta. This represents poststenotic dilation. In many instances, dilation to the degree seen here may be due to both disease of the aortic valve and concurrent aortic aneurysm. Ao, aorta; LA, left atrium; LV, left ventricle.

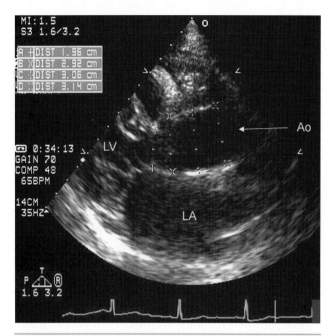

FIGURE 20.12. Parasternal long-axis view of the left ventricle and aorta demonstrates a dilated ascending aorta with effacement of the sinotubular junction. There is classic effacement, with the sinotubular junction having the same dimension as the Valsalva sinus. The dimension at each segment of the aorta is as noted. Effacement of the sinotubular junction often results in aortic insufficiency due to malcoaptation of the aortic cusps. Ao, aorta; LA, left atrium; LV, left ventricle.

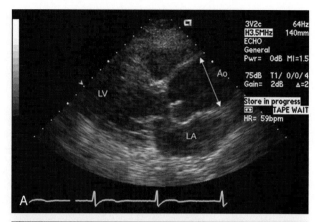

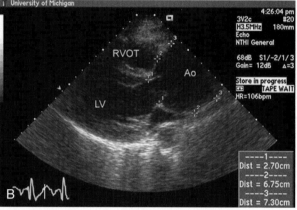

FIGURE 20.13. Parasternal long axis thoracic echocardiograms recorded in patients with ascending aortic aneurysms. **A:** Note the relatively normal dimension of the anulus and sinuses with maximal dilation in true ascending aorta (Ao) which measures approximately 43 mm in greatest dimension. **B:** There is more diffuse dilation that begins at the sinuses and continues at the level of the sinotubular junction. The maximal dimension is 73 mm, as noted by the measurement bar in the lower right. LA, left atrium; LV, left ventricle; RVOT, right ventricular outflow tract.

tion. Additionally, a rapid change in the degree of dilation, usually defined as more than 5 mm per year is often used as an indication for surgery. As operation success and outcomes have improved and risk reduced with advances in technique, many centers are using a lower threshold (typically >50 mm) as an indication for surgery.

Aneurysms of the arch and descending thoracic aorta can also be accurately diagnosed and followed using transesophageal echocardiography. Aneurysms of the descending thoracic aorta frequently coexist with substantial atherosclerotic involvement, which can include protruding and mobile components as well as laminar thrombus. Figures 20.15 through 20.19 were recorded in patients with arch and descending thoracic aortic aneurysms. The same considerations regarding size and likelihood of rupture and need for prophylactic surgical repair pertain to the descending thoracic aorta as for the ascending thoracic aorta.

MARFAN SYNDROME

Marfan Syndrome is a heritable disorder of connective tissue that is associated with characteristic cardiac abnormalities. These include marked dilation of predominantly the ascending aorta where the sinuses typically are disproportionately involved. Early cases may have only

mild dilation of the sinus with sinotubular effacement. The sinotubular effacement results in malcoaptation of the aortic valve and secondary aortic insufficiency. Figures 20.20 through 20.23 were recorded in individuals with Marfan syndrome and proximal aortic involvement. The range of aortic dilation can be relatively mild, as seen in Figure 20.20A, or massive, as seen in Figures 20.20B and 20.21. Aortic insufficiency occurs in Marfan syndrome due to dilation of the sinotubular junction, which results in loss of normal aortic valve coaptation. Figures 20.22 and 20.23 were recorded in patients with significant aortic insufficiency due to sinotubular dilation.

Typically, transthoracic echocardiography suffices for monitoring the size and change in proximal aortic dimensions. Once aortic abnormalities have been noted in a patient with suspected Marfan syndrome, it is important to further characterize cardiac anatomy because there is a high prevalence of mitral valve prolapse as well. Be-

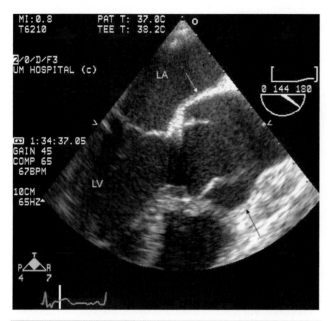

FIGURE 20.14. Transesophageal echocardiogram recorded in a patient with an ascending aortic aneurysm. Recorded in a longitudinal (144-degree probe angle) view demonstrating the marked dilation of the ascending aorta beginning at the Valsalva sinuses. The outer boundary of the sinuses is noted by the arrows.

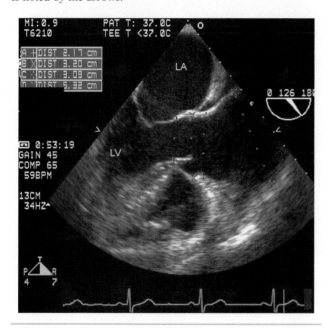

FIGURE 20.15. Transesophageal echocardiogram reveals a large aneurysm of the ascending aorta. Note the somewhat asymmetric dilation with a maximal dimension of 53 mm in the ascending aorta, distal to the sinotubular junction. LA, left atrium; LV, left ventricle.

cause of its noninvasive nature, transthoracic echocardiography should be considered the initial screening tool for patients or first-degree relatives with suspected Marfan syndrome and transesophageal echocardiography reserved only for further specific characterization.

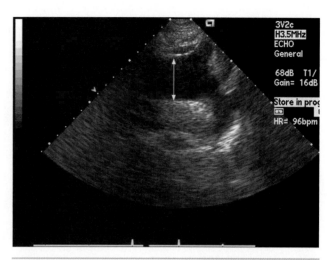

FIGURE 20.16. Transthoracic suprasternal notch view of the aortic arch recorded in a patient with an ascending and arch aneurysm. Note the pathologically dilated arch (38 mm), which was contiguous with a more proximal ascending aortic aneurysm.

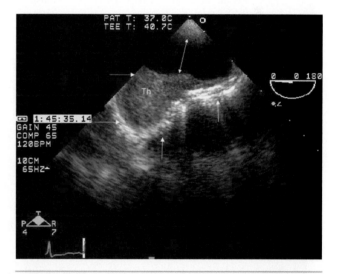

FIGURE 20.17. Transesophageal echocardiogram of the aortic arch shows a discrete aneurysm of the arch. The lumen of the arch is noted by the *double-headed arrow*. The remaining *horizontal and vertical arrows* outline the boundary of the discrete aneurysm, which is filled with a thrombus (*Th*).

VALSALVA SINUS ANEURYSM

Aneurysms can form from any of the three Valsalva sinuses but most often arise from the right sinus. They can be highly variable in size and by definition communicate with the sinus by a relatively wide mouth. The overall length of a Valsalva sinus aneurysm can reach substantial portions, and Valsalva sinus aneurysms 5 to 8 cm in length have been described. Aneurysms arising from the right Valsalva sinus typically protrude down into the right atrium where they are often initially visualized as a fila-

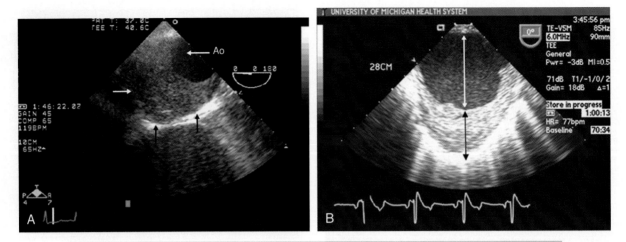

FIGURE 20.18. Transesophageal echocardiogram of a descending thoracic aortic aneurysm. **A:** In the upper right, one can appreciate the actual flow containing lumen of the aorta (*Ao*). The *black vertical and remaining horizontal white arrow* delineate the absolute external boundary of the aorta and the maximal dimensions of the aneurysm, which is largely filled with a thrombus and atheroma. **B:** A descending thoracic aortic aneurysm is depicted. The *double-headed white arrow* outlines the dimension of the aortic lumen. The *double-headed black arrow* denotes a thrombus and atheroma filling an aneurysmal cavity. The total dimension of the aorta would be the summed lengths of *black and white arrows*.

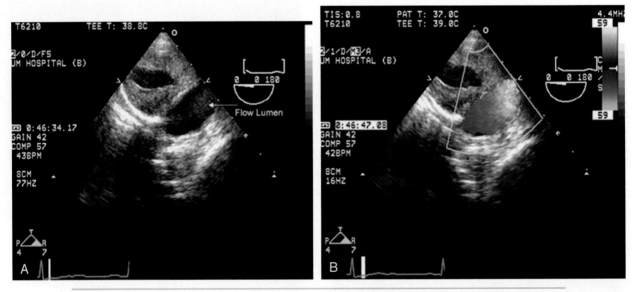

FIGURE 20.19. Short-axis view of a descending thoracic aorta with aneurysm and chronic dissection. **A:** Short-axis view of the aorta at the mid-thoracic level. Note the maximal dimension, which exceeds 4 cm. Note also that a substantial portion of the lumen is filled with thrombus, which in turn contains a lucent nonflow cavity. The flow containing lumen is at the lower right of the image. **B:** Color flow Doppler has been employed to demonstrate flow in the larger lumen.

mentous or "windsock" structure in the right atrium. A Valsalva sinus aneurysm arising from the noncoronary sinus can dissect inferiorly into the interventricular septum where it is noted as a cystic structure in the ventricular septum. The differential of a cystic structure in the proximal septum would include an echinococcal cyst as well. Less frequently, Valsalva sinus aneurysms protrude into the left atrium.

Figures 20.24 through 20.27 were recorded in patients with Valsalva sinus aneurysms. Note in Figure 20.26 the Valsalva sinus aneurysm arising from the right sinus, which protrudes into the right atrium. With only grayscale imaging, it appears as a highly mobile, filamentous mass in the right atrium. The addition of color Doppler often provides definitive clues as to the nature of these echos because the "windsock" anatomy of the aneurysm

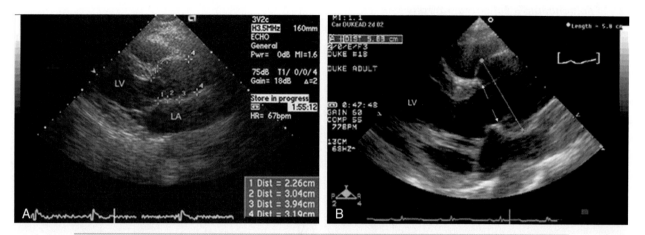

FIGURE 20.20. A: Parasternal long-axis transthoracic echocardiogram recorded in patients with Marfan syndrome. Notice the pathologic dilation of the aorta comparing the anulus (point 1) to the Valsalva sinuses (point 2) and the sinotubular junction (point 3). The aorta narrows to a nearly normal dimension in its ascending portion (point 4). **B:** Recorded in a patient with substantially greater dilation at the level of the sinuses, which measure 5.8 cm compared with 2.8 cm at the anulus. LA, left atrium; LV, left ventricle.

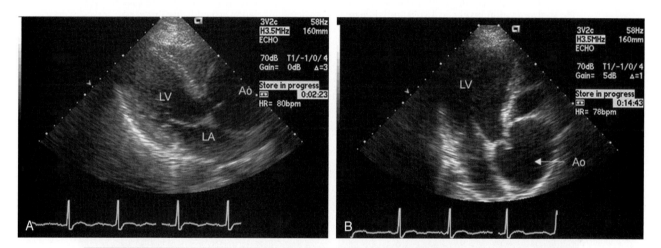

FIGURE 20.21. Parasternal long-axis **(A)** and apical transthoracic **(B)** views in a patient with Marfan syndrome. In each instance, note the marked dilation of the proximal aorta (*Ao*), which is maximal at the level of the Valsalva sinuses. **B:** Often the dilated proximal aorta may compress the right atrium. LA, left atrium; LV, left ventricle.

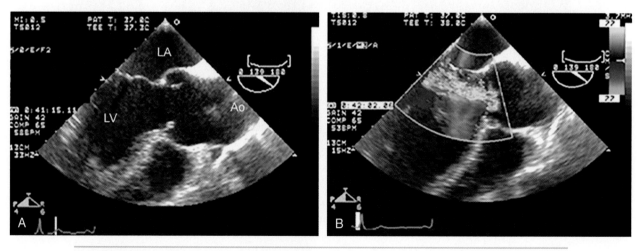

FIGURE 20.22. A: Longitudinal plane transesophageal echocardiogram recorded in a patient with Marfan syndrome and proximal aortic dilation. Again, note the effacement of the sinotubular junction, which has resulted in malcoaptation of the aortic cusps and significant aortic regurgitation as noted in the color flow Doppler image **(B)**. Ao, aorta; LA, left atrium; LV, left ventricle.

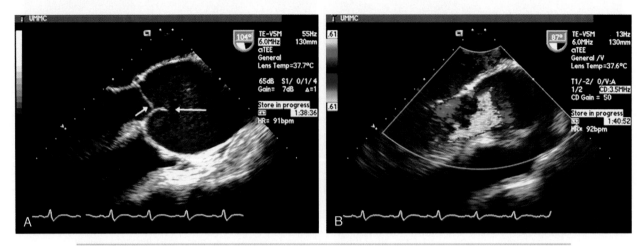

FIGURE 20.23. Transesophageal longitudinal view of the ascending aorta recorded in a patient with Marfan syndrome. Note the marked dilation of the aortic sinuses with some tapering at the level of the sinotubular junction. Note, however, that the sinotubular junction dimension still exceeds the anular dimension by a substantial degree. Note also the malcoaptation of the aortic cusps with the normal position of the left cusp (*horizontal arrow*) and malcoaptation of the noncoronary cusp (*angled arrow*). The malcoaptation results in a substantial degree of aortic insufficiency, which is highly eccentric, the initial portion of which is directed posteriorly to anteriorly (top to bottom) on the accompanying color flow Doppler image.

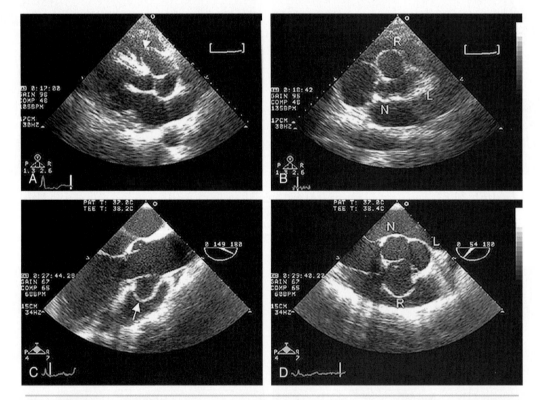

FIGURE 20.24. Valsalva sinus aneurysm recorded from a transthoracic echocardiogram (**A, B**) and transesophageal echocardiogram (**C, D**). All images are from the same patient. **A:** Note the marked asymmetric bulging of the right Valsalva sinus into the right ventricular outflow tract (*arrow*). This is appreciable both on the parasternal long-axis view (upper left) and parasternal short-axis view (upper right). Virtually identical anatomy is seen in the longitudinal and short-axis views of the ascending aorta recorded from the transesophageal approach (**C, D**). L, N, R; left, non-, and right Valsalva sinuses.

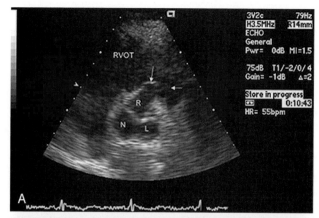

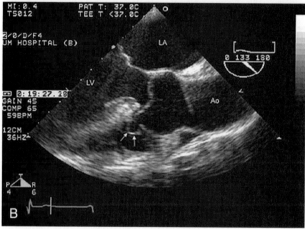

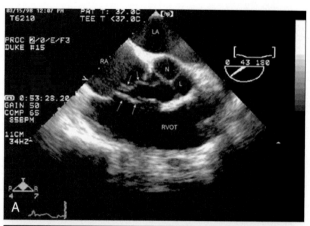

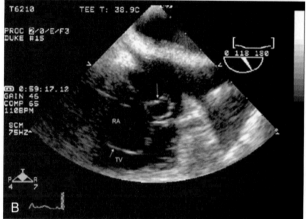

FIGURE 20.25. Short-axis transthoracic echocardiogram at the base of the heart. Note the marked asymmetric bulging of the Valsalva sinus into the right ventricular outflow tract (RVOT) (*arrows*). **B:** Longitudinal transesophageal view image of the aorta from the same patient. Note the aneurysm of the right sinus prolapsing along the ventricular septum into the right ventricular outflow tract (*arrows*). Ao, aorta; LA, left atrium; LV, left ventricle; RVOT, right ventricular outflow tract; L, N, R, left, non-, and right Valsalva sinuses.

FIGURE 20.26. Transesophageal echocardiogram of a Valsalva sinus aneurysm arising from the right coronary sinus. **A:** Recorded at 43-degree probe rotation. Note the normal size and geometry of the left (*L*) and non- (*N*) coronary sinuses and the elongated windsock aneurysm rising off the right coronary sinus (*arrows*) and protruding into the right atrium (RA). **B:** Recorded at a 118-degree image plane (orthogonal to that in **A**), and the aneurysm now appears as a circular or cystic, highly mobile structure in the right atrium (*arrow*). Note the position of the tricuspid valve (*TV*) as well. RVOT, right ventricular outflow tract.

can be more fully appreciated when it contains the abnormal color flow signal (Fig. 20.27). The major complication of a Valsalva sinus aneurysm is spontaneous rupture. The most common location for a Valsalva sinus aneurysm to rupture is into the right atrium where it results in instantaneous elevation of right heart pressures, jugular venous distention, and a loud continuous murmur. Other complications of a Valsalva sinus aneurysm include distortion of normal coronary sinus anatomy, which can result in malcoaptation of the aortic valve cusps and subsequent aortic insufficiency. Although a Valsalva sinus aneurysm can be suspected from transthoracic imaging, when a highly mobile echo is noted in the right atrium with color flow contained within it, transesophageal echocardiography provides a definitive diagnosis and is probably essential in all cases for full characterization of the aneurysm (Fig. 20.27).

An abnormality closely related to the Valsalva sinus aneurysm is the fibrosa aneurysm. This is an exception-

ally rare entity in which an aneurysm forms in the fibrous skeleton of the heart and communicates with one of the Valsalva sinuses via a relatively narrow neck. These frequently are seen as a cystic space between the aorta and left atrium. As with the Valsalva sinus aneurysm, transesophageal echocardiography is probably essential for the definitive diagnosis of this entity.

AORTIC DISSECTION

Acute aortic dissection occurs with an incidence of 10 to 20 per million population. It is a syndrome that results in sudden onset of severe chest and/or back pain with a wide range of secondary cardiovascular and physiologic abnormalities. It typically occurs in the setting of preexisting aortic dilation, cystic medial fibrosis due to Marfan syn-

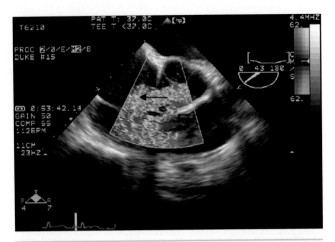

FIGURE 20.27. Transesophageal echocardiogram with color flow Doppler imaging in a patient with a Valsalva sinus aneurysm. This image was recorded at 43 degrees, providing a short-axis view of the Valsalva sinus aneurysm. This image was recorded from the same transducer position and probe rotation as that in Figure 20.26A. Note the high volume and highly turbulent flow from the right Valsalva sinus into and through the aneurysmal cavity before emerging in the right atrium and right ventricular outflow tract.

The classic type of aortic dissection typically begins either at the area of the *ligamentum arteriosum* and propagates proximally through the arch and into the ascending aorta or starts in the ascending aorta and propagates distally. On occasion, patients may present with a limited intimal tear without dissection. This variant may be associated with only very subtle abnormalities on transesophageal echocardiography or other imaging techniques.

The second pathophysiology for aortic dissection is the spontaneous intramural hematoma. The clinical presentation with respect to the nature of symptoms is virtually identical to that of classic dissection, and most authorities believe that it requires the same approach with respect to therapy. The hemorrhage into the medial layer then dissects proximally or distally to a variable degree, without rupturing into the lumen. Intramural hemorrhage may progress to rupture into the adventitia, resulting in typical aortic dissection. The clinical presentation, prognosis, and forms of therapy for these two different mechanisms of acute aortic pathology are similar. A more recently recognized variant of acute aortic pathology is the so-called intramural hematoma without dissection. In this instance, a relatively limited area of acute hemorrhage occurs in the medial layer but does not propagate.

Aortic dissections are characterized by their location using either the Stanford or DeBakey schemes. Figure 20.29 schematizes the two different characterization schemes. The crucial factor in aortic dissection is whether it involves the ascending aorta (Stanford A or DeBakey I or II). These patients have a greater likelihood of subsequent rupture, pericardial effusion, aortic insufficiency, and coronary involvement, all of which may be lethal complications of acute dissection. Ascending aortic dis-

drome, or long-standing hypertension. Any aspect of the aorta can dissect. Aortic dissection is typically characterized as one of two basic variants, each of which has a similar presentation with respect to symptoms (Fig. 20.28).

Classic aortic dissection consists of a tear from the lumen through the intima into the medial layer with subsequent propagation of a column of blood, which then further dissects the intima away from the media. Propagation can be both proximal and distal to the initial intimal tear.

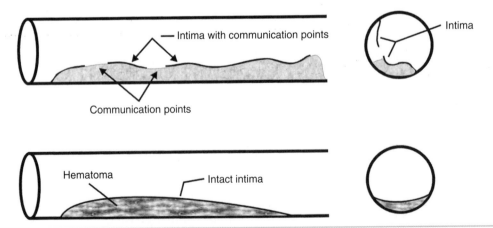

FIGURE 20.28. Schematic representation depicts the forms of acute aortic pathology. **A:** Depicts classic aortic dissection in which there is a tear of the intima from the media. The column of blood propagates proximally and distally, and there may be multiple communication points between the lumen and the intima media space. **B:** The spontaneous intramural hematoma variant of aortic dissection in which there is rupture of the vasa vasorum resulting in hematoma in the medial space without communication between the lumen and the hematoma is depicted. The two right-hand schematics depict the same phenomenon in a short-axis view of the aorta.

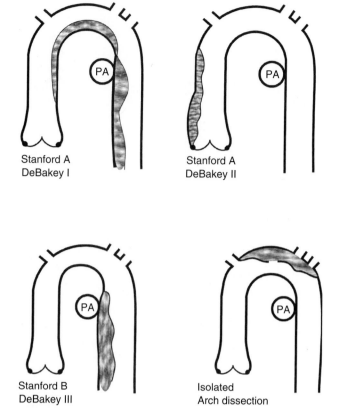

FIGURE 20.29. Schematic representation of categorization schemes for aortic dissection. The schematics include the typical distinction of proximal ascending dissection as well as distal dissection. Additionally, the more recently appreciated isolated arch dissection is likewise depicted. PA, pulmonary artery.

section is considered a surgical emergency for which rapid, accurate diagnosis is essential and in which transesophageal echocardiography plays a crucial role. Dissection isolated to the descending thoracic aorta (Stanford type B or DeBakey III) is best managed medically unless complications occur.

Echocardiographic Diagnosis

Because transthoracic echocardiography visualizes only a limited area of the ascending aorta, it generally is not considered an adequate diagnostic tool for detection of aortic dissection. Only a minority of ascending aortic dissections will be detected from the transthoracic window. Figures 20.30 and 20.31 are transthoracic echocardiograms recorded in patients with documented aortic dissection in which the proximal dissection flap can be identified. Additional imaging from the aortic arch and imaging of the descending thoracic aorta can supplement these views. The transthoracic echocardiogram can provide additional confirmatory information such as detection of proximal aortic dilation or aortic insufficiency (Fig. 20.30). Proxi-

mal aortic dilation is usually present in patients with ascending aortic dissection. Identification of normal aortic dimensions and geometry and the absence of aortic insufficiency from a transthoracic echocardiogram are strong evidence against the presence of an aortic dissection in the ascending aorta.

Transesophageal echocardiography has emerged as a primary diagnostic tool in the detection of aortic dissection, and large series have suggested that it is used in approximately two-thirds of patients with suspected acute aortic dissection. It can be performed in critically ill patients in intensive care units, the emergency department, and the operating room and provides a definitive diagnostic methodology. Additionally, complications such as pericardial effusion, aortic insufficiency, pseudoaneurysm, adventitial hematoma, and rupture can all be identified.

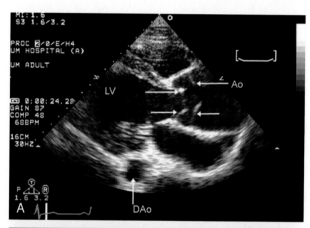
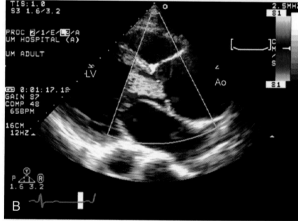

FIGURE 20.30. Transthoracic echocardiogram in a patient with acute type A dissection. **B:** Images are recorded in a parasternal long-axis view with color flow Doppler imaging. **A:** Note the marked dilation of the ascending aorta, which is nearly ubiquitous in type A dissection. The *rightward-pointing arrows* in the left ventricular outflow tract outline the actual aortic valve. The *leftward-pointing echoes* denote portions of the intimal flap. **B:** Note the significant amount of aortic regurgitation, which is due to malcoaptation of the aortic valve. DAo, descending aorta; LV, left ventricle.

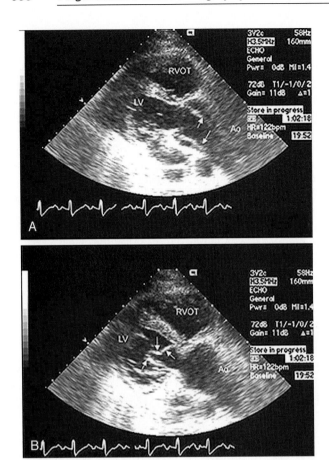

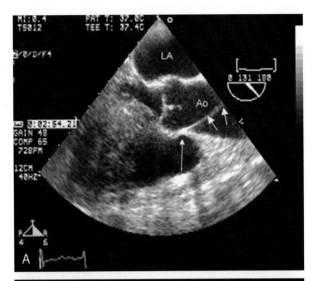

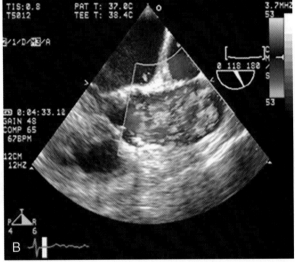

FIGURE 20.31. Parasternal long-axis view in systole **(A)** and diastole **(B)** in a patient with a type A dissection. **A:** Note the remnants of the intimal flap within the lumen of the dilated ascending aorta (*arrows*). In diastole, the intimal flap prolapses through the aortic valve into the left ventricular outflow tract. This is one of the several mechanisms for developing aortic insufficiency in acute aortic dissection. Ao, aorta; LV, left ventricle; RVOT, right ventricular outflow tract.

FIGURE 20.32. Transesophageal echocardiogram recorded in a longitudinal plane of the ascending aorta (Ao). This image shows a common artifact that could be confused with a dissection. This is a classic side lobe artifact arising (*small arrows*) from a rather bright echo at the sinotubular (*vertical arrow*) resulting in an unnaturally curvilinear echo extending along the direction of the scan plane lines within the lumen of the aorta. **B:** Color flow imaging has been superimposed. Note the lack of any margination of flow by the linear echo, helping to confirm that this is artifact rather than a true dissection flap. LA, left atrium.

When evaluating the ascending aorta, it is not uncommon to encounter artifactual echos within the aortic lumen. A skilled echocardiographer should not have difficulty in separating these from aortic dissection. Clues to artifact versus true dissection include random mobility of a true dissection flap as opposed to a more rigid and fixed location with respect to the aortic wall seen in artifact. Artifacts not infrequently will arise as a side lobe from the sinotubular junction, and their intensity will progressively diminish in the lumen, whereas a true dissection flap will not lose its echo intensity along its course (Fig. 20.32). Color flow imaging can be very useful for demonstrating margination of flow by a true dissection flap, whereas an artifact will not affect the distribution of the color flow signal (Fig. 20.32B).

An additional confusing echo can be a superimposed venous structure coursing adjacent to the aorta. Typically, this represents the left brachiocephalic vein as it courses adjacent to the arch. The combination of the brachial cephalic vein and aorta creates a tubular echo, larger than that of the normal aorta with a linear solid structure running longitudinally. This can occasionally be confused with a dilated aorta with a dissection flap. Color flow imaging will reveal a color flow signal on both sides of the linear echo. Careful scrutiny of the color flow signal will clearly demonstrate that the larger lumen contains pulsatile flow representing the true aorta, and the smaller lumen contains continuous flow in a typical venous pattern (Figure 20.33). An additional method for identifying this as a venous structure is to inject agitated saline contrast into the

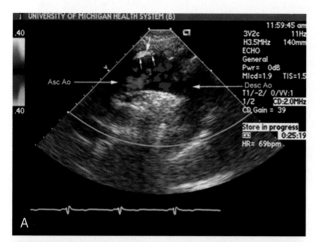

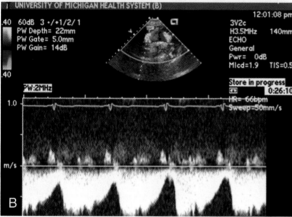

FIGURE 20.33. Venous flow adjacent to the aortic arch, mimicking aortic dissection (*arrow*). This represents normal venous communication from the superior vena cava with flow toward the heart. It is common to encounter this space, which can occasionally be confused for aortic dissection. As the structure contains normal venous flow, color flow Doppler will demonstrate a continuous color signal that should not be confused with flow into a false lumen. Use of spectral Doppler imaging will typically demonstrate a normal venous flow pattern (**B**). Contrast injection into an upper extremity vein will likewise demonstrate the true origin of this structure.

left upper extremity, at which point one can see the contrast confined to the smaller venous structure thereby definitively identifying it as the brachiocephalic vein.

It can occasionally be difficult to separate the true from the false lumen. Several clues enable accurate distinction of the two. In the ascending aorta, there is usually little confusion because one can appreciate the outlet of blood through the aortic valve, which, by definition, will be into the true lumen. Distinction between the true and false lumens may sometimes be more problematic in a short-axis view or in the descending thoracic aorta. Clues that enable accurate identification of the true lumen include the fact that it will expand with systole as blood is ejected into it. It often has a more regular shape, which may be either circular or oval. Often in the descending

thoracic aorta, the true lumen is the smaller of the two lumens. The false lumen is often filled with swirling homogeneous echoes, representing stasis of blood or occasionally with frank thrombus. Finally, the shearing of the intima from the media often results in small fibrinous tags of tissue in the false lumen, which represent small muscle remnants where the intima has been sheared from the media.

Figures 20.34 through 20.42 were recorded in patients with acute aortic dissections. Figure 20.34 is an example

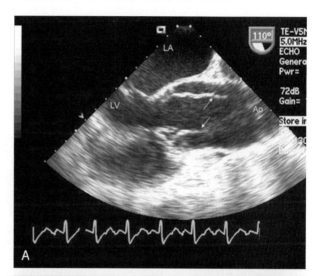

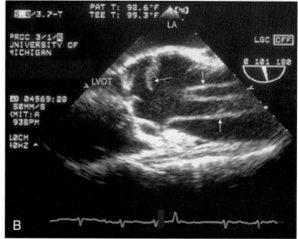

FIGURE 20.34. Transesophageal echocardiograms recorded in a longitudinal plane in two patients with a type A dissection. **A:** Note the two linear echos within the lumen of the aorta that represent margins of a nearly circumferential aortic dissection that extended from below the sinotubular junction into the ascending aorta (*arrows*). **B:** Recorded in a longitudinal plane in a patient with a greater degree of aortic dilation in a far more complex intimal flap. Note the multiple linear serpiginous echoes (*arrows*) within the lumen of the aorta that represent almost complete shearing off of the aortic intima. In real time, these echoes take on a highly mobile, undulating motion pattern in the blood flow. Ao, aorta; LA, left atrium; LV, left ventricle; LVOT, left ventricular outflow tract.

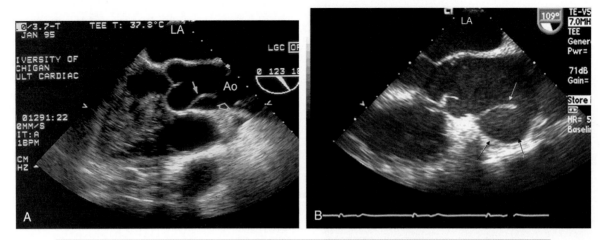

FIGURE 20.35. Transesophageal echocardiogram recorded in a longitudinal plane in two patients with type A dissection. **A:** Note the relatively normal aortic dimensions and the very limited dissection flap (*arrow*). A single communication point (*open arrowhead*) can be seen as well. **B:** A similarly localized aortic dissection (*white arrow*) is revealed. In this instance, however, note the fairly discrete aneurysmal bulge of the anterior wall of the aorta (*black arrows*). This was subsequently confirmed at the time of corrective surgery to represent a partial rupture of the aortic wall and small aortic pseudoaneurysm. Ao, aorta; LA, left atrium.

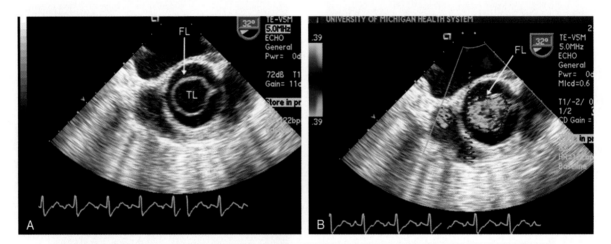

FIGURE 20.36. Transesophageal echocardiogram recorded in a short-axis view of the proximal ascending aorta in a patient with a circumferential type A dissection. Note the circular aorta containing a second circular structure that is the intimal flap, which now defines a circular true lumen (*TL*), surrounded by a ring shape and completely circumferential false lumen (*FL*). **B:** Note that color flow in systole is confined only to the smaller inner true lumen.

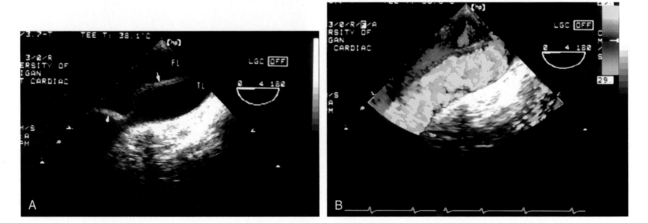

FIGURE 20.37. Transesophageal echocardiogram recorded in a patient with an aortic arch dissection. This image was recorded approximately 25 cm from the incisors at a 0-degree imaging plane and with clockwise rotation of the probe. Note the dilation of the aortic arch with the linear intimal flap running the length of the arch (*arrows*). Separating the true (*TL*) and false lumens (*FL*). **B:** Note the higher velocity systolic flow in the lower true lumen.

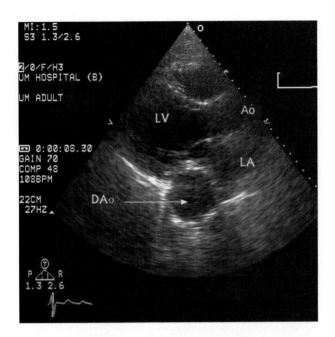

FIGURE 20.38. Parasternal long-axis transthoracic echocardiogram shows a markedly dilated descending aorta. Occasionally, the transthoracic echocardiogram revealing a dilated descending thoracic aorta (*DAo*) can be the first clue to the presence of a descending thoracic aneurysm or dissection. Ao, ascending aorta; LA, left atrium; LV, left ventricle.

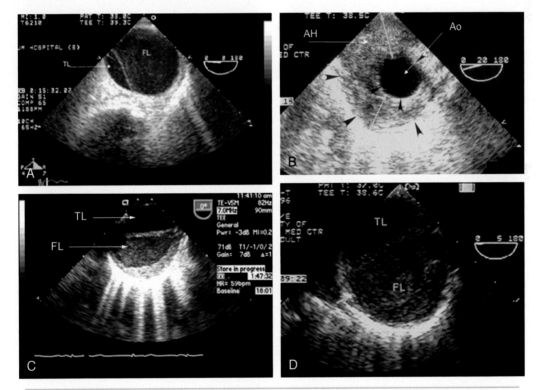

FIGURE 20.39. Transesophageal short-axis views of aortic dissection from four different patients. **A:** Note the relatively preserved circular geometry of the aorta, which is separated into a true lumen (*TL*) and substantially larger false lumen (*FL*). Note that the false lumen is filled with stagnant swirling blood. **C:** A type B dissection in which the true lumen and false lumen are of more equal size is demonstrated. Note also in this instance the atheromatous involvement of the anterior wall of the aorta. **B:** Recorded in a patient with a type B dissection. This image was recorded at a site in the aorta not involved by the dissection. Note the normal size circular aortic lumen (*Ao*) and the much larger homogeneous mass (*black arrowheads*) circumferentially surrounding the aorta. This represents a dissecting adventitial hematoma (AH) external to the aorta at this point. **D:** A type B dissection with a smaller, upper true lumen and a much larger false lumen. Note that the false lumen again contains stagnant swirling blood with some areas of lucency.

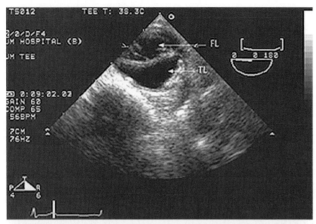

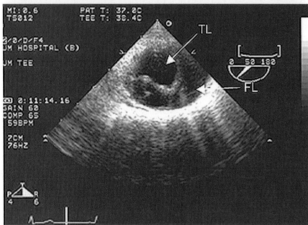

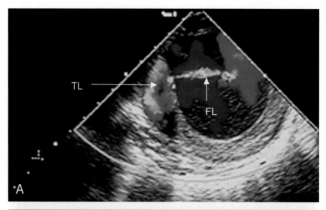

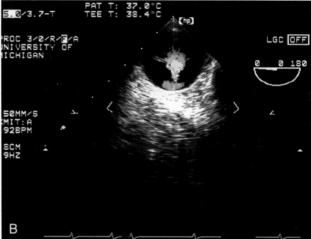

FIGURE 20.40. Transesophageal echocardiogram recorded in the descending thoracic aorta at two different levels with slightly different angulation. In each instance, notice the true and false lumens (TL and FL) and the ragged echoes present within the false lumen that represent combinations of organizing thrombus and aortic wall components that have been disrupted as part of the dissection.

FIGURE 20.41. Short-axis views of the aorta in two patients with type B dissection. **A:** Recorded in a patient with a chronic type B dissection and significant atheromatous involvement. Note the marked aortic dilation and the relatively small true lumen and much larger false lumen. A single entry point can be noted connecting the true and false lumens by a distinct color jet in systole (*vertical arrow*). **B:** Recorded in a patient with an acute type A dissection that extended into the descending thoracic aorta. Note the relatively normal aortic size at this point and the single fairly large communication point denoted by color flow Doppler imaging.

of a classic type A dissection in which multiple imaging planes reveal the pathology. Color flow imaging can be used to identify the communication points between the true and false lumens. It should be emphasized that the earlier concept of an entry and exit point with the dissection extending between these two points is not accurate. Most dissections will have multiple communication points between the true and false lumens at areas where intima has been sheared from the media. It is important to recognize the larger communication points because they have relevance for surgical repair.

Figures 20.38 through 20.42 were recorded in patients with type B dissections. In this location, there is frequently a substantial atherosclerotic component as well. On occasion, a dilated, descending aorta can be identified behind the atrioventricular groove in a parasternal long-axis view (Fig. 20.38). Detection of such an abnormality from the transthoracic echocardiogram may be the first clue to the presence of an aneurysm or dissection in the

descending aorta. In Figure 20.39B, note the substantial adventitial hematoma surrounding the otherwise normal segment of the aorta. In many instances, the adventitial hematoma can propagate along the course of the aorta in a manner similar to that of the dissection. It is often the adventitial hematoma that results in the abnormal aortic contour seen in chest radiography.

Intramural hematoma can occur at any point along the aorta but is more common in the descending aorta and arch. When visualized with transesophageal echocardiography, it appears as a smooth homogeneous crescentic thickening of the wall, typically more than 7 mm in thickness. By definition, there is no active flow within the "lumen" and no tear in the intima. It may extend a variable distance along the aortic length (Figs. 20.43 and 20.44).

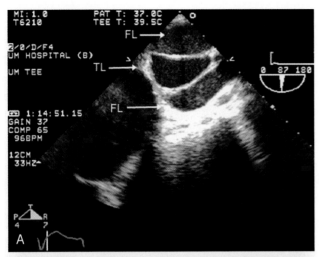

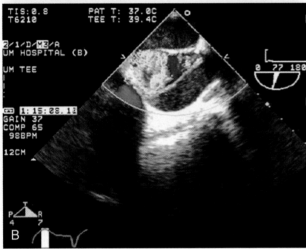

FIGURE 20.42. Transesophageal echocardiogram recorded in a patient with arch involvement of a dissection that extended from the sinotubular junction through the arch. These images were recorded in a short-axis view of the arch. Note the total dimension of the arch, which is approximately 6 cm. There is a complex dissection present with the appearance of one true (*TL*) and two false lumens (*FL*). **B:** With color flow Doppler imaging, notice that flow is confined only to the central true lumen and is excluded from the more peripheral false lumens.

A number of complications of aortic dissection can be identified including aortic insufficiency. Echocardiography has identified several different mechanisms for aortic insufficiency that have relevance for surgical correction (Fig. 20.45). Aortic insufficiency can occur when the dissection protrudes down into the Valsalva sinus and disrupts the base of an aortic cusp. This results in abnormal aortic valve coaptation. Figure 20.46 is an example of a patient with this type of aortic insufficiency. Commonly, aortic dissection results in dilation of the sinotubular junction and valve cusp malcoaptation on this basis. Figures 20.22, 20.23, and 20.46 are examples of sinotubular dilation with secondary aortic insufficiency. This mecha-

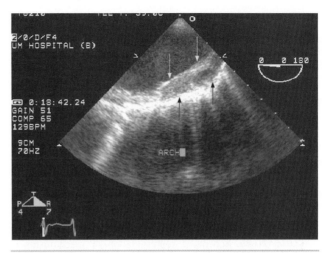

FIGURE 20.43. Transesophageal echocardiogram of the aortic arch shows an intramural hematoma. The *black arrows* denote the external wall of the aorta, and the *downward-pointing white arrows* denote the boundary of the intramural hematoma and lumen. Notice the space between the two is approximately 1 cm in distance, filled with a homogeneous organizing thrombus and does not communicate with the lumen.

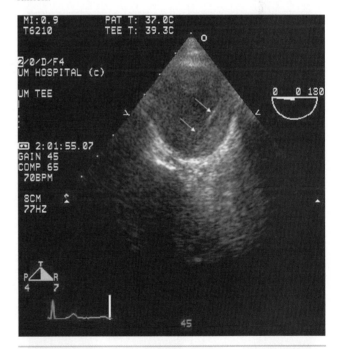

FIGURE 20.44. Transesophageal echocardiogram recorded in the descending thoracic aorta in a patient with a spontaneous intramural hematoma. This image was recorded at a 0-degree imaging plane of the descending thoracic aorta in a patient presenting with acute chest and back pain. Notice the relatively normal circular aortic geometry and the crescent-shaped filling defect distending from approximately 2 o'clock to 6 o'clock. With close scrutiny, one can appreciate the intima (*arrows*), which has lifted off the medial layers with the hematoma within the intima/medial space. There was no evidence of communication between the lumen and intima.

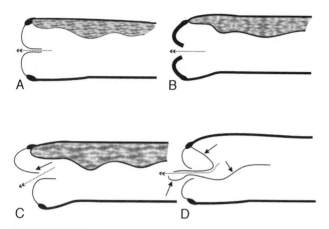

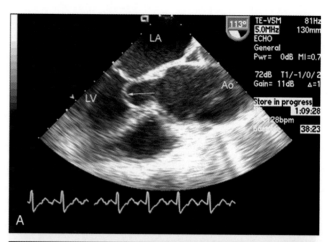

FIGURE 20.45. Schematic representation of mechanisms of aortic insufficiency in acute aortic dissection and disease of the proximal aorta. Multiple mechanisms can be responsible for aortic insufficiency including effacement of dilation of the sinotubular junction resulting in malcoaptation of the aortic valve **(A)**, aortic dissection in the presence of intrinsic aortic valve disease **(B)**, actual disruption of the insertion of an aortic cusp **(C)**, and prolapse of a portion of the intimal dissection flap through the aortic valve, which serves as a conduit for aortic regurgitation **(D)**.

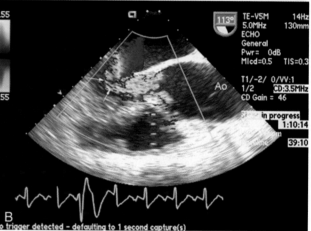

FIGURE 20.47. Transesophageal echocardiogram recorded in a patient with acute type A dissection and severe aortic insufficiency. **A:** Recorded in a longitudinal (113-degree) view of the ascending aorta in diastole. Note the portion of the dissection flap (*white arrow*) that is prolapsing through the aortic anulus into the left ventricular outflow tract. **B:** The accompanying color flow image was recorded in diastole. Note the color flow jet that fills the entire left ventricular outflow tract and is flowing through the prolapsing intimal flap. There is a communication point within the intimal flap resulting in flow of blood directly into the left ventricle (*white arrows*). Note that the amount of blood escaping from the prolapsing flap (*arrows*) is substantially less than that confined by the flap in the left ventricular outflow tract. Ao, aorta; LA, left atrium; LV, left ventricle.

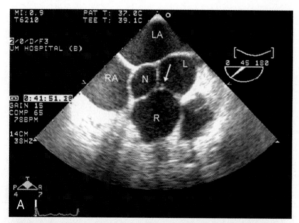

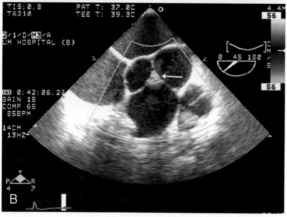

FIGURE 20.46. Transesophageal echocardiogram recorded in a patient with dilation of the proximal aorta resulting in malcoaptation of an otherwise normal three-cusp aortic valve. **A:** Recorded in diastole, note the failure of the three cusps to completely coapt at their center (*arrow*). **B:** The aortic insufficiency jet can be visualized as confined to the area of malcoaptation (*arrow*).

nism of aortic insufficiency is usually amenable to valve-sparing surgery in which restoration of the normal sinotubular junction results in correction of aortic insufficiency. A final mechanism that is uniquely identified by transesophageal echocardiography consists of prolapse of an aortic dissection flap through the aortic orifice (Figs. 20.31 and 20.47). The flap then becomes a conduit for insufficiency of the aortic valve.

In skilled hands, the accuracy of transesophageal echocardiography for detection of aortic dissection is exceptionally high and equivalent to that of the competing techniques of computed tomography and magnetic resonance imaging. Table 20.2 outlines results of studies that

▶ **TABLE 20.2** Accuracy of Transesophageal Echocardiography for Detection of Aortic Dissection

Ref.	N	Sensitivity	Specificity	Probe
Erbel et al., 1987	21	21/21 (100%)	N/C	SP
Erbel et al., 1989	164	81/82 (98.7%)	78/80 (97.5%)	SP
Hashimoto et al., 1989	22	22/22 (100%)	N/C	BP
Adachi et al., 1991	45	44/45 (97.7%)	N/C	SP, BP
Ballal et al., 1991	61	33/34 (97%)	27/27 (100%)	SP, BP
Simon et al., 1992	32	28/28 (100%)	4/4 (100%)	SP, BP
Nienaber et al., 1993	70	43/44 (97.7%)	20/26 (76.9%)	BP
Keren et al., 1996	112	48/49 (98%)	60/63 (95%)	BP, MP
Total	527	320/325 (98.5%)	189/200 (94.5%)	

BP, biplane probe; MP, multiplane probe; N/C, not calculated; study contained only patients with confirmed dissection; SP, single-plane probe.

have evaluated the accuracy of transesophageal echocardiography. In actual practice, false positives most commonly occur when using older generation single or biplane probes or when confusion exists between an artifactual echo protruding into the aorta and a true dissection flap (Fig. 20.32). False-negative examinations are exceedingly uncommon but occasionally occur near the inferior portion of the arch, which represents a relative blind spot for transesophageal echocardiography. Most aortic dissections, however, extend for a fairly long portion of the aorta, and a dissection localized only to this limited blind spot is quite uncommon.

Echocardiography has been used to follow the status of surgical repair of aortic dissection. The goal of surgery for aortic dissection is to arrest further propagation of the aortic dissection. This often includes prosthetic graft and/or prosthetic valve implantation. For ascending aorta graft placement, the ostia of the left main coronary and right coronary arteries are resected from the native aorta and sutured to the aortic graft. Therefore, it is important to evaluate left ventricular function in the operating room, looking for wall motion abnormalities after repair. In some aortic dissection repairs, the aortic valve is preserved. In these cases, postoperative transesophageal echocardiography is important to confirm aortic valve competence. After surgery, a false lumen frequently persists, especially in the descending thoracic aorta. In a substantial number of these patients, chronic thrombosis of the false lumen occurs. Limited communication points may still be visualized after surgical repair. Figure 20.48 contains examples of patients after surgical correction of an acute aortic dissection.

Therapy for aortic dissection typically involves surgical correction. More recently, a number of high-volume centers have engaged in a protocol of temporizing with percutaneous fenestration of the intimal flap and intravascular stents. Fenestration is a procedure in which communication points are created between the true and false lumens using balloon dilation techniques. This has the result of equalizing pressure and flow in the true and

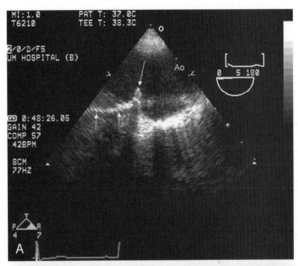

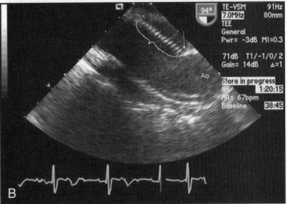

FIGURE 20.48. Transesophageal echocardiograms recorded in patients after aortic dissection repair. **A:** Transesophageal echocardiogram of the aortic arch in a patient with a graft repair of dissection. The margin of the native aorta and graft is depicted by the *longer downward-pointing arrow* and actual graft tissue is noted by the *upward-pointing arrows.* Notice the linear striping of the prosthetic material that is characteristic of a graft. **B:** Recorded in a patient after graft repair of a descending thoracic aneurysm. The image was recorded in a longitudinal view of the aorta. The *downward-pointing arrow* denotes the margin of the native aorta and graft, which in turn is noted by the brackets. Again note the striped pattern of the graft material that is characteristic of a prosthetic material.

false lumens and can restore and protect blood flow to vital organs. Intravascular ultrasound is frequently used at the time of performing this procedure to determine the relative size and flow status of the true and false lumens. It is also used to confirm flow in aortic branches, whether arising from the true or false lumen.

AORTIC ATHEROMA

Atherosclerosis of the aorta is frequently encountered during transesophageal echocardiography. It can also be identified from a suprasternal notch view (Fig. 20.49). It is most common with advanced age, hypertension, and elevated cholesterol and, as noted previously, may be an integral component of atherosclerotic aneurysm and intramural hematoma of the aorta. It is also not infrequently encountered in patients in whom a cardiovascular source of embolus is suspected. Atheroma of the aorta is characterized by its location and topographic characteristics. It is most common in the descending thoracic aorta and arch and less frequently encountered in the ascending aorta.

Atheroma can be characterized as symmetric and crescentic, in which case it creates a smooth homogeneous crescent filling a portion of the aortic lumen, protruding or complex. Symmetric atheroma can be confused for intramural hemorrhage; however, the former is more likely to have intimal thickening and areas of calcification. Complex atheroma is defined as atherosclerotic disease with pedunculated or mobile components. Typically, a threshold of 4 mm of protrusion into the lumen has been used for this

definition. Atherosclerotic disease with protruding and mobile components is more likely to be associated with cardioembolic disease than is smooth, crescentic atherosclerotic involvement. Complications of significant atherosclerosis of the aorta include aneurysm formation and penetrating ulcer of the aorta, which presents in a manner similar to that of aortic dissection. Figures 20.49 through 20.52 depict aortas with varying degrees and types of atherosclerotic involvement. On occasion, a penetrating ulcer may be detected either on the surface or within an atherosclerotic plaque (Fig. 20.53).

With advancing age and varying degrees of atherosclerosis, the distensibility and pulsatility of the aorta diminishes. Several studies have confirmed the ability of transesophageal echocardiographic imaging either with manual tracing of the aortic contour throughout the cardiac cycle or automatic edge detection contouring to demonstrate changes in aortic distensibility during systole. These changes have been suggested as an early pre-

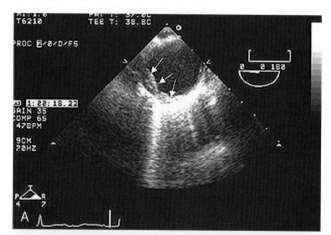

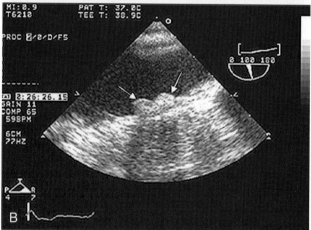

FIGURE 20.50. Transesophageal echocardiograms from two different patients with varying degrees of atheroma of the descending thoracic aorta. **A:** Note the rather laminar atheroma of the aorta extending from approximately 6 o'clock to 9 o'clock (*arrows*). **B:** Note the more pedunculated bilobed atheroma protruding into the lumen of the aorta (*arrows*).

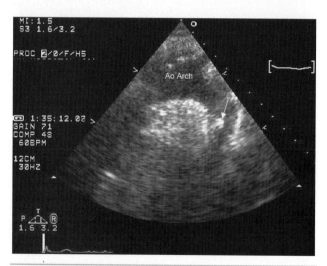

FIGURE 20.49. Suprasternal notch transthoracic echocardiogram recorded in a patient with atheromatous involvement of the proximal descending thoracic aorta. Notice the relatively normal aortic (Ao) arch and the distinct echo density protruding into the lumen of the proximal descending thoracic aorta (*arrow*) that represents focal pedunculated atheroma.

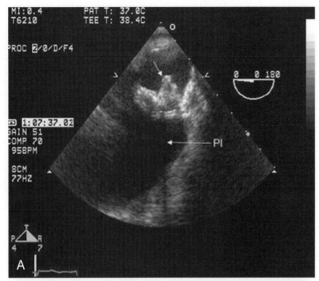

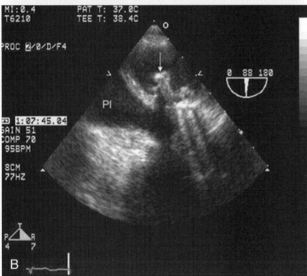

FIGURE 20.51. Transesophageal echocardiogram recorded in short-axis and longitudinal views of the descending thoracic aorta. **A:** Note the relatively circular aorta into which there is marked protrusion by pedunculated atheroma (*arrow*). **B:** Recorded at the same depth of imaging but in an orthogonal view where the complex pedunculated nature of the atheroma can again be appreciated. An incidental pleural effusion (*Pl*) is also noted.

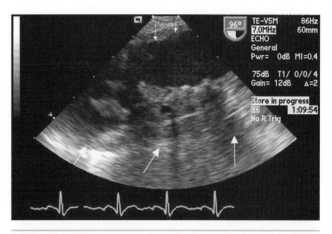

FIGURE 20.52. Transesophageal echocardiogram recorded in the longitudinal plane of a descending thoracic aorta with aneurysm. The *arrows* outline the external boundary of the aorta with all space in between representing an aneurysm with complex atheroma. Note the markedly complex atheroma with multiple pedunculated and mobile components filling the dilated lumen.

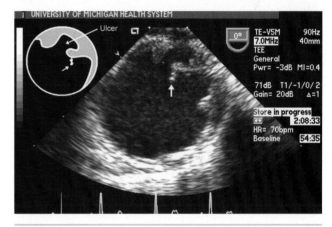

FIGURE 20.53. Transesophageal echocardiogram recorded in a patient with acute chest and back pains suggesting acute aortic pathology. In this instance, no typical dissection or intramural hematoma could be detected. There was substantial atheroma with a distinct area of ulceration (*arrow*) into the atheroma. This is a typical ulceration of an atheromatous plaque that can present with symptoms virtually identical to acute aortic dissection.

dictor of atherosclerosis and thought to represent end-organ effects of hypertension and atherosclerosis.

MISCELLANEOUS CONDITIONS

Aortic Pseudoaneurysm

Aortic pseudoaneurysm represents a contained rupture of the aorta and, as with left ventricular pseudoaneurysm, is characterized by an extraluminal aneurysmal sack communicating with the true lumen by a relatively narrow neck.

Aortic pseudoaneurysms occur in several situations, including spontaneous rupture of an aortic aneurysm with subsequent sealing off of the hemorrhage, or as a sequelae of aortic dissection, in which there is further rupture through the adventitial layers (Figs. 20.54 and 20.55). On rare occasions, pseudoaneurysm is the result of iatrogenic injury.

Aortic Trauma

Aortic transection is a catastrophic sequela of blunt chest injury, typically after a high-speed impact injury such as

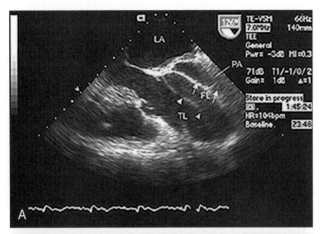

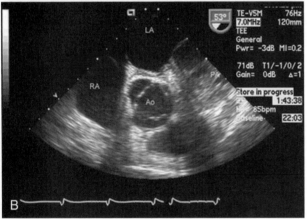

FIGURE 20.54. Transesophageal echocardiogram recorded in a patient with a complex dissection and subsequent pseudoaneurysm of the ascending aorta. **A:** Longitudinal view of the ascending aorta in which the true (TL) and false lumens (FL) of the aorta can be appreciated. The intimal flap is denoted by *arrowheads*. External to the posterior wall of the aorta is a space bounded by the true wall of the aorta (*upward-pointing arrows*) and the left atrium (LA), which represents a pseudoaneurysm (*PA*). **B:** Short-axis view representing the same anatomy in which the relatively circular aorta (Ao) can be noted. Lateral to this is a large complex space partially filled with hematoma representing the pseudoaneurysm. RA, right atrium.

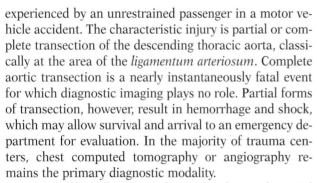

experienced by an unrestrained passenger in a motor vehicle accident. The characteristic injury is partial or complete transection of the descending thoracic aorta, classically at the area of the *ligamentum arteriosum*. Complete aortic transection is a nearly instantaneously fatal event for which diagnostic imaging plays no role. Partial forms of transection, however, result in hemorrhage and shock, which may allow survival and arrival to an emergency department for evaluation. In the majority of trauma centers, chest computed tomography or angiography remains the primary diagnostic modality.

Transesophageal echocardiography has substantial promise for the detection of aortic trauma. It should be emphasized that there are several different manifestations

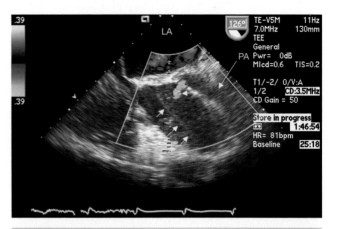

FIGURE 20.55. Longitudinal transesophageal echocardiogram recorded in the same patient as depicted in Figure 20.54. The *shorter arrows* denote the intimal flap. The pseudoaneurysm (*PA*) is denoted by the *longer arrow*. Distinct color flow (*horizontal arrow*) can be seen through a communication point between the aorta and pseudoaneurysm. LA, left atrium.

of aortic trauma, many of which are remarkably subtle. Because most patients with complete or nearly complete aortic transection do not survive, it is uncommon to document this fatal complication. For any form of aortic trauma in which there has been at least partial disruption through the media into the adventitia, one will frequently encounter a periadventitial hematoma. This hematoma may distort the shape of the aorta so that it is no longer imaged as a circular structure and may also deviate either the aorta or esophagus out of position so that when withdrawing the probe to scan from the gastroesophageal junction superiorly, the aorta moves out of the imaging plane. When examining the lumen of the aorta itself, varying degrees of dissection and intimal tear may be seen, some of which may be subtle and represent a limited intimal tear without actual dissection. On occasion, a focal area of the aorta is encountered where circular geometry is transiently lost and a limited ridge may be seen protruding into the aortic lumen. This is indirect evidence of partial thickness trauma at that site. On occasion, limited trauma results in formation of a thrombus within the medial space or in the lumen of the aorta itself, and if an apparent thrombus is detected in a relatively young patient after blunt chest trauma, aortic trauma rather than atheroma should be considered as the major diagnosis.

Intravascular ultrasound has been used with a high degree of success to document the presence of aortic trauma after blunt chest injury (Fig. 20.56). Because of the high-frequency resolution of this technique, more limited areas of intimal tear and disruption of the aortic wall integrity can be detected, which may not be seen with either transesophageal echocardiography or other imaging techniques such as computed tomography. A limitation of this technique is its relatively shallow penetration, which pre-

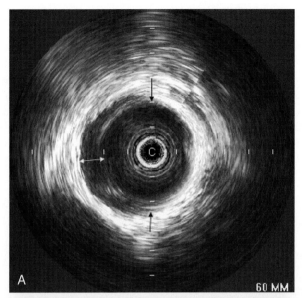

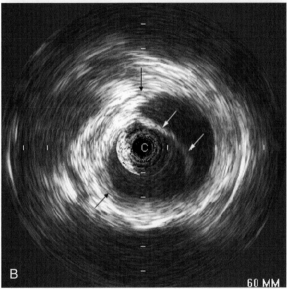

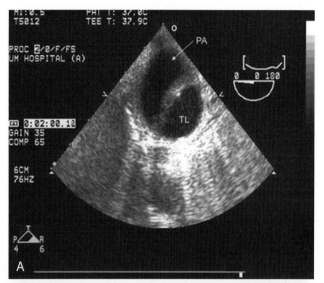

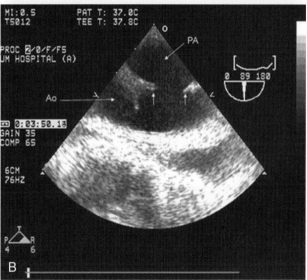

FIGURE 20.56. Intravascular ultrasound (*IVUS*) recorded in a patient with traumatic aortic injury. **A:** Recorded in the same patient depicted in Figure 20.10 who is a 38-year-old man involved in a motor vehicle accident and suspected of having aortic trauma. For comparison, refer to Figure 20.10, which was recorded in a noninvolved area of the lower thoracic aorta. **A:** Note the central position of the imaging catheter (*C*) and the relatively circular aortic geometry. From roughly the 6 o'clock to 12 o'clock position (*black arrows*) there is a distinct area of crescentic thickening in the wall, the maximal dimension of which is denoted by the *double-headed white arrow*. This represents intramural thrombus formation as a result of aortic trauma. This image was recorded at the level of the *ligamentum arteriosum*. **B:** Recorded in a 23-year-old patient after a motor vehicle accident. Note the noncircular shape of the overall aorta with marked irregularity of the inner wall from approximately the 7 o'clock to 12 o'clock position (*black arrows*). There is also a limited dissection flap (*white arrows*) within the lumen.

FIGURE 20.57. Transesophageal echocardiogram recorded in a patient 2 weeks after a high-speed motor vehicle accident in whom an aortic pseudoaneurysm formed at the site of rupture. **A:** Recorded in the short-axis view in which the true aortic lumen (*TL*) can be seen. There is additional space that represents the pseudoaneurysm posterior to the aorta (*PA*). The nature of the pseudoaneurysm is better appreciated in **B**, which is a longitudinal view recorded in the same area. The lumen of the aorta is noted (*Ao*) as well as 1-cm long break in its continuity (*arrowheads*) communicating to the pseudoaneurysm (*PA*).

cludes defining the presence and extent of an adventitial hematoma to the same degree that can be done with transesophageal echocardiography.

Occasional patients may experience a partial-thickness tear of the aortic wall that is not immediately fatal. This complication can then lead to formation of an aortic pseudoaneurysm, which can be detected with a number of imaging techniques, including transesophageal echocardiography (Fig. 20.57).

Other sequelae of aortic trauma include acute rupture of a Valsalva sinus, typically into the right atrium. Whether this occurs in a structurally normal aorta or requires a preexisting Valsalva sinus aneurysm is uncertain. Other less common forms of aortic trauma have included formation of aortovena caval fistulae, which can be suspected on the basis of high-volume turbulent flow in the inferior vena cava.

Infections of the Aorta

Bacterial or fungal infections of the aorta are uncommon but do represent a subset of infectious endocarditis (Fig. 20.58). They typically will arise at an area of atherosclerotic involvement or at the area of the ligamentum arteriosum on the aortic side of a persistent ductus. They will manifest as a pedunculated mobile mass in the area for which the differential obviously includes complex mobile atherosclerotic disease. Rarely encountered in contemporary practice is syphilitic aortitis, which results in inflammatory thickening of the proximal aorta. The infectious nature of the mass may be suggested by the overall clinical situation but obviously only proven by direct inspection.

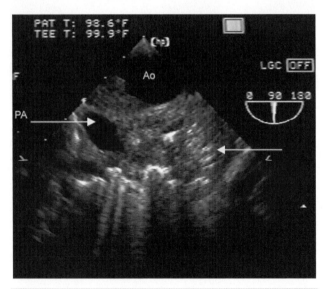

FIGURE 20.58. Longitudinal axis transesophageal echocardiogram recorded in an immunocompromised patient with a fungal infection. In this instance, there has been involvement of the lung by aspergillosis, which has subsequently invaded both the pulmonary artery (*PA*) and aorta (*Ao*). Note the irregular intraluminal echos in both the pulmonary artery and aorta, which represent direct extension of the infection into the vascular structures. The *long leftward-pointing arrow* denotes a area of pulmonary consolidation due to this infection.

Aortic Thrombus

In rare instances, a bland mobile thrombus can form within the thoracic aorta. This is more common in the proximal descending thoracic aorta and often has been associated with evidence of peripheral embolization. Such thrombi are noted as highly mobile echo-dense masses within the lumen, which frequently appear to be attached to the aortic wall by a fairly thin stalk. Figures 20.59 and 20.60 were recorded in patients with peripheral

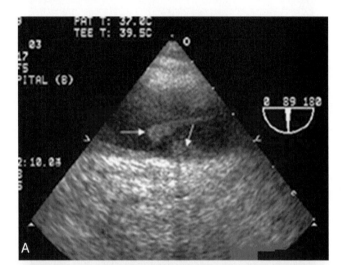

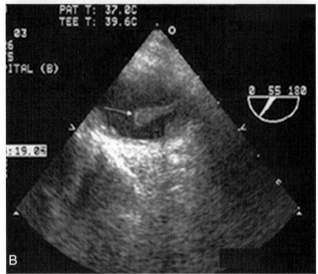

FIGURE 20.59. Transesophageal echocardiogram recorded in a patient with a recent embolic event to the kidney. **A:** Longitudinal view of the aorta in which there is focal protruding atheroma and/or a thrombus (*vertical arrow*) protruding into the lumen. Additionally, there is an elongated soft tissue density mass within the lumen of the aorta (*horizontal arrow*) that in real time is highly mobile. **B:** The same patient at the same level of the aorta recorded in the short axis in which the elongated, highly mobile soft thrombus can again be appreciated.

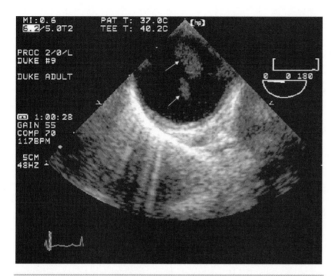

FIGURE 20.60. Transesophageal echocardiogram recorded in a patient with an embolic event to the lower extremity. Note the relatively normal appearing circular aorta in which there were two highly mobile echo densities consistent with a mobile thrombus that arose from the surface of a complex atheroma (not in view in this image).

embolization who underwent transesophageal echocardiography in a search for the source of an embolus. Note the highly mobile echo densities within the aorta that are consistent with a thrombus. Appropriate therapy for intraaortic thrombus is controversial, and the relative roles of aggressive anticoagulation versus surgical removal have not been fully elucidated.

Takayasu Arteritis

Takayasu arteritis is an inflammatory disease of the aorta and its proximal branches. By definition, it occurs in patients younger than 40 years of age. It results in marked, irregular intimal thickening and accumulation of inflammatory tissue in the proximal aorta and ostia of major branches including the coronary arteries. Echocardiographically, its appearance is similar to that of atherosclerotic disease (Fig. 20.61). On very rare occasions, other forms of arteritis, such as giant cell arteritis, can involve the aorta.

The reader is directed to Chapters 10 and 22 for additional discussion of aortic pathology.

SUGGESTED READINGS

Adachi H, Omoto R, Kyo S, et al. Emergency surgical intervention of acute aortic dissection with the rapid diagnosis by transesophageal echocardiography. Circulation 1991;84(5 Suppl): III14–III19.

Appelbe AF, Walker PG, Yeoh JK, et al. Clinical significance and origin of artifacts in transesophageal echocardiography of the thoracic aorta. J Am Coll Cardiol 1993;21:754–760.

Armstrong WF, Bach DS, Carey LM, et al. Spectrum of acute dissection of the ascending aorta: a transesophageal echocardiographic study. J Am Soc Echocardiogr 1996;9:646–656.

Armstrong WF, Bach DS, Carey LM, et al. Clinical and echocardiographic findings in patients with suspected acute aortic dissection. Am Heart J 1998;136:1051–1060.

Ballal RS, Nanda NC, Gatewood R, et al. Usefulness of transesophageal echocardiography in assessment of aortic dissection. Circulation 1991;84:1903–1914.

Brown OR, DeMots H, Kloster FE, et al. Aortic root dilatation and mitral valve prolapse in Marfan's syndrome: an echocardiographic study. Circulation 1975;52:651–657.

Cohen A, Tzourio C, Bertrand B, et al. Aortic plaque morphology and vascular events: a follow-up study in patients with ischemic stroke. FAPS Investigators. French Study of Aortic Plaques in Stroke. Circulation 1997;96:3838–9841.

Come PC, Fortuin NJ, White RI Jr, et al. Echocardiographic assessment of cardiovascular abnormalities in the Marfan syndrome. Comparison with clinical findings and with roentgenographic estimation of aortic root size. Am J Med 1983;74:465–474.

Erbel R, Borner N, Steller D, et al. Detection of aortic dissection by transoesophageal echocardiography. Br Heart J 1987;58:45–51.

Erbel R, Engberding R, Daniel W, et al. Echocardiography in diagnosis of aortic dissection. Lancet 1989;1:457–461.

Erbel R, Oelert H, Meyer J, et al. Effect of medical and surgical therapy on aortic dissection evaluated by transesophageal echocardiography. Implications for prognosis and therapy. The European Cooperative Study Group on Echocardiography. Circulation 1993;87:1604–1615.

Fann JI, Smith JA, Miller DC, et al. Surgical management of aortic dissection during a 30-year period. Circulation 1995;92(9 Suppl):II113–II121.

Hagan PG, Nienaber CA, Isselbacher EM, et al. The International Registry of Acute Aortic Dissection (IRAD): new insights into an old disease. JAMA 2000;283:897–903.

Hashimoto S, Kumada T, Osakada G, et al. Assessment of transesophageal Doppler echography in dissecting aortic aneurysm. J Am Coll Cardiol 1989;14:1253–1262.

Ishikawa K. Diagnostic approach and proposed criteria for the clinical diagnosis of Takayasu's arteriopathy. J Am Coll Cardiol 1988;12:964–972.

Jones EF, Kalman JM, Calafiore P, et al. Proximal aortic atheroma. An independent risk factor for cerebral ischemia. Stroke 1995;26:218–224.

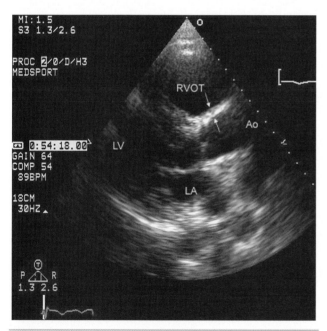

FIGURE 20.61. Parasternal long-axis transthoracic echocardiogram recorded in a patient with Takayasu arteritis. Note the abnormally bright echo within the anterior and posterior wall of the aorta in the young female patient in whom atherosclerotic disease would not be expected. Ao, aorta; LA, left atrium; LV, left ventricle.

Karalis DG, Chandrasekaran K, Victor MF, et al. Recognition and embolic potential of intraaortic atherosclerotic debris. J Am Coll Cardiol 1991;17:73–78.

Katz ES, Tunick PA, Rusinek H, et al. Protruding aortic atheromas predict stroke in elderly patients undergoing cardiopulmonary bypass: experience with intraoperative transesophageal echocardiography. J Am Coll Cardiol 1992;20:70–77.

Keane MG, Wiegers SE, Yang E, et al. Structural determinants of aortic regurgitation in type A dissection and the role of valvular resuspension as determined by intraoperative transesophageal echocardiography. Am J Cardiol 2000;85:604–610.

Keren A, Kim C, Hu B, et al. Accuracy of biplane and multiplane transesophageal echocardiography in diagnosis of typical acute aortic dissection and intramural hematoma. J Am Coll Cardiol 1996;28:627–636.

Losi MA, Betocchi S, Briguori C, et al. Determinants of aortic artifacts during transesophageal echocardiography of the ascending aorta. Am Heart J 1999;137:967–972.

Maraj R, Rerkpattanapipat P, Jacobs LE, et al. Meta-analysis of 143 reported cases of aortic intramural hematoma. Am J Cardiol 2000;86:664–668.

Mehta RH, Suzuki T, Hagan PG, et al. Predicting death in patients with acute type a aortic dissection. Circulation 2002;105:200–206.

Mohr-Kahaly S, Erbel R, Kearney P, et al. Ambulatory follow-up of aortic dissection by transesophageal two-dimensional and color-coded Doppler echocardiography. Circulation 1989;80:24–33.

Mohr-Kahaly S, Erbel R, Kearney P, et al. Aortic intramural hemorrhage visualized by transesophageal echocardiography: findings and prognostic implications. J Am Coll Cardiol 1994;23:658–664.

Montgomery DH, Ververis JJ, McGorisk G, et al. Natural history of severe atheromatous disease of the thoracic aorta: a transesophageal echocardiographic study. J Am Coll Cardiol 1996;27:95–101.

Movsowitz HD, Levine RA, Hilgenberg AD, et al. Transesophageal echocardiographic description of the mechanisms of aortic regurgitation in acute type A aortic dissection: implications for aortic valve repair. J Am Coll Cardiol 2000;36:884–890.

Nienaber CA, von Kodolitsch Y, Nicolas V, et al. The diagnosis of thoracic aortic dissection by noninvasive imaging procedures. N Engl J Med 1993;328:1–9.

Nienaber CA, von Kodolitsch Y, Nicolas V, et al. Intramural hemorrhage of the thoracic aorta. Diagnostic and therapeutic implications. Circulation 1995;92:1465–1472.

Schwammenthal E, Schwammenthal Y, Tanne D, et al. Transcutaneous detection of aortic arch atheromas by suprasternal harmonic imaging. J Am Coll Cardiol 2002;39:1127–1132.

Simon P, Owen AN, Havel M, et al. Transesophageal echocardiography in the emergency surgical management of patients with aortic dissection. J Thorac Cardiovasc Surg 1992;103:1113–1118.

Smith MD, Cassidy JM, Souther S, et al. Transesophageal echocardiography in the diagnosis of traumatic rupture of the aorta. N Engl J Med 1995;332:356–362.

Song JK, Kim HS, Kang DH, et al. Different clinical features of aortic intramural hematoma versus dissection involving the ascending aorta. J Am Coll Cardiol 2001;37:1604–1610.

Song JK, Kim HS, Kang DH, et al. Outcomes of medically treated patients with aortic intramural hematoma. Am J Med 2002;113:181–187.

Spangler RD, Nora JJ, Lortscher RH, et al. Echocardiography in Marfan's syndrome. Chest 1976;69:72–78.

Sutsch G, Jenni R, von Segesser L, et al. Predictability of aortic dissection as a function of aortic diameter. Eur Heart J 1991;12:1247–1256.

Svensson LG, Labib SB, Eisenhauer AC, et al. Intimal tear without hematoma: an important variant of aortic dissection that can elude current imaging techniques. Circulation 1999;99:1331–1336.

Triulzi M, Gillam LD, Gentile F, et al. Normal adult cross-sectional echocardiographic values: linear dimensions and chamber areas. Echocardiography 1984;1:403–426.

Tunick PA, Kronzon I. Atheromas of the thoracic aorta: clinical and therapeutic update. J Am Coll Cardiol 2000;35:545–554.

Vasan RS, Larson MG, Benjamin EJ, et al. Echocardiographic reference values for aortic root size: the Framingham Heart Study. J Am Soc Echocardiogr 1995;86:793–800.

Vilacosta I, San Roman JA, Ferreiros J, et al. Natural history and serial morphology of aortic intramural hematoma: a novel variant of aortic dissection. Am Heart J 1997;134:495–507.

Vilacosta I, San Roman JA, Ferreiros J, et al. Penetrating atherosclerotic aortic ulcer: documentation by transesophageal echocardiography. J Am Coll Cardiol 1998;321:83–89.

Willens H, Kessler K. Transesophageal echocardiography in the diagnosis of diseases of the thoracic aorta: Part 1. Aortic dissection, aortic intramural hematoma, and penetrating atherosclerotic ulcer of the aorta. Chest 1999;116:1772–1779.

Willens HJ, Kessler KM. Transesophageal echocardiography in the diagnosis of diseases of the thoracic aorta. Part II. Atherosclerotic and traumatic diseases of the aorta. Chest 2000;117:233–243.

Masses, Tumors, and Source of Embolus

NORMAL VARIANTS AND ARTIFACTS: SOURCES OF FALSE-POSITIVE FINDINGS

The echocardiographic evaluation of intracardiac masses is critically dependent on the ability to distinguish normal from abnormal findings. Ultrasound artifacts are common, even in high-quality studies, and may be mistaken for pathologic conditions. Near-field clutter and reverberations are examples of artifacts often confused with pathology (e.g., apical thrombi) on two-dimensional echocardiography. Such artifacts, which are covered in Chapter 2, must be avoided whenever possible and correctly identified when present. Proper transducer selection and the use of multiple acoustic windows are among the strategies that can be used to avoid potential misinterpretations.

Anatomic variants are ubiquitous, may involve any chamber or valve structure, and are potentially confused with pathologic structures. A list of commonly encountered normal structures that often are interpreted as pathologic is provided in Table 21.1. The right atrium is the chamber that is most often a source of anatomic variants leading to inaccurate interpretation. The Chiari network, eustachian valve, and crista terminalis are examples of structures normally found in the right atrium that, due to individual variation, are frequently confused with pathologic entities. Fatty infiltration in the atrioventricular groove, especially around the tricuspid valve, is a common source of confusion. A benign condition, this fatty deposit is frequently mistaken for tumor or fluid. False tendons in the left ventricular apex are common and occasionally misinterpreted as thrombi (Fig. 21.1). In this example, the diagnosis of a false tendon is relatively straightforward. In some cases, the tendon can be mistaken for the surface of an apical thrombus. Color flow imaging or contrast echocardiography, by demonstrating flow on either side of the linear structure, can be helpful to make this distinction. Additional sources of confusion can be iatrogenic. For example, the suture line in the posterior atrial wall after cardiac transplantation and in-

▶ TABLE 21.1 Normal Variants and Benign Conditions Often Misinterpreted as Pathologic

Right atrium
  Chiari network
  Eustachian valve
  Crista terminalis
  Catheters/pacemaker leads
  Lipomatous hypertrophy of interatrial septum
  Pectinate muscles
  Fatty material (surrounding the tricuspid anulus)
Left atrium
  Suture line following transplant
  Fossa ovalis
  Calcified mitral anulus
  Coronary sinus
  Ridge between LUPV and LAA
  Lipomatous hypertrophy of interatrial septum
  Pectinate muscles
  Transverse sinus
Right ventricle
  Moderator band
  Muscle bundles/trabeculations
  Catheters and pacemaker leads
Left ventricle
  False chords
  Papillary muscles
  LV trabeculations
Aorta
  Brachiocephalic vein
  Innominate vein
  Pleural effusion

LAA, left atrial appendage; LUPV, left upper pulmonary vein; LV, left ventricle

dwelling pacemaker leads or catheters are examples of "normal" structures that may be misinterpreted as pathologic. Figure 21.2 is an example of a right ventricular moderator band, another normal cardiac structure that can be confused with abnormal masses, such as thrombi.

Recognition of such normal variants depends on image quality and technique as well as experience. The use of

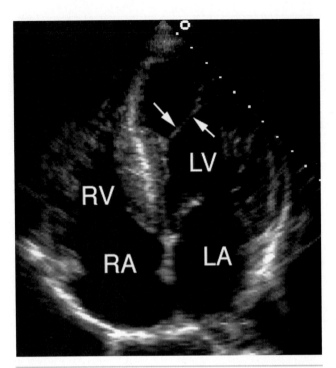

FIGURE 21.1. An apical four-chamber view demonstrates a false tendon (*arrows*) in the left ventricular (*LV*) apex. LA, left atrium; RA, right atrium; RV, right ventricle.

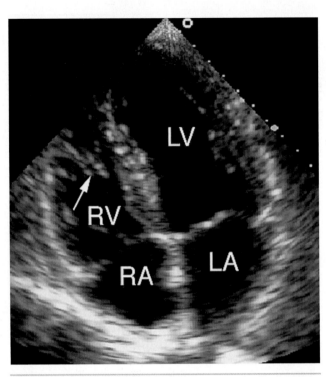

FIGURE 21.2. A moderator band (*arrow*) is seen in the apex of the right ventricle (*RV*). LA, left atrium; LV, left ventricle; RA, right atrium.

multiple imaging windows and transducers of different frequency are additional strategies to ensure an accurate diagnosis. The availability of clinical information (such as whether the patient has a pacemaker) can be extremely valuable in avoiding errors.

CARDIAC TUMORS

Primary Tumors

A list of indications for echocardiography in patients with cardiac masses and tumors is provided in Table 21.2.

Echocardiography is useful to identify conditions in which masses may develop, is an accurate technique to detect and characterize masses once they occur, and provides a noninvasive means for surveillance after treatment or removal. Most tumors in the heart are the result of direct spread from adjacent malignancies or metastatic disease; *primary* cardiac tumors account for a small percentage of the total number. Primary tumors can be either benign or malignant and can occur in all age groups. The most common primary cardiac tumors are listed in Table 21.3. Of these, benign tumors outnumber malignant ones by a ratio of approximately 3 to 1.

▶ TABLE 21.2 **Echocardiography in Patients with Cardiac Masses and Tumors**

Indications	Class
1. Evaluation of patients with clinical syndromes and events suggesting an underlying cardiac mass.	I
2. Evaluation of patients with underlying cardiac disease known to predispose to mass formation for whom a therapeutic decision regarding surgery or anticoagulation will depend on the results of echocardiography.	I
3. Follow-up or surveillance studies after surgical removal of masses known to have a high likelihood of recurrence (i.e., myxoma).	I
4. Patients with known primary malignancies when echocardiographic surveillance for cardiac involvement is part of the disease staging process.	I
5. Screening persons with disease states likely to result in mass formation but for whom no clinical evidence for the mass exists.	IIb
6. Patients for whom the results of echocardiography will have no impact on diagnosis or clinical decision making.	III

Adapted with permission from Cheitlin MD, Alpert JS, Armstrong WF, et al. ACC/AHA Guidelines for the Clinical Application of Echocardiography: a report of the American College of Cardiology/American Heart Association Task Force on Practice Guidelines (Committee on Clinical Application of Echocardiography) developed in collaboration with the American Society of Echocardiography. Circulation 1997;95:1686–1744.

▶ **TABLE 21.3 Relative Frequency of Primary Cardiac Tumors**

Type	%
Benign	
Myxoma	30
Lipoma	10
Papillary fibroelastoma	8
Rhabdomyoma	6
Fibroma	3
Hemangioma	2
Teratoma	1
Malignant	
Angiosarcoma	8
Rhabdomyosarcoma	5
Fibrosarcoma	3
Mesothelioma	3
Lymphoma	2
Leiomyosarcoma	1

By far, the most common benign primary tumor of the heart is the myxoma, accounting for approximately 30% of all primary cardiac tumors. Myxomas are usually single and occur in the left atrium in 75% of cases where they most often arise from the area of the fossa ovalis (Fig. 21.3A). Their size, shape, and texture can be quite varied. Myxomas may be smooth surfaced but are more often irregularly shaped with filamentous fronds or have the appearance of a "cluster of grapes." They are typically non-homogeneous in texture with lucent centers or areas of calcification. Myxomas can be quite large, occupying most of the left atrium and resulting in obstruction to left ventricular filling. A large atrial myxoma is shown in Figure 21.3B. In this patient, the tumor nearly occludes the mitral orifice during diastole. The most important clue to the diagnosis is their location in the left atrium and origin from the midportion of the atrial septum. Given a typical presentation, echocardiography is virtually diagnostic of myxoma. Transthoracic imaging is usually sufficient, although small tumors or those that involve the right heart may require transesophageal echocardiography for diagnosis. Three-dimensional echocardiography has also been used to more fully characterize atrial myxomas (Fig. 21.4). Myxomas sometimes involve the right atrium (15%) or the left or right ventricle (5% each) (Fig. 21.5). In 5% of cases, they are multiple. They are most often confused with thrombi, although their characteristic location and attachment site is generally helpful in the differential diagnosis. After surgical excision, myxomas can recur. Therefore, surveillance echocardiograms should be obtained annually for several years to guard against this possibility.

Papillary fibroelastoma accounts for approximately 10% of all primary tumors. These are usually found in older patients and arise from either the aortic or mitral valve (Fig. 21.6). Because tumors arising from the heart valves are rare and often asymptomatic, establishing a diagnosis can be challenging and often relies on echocardiography. Among tumors that affect the valves, papillary

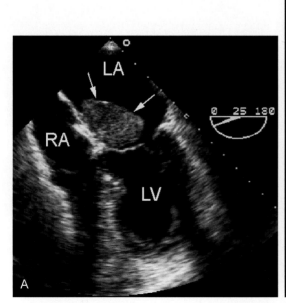

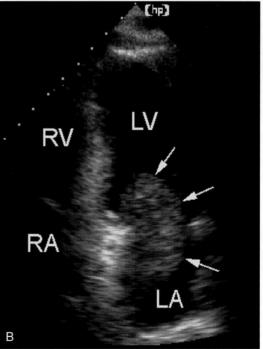

FIGURE 21.3. A: A myxoma (*arrows*) is seen in the left atrium (*LA*) on transesophageal imaging. The mass is attached to the fossa ovalis. **B:** A four-chamber view demonstrates a large myxoma within the left atrium partially obstructs the mitral orifice during diastole. LV, left ventricle; RA, right atrium; RV, right ventricle.

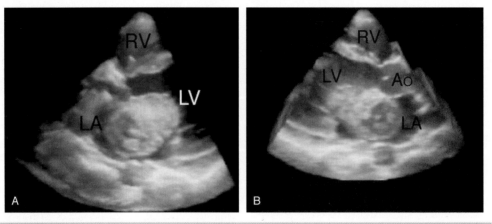

FIGURE 21.4. A large left atrial myxoma is demonstrated using three-dimensional imaging. The advantages of this modality are best appreciated when viewed in a cine loop format. LA, left atrium; LV, left ventricle; RA, right atrium; RV, right ventricle.

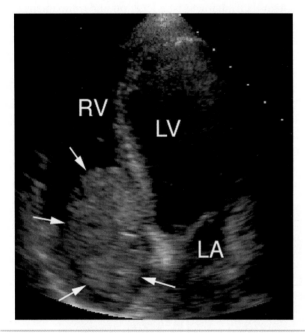

FIGURE 21.5. A large right atrial myxoma (*arrows*) is indicated by the *arrows*. The mass extends through the tricuspid valve into the right ventricle (*RV*). LA, left atrium; LV, left ventricle.

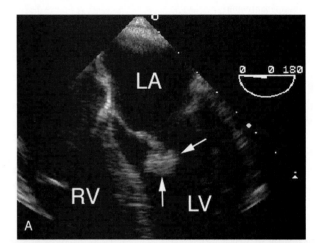

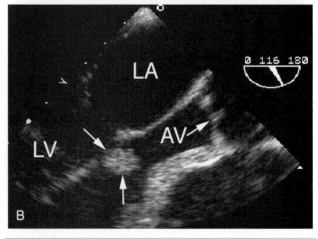

FIGURE 21.6. A, B: A papillary fibroelastoma of the mitral valve is demonstrated. The tumor was attached by a small pedicle to the anterior leaflet and was highly mobile. AV, aortic valve; LA, left atrium; LV, left ventricle; RV, right ventricle.

fibroelastomas are by far the most common, accounting for more than 85% of valve-associated tumors. Myxomas and fibromas account for the remainder, whereas malignant tumors involving the valves are very rare.

Papillary fibroelastomas are small, generally 0.5 to 2.0 cm in diameter, and are often confused with vegetations. Making this distinction is difficult because of the similarity in the echocardiographic appearance. A correct diagnosis therefore depends on the clinical setting, i.e., the presence or absence of signs of infection. These tumors usually attach to the downstream side of the valve by a small pedicle and are irregularly shaped with delicate frond-like surfaces

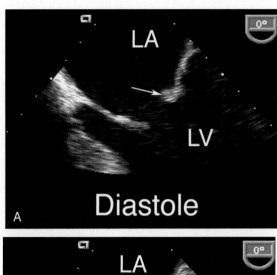

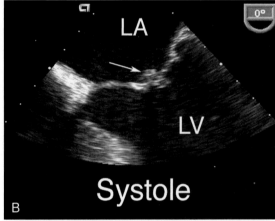

FIGURE 21.7. A small papillary fibroelastoma is seen in a patient who had a stroke. The mass (*arrow*) is seen on the posterior leaflet in diastole (**A**) and systole (**B**). LA, left atrium; LV, left ventricle.

(Figs. 21.7 and 21.8). Mobility is common and generally considered a risk factor for embolization. Significant valvular regurgitation is rare. There is some confusion as to whether fibroelastomas are distinct from Lambl's excrescences, which are smaller and frequently seen on otherwise normal valves in elderly patients (Fig. 21.9). Whether the two represent the distinct entities remains controversial. Fibroelastomas are also confused with blood cysts, which are unusual blood-containing cystic structures that develop within mitral leaflets (Fig. 21.10). Blood cysts have a broader base, are sessile, and are less mobile than fibroelastomas. Papillary fibroelastomas may be detected as an incidental finding on echocardiography. Because tumors can act as a nidus for the formation of fibrin-platelet aggregates, embolic events have been attributed to papillary fibroelastomas.

Lipomas are uncommon benign tumors involving the heart. Lipomatous hypertrophy of the atrial septum is one presentation. In this condition, the atrial septum is infiltrated by lipomatous material that results in dramatic thickening and increased echogenicity of its inferior and

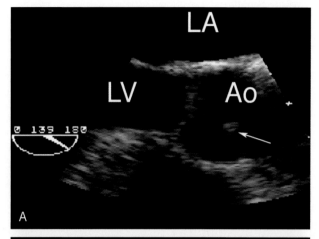

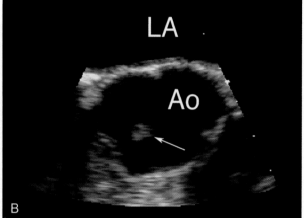

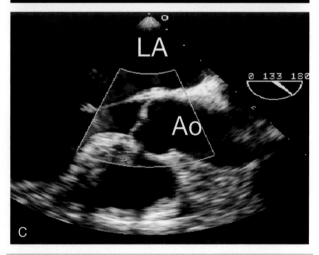

FIGURE 21.8. A papillary fibroelastoma involving the aortic valve is shown. **A:** A small spherical mass (*arrow*) is seen attached by a pedicle to the aortic valve. **B:** Short-axis view demonstrates the tumor (*arrow*). **C:** Color Doppler imaging reveals no evidence of aortic regurgitation. Ao, aorta; LA, left atrium; LV, left ventricle.

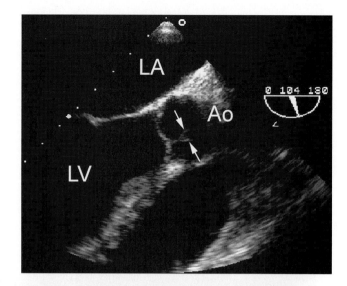

FIGURE 21.9. An example of Lambl's excrescence of the aortic valve is demonstrated (*arrows*). Ao, aorta; LA, left atrium; LV, left ventricle.

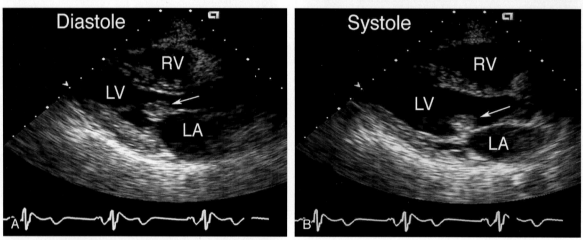

FIGURE 21.10. A blood cyst (*arrow*) within the anterior mitral leaflet is shown. The cyst is relatively immobile and the attachment is broad based. The mass is seen during diastole (**A**) and systole (**B**). LA, left atrium; LV, left ventricle; RV, right ventricle.

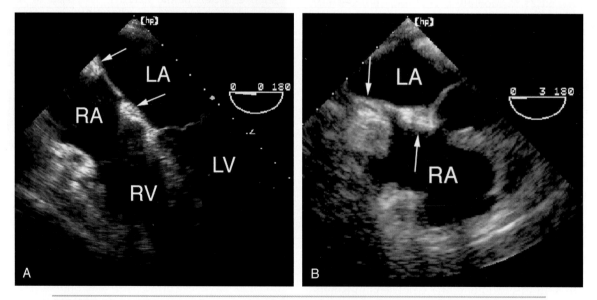

FIGURE 21.11. Lipomatous hypertrophy of the atrial septum is demonstrated. **A:** A mild degree of accumulation of lipomatous material is present (*arrows*). The fossa ovalis is characteristically spared. **B:** A more extreme form of lipomatous hypertrophy is demonstrated (*arrows*). LA, left atrium; LV, left ventricle; RA, right atrium; RV, right ventricle.

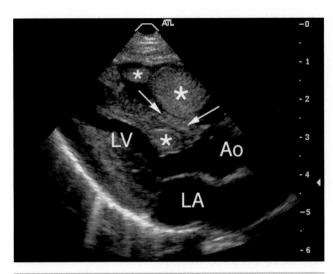

FIGURE 21.12. Rhabdomyoma is a common pediatric tumor. In this 12-year-old patient, multiple tumors are seen within the left and right ventricle (*asterisks*) and interventricular septum (*arrows*). Ao, aorta; LA, left atrium; LV, left ventricle.

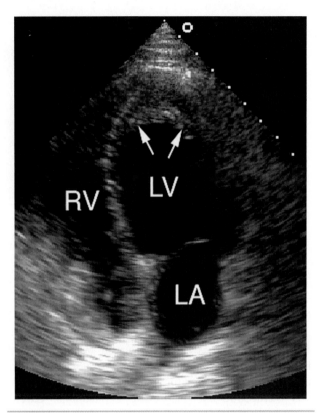

FIGURE 21.13. An example of endocardial fibroelastosis is shown. Endocardial thickening in the left ventricular apex is present. Thrombus overlies the thickened endocardium (*arrows*). LA, left atrium; LV, left ventricle; RV, right ventricle.

superior portions with sparing of the fossa ovalis (Fig. 21.11). The fatty infiltrate is highly echogenic and results in a "dumbbell-shaped" appearance on two-dimensional echocardiography. The condition is thought to be benign and rarely associated with clinical manifestations.

Rhabdomyomas are among the most common benign pediatric tumors (Fig. 21.12). They occur either within a cavity, sometimes as a pedunculated mass, or embedded within the myocardium. Such tumors can grow quite large and can obstruct blood flow within the heart. Fibromas are uncommon benign tumors, most often seen in children, that usually involve the left ventricular free wall. On echocardiography, they appear as distinct, highly echogenic, and well-demarcated masses that often extend into the cavity of the ventricle. Although benign, they occasionally result in obstruction to left ventricular filling and have been associated with ventricular arrhythmias. A rare condition that can be confused with a fibroma (or a thrombus) is endocardial fibroelastosis. This disease is usually seen in young children and is characterized by fibrous thickening of the left ventricular endothelium, probably as a nonspecific response to inflammation or infection. An example of endocardial fibroelastosis is provided in Figure 21.13. Unlike fibromas, the mass is endocardial rather than intramyocardial.

Malignant primary tumors of the heart are quite rare and include angiosarcoma, rhabdomyosarcoma, and fibrosarcoma. Figure 21.14 is an example of a fibrosarcoma that occupies the right ventricular outflow tract. Its size and location combine to produce a significant outflow tract gradient, as evidenced by the Doppler record-

ing. Such tumors tend to invade or replace myocardial tissue and thereby dramatically alter the appearance and/or function of the heart. As opposed to the well-circumscribed appearance of benign tumors, cardiac malignancies appear to infiltrate the tissues, disrupting normal anatomic planes, and invade or obliterate contiguous structures. The heart often appears tethered and relatively immobile, without the normal translational motion (Fig. 21.15).

The echocardiographic assessment of these patients has several components. Because primary cardiac malignancy is so much less common than metastatic involvement, the echocardiographic demonstration of an invasive cardiac tumor should suggest the possibility of metastatic disease. In addition, the exact location and extent of a cardiac malignancy must be thoroughly assessed to determine whether resection might be possible. Some malignancies are likely to affect a given chamber or location within the heart. Angiosarcomas, for example, usually involve the right atrium, whereas rhabdomyosarcomas may occur anywhere. Associated pericardial effusion is common, sometimes leading to tamponade.

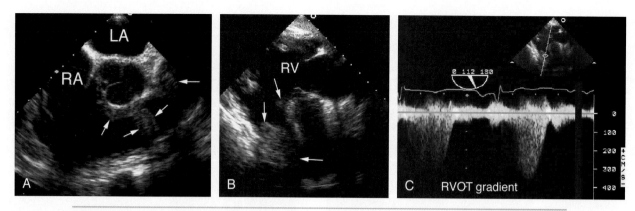

FIGURE 21.14. A primary fibrosarcoma is demonstrated in the right heart. **A:** The tumor involves the right ventricular outflow tract and pulmonary artery. **B:** Narrowing of the right ventricular outflow tract is indicated by the *arrows*. **C:** Doppler imaging demonstrates an RVOT gradient of approximately 50 mm Hg. LA, left atrium; RA, right atrium; RV, right ventricle; RVOT, right ventricular outflow tract.

Metastatic Tumors to the Heart

Echocardiography is often performed in patients with known or suspected malignancy. Among patients with cardiac symptoms, looking for evidence of metastatic spread has therapeutic and prognostic implications. Cardiac function helps to determine whether a given patient may be a candidate for particular therapies, such as doxorubicin (Adriamycin). In patients who have already received cancer therapy, echocardiography is useful to evaluate for side effects. Adriamycin, for example, can cause cardiomyopathy. Chest irradiation can result in constrictive pericarditis or scarring and fibrosis of the epicardial coronary arteries. In unstable or critically ill patients, the portability and noninvasive nature of ultrasound represent a significant advantage.

The heart is affected relatively less often by metastatic disease compared with other organs. Some investigators speculate that blood-borne malignant cells are destroyed by the contraction of the heart before they become established. Malignant tumors can spread to the heart through direct invasion from adjacent tumors, from propagation through the venous system, or by hematogenous spread (Table 21.4). Melanoma, for example, has a high propen-

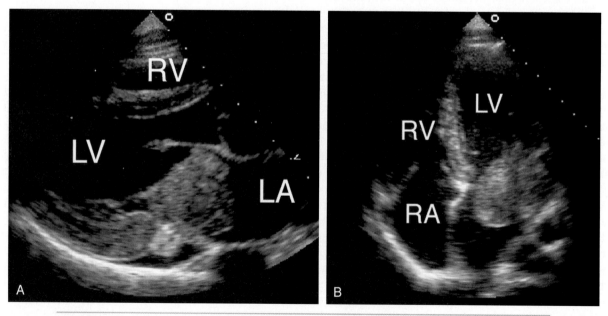

FIGURE 21.15. **A, B:** An example of angiosarcoma is provided. The mass had infiltrated the lateral wall of the left atrium (*LA*) and left ventricle (*LV*) and invaded the mitral valve. Obstruction to mitral inflow was present. In real time, the heart appeared fixed due to infiltration by the malignancy. A pericardial effusion is also present. RA, right atrium; RV, right ventricle.

▶ **TABLE 21.4 Metastatic Tumors to the Heart:**
Source and Cardiac Manifestations

Original Source	Cardiac Effect
Lung	Direct extension, often via pulmonary veins; effusion common
Breast	Hematogenous or lymphatic spread; effusion common
Lymphoma	Lymphatic spread, varied manifestations
Gastrointestinal	Variable manifestations
Melanoma	Intracardiac or myocardial involvment
Renal cell carcinoma	IVC to RA to RV; confused with thrombus
Carcinoid	Tricuspid and pulmonic valve thickening

IVC, inferior vena cava; RA, right atrium; RV, right ventricle.

sity for metastasizing to the pericardium and/or myocardium, involving the heart in more than 50% of cases. Intracardiac masses are frequently seen as a manifestation of malignant melanoma. Figure 21.16 is an example of a melanoma that has metastasized to the left ventricular apex. The presence of a mass is suggested on the transthoracic study but is best visualized after injection of a contrast agent. Although the appearance of the mass is similar to that of a thrombus, preserved apical contractility makes a thrombus unlikely and should suggest the possibility of alternative diagnoses. Figure 21.17 is from another patient with metastatic melanoma, this time to the right ventricular apex. Some leukemias also have a

similarly high rate of cardiac spread. However, more common malignancies, such as breast or lung cancer, account for the greatest percentage of nonprimary cardiac tumors. There is also a high incidence of cardiac involvement among patients with lymphoma secondary to acquired immunodeficiency syndrome.

The location of involvement of metastatic disease is frequently the pericardium, resulting in a pericardial effusion and epicardial involvement (Fig. 21.18). The usual signs and symptoms of pericarditis are often absent. In patients with known malignancies, the detection of a pericardial effusion should raise concern about cardiac metastases. However, it is almost impossible, based on echocardiographic findings alone, to establish the cause of a pericardial effusion. Patients with cancer may develop pericardial effusion for any of several reasons. For example, particular chemotherapies can cause pericardial effusion. In most cases, confirming that the effusion is malignant often has therapeutic implications. Pericardiocentesis, usually with biopsy, is generally appropriate. When the pericardial involvement is due to metastatic disease, the prognosis is uniformly poor. Figure 21.19 is a case of metastatic disease involving the posterior left ventricular wall and pericardium. Over a period of several weeks, the tumor eroded through the myocardium, resulting in formation of a pseudoaneurysm that gradually increased in size until the time of the patient's death. Intramyocardial involvement is less common than pericardial metastases and usually occurs secondary to lymphoma or melanoma. Heart failure, obstruction to flow,

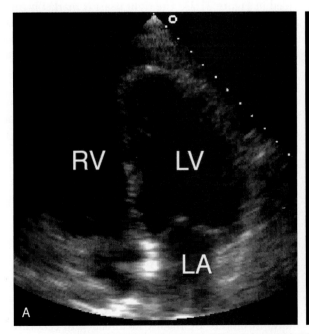
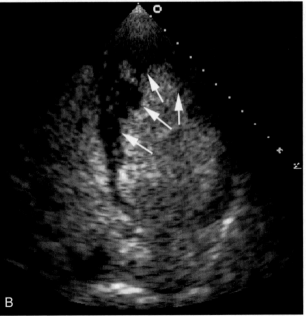

FIGURE 21.16. Metastatic melanoma often involves the heart. **A:** Image quality prevents visualization of the apical mass. **B:** After contrast injection, the outline of the apical mass (*arrows*) is apparent. LA, left atrium; LV, left ventricle; RV, right ventricle.

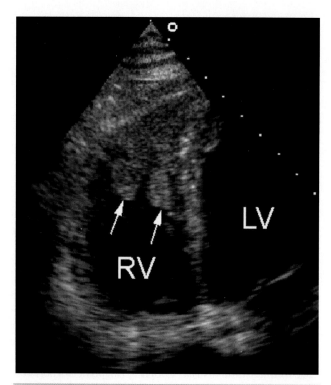

FIGURE 21.17. Metastatic melanoma involving the right ventricular apex (*arrows*) is shown. LV, left ventricle; RV, right ventricle.

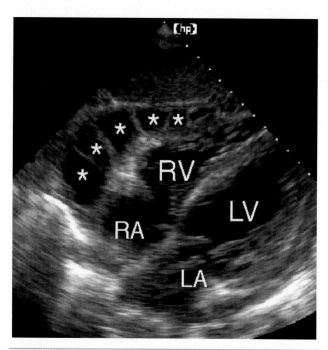

FIGURE 21.18. A malignant pericardial effusion (*asterisks*) demonstrated in a patient with bronchogenic carcinoma. LA, left atrium; LV, left ventricle; RA, right atrium; RV, right ventricle.

and arrhythmias may develop as a result. Cardiac involvement is often established at autopsy as an incidental finding in patients with widely metastatic disease. Figure 21.20 is an example of a pericardial mesothelioma. The mass is huge and grossly distorts the right heart. Figure 21.21 shows a patient with lymphoma, before and after chemotherapy. The tumor involved the aortic root and posterior wall of the heart, including the area of the coronary sinus. After successful chemotherapy, normal anatomy is restored. In this case, serial echocardiography was critical to follow the progress of therapy and the reduction in tumor burden.

Intravascular extension of tumor is a common manifestation of renal cell carcinoma (Fig. 21.22). Extension of the cancer into the inferior vena cava can lead to right atrial involvement. Pulmonary embolization can occur and occasionally can be recorded with echocardiography. In some cases, the initial diagnosis of this tumor is made after detection of a right atrial mass on echocardiography. Distinguishing tumor from thrombi or other etiologies depends on demonstration of extension into the inferior vena cava, retrograde to the kidneys.

Carcinoid tumors secrete a variety of vasoactive substances, such as serotonin, into the venous system that are usually inactivated by the liver and lung. When metastatic disease allows these tumor products to reach the right heart, they produce characteristic abnormalities that affect the tricuspid and pulmonary valves. The valve pathology involves fibrosis, smooth muscle proliferation, and endocardial thickening. Echocardiographically, the valves appear thickened, retracted, and immobile. A typical but advanced case of carcinoid heart disease is provided in Figure 21.23. The right heart is markedly dilated and the tricuspid valve is thickened and rigid. It appears nearly fixed in a position midway between open and closed. As a result, severe tricuspid regurgitation is present. In most patients with carcinoid heart disease, the tricuspid valve is the predominant site of involvement. Although some degree of stenosis may be present, the main hemodynamic abnormality is usually regurgitation and is often severe. In contrast, when the pulmonary valve is affected, stenosis tends to predominate. An example of this is shown in Figure 21.24. Involvement of the left-sided valves occurs in less than 10% of cases and suggests the possibility of a patent foramen ovale (PFO) with right-to-left shunting.

INTRACARDIAC THROMBI

Left Ventricular Thrombi

Patients at risk of the development of a left ventricular mural thrombus are readily identified with echocardiography. Predisposing factors include recent myocardial infarction, left ventricular aneurysm, and dilated cardiomyopathy. Thrombi generally involve the apex of the left

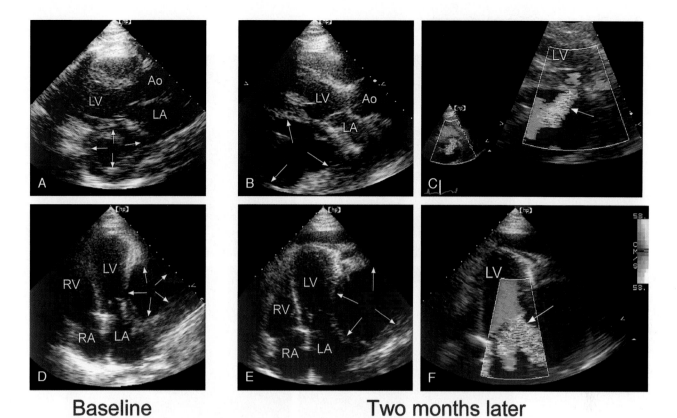

FIGURE 21.19. Progression of disease over time in a patient with metastatic melanoma is shown. **A–C:** Long-axis views. **D–F:** Four-chamber views. On the initial echocardiogram, a large cystic mass (*arrows*) was present posterior and lateral to the left heart. Two months later, the mass had increased in size and color Doppler imaging demonstrated flow communication between this structure and the left ventricle (*LV*). This was due to free wall rupture and pseudoaneurysm formation. Note how the pseudoaneurysm compresses the left heart. Ao, aorta; LA, left atrium; RA, right atrium; RV, right ventricle.

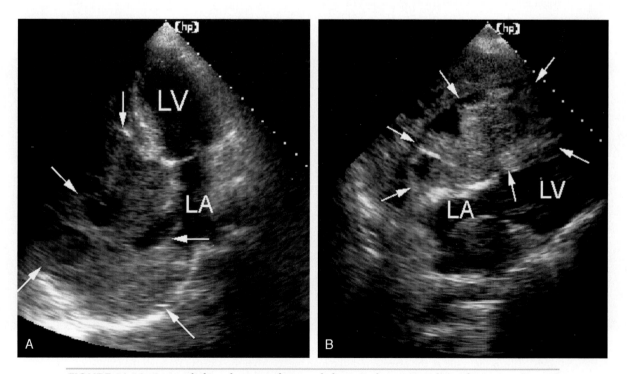

FIGURE 21.20. Pericardial involvement of a mesothelioma is demonstrated. **A:** A large mass (*arrows*) completely obscures the right heart and encroaches on the left atrium (*LA*). **B:** Subcostal image demonstrates the extent of the malignancy (*arrows*) and the mass effect that it creates on the left heart. LV, left ventricle.

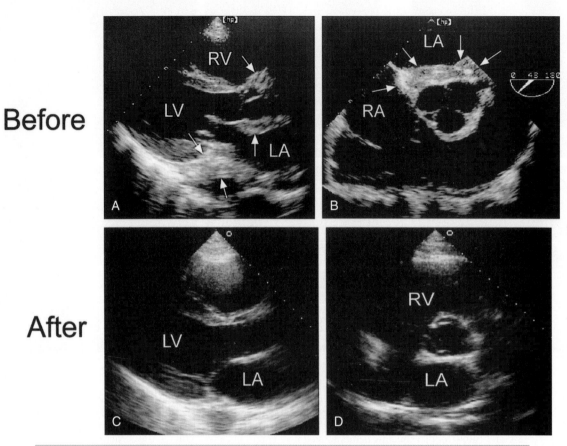

FIGURE 21.21. A, B: A lymphoma invading the heart and great vessels is shown. The tumor can be seen encasing the aortic root and the posterior atrioventricular groove (*arrows*). After successful chemotherapy, the echocardiogram appears essentially normal **(C, D)**. LA, left atrium; RA, right atrium; LV, left ventricle; RV, right ventricle.

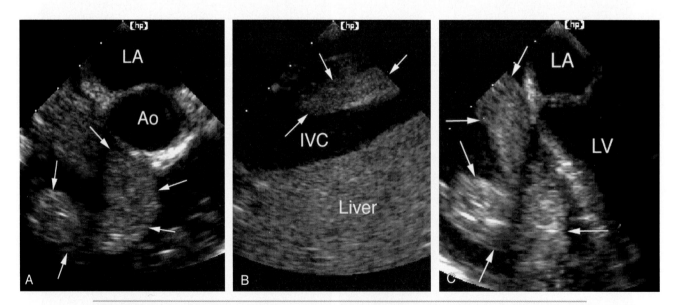

FIGURE 21.22. Renal cell carcinoma often affects the right heart. **A:** Tumors fill the right atrium (*arrows*). This is the result of the extension of the malignancy from the kidneys through the inferior vena cava (*IVC*) **(B)**. **C:** The tumor is seen invading the right ventricle. Ao, aorta; LA, left atrium; LV, left ventricle.

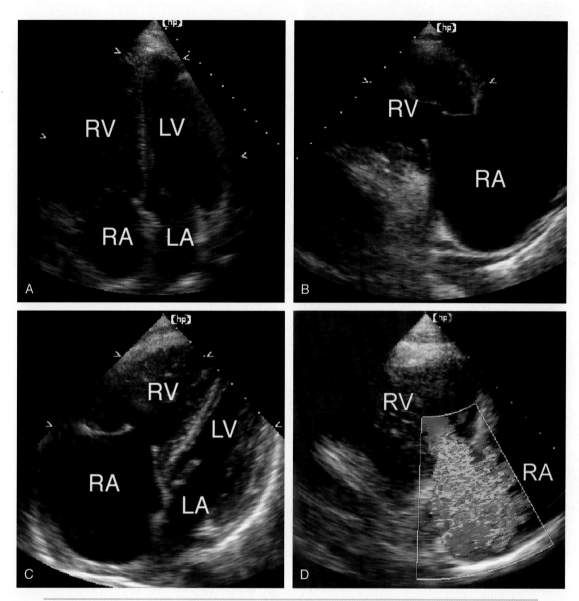

FIGURE 21.23. An example of carcinoid heart disease is shown. **A:** The right heart is dilated and the tricuspid valve is thickened, fibrotic, and immobile. The tricuspid leaflets are fixed **(B)** and do not coapt in systole **(C)**. **D:** Color Doppler imaging demonstrates severe tricuspid regurgitation. LA, left atrium; LV, left ventricle; RA, right atrium; RV, right ventricle.

ventricle, most often in the presence of akinesis or dyskinesis. Infarcts that do not result in an apical wall motion abnormality are less likely to be associated with thrombus formation. Although myocardial infarction is the most common predisposing cause of left ventricular thrombi, they can develop in any situation in which low flow and blood stasis occur, such as a chronic left ventricular aneurysm. In patients with dilated cardiomyopathy, low-velocity swirling of blood within the left ventricle also predisposes to the development of a thrombus. With color flow imaging from the apical four-chamber view, a slow, counterclockwise flow of blood during diastole may be present.

Left ventricular thrombi are best detected using transthoracic echocardiography. Apical views that position the left ventricular apex in the near field are optimal for this purpose. To enhance sensitivity, a high-frequency transducer with a short focal length is optimal. Thrombi are typically amorphous, echogenic structures with variable shape and are adherent to the endocardium (Fig. 21.25). Thrombi may be multiple and mobile and may protrude into the left ventricular cavity. In most cases, they have a texture and appearance that are distinct from the adjacent myocardium. An echo-lucent center may be present and suggests that the thrombus is relatively new and actively growing. In some patients, differentiating be-

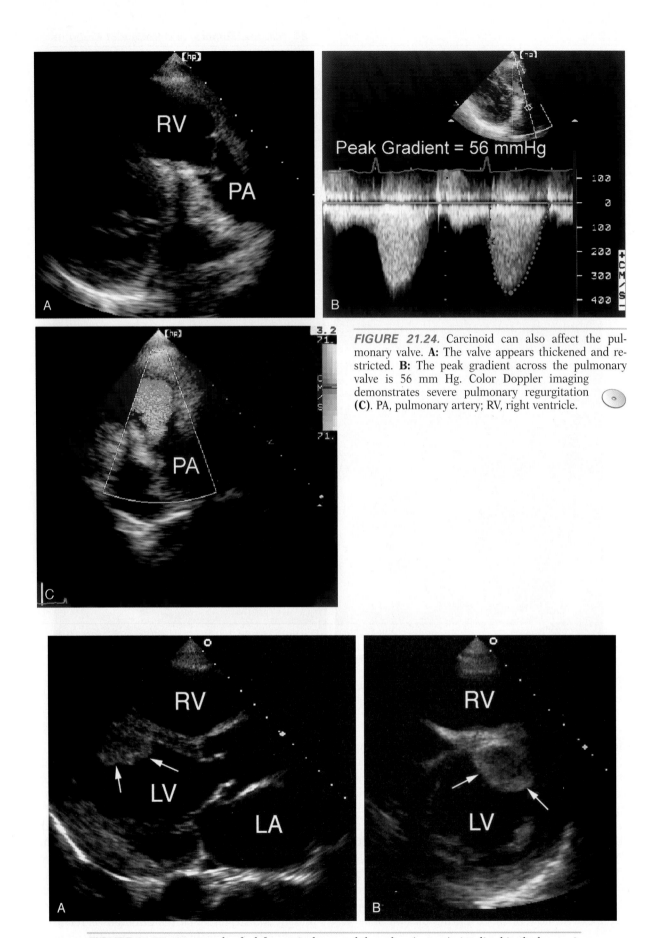

FIGURE 21.24. Carcinoid can also affect the pulmonary valve. **A:** The valve appears thickened and restricted. **B:** The peak gradient across the pulmonary valve is 56 mm Hg. Color Doppler imaging demonstrates severe pulmonary regurgitation **(C)**. PA, pulmonary artery; RV, right ventricle.

FIGURE 21.25. An example of a left ventricular mural thrombus (*arrows*) visualized in the long-axis **(A)** and short-axis **(B)** views. LA, left atrium; LA, left atrium; LV, left ventricle; RV, right ventricle.

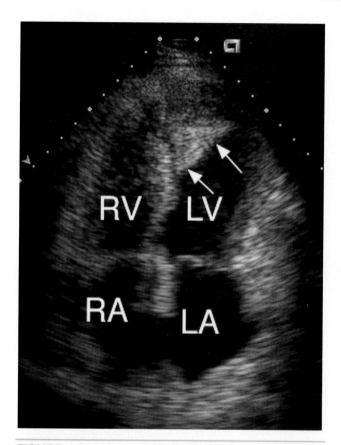

FIGURE 21.26. A large apical left ventricular thrombus is seen filling an apical aneurysm. In real time, the thrombus demonstrated little mobility. LA, left atrium; LV, left ventricle; RA, right atrium; RV, right ventricle.

tween thrombus and myocardium may be difficult. In Figure 21.26, a large thrombus can be seen within an apical aneurysm. Despite its size, the thrombus is immobile and does not extend into the cavity of the left ventricle. Figure 21.27 demonstrates a smaller thrombus but one that exhibits mobility and protrusion.

The sensitivity of transthoracic echocardiography for detecting left ventricular thrombi is between 75% and 95%. Small, laminar thrombi that do not protrude into the cavity are most likely to be missed. Poor image quality greatly affects accuracy and may produce both false-negative and false-positive results. To avoid false-negative results, appropriate transducer selection is critical. A high-frequency (e.g., 5 MHz), short-focus transducer is optimal in most cases. In addition, the use of modified apical transducer positions allows a thorough interrogation and improves accuracy. Large, protruding thrombi are readily seen from the apical window (Fig. 21.26 and 21.27). Figure 21.28 illustrates a relatively large apical thrombus that was not apparent using "standard" apical views. Only when tangential or off-axis views were obtained was the mass evident. Contrast can also be used to improve detection thrombi in cases of poor image quality. Figure 21.29 is an example of an apical thrombus that could not be visualized on routine transthoracic imaging. After administration of contrast, the apical mass is clearly recorded. Thrombi may involve more than one cardiac chamber. Figure 21.30 is from a patient with alcoholic cardiomyopathy and atrial fibrillation. Thrombi were detected in both left and right ventricular apices as well as the right atrium.

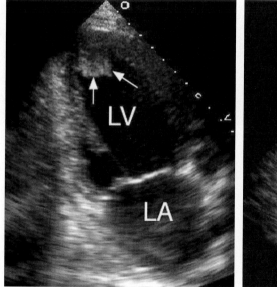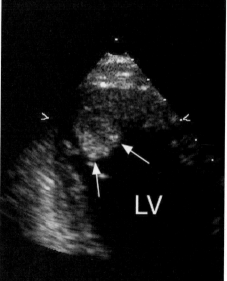

FIGURE 21.27. A small left ventricular apical thrombus (*arrows*) is recorded. From the apical two-chamber view (*left*), the thrombus protrudes into the cavity and demonstrates mobility on real-time imaging (*right*). LA, left atrium; LV, left ventricle.

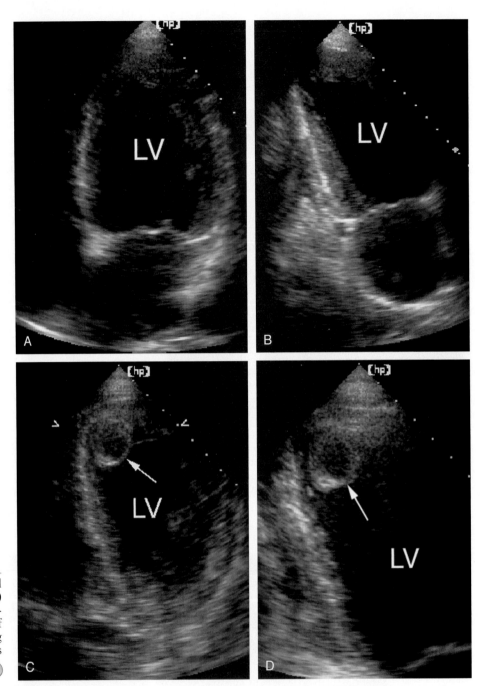

FIGURE 21.28. Standard apical four- (A) and two-chamber (B) views, respectively. From this window, the apex appears free of thrombi. C, D: Off-axis imaging demonstrates a large, circular mass (*arrow*) consistent with a thrombus. LV, left ventricle.

False-positive results also occur, most often as a result of improper imaging technique leading to foreshortening of the true apex. In most cases, the diagnosis can be made based on the presence or absence of an apical wall motion abnormality. Apical hypertrophy is occasionally misdiagnosed as a mural thrombus. Figure 21.13 is an example of endocardial fibroelastosis, which is a rare condition that can mimic an apical thrombus. Other left ventricular conditions that may be confused with thrombi include

hypereosinophilic syndrome (Fig. 21.31). This produces dense endocardial fibrosis that has a characteristic echogenicity or brightness on the echocardiogram. In the example shown, note the bright appearance of both the apical mass and the underlying myocardium. This is likely due to fibrosis and infiltration within the tissue. Mural thrombi often form over the thickened endocardium, thus distinguishing a thrombus from fibrosis may be difficult.

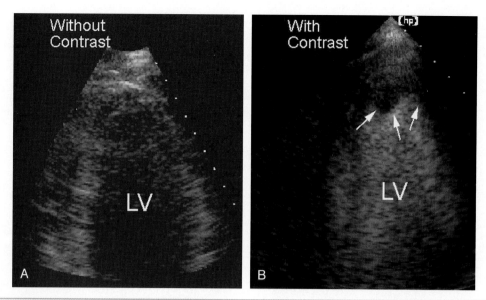

FIGURE 21.29. In patients with poor acoustic windows, contrast injection can be useful to outline a mural thrombus. **A:** Without contrast, the thrombus is not visualized. **B:** The presence of contrast within the left ventricle (*LV*) outlines the apical mass (*arrows*).

Myocardial noncompaction is a rare congenital form of cardiomyopathy in which the apical portion of the left (and sometimes right) ventricle is involved (Fig. 21.32). Due to failure of normal "compaction" *in utero*, the involved myocardium is characterized by a spongy appearance with prominent trabeculations and deep intertrabecular recesses. In some cases, color flow imaging will demonstrate flow within these spongiform recesses, creating a "Swiss cheese-like" appearance.

Thrombi rarely form in the absence of apical dyskinesis, so masses seen in the setting of normal wall motion should suggest other possibilities. Figure 21.33 is an example of an apical mass in a patient with normal wall motion. This most likely represents a muscle bundle or trabeculation. Tumors or vegetations may also occur in this location, and the final diagnosis can rarely be made solely on the basis of the echocardiogram. Transesophageal echocardiography offers few advantages over transthoracic imaging for assessing the apex and detecting left ventricular thrombi. However, the use of multiplane imaging from the gastric views does permit a thorough evaluation of the apex. This is particularly

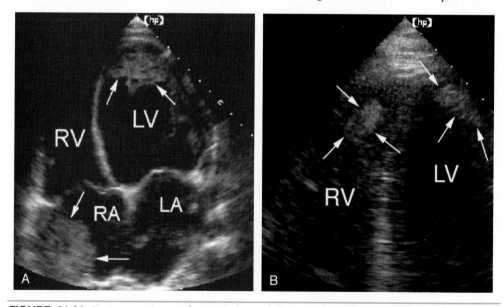

FIGURE 21.30. From a patient with severe heart failure due to dilated cardiomyopathy, multiple thrombi are recorded. **A:** A left ventricular apical thrombus and a large right atrial thrombus are indicated by the *arrows*. **B:** A modified apical view demonstrates thrombi in both the left and right ventricle (*arrows*). LA, left atrium; LV, left ventricle; RA, right atrium; RV, right ventricle.

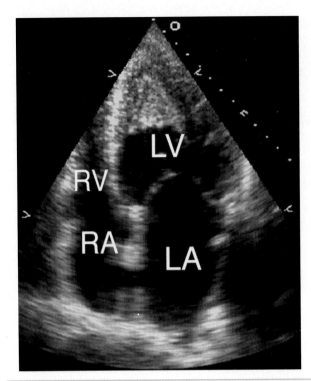

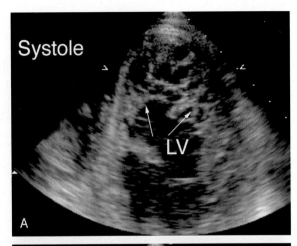

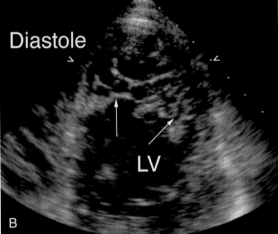

FIGURE 21.31. Endocardial thickening and fibrosis are characteristics of hypereosinophilic syndrome. The highly echogenic mass within the left ventricular apex is the result of this process. LA, left atrium; LV, left ventricle; RA, right atrium; RV, right ventricle.

FIGURE 21.32. An example of noncompaction of the left ventricular myocardium is illustrated. Systolic **(A)** and diastolic **(B)** images are provided. The left ventricle (*LV*) apex has a thickened, spongiform appearance (*arrows*).

helpful in the presence of poor transthoracic image quality.

Echocardiography can also identify thrombi that are most likely associated with embolic risk (Fig. 21.27). Risk factors include large size, mobility, and protrusion into the left ventricular cavity. Other less well established risk factors are hyperkinetic wall motion adjacent to the thrombus and an echo-lucent center (presumably identifying an actively growing thrombus). Assessment of these various characteristics may be helpful in guiding the use of anticoagulation in some patients. Echocardiography can also be used to follow known ventricular thrombi, particularly after myocardial infarction, to detect changes over time and ultimate resolution.

Left Atrial Thrombi

Although thrombi may form anywhere within the left atrium, the appendage is by far the most likely site. Any condition leading to stasis of blood within the left atrium predisposes to thrombus formation. These include mitral stenosis, atrial fibrillation, and left ventricular failure. On the other hand, significant mitral regurgitation, by increasing flow velocity within the left atrium during systole, may reduce the risk of thrombus formation. Figure 21.34 demonstrates a very large left atrial thrombus from a patient with rheumatic mitral valve disease and a huge

left atrium. In this extreme case, the thrombus most likely originated in the atrial appendage but grew in size and eventually spread to the body of the left atrium. The left atrial appendage is difficult to image using the transthoracic approach. The basal short-axis view can be manipulated to visualize the left atrial appendage just below the pulmonary artery in some patients. In other cases, the apical two-chamber view will permit recording of the appendage (Fig. 21.35). Because this is feasible in only a minority of patients, however, transthoracic imaging should rarely be relied on to exclude left atrial thrombi. In most cases, transesophageal imaging is necessary to visualize the entire left atrium, including the appendage, and thus to exclude the possibility of a thrombus. The approach to interrogation of the left atrium using transesophageal echocardiography is discussed in detail in Chapters 5 and 7. It should be emphasized that the appendage is multilobed in as many as 70% of patients and is lined by pectinate muscles, which can be confused with thrombus (Fig. 21.36). Despite this, the sensitivity of transesophageal imaging for the detection of left atrial thrombus is approxi-

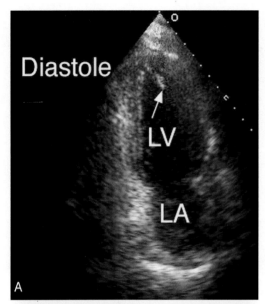

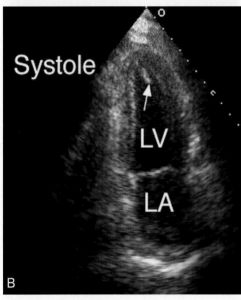

FIGURE 21.33. An echogenic, small apical mass (*arrow*) is recorded in a patient with normal left ventricular wall motion. The two-chamber view is shown in diastole **(A)** and systole **(B)**. This likely represents a trabeculation or muscle bundle within the cavity. LA, left atrium, LV, left ventricle.

mately 95% and in some series has been 100%. Specificity is similarly high. Once visualized, thrombi should be assessed for their size and mobility, and whether they extend into the body of the left atrium. Figure 21.37 is an example of a mobile and protuberant appendage thrombus. Figure 21.38 includes two examples of larger thrombi in the left atrial appendage. A small thrombus associated with spontaneous echo contrast is shown in Figure 21.39.

Echocardiography also allows detection of spontaneous echo contrast within the left atrium, possibly a precursor to the development of thrombus formation and certainly a risk factor for embolization (this topic is cov-

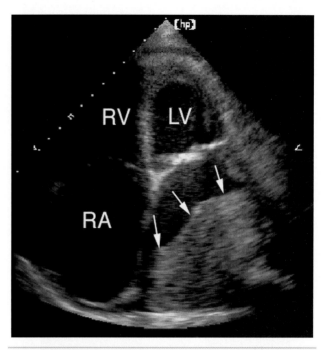

FIGURE 21.34. In a patient with untreated rheumatic heart disease, a very large left atrial thrombus (*arrows*) is seen. The right atrium (*RA*) is also severely dilated. LV, left ventricle; RV, right ventricle.

ered later in this chapter). The most direct evidence of embolic risk is visualization of the thrombus with two-dimensional echocardiography. In addition, pulsed Doppler imaging should also be performed to assess flow velocity within the appendage. Low left atrial appendage empty-

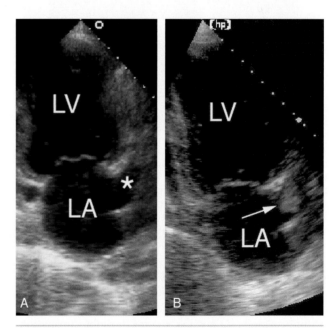

FIGURE 21.35. The left atrial appendage (*asterisk*) sometimes can be recorded using transthoracic echocardiography from the apical two-chamber view **(A)**. **B:** A thrombus within the appendage is indicated by the *arrow*. LA, left atrium; LV, left ventricle.

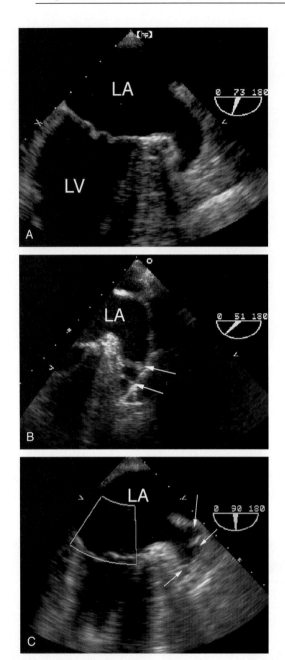

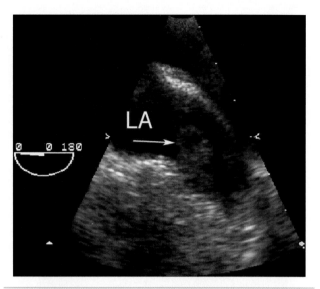

FIGURE 21.37. This magnified view of the left atrial appendage demonstrates a small mobile thrombus (*arrow*). LA, left atrium.

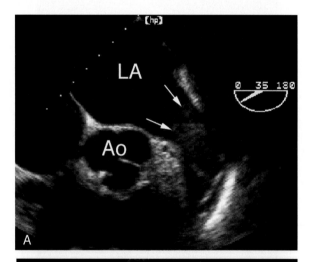

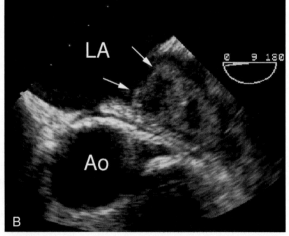

FIGURE 21.36. Transesophageal echocardiography is used to assess the left atrial appendage for thrombus. **A:** A normal left atrial appendage is demonstrated. **B:** The *arrows* indicate small pectinate muscles within the appendage. These are normal structures that are sometimes confused with thrombi. **C:** A multilobed appendage is illustrated, the different lobes indicated by the *arrows*. LA, left atrium; LV, left ventricle.

ing velocity (<20 cm/sec) has been reported to significantly increase the embolic risk (Fig. 21.40). Once the left atrial appendage is assessed, the atrial septum should also be interrogated as a possible site for thrombus formation in the presence of an atrial septal aneurysm and/or a PFO. These aneurysms are the result of redundancy of atrial septal tissue leading to a "windsock" appearance within which thrombi may form. In rare instances, echocardiog-

FIGURE 21.38. Two examples of left atrial appendage thrombi are included. **A:** A relatively small, nonmobile thrombus is indicated by the *arrows*. **B:** A larger thrombus is present (*arrows*) and appears to fill most of the appendage. Ao, aorta; LA, left atrium.

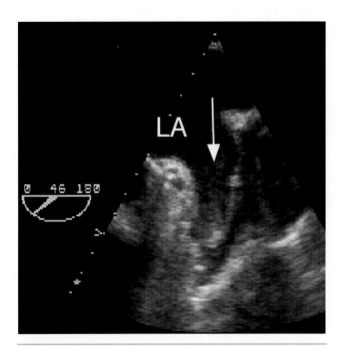

FIGURE 21.39. An example of a small thrombus within the left atrial appendage is demonstrated (*arrow*). LA, left atrium.

raphy may demonstrate thrombus crossing a PFO, from the right atrium to the left atrium. Figure 21.41 illustrates a thrombus that probably originated in the lower extremity veins and can be seen straddling the atrial septum through a PFO. This patient had presented with dyspnea, the result of recurring pulmonary emboli. Figure 21.42 is another example of a very mobile thrombus that can be seen crossing the atrial septum via a large PFO.

Right Atrial Thrombi

Although less common, patients with atrial fibrillation may develop thrombi within the right atrium. The right atrial appendage has a different shape compared with its left-sided counterpart (Fig. 21.43), and echocardiographers are generally less adept at visualizing this structure. However, a right atrial thrombus in the setting of atrial fibrillation is well documented and has been associated with the potential for pulmonary embolus. Thrombi have also been recorded within the right atrium "in transit" (Figs. 21.44 and 21.45). In such cases, the detection of mobile thrombi within the body of the right atrium most likely represents a stage in the development of pulmonary embolus in which thrombi have migrated from lower extremity or pelvic veins into the right heart before embolization to the lungs. Finally, a common source of thrombus formation within the right atrium involves the presence of indwelling catheters or pacemaker leads (Figs. 21.46 and 21.47). In such patients, transesophageal echocardiography is most useful for detecting amorphous and irregularly shaped masses attached to catheters. Such thrombi may become infected or lead to right-sided embolic events.

Spontaneous Echo Contrast

Spontaneous echo contrast (SEC), or "smoke," is the swirling, hazy echocardiographic appearance associated with low blood flow. The development of SEC has been attributed to a variety of low-flow states and the associated red blood cell–protein interactions (e.g., rouleau formation) that characterize such conditions. To occur, therefore, two conditions must be met. First, there must be a

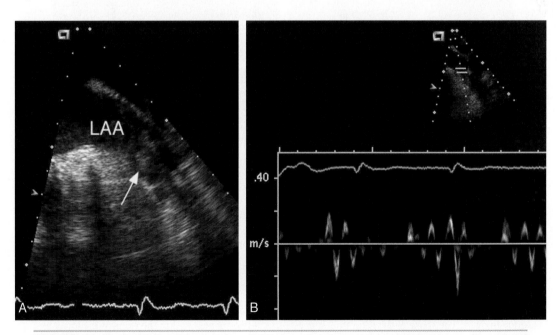

FIGURE 21.40. **A:** A left atrial appendage (*LAA*) thrombus (*arrow*) is recorded with two-dimensional imaging. **B:** Pulsed Doppler imaging records low (<20 cm/sec) atrial appendage emptying velocity. Spontaneous echo contrast was also present within the left atrium.

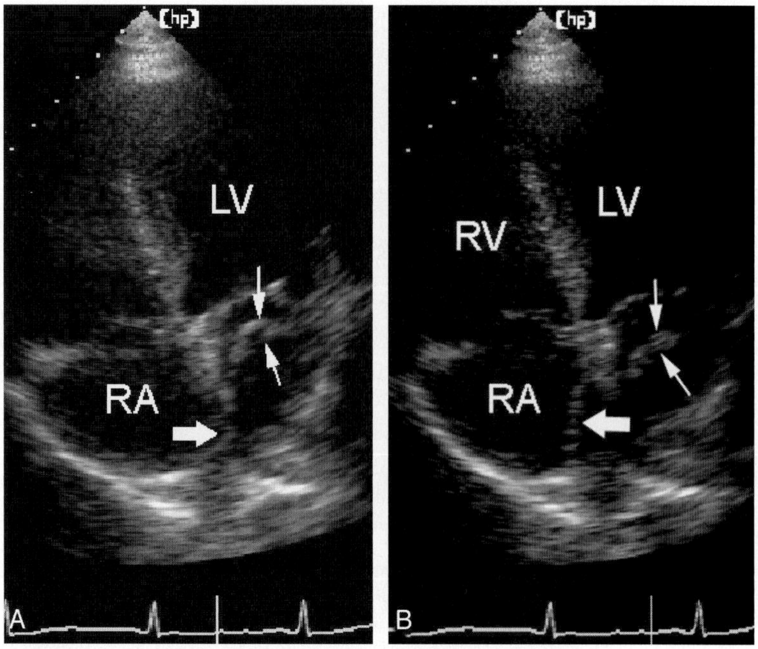

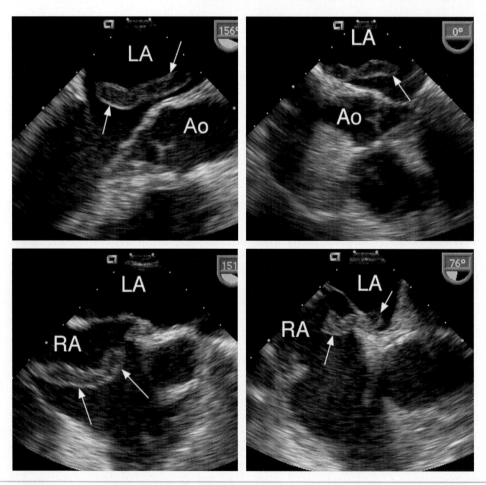

FIGURE 21.41. A, B: A thrombus is recorded straddling the interatrial septum through a patent foramen ovale and extending into the left atrium (*small arrows*). The thrombus was highly mobile and likely originated in the lower extremities. Increased mobility of atrial septal tissue is indicated by the *large arrow.* LV, left ventricle; RA, right atrium; RV, right ventricle.

FIGURE 21.42. A large, tubular-shaped thrombus (*arrows*) is demonstrated as it crosses a patent foramen ovale. The shape of the thrombus suggests that it was formed within the veins of the lower extremities. Its presence within the left heart greatly increases the likelihood of systemic embolization. The four images were recorded over several minutes, demonstrating the thrombus in the right and left atrium, and straddling the patent foramen ovale (lower right panel). Ao, aorta; LA, left atrium; RA, right atrium.

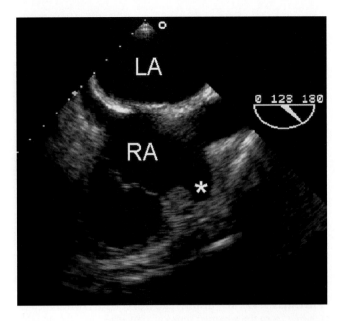

FIGURE 21.43. With transesophageal echocardiography, the bicaval view can be adjusted to record the right atrial appendage (*asterisk*). LA, left atrium; RA, right atrium.

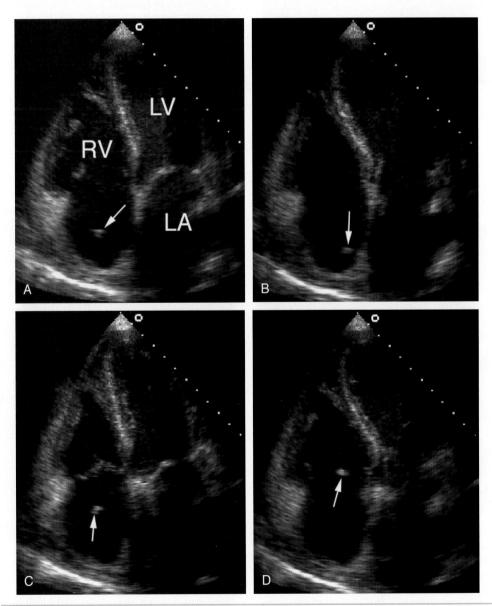

FIGURE 21.44. Thrombi can occasionally be recorded during transit through the right heart. **A–D:** Small thrombi are recorded at various locations within the right atrium and right ventricle (*RV*) (*arrows*). These will most likely lead to a pulmonary embolism. LA, left atrium; LV, left ventricle.

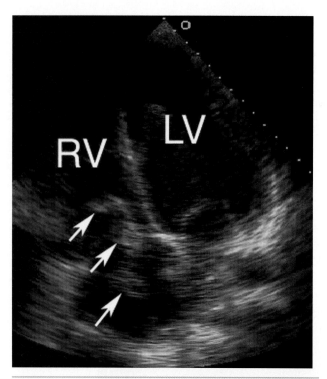

FIGURE 21.45. This apical four-chamber view demonstrates a large, multilobed thrombus straddling the tricuspid valve (*arrows*). The thrombus could be traced to the inferior vena cava. LV, left ventricle; RV, right ventricle.

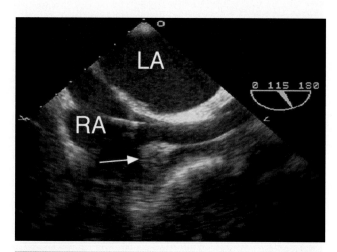

FIGURE 21.47. Two distinct pacemaker leads are recorded extending from the superior vena cava into the right atrium (*RA*). A large mass is attached to one lead (*arrow*). This most likely represents thrombus formation. LA, left atrium.

location, usually in the left atrium, right atrium, or left ventricle, where stasis or low-flow velocity is present. Then, as a result, some interaction between blood cells and plasma proteins, specifically fibrinogen, must occur (Fig. 21.48). Some investigators have considered SEC a prethrombotic condition, although whether SEC actually leads to thrombus formation is not clearly established. Regardless of cause and effect, the presence of SEC has been consistently associated with increased risk of throm-

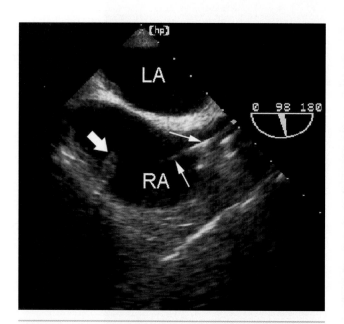

FIGURE 21.46. The bicaval view is useful to interrogate indwelling catheters and pacemaker leads for the presence of thrombi and/or vegetations. In this example, a pacemaker lead extends from the superior vena cava into the right atrium (*RA*) (*small arrows*). A mass within the lower portion of the right atrium (*large arrow*) represents thrombus attached to the lead. LA, left atrium.

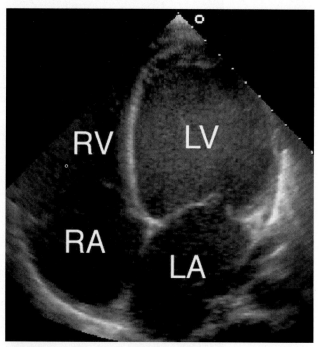

FIGURE 21.48. This apical four-chamber view from a patient with dilated cardiomyopathy demonstrates spontaneous echo contrast within the left ventricle (*LV*). This is due to low blood flow. LA, left atrium; RA, right atrium; RV, right ventricle.

boembolism. SEC is difficult to quantify, and its detection is also dependent on instrument settings. A higher frequency transducer and increased gain settings are sometimes necessary to visualize SEC. One final cautionary note is in order. With modern equipment, using higher frequency transducers and tissue harmonics, SEC may occasionally be seen in normal individuals. This is simply a consequence of highly sensitive instrument settings. The distinction between pathologic and artifactual SEC should be obvious from other echocardiographic clues. For example, if SEC is recorded in the absence of left ventricular failure, mitral stenosis, or atrial fibrillation, it is most likely attributable to machine settings.

ROLE OF ECHOCARDIOGRAPHY IN ATRIAL FIBRILLATION AND CARDIOVERSION

Atrial fibrillation is a risk factor for stroke, and there is strong evidence that this risk is reduced by long-term anticoagulation or restoration of normal rhythm. Transthoracic echocardiography is useful in patients with atrial fibrillation for several reasons. It defines cardiac anatomy that predisposes to arrhythmia and permits an assessment of left ventricular wall thickness, mass, and function. The decrease in global left ventricular function that is often seen in atrial fibrillation can be visually assessed. Echocardiography also can be used to document the improvement in ventricular function after cardioversion. Finally, a transthoracic study allows a direct measurement of left and right atrial size. Although left atrial size is often used to help determine the likelihood of successfully maintaining sinus rhythm, it does not correlate well with the risk of thromboembolism. Thus, a transthoracic echocardiogram can be used to determine the underlying factors responsible for atrial fibrillation, the risk of thromboembolism, and the likelihood of successful cardioversion. However, transthoracic echocardiography is unable to reliably detect left atrial thrombi that are causative in most cases of thromboembolic stroke. To do so requires transesophageal imaging.

The major advantage offered by transesophageal echocardiography in patients with atrial fibrillation is the ability to interrogate the atrial appendage for thrombus. The risk of stroke after successful direct current cardioversion is increased in the presence of left atrial thrombi. In addition, reduced appendage emptying velocity (<20 cm/sec), dense left atrial spontaneous contrast, and complex aortic plaque are findings on transesophageal echocardiography that also increase thromboembolic risk. Because of its high sensitivity, transesophageal echocardiography is frequently used before elective cardioversion to detect atrial thrombi. Although the left atrium is of primary interest in this assessment, the operator should always examine the right atrial appendage as well because thrombi also occur there.

In recent years, considerable research has focused on the potential role of transesophageal echocardiography in guiding the management of patients with atrial fibrillation. For most patients, conventional therapy involves 3 to 4 weeks of oral anticoagulation before cardioversion, followed by 3 to 6 months of warfarin after restoration of sinus rhythm. The institution of 3 to 4 weeks of warfarin before cardioversion will reduce the likelihood of thromboembolism from 4%–6% to 0%–1.6%. If low-risk status could be determined using echocardiography, cardioversion could be performed immediately, thereby reducing the risks associated with anticoagulation and perhaps increasing the likelihood of successful cardioversion. Specifically, it was postulated that, in the absence of echocardiographic evidence of left atrial thrombus, elective cardioversion could proceed with a low risk of an embolic event (provided that patients were adequately anticoagulated at the time of the procedure and anticoagulation was maintained for several weeks afterward). The need for continued anticoagulation after cardioversion is predicated on the likelihood of transient left atrial appendage "stunning," which has been documented echocardiographically and is a risk factor for thrombus formation. This strategy shortens the duration of atrial fibrillation and promotes more rapid recovery of mechanical atrial function (i.e., reduced left atrial appendage stunning). If this rate were comparable with the reduction in risk provided by 3 to 4 weeks of precardioversion anticoagulation, the echocardiography-guided strategy would be very attractive. Alternatively, if a thrombus were present, the conventional strategy could be followed. That is, cardioversion would be delayed and oral anticoagulation instituted for several weeks before attempting to restore sinus rhythm.

A multicenter clinical trial has examined the role of transesophageal echocardiography in guiding management of atrial fibrillation (Klein et al., 2001). In the Assessment of Cardioversion Using Transesophageal Echocardiography (ACUTE) study, patients were randomized to either transesophageal echocardiography or conventional therapy. Patients who underwent echocardiography were anticoagulated and either cardioverted within 24 hours (in the absence of thrombus) or anticoagulation was continued for 3 weeks before a repeat transesophageal echocardiogram.

Conventional therapy consisted of 3 to 4 weeks of anticoagulation before cardioversion. The flow chart provided in Figure 21.49 indicates the number of patients in each treatment arm and the end points achieved. The success or failure to restore sinus rhythm with cardioversion is also provided for each strategy. The study demonstrated a similar rate of embolic events in the two groups (0.8 % in the transesophageal echocardiography group and 0.5% in the conventional treatment group). Hemorrhagic events were significantly lower among patients whose management was guided by echocardiography. This group also had a shorter time to cardioversion and a higher initial success rate for restoration of sinus rhythm compared

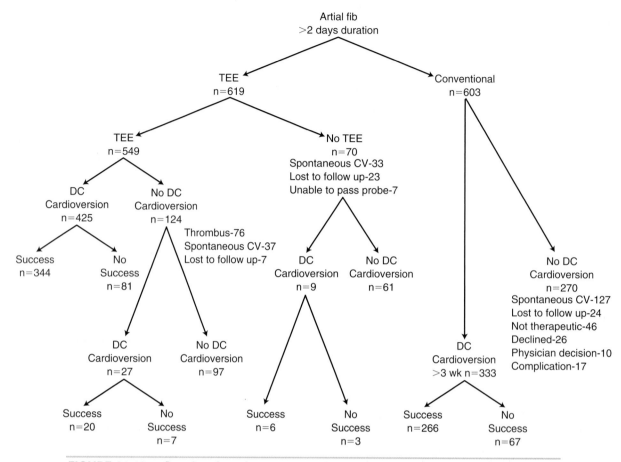

FIGURE 21.49. A flow chart from the Assessment of Cardioversion Using Transesophageal Echocardiography (ACUTE) trial is shown. Patients were randomized to conventional or transesophageal echocardiography–guided therapy. "Success" refers to the restoration of sinus rhythm after cardioversion. See text for details. Atrial fib, atrial fibrillation; CV, cardioversion; DC, direct current; TEE, transesophageal echocardiography. (Modified from Klein AL, Grimm RA, Murray RD, et al. Use of transesophageal echocardiography to guide cardioversion in patients with atrial fibrillation. N Engl J Med 2001;344:1411–1420, with permission.)

with conventional management. However, the rate at which sinus rhythm was maintained at 8 weeks was similar in the two groups.

In summary, a growing body of evidence supports the use of transesophageal echocardiography to identify patients with atrial fibrillation who might be candidates for early cardioversion. The sensitivity and specificity of the test to detect atrial thrombi and the link between the presence of thrombus and the risk of stroke underscore the utility of this approach. Some guidelines regarding accepted indications for echocardiography before elective cardioversion are listed in Table 21.5.

ROLE OF ECHOCARDIOGRAPHY IN SYSTEMIC EMBOLUS

One of the most frequent reasons to request an echocardiogram involves the search for a potential cardiac source of embolus. In many large laboratories, this is the single

most common indication for transesophageal echocardiography. Embolic events, particularly strokes, can be devastating. Because the cause of a stroke can be difficult to establish on clinical grounds and because embolic strokes are often recurrent, an aggressive attempt to identify potential cardiac sources of emboli is understandable.

Unfortunately, the proper use of echocardiography in this setting remains controversial. It is estimated that approximately one-fourth of all strokes are due to a cardiac source of embolus, although the rate is significantly higher in younger patients. A list of potential cardiac sources of embolus is provided in Table 21.6. It is apparent that many of these potential cardiac sources can be identified with echocardiography. In most series, the yield of transesophageal echocardiography is significantly higher than that of transthoracic echocardiography (Table 21.7). For example, atrial thrombi are rarely seen by transthoracic echocardiography but readily detected using transesophageal techniques (Fig. 21.41). Using the transthoracic method, only approximately 15% of pa-

▶ TABLE 21.5 **Echocardiography Before Cardioversion**

Indications	Class
1. Patients requiring urgent (not emergent) cardioversion for whom extended precardioversion anticoagulation is not desirable.[a]	I
2. Patients who have had prior cardioembolic events thought to be related to intraatrial thrombus.[a]	I
3. Patients for whom anticoagulation is contraindicated and for whom a decision about cardioversion will be influenced by TEE results.[a]	I
4. Patients for whom intraatrial thrombus has been demonstrated in previous TEE.[a]	I
5. Evaluation of patient for whom a decision concerning cardioversion will be impacted by knowledge of prognostic factors (such as LV function, coexistent mitral valve disease, etc.).	I
6. Patients with atrial fibrillation of <48 hours' duration and other heart disease.[a]	IIa
7. Patients with atrial fibrillation of <48 hours' duration and no other heart disease.[a]	IIb
8. Patients with mitral valve disease or hypertrophic cardiomyopathy who have been on long-term anticoagulation at therapeutic levels before cardioversion unless there are other reasons for anticoagulation (e.g., prior embolus or known thrombus on previous TEE).[a]	IIb
9. Patients undergoing cardioversion from atrial flutter.	IIb
10. Patients requiring emergent cardioversion.	III
11. Patients who have been on long-term anticoagulation at therapeutic levels and who do not have mitral valve disease or hypertrophic cardiomyopathy before cardioversion unless there are other reasons for anticoagulation (e.g., prior embolus or known thrombus on previous TEE).	III
12. Precardioversion evaluation of patients who have undergone previous TEE and with no clinical suspicion of a significant interval change.	III

[a]TEE only. TEE, transesophageal echocardiography.
Adapted with permission from Cheitlin MD, Alpert JS, Armstrong WF, et al. ACC/AHA Guidelines for the Clinical Application of Echocardiography: a report of the American College of Cardiology/American Heart Association Task Force on Practice Guidelines (Committee on Clinical Application of Echocardiography) developed in collaboration with the American Society of Echocardiography. Circulation 1997;95:1686–1744.

▶ TABLE 21.6 **Potential Sources of Embolus and Associated Echocardiographic Findings**

Actual Source	Echocardiographic Findings
LV thrombus	Apical aneurysm, presence of thrombus, dilated CM
LA thrombus	Presence of thrombus in LAA, spontaneous echo contrast, LAA emptying velocity, mitral stenosis, interatrial septal low aneurysm
Pelvic veins or LE thrombus	ASD, atrial septal aneurysm, PFO
Native valves	Vegetation, tumor, MVP, mitral annular calcification, sclerotic aortic valve
Prosthetic valves	Thrombus, vegetation
Cardiac tumor	LA myxoma, papillary fibroelastoma
Aorta	Complex aortic plaque, atheroma

ASD, atrial septal defect; CM, cardiomyopathy; LA, left atrium; LAA, left atrial appendage; LE, lower extremity; LV, left ventricle; PFO, patent foramen ovale; MVP, mitral valve prolapse.

tients with a suspected embolic event have an identifiable cardiac source. This low incidence may be explained in part by the fact that the echocardiogram is performed after the event so that the cause is no longer present within the heart. More importantly, many of the potential cardiac sources of emboli are not easily evaluated from the transthoracic approach. If patients with evidence of cardiovascular disease (by history and physical examination or electrocardiography) are evaluated with transthoracic echocardiography, the yield is higher, approaching 50%. In all published series, however, transesophageal echocardiography identified a higher percentage of patients with a potential source of embolus. It should be emphasized that although a potential source of embolus may be detected, its presence does not establish a cause-and-effect relationship between the echocardiographic abnormality and the clinical event.

▶ TABLE 21.7 **Comparing the Yield of TTE versus TEE for Identifying Possible Source of Embolus**

Author/year	n	TTE %	TEE %
Pop/1990	72	8	15
Hofman/1990	153	36	58
Cujec/1991	63	14	41
Lee/1991	50	0	52
De Belder/1992	131	55	70
Comess/1994	145	ND	45

TEE, transesophageal echocardiography; TTE, transthoracic echocardiography; ND, not done.

Therefore, most cardiac findings are nonspecific, i.e., they are seen with similar frequency in patients with and without embolic events. For example, valve excrescences are seen so commonly in normal, asymptomatic elderly individuals that their detection in patients who have suffered an embolic event is of questionable significance. Aortic atheromas are also seen with regularity on transesophageal imaging (Fig. 21.50). Although they can embolize, their mere presence is usually insufficient proof of cause and effect. A PFO is present in approximately one-third of unselected patients. It can be detected with either transthoracic or transesophageal imaging, using color flow Doppler imaging, or injection of agitated saline (Figs. 21.51 and 21.52). The atrial septum often shows increased mobility or redundancy. A PFO is defined (and differentiated from an atrial septal defect) by the demonstration of atrial shunting in the absence of an anatomic defect or gap in the secundum septum. With transesophageal echocardiography, however, some separation between the overlapping primum and secundum septa may be seen. This is often respiratory cycle dependent. Once a PFO is demonstrated, estimating its size and the magnitude of shunting has practical implications. In general, separation of the overlapping septal planes by more than 2 mm is consistent with a large PFO. With injection of contrast, the presence of more than 10 microbubbles in the left atrium within three cardiac cycles is also consistent with a large PFO, and it has been suggested that this may confer a stronger link to clinical events.

Although the incidence of PFO may be higher in young patients who have suffered cerebrovascular events, compared with the general population, the frequency of the finding in the unselected population and the difficulty in establishing cause and effect, renders the presence of a PFO inconclusive in many cases. In contrast, the combination of PFO and atrial septal aneurysm appears to be associated

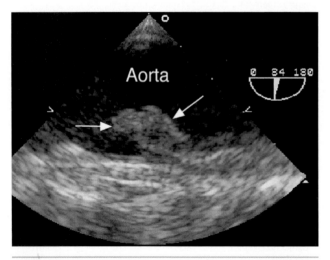

FIGURE 21.50. Complex aortic atheroma (*arrows*) is demonstrated using transesophageal echocardiography. The walls of the aorta are thickened and a mobile atheroma is present.

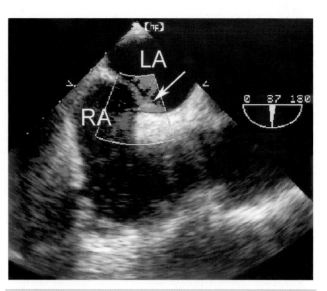

FIGURE 21.51. Detecting the presence of a patent foramen ovale often relies on color flow imaging. In this example, a small degree of shunting between the right (*RA*) and left atrium (*LA*) is present.

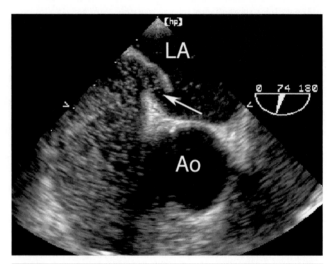

FIGURE 21.52. More extensive shunting is present in this example and is demonstrated using injection of agitated saline through a peripheral vein. The interatrial septum shows excessive mobility, and a clear tunnel-like defect is present. The degree of shunting can be estimated by virtue of the number of bubbles that appear within the left atrium (*LA*). Ao, aorta.

with a significant increase in risk (Fig. 21.53). In a prospective, multicenter study of patients who had had an ischemic stroke (Mas et al., 2001), the rate of recurrence was increased in the presence of both PFO and an atrial septal aneurysm compared with either condition alone.

An additional difficulty in this area is the challenge of demonstrating that echocardiographic findings alter management after an embolic event. In the Value of Transesophageal Echocardiography (VOTE) study (Goldman et al., 1994), among the subset of patients who were

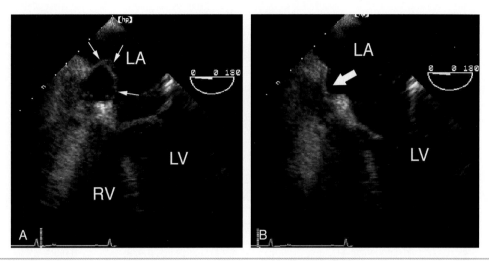

FIGURE 21.53. An example of an atrial septal aneurysm is shown. **A:** The aneurysm billows into the left atrium (*LA, arrows*). **B:** The redundant tissue billows into the right atrium (*large arrow*). Injection of contrast into the right heart confirms an associated patent foramen ovale by demonstrating right-to-left shunting. LV, left ventricle; RV, right ventricle.

studied because of a cerebrovascular event, the results of the echocardiogram affected clinical management in 27% and led to a change in drug therapy in 16%. In most cases, the altered management involved the decision to anticoagulate or close a PFO. It is clear, however, that many patients referred for echocardiography after an embolic event will not see their management altered substantially by the results of the imaging study.

Although the potential for overuse of echocardiography in search of a cardiac source of embolus exists, some studies have supported the cost-effectiveness of this approach. In one investigation (McNamara et al., 1997) in which clinical practice was simulated using a Markov decision model, the cost-effectiveness of different strategies, with and without echocardiography, were compared (Fig. 21.54). Using a hypothetical patient in sinus rhythm who suffers a first stroke, several strategies were tested for the likelihood of establishing a diagnosis and affecting the decision to anticoagulate. The different strategies included various combinations of cardiac history, transthoracic echocardiography, and transesophageal echocardiography, performed in different sequences. Assumptions were made about diagnostic yield, risk of recurrence, likelihood of complications, and outcome, and the cost of each strategy was compared with its utility. Cost-effectiveness was expressed as total cost per quality-adjusted life-year ($/QALY). Transthoracic echocardiography was not cost-effective under any circumstances. In contrast, strategies employing transesophageal imaging were found to be most efficient. Specifically, the two most cost-effective approaches were (1) transesophageal echocardiography performed only in patients with a history of cardiac problems (most cost-effective, at $8,700 per QALY) and (2) transesophageal echocardiography in all patients ($20,000 per

QALY). This was largely based on the ability to detect atrial thrombi and to prevent recurrent strokes by selectively initiating anticoagulation in such patients. The authors concluded that transesophageal echocardiography should be performed in all patients with acute stroke.

Although formal guidelines for this application of echocardiography do not yet exist, some general recommendations can be provided. A list of possible indications for the proper use of echocardiography in patients experiencing an embolic event is offered in Table 21.8. Among patients with a strong clinical suspicion of an embolic event, the yield of echocardiography (especially transesophageal imaging) is reasonable and the test should be considered. Echocardiographic imaging is more likely to provide a diagnosis in younger patients (<50 years) or in patients with known risk factors such as congenital heart disease or a PFO. In most instances, the greater diagnostic yield provided by transesophageal imaging compared with transthoracic echocardiography makes this the technique of choice to search for a potential source of embolus. Finally, the use of echocardiography in this complicated setting should be reserved for those instances in which the results are likely to alter management or to affect therapy. In older patients without clinical evidence of predisposing heart disease who are likely to have cerebrovascular disease, the very low yield of echocardiography argues against its use in this setting.

PSEUDOTUMORS AND OTHER CARDIAC MASSES

In addition to the false-positive results describe earlier in this chapter that represent normal variants (Table 21.1),

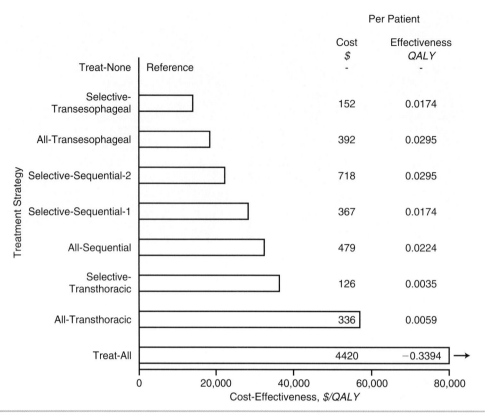

FIGURE 21.54. The cost-effectiveness of the different treatment strategies are compared with the treat-none approach. Both the cost per patient and the effectiveness [in quality-adjusted life-years (QALYs)] are listed for each strategy. See text for details. (From McNamara RL, Lima JA, Whelton PK, et al. Echocardiographic identification of cardiovascular sources of emboli to guide clinical management of stroke: a cost-effectiveness analysis. Ann Intern Med 1997;127:775–787, with permission.)

▶ **TABLE 21.8 Echocardiography in Patients with Neurologic Events or Other Vascular Occlusive Events**

Indications	Class
1. Patients of any age with abrupt occlusion of a major peripheral or visceral artery.	I
2. Younger patients (typically <45 years) with cerebrovascular events.	I
3. Older patients (typically >45 years) with neurologic events without evidence of cerebrovascular disease or other obvious cause.	I
4. Patients for whom a clinical therapeutic decision (anticoagulation, etc.) will depend on the results of echocardiography.	I
5. Patients with suspicion of embolic disease and with cerebrovascular disease of questionable significance.	IIa
6. Patients with a neurologic event and intrinsic cerebrovascular disease of a nature sufficient to cause the clinical event.	IIb
7. Patients for whom the results of echocardiography will not impact a decision to institute anticoagulant therapy or otherwise alter the approach to diagnosis or treatment.	III

Adapted with permission from Cheitlin MD, Alpert JS, Armstrong WF, et al. ACC/AHA Guidelines for the Clinical Application of Echocardiography: a report of the American College of Cardiology/American Heart Association Task Force on Practice Guidelines (Committee on Clinical Application of Echocardiography) developed in collaboration with the American Society of Echocardiography. Circulation 1997;95:1686–1744.

extracardiac masses may impinge on or compress the heart, creating the illusion of a mass effect. These include tumors within the mediastinum, coronary aneurysms, or hiatal hernias. An example of a hiatal hernia is illustrated in Figure 21.55. The mass appears to be within the atrium but is actually a portion of the stomach. The diagnosis can be clarified by having the patient drink a carbonated beverage during transthoracic imaging. After heart sur-

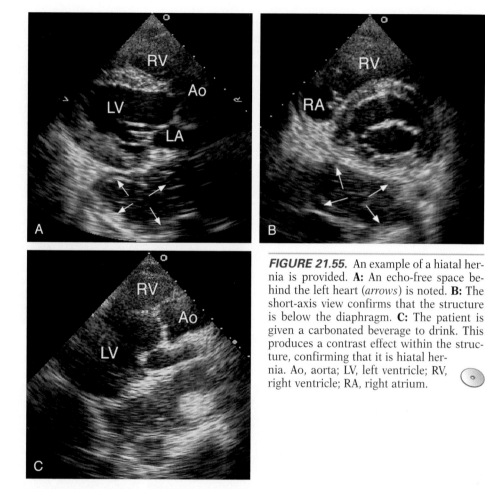

FIGURE 21.55. An example of a hiatal hernia is provided. **A:** An echo-free space behind the left heart (*arrows*) is noted. **B:** The short-axis view confirms that the structure is below the diaphragm. **C:** The patient is given a carbonated beverage to drink. This produces a contrast effect within the structure, confirming that it is hiatal hernia. Ao, aorta; LV, left ventricle; RV, right ventricle; RA, right atrium.

gery, accumulation of blood and hematoma within the mediastinum or pericardial space can result in external cardiac compression and the illusion of a mass (Figs. 21.56 and 21.57). These usually impinge on the right side of the heart and may affect right ventricular filling or pulmonary blood flow. Although the effects may resolve spontaneously, surgical evacuation is sometimes required.

The development of myocardial cysts is an uncommon complication of echinococcal infection. Although echo-

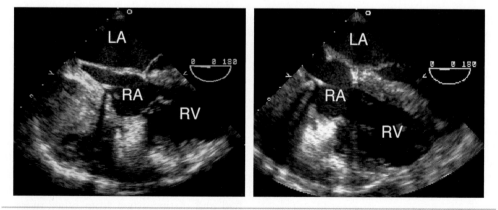

FIGURE 21.56. These transesophageal images were recorded from a patient 2 days after coronary artery bypass surgery. A systolic (left) and diastolic (right) image are provided. The patient had become hypotensive. A large, amorphous mass within the pericardial space can be seen to impinge on the right atrium (*RA*) and right ventricle (*RV*). This represents a hematoma that compressed the right heart and contributed to the hypotension. LA, left atrium; LV, left ventricle.

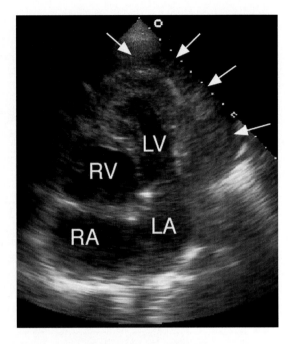

FIGURE 21.57. This transthoracic echocardiogram was recorded in a patient 1 week after open-heart surgery. A mass (*arrows*) is present adjacent to the apex and lateral wall of the left ventricle (*LV*). This likely represents a pericardial hematoma. The patient was clinically stable, and the mass gradually resolved. LA, left atrium; RA, right atrium; RV, right ventricle.

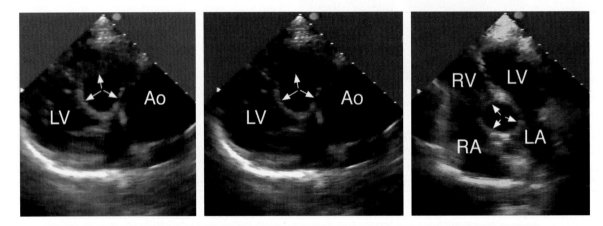

FIGURE 21.58. An echinococcal cyst (*arrows*) within the interventricular septum is demonstrated in a patient who had recently emigrated from the Middle East. The mass is seen in the long-axis (left), modified long-axis (middle) and four-chamber (right) views. The large hydatid cyst is typical of cardiac involvement of echinococcal infection. Ao, aorta; LA, left atrium; LV, left ventricle; RA, right atrium; RV, right ventricle.

cardiography is an accurate means of diagnosis, the rarity of the disease contributes to frequent misinterpretation. These cysts most often involve the left ventricular free wall and may project into the chamber or the pericardial space. They tend to be large, thin walled, and septated (Fig. 21.58). Such an appearance is considered classic, and, when present, the echocardiographic diagnosis is straightforward. Color Doppler imaging can be used to confirm the lack of blood flow within the cystic spaces. Rupture can occur and have catastrophic consequences.

A more benign condition is the pericardial cyst (Fig. 21.59). These cysts are simple, thin-walled, fluid-filled structures that typically are located within the right costophrenic angle. Because they are benign and usually do not produce symptoms, they must be correctly identified and distinguished from other more serious conditions. Unlike echinococcal cysts, they are extramyocardial and their interior is devoid of loculations or septa. These characteristics, in addition to their typical location, help to identify them and distinguish them from malignancy.

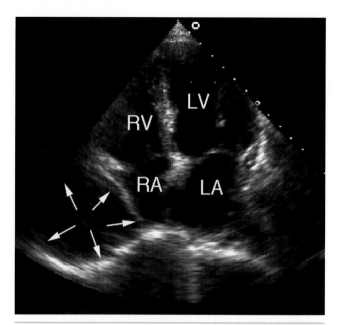

FIGURE 21.59. A large pericardial cyst (*arrows*) is demonstrated from the apical four-chamber view. These cysts are typically circular, thin walled, and echo free. They are often located near the right costophrenic angle. LA, left atrium; RA, right atrium; LV, left ventricle; RV, right ventricle.

SUGGESTED READINGS

Abraham KP, Reddy V, Gattuso P. Neoplasms metastatic to the heart: review of 3314 consecutive autopsies. Am J Cardiovasc Pathol 1990;3: 195–198.

Alam M. Pitfalls in the echocardiographic diagnosis of intracardiac and extracardiac masses. Echocardiography 1993;10:181–191.

Aschenberg W, Schluter M, Kremer P, et al. Transesophageal two-dimensional echocardiography for the detection of left atrial appendage thrombus. J Am Coll Cardiol 1986;7:163–166.

Cheitlin MD, Alpert JS, Armstrong WF, et al. ACC/AHA Guidelines for the Clinical Application of Echocardiography: a report of the American College of Cardiology/American Heart Association Task Force on Practice Guidelines (Committee on Clinical Application of Echocardiography) developed in collaboration with the American Society of Echocardiography. Circulation 1997;95:1686–1744.

Come PC, Riley MF, Bivas NK. Roles of echocardiography and arrhythmia monitoring in the evaluation of patients with suspected systemic embolism. Ann Neurol 1983;13:527–531.

Comess KA, DeRook FA, Beach KW, et al. Transesophageal echocardiography and carotid ultrasound in patients with cerebral ischemia: prevalence of findings and recurrent stroke risk. J Am Coll Cardiol 1994;23:1598–603.

Cujec B, Polasek P, Voll C, et al. Transesophageal echocardiography in the detection of potential cardiac source of embolism in stroke patients. Stroke 1991;22:727–733.

de Belder MA, Lovat LB, Tourikis L, et al. Limitations of transoesophageal echocardiography in patients with focal cerebral ischaemic events. Br Heart J 1992;67:297–303.

De Rook FA, Comess KA, Albers GW, et al. Transesophageal echocardiography in the evaluation of stroke. Ann Intern Med 1992;117:922–932.

Ezekowitz MD, Wilson DA, Smith EO, et al. Comparison of Indium-111 platelet scintigraphy and two-dimensional echocardiography in the diagnosis of left ventricular thrombi. N Engl J Med 1982;306:1509–1513.

Farfel Z, Shechter M, Vered Z, et al. Review of echocardiographically diagnosed right heart entrapment of pulmonary emboli-in-transit with emphasis on management. Am Heart J 1987;113:171–178.

Fatkin D, Kelly RP, Feneley MP. Relations between left atrial appendage blood flow velocity, spontaneous echocardiographic contrast and thromboembolic risk in vivo. J Am Coll Cardiol 1994;23:961–969.

Fisher DC, Fisher EA, Budd JH, et al. The incidence of patent foramen ovale in 1,000 consecutive patients. A contrast transesophageal echocardiography study. Chest 1995;107:1504–1509.

Fowles RE, Miller DC, Egbert BM, et al. Systemic embolization from a mitral valve papillary endocardial fibroma detected by two-dimensional echocardiography. Am Heart J 1981;102:128–130.

Fyke FE III, Tajik AJ, Edwards WD, et al. Diagnosis of lipomatous hypertrophy of the atrial septum by two-dimensional echocardiography. J Am Coll Cardiol 1983;1:1352–1357.

Goldman M, Kronzon I, Goldstein M, et al. Value of Transesophageal Echo (VOTE): results in 3001 patients. Circulation 1994;90:I-20.

Gowda RM, Khan IA, Nair CK, et al. Cardiac papillary fibroelastoma: a comprehensive analysis of 725 cases. Am Heart J 2003;146:404–410.

Grenadier E, Lima CO, Barron JV, et al. Two-dimensional echocardiography for evaluation of metastatic cardiac tumors in pediatric patients. Am Heart J 1984;107:122–126.

Grimm RA, Stewart WJ, Black IW, et al. Should all patients undergo transesophageal echocardiography before electrical cardioversion of atrial fibrillation? J Am Coll Cardiol 1994;23:533–541.

Hofman T, Kasper W, Meinertz T, et al. Echocardiographic evaluation of patients with clinically suspected arterial emboli. Lancet 1990;336: 1421–1424.

Hwang JJ, Chen JJ, Lin SC, et al. Diagnostic accuracy of transesophageal echocardiography for detecting left atrial thrombi in patients with rheumatic heart disease having undergone mitral valve operations. Am J Cardiol 1993;72:677–681.

Johnson MH, Soulen RL. Echocardiography of cardiac metastases. Am J Roentgenol 1983;141:677–681.

Khandheria BK, Seward JB, Tajik AJ. Critical appraisal of transesophageal echocardiography: limitations and pitfalls. Crit Care Clin 1996;12:235–251.

Kindman LA, Wright A, Tye T, et al. Lipomatous hypertrophy of the interatrial septum: characterization by transesophageal and transthoracic echocardiography, magnetic resonance imaging, and computed tomography. J Am Soc Echocardiogr 1988;1:450–454.

Klarich KW, Enriquez-Sarano M, Gura GM, et al. Papillary fibroelastoma: echocardiographic characteristics for diagnosis and pathologic correlation. J Am Coll Cardiol 1997;30:784–790.

Klein AL, Grimm RA, Black IW, et al. Cardioversion guided by transesophageal echocardiography: the ACUTE Pilot Study. A randomized, controlled trial. Assessment of cardioversion using transesophageal echocardiography. Ann Intern Med 1997;126: 200–209.

Klein AL, Grimm RA, Murray RD, et al. Use of transesophageal echocardiography to guide cardioversion in patients with atrial fibrillation. N Engl J Med 2001;344:1411–1420.

Labovitz AJ, Bransford TL. Evolving role of echocardiography in the management of atrial fibrillation. Am Heart J 2001;141:518–527.

Laupacis A, Albers G, Dalen J, et al. Antithrombotic therapy in atrial fibrillation. Chest 1995;108:352S–359S.

Lee RJ, Bartzokis T, Yeoh TK, et al. Enhanced detection of intracardiac sources of cerebral emboli by transesophageal echocardiography. Stroke 1991;22:734–739.

Leung DY, Black IW, Cranney GB, et al. Prognostic implications of left atrial spontaneous echo contrast in nonvalvular atrial fibrillation. J Am Coll Cardiol 1994;24:755–762.

Leung DY, Davidson PM, Cranney GB, et al. Thromboembolic risks of left atrial thrombus detected by transesophageal echocardiogram. Am J Cardiol 1997;79:626–629.

Manning WJ, Silverman DI, Gordon SP, et al. Cardioversion from atrial fibrillation without prolonged anticoagulation with use of transesophageal echocardiography to exclude the presence of atrial thrombi. N Engl J Med 1993;328:750–755.

Manning WJ, Silverman DI, Katz SE, et al. Impaired left atrial mechanical function after cardioversion: relation to the duration of atrial fibrillation. J Am Coll Cardiol 1994;23:1535–1540.

Manning WJ, Weintraub RM, Waksmonski CA, et al. Accuracy of transesophageal echocardiography for identifying left atrial thrombi. A prospective, intraoperative study. Ann Intern Med 1995;123:817–822.

Mas JL, Arquizan C, Lamy C, et al. Recurrent cerebrovascular events associated with patent foramen ovale, atrial septal aneurysm, or both. N Engl J Med 2001;345:1740–1746.

McAllister HA Jr, Fenoglio JJ Jr. Atlas of Tumor Pathology. Second Series, Fascicle 15, 1978.

McNamara RL, Lima JA, Whelton PK, et al. Echocardiographic identification of cardiovascular sources of emboli to guide clinical management of stroke: a cost-effectiveness analysis. Ann Intern Med 1997;127:775–787.

Meltzer RS, Visser CA, Fuster V. Intracardiac thrombi and systemic embolization. Ann Intern Med 1986;104:689–698.

Narang J, Neustein S, Israel D. The role of transesophageal echocardiography in the diagnosis and excision of a tumor of the aortic valve. J Cardiothorac Vasc Anesth 1992;6:68–69.

Nishide M, Irino T, Gotoh M, et al. Cardiac abnormalities in ischemic cerebrovascular disease studied by two-dimensional echocardiography. Stroke 1983;14:541–545.

Nomeir AM, Watts LE, Seagle R, et al. Intracardiac myxomas: twenty-year echocardiographic experience with review of the literature. J Am Soc Echocardiogr 1989;2:139–150.

Pearson AC, Labovitz AJ, Tatineni S, et al. Superiority of transesophageal echocardiography in detecting cardiac source of embolism in patients with cerebral ischemia of uncertain etiology. J Am Coll Cardiol 1991;17:66–72.

Pollick C, Taylor D. Assessment of left atrial appendage function by transesophageal echocardiography. Implications for the development of thrombus. Circulation 1991;84:223–231.

Pop G, Sutherland GR, Koudstaal PJ, et al. Transesophageal echocardiography in the detection of intracardiac embolic sources in patients with transient ischemic attacks. Stroke 1990;21:560–565.

Predictors of thromboembolism in atrial fibrillation: I. Clinical features of patients at risk. The Stroke Prevention in Atrial Fibrillation Investigators. Ann Intern Med 1992;116:1–5.

Rastegar R, Harnick DJ, Weidemann P, et al. Spontaneous echo contrast videodensity is flow-related and is dependent on the relative concentrations of fibrinogen and red blood cells. J Am Coll Cardiol 2003;41:603–610.

Raymond RJ, Lee AJ, Messineo FC, et al. Cardiac performance early after cardioversion from atrial fibrillation. Am Heart J 1998;136:435–442.

Rey M, Alfonso F, Torrecilla EG, et al. Diagnostic value of two-dimensional echocardiography in cardiac hydatid disease. Eur Heart J 1991;12:1300–1307.

Reynen K. Cardiac myxomas. N Engl J Med 1995;333:1610–1617.

Roijer A, Lindgren A, Rudling O, et al. Potential cardioembolic sources in an elderly population without stroke. A transthoracic and transoesophageal echocardiographic study in randomly selected volunteers. Eur Heart J 1996;17:1103–1111.

Roldan CA, Shively BK, Crawford MH. Valve excrescences: prevalence, evolution and risk for cardioembolism. J Am Coll Cardiol 1997;30:1308–1314.

Sansoy V, Abbott RD, Jayaweera AR, et al. Low yield of transthoracic echocardiography for cardiac source of embolism. Am J Cardiol 1995;75:166–169.

Shub C, Tajik AJ, Seward JB, et al. Cardiac papillary fibroelastomas. Two-dimensional echocardiographic recognition. Mayo Clin Proc 1981;56:629–633.

Stoddard MF, Dawkins PR, Prince CR, et al. Left atrial appendage thrombus is not uncommon in patients with acute atrial fibrillation and a recent embolic event: a transesophageal echocardiographic study. J Am Coll Cardiol 1995;25:452–459.

Stoddard MF, Liddell NE, Longaker RA, et al. Transesophageal echocardiography: normal variants and mimickers. Am Heart J 1992;124:1587–1598.

Stollberger C, Chnupa P, Kronik G, et al. Transesophageal echocardiography to assess embolic risk in patients with atrial fibrillation. ELAT Study Group. Embolism in Left Atrial Thrombi. Ann Intern Med 1998;128:630–638.

Stratton JR, Lighty GW Jr, Pearlman AS, et al. Detection of left ventricular thrombus by two-dimensional echocardiography: sensitivity, specificity, and causes of uncertainty. Circulation 1982;66:156–166.

Stratton JR, Nemanich JW, Johannessen KA, et al. Fate of left ventricular thrombi in patients with remote myocardial infarction or idiopathic cardiomyopathy. Circulation 1988;78:1388–1393.

Tazelaar HD, Locke TJ, McGregor CG. Pathology of surgically excised primary cardiac tumors. Mayo Clin Proc 1992;67:957–965.

Thomas MR, Jayakrishnan AG, Desai J, et al. Transesophageal echocardiography in the detection and surgical management of a papillary fibroelastoma of the mitral valve causing partial mitral valve obstruction. J Am Soc Echocardiogr 1993;6:83–86.

Tunick PA, Rosenzweig BP, Katz ES, et al. High risk for vascular events in patients with protruding aortic atheromas: a prospective study. J Am Coll Cardiol 1994;23:1085–1090.

van Kuyk M, Mols P, Englert M. Right atrial thrombus leading to pulmonary embolism. Br Heart J 1984;51:462–464.

Verhorst PM, Kamp O, Welling RC, et al. Transesophageal echocardiographic predictors for maintenance of sinus rhythm after electrical cardioversion of atrial fibrillation. Am J Cardiol 1997;79:1355–1359.

Visser CA, Kan G, Meltzer RS, et al. Embolic potential of left ventricular thrombus after myocardial infarction: a two-dimensional echocardiographic study of 119 patients. J Am Coll Cardiol 1985;5:1276–1280.

Zabalgoitia M, Halperin JL, Pearce LA, et al. Transesophageal echocardiographic correlates of clinical risk of thromboembolism in nonvalvular atrial fibrillation. Stroke Prevention in Atrial Fibrillation III Investigators. J Am Coll Cardiol 1998;31:1622–1626.

Zackai AH, Weber DJ, Ramsby G, et al. Recurrence of left atrial myxoma. J Cardiovasc Surg (Torino) 1974;15:467–471.

Echocardiography in Systemic Disease and Clinical Problem Solving

There are a number of systemic diseases with cardiovascular manifestations in which echocardiography plays a valuable role for surveillance and follow-up of anticipated cardiovascular abnormalities (Table 22.1). Similarly, there are several clinical scenarios in which echocardiography plays an instrumental role and is regarded as a first-line investigative technique. The specific use of echocardiography for some of these diseases such as cardioembolic disease is addressed in previous chapters. This chapter discusses the integrated approach of clinical and echocardiographic information in patients with a variety of clinical presentations.

ECHOCARDIOGRAPHY AND SYSTEMIC DISEASE

Hypertension

The role of echocardiographic imaging in patients with hypertension is briefly discussed in Chapter 6. From a clinical perspective, the role of echocardiography is to detect cardiac end-organ damage due to systemic hypertension. This includes the obvious sequelae of left ventricular hypertrophy (Fig. 22.1), diastolic dysfunction (Fig. 22.2), and later systolic dysfunction.

The precise methodology for determining left ventricular mass and thereby quantifying left ventricular hypertrophy is discussed in Chapter 6. Numerous algorithms have been proposed. The M-mode–derived Teichholz or cubed formula, which assumes spherical geometry of the left ventricle, was used in most of the early serial hypertension studies. Because the left ventricle does not adhere to spherical geometry, the absolute accuracy of this technique is relatively low compared with two-dimensional imaging. Second, the absolute measurements are often inaccurate due to tangential imaging planes. Nevertheless, in any given patient, assuming no intervening event such as myocardial infarction, this methodology provides a relatively stable determination of left ventricular mass over time and has been used successfully for tracking left ven-

▶ **TABLE 22.1 Systemic Diseases and Clinical Presentations in Which Echocardiography Plays a Valuable Role**

Systemic Disease Conditions with Cardiovascular Manifestations
    Hypertension
    Diabetes mellitus
    Pregnancy
    Chronic renal insufficiency
  Connective tissue disease
    Systemic lupus erythematosus
    Scleroderma
    Marfan syndrome
  Chronic hepatic disease
  Pulmonary arterial hypertension
  Miscellaneous Diseases
    Thyroid disease
    Sarcoidosis
    Hemachromatosis
    Muscular dystrophies
    Friedreich ataxia
    Carcinoid syndrome
    Ergotamine toxicity
Clinical presentations
    Congestive heart failure
    Dyspnea
    Pulmonary embolus
    Atrial fibrillation
    Cardioembolic disease
    Radiation therapy
    Syncope
    Athletic screening
    Pregnancy

tricular mass regression during therapeutic trials of antihypertensive agents.

Other cardiac anomalies, which have a relatively greater prevalence in the hypertensive population, include calcification of the mitral anulus and mild degrees of aortic thickening as well as dilation of the ascending aorta (Fig. 22.3). With long-standing hypertension, there is secondary dila-

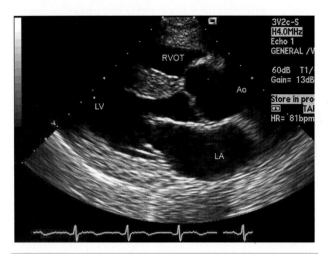

FIGURE 22.1. Parasternal long-axis view recorded in a 30-year-old patient with essential hypertension. In this diastolic frame, note the mild degree of left ventricular hypertrophy but otherwise normal cardiac structures and preserved systolic function in the real time image. Ao, aorta; LA, left atrium; LV, left ventricle; RVOT, right ventricular outflow tract.

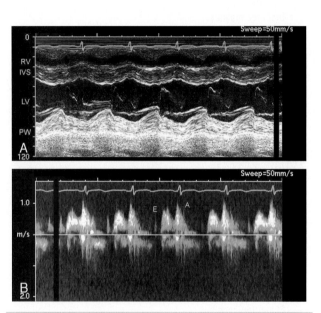

FIGURE 22.2. M-mode echocardiogram **(A)** recorded in the same patient presented in Figure 22.1 reveals left ventricular hypertrophy and normal systolic function of the left ventricle. **B:** The mitral valve inflow pattern shows a reduced to E/A ratio, which would be unexpected in a 30-year-old patient and is indicative of early diastolic dysfunction.

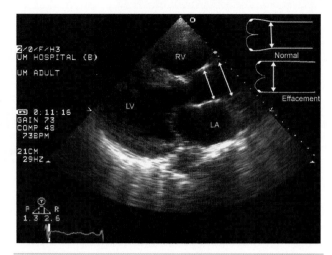

FIGURE 22.3. Parasternal long-axis image recorded in a patient with severe long-standing and poorly controlled hypertension. Note the significant left ventricular hypertrophy and the mild left atrial dilation. In the real-time image, note the global hypokinesis of the left ventricle (*LV*). Also note the dilation of the ascending aorta with effacement at the sinotubular junction, which results in aortic regurgitation due to malcoaptation of the aortic cusps (Fig. 22.4). LA, left atrium; RV, right ventricle.

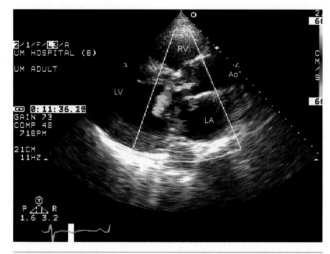

FIGURE 22.4. Parasternal long-axis echocardiogram with color Doppler flow imaging recorded in the same patient presented in Figure 22.3. Note the effacement of the sinotubular junction, which results in malcoaptation of the aortic cusps and a central aortic regurgitation jet. Ao, aorta; LA, left atrium; LV, left ventricle; RV, right ventricle.

tion of the ascending aorta with effacement of the sinotubular junction. This has the effect of splaying the closure of the three aortic cusps and secondarily resulting in aortic insufficiency (Fig. 22.4). The degree to which aortic insufficiency is attributable to hypertension alone has been debated; however, there appears to be a fairly strong correlation between this type of functional aortic insufficiency due

to effacement of the sinotubular junction and chronic hypertension. Additional abnormalities associated with long-standing hypertension include advanced atherosclerosis of the aorta, which can be detected with transesophageal echocardiography, and peripheral vascular disease.

Diastolic dysfunction is one of the earliest manifestations of hypertensive heart disease. Generally speaking, this is mild at first, but in advanced cases of severe untreated hypertension, it may progress to the point of being the predominant contributor to congestive heart failure symptoms. Methods by which diastolic dysfunction is evaluated in hypertensive patients are the same as for other diseases. Generally, in early hypertension, there is delayed relaxation of the myocardium due to hypertrophy and mild degrees of stiffening, which is manifested as a reduced E/A ratio of mitral valve inflow (Fig. 22.2). If left ventricular hypertrophy remains uncomplicated by concurrent systolic dysfunction, no other changes are anticipated. In severe long-standing hypertension, the left ventricle may develop systolic dysfunction as well (Fig. 22.3). At this point, there may be development of more worrisome mitral inflow patterns such as a restrictive pattern with a high E/A ratio. Other echocardiographic modalities, including Doppler tissue imaging, have been employed in the hypertensive population. Generally, results of Doppler tissue imaging of the anulus parallel the abnormalities seen in the mitral valve inflow and consist of reduced early diastolic relaxation velocities.

Diabetes Mellitus

Diabetes mellitus is associated with what can be viewed as both primary and secondary cardiovascular abnormalities. For patients with predominantly type 1 but also type 2 diabetes, the metabolic derangement results in premature coronary artery disease, sometimes in a very aggressive manner. It is not unusual to encounter an individual with type 1 diabetes in the third decade of life with advanced atherosclerotic coronary artery disease. There is also an increased prevalence of lipid disorders and hypertension, which exacerbates this phenomenon.

The long-term effect of diabetes on the coronary vasculature is similar to that of coronary disease in those without diabetes; however, diabetes tends to result in more diffuse atherosclerotic involvement. There are numerous clinical scenarios in which it is well recognized that patients with diabetes behave in a different manner and probably should undergo different forms of therapy and evaluation than those without diabetes. Detection of coronary disease in the population with diabetes is done in a manner identical to that of the population without coronary disease, including the use of rest and stress echocardiography. From a clinical standpoint, it should be recognized that because of the autonomic neuropathy associated with diabetes, typical symptoms may not be present. As such, the indications for proceeding with provocative cardiovascular stress testing and the end points for termination of a cardiovascular stress test, including stress echocardiography, may not be the same as they are in the population of patients without diabetes. Because the likelihood of rapid progression of disease is

substantially greater in patients with diabetes, the time frame during which one can anticipate a benign prognosis after a negative test ("the warranty period") is substantially shorter than it is in the patient without diabetes. Patients with diabetes comprise the largest single subset of patients presenting for renal transplantation, and dobutamine stress echocardiography has had substantial acceptance as a screening tool to identify high-risk patients before renal transplantation.

In addition to these secondary sequelae of diabetes that behave in a manner similar to that for the patient population without diabetes, but in a more aggressive fashion, there are subtle, less clinically obvious cardiovascular manifestations of diabetes. A well-recognized one is a tendency to develop diastolic dysfunction even in the absence of "significant" hypertension or coronary artery disease. This is presumed to be due to accumulation of metabolic byproducts within the myocardial interstitium, which results in stiffening of the myocardium and delayed relaxation. This is manifested as a reduced E/A ratio of mitral valve inflow. It has been well recognized that the mitral valve E/A ratio diminishes with age; however, in the population with diabetes, the rate at which it diminishes exceeds that in the population without diabetes due to occult diastolic dysfunction. The degree to which aggressive control of even borderline hypertension and scrupulous control of blood glucose levels will mitigate against these structural changes is yet to be determined.

Management of the patient with diabetes requires a different set of guidelines than for the patient without diabetes. For a patient with type 1 diabetes requiring a major noncardiac surgical procedure, such as renal transplantation or valvular surgery, provocative stress testing to identify occult obstructive coronary artery disease is typically warranted for any major procedure, even in the absence of classic symptoms for the reasons alluded to previously. Similarly, the frequency with which diagnostic testing should be undertaken to ensure stability of the underlying substrate is greater than it is for the population without diabetes. After coronary artery bypass surgery, guidelines for routine postoperative stress testing have suggested that within the first 5 years, those patients without diabetes do not require routine testing. However, the likelihood of rapid progression is substantially greater in patients with diabetes, and many authorities have recommended earlier and more frequent provocative stress testing, including stress echocardiography, in the population with diabetes than in the population without diabetes.

Thyroid Disease

Both hyperthyroidism and hypothyroidism result in clinical cardiovascular disease. Hyperthyroidism results in an increase in total blood volume as well as an increase in left ventricular contractility and a decrease in systemic vascular resistance. This results in a high-output state with an increased left ventricular stroke volume. In addition to these hemodynamic effects, hyperthyroidism results in sinus tachycardia and on occasion may trigger atrial fibrillation. In patients with underlying structural heart disease, the increase in heart rate and stroke volume may precipitate heart failure or unmask previously compensated congestive heart failure or angina pectoris. Extreme hyperthyroidism may result in a high-output state sufficient to cause a picture identical to that of dilated cardiomyopathy (Fig. 22.5). The cardiomyopathy of hyperthyroidism typically reverses after successful treatment of the metabolic disorder.

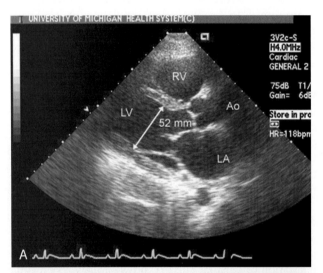

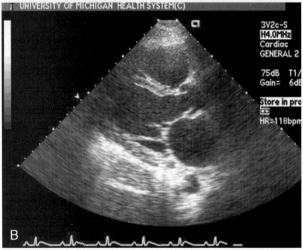

FIGURE 22.5. Parasternal long-axis echocardiogram recorded in a patient with severe thyrotoxicosis who presented with nonsustained ventricular tachycardia and congestive heart failure. Note the relatively preserved left ventricular internal dimension (52 mm) **(A)** but the severe hypokinesis in systole **(B)**. Ao, aorta; LA, left atrium; LV, left ventricle; RV, right ventricle.

Hypothyroidism results in directionally opposite changes in left ventricular performance and cardiac output. Pericardial effusion occurs frequently but is an uncommon cause of hemodynamic compromise. In advanced cases of myxedema, which are rarely seen in contemporary practice, there may be increased myocardial thickness with abnormal texture and reduced systolic function.

Chronic Renal Insufficiency

Chronic renal insufficiency results in a characteristic constellation of cardiac abnormalities. First, it should be recognized that patients with chronic renal insufficiency are often either elderly and hence at high risk of cardiovascular disease in general or frequently have renal disease based on hypertension or diabetes, which, as discussed previously, results in premature coronary artery disease and other anatomic cardiac abnormalities. In addition to the above secondary features, the metabolic derangement in chronic renal insufficiency, including hyperparathyroidism, results in ectopic calcification, predominantly of the fibrous skeleton of the heart. This is most often manifest as calcification of the mitral anulus. The degree of anular calcification appears directly related to the magnitude of hyperparathyroidism and can range from small focal deposits of calcium in the mitral anulus to extensive circumferential deposits of calcium in the anulus, which then invade the proximal portions of the mitral valve leaflets, resulting in functional mitral stenosis. In advanced cases, there may be involvement of the aortic valve as well. The secondary features of chronic renal insufficiency include left ventricular hypertrophy due to longstanding hypertension and an abnormal texture to the hypertrophied myocardium that mimics that seen in cardiac amyloid. Figures 22.6 and 22.7 are echocardiograms recorded in patients with chronic renal insufficiency and illustrate these classic abnormalities seen in advanced renal disease. On occasion, patients with chronic renal insufficiency on dialysis develop systolic dysfunction, which cannot be related to uncontrolled hypertension, identifiable coronary artery disease, or other inciting factors. The presumed etiology of the dysfunction is metabolic, and numerous anecdotal cases have been reported in which systolic function recovers after institution of more aggressive dialysis or renal transplantation.

Other abnormalities seen in chronic renal insufficiency include pericardial effusion, which may range from small chronic effusions to presentation with cardiac tamponade. Uremia results in a relatively inflammatory and occasionally hemorrhagic pericarditis in which there is often evidence of "stranding" on the visceral pericardium (Fig. 22.8).

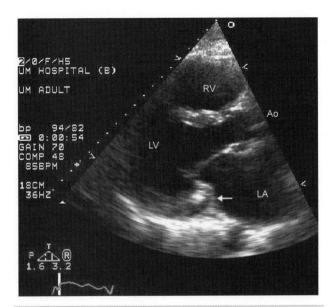

FIGURE 22.6. Parasternal long-axis echocardiogram recorded in a patient with end-stage renal disease on hemodialysis and secondary abnormalities including calcification of the mitral anulus (*arrow*). Note the dilation of the left ventricle (*LV*) and left atrium (*LA*) due to a combination of hypertension and anemia with high output. Ao, aorta; RV, right ventricle.

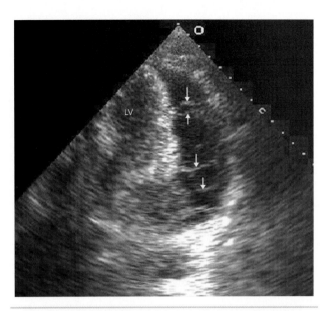

FIGURE 22.8. Apical view is recorded in a patient with end-stage renal disease and uremic pericarditis. Note the stranding within the pericardial space (*arrows*), which can also be seen in pericardial effusion of any type with a marked inflammatory component. LV, left ventricle.

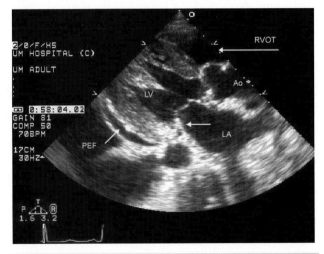

FIGURE 22.7. Parasternal long-axis echocardiogram recorded in a patient with end-stage renal disease. Again note the calcification of the mitral anulus (*arrow*) and the small pericardial effusion (*PEF*). Left ventricular hypertrophy and aortic valve thickening are also present. Ao, aorta; LA, left atrium; LV, left ventricle.

CONNECTIVE TISSUE/AUTOIMMUNE DISEASE

Systemic Lupus Erythematosus

Systemic lupus erythematosus (SLE) has long been known to be associated with cardiovascular disease. There is substantial crossover among many of the connective tissue diseases such as mixed connective tissue disease, SLE, Raynaud phenomenon, and scleroderma. A

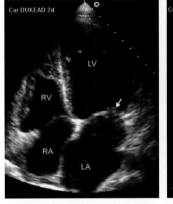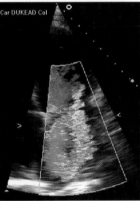

FIGURE 22.9. Apical four-chamber view recorded in a patient with systemic lupus and Libman-Sacks lesions of the mitral valve (*arrow*), associated with moderate to severe regurgitation as noted in the color flow image. LA, left atrium; LV, left ventricle; RA, right atrium; RV, right ventricle.

classic lesion encountered in patients with SLE is noninfectious endocarditis with the so-called Libman-Sacks vegetation (Figs. 22.9 and 22.10). These are most commonly encountered on the mitral valve and more frequently are on the atrial side of the leaflet. Unlike infectious vegetations, they usually are not mobile. They may have an inflammatory component that can result in leaflet deformity and valvular regurgitation.

Other manifestations of SLE include coronary vasculitis, which can result in regional or global dysfunction and

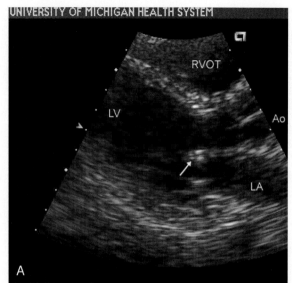

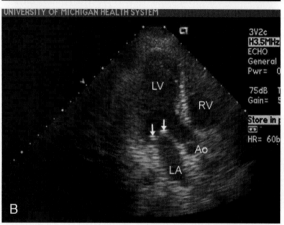

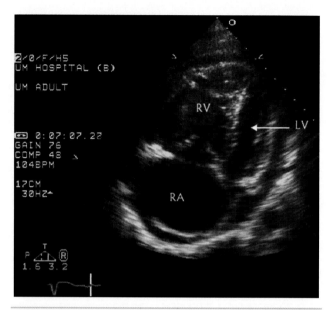

FIGURE 22.11. Apical four-chamber view recorded in a patient with systemic scleroderma and Raynaud phenomenon who has the complication of severe pulmonary arterial hypertension. Note the massive dilation of the right atrium (*RA*) and right ventricle and the small underfilled left ventricle (*LV*). A small pericardial effusion is also present that is indicative of advanced pulmonary hypertension. In the real-time image, also note the hypertrophy and reduced function of the right ventricle (*RV*).

FIGURE 22.10. Parasternal long-axis (**A**) and apical long-axis (**B**) views recorded in a patient with long-standing lupus erythematosus and Libman-Sacks lesions involving the mitral valve. In both images, note the nodular thickening at the tips of the mitral valve (*arrows*). Ao, aorta; LA, left atrium; LV, left ventricle; RV, right ventricle; RVOT, right ventricular outflow tract.

thereby mimic either an acute coronary syndrome or cardiomyopathy. A final manifestation of SLE may be acute pericarditis. Other than detection of pericardial fluid in a patient with well-defined SLE and concurrent elevation of erythrocyte sedimentation rate, there are no characteristic features of the pericarditis or pericardial infusion seen in SLE. On rare occasion, SLE has been associated with pulmonary hypertension, although this association is far more common with scleroderma.

Scleroderma/Raynaud Phenomenon

Many other connective tissue diseases can have cardiovascular manifestations. Diseases closely related to SLE

such as mixed connective tissue disease represent an obvious crossover category for which all the different manifestations of SLE may be seen. Patients with Raynaud phenomenon or with the full complex of scleroderma have a greater than usual prevalence of pulmonary arterial hypertension. In patients with scleroderma, the pulmonary hypertension anatomically and physiologically is similar to primary pulmonary hypertension with an increase in pulmonary vascular resistance at the arteriolar level (Fig. 22.11). The manifestations of pulmonary hypertension in connective tissue disease are identical to those seen in any other form of pulmonary hypertension that is not the result of an intracardiac shunt. The manifestations of pulmonary hypertension as a distinct entity are discussed further in this chapter, and the echocardiographic features of right ventricular pressure overload have been discussed in Chapters 7, 8, and 12.

Marfan Syndrome

The Marfan syndrome is a heritable disorder of connective tissue disease that has been long known to be associated with multiple cardiovascular abnormalities. Before the advent of corrective surgery, cardiovascular complications, especially aortic dissection and proximal aortic rupture, were the leading causes of mortality in patients with Marfan syndrome, resulting in an average age at death in the fourth decade. The cardiovascular manifestations of Marfan syndrome include cystic medial necrosis, which is a degeneration of the medial layer of the aorta. This results in dilation of virtually any portion of the aorta and as such should be considered a disease of the entire aorta. Clinically, the most prominent areas of dilation frequently are in the proximal aorta and may be confined to the aortic sinuses. Figures 22.12 and 22.13 were recorded in patients with characteristic features of Marfan syndrome. Although the sinuses are the most common site of dilation, it should be recognized that the underlying pathologic process extends throughout the entire aorta, and patients with Marfan syndrome are at risk of aneurysm formation, dissection, and rupture at any point along the course of the aorta. For the majority of patients, initial screening can be undertaken with transthoracic echocardiography. Evaluation of the proximal aorta should be undertaken in a systematic fashion and measurements made at the level of the anulus, sinuses, sinotubular junction, and proximal ascending aorta (Fig. 22.14). Many laboratories have adopted a policy of giving only a single measurement of the aorta without specifying its location. The anatomy of the normal aorta is relatively well defined and consists of a relatively small anulus with gradual dilation at the level of the sinuses, with the sinuses typically measuring 6 mm/M² more than the anulus. The aorta then narrows to within 2 to 3 mm of the anular dimension at the sino-

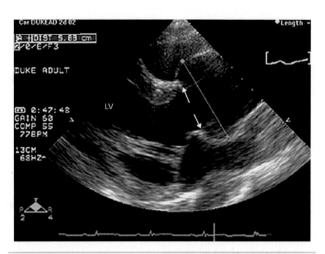

FIGURE 22.13. Parasternal long-axis view recorded in a patient with marked dilation of the ascending aorta, most prominent at the level of the Valsalva sinuses. In this patient, the Valsalva sinuses measure 5.8 cm, which exceeds the typical threshold for recommending prophylactic aortic root replacement. LV, left ventricle.

tubular junction and tapers very slightly throughout its course distally. Failure to narrow at the level of the sinotubular junction is referred to as effacement. The aortic cusps actually insert at the level of the sinotubular junction, and effacement or frank dilation of the sinotubular junction will result in malcoaptation and subsequent aortic regurgitation (Fig. 22.15). In patients with Marfan syndrome, this is the most common etiology of aortic regurgitation. Much of the older literature has referred to dilation of the anulus of the aorta as a cause of aortic insufficiency. Dilation of the true anulus is uncommon, and the majority of the patients with aortic insufficiency have it because of effacement of the sinotubular junction and not an abnormality of the anulus.

Management of patients with Marfan syndrome involves serial imaging to evaluate aortic size and progression of dilation. Most authorities believe that, at the time of detection, a patient should undergo an evaluation of the entire extent of at least the thoracic aorta, which can be performed with transesophageal echocardiography, computed tomography, or magnetic resonance imaging. If there is no evidence of distal aortic dilation, follow-up usually can be performed with transthoracic echocardiography because the proximal ascending aorta is the single most likely site to be involved in subsequent dilation. It should be emphasized that follow-up should include serial measurements as noted previously for comparison. The threshold level of dilation or change in diameter for which prophylactic aortic surgery is recommended varies with the experience and expertise of the operative center. Generally, an aortic dimension of 55 mm is considered an indication for elective surgical intervention, as is an in-

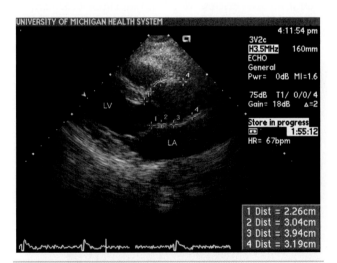

FIGURE 22.12. Parasternal long-axis echocardiogram recorded in a patient with Marfan syndrome and dilation of the proximal aorta. In this image, the aorta has been measured at four points including the anulus (*1*), Valsalva sinus (*2*), sinotubular junction (*3*), and the ascending aorta (*4*). Measurements are as noted at the lower right. See Figure 22.14 for further measurement details. LA, left atrium; LV, left ventricle.

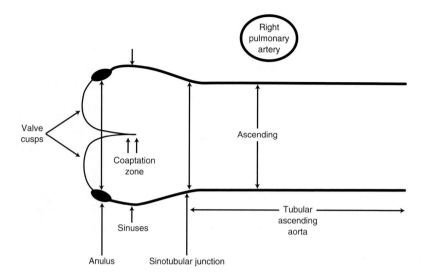

FIGURE 22.14. Schematic representation of normal aortic anatomy and the different components of the proximal aorta as well as recommended sites for making measurements.

crease of 1.0 cm over a period of 12 months or less. In many high-volume centers, with a track record of excellent surgical results, prophylactic aortic replacement is being recommended at an aortic dimension of 50 mm (and occasionally less). The need to index aortic size to body size is less well recognized than it is for some other entities; however, the implications of dilation less than 50 mm in a small-statured individual are obvious. Aortic dilation associated with clinically relevant aortic insufficiency has been considered an indication for surgery as well. After surgical repair, continued surveillance is crucial because this is a systemic process involving all portions of the aorta. However, after replacement of the ascending aorta in a patient with Marfan syndrome,

follow-up may require transesophageal echocardiography, computed tomography, or magnetic resonance imaging because additional disease will typically not be in the range of view of transthoracic echocardiography.

The full spectrum of cardiovascular abnormalities in Marfan syndrome includes not only disease of the aorta but also an increased prevalence of myxomatous degeneration of the mitral valve with mitral valve prolapse (Fig. 22.16). When present, it has the same appearance and clinical implications of myxomatous degeneration and prolapse occurring in the patient without Marfan syndrome. Typically, the leaflets are diffusely thickened and redundant and have characteristic buckling or prolapse behind the plane of the mitral anulus. Because of the myxomatous degeneration,

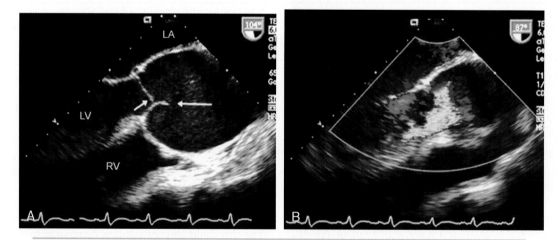

FIGURE 22.15. Transesophageal echocardiogram recorded in a patient with Marfan syndrome and proximal aortic dilation. There is significant effacement of the sinotubular junction resulting in malcoaptation of the aortic cusps. Note the relatively normal position in diastole of the right aortic cusp (*horizontal arrow*) and the abnormal closure position of the noncoronary cusp, which fails to contact the opposing cusp, resulting in functional regurgitation, which is highly eccentric **(B)**. LA, left atrium; LV, left ventricle; RV, right ventricle.

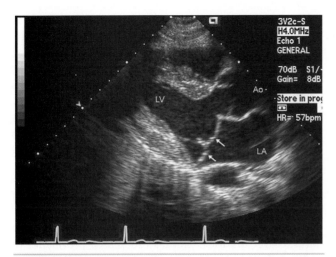

FIGURE 22.16. Parasternal long-axis echocardiogram recorded in a young patient with Marfan syndrome and only mild dilation of the ascending aorta. This patient also has classic mitral valve prolapse. Note the distinct bowing of both the anterior and posterior mitral leaflets into the left atrium (*LA*) in systole (*arrows*). LV, left ventricle; Ao, aorta.

there is a greater incidence of spontaneous chordal rupture and secondary mitral regurgitation. Echocardiographic imaging in clinical management of mitral valve disease is similar to that of patients discussed in Chapter 11.

Aortic insufficiency may result in left ventricular dilation, which may mask underlying mitral valve prolapse. In many cases, mitral valve prolapse with mitral regurgitation and aortic insufficiency may both be noted. However, if aortic regurgitation is the predominant lesion, the left ventricle may dilate, resulting in reduction of the anatomic appearance of mitral valve prolapse and occasionally in a reduction in the amount of visualized mitral regurgitation. After aortic valve replacement, ventricular size diminishes, at which point mitral valve prolapse again becomes apparent and mitral regurgitation of a clinical relevant degree may again be appreciated. For patients undergoing aortic valve replacement, who have mitral valve anatomy that is suspicious for myxomatous change, or in whom this lesion complex is suspected, repeat intraoperative evaluation of mitral valve prolapse and regurgitation should be undertaken after aortic valve replacement so that a combined aortic and mitral valve procedure can be performed if necessary.

A final complication of Marfan syndrome involves spontaneous coronary artery dissection. Cystic medial necrosis can also involve proximal coronary arteries, and patients with Marfan syndrome are more likely to develop an acute coronary syndrome secondary to spontaneous dissection of a proximal coronary artery than is the otherwise healthy patient population. Spontaneous coronary dissection may occur in association with pregnancy or in the postpartum period. These patients will present with an acute chest pain syndrome and electrocardiographic

and enzymatic evidence of myocardial infarction that is associated with regional wall motion abnormalities in the distribution of involvement. Because the proximal coronary arteries are involved, it is not infrequently the left main coronary artery that dissects, resulting in a nearly instantaneous fatal event in many instances. From an echocardiographic standpoint, identification of a regional wall motion abnormality in a patient with Marfan syndrome or a closely related connective tissue disease who is otherwise not at risk of atherosclerotic coronary artery disease should heighten the awareness of spontaneous coronary dissection as a possible etiology.

CHRONIC LIVER DISEASE AND CIRRHOSIS

The relationship between cardiac and renal disease has been well appreciated, whereas the relationship between hepatic and cardiac disease is less well clinically recognized. There are numerous clinical situations in which cardiac disease results in hepatic dysfunction and similarly several hepatic diseases that secondarily result in cardiac disease (Table 22.2).

Clinical liver disease can occur as a result of cardiovascular disease when either poor cardiac output with malperfusion occurs or there is long-standing right ventricular dysfunction with elevated systemic venous pressures. Poor perfusion due to low cardiac output results in multisystem organ dysfunction, and typically the liver is only one of several organs involved. In this instance, there will be biochemical evidence of both synthetic dysfunction and reduced clearance of toxic metabolites. In rare occasions either poor hepatic perfusion or elevated venous pressures resulting in hepatic congestion result in an obstructive biochemical pattern mimicking biliary disease.

In patients with chronic right heart failure, systemic venous pressures are chronically elevated, which results in passive hepatic venous congestion. Chronically, this results in the syndrome of "cardiac cirrhosis," which has several distinct histologic features. This syndrome should be suspected when there is evidence of either acute or

▶ **TABLE 22.2 Heart and Liver Disease**

Cardiac disease with an impact on hepatic function
Malperfusion (hypotension/low-output state)
Passive venous congestion
Pericardial constriction
Pulmonary hypertension
Severe tricuspid regurgitation
Cardiovascular sequelae of chronic liver disease
Lowered systemic vascular resistance
Fluid retention
High-output state
Pulmonary hypertension
Pulmonary arteriovenous malformations

chronic hepatic dysfunction and cardiac disease is present, which is likely to have resulted in marked elevation of hepatic venous pressure. The cardiovascular diseases that may result in this syndrome are constrictive pericarditis, primary pulmonary hypertension, and chronic mitral stenosis or dilated cardiomyopathy with secondary pulmonary hypertension. It is occasionally seen in instances of severe tricuspid regurgitation without pressure elevation, such as after tricuspid valve resection.

There are also secondary effects of liver disease on the cardiovascular system. Advanced cirrhosis of any etiology is frequently associated with pathologically low systemic vascular resistance. This results in a chronic high-output state in which the resting cardiac output may exceed 10 L/min. In this situation, the normal heart has hyperdynamic left ventricular function with a resting ejection fraction exceeding 65% (Fig. 22.17). Additionally, because of the elevated flow volumes, pulmonary artery pressures of 35 to 50 mm Hg may be seen with normal pulmonary vascular resistance (Fig. 22.18). This is analogous to the elevation in pulmonary artery systolic pressure seen in a left-to-right shunt such as atrial septal defect or in the high-output state of pregnancy. Mild elevation of pulmonary artery systolic pressure in chronic liver disease is not necessarily an indication of intrinsic abnormalities of the pulmonary vasculature.

Other anomalies that can be seen in patients with chronic liver disease include an increased prevalence of pulmonary arteriovenous malformations (AVM). These can be detected with contrast echocardiography and result in a delayed right-to-left shunt compared with an instantaneous or phasic shunt seen with a true anatomic

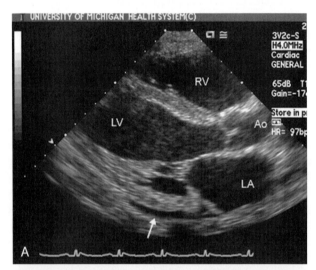

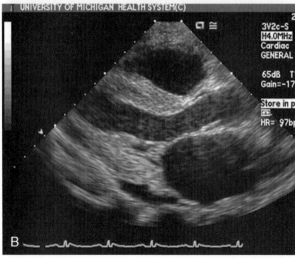

FIGURE 22.17. Apical four-chamber view recorded in diastole (upper panel) and systole (lower panel) of a patient with end-stage liver disease and a high-output state. Resting cardiac output was measured as 16 L/min in the catheterization laboratory in this patient. Note the mild dilation of the left atrium (*LA*) and left ventricle (*LV*) and the hyperdynamic motion of the left ventricle at rest. Incidental note is made of a small pericardial effusion (*arrow*). Ao, aorta; RV, right ventricle.

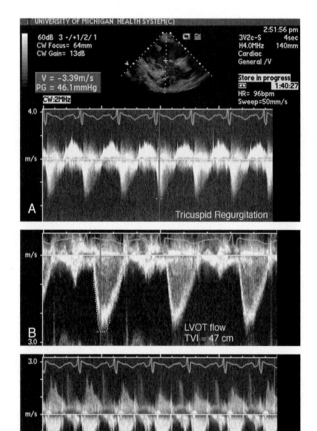

FIGURE 22.18. Spectral Doppler imaging recorded in the patient presented in Figure 22.17 with end-stage liver disease and a high-output state. Note the peak velocity of 3.4 m/sec for the tricuspid regurgitation jet **(A)** and the greater than usual time velocity integral (*TVI*) **(B)** of both the left ventricular outflow tract (LVOT) and right ventricular outflow tract (RVOT) flows **(C)**.

atrial defect (Fig. 22.19). Additional features of the pulmonary AVM include a gradual increase in the amount of contrast appearing in the left heart over time and identification of saline contrast in the pulmonary veins. In the presence of a large pulmonary AVM, the contrast intensity in the left heart will progressively increase over time and may, after a substantial delay, exceed the intensity in the right heart. For patients with chronic liver disease presenting with hypoxia, contrast echocardiography should be performed to identify any pathologic right-to-left shunt due to pulmonary AVMs. If the magnitude of shunting is significant, percutaneous closure of the pulmonary AVM may be beneficial. Identification

of such a shunt also assists in clinical management because it may provide an explanation for otherwise undefined arterial desaturation.

Pulmonary hypertension with elevated pulmonary vascular resistance (not as a result of high flow) also has been associated with chronic liver disease. There may be slightly greater prevalence of this syndrome in chronic liver disease due to hepatitis C, suggesting a common autoimmune pathophysiology. For patients with chronic liver disease presenting for echocardiographic evaluation, the examiner should be cognizant of the anticipated supernormal left ventricular function and the relatively high ejection fraction. A normal or low normal ejection fraction in the presence of chronic liver disease is indirect evidence that an occult cardiomyopathy may be present.

Patients with chronic liver disease not infrequently have abdominal distention due to either an enlarged liver or ascites. The effect of this is to elevate the diaphragm and compress the cardiac structures from below. This can result in the need for atypical imaging windows. Because the posterior wall is frequently compressed, pseudodyskinesis of the posterior wall may be noted. The genesis of this phenomenon is illustrated in Figure 22.20. In this situation, the posterior wall is compressed anteriorly by the diaphragm and hence assumes abnormal geometry in the short axis in diastole. With active myocardial contraction, the ventricle actively reassumes a circular geometry and normal thickening and contraction then ensue. The genesis of this phenomenon is analogous to the right ventricular volume overload pattern with paradoxical septal motion. It is important to recognize the origin of this wall motion abnormality to avoid confusing it with a primary wall motion abnormality attributable to ischemic heart disease.

Occasionally, when performing transesophageal echocardiography in a patient with end-stage liver disease, one encounters large cystic vascular structures adjacent to the esophagus (Fig. 22.21). These represent dilated venous collaterals due to portal hypertension, analogous to true esophageal varices.

Finally, patients with chronic liver disease not infrequently are evaluated for liver transplantation. Whereas dobutamine stress echocardiography has had substantial success at identifying low- and high-risk patients presenting for renal transplantation, the success rate for accurate identification of patients likely to have perioperative complications after liver transplantation is less well established. Many cases of cardiovascular compromise after liver transplantation may relate to an underlying cardiomyopathy that was masked by low peripheral vascular resistance and would not be expected to be detected with dobutamine stress echocardiography. Immediately after liver transplantation, there is an acute increase in systemic vascular resistance (to normal or above), commonly in association with substantial volume loading due to

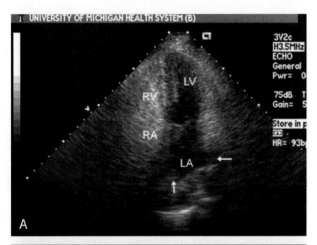

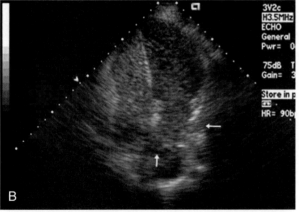

FIGURE 22.19. Apical four-chamber view with intravenous saline contrast recorded in a patient with end-stage liver disease and pulmonary arterial venous malformations. **A:** Contrast is present in the right atrium (*RA*) and right ventricle (*RV*) but has not yet appeared in the left atrium (*LA*) or left ventricle (*LV*). **A:** Note the position of two pulmonary veins that are free of contrast (*arrows*). **B:** Recorded 27 seconds after image **A** and shows nearly complete opacification of the left atrium and left ventricle, with intensity of the contrast being almost equal in the four chambers. Note also that the contrast can be clearly seen in the pulmonary veins (*arrows*), documenting that the level of shunt is not directly at the atrial level but rather due to a pulmonary arteriovenous malformation.

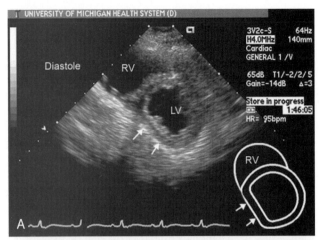

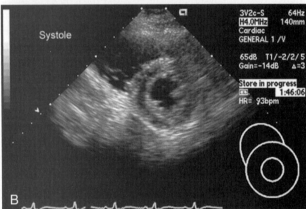

FIGURE 22.20. Parasternal short-axis view recorded in a patient with end-stage liver disease and significant hepatomegaly, which has elevated the diaphragm. This has resulted in compression of the inferior wall resulting in a noncircular geometry of the left ventricle (*LV*) in diastole **(A)**. **B:** In early systole, with active ventricular contraction, the ventricle reassumes a circular position, giving the appearance of paradoxic motion in the inferior wall. Note that systolic thickening is preserved. A similar pattern of inferior wall pseudodyskinesis can be seen in any entity that results in sufficient abdominal distention to compress the left ventricle inferiorly including significant hepatomegaly, ascites, or pregnancy. RV, right ventricle.

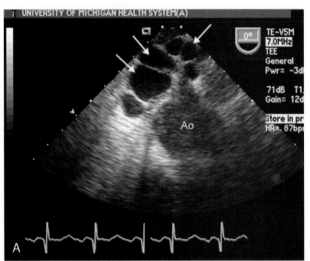

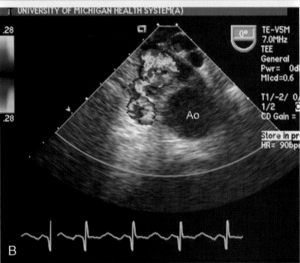

FIGURE 22.21. Transesophageal echocardiogram recorded in a patient with end-stage liver disease and large venous malformations. This image was recorded at approximately 40 cm from the incisors. **A:** Note the position of the aorta (*Ao*) and multiple large cystic spaces surrounding it. **B:** Note the continuous venous flow in the spaces documenting their nature as large venous collaterals.

massive transfusion. This may precipitate acute decompensation of left ventricular function and severe congestive heart failure in the absence of ischemic heart disease.

CHRONIC OBSTRUCTIVE PULMONARY DISEASE

Chronic lung disease, either obstructive or restrictive, can be associated with significant cardiovascular changes, predominantly due to elevation in pulmonary arterial pressure. This leads to right ventricular hypertension with secondary right ventricular hypertrophy and/or dilatation. From a cardiac perspective, the appearance is similar to that of any pulmonary arterial hypertension, and it frequently includes variable degrees of tricuspid regurgitation

with elevated tricuspid regurgitation velocity consistent with high right ventricular systolic pressure. Patients with chronic obstructive lung disease frequently have limited parasternal and apical windows because of interference with ultrasound transmission due to intervening lung tissue and a more vertical and inferior position of the heart. They often can be better imaged from a subcostal transducer position (Fig. 22.22) from which virtually all cardiac chambers are sometimes visualized in excellent detail.

PULMONARY HYPERTENSION

Pulmonary hypertension occurs either as a primary pulmonary arterial process or as secondary to other (usually

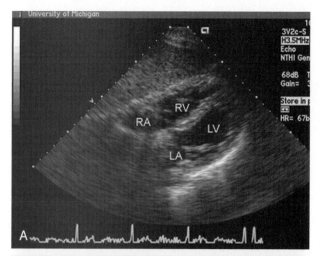

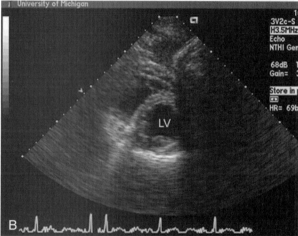

FIGURE 22.22. Subcostal echocardiogram recorded in a four-chamber view **(A)** and a short-axis view **(B)** in a patient with chronic obstructive lung disease. LA, left atrium; LV, left ventricle; RA, right atrium; RV, right ventricle.

▶ **TABLE 22.3 Etiologies of Pulmonary Hypertension**

Shunt related
  Ventricular septal defect
  Atrial septal defect
  Patent ductus arteriosus
Related to elevated pulmonary venous pressure
  Mitral stenosis
  Mitral regurgitation
  Left ventricular systolic dysfunction
  Left ventricular diastolic dysfunction
  Restrictive cardiomyopathy
  Pulmonary vein stenosis/thrombosis
Pulmonary embolus
  Acute
  Chronic
Pulmonary
  Obstructive lung disease
  Restrictive lung disease
  High altitude
Obesity/hypoventilation
Primary pulmonary hypertension
  Pulmonary arterial hypertension
  Toxins
  Anorexigens

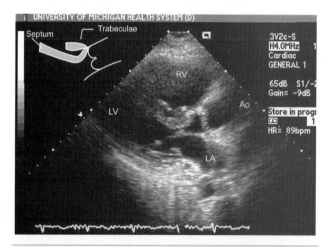

FIGURE 22.23. Parasternal long-axis view recorded in a patient with severe primary pulmonary arterial hypertension. Note the marked dilation of the right ventricle (*RV*) and the abnormal configuration of the proximal ventricular septum which, in this diastolic frame, bows into the left ventricular outflow tract. Note also (see schematic) the hypertrophied right ventricular trabeculation that lies along the right side of the ventricular septum. On occasion, hypertrophied right ventricular muscle bundles are mistaken for a portion of the actual ventricular septum and included in the measurement of septal thickness, resulting in an artifactual diagnosis of asymmetric septal hypertrophy and hypertrophic cardiomyopathy. In the real-time image, note the abnormal ventricular septal motion in both diastole and systole. Ao, aorta; LA, left atrium; LV, left ventricle.

left-sided) cardiovascular disease. Table 22.3 outlines the primary and secondary etiologies of pulmonary hypertension. Echocardiography plays a valuable role in identifying cardiac disease that has resulted in elevation in pulmonary arterial pressure. Examples include detection of shunt lesions such as atrial septal defect, mitral stenosis, or severe left ventricular systolic or diastolic dysfunction. The echocardiographic manifestations of right heart hypertension on an echocardiogram are similar irrespective of the pressure elevation (Figs. 22.11, 22.23–22.26). Basically any disease that results in a right ventricular volume or pressure overload results in dilation and eventual hypertrophy of the right ventricle. The ventricular septum, because it is a shared wall between the right and left ventricles, reflects the magnitude of hemodynamic derangement whether it is a volume or pressure overload.

When a patient is encountered with pulmonary hypertension, echocardiography plays a crucial role in identify-

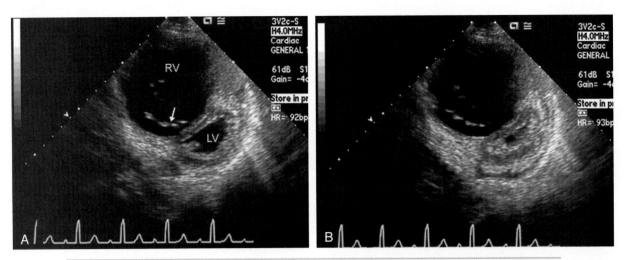

FIGURE 22.24. Parasternal short-axis view recorded in a patient with severe primary pulmonary hypertension. **A:** Note the massively dilated right ventricle (RV) with components of the tricuspid valve (*arrow*) visible in the cavity. In diastole, the left ventricle (LV) is compressed with flattened septal geometry and frank reversal of curvature in systole **(B)**, suggesting systemic right ventricular systolic pressures.

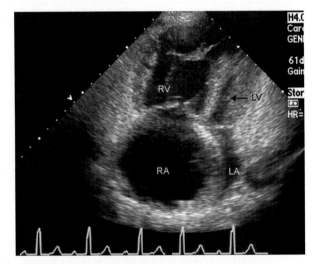

FIGURE 22.25. Apical four-chamber view recorded in a patient with severe primary pulmonary hypertension. Note the massive dilation of the right ventricle (*RV*) and right atrium (*RA*) and the small compressed slit-like left atrium (*LA*) and left ventricle (*LV*).

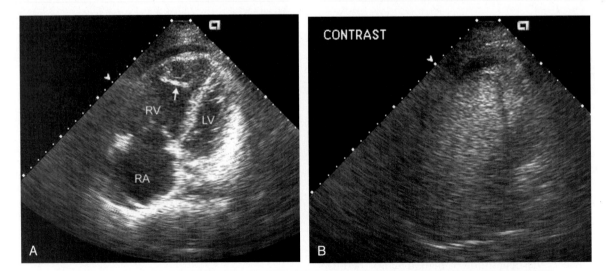

FIGURE 22.26. Apical four-chamber view recorded in a patient with severe pulmonary arterial hypertension. **A:** Note the marked dilation of the right atrium (*RA*) and right ventricle (*RV*) and the mass of echos in the right ventricular apex. The left ventricle (*LV*) is small and underfilled and has been compressed out of view. On occasion, the echos in the apex can be confused for thrombus or other mass. With significant right ventricular hypertrophy, the moderator band and other right ventricular trabecular structures hypertrophy as well and can assume a mass-like appearance. **B:** Recorded after injection of intravenous contrast and demonstrates that the contrast fills the apex completely documenting that these "masses" are muscle bundles and not a pathologic mass.

ing any underlying cardiovascular abnormality that may have resulted in secondary pulmonary hypertension. Echocardiography is less valuable for making a definitive diagnosis of primary pulmonary arterial hypertension, which is by definition a diagnosis of exclusion.

For patients with pulmonary hypertension, the echocardiographic examination should be tailored to identification of any cardiac entity likely to have resulted in secondary pulmonary hypertension, such as an atrial (Fig. 22.27) or ventricular septal defect. This is typically easily accomplished with transthoracic echocardiography, combined with detailed color flow imaging. Detailed attention should be paid to the right ventricular outflow tract for detection of subvalvular obstruction and to the right ventricular outflow tract spectral flow profile with respect to parameters such as acceleration time, which can be used as a indirect measure of pulmonary artery pressure.

Contrast echocardiography is commonly employed to detect the presence of a significant right-to-left shunt and hence, by inference, make the diagnosis of an atrial septal defect. In a large number of patients with significant pulmonary hypertension, right atrial dilation will result in stretching of the foramen ovale, and mild right-to-left shunting is very common in severe pulmonary hypertension. Separation of the small secondary right-to-left shunt due to a patent foramen ovale from a shunt attributable to an atrial septal defect is occasionally problematic (Figs. 22.28 and 22.29). Typically, however, if significant pul-

monary hypertension is present and is secondary to an atrial septal defect, the magnitude of the shunt will be substantial and the appearance of contrast in the left atrium nearly instantaneous and continuous throughout the cardiac cycle. Conversely, shunting through a small

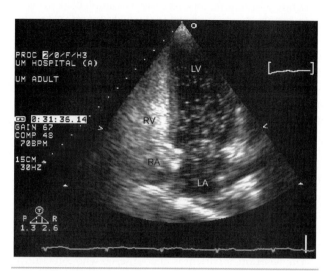

FIGURE 22.28. Apical four-chamber view with intravenous saline contrast recorded in a patient with significant pulmonary arterial hypertension. Note the modest amount of contrast appearing in the left atrium (*LA*) and left ventricle (*LV*) consistent with a patent foramen ovale. In the presence of a large atrial septal defect and severe pulmonary arterial hypertension, one would anticipate a significantly greater degree of right-to-left shunting (Fig. 22.29). RA, right atrium; RV, right ventricle.

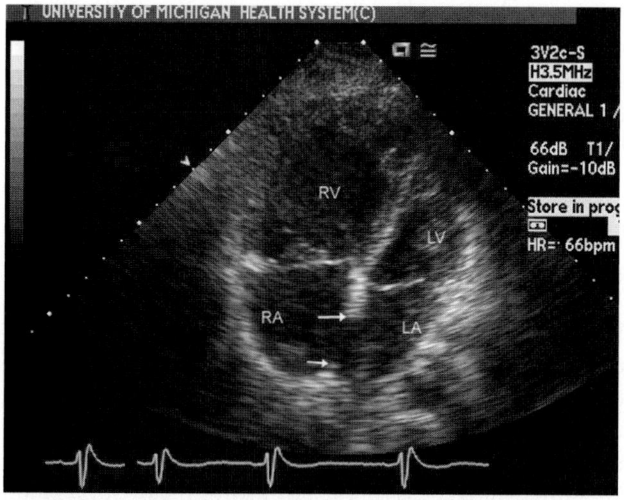

FIGURE 22.27. Apical four-chamber view recorded in a patient with severe pulmonary arterial hypertension who was subsequently documented to have a large secundum atrial septal defect. Note that the appearance of the right heart is virtually identical to that presented in Figures 22.23 through 22.26. There is a distinct dropout of echoes in the atrial septum (noted between the *two arrows*) consistent with a secundum atrial septal defect. LA, left atrium; LV, left ventricle; RA, right atrium; RV, right ventricle.

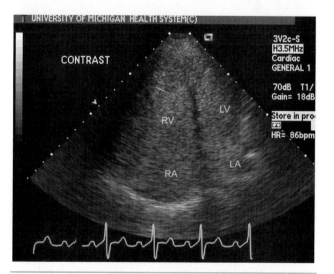

FIGURE 22.29. Apical four-chamber view after intravenous saline injection in a patient with pulmonary arterial hypertension and an atrial septal defect. Note the equal opacification by saline contrast of all four cardiac chambers, suggesting a greater degree of interatrial shunting than seen in Figure 22.28. LA, left atrium; LV, left ventricle; RA, right atrium; RV, right ventricle.

patent foramen ovale often occurs phasically with the respiratory cycle.

With two-dimensional echocardiography, the majority of patients with significant pulmonary hypertension will have evidence of right atrial and/or right ventricular dilation. Concurrent tricuspid regurgitation is nearly ubiquitous and may range from mild to severe. Interrogation of the tricuspid regurgitation velocity allows calculation of right ventricular systolic pressures. This is occasionally problematic in patients with eccentric regurgitation jets or in whom the regurgitation is not holosystolic. In the absence of obstruction of right ventricular outflow, this equals systolic pressure in the pulmonary artery (Fig. 22.30). The echocardiographic methodology for determination of right ventricular pressure is discussed in Chapters 8 and 12. Finally, many patients with significant pulmonary hypertension will have evidence of abnormal left ventricular filling (reduced mitral valve E/A ratio), presumably as an indirect effect of septal hypertrophy and right ventricular pressure overload or reduced left atrial filling pressure (Fig. 22.31). The mitral inflow pattern will often revert to normal with reduction in the pulmonary hypertension.

On occasion, a patient is encountered who, on clinical grounds, is suspected to have pulmonary hypertension but in whom the right ventricular systolic pressure is calculated to be relatively low. In these cases, reassessing the pressure during exercise (supine bicycle) may unmask

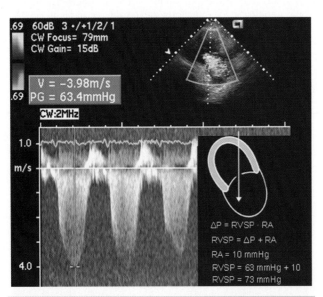

FIGURE 22.30. Calculation of right ventricular systolic pressure from a tricuspid regurgitation jet in a patient with pulmonary arterial hypertension. This jet was recorded from the right ventricular inflow tract view and reveals a tricuspid valve V_{max} of approximately 4.0 m/sec, from which right ventricular systolic pressure (*RVSP*) can be calculated using the formula noted in the superimposed schematic. In this example, right atrial pressure has been estimated to be 10 mm Hg based on right atrial size, severity of tricuspid regurgitation, and the appearance of the inferior vena cava. RA, right atrium.

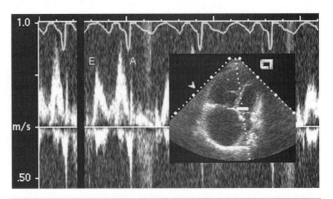

FIGURE 22.31. Pulsed Doppler recording of mitral inflow in a young female patient with severe primary pulmonary hypertension. In a patient at this age, without left ventricular disease or hypertension, one would anticipate an E/A ratio of more than 1.2. Note the reversed E/A ratio in this patient with severe primary pulmonary hypertension due to adverse diastolic interaction of the ventricles, which impedes left ventricular filling, resulting in the appearance of left ventricular diastolic dysfunction.

substantial exercise-induced pulmonary hypertension, which is more consistent with the patient's presenting clinical symptoms (Fig. 22.32).

There are several echocardiographic features in patients with pulmonary hypertension that confer a worse prognosis. These include more marked degrees of right atrial enlargement, the presence of pericardial effusion, and greater degrees of left ventricular compression due to right ventricular enlargement. In this setting, the pericardial effusion typically does not result in hemodynamic compromise but is simply a manifestation of more marked elevation of right heart pressures. Patients who have marked reversal of septal curvature with a small slit-like left ventricle are also more prone to develop significant, and occasionally fatal, hypotension if given vasodilators.

MISCELLANEOUS DISEASES

Sarcoidosis

Sarcoidosis is an inflammatory multisystem disease of uncertain etiology. Histologically, the hallmark is noncaseating granulomas in multiple organs. The predominant sites for involvement are the lungs and lymphatic system. Cardiac structures may be involved in as many as 40% of advanced cases. Cardiac involvement can include the pericardium, conducting system or myocardium and result in either diffuse microscopic focal infiltrates or larger nodules within the myocardium. Involvement seems to predominate in the posterior wall (Fig. 22.33), and mitral regurgitation is not uncommon. On occasion, patients with disseminated sarcoidosis present with global left ventricular dysfunction and malignant ventricular arrhythmias, mimicking dilated cardiomyopathy.

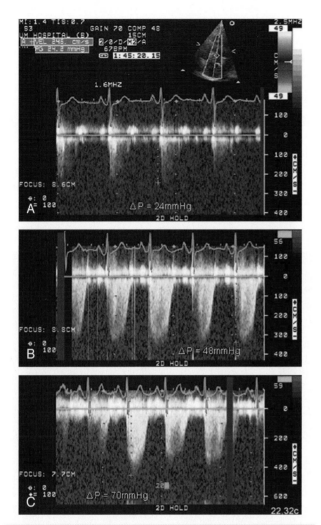

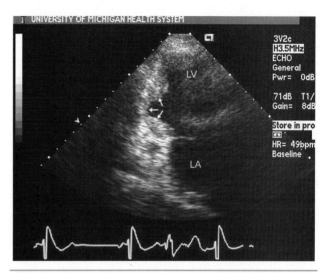

FIGURE 22.33. Apical two-chamber view recorded in a patient with documented cardiac sarcoidosis. Note the discrete aneurysm in the proximal third of the inferior wall, which is a common site of involvement by cardiac sarcoid. LA, left atrium; LV, left ventricle.

dilated cardiomyopathy, which is indistinguishable from cardiomyopathy of other etiologies. The diagnosis should be suspected in patients with other manifestations of hemochromatosis such as diabetes and abnormal skin coloring who simultaneously present with a dilated cardiomyopathy. Figure 22.34 was recorded in a patient who had previously undergone cardiac transplantation for end-stage dilated cardiomyopathy due to hemochromatosis and subsequently developed biopsy-proven hemochromatosis in the transplanted heart. Note the thickened ventricular walls with abnormal myocardial texture.

FIGURE 22.32. Continuous wave Doppler imaging of the tricuspid regurgitation jet recorded from the apical view in a patient with limiting dyspnea but no evidence of significant pulmonary arterial hypertension at rest. **A:** Image recorded at rest reveals a tricuspid valve V_{max} of approximately 2.5 m/sec, corresponding to a gradient of 24 mm Hg between the right ventricle and right atrium. This would be at the upper limits of normal. **B:** Recorded at 50 W of exercise on a supine bicycle at which point the spectral density has increased, suggesting an increase in the severity of tricuspid regurgitation, and the tricuspid valve gradient has increased to 48 mm Hg. **C:** Image recorded at 75 W of exercise shows a further increase in spectral density and increase in the RV-RA gradient to 70 mm Hg, suggesting significant exercise-induced pulmonary hypertension.

Therapy for cardiac sarcoidosis most often includes high-dose steroid therapy and may result in improvement in global systolic function.

Hemochromatosis

Hemochromatosis involves the heart in the majority of advanced cases and results in either an infiltrative pattern, similar to that seen with amyloidosis, or more commonly a

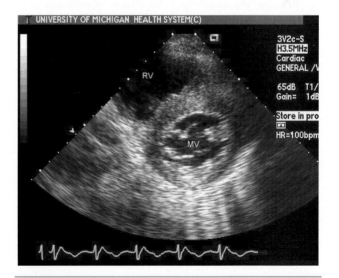

FIGURE 22.34. Parasternal short-axis view recorded in a patient with documented cardiac hematochromatosis. Note the increased wall thickness and the abnormal myocardial texture with modest reduction in systolic function. MV, mitral valve; RV, right ventricle.

Muscular Dystrophy

Several of the muscular dystrophies as well as Friedreich ataxia may have cardiac involvement. The cardiac involvement typically mimics hypertrophic or dilated cardiomyopathy, and there may be greater regional variation in left ventricular dysfunction than with typical cardiomyopathy. The classic abnormality in Friedreich ataxia is a posterior wall motion abnormality.

Hypereosinophilia

Hypereosinophilia due to eosinophilic leukemia, tropical hypereosinophilia, or idiopathic eosinophilia results in characteristic abnormalities detected with echocardiography. The most classic abnormality is obliteration of the left or right ventricular apex by laminar thrombus (Fig. 22.35A). Pathologically, the thrombus is composed of inflammatory tissue, thrombus, and eosinophilic infiltrates. It results in a reduction of ventricular chamber size and increasing stiffness, resulting in a restrictive cardiomyopathic picture. Additionally, hypereosinophilic syndrome has a propensity to involve the posterior left ventricular wall and posterior mitral valve leaflet and result in mitral regurgitation (Fig. 22.35B).

Carcinoid Syndrome

Carcinoid syndrome is an endocrinologic syndrome resulting in release of active metabolites of serotonin and tryptophan that have a toxic effect on the endothelium of the heart. The toxic metabolites are deactivated in the lung, and, as such, left-sided involvement is less common unless there are concurrent pulmonary metastases or a right-to-left shunt. The classic abnormality in carcinoid syndrome is diffuse thickening and immobility of the tricuspid and less commonly the pulmonary valve (Fig. 22.36). This results in a combination of stenosis and regurgitation. In advanced cases, the entire length of the tricuspid valve leaflet will appear to be thickened and rigid as opposed to a more domed appearance in rheumatic tricuspid valve disease. Rheumatic involvement can also be separated from carcinoid syndrome because the vast majority of patients with rheumatic tricuspid valve disease will have concurrent mitral valve disease.

Sickle Cell Anemia

Sickle cell anemia (hemoglobin SS) has been associated with a number of cardiovascular abnormalities. It should be recognized that any severe, chronic anemia (including thalassemia) results in a high-output state, which in turn may lead to left ventricular dilation and, if severe and long-standing, to the appearance of a dilated cardiomyopathy. Sickle cell anemia may also be associated with mi-

croinfarction and ventricular dysfunction (Fig. 22.37). Through a presumed similar mechanism, these patients may also develop pulmonary arterial hypertension.

Human Immunodeficiency Virus

Infection with human immunodeficiency virus or acquired immunodeficiency syndrome has been associated with a variety of cardiovascular manifestations, none of which is specific to the syndrome. Because of their immunocompromised state, patients are prone to infections, including endocarditis with unusual organisms. Addition-

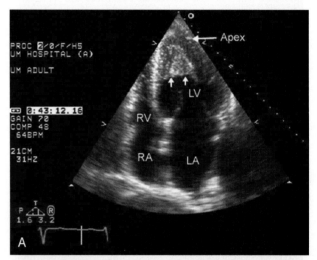

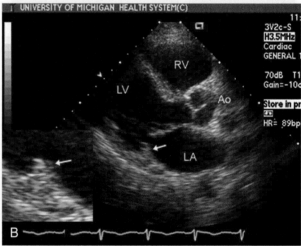

FIGURE 22.35. Apical four-chamber view **(A)** recorded in a patient with the hypereosinophilic syndrome and obliteration of the left ventricular apex. Note the abnormal texture of the mass that homogeneously fills the left ventricular apex and its distinct margin with the blood pool cavity (*arrows*). **B:** Parasternal long-axis view shows involvement of the posterior mitral valve, which is markedly thickened and tethered to the wall. The inset is an expanded view of the posterior mitral valve leaflet. Ao, aorta; LA, left atrium; LV, left ventricle; RA, right atrium; RV, right ventricle.

ally pericarditis, pulmonary hypertension, and dilated cardiomyopathy have all been described. The mechanism by which the human immunodeficiency virus results in these manifestations is not fully understood.

Diet Drug Valvulopathy

In the late 1990s, it became apparent that a number of patients who had been exposed to anorexigens, especially the combination of fenfluramine and phentermine, developed an unusual form of valvular heart disease. Anatomically, the most obvious lesion was of the mitral valve. In advanced cases, the mitral valve and its chordae appeared encased in a matrix (Fig. 22.38), similar to that seen in the

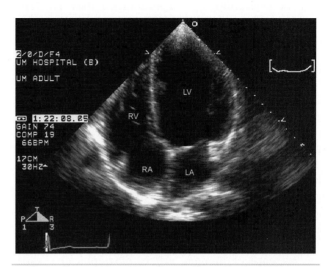

FIGURE 22.37. Apical four-chamber view recorded in a patient with sickle cell anemia (hemoglobin SS) and a chronic hemoglobin of approximately 6 g/dL. This echocardiogram was recorded in a 19-year-old female patient (weight, 110 lb; height, 5 ft 6 in.) and reveals obvious left ventricular dilation for an individual of that size. Note the global hypokinesis of the left ventricle (*LV*), which may be due to a combination of microinfarcts and long-standing high-output state. LA, left atrium; RA, right atrium; RV, right ventricle.

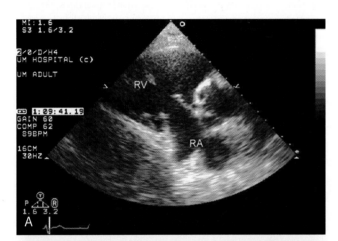

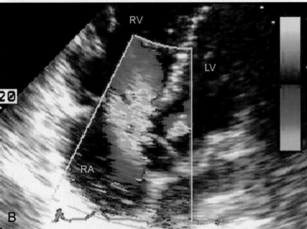

FIGURE 22.36. Right ventricular inflow tract view recorded in a patient with carcinoid syndrome and involvement of the tricuspid leaflets. In the still image (**A**), recorded in early systole, note the rigid appearance of the tricuspid valve, which has remained in a nearly fully opened position. In the real-time image, note that the valve is thickened along its entire extent and fails to coapt at any point during systole. **B:** Severe tricuspid regurgitation due to a complete failure of the leaflets to coapt in systole is revealed. LV, left ventricle; RA, right atrium; RV, right ventricle.

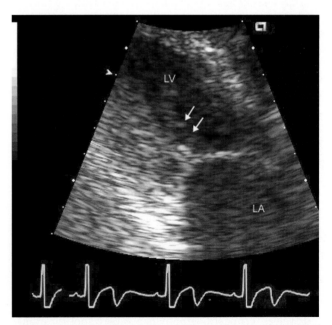

FIGURE 22.38. Apical long-axis view recorded in a patient with previous exposure to anorexigens and diffuse distal leaflet and chordal (*arrows*) thickening of the mitral valve. This appearance is not specific to diet-drug exposure, and the relationship to drug exposure is only presumptive and made in the absence of any other potential etiology for the leaflet thickening. LA, left atrium; LV left ventricle.

carcinoid syndrome; however, the tricuspid valve was not involved. Aortic insufficiency was likewise noted; however, the echocardiographic appearance of the aortic valve was most often unremarkable. Initial reports suggesting an incidence of diet drug valvulopathy of 16% to 40% were clearly erroneous. More well-done surveillance studies demonstrated an incidence between 3% and 15%, with the more prevalent lesion being aortic insufficiency rather than mitral insufficiency. There was a definite relationship between duration of exposure to the drugs and the prevalence of valve disease. Most studies suggested that valve involvement was rare with less than 6 months of drug exposure and the majority of valvular lesions were mild. It should be emphasized that substantial controversy continues to surround this issue, and the true prevalence of diet drug valvulopathy will probably never be known. Many patients presumed to have direct drug valvulopathy have evidence of valvular regurgitation in the presence of minimal echocardiographically visible anatomic changes. It should be emphasized that there are no universally agreed on echocardiographic findings specific to this syndrome. Several small follow-up studies have suggested that, in many patients, the severity of valvular regurgitation may regress over time and that it is highly unlikely to worsen.

Obesity

Morbid obesity has long been associated with significant cardiovascular changes. It has been very difficult to identify the independent contribution of obesity to cardiac disease because of a high prevalence of concurrent hypertension and diabetes. Morbid obesity has been associated with a high-output state, which in its extreme forms may result in congestive heart failure. More moderate degrees of obesity typically have been associated with a slight increase in left ventricular mass and internal dimension; however, after correcting for either height and/or lean body mass, the relationship is relatively weak. Using recently developed, more detailed techniques for evaluation of systolic and diastolic function, some investigators have suggested subtle systolic and diastolic dysfunction in patients with significant obesity.

CLINICAL PRESENTATIONS AND PROBLEMS

Because it evaluates all four cardiac chambers and all four valves, echocardiography is a superb tool for evaluating the vast majority of cardiac problems that arise in the practice of medicine. There are several distinct clinical presentations for which echocardiography plays the primary diagnostic and management role and has a direct and relevant impact on the management of patients. Table 22.1 lists many of the clinical syndromes or presentations

for which echocardiography plays an instrumental role. For many of these presentations, echocardiography carries a class I recommendation as a primary diagnostic tool in the respective American College of Cardiology/American Heart Association guidelines for management of that particular disease.

Peripheral Vascular Disease

Patients with peripheral vascular occlusive disease represent a population at high risk of concurrent coronary artery disease. Many surveillance studies have suggested that the presence of peripheral vascular disease is an excellent marker for underlying coronary artery disease. Peripheral vascular disease develops as a sequela of many of the same risk factors leading to coronary disease including tobacco use, hypertension, and lipid disorders, so this association is not unexpected. Concurrent diabetes obviously plays a significant role in development of simultaneous coronary and peripheral vascular disease. For many of these patients, exercise tolerance is limited by the peripheral disease and as such they may not experience episodes of spontaneous angina.

Echocardiography plays a valuable role in the evaluation of patients with clinically relevant peripheral vascular disease. The resting echocardiogram can be used to assess end-organ damage from concurrent hypertension or diabetes and determine left ventricular systolic and diastolic function. Additionally, pharmacologic stress testing with dobutamine stress echocardiography can be used to identify occult coronary artery disease in a patient population that frequently has limited exercise capacity. Dobutamine stress echocardiography plays a major role in identifying high- and low-risk subsets of patients before surgical intervention for peripheral vascular disease.

Congestive Heart Failure

Congestive heart failure is one of the most rapidly increasing diagnoses encountered in today's practice of medicine. The anatomic and physiologic substrate underlying congestive heart failure is quite diverse and includes valvular heart disease, ischemic heart disease, and primary myocardial disease. Between 30% and 40% of patients presenting with congestive heart failure have preserved systolic function and have heart failure based on diastolic dysfunction. Indices of systolic function such as fractional shortening and fractional area change as well as left ventricular diastolic and systolic volumes and ejection fraction can be determined with echocardiography and are instrumental in stratifying patients into predominantly systolic versus diastolic dysfunction (Figs. 22.39 and 22.40). Echocardiography can identify the underlying anatomic substrate in the majority of patients presenting

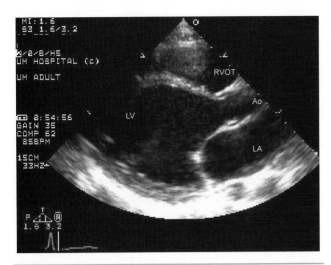

FIGURE 22.39. Parasternal long-axis view recorded in a 30-year-old patient with a previously undiagnosed severe dilated cardiomyopathy (presumably familial). Note the marked dilation of the left ventricle (*LV*), and the spherical geometry with severe global hypokinesis and a marked reduction in systolic function. Ao, aorta; LA, left atrium; RVOT, right ventricular outflow tract.

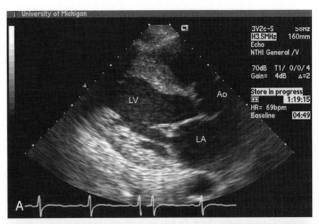

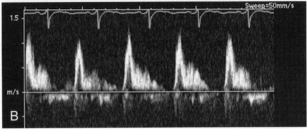

FIGURE 22.40. **A:** Parasternal long-axis view recorded in a patient with an idiopathic restrictive cardiomyopathy. Note the slightly increased left ventricular wall thickness, the left atrial enlargement, and the mildly reduced left ventricular systolic function. In the accompanying spectral Doppler imaging **(B)**, note the pathologically elevated mitral E/A ratio, suggesting significant (grade 3) diastolic dysfunction. Ao, aorta; LA, left atrium; LV, left ventricle.

with congestive heart failure. Performance of echocardiography is considered a class I indication in the American College of Cardiology/American Heart Association guidelines for clinical management of patients with congestive heart failure. In modern practice, virtually 100% of patients initially presenting with congestive heart failure, whether chronic or acute, should undergo echocardiography to determine the underlying anatomic substrate.

On the basis of echocardiographic findings, heart failure can be stratified into diseases requiring surgical management such as valvular heart disease and those requiring medical management such as dilated cardiomyopathy. The complete evaluation of patients with congestive heart failure typically can be performed with transthoracic echocardiography. Exercise and dobutamine stress echocardiography can play an incremental role in identifying an ischemic substrate and viable myocardium in patients with chronic ischemic dysfunction. For patients with primary myocardial dysfunction or secondary ventricular dysfunction due to valvular heart disease, serial echocardiography can be used to evaluate recovery of function and screen for complications of heart failure.

There are several echocardiographic features to be noted in patients with heart failure that have direct prognostic relevance (Table 22.4). As with other imaging techniques, there is a direct and inverse relationship between left ventricular systolic function and clinical outcome. Additional features to be noted in patients with congestive heart failure include the presence of concurrent mitral or tricuspid regurgitation or secondary pulmonary hyper-

▶ **TABLE 22.4 Prognostic Markers in Congestive Heart Failure**

Left ventricular systolic function
  Chamber size
  Ventricular volume
  Ventricular geometry
  Ejection fraction
  Myocardial performance index
Left ventricular diastolic function
  Delayed relaxation
  "Restrictive" filling pattern
  Pseudonormal filling
  Mitral anular diastolic velocity
  Left atrial volume
Mitral regurgitation
Tricuspid regurgitation
Pulmonary hypertension
Right ventricular function

tension, each of which has been shown to confer a worse prognosis in patients with systolic dysfunction and congestive heart failure. Concurrent right ventricular dysfunction also confers a worsened prognosis.

Evaluation of diastolic properties of the heart using Doppler echocardiography also provides important prognostic information. Patients with a high E/A ratio and short deceleration time (the so-called restrictive pattern) have a worse prognosis compared with those with a pattern of delayed relaxation and an E/A ratio less than 1 (Table 22.5). In the setting of systolic dysfunction, the exaggerated E/A ratio represents pathologic stiffening of the ventricle with concurrent elevation of left ventricular diastolic pressures. It generally implies a component of volume overload and diastolic dysfunction. Recent data have suggested that the intermediate pattern of pseudonormalization confers a similar prognosis. Evaluation of pulmonary vein flow and Doppler tissue imaging of the mitral anulus can assist in identifying patients with the pseudonormal pattern and hence an adverse prognosis. As noted in Chapters 6 and 8, many of the newer indices of ventricular function such as the myocardial performance index, Doppler tissue imaging with myocardial displacement, and strain and strain rate imaging are playing an increasing role in the evaluation of patients with congestive heart failure.

Evaluation of Dyspnea

Exertional and resting dyspnea is a common clinical presentation with multiple and diverse etiologies ranging from metabolic disorders to primary pulmonary disorders to cardiovascular disorders. Many patients have dyspnea for multifactorial reasons, a classic example being cardiac disease with congestive heart failure and concurrent obstructive lung disease. Echocardiography should be an initial diagnostic tool in patients presenting with unexplained dyspnea. As discussed previously in the section on congestive heart failure, a transthoracic echocardiogram will typically identify any relevant cardiac contribution to a patient's breathlessness and help direct appropriate cardiac-specific therapy. Similarly, when a normal echocardiogram is encountered, the etiology of

▶ TABLE 22.5 Outcome in Heart Failure: Impact of Diastolic Dysfunction

Ref.	Total N	Entry Criteria	Diastolic Pattern	n	F/U (mo)	Outcome	Marker Present (%)	Marker Absent (%)
Faris et al., 2002	337	DCM	E/A >1.2, DT <140 ms	195	36	Survival	77	92
Aurigemma et al., 2001	2,671	Longitudinal study	E/A <0.7		60	CHF (new)	14.4	—
			E/A 0.7–1.5		60	CHF (new)	4.6	—
			E/A >1.5		60	CHF (new)	11.0	—
Dujardin et al., 1998	75	DCM	MPI >0.77	38	33	Survival	36	83
Temporelli et al., 1998	144	CHF	DT ≤125 ms, NR	80	48	Survival	52	86
Rihal et al., 1994	102	DCM	DT >130 ms, EF >0.25	26	24	Survival	95	—
			DT <130 ms, EF >0.25	29	24	Survival	100	—
			DT >130 ms, EF <0.25	37	24	Survival	72	—
			DT <130 ms, EF <0.25	10	24	Survival	35	—
Pinamonti et al., 1993	0	DCM	DT <115 ms	36	22	Survival	61	100
Florea et al., 2000	144	CHF, age > 67 y	IVRT ≤30 ms	79	36	Survival	52	78
Whalley et al., 2002	115	CHF on admission	E/A >1.0, DT >230 ms	46	12	Death	17	—
			Pseudonormal			Readmission	15	—
			E/A >2.0, DT <140 ms	42	12	Death	23	—
						Readmission	31	—
				27	12	Death	37	—
						Readmission	41	—
Pinamonti et al., 1997	110	DCM	DT ≤115 ms	57	48	Death/txp	87	—
			DT <115 ms	24	48	Death/txp	4	—
			DT <115, REV	29	48	Death/txp	3	—

CHF, congestive heart failure; DCM, dilated cardiomyopathy; DT, deceleration time; DR, delayed relaxation; EF, ejection fraction; IVRT, isovolumic relation time; MFP, mitral filling pattern; MPI, myocardial performance index; NR, no reversal with therapy; txp, heart transplant.

the dyspnea is far less likely to be cardiac and the clinician's attention can appropriately be turned to pulmonary or other medical illnesses. It is not uncommon, in an adult population, to encounter patients in whom the magnitude of the dyspnea appears to exceed that which can be attributed to identifiable cardiovascular disease. In these instances, reevaluation of cardiac hemodynamics including pulmonary artery systolic pressure with exercise echocardiography may provide valuable diagnostic information. Additionally, detailed cardiopulmonary stress testing is often useful in separating cardiac from noncardiac dyspnea.

Acute Pulmonary Embolus

Acute pulmonary embolus occurs both in a background of major medical illnesses and in previously healthy individuals with a precipitating risk factor such as immobilization. The classic symptoms of a pulmonary embolus include acute onset of pleuritic chest pain and breathlessness; however, many patients with a pulmonary embolus have atypical presentations or may be asymptomatic. The degree of hemodynamic compromise and presumably symptomatic status are directly related to the embolic burden and ranges from trivial and inconsequential hemodynamic derangement, as is seen in a small pulmonary embolus, to instantaneously fatal events with a large proximal "saddle" embolus. For patients presenting with the acute onset of dyspnea, echocardiography can be a helpful tool, but a normal echocardiogram should not be used to exclude the presence of a pulmonary embolus in a patient whose symptoms otherwise warrant evaluation of that entity.

Echocardiographic Findings

Echocardiographic findings in a pulmonary embolus are directly related to the magnitude of the embolus. The degree to which there has been preexisting cardiovascular disease must also be factored into this analysis. With large hemodynamically significant pulmonary emboli, typically a right heart pressure and/or volume overload pattern will develop (Fig. 22.41). Assuming a previously normal cardiovascular system with normal pulmonary artery pressures, the right ventricle is not conditioned to generate pressures in excess of 60 to 70 mm Hg. Therefore, if one encounters pressures of 70 mm Hg or more in a suspected pulmonary embolus, one must consider the scenario of acute on chronic thromboembolic disease or a pulmonary embolus superimposed on previously existing pulmonary hypertension. For a patient presenting with acute breathlessness and chest pain and in whom right ventricular dilation with tricuspid regurgitation and mild elevation of the pulmonary artery pressure is noted, a pulmonary em-

bolus should be one of the initial diagnoses to be considered. Evaluation of left ventricular function is obviously crucial because inferior infarct, complicated by right ventricular infarction, may have a similar echocardiographic appearance but would not be expected to be seen in conjunction with elevated pulmonary artery pressure. For smaller pulmonary emboli, the echocardiographic findings are often more subtle. In many patients, even with relatively small pulmonary emboli, a subtle degree of right heart dilation with mild tricuspid regurgitation may be noted and result in subtle nonspecific abnormalities of ventricular septal motion. For small pulmonary emboli, it is not uncommon to see an entirely normal echocardiogram, thus a normal echocardiogram should not be used to exclude the diagnosis of an acute pulmonary embolus.

On occasion, one can directly visualize a pulmonary embolus in a proximal pulmonary artery (Fig. 22.42). This is best accomplished with transesophageal echocardiography (Fig. 22.43), which is not usually performed for the routine evaluation of a suspected pulmonary embolus. On occasion, one identifies thromboembolism in transit, which represents a large thrombus, typically from a deep venous structure in the pelvis or lower extremities that has become entangled in the tricuspid valve apparatus. This thrombus takes on a serpiginous and highly mobile appearance on echocardiography and appears to curl on itself. Figures 22.44 through 22.46 were recorded in a patient with such thromboembolism in transit. Notice in Figure 22.45 that a portion of the thrombus has actually

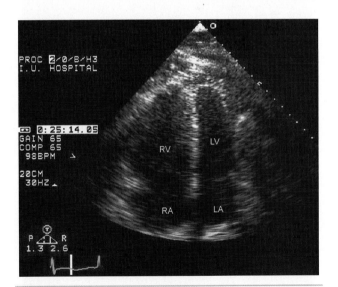

FIGURE 22.41. Apical four-chamber view recorded in a patient with an acute massive pulmonary embolus. Note the dilation of the right atrium (*RA*) and right ventricle (*RV*), suggesting a degree of pre-existing pulmonary arterial hypertension or dysfunction. Also note the reduced systolic function of the right ventricle in the real-time image. LA, left atrium; LV, left ventricle.

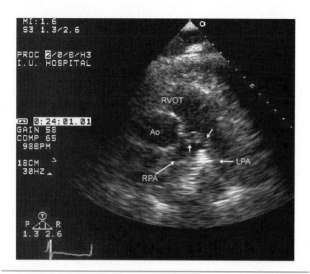

FIGURE 22.42. Parasternal short-axis view recorded in the same patient presented in Figure 22.41. Note the tubular mass at the bifurcation of the pulmonary artery into the right-and-left pulmonary artery (*RPA, LPA*). In the real-time image, note the mobile nature of this mass, which has the classic appearance of a "saddle" embolus. Ao, aorta; RVOT, right ventricular outflow tract.

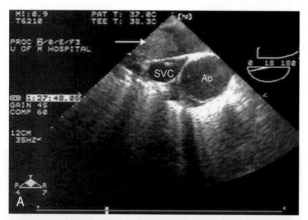

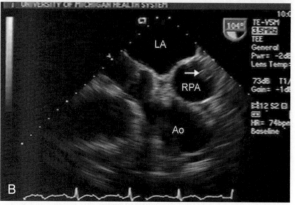

FIGURE 22.43. Transesophageal echocardiogram recorded in patients with acute pulmonary emboli. **A:** Note the mass (*arrow*) occluding a significant portion of the proximal right pulmonary artery consistent with large pulmonary embolism. **B:** Recorded in a patient with a smaller embolus visible as a circular density (*arrow*) in the right pulmonary artery (*RPA*). Ao, aorta; LA, left atrium; SVC, superior vena cava.

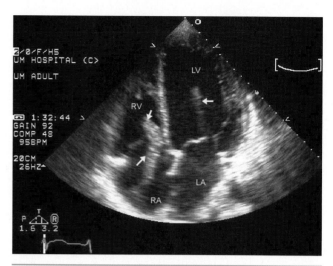

FIGURE 22.44. Apical four-chamber view recorded in a patient with new-onset dyspnea. Note the long serpiginous mass in the right atrium (*RA*), which crosses the tricuspid valve (*arrows in the right heart*). Note the serpiginous nature of this mass and its highly mobile nature in the real-time image. This represents the cast of a deep vein thrombus that has migrated to the heart and become entrapped in the tricuspid valve chordae. The linear echo in the cavity of the left ventricle (*LV*) (*arrow*) is an artifact that can be appreciated on the real-time image. LA, left atrium; RV, right ventricle.

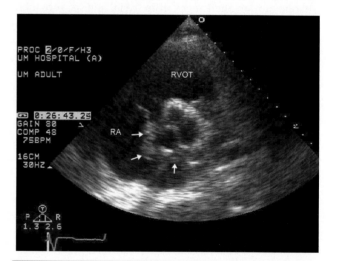

FIGURE 22.45. Parasternal short-axis view recorded in a patient with thromboembolism in transit. Note the serpiginous mass in the right atrium (*RA*) (*arrows*), a portion of which crosses the atrial septum and protrudes through a patent foramen ovale into the left atrium. This patient presented with a combination of acute pulmonary embolus and a neurologic event. RVOT, right ventricular outflow tract.

protruded through a patent foramen ovale into the left atrium, hence placing the patient at risk of paradoxical systemic embolization. Treatment of thromboembolism in transit remains somewhat controversial, with most authorities arguing for immediate surgical removal of the thrombus and others recommending either lytic therapy

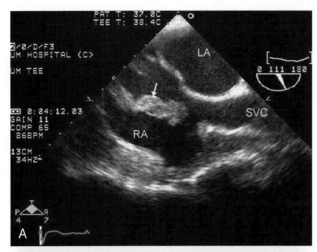

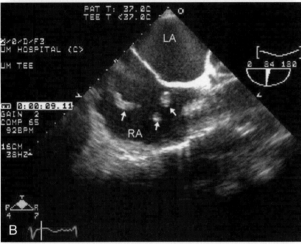

FIGURE 22.46. Transesophageal echocardiogram recorded in a patient with a thromboembolism in transit. **A:** Note the bulky serpiginous mass that appears to arise from the area of the inferior vena cava. Note the marked mobility of this mass in the real-time image. **B:** Because of the manner in which this elongated mass folds on itself, it appears as three distinct masses in the right atrium (*RA*) (*arrows*), which in the real-time image can be seen to be connected as one continuous tubular mass. LA, left atrium; SVC, superior vena cava.

or aggressive heparinization. Detection of thromboembolism in transit represents a remarkably high risk subset of patients with mortality exceeding 75% if not treated.

Saline contrast echocardiography should be employed as part of the evaluation in a suspected pulmonary embolus. Detection of right-to-left shunting attributable to a patent foramen ovale is additional circumstantial evidence that right heart pressures may be elevated above the patient's baseline, thereby suggesting an acute process. Additionally, attention should be paid to curvature of the interatrial septum. If there is elevation of right heart pressure, often the interatrial septum will bow persistently from right-to-left rather than having normal phasic variation in both directions. Several echocardio-

graphic features have been associated with a worsened prognosis in patients with an acute pulmonary embolus, the detection of which has been suggested as an indication for more aggressive therapy with lytics. These include the detection of thromboembolism in transit as noted previously and evidence of significant right heart dilation and right ventricular systolic dysfunction.

ATRIAL FIBRILLATION AND CARDIOVERSION

Atrial fibrillation is a common arrhythmia to encounter and is present in 6% to 10% of patients over the age of 70. It may exist in isolation, in the presence of a structurally normal heart (lone atrial fibrillation), or more commonly in association with underlying structural cardiovascular disease. There are several classic cardiovascular diseases associated with atrial fibrillation, most notably rheumatic mitral stenosis. Based on clinical and echocardiographic criteria, patients with atrial fibrillation are often classified as having valvular versus nonvalvular atrial fibrillation. Echocardiography should be performed in all patients with atrial fibrillation. Detection of a structurally normal heart identifies a subset of patients more likely to have spontaneous conversion to sinus rhythm and, when combined with a relatively young age, identifies a subset at relatively low risk of embolic complications. Conversely, detection of previously unsuspected cardiomyopathy or mitral stenosis implies less likelihood of spontaneous restoration of sinus rhythm and an increased likelihood of cardioembolic complications. Guidelines for long-term anticoagulation in patients with chronic atrial fibrillation are based in large part on patient age and evidence of underlying structural heart disease, which can be easily assessed with transthoracic echocardiography.

Thromboembolism occurs in patients with atrial fibrillation because of stasis of blood in the left atrium leading to thrombus formation (Figs. 22.47 and 22.48). More than 90% of thrombi forming in the presence of atrial fibrillation will be noted in the left atrial appendage. The prevalence of thrombus in atrial fibrillation has been described in several relatively large studies of patients with atrial fibrillation and ranges from 6% to 30%. The likelihood of finding thrombus is directly related to the nature of underlying cardiac disease and the duration of atrial fibrillation, which explains the broad range in prevalence. It should be emphasized that detection of dense "smoke" or spontaneous contrast (Fig. 22.48) in the left atrium or left atrial appendage may be associated with a risk of thromboembolic events similar to that of thrombus.

Most clinicians believe that restoration of sinus rhythm is beneficial, and hence patients with atrial fibrillation are often referred for electrical or chemical cardioversion. Electrical cardioversion has long been known to be associated with embolic events after successful

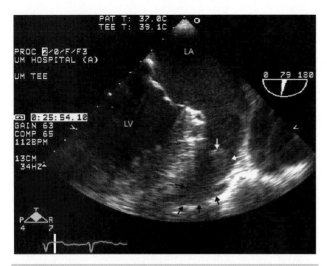

FIGURE 22.47. Transesophageal echocardiogram of the left atrial appendage in a patient with atrial fibrillation and a recent neurologic event. The outer border of the atrial appendage is noted by the *black arrows*. Note the vague homogeneous echo density filling approximately 50% of the left atrial appendage (*white arrows*). In the real-time image, note the spontaneous echo contrast or "smoke" arising from the mouth of the left atrial appendage. LA, left atrium; LV, left ventricle.

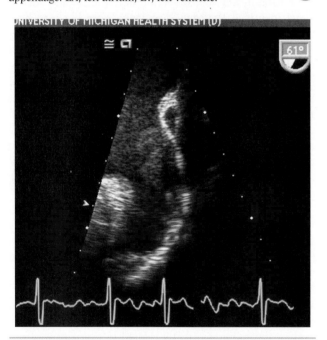

FIGURE 22.48. Expanded view of the left atrial appendage in a patient with atrial fibrillation. In this example, there is no distinct thrombus but vague swirling smoke-like echoes suggesting stagnant blood in the body of the left atrial appendage.

restoration of sinus rhythm. Traditional teaching had been that embolic events occurred because of a preexisting thrombus in the atrial appendage that had remained localized to the atrial appendage during atrial fibrillation. After restoration of sinus rhythm, atrial contractility increased and the thrombus was ejected into the systemic

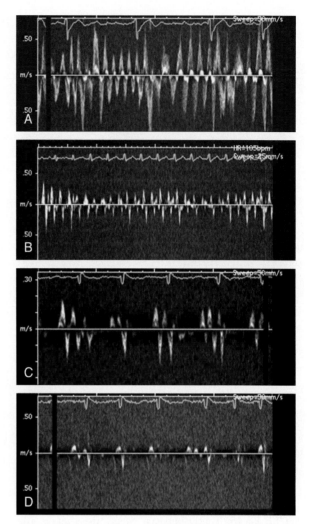

FIGURE 22.49. Pulsed wave Doppler recordings from patients with atrial fibrillation demonstrate the broad range in left atrial appendage emptying and filling velocities. Note the variation over time in the velocities. For a disease-free individual in sinus rhythm, these velocities frequently exceed 80 to 100 cm/sec and are timed with atrial contraction (P wave). Note the near-normal atrial appendage velocities (**A**), the significant reduction (**B**), and the near absence (**C, D**) of atrial activity. Subjects with more well preserved atrial appendage velocities appear less likely to have spontaneous echo contrast or to form atrial thrombus and may represent a group with a lower likelihood of embolic events.

circulation. This scenario is not accurate. Transesophageal echocardiography has clearly demonstrated that there is a broad range of mechanical atrial transport activity in patients with atrial fibrillation. By placing a pulsed sample volume in the mouth of the atrial appendage, one can measure velocity of blood flow into and out of the atrial appendage and identify mechanical contraction of the atrial appendage with a frequency of 200 to 300 Hz. This can be associated with near-normal velocities, which prevent stasis, or with pathologically low velocities, which are the precursor of stasis and thrombus formation (Fig. 22.49).

Several studies have demonstrated that immediately after successful electrical cardioversion, a phenomenon of atrial stunning occurs. Although electrical activity may have been restored, mechanical activity of the atrium and atrial appendage may be delayed in its recovery by several days to weeks. Acutely after successful cardioversion, emptying velocities of the atrial appendage decline in the majority of patients, hence increasing the likelihood of blood stasis and thrombus formation (Figs. 22.50 and 22.51). Emboli occurring after cardioversion are more likely to have arisen *de novo* than to represent ejection of a previously existing thrombus that may be relatively well endothelialized in the atrial appendage.

There are several strategies for cardioversion of patients with atrial fibrillation. The conventional approach has been anticoagulation therapy for 6 weeks followed by cardioversion and then continued anticoagulation therapy for 6 weeks to 6 months. The second approach, which has been more recently popularized, is transesophageal echocardiography–guided cardioversion. With this strategy, patients are acutely anticoagulated with heparin and undergo transesophageal echocardiography. If no thrombus is present, electrical cardioversion is undertaken at that time, thereby reducing the patient exposure to pre-cardioversion anticoagulation. If thrombus is present, cardioversion is deferred. In theory, the transesophageal echocardiographic–guided approach reduces the patient's total exposure to anticoagulation and hence bleeding risk. It was also postulated that earlier cardioversion may result in more successful long-term maintenance of sinus rhythm. Several large-scale studies have clearly demonstrated that the outcome at 1 year with respect to maintenance of sinus rhythm and the embolic rate after cardioversion is virtually identical with either approach.

NEUROLOGIC EVENTS AND CARDIAC SOURCE OF EMBOLUS

For patients who present with evidence of abrupt arterial occlusion, an embolic etiology is a relevant clinical consideration. This includes patients with sudden loss of flow

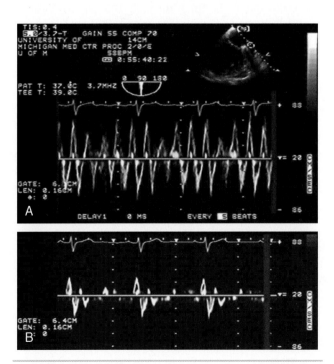

FIGURE 22.50. Pulsed wave Doppler image recorded in the left atrial appendage in a patient during atrial fibrillation (**A**) and immediately after cardioversion to sinus rhythm (**B**). **A:** Note the rapid velocities of 40 to 60 cm/sec. **B:** Sinus rhythm has been restored, and atrial appendage velocities occur only timed with the P wave on the electrocardiogram. Note the marked reduction in velocity to less than 30 cm/sec. This phenomenon of atrial appendage stunning may result in an increased propensity to thrombus formation after cardioversion compared with precardioversion when there are relatively preserved emptying velocities.

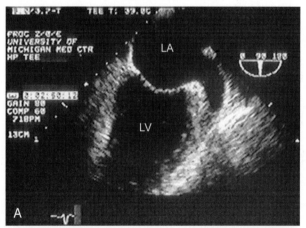

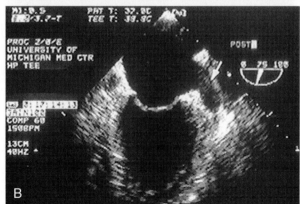

FIGURE 22.51. Transesophageal echocardiogram of the left atrial appendage in a patient during atrial fibrillation (**A**) and immediately after cardioversion to sinus rhythm (**B**). **A:** Note the absence of spontaneous contrast in the atrial appendage and its almost immediate appearance (*arrow*) after conversion to sinus rhythm (**B**). LA, left atrium; LV, left ventricle.

to an extremity, major organ, or, perhaps most commonly, the cerebrovascular system. There is a broad range of cardiovascular abnormalities that have been associated with subsequent embolization. For complete evaluation of potential cardiac embolic sources, transesophageal echocardiography is required because many of the entities such as left atrial appendage thrombus can be detected only with this technique. Identification of appropriate patients for evaluation with transesophageal echocardiography is somewhat controversial. Table 22.6 lists a number of clinical situations in which a cardiac source of embolus should be investigated as the etiology of a neurologic or other presumed embolic event.

Numerous studies have outlined the prevalence of different cardiovascular anomalies encountered in patients with neurologic events. Often patients have multiple potential etiologies. Demonstrating cause and effect between entities such as aortic atheroma or a patent foramen ovale and an antecedent event has been problematic. Many patients who are investigated for a potential cardiac source of embolus have noncardiac etiologies such as atherosclerotic disease of the extracranial vasculature or long-standing hypertension. A decision to proceed with transesophageal echocardiography should be based on the likelihood of finding unique information identifying a causative anomaly for the embolic event and the likelihood that identification of such an abnormality will result in a change in therapy. Tables 22.7 and 22.8 outline the relative frequency with which potential cardiac sources of embolus are noted in patients presenting with cerebrovascular accidents. One of the more common anomalies found are aortic atheromas (Fig. 22.52). There is a tremendous range in the appearance of atheroma. Most authorities believe that it is the mobile pedunculated and complex atheroma that confers the greatest potential embolic risk. Atheromas exceeding 4 mm in thickness have been more closely associated with presumed cardioembolism phenomena.

A patent foramen ovale has been associated with cardioembolic events. The proposed mechanism is paradoxical right-to-left shunting through the patent foramen ovale. A patent foramen ovale can easily be documented with transesophageal echocardiography (Figs. 22.53 and 22.54) or intravenous saline echocardiography (Fig. 22.55). There is a range in the magnitude of size and shunt of a patent foramen ovale, and trivial right-to-left shunt with saline contrast echocardiography during the Valsalva maneuver is noted in a substantial portion of the population. It appears that a patent foramen with 5 mm or more of separation of the foraminal tissue from the atrial septum or those that are associated with more significant right-to-left shunts confer the greatest risk of em-

▶ TABLE 22.6 Clinical Events with Potential Embolic Source

Reasonable likelihood of causative cardiac etiology
  Abrupt peripheral artery occlusion
  Abrupt occlusion of organ vasculature (renal, mesenteric, etc.)
  Cerebrovascular/transient ischemic accident in young patient (age <45 y)
  Cerebrovascular/transient ischemic accident in older patient without "significant" cerebrovascular disease
Low likelihood of causative cardiac embolic source
  Seizure
  Syncope
  Dizziness
  Headache
  Nonfocal events

▶ TABLE 22.7 Prevalence of Cardiac Abnormalities in Patients with and without Presumed Embolic Events Derived from General Surveillance Studies

Evaluated Pacemaker	Event Patients[a] (n =)	Echo Positive			Control Patients[a] (n =)	Echo Positive		
		n	%	Range[b]		n	%	Range[b]
No potential source of embolus	1,530	772	50.5	32–85	—	—	—	—
Any potential source of embolus	1,530	758	49.5	15–68	—	—	—	—
Left atrial thrombus	1,153	98	8.5	3–17	877	28	3.2	2–81
Spontaneous contrast	1,081	187	17.3	11–23	1,105	63	5.7	5–6
Patent foramen ovale	1,292	247	19.1	8–45	1,043	87	8.3	2–23
Atrial septal aneurysm	1,131	150	13.3	3–28	1,204	85	7.1	3–12
Aortic atheroma	348	49	14.1	4–44	n/a	—	—	—
Mitral valve prolapse	1,131	57	5.0	2–9	927	83	8.9	5–9

Lesions not tabulated above, such as vegetations, myxoma, other tumors, and mitral valve strands, were too few in number and in too few studies to derive meaningful conclusions.
[a]Control patient population derived from studies in which lesion was specifically sought. The control subjects were not necessarily age and risk factor matched.
[b]Range refers to minimal and maximal prevalence of abnormalities reported for the cited references.
n/a, reliable extraction data not available.
From Cheitlin et al, ACC/AHA/ASE 2003 Guideline Update for the Clinical Application of Echocardiography. J Am Coll Cardiol 2003;42:954–970, with permission.

▶ **TABLE 22.8** Prevalence of Echocardiographic Findings in Cryptogenic and Non-Cryptogenic Stroke

	Cryptogenic (n = 308)			Non-Cryptogenic (n = 263)		
	Total[a]	Echo[b]	Echo %	Total[a]	Echo[†]	Echo %
PFO	308	100	32.5	263	64	24.3
SC	104	17	16.3	74	10	13.5
ASA	168	38	22.6	110	14	12.7

[a]Total indicates number of patients in each subgroup for whom each entity was specifically tabulated in the referenced studies. Not all studies tabulated data for each entity.
[†]Presence of specific abnormality on the echocardiogram.
ASA, atrial septal aneurysm; PFO, patient foramen ovale; SC, spontaneous contact.
From Cheitlin et al. ACC/AHA/ASE 2003 Guideline Update for the Clinical Application of Echocardiography. J Am Coll Cardiol 2003;42:954–970, with permission.

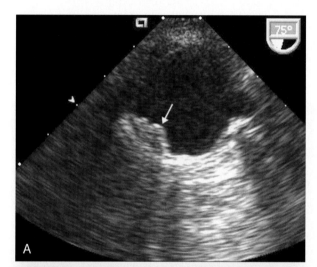

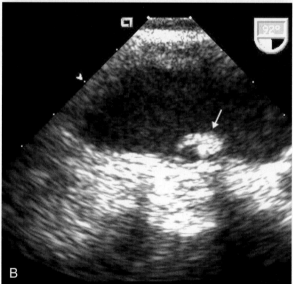

FIGURE 22.52. Transesophageal echocardiogram recorded in two patients with cryptogenic stroke identified as having significant aortic atheroma (*arrows*) on transesophageal echocardiography. **A:** Note the broad-based but pedunculated atheroma in the proximal descending aorta, with a thickness exceeding 4 mm. **B:** Note the mobile nature of the atheroma in the real-time image.

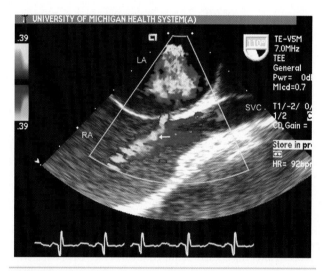

FIGURE 22.53. Transesophageal echocardiogram recorded in a 20-year-old patient with a neurologic event. Note the patent foramen ovale (vs. very small atrial septal defect) documented by color flow imaging (*arrow*). LA, left atrium; RA, right atrium; SVC, superior vena cava.

bolic events. An atrial septal aneurysm is defined as a phasic protrusion of the tissue of the foramen ovale with 1.5-cm excursion. Typically, the aneurysm bulges from the right to the left atrium in phase with the respiratory cycle (Fig. 22.56). Aneurysms have been associated with cardioembolic events. The presumed mechanism is either due to formation of small fibrin/clot masses in the aneurysmal invaginations, which then embolize, or, far more likely, shunting through an associated patent foramen ovale. Several recent studies have suggested a link between a patent foramen ovale and migraine headaches, presumably via the mechanism of vasospasm triggered by paradoxical microemboli.

Other embolic etiologies, such as a previously unsuspected tumor or vegetation, occur very infrequently. In the absence of mitral stenosis or atrial fibrillation, the likelihood of finding a left atrial thrombus is low but has obvious therapeutic implications (Fig. 22.57).

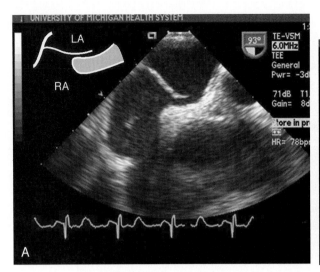

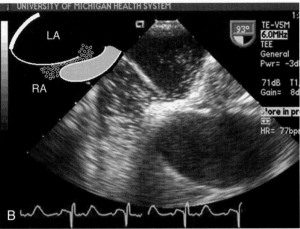

FIGURE 22.54. Transesophageal echocardiogram recorded in a young patient with cryptogenic stroke documenting the presence of a patent foramen ovale. **A:** Note the redundancy of the foraminal tissue and the "liftoff" of the tissue from the primum portion of the septum of approximately 3 to 4 mm. **B:** Note the right-to-left shunting of saline contrast through the patent foramen ovale. LA, left atrium; RA, right atrium.

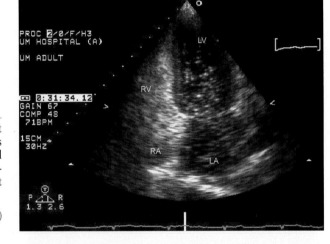

FIGURE 22.55. Apical four-chamber view recorded in a patient being evaluated for cardioembolic disease. This image was recorded after injection of saline contrast, which can be seen to fill the right atrium (*RA*) and right ventricle (*RV*). Note the appearance of a mild amount of contrast in the left atrium (*LA*) and left ventricle (*LV*) and the normal size of the right atrium and right ventricle leading to a presumptive diagnosis of a patent foramen ovale with right-to-left shunting.

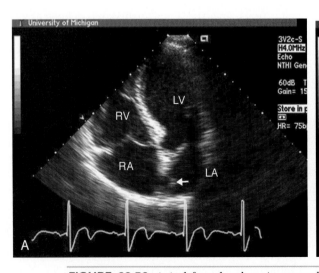

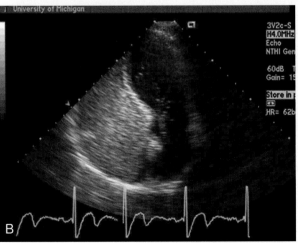

FIGURE 22.56. Apical four-chamber view recorded in a patient with an atrial septal aneurysm. **A:** Note the discrete bulging of a portion of the atrial septum into the left atrium (*LA*) (*arrow*). **B:** Recorded after injection of saline contrast. Note the complete filling of the right atrium and right ventricle and the small amount of shunting consistent with a patent foramen ovale associated with the atrial septal aneurysm. LV, left ventricle; RA, right atrium; RV, right ventricle.

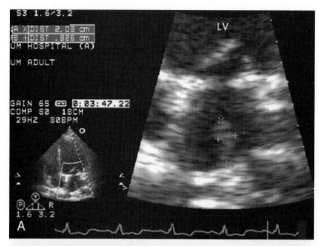

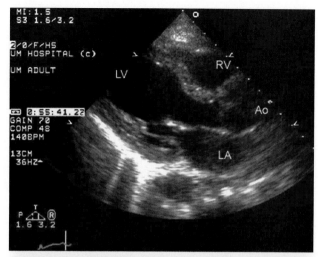

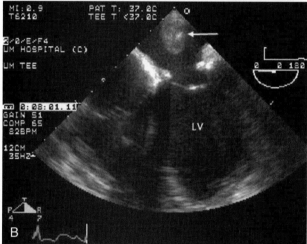

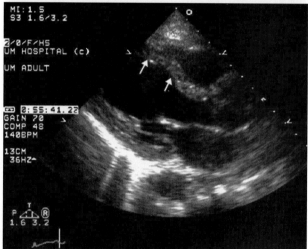

FIGURE 22.57. Expanded view of an apical four-chamber view in a patient who had previously undergone mitral anular ring placement for mitral regurgitation. **A:** Note the vague pedunculated mass arising from the back wall of the left atrium. **B:** A transesophageal echocardiogram recorded in the same patient, confirming the presence of a large thrombus in the body of the left atrium. LV, left ventricle.

FIGURE 22.58. Parasternal long-axis view recorded in diastole (upper panel) and systole (lower panel) in a 58-year-old patient after an intracranial hemorrhage. Note the marked dyskinesis of the distal three-fourths anterior septum (*arrows*). In the real-time image, note the significant hypokinesis of the remaining walls of well. This echocardiogram was associated with deep symmetric T-wave inversion on the electrocardiogram but no significant leak of cardiac enzymes. This patient was subsequently demonstrated to be free of obstructive coronary disease (see Figure 22.59 for follow-up). Ao, aorta; LA, left atrium; LV, left ventricle; RV, right ventricle.

NEUROGENIC MYOCARDIAL STUNNING

Occasionally after an acute severe neurologic event, classically intracerebral hemorrhage, a phenomenon of myocardial neurogenic stunning occurs. It has also been reported after severe emotional stress (the apical ballooning syndrome). The syndrome is characterized by deep T-wave inversion in the anterior precordial leads of the electrocardiogram. On echocardiography, these patients have a significant wall motion abnormality, most often mimicking ischemia or infarction in the left anterior descending coronary artery territory (Fig. 22.58). The wall motion abnormality is not associated with a significant elevation in cardiac enzymes and typically reverses to normal over a 3- to 14-day period (Fig. 22.59). The etiology of this phenomenon is not fully known but appears related to auto-

nomic discharge and experimentally can be mimicked by stellate ganglion stimulation.

SYNCOPE

Evaluation of patients with syncope is often problematic, and the incremental yield and overall utility of echocardiographic screening of otherwise healthy individuals with a single episode of syncope is controversial. There are obvious cardiovascular diseases that can result in syncope such as critical aortic stenosis, hypertrophic cardiomyopathy,

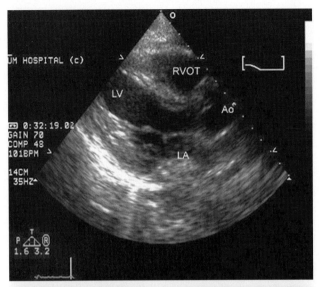

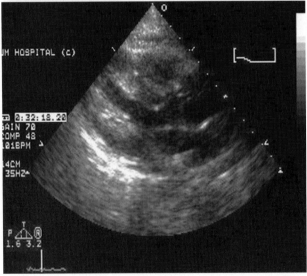

FIGURE 22.59. Parasternal long-axis view recorded in diastole (upper panel) and systole (lower panel) in the same patient presented in Figure 22.58 10 days after the initial presentation. Note the significant reduction left ventricular size and the restoration of normal left ventricular systolic function. Ao, aorta; LA, left atrium; LV, left ventricle; RVOT, right ventricular outflow tract.

and other cardiovascular diseases associated with arrhythmia such as dilated cardiomyopathy and mitral valve prolapse. The yield of echocardiographic screening for detection of these abnormalities in a patient with a normal physical examination and a normal resting 12-lead electrocardiogram is relatively low, and the need for two-dimensional echocardiography in all patients presenting with a single episode of syncope has not been established.

EVALUATION OF CARDIAC ARRHYTHMIAS

For patients presenting with symptomatic cardiac arrhythmias or arrhythmias known to be associated with adverse events such as atrial fibrillation, ventricular tachycardia, and pathologic heart block, echocardiography may play a role in identifying underlying anatomic heart disease. For an overtly healthy individual with a normal cardiovascular examination and a normal 12-lead electrocardiogram, echocardiographic evaluation of a patient with isolated unifocal premature ventricular or atrial contractions is generally not warranted. Conversely, arrhythmias such as atrial fibrillation have a high prevalence of associated underlying cardiovascular disease, which often has specific therapeutic implications. In this subset, surveillance echocardiography is indicated. Similarly for patients with ventricular tachycardia, identification of the subset of patients with underlying structural heart disease is crucial for management because the prognosis of isolated, asymptomatic, nonsustained ventricular tachycardia with a structurally normal heart is relatively benign compared with ventricular tachycardia in the presence of left ventricular dysfunction.

EVALUATION OF PATIENTS BEFORE AND DURING CHEMOTHERAPY

Several commonly used chemotherapeutic agents are associated with well-known cardiotoxicity. The most widely appreciated are the anthracycline class of agents typified by doxorubicin. Typically, doxorubicin results in left ventricular systolic dysfunction and a cardiomyopathy, indistinguishable from cardiomyopathy of other etiologies. There is a less well recognized acute and transient decrease in left ventricular systolic function that is occasionally seen at the time of acute infusion and does not necessarily imply long-term systolic dysfunction. In many centers, patients at risk of having preexisting cardiovascular disease undergo surveillance echocardiography to ensure normal left ventricular systolic function before institution of chemotherapy. If, during the course of chemotherapy, a patient develops symptoms suggestive of congestive heart failure, repeat echocardiography is clinically indicated to reassess left ventricular function. There are no specific echocardiographic markers that allow identification of patients likely to develop chemotherapy-related cardiotoxicity, nor are there any specific echocardiographic markers that detect it in its preclinical phase. Chemotherapy agents other than anthracyclines can also result in acute cardiac decompensation, including high-dose Cytoxan. The frequency with which this occurs is substantially less than that with doxorubicin and the dysfunction usually is transient.

RADIATION-INDUCED CARDIAC DISEASE

Mediastinal radiation has been associated with both acute and chronic cardiac pathology. Fortunately, modern techniques of radiation therapy have resulted in more precise "aiming" of the radiation beam, which has reduced the magnitude of this problem. Acutely, if the heart is not fully shielded, radiation-induced pericarditis may be seen. It has all the characteristics of other forms of pericarditis but may have a more inflammatory component (Fig. 22.60). The time course for resolution of this form of pericarditis may be months. An obvious clinical dilemma when one encounters a new pericardial effusion in a patient who has undergone radiation therapy for malignancy is whether the effusion is related to the malignancy or the radiation therapy. This distinction needs to be made on clinical grounds.

Radiation therapy also affects the heart in a delayed manner. Occasionally, patients will develop manifestations 5 to 15 years after mediastinal radiation, which may present either as chronic constrictive or effusive constrictive pericarditis. Radiation may also result in direct myocardial damage. Assuming an anterior portal, the right ventricle may be disproportionately affected and may result in the appearance of a restrictive cardiomyopathy.

Finally, cardiac valves may be damaged by radiation. Most commonly, this involves the aortic valve and anterior mitral valve leaflet (Fig. 22.61). The usual lesion is valvular regurgitation with valvular stenosis being less common. The likelihood of valvular damage from radiation is dose dependent, and there is usually a 3- to 5-year delay in its appearance from the time of radiation.

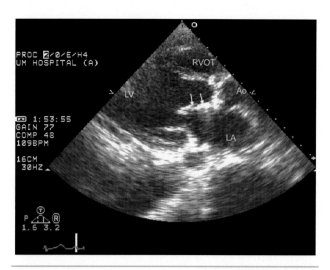

FIGURE 22.61. Parasternal long-axis view recorded in a 27-year-old patient 15 years after radiation therapy for lymphoma. Note the thickening of the aortic valve and the marked thickening and rigidity of the proximal anterior mitral valve leaflet (*arrows*). Ao, aorta; LA, left atrium; LV, left ventricle; RVOT, right ventricular outflow tract.

SCREENING FOR ATHLETIC COMPETITION AND THE ATHLETE'S HEART

Before competitive athletic activity, potential participants often undergo a general health evaluation. From a standpoint of cardiovascular disease, this generally consists only of recording blood pressure, heart rate, and auscultation of the heart. In an asymptomatic individual with a normal cardiovascular physical examination and no family history of heritable cardiovascular disorders, the likelihood of finding significant underlying cardiovascular disease that would adversely affect the suitability for competitive sports is low. In this setting, further evaluation with echocardiography has not been shown to be cost-effective. Individuals for whom an echocardiogram may be indicated include those with a family history of exertional syncope or sudden cardiac death and those who have symptoms. Table 22.9 lists a number of cardiovascular abnormalities that have relevance for competitive sports. Many, such as aortic stenosis, should be detected on physical examination, and a combination of a thorough physical examination and 12-lead electrocardiogram generally suffices for detection of the majority of relevant abnormalities. In individuals in whom surveillance echocardiography is indicated before participation in competitive sports, the examination should be tailored to exclude disease of the proximal aorta that would predispose to dissection or rupture, hypertrophic cardiomyopathy, and occult valvular heart disease. Additionally, the origin of both coronary arteries should be identified because anomalous origin of the coronary artery has been associated with sudden cardiac death at the time of physical exertion. This rare anomaly obviously will not be de-

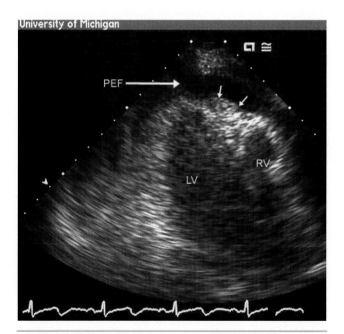

FIGURE 22.60. Apical view recorded in a patient with esophageal cancer, status post-radiation therapy. Note the anterior pericardial effusion (*PEF*) and the nodular densities in the interventricular groove (*arrows*). See text for further discussion. LV, left ventricle; RV, right ventricle.

▶ **TABLE 22.9** Athletic Screening: Relevant Abnormalities Conferring Increased Risk for Participation

Moderate and high risk
- Marfan syndrome
- Other aortic dilation
- Hypertrophic cardiomyopathy
- Occult dilated cardiomyopathy
- Valvar aortic stenosis (moderate or worse)
- Pulmonary hypertension
- Anomalous coronary artery origin

Low risk
- Mitral valve prolapse with ≤ mild regurgitation
- Bicuspid aortic valve with gradient ≤25 mm Hg (peak)
- Mild mitral stenosis (New York Heart Association Class I)
- Uncomplicated atrial septal defect
- Mild pulmonary stenosis
- Small, restrictive ventricular septal defect

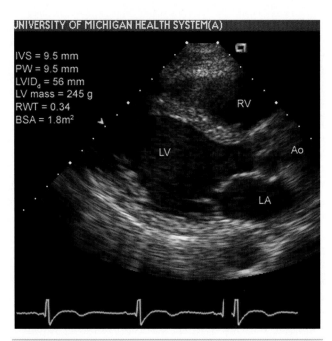

FIGURE 22.62. Parasternal long-axis echocardiogram recorded in a marathon runner (height, 5 ft 10 in.; weight, 150 lb, BSA = 1.9 M²). Note the mild degree of left ventricular dilation for a subject of this body size and the wall thickness, which is at the upper normal range. Relative wall thickness (*RWT*) is preserved at 0.34. Left ventricular mass index is at the upper range of normal. Ao, aorta; BSA, body surface area; IVS, interventricular septum; LA, left atrium; LV, left ventricle; LVID$_d$, left ventricular end-diastolic internal diameter; RV, right ventricle.

tected by a history, physical examination, or 12-lead electrocardiogram. Its overall prevalence in the population is probably too low to warrant routine echocardiographic screening solely for that purpose.

Vigorous athletic training results in compensatory changes in cardiac anatomy, most of which are confined to the left ventricle. The degree of athletic training required to result in the so-called "athletes heart" is substantial, and changes are typically not seen in casual recreational athletes. The type of athletic activity has an impact on the nature of left ventricular remodeling. Classically, vigorous endurance training such as long-distance running or cycling results in mild hypertrophy with an elevation in left ventricular mass due to chamber enlargement and, to a lesser degree, in wall thickness (Fig. 22.62). Conversely, intense isotonic training (weight lifting) results in more concentric hypertrophy. Table 22.10 outlines the anticipated changes in left ventricular wall thickness, internal dimension, and mass for different types of highly trained athletes. An additional factor to consider is that most modern athletes train with a combination of resistance and endurance exercise, and, as such, the "pure" categories of athletic heart anatomy are relatively uncommon. Posterior wall thickness rarely exceeds 13 mm in the "athlete's heart," and the posterior wall/left ventricular dimension ratio remains normal. A posterior wall dimension exceeding 16 mm has not been reported due to athletic training alone, and a wall thickness exceeding 16 mm should raise the consideration of a hypertrophic cardiomyopathy. An unfortunate social and medical consequence of intense competition has been the use of anabolic steroid supplements, which may result in substantial pathologic hypertrophy.

THE HEART IN PREGNANCY

Pregnancy results in substantial physiologic and hemodynamic changes that have manifestations on the echocardiogram (Table 22.11). By the third trimester of pregnancy, there is an increase in blood volume of 50%, a decline in peripheral vascular resistance, and an increase in cardiac output. These changes reach their maximum at the end of the second trimester. From an anatomic and echocardiographic perspective, this results in a mild increase in chamber dimensions and the appearance of a high-output state with an increased stroke volume. Typically, the left atrium increases in size by 10% to 15% and the left ventricle by 5% to 10%. Dilation of the right atrium and right ventricle is often more obvious (Fig. 22.63). The increased stroke volume manifests as an increased time velocity integral of aortic and pulmonary flow (Fig. 22.64). Mild degrees of tricuspid insufficiency are commonly encountered.

Other features of pregnancy include small pericardial effusions, which can be seen in 20% of patients. Effusions resulting in hemodynamic compromise do not occur due to uncomplicated pregnancy, and if there is evidence of hemodynamic compromise, an alternate etiology for the effusion should be considered.

▶ TABLE 22.10   Cardiac Structure and Function in Endurance-Trained Athletes, Combined
Endurance and Strength-Trained Athletes, Strength-Trained Athletes, and
Control Subjects

	Endurance-Trained Athletes	Combined Endurance-and Strength-Trained Athletes	Strength-Trained Athletes	Control Subjects	P
LVID$_d$ (mm)	53.7	56.2	52.1	49.6	<0.001
PWT$_d$, mm	10.3	11.0	11.0	8.8	<0.001
RWT	0.389	0.398	0.442	0.356	<0.001
LVM (g)	249	288	267	174	<0.001

LVID$_d$, left ventricular end-diastolic internal diameter; LVM, left ventricular mass; PWTd, diastolic posterior wall thickness; RWT, relative wall thickness.
From Pluim BM, Zwinderman AH, van der Laarse A, et al. Correlation of heart rate variability with cardiac functional and metabolic variables in cyclists with training induced left ventricular hypertrophy. Heart 1999;81:612–617, with permission.

▶ TABLE 22.11   Cardiovascular and Echocardiographic Changes in Pregnancy

Physiologic Sequelae	Echocardiographic Findings
Increased blood volume	Dilation of LA, LV
Decreased systemic vascular resistance	Increased LV stroke volume
Increased stroke volume and cardiac output	Altered MV coaptation
	Mild tricuspid regurgitation
	Elevated TR velocity (mild)
Other	
Pericardial effusion	
Increased prevalence of benign arrhythmias (PVCs, PACs, PSVT)	

LA, left atrium; LV, left ventricle; MV, mitral valve; TR, tricuspid regurgitation; PVC, premature ventricular contraction; PAC, premature atrial contraction; PSVT, paroxysmal supraventricular tachycardia.

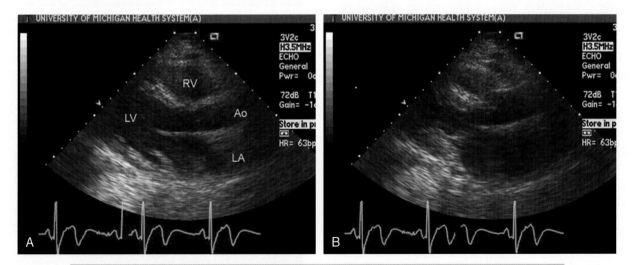

FIGURE 22.63.   A, B: Parasternal long-axis view echocardiogram recorded in diastole (left) and systole (right) in a healthy female patient in the third trimester of pregnancy. Note the mild dilation of the left atrium (*LA*) and the left ventricular systolic function, which is at the upper normal range. Ao, aorta; LV, left ventricle; RV, right ventricle.

The mild left ventricular dilation can secondarily result in a change in the appearance of the mitral valve. On occasion, one encounters a female patient with mitral valve prolapse and mitral regurgitation in whom the prolapse becomes less apparent during pregnancy. The mechanism underlying this phenomenon is the more ideal mitral valve coaptation, which occurs as a result of an increase in left ventricular volume and internal dimensions.

In late pregnancy, the enlarged uterus results in compression of thoracic structures, including the heart. This may result in a pseudo wall motion abnormality in the posterior wall, similar to that seen in chronic liver disease with significant ascites (Fig. 22.20).

Rarely after pregnancy does an acute cardiomyopathy develop, referred to as peripartum cardiomyopathy. The echocardiographic appearance of peripartum cardiomyopathy is identical to dilated cardiomyopathy of any etiology, as discussed in Chapter 17. Finally, the peripartum period may represent a period of vascular "laxity," and both aortic and spontaneous coronary artery dissection is more common at this time. If a pregnant or peripartum patient presents with acute chest pain, consideration should be given to these entities.

EFFECTS OF ADVANCED AGE

With age, there are predictable changes that are commonly seen in the heart. One of the most common is a progressive angulation between the ascending aorta and left ventricular outflow tract often in conjunction with localized proximal septal hypertrophy (Fig. 22.65). This re-

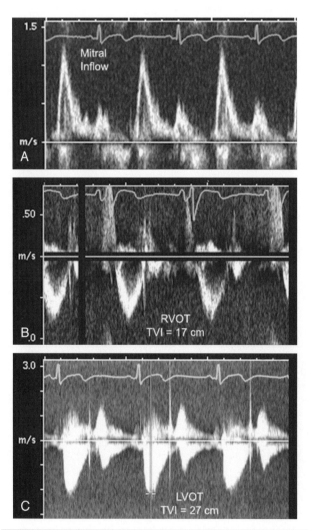

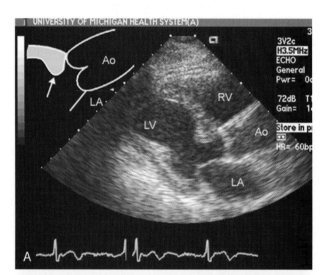

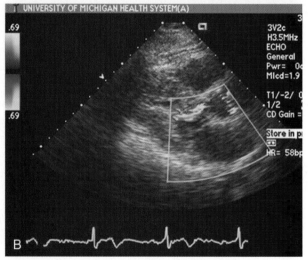

FIGURE 22.64. Spectral Doppler recordings from the same patient presented in Figure 22.63. **A:** Note the mitral inflow pattern with an E/A ratio of 2.2. **B:** Recorded from the right ventricular outflow tract (*RVOT*) and reveals a time velocity integral (*TVI*) of 17 cm. **C:** Recorded through the left ventricular outflow tract (*LVOT*) and reveals an elevated peak velocity of 2 m/sec and an increased time velocity integral of 27 cm. Note in Figure 22.63 that there is no evidence of aortic stenosis or other outflow tract obstruction and the elevated velocities are the result of high cardiac output and not obstruction.

FIGURE 22.65. Parasternal long-axis echocardiogram recorded in an 87-year-old patient with a systolic murmur. **A:** Note the angulated septum with proximal septal hypertrophy (*arrow* in the schematic) and the mild thickening of the aortic valve. **B:** The image was recorded with color flow Doppler imaging and reveals the marked acceleration of flow around the sigmoid septum, which is the cause of a systolic murmur in this patient. Ao, aorta; LA, left atrium; LV, left ventricular, RV, right ventricular.

sults in a "sigmoid" shape to the proximal ventricular septum. The hypertrophy may be quite focal and result in a localized area of turbulence in the outflow tract that may be the source of the ejection murmur often heard in elderly patients (Fig. 22.66). Additionally, characteristic changes will be seen in the wall of the aorta due to progressive thickening. Mild focal degrees of thickening are common in the aortic and mitral valves as well as the mitral valve chordae (Fig. 22.67). There is a progressive increase in the likelihood of anular calcium with age. With advanced age, even in the absence of sustained hypertension, myocardial stiffness increases, presumably due to mild degrees of progressive fibrosis. This results in chronic diastolic dysfunction that can be detected with standard Doppler techniques and that often results in modest left atrial dilation. Finally, with advanced age combined with long-standing hypertension (especially if poorly controlled), a pattern mimicking (genetically determined) hypertrophic cardiomyopathy may develop (Fig. 22.68).

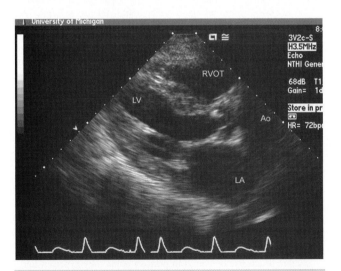

FIGURE 22.66. Apical four-chamber view recorded in an elderly patient with a marked increase in the angle between the left ventricular outflow tract and the aorta (*Ao*). LA, left atrium; LV, left ventricle; RV, right ventricle.

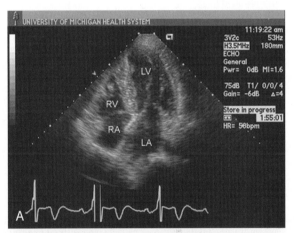

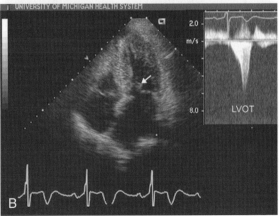

FIGURE 22.68. Apical four-chamber view recorded in an elderly hypertensive patient with the hypertensive hypertrophic cardiomyopathy of the elderly. **A:** In the apical four-chamber view, note the relatively small cavity size and evidence of left ventricular hypertrophy. **B:** In systole, note the systolic left anterior motion of the mitral valve (*arrow*). The inset is a continuous wave Doppler image recorded through the left ventricular outflow tract (*LVOT*) showing a characteristic late peaking velocity consistent with dynamic outflow tract obstruction. LA, left atrium; LV, left ventricle; RA, right atrium; RV, right ventricle.

FIGURE 22.67. Parasternal long-axis echocardiogram recorded in a 95-year-old patient with no significant chronic medical diseases including hypertension. Note the left atrial dilation, the modest degree of proximal septal hypertrophy, and the diffuse thickening and fibrosis of the mitral valve and chordae as well as the aortic valve. Ao, aorta; LA, left atrium; LV, left ventricle; RVOT, right ventricular outflow tract.

SUGGESTED READINGS

Agmon Y, Khandheria BK, Meissner I, et al. Frequency of atrial septal aneurysms in patients with cerebral ischemic events. Circulation 1999;99:1942–1944.

Alizad A, Seward JB. Echocardiographic features of genetic diseases: part 4. Connective tissue. J Am Soc Echocardiogr 2000;13:325–330.

Alizad A, Seward JB. Echocardiographic features of genetic diseases: part 2. Storage disease. J Am Soc Echocardiogr 2000;13:164–170.

Applefeld MM, Wiernik PH. Cardiac disease after radiation therapy for Hodgkin's disease: analysis of 48 patients. Am J Cardiol 1983;51:1679–1681.

Asinger RW, Koehler J, Pearce LA, et al. Pathophysiologic correlates of thromboembolism in nonvalvular atrial fibrillation: II. Dense spontaneous echocardiographic contrast (The Stroke Prevention in Atrial Fibrillation [SPAF-III] study). J Am Soc Echocardiogr 1999;12;1088–1096.

Aurigemma GP, Gottdiener JS, Shemanski L, et al. Predictive value of systolic and diastolic function for incident congestive heart failure in the elderly: the cardiovascular health study. J Am Coll Cardiol 2001;37:1042–1048.

Barbaro G. Cardiovascular manifestations of HIV infection. Circulation 2002;106:1420–1425.

Cabell CH, Trichon BH, Velazquez EJ, et al. Importance of echocardiography in patients with severe nonischemic heart failure: the second Prospective Randomized Amlodipine Survival Evaluation (PRAISE-2) echocardiographic study. Am Heart J 2004;147:151–157.

Cheitlin MD, Armstrong WF, Aurigemma GP, et al. ACC/AHA/ASE 2003 guideline update for the clinical application of echocardiography—summary article: a report of the American College of Cardiology/American Heart Association Task Force on Practice Guidelines (ACC/AHA/ASE Committee to Update the 1997 Guidelines for the Clinical Application of Echocardiography). J Am Coll Cardiol 2003;42:954–970.

Collis T, Devereux RB, Roman MJ, et al. Relations of stroke volume and cardiac output to body composition: the Strong Heart study. Circulation 2001;103:820–825.

Curtis JP, Sokol SI, Wang Y, et al. The association of left ventricular ejection fraction, mortality, and cause of death in stable outpatients with heart failure. J Am Coll Cardiol 2003;42:736–742.

Di Salvo TG, Mathier M, Semigran MJ, et al. Preserved right ventricular ejection fraction predicts exercise capacity and survival in advanced heart failure. J Am Coll Cardiol 1995;25:1143–1153.

Dujardin KS, Tei C, Yeo TC, et al. Prognostic value of a Doppler index combining systolic and diastolic performance in idiopathic-dilated cardiomyopathy. Am J Cardiol 1998;82:1071–1076.

Eckel RH, Barouch WW, Ershow AG. Report of the National Heart, Lung, and Blood Institute–National Institute of Diabetes and Digestive and Kidney Diseases Working Group on the pathophysiology of obesity-associated cardiovascular disease. Circulation 2002;105:2923–2928.

Fang ZY, Yuda S, Anderson V, et al. Echocardiographic detection of early diabetic myocardial disease. J Am Coll Cardiol 2003;41:611–617.

Faris R, Coats AJ, Henein MY. Echocardiography-derived variables predict outcome in patients with nonischemic cardiomyopathy with or without a restrictive filling pattern. Am Heart J 2002;144:343–350.

Florea VG, Henein MY, Cicoira M, et al. Echocardiographic determinants of mortality in patients >67 years of age with chronic heart failure. Am J Cardiol 2000;86:158–161.

Gardin JM, Schumacher D, Constantine G, et al. Valvular abnormalities and cardiovascular status following exposure to dexfenfluramine or phentermine/fenfluramine. JAMA 2000;283:1703–1709.

Gardin JM, Weissman NJ, Leung C, et al. Clinical and echocardiographic follow-up of patients previously treated with dexfenfluramine or phentermine/fenfluramine. JAMA 2001;286:2011–2014.

Ghio S, Gavazzi A, Campana C, et al. Independent and additive prognostic value of right ventricular systolic function and pulmonary artery pressure in patients with chronic heart failure. J Am Coll Cardiol 2001;37:183–188.

Goldman ME, Pearce LA, Hart RG, et al. Pathophysiologic correlates of thromboembolism in nonvalvular atrial fibrillation: I. Reduced flow velocity in the left atrial appendage (The Stroke Prevention in Atrial Fibrillation [SPAF-III] Study). J Am Soc Echocardiogr 1999;12:1080–1087.

Grimm RA, Stewart WJ, Arheart K, et al. Left atrial appendage "stunning" after electrical cardioversion of atrial flutter: an attenuated response compared with atrial fibrillation as the mechanism for lower susceptibility to thromboembolic events. J Am Coll Cardiol 1997;29:582–589.

Heidenreich PA, Hancock SL, Lee BK, et al. Asymptomatic cardiac disease following mediastinal irradiation. J Am Coll Cardiol 2003;42:743–749.

Hogg K, Swedberg K, McMurray J. Heart failure with preserved left ventricular systolic function; epidemiology, clinical characteristics, and prognosis. J Am Coll Cardiol 2004;43:317–327.

Jollis JG, Landolfo CK, Kisslo J, et al. Fenfluramine and phentermine and cardiovascular findings: effect of treatment duration on prevalence of valve abnormalities. Circulation 2000;101:2071–2077.

Katz R, Karliner JS, Resnik R. Effects of a natural volume overload state (pregnancy) on left ventricular performance in normal human subjects. Circulation 1978;58:434–441.

Kimura BJ, Bocchicchio M, Willis CL, et al. Screening cardiac ultrasonographic examination in patients with suspected cardiac disease in the emergency department. Am Heart J 2001;142:324–330.

Klein AL, Grimm RA, Murray RD, et al. Use of transesophageal echocardiography to guide cardioversion in patients with atrial fibrillation. N Engl J Med 2001;344:1411–1420.

Klein AL, Murray RD, Grimm RA. Role of transesophageal echocardiography-guided cardioversion of patients with atrial fibrillation. J Am Coll Cardiol 2001;37:691–704.

Koelling TM, Aaronson KD, Cody RJ, et al. Prognostic significance of mitral regurgitation and tricuspid regurgitation in patients with left ventricular systolic dysfunction. Am Heart J 2002;144:524–529.

Kuperstein R, Hanly P, Niroumand M, et al. The importance of age and obesity on the relation between diabetes and left ventricular mass. J Am Coll Cardiol 2001;37:1957–1962.

Leibowitz D. Role of echocardiography in the diagnosis and treatment of acute pulmonary thromboembolism. J Am Soc Echocardiogr 2001;14:921–926.

Meacham RR 3rd, Headley AS, Bronze MS, et al. Impending paradoxical embolism. Arch Intern Med 1998;158:438–448.

Miniati M, Monti S, Pratali L, et al. Value of transthoracic echocardiography in the diagnosis of pulmonary embolism: results of a prospective study in unselected patients. Am J Med 2001;110:528–535.

Naschitz JE, Slobodin G, Lewis RJ, et al. Heart diseases affecting the liver and liver diseases affecting the heart. Am Heart J 2000;140:111–120.

Pelliccia A, Maron BJ, Spataro A, et al. The upper limit of physiologic cardiac hypertrophy in highly trained elite athletes. N Engl J Med 1991;324:295–301.

Peterson LR, Waggoner AD, Schechtman KB, et al. Alterations in left ventricular structure and function in young healthy obese women: assessment by echocardiography and tissue Doppler imaging. J Am Coll Cardiol 2004;43:1399–1404.

Pinamonti B, Di Lenarda A, Sinagra G, et al. Restrictive left ventricular filling pattern in dilated cardiomyopathy assessed by Doppler echocardiography: clinical, echocardiographic and hemodynamic correlations and prognostic implications. Heart Muscle Disease Study Group. J Am Coll Cardiol 1993;22:808–815.

Pinamonti B, Zecchin M, Di Lenarda A, et al. Persistence of restrictive left ventricular filling pattern in dilated cardiomyopathy: an ominous prognostic sign. J Am Coll Cardiol 1997;29:604–612.

Pluim BM, Zwinderman AH, van der Laarse A, et al. Correlation of heart rate variability with cardiac functional and metabolic variables in cyclists with training induced left ventricular hypertrophy. Heart 1999;81:612–617.

Rahman JE, Helou EF, Gelzer-Bell R, et al. Noninvasive diagnosis of biopsy-proven cardiac amyloidosis. J Am Coll Cardiol 2004;43:410–415.

Raymond RJ, Hinderliter AL, Willis PW, et al. Echocardiographic predictors of adverse outcomes in primary pulmonary hypertension. J Am Coll Cardiol 2002;39:1214–1219.

Ribeiro A, Lindmarker P, Juhlin-Dannfelt A, et al. Echocardiography Doppler in pulmonary embolism: right ventricular dysfunction as a predictor of mortality rate. Am Heart J 1997;134:479–487.

Ribeiro A, Lindmarker P, Johnsson H, et al. Pulmonary embolism: one-year follow-up with echocardiography Doppler and five-year survival analysis. Circulation 1999;99:1325–1330.

Rihal CS, Nishimura RA, Hatle LK, et al. Systolic and diastolic dysfunction in patients with clinical diagnosis of dilated cardiomyopathy. Relation to symptoms and prognosis. Circulation 1994;90:2772–2779.

Rubler S, Damani PM, Pinto ER. Cardiac size and performance during pregnancy estimated with echocardiography. Am J Cardiol 1977;40: 534–540.

Savage DD, Levy D, Dannenberg AL, et al. Association of echocardiographic left ventricular mass with body size, blood pressure and physical activity (the Framingham Study). Am J Cardiol 1990;65: 371–376.

Schuchlenz HW, Weihs W, Horner S, et al. The association between the diameter of a patent foramen ovale and the risk of embolic cerebrovascular events. Am J Med 2000;109:456–462.

Silverman DI, Manning WJ. Role of echocardiography in patients undergoing elective cardioversion of atrial fibrillation. Circulation 1998;98:479–486.

Svenungsson E, Jensen-Urstad K, Heimburger M, et al. Risk factors for cardiovascular disease in systemic lupus erythematosus. Circulation 2001;104:1887–1893.

Temporelli PL, Corra U, Imparato A, et al. Reversible restrictive left ventricular diastolic filling with optimized oral therapy predicts a more favorable prognosis in patients with chronic heart failure. J Am Coll Cardiol 1998;31:1591–1597.

Transesophageal echocardiographic correlates of thromboembolism in high-risk patients with nonvalvular atrial fibrillation. The Stroke Prevention in Atrial Fibrillation Investigators Committee on Echocardiography. Ann Intern Med 1998;128:639–647.

Tsang TS, Barnes ME, Gersh BJ, et al. Prediction of risk for first age-related cardiovascular events in an elderly population: the incremental value of echocardiography. J Am Coll Cardiol 2003;42: 1199–1205.

Whalley GA, Doughty RN, Gamble GD, et al. Pseudonormal mitral filling pattern predicts hospital re-admission in patients with congestive heart failure. J Am Coll Cardiol 2002;39:1787–1795.

Zabalgoitia M, Halperin JL, Pearce LA, et al. Transesophageal echocardiographic correlates of clinical risk of thromboembolism in nonvalvular atrial fibrillation. Stroke Prevention in Atrial Fibrillation III Investigators. Am Coll Cardiol 1998;31:1622–1626.

Zaroff JG, Rordorf GA, Ogilvy CS, et al. Regional patterns of left ventricular systolic dysfunction after subarachnoid hemorrhage: evidence for neurally mediated cardiac injury. J Am Soc Echocardiogr 2000;13:774–779.

Index

Page numbers followed by *f* refer to figures; page numbers followed by *t* refer to tables.

A